SOLVED MULTIPLE CHOICE QUESTIONS

UPSC & MD
ENTRANCE EXAMINATION
(HOMEOPATHY)

MCQ's From: UPSC, KPSC, PG Entrance (Hom.), AIIMS,
ALL INDIA ENTRANCE EXAMINATIONS

PART-I

SECOND EDITION

Dr V. K. Chauhan, MD (Hom.)
Principal
Dr B. R. Sur Homoeopathic Medical College
and Hospital Nanak Pura, New Delhi
WHO Fellow
Royal London Homoeopathic Hospital (UK)
New England School of Homoeopathy Connecticut (USA)
Management Science for Health, Arlington (USA)
Recipient: State Award 2006, Delhi.

B. Jain Publishers (P) Ltd.
USA—Europe—India

SOLVED MULTIPLE CHOICE QUESTIONS
UPSC & MD ENTRANCE EXAMINATION (HOMEOPATHY)

First Edition : 2008
6th Impression : 2010
Second Edition : 2011
14th Impression: 2017

All rights reserved. No part of this book may be reproduced, stored in a retrieval system or transmitted, in any form or by any means, mechanical, photocopying, recording or otherwise, without any prior written permission of the publisher.

© with the Author

Published by Kuldeep Jain for
B. Jain PUBLISHERS (P) LTD.
B. Jain House, D-157, Sector-63,
NOIDA-201307, U.P. (INDIA)
Tel.: +91-120-4933333 • *Email:* info@bjain.com
Website: www.bjain.com

Printed in India by
Printed at : **L.B. Enterprises**

ISBN: 978-81-319-1166-2

PUBLISHER'S NOTE TO FIRST EDITION

At this time of the year when all the aspirants for UPSC and MD Entrance Examinations are planning their preparation for the exams, B. Jain is there to help the aspirants to achieve their dreams.

This book of Dr V. K. Chauhan which has been in the making since last two years is being released at just the appropriate hour. Dr Chauhan has been working day and night on this book for the last two years.

We hope that this book is useful for the students and doctors appearing for the entrance examinations. The final checking of this book was done in the shortest time possible to make it available to you in time.

Some mistakes in spelling might remain, the responsibility of which is on our shoulders. As far as the answers are concerned the book has been checked three times to correct all such errors and is as near perfection as any book on MCQs could be.

We hope that you find it as a useful tool for your preparation and look forward to your feedback about the book.

Kuldeep Jain
C.E.O., B. Jain Publishers (P) Ltd.

PUBLISHER'S NOTE TO SECOND EDITION

All what was left unchecked in previous editions has been taken care of. The editorial team of the book has corrected all mistakes of the previous edition. The book has been enhanced with new questions asked in various competitive examinations since 2008. The book was a bestseller for the past 3 years and we thank our readers for the same. We wish all new aspirants make the maximum out of this new effort.

Kuldeep Jain
C.E.O., B. Jain Publishers (P) Ltd.

PREFACE

In recent times there has been a growing need for objective assessment of knowledge and it is best done with good Multiple Choice Question Papers. The MCQ's help in discriminating accurately between candidates on the basis of their knowledge of the topics being tested in shortest possible time. The most important function of any MCQ is to rank candidates accurately and fairly according to their performance in that paper.

Keeping in view the above objective, this work has been undertaken. It mainly contains the MCQ's from the test papers of UPSC and State Public Service Commission as well as from PG Entrance Examinations in Homeopathic and Allopathic Institutions.

One should remember that the Multiple Choice Questions are not designed to trick or confuse any anyone but they are designed to test the knowledge in the subject concerned. Therefore, one should not try to look for the problems that aren't there.

While attempting to solve MCQ's one should follow the five most important points:

1. Read the questions carefully and be sure that you understand it.
2. Mark your responses clearly, correctly and accurately.
3. Use reasoning to work out answers, but if you do not know the answer it is better to leave it, especially when there is a provision of negative marking for wrong answers.
4. Good marks can only be obtained by having a basic and wide knowledge in the subject concerned.
5. One should be aware of the time constrain while solving the MCQ's.

All efforts were taken to make this book as error free as possible; however, many inadvertently might have crept in. I request all our readers and critics to kindly inform about any deficiencies. Suggestions to improve are welcome. I wish all the users make best possible use of this compilation and succeed in their endeavor.

Dr V. K. Chauhan

ACKNOWLEDGMENTS

At first I would like to sincerely thank Dr K.R. Mansoor Ali, BHMS, MD (Hom.) for his great contribution to the cause of homeopathy & his website www.similima.com for exhaustive information on Homeopathy and collection of questions asked in UPSC, MD Entrance, other State Service Examinations and Model Question Papers of Indian Homoeopathic Medical Association. This website is highly recommended to all the aspirants of UPSC and other competitive examinations.

I would also like to thank the creators of world renowned software(s) RADAR & Hompath for numerous valuable references taken from them for this book wherever needed.

I would like to express my gratitude and sincere thanks to my teachers, without whose help, guidance and blessings, this work would not have seen the light of the day. I sincerely wish to thank: Late Dr B.K. Bhatnagar, Ex. Principal NHMC & H; Dr K.K. Shrivastava, MD; Late Dr D.P. Rastogi, Ex. Principal NHMC & H; Dr V.K. Gupta, Ex. Principal NHMC & H; Dr V.K. Khanna, Ex. Principal NHMC & H, New Delhi.

I extend my sincere thanks to Dr Vimal Kumar Bhardwaj for helping me with his useful suggestions and contributing long hours towards the completion of this project. I would also like to thank interns Dr Shweta Garg, Dr Neetu Garg, Dr Namita Amawate, Dr Nirmal Yadav, Dr Anjali Sirpal from Nehru Homoeopathic Medical College and Hospital.

I would also like to thank Assistant Professors; Dr K.G. Mahabole, Dr Asha Choudhary, Dr Neena Mehan and interns Dr Uttara Jain, Dr Vandana Gulati, Dr Gufrana Kamal, Dr Uttam Singh, Dr Aditi Khurana, Dr Meenakshi Dubey of Dr B.R. Sur Homoeopathic Medical College and Hospital for reviewing the literature and helping me in finding suitable references.

From the deepest core of my heart I would like to thank Mr. Kuldeep Jain C.E.O., B. Jain Publishers for his consistent motivation and support for bringing out this book.

Last but not the least, I express my thanks to my wife Rekha and other family members for their unconditional support.

Dr V. K. Chauhan

GUIDELINES FOR PREPARATION

The Union Public Service Commission and various other government organizations conduct recruitment examinations for filling up the vacancies in homeopathic departments; similarly various Indian universities conduct entrance examinations for admission to various MD courses in homeopathy. It is best done with Multiple Choice Question Papers. The MCQs helps in discriminating accurately between candidates on the basis of their knowledge of the topics; being tested in shortest possible time. Most of the MCQs are based on practical and real life situations which a homeopathic medical practitioner is likely to encounter. Therefore, Multiple Choice Questions are structured to test the intellectual ability of the candidates in different dimentions that is, subject knowledge, logical reasoning, inductive and deductive inference, perceptual speed and quantitative aptitude. About 200 MCQs are to be answered in 2 hours time.

Following is the breakup of approximate number of MCQs in each subject:

Serial No		Subjects	Number of MCQ's
Group A	**Major Subject**		
	1	Materia Medica	30-35
	2	Practice of Medicine	25-30
	3	Organon & Chronic Diseases	20-25
Group B	**Minor Subjects**		
	4	Anatomy	03-05
	5	Physiology	03-05
	6	Pharmacy	03-05
	7	Pathology	05-08
	8	Forensic Medicine	02-05
	9	Community Medicine	02-05
	10	Surgery	08-10
	11	Gynecology & Obstetrics	08-10
	12	Case taking & Repertorisation	10-15

Generally a candidate will encounter in most of the test paper following basic types of MCQs:

Type A
The Simple MCQ
Usually there are four choices given. In this type only one is the correct choice and rest three are distractors. Its example is as under:

Q. The Modus operandi of homeopathic medicines is explained in Organon of Medicine, in Aphorism? (UPSC-2004)
   (a) § 26
   (b) § 25
   (c) § 29
   (d) § 39

Ans: (c)

Note

The Modus operandi of homeopathic medicines is explained in Organon of Medicine, in Aphorism '29'.

Type B
The Multiple Selection Type MCQ

In this type of MCQ only one is correct answer and rest three are distractors. It's example as as under:
Consider the following symptoms regarding hemorrhagic diathesis: (UPSC-02)
   (I) Hamamelis virginiana - Prostration out of proportion to the amount of blood loss.
   (II) Secale cornutum - Continuous oozing of sanguinous liquid blood.
   (III) Lachesis mutus - Haemorrhage from left side of the body, bright red and coaguable.
   (IV) Cinchona officinalis - Aversion to sour things during haemorrhage.

Which of these statements is / are correct?
   (a) (I) only.
   (b) (I) and (II)
   (c) (II), (III), and (IV).
   (d) (III) and (IV).

Ans: (a)

Note:

The statement- (I) Hamamelis virginiana - Prostration out of proportion to the amount of blood loss is correct

Type C
Matching type MCQ

In this type of MCQ, the list I is to be matched with list II by selecting the answer using the given codes. It's example is as under:

Match list – I (Medicines) with list-II (symptoms in a case of prolapse uterus) and select the correct answer using the codes given below the lists: (UPSC-02)

List I (Homeopathic Medicine)	List II (Symptoms in case of prolapsed uterus)
A. Stannum metallicum	1. Worse during stool
B. Belladona	2. Better standing and sitting erect
C. Sepia	3. Better supporting vulva with hands
D. Lilium tigrinum	4. Better by sitting close

Code:

Code	A	B	C	D	Code	A	B	C	D
(a)	1	2	4	3	(b)	2	3	4	1
(c)	3	4	1	2	(d)	4	1	2	3

Ans: (a)

Guidelines for preparation

Type D:
The Sequencing Type MCQ
In this type of MCQ only one is the correct answer and rest of the three are disctractors. It's example is as under:

Which of the following is the correct order that matches with the sequential order of 'desire for sweets', 'aversion to sweets' and 'aggravation from sweets'? (UPSC-02)

(a) Argentum nitricum; Cinchona officinalis; Graphites
(b) Cinchona officinalis; Argentum nitricum; Graphites
(c) Graphites; Argentum nitricum; Cinchona officinalis
(d) Cinchona officinalis; Graphites; Argentum nitricum

Ans: (d)

Note
The correct order that matches with the sequential order of 'desire for sweets', 'aversion to sweets' and 'aggravation from sweets' is (d)

Type E
The Assertion and Reason Type MCQ
In this type of MCQ only one choice is correct and rest of the three are distractors. It's example is as under:
Assertion (A): Magnesium phosphoricum is preferred to Belladonna in spasmodic pains.
Reason (R): In Belladonna congestion is marked and pain appears and disappears suddenly.

Answer Code:
(a) Both A and R is true and R is the correction explanation of A.
(b) Both A and R is true but R is NOT a correct explanation of A.
(c) A is true but R is false.
(d) A is false but R is true.

Ans: (b)

Contents

Publisher's Note.. *iii*
Preface .... *v*
Acknowledgements .... *vii*
Guidelines for Preparation .... *ix*

CHAPTERS

1. Organon of Medicine & Homeopathic Philosophy 1
2. Materia Medica 101
3. Anatomy 244
4. Physiology and Biochemistry 261
5. Homeopathic Pharmacy 313
6. Pathology including Microbiology and Parasitology 360
7. Forensic Medicine and Toxicology 409
8. Community Medicine 466
9. Surgery, Orthopedic, Eye, ENT and Dental 522
10. Obstetrics and Gynecology 644
11. Practice of Medicine, Pediatrics and Radiology 707
12. Case Taking and Repertory 1018
13. Screening Test – UPSC 2001 Solved Questions 1085
14. History of Homeopathy in India 1098
15. Various Institutes and Organizations of Homeopathy in India 1103

Chapter 1
ORGANON

Q. 1. The fundamental cause of congenital idiosyncrasy is (UPSC-02)
    (a) Psoric miasm
    (b) Syphilitic miasm
    (c) Sycotic miasm
    (d) Tubercular miasm

Ans. (a)

Note
The fundamental cause of congenital idiosyncrasy is 'Psoric Miasm'.

Also see
References for idiosyncrasy from Organon
§ 116. Some drug symptoms appear with tolerably uniform regularity in each of the several provers, other symptoms appear rarely and with only isolated provers.
§ 117. This latter class may possess, so-called, idiosyncrasies, however, this peculiarity is more apparent than real, since drugs, when indicated by similarity of symptoms never fail to produce curative reactions. However there are certain constitutions that seem to be morbidly affected by certain things that produce no impressions on others. It is a question whether the susceptibility or the immunity is peculiar.
In reference to Congenital or Acquired miasmatic dyscrasia see following:
§ 206. ....the internal itch dyscrasia (the psora) is far the *most frequent* (most certain) *fundamental cause of chronic diseases*, either united (complicated) with syphilis or with sycosis, if the latter infections have avowedly occurred; or, as is much more frequently the case, *psora is the sole fundamental cause of all other chronic maladies, whatever names they may bear,* which are, moreover, so often bungled, increased and disfigured to a monstrous extent by allopathic unskillfulness.
Ref: Organon – By B.K. Sarkar

Extended information
From above the inference
    a. Idiosyncrasy is genetic in origin.
    b. Idiosyncrasy may not present any other manifestation of deranged health.
    c. Idiosyncrasy is difficult to treat.
IDIO = Self; SYN = with, along with; CRASY = make up, constitution. It is a habit or quality peculiar to any person or an abnormal susceptibility to some drug or protein peculiar to a person. Idiosyncrasy as an over sensitiveness and Psora is at the bottom of these idiosyncrasies.

Q. 2. 'Cessat Effectus Cessat Causa' is applicable to (UPSC-02)
    (a) Isopathy
    (b) Homeopathy
    (c) Naturopathy
    (d) Allopathy

Ans. (b)

Note
'Cessat Effectus Cessat Causa' is applicable to 'Homeopathy'.

Extended information
It is impossible to know all the antecedents' causative of disease consequents.
Tolle causam is easier said than done. How, then, shall we remove or palliate these effects by medical substances? Here, Hahnemann steps in to say, for the first time in all history: Remove the effects and you remove the disease, the cause of the effects. Cessat effectus cessat causa. Empiric medicine guesses, recommends, tries, hits and misses, misses and hits again. Scientific medicine does not guess. Scientific medicine, like any other scientific art, compares effects, sensations and motions with corresponding effects, corresponding sensations

and motions. Only the mountebanks in medicine decry methods of comparison as unscientific. All that we can humanly do, and scientifically do, is to observe and classify, to compare and infer. Hahnemann says, we must apply medicinal substances on the basis of knowledge of their actual effects. Since it is impossible to know all the antecedents' causative of disease consequents, we must treat the disease effects which we do know by medicinal effects which we have ascertained and know. Disease effects are removed by the application of medicines having corresponding medicinal effects. If the disease effects are removed *in toto*, we have a cure. If the disease effects are removed in part, we have palliation.

Ref: Introduction (to Dr. Boericke's translation of the sixth Edition) of Hahnemann's Organon by James Krauss MD, Sept 30, 1930.

Q. 3. The phrase 'Aude Sapere' was coined by (UPSC-02), (KPSC-Lect/Org-05)- 78, 121,
- (a) Hahnemann
- (b) Horace
- (c) Huffeland
- (d) Hippocrates

Ans. (b)
Note
The phrase 'Aude Sapere' was coined by 'Horace'.
Also see

'Aude' has originated from Latin word, 'Audthere' which means 'to dare'; 'Sapere' means 'to be wise'. So 'Aude Sapere' means 'dare to be wise'. This quotation of Horace was used by Hahnemann for his 'Medicine of Experience'.

Q. 4. When vital force is suddenly overpowered by the disease, which one the following modes of treatment is useful (UPSC-02)
- (a) Allopathy
- (b) Isopathy
- (c) Homeopathy
- (d) Antipathy

Ans. (d)
Note
When vital force is suddenly overpowered by the disease, the 'Antipathic' modes of treatment is useful.
Also see
Foot note at § 67

Only in the most urgent cases, *where danger to life and imminent death allow no time for action of a homeopathic remedy – not hours, sometimes not even quarter-hours, and scarcely minutes – in sudden accidents occurring to previously healthy individuals – for example in asphyxia and suspended animation from lightning, from suffocation, freezing, drowning, etc. – is it admissible and judicious*, at all events as a preliminary measure, to stimulate the irritability and sensibility (the physical life) with a palliative, as for instance, with gentle electrical shocks, with clysters of strong coffee, with a stimulating odour, gradual application of heat etc. when this stimulation is effected, the play of the vital organs again goes on in its former healthy manner, for there is here no disease to be removed, but merely an obstruction and suppression of the healthy vital force. To this category belong various antidotes to sudden poisonings: alkalies for mineral acids, hepar sulphuric for metallic poisons, coffee and camphor (and ipecacuanha) for poisoning by opium, etc.
Ref: Organon – By B.K. Sarkar

Q. 5. Who is the worst patient among the following to treat? (UPSC-02)
- (a) Hypochondriac patient
- (b) Idiosyncratic patient
- (c) Hysterical patient
- (d) Non co-operative patient

Ans. (d)
Note
Worst patient among the above to treat 'Non co-operative patient'.

Also see
a. Hypochondriac patient; they have a peculiar nature of seeking reassurance from physician that there sickness may not be a serious one.
b. Idiosyncratic patient; these have a peculiar constitution, which do not require any treatment.
c. Hysterical patient; who has hysterical personality traits can be managed.
d. Non-cooperative patient; whether afflicted by mild or severe disease is a worst patient as he do not follow the instructions as well as medication prescribed by physician.

Q. 6. Causa Occasionalis means (UPSC-02)
   (a) Exciting cause and maintaining cause
   (b) Maintaining cause
   (c) Miasmatic cause
   (d) Fundamental cause

Ans. (a)
Note
Causa occasionalis means exciting and maintaining cause. References from § 7 and Foot note of § 7.
Also see
§ 7
Now, as in a disease, from which no manifest exciting or maintaining cause (*causa occasionalis*) has to be removed². We can perceive nothing but morbid symptoms, it must (regard being had to the possibility of a miasm, and attention paid to the accessory circumstances § 5), be the symptoms alone by which the disease demands and points to the remedy suited to relieve it.

Foot note of § 7
2. It is necessary to say that every intelligent physician would first remove this where it exists; the indisposition thereupon generally ceases spontaneously. He will remove from the room strong smelling flowers, which have a tendency to cause syncope and hysterical suffering; extract from the cornea the foreign body that excites inflammation of the eye; loosen the over tight bandage on a wounded limb that threatens to cause mortification, and apply a more suitable one, lay bare and put a ligature on the wounded artery that produces fainting; endeavour to promote the expulsion by vomiting of belladonna berries, etc., that may have been swallowed; extract foreign substances that may have got into the orifices of the body (the nose, gullet, ears, urethra, rectum, vagina); crush the vesical calculus; open the imperforated anus of the new born infant, etc.¹
Ref: Organon By B.K. Sarkar

Q. 7. The 'cure' is possible by Homeopathy if (UPSC-02)
   (a) Exciting and maintaining causes are removed
   (b) Disease is removed
   (c) Miasms are removed
   (d) Idiosyncrasy is removed

Ans. (b)
Note
The 'cure' is possible by Homeopathy if 'disease is removed'.
Also see
In disease, the totality of symptoms is the outward image of the inner disease, of the suffering vital force, related as cause and effect. These symptoms alone must constitute the medium through which the disease demands and points out its curative agent. In each case of 'disease' only this 'totality of symptoms' is to be recognized and removed, by the art of healing, that it may be cured and converted into health. When all the symptoms disappear, health remains. The cause removed the effects cease.

Extended information
§ 7
Now, as in a disease, from which no manifest exciting or maintaining cause (*causa occasionalis*) has to be removed, we can perceive nothing but morbid symptoms, it must (regard being had to the possibility of a miasm, and attention paid to the accessory circumstances § 5) be the symptoms alone by which the disease demands and points to the remedy suited to relieve it – and, moreover, the totality of these symptoms, *of this outwardly reflected picture of the internal essence of the disease, that is, of the affection of the vital force,* (a) must be the principal, or the sole means, whereby the disease makes known what remedy it requires – the

only thing that can determine the choice of the most appropriate remedy – and thus, in a word, the totality of the symptoms must be the principal, indeed that only thing the physician has to take note of in every case of disease and to *remove* by means of his art, in order that it shall be cured and transformed into health.(a)
Ref: Organon By B.K. Sarkar

Q. 8. Name the chronic miasm of the following symptom "Complaints better by abnormal discharges e.g. leucorrhea, coryza etc. Discharges acrid; corroding the parts with characteristic odour." (UPSC-02)
    (a) Psora
    (b) Tuberculous
    (c) Sycotic
    (d) Syphilitic

Ans. (c)
Note
Chronic miasm of the symptom "Complaints better by abnormal discharges e.g. leucorrhea, coryza etc. Discharges acrid; corroding the parts with characteristic odour" is 'sycotic miasm'.

Also see
a. Psoric discharges are characterised by- functional (normal e.g., sweat, urine, saliva) discharges.
b. Tubercular discharges are characterised by- offensive (musty, fetid, sour and carrion like) debilitating.
c. Sycotic discharges are characterised by- yellow, greenish fish brine, acrid corroding. Amelioration by unnatural elimination, through mucous surfaces, e.g. leucorrhea, nasal discharge etc.
d. Syphilitic discharges are characterised by bloody purulent offensiveness.

Q. 9. For the treatment of intermittent fever, Dr. Hahnemann has advised to prescribe to the patient (UPSC-02)
    (a) Highly potentised solution of Cinchona bark
    (b) Thuja occidentalis in crude form
    (c) Anti-psoric medicine in low potency
    (d) Solution of Sulphur

Ans. (c)
Note
For the treatment of intermittent fever, Dr. Hahnemann has advised to prescribe to the patient 'Anti-psoric medicine in low potency'.

Also see
§- 242
If, however, in such an epidemic intermittent fever the first paroxysms have been left uncured, or if the patients have been weakened by improper allopathic treatment; then the inherent psora that exists, alas! in so many person, although in a latent state, becomes developed, takes on the type of intermittent fever, and to all appearance continues to play the part of the epidemic, intermittent fever, so that the medicine, which would have been useful in the first paroxysms (rarely an Antipsoric) is now no longer suitable and cannot be of any service. We have now to do with a Psoric intermittent fever only and this will generally be subdued by minute and rarely repeated doses of sulphur or hepar sulphuric in a high potency.
Ref: Organon By B.K. Sarkar

Q. 10. The peculiar constitution which although otherwise healthy, possesses a disposition to be brought into a more or less morbid state by certain things which seem to produce no change in many other individuals this condition is called (UPSC-02)
    (a) Susceptibility
    (b) Indisposition
    (c) Diathesis
    (d) Idiosyncrasy

Ans. (d)
Note
This condition is called 'Idiosyncrasy'

Also see
§ 117
To the latter category belong the so-called idiosyncrasies, by which are meant peculiar corporeal constitutions which, although otherwise healthy, possess a disposition to be brought into a more or less morbid state by certain things which seem to produce no impression and no change in many other individuals.
Foot note 1
Some few persons are apt to faint from the smell of roses etc.
Ref: Organon By B.K. Sarkar

Q. 11. Psoro-sycotic patient is to be treated as (UPSC-02)
    (a)   Mixed miasmatic case
    (b)   Non-miasmatic
    (c)   Pseudo psoric
    (d)   Pseudo sycotic

Ans. **(a)**
Note
Psoro-sycotic patient is to be treated as 'Mixed miasmatic case'.
Also see

Psoric miasm is probably as old as the human race and manifests mostly in a tendency to skin lesions and catarrhal conditions of the nose, throat and respiratory organs. The superimposed sycotic miasm results from a suppressed or partly cured attack of acute gonorrhea. This condition is usually expressed in the body in some form of warts, moles or tumours, and in some cases arthritis; and there may be a tendency to suicide in those markedly affected by this miasm. Therefore such a patient having psoro-sycotic background is to be treated as mixed miasmatic case.

Extended information
Chronic diseases
The chronic diseases tend to a chronic course. Its start is insidious, the continuation sustained, the outcome hopeless. It is caused due to some internal dyscrasia called the miasm, according to Dr. Hanhemanns writings. The main miasms are three:
Mono-Miasmatic chronic disease
Having single miasmatic preponderance:
    - Psora
    - Sycosis
    - Syphilis
Mixed Miasmatic Chronic diseases:
    -Psoro-sycosis
    -Psoro-syphilitic
    -Syco-syphilitic
    -Psoro-syco-syphilitic

Q. 12. Treatment of the so called mental or emotional diseases is mentioned in which § of Organon of medicine? (UPSC-02)
    (a)   § 105 – 145
    (b)   § 185 – 203
    (c)   § 210 – 230
    (d)   § 212 – 232

Ans. **(c)**
Note
Treatment of the so called mental or emotional diseases is mentioned in § 210 – 230 of Organon of medicine.
Also see
§ 210 – 230
Treatment of so-called mental or emotional diseases.
Ref: Organon By B.K. Sarkar

Q. 13. Which one of following is considered the landmark books in Homeopathy (UPSC-02)
    (a)   Rene Arzneimittellelere
    (b)   Fragmenta de viribus medicamentorum positivis sive in sano Corpore Humano Observatis
    (c)   Systematic Materia-Medica
    (d)   Red lines Symptoms

Ans. (a)
Note
From above the 'Rene Arzneimittellelere' is considered as a landmark book in homeopathy.
Also see
§ 109
I was the first that opened this path, which I have pursued with a perseverance that could only arise and be kept up in a perfect conviction of the great truth, fraught with such blessings to humanity, that it is only by the homeopathic employment of medicines that the certain cure of human maladies is possible.
Foot note to § 109

2. The first fruits of these labours, as perfect as they could be at that time, I recorded in the *Fragmenta de viribus medicamentorum positivis, sive in sano corpore humano observatis pts.* i ii, Lipsiae, 8: 805, ap. J. A. Barth; the more mature fruits in the *Reine Arzneimittellehre,* I Th., Dritte Ausg.; II th, dritte Ausg; 1833; II Th., zweite Ausg., 1825 ; IV T., zw. Ausg., 1825;V Th., zw. Ausg., 1826; Vi Th., zw. Ausg., 1827 English translation, Materia Medica Pura, Vol. i and ii); and in the second, third, and fourth parts of *Di chronishem Krankheiten,* 1828, 1830, Dresden bei Arnold (2nd edit, with a fifth part, Dresseldorf bei Schaub, 1835, 1839).
Ref: Organon By B.K. Sarkar

Q. 14. Which of the above in Q. 13 are authored by Dr. Hahnemann? (UPSC-02)
    (a)   a, b, c and d
    (b)   b, c and d
    (c)   a and b
    (d)   a, c and d

Ans. (c)
Note
Of the above
(a)   Rene Arzneimittellelere
(b)   Fragmenta de viribus medicamentorum positivis sive in sano Corpore Humano Observatis
Were authored by Dr. Hahnemann.

Q. 15. To treat pseudosyphilis cases successfully, Hahnamann advised to begin treatment with (UPSC-04)
    (a)   Anti-syphilitic remedy
    (b)   Anti-Psoric remedy
    (c)   Anti-sycotic remedy
    (d)   Anti-tubercular remedy

Ans. Use your own discretion
Note
In case of Pseudo-syphilis no medication is to be given as it is an 'Iatrogenic Disease'.
Also see
The idiopathic character of syphilitic phenomenon, as a general rule, the morbid dispositions which syphilis excites into active manifestation, do not break forth until sometime after the syphilis is cured; very frequently, however, they become manifest towards the termination of the cure, or perhaps do not owe their awakening to syphilis, but to the insensate masses of Mercury, Iodine, Iodide of Potassium, and other powerful agents with which old-School physicians sometimes drench their patients, as if they were chemical resorts; it is even possible that many of the so-called sequelae of syphilis, which likewise occur under improper homeopathic treatment, are caused by excessive doses of Mercurial Iodides, Phosphorus, Nitric acid, etc.; such sequelae may constitute a sort of pseudo syphilis, and, in reality, may be nothing else than medicinal diseases. However, in whatsoever manner certain original morbid dispositions become roused, be it by the syphilis itself, or by the tumultuous manner in which this disease is treated, the disease thus roused into action, such as tubercular suppurations of the lungs, scrofulous glandular, swellings, affections of bones, cancerous ulcerations, etc.,

continue to exist, by virtue of their own specific cause, long after the syphilis had been cured; but, in such a case, will only manifest their own special characteristic properties, and none of those of the syphilitic disease. Even if this disease should not have been entirely eradicated, but should continue to betray its existence by the occasional outbreak of constitutional symptoms, these latter will always appear perfectly distinct from the symptoms of scrofula, and will be clearly recognizable by their own specific forms.(venereal pathology – from archives windows application)According to the teachings of Hahnemann – no medical intervention like anti-psoric, anti-sycotic, anti-syphilitic or anti-tubercular is to be given as such, but we should be guided by § 76.

§ 76

Only for natural diseases has the beneficent Deity granted us, in homeopathy, the means of affording relief; but those devastations and maintaining of human organism exteriorly and interiorly, effected by years, frequently of the unsparing exercise of a false art, with its hurtful drugs and treatment, *must be removed by the vital force itself.*
Ref: Organon By B.K. Sarkar

Q. 16. Homeopathic aggravation is due to (UPSC-04) & (KPSC-Lect/Org/2005) Q No-98
    (a)   Primary action of medicine
    (b)   Secondary action of medicine
    (c)   Large doses of medicine
    (d)   Incorrect selection of medicine

Ans. (a)
Note
Homeopathic aggravation is due to 'Primary action of medicine'.
Also see
This so called homeopathic aggravation occurs due to the primary action of the homeopathic medicine administered.

Extended information
Ref: § 161
When I here limit the so-called homeopathic aggravation, or rather the primary action of the homeopathic medicine that seems to increase somewhat the symptoms of the original disease.
Ref: Organon By B.K. Sarkar

Q. 17. A person comes with a small piece of straw (foreign body) in one of his eyes. Which one of the following is correct? (UPSC-04)
    (a)   He should be prescribed Aconitun napellus.
    (b)   The case should be managed as per instructions in foot note to § 7 of Organon of Medicine related to causa occasionalis.
    (c)   The repertory should be consulted and indicated drug should be given.
    (d)   Belladonna should be prescribed.

Ans. (b)
Note
In the above situation the 'case should be managed as per instructions in foot note to § 7 of Organon of Medicine.
Also see
§ 7. Foot Note
The cause that manifestly produces and maintains the disease should be removed. (Causa occasionalis).
Ref: Organon – By B.K. Sarkar

Q. 18. 50 Millisimal scale is described in which edition of 'Organon of Medicine'? (UPSC-04)
    (a)   Ist edition
    (b)   IInd edition
    (c)   IIIrd edition
    (d)   VIth edition

Ans. (d)

Note
50 Millisimal scale is described in VIth edition of 'Organon of Medicine'.

Also see
After a long experiment and verification Hahnemann introduced his 'New Altered but Perfect method' of Dynamisation – LM potencies or The Fifty Millesimal Scale potency, which he mentioned in the sixth edition of Organon of Medicine (Aphorism 270). This manuscript was completed in 1842 but published well after death of Hahnemann. It is claimed that Madam Hahnemann was not ready to part when it unless she was paid a very large and handsome royalty. After her death, from her heirs, Dr. Richard Haehl procured the manuscript and published it in German language in 1920. Dr. William Boericke published its English version in 1921.

Q. 19. Hering's law of cure is depicted in Kent's Philosophy under (UPSC-04)
    (a)   8th Observation
    (b)   9th Observation
    (c)   10th Observation
    (d)   11th Observation

Ans. (d)

Note
Hering's law of cure is depicted in Kent's Philosophy under 11th Observation.

Also see
Hering's law of cure *states that: at the time of cure the symptoms will disappear in the following order:*
a.   From within outwards
b.   From above downwards
c.   In the reverse order of their appearance, the first to appear being the last to disappear.

Kent's observations
8th Observation: Some patients prove every remedy they get.
    – Not related to Hering's law of cure.
9th Observation: The action of medicines upon provers.
    – Not related to Hering's law of cure.
10th Observation: New symptoms appearing after the remedy.
    – Not related to Hering's law of cure.
11th *Observation:* When old symptoms are observed to reappear.
    – It is related to Hering's law of cure.

Interpretation
Patient is on the road of recovery, when symptoms are disappearing in the reverse order of their appearance.

Comment
Case is showing a classical recovery.

Intervention
When old symptoms comeback and disappear, stop the medication. Keep watch on the development and if old symptoms come back to stay; repetition of the dose is necessary.

Q. 20. The interpretation of Kent's twelfth observation states that (UPSC-04)
    (a)   The medicine must be left alone.
    (b)   The medicine must be antidoted at once.
    (c)   The medicine was only a superficial remedy.
    (d)   The medicine has been too late.

Ans. (b)

Note
The interpretation of Kent's twelfth observation states that 'the medicine must be antidoted at once'

Also see
The 12th Observation
    – Symptoms take the wrong direction.
Interpretation
    a.   The medicine was wrong.
    b.   The prognosis is bad.

Intervention
Medicine must be antidoted at once.

Q. 21. What happens when the two dissimilar diseases of different strength meet in a living organism? (UPSC-04)
    (a)   The weaker one will suspend the stronger one.
    (b)   Both of them will co-exist with their manifestation.
    (c)   They will be curing each other.
    (d)   The stronger one will suspend the weaker one.

Ans. (d)
Note
When the two dissimilar diseases of different strength meet in a living organism the stronger one will suspend the weaker one.

Also see
Acc to § 38 II
A new dissimilar disease, if of greater intensity, suspends the weaker, or old disease, which reappears when the new disease runs its course.

Ref: Organs of art of healing by Baldwin

Extended information
§ 36
If the two dissimilar diseases meeting together in the human being be of equal strength, or still more if the older one be the stronger, the new disease will be repelled by the old one from the body and not allowed to affect it. A patient suffering from a severe chronic disease will not be infected by moderate autumnal dysentery or other epidemic disease. The plague of the Levant, according to Larry, {"Memoires et Observations", in the Description de l' Egypte, tom.i} does not break out where scurvy is prevalent, and persons suffering from eczema are not infected by it. Rachitis, Jenner alleges, prevents vaccination from taking effect. Those suffering from pulmonary consumption are not liable to be attacked by epidemic fevers of not a very violent character, according to Von Hildenbrand.
Ref: Organon By B.K. Sarkar

Q. 22. The highest ideal of cure is (UPSC-04)
    (a)   Slow, gentle and permanent restoration of health.
    (b)   Slow; vigorous and temporary restoration of health.
    (c)   Rapid, gentle and temporary restoration of health.
    (d)   Rapid, gentle and permanent restoration of health.

Ans. (d)
Note
The highest ideal of cure is 'Rapid, gentle and permanent restoration of health'.

Also see
§ 2
The highest ideal of cure is rapid, gentle and permanent restoration of the health, or removal and annihilation of the disease in its whole extent, in the shortest, most harmless way, and easily comprehensible principles.
Ref: Organon – By B.K. Sarkar

Q. 23. Removal of the totality of symptoms means the removal of disease. This concept is reflected in (UPSC-04)
    (a)   § 10 of Organon of Medicine
    (b)   § 15 of Organon of Medicine
    (c)   § 17 of Organon of Medicine
    (d)   § 20 of Organon of Medicine

Ans. (c)
Note
Removal of the totality of symptoms means the removal of disease. This concept is reflected in § '17' of Organon of Medicine.

Also see
§17
Now, as in the cure effected by the removal of the whole of the perceptible signs and symptoms of the disease the internal alterations of the vital force to which the disease is due – consequently the whole of the disease – is at the same time removed, it follows that the physician has only to remove the whole of the symptoms in order, at the same, to abrogate and annihilate the internal change, that is to say, the morbid derangement of the vital force – consequently the totality of the disease, the disease itself. But when the disease is annihilated the health is restored, and this is the highest, the sole aim of the physician who knows the true object of his mission, which consists not in learned-sounding prating, but in giving aid to the sick.
Ref: Organon By B.K. Sarkar

Q. 24. What is the need to repeat the first prescription? (UPSC-04) &(KPSC/Lect/Org-05)
    (a)   When there is aggravation of existing symptoms.
    (b)   When there is presence of additional new symptoms.
    (c)   When there is amelioration of the symptoms.
    (d)   When amelioration comes to a standstill.

Ans. (d)
Note
The need of repeat of first prescription is when amelioration comes to standstill.
Also see
Repetition of the first prescription
a.   After initial relief following the first prescription, the original symptoms return having the same general and particulars.
b.   After some improvement, the action of medicine stops, the case comes to a standstill position even after waiting for a considerable period.

Mode of using the remedies foot note- Repetition of doses is discussed in 245 – 251 § of Organon. The important ones are as under:

§ 245
Having thus seen what attention should in the homeopathic treatment, be paid to the chief varieties of disease and to the peculiar circumstance connected with them, we now pass on to what we have to say *respecting the remedies and the modes of employing them, together with the diet and regimen to the observed during their use*. Every perceptible progressive to be observed during their use. Every perceptible progressive and strikingly increasing amelioration in a transient (acute) or persistent(chronic) disease, is a condition which as long as it lasts, completely precludes every repetition of the administration of any medicine whatsoever, because all the good medicine taken continues to effect is now *hastening* towards its completion. Every new dose of any medicine whatsoever, even of the one last administered, that the hitherto shown itself to be salutary, would in this case disturb the work of amelioration.

§ 248
The dose of the same medicine may be repeated several times according to the circumstances, but only so long as until either recovery ensues, or the same remedy ceases to do good and the rest of the disease, presenting a different group of symptoms, demands a different homeopathic remedy.
Ref: Organon By B.K. Sarkar

Q. 25. Which of the following miasms has the symptom- 'desire for cold food'? (UPSC-04)
    (a)   Psora
    (b)   Sycosis
    (c)   Syphilis
    (d)   Tubercular

Ans. (c)
Note
The subjects with syphilitic miasmatic trait presents with 'desire for cold food'.
Also see
Psoric patients like: Sweets, sour, fatty, fried, indigestible, spicy, oily, hot food.
Sycotic patients like: Table salt, alcohol, coconut, fat meat, well seasoned foods, peppers, pungent, salty foods.

Syphilitic patients like: Stimulants, alcohol, tea coffee, smoking, very spicy meat, cold food, and drinks.
Ref: Organon of Medicine, Commentary by B.K. Sarkar Pg-371.
Tubercular patients like: Clay, potato, salt, fatty greasy and salty foods etc. Craves things which make them sick. Desires tea, tobacco, meat, craving for salt. Extremes like hot or really cold things.
Some other characteristics of the *syphilitic* patient are:
    a. Diseases associated with ulceration and destruction of tissues.
    b. Silent type of patient that goes out and commits suicide.
    c. Pains are < from cooling.
    d. Dull, stupid, stubborn, sullen, moves and usually suspicious; sulky.
    e. Fixed ideas and one cannot reason with them.
    f. Melancholic and condemn themselves.
    g. Slow comprehension and forgetful.
    h. Complaints < at night, restless and anxious.
    i. Complaints < at summer and > in winters.
    j. Ulcerations and discharge of pus with offensive odour but it ameliorates the complaints.
    k. Eruptions crusty and oozing pus.
    l. Skin greasy and sweaty; much offensive odour.
    m. Hair tends to fall out.
    n. *Desires cold food* – aversion to meat.
    o. Bone pains – deformities – gangrenous conditions.
Ref: Organon of Medicine, Commentary by B.K. Sarkar. Pg no. 371, Edi. 7.

Q. 26. In case of homeopathic aggravation, we should (UPSC-04, 06), (KPSC-Lect/Org-05)
    (a) Antidote the medicine
    (b) Wait and watch
    (c) Prescribe a complementary medicine
    (d) Repeat the medicine immediately in lower potency

Ans. (b)
Note
In case of homeopathic aggravation, we should 'wait and watch'.

Also see
Homeopathic aggravation is an essential phenomenon in the process of homeopathic cure. It is produced by artificial disease which exhibits its dominancy over the natural disease.
§ 161
When I here limit the so-called homeopathic aggravation, or rather the primary action of the homeopathic medicine that seems to increase somewhat the symptoms of the original disease, to the first or few first hours, this is certainly true with respect to diseases of a more acute character and of recent origin; but where medicines of long action have to combat a malady of considerable or of very long standing, (where no such apparent increase of the original disease ought to appear during treatment and it doses not so appear if the accurately chosen medicine was given in proper small, gradually higher doses, each somewhat modified with renewed Dynamisation (§ 247) Such increase of the original symptoms of a chronic disease can appear only at the end of treatment when the cure is almost or quite finished.)
Assessment
    a) Remedy is correct
    b) Potency is correct
    c) Reaction wholesome
    d) No irreversible organic changes
    e) Prognosis good
Implication
It implies that; patient is on the road of recovery. (Approaching cure). After the aggravation period is over, the convalescence period will progress simultaneously to final and complete cure. In such a situation best strategy is wait and watch.

Extended information
Kent's Observations related to aggravation are as under:
1. Kent's 1ˢᵗ Observation: A prolonged aggravation and final decline of the patient.
    Interpretation: Case is incurable (advanced pathology).

Comment: Advanced pathological changes acting as obstruction to recovery.
Intervention: Use low or moderately low potency to provide symptomatic relief.
2. Kent's 2nd Observation: Long aggravation, but final and slow improvement.
Interpretation: Early stage having some tissue change in some organs.
Comment: Pathological changes are in early reversible stage.
Intervention: Keep watches for the improvement, do not repeat the medicine.
3. Kent's 3rd Observation: Aggravation is quick, short and strong with rapid improvement of the patient.
Interpretation: Remedy and potency both correct.
Comment: No irreversible or any structural changes in vital organs.
Intervention: Stop the medicine and observe till improvement takes place.
4. Kent's 4th Observation: No aggravation, but steady improvement.
Interpretation: Assessment and potency selection is extremely well.
Comment: No tissue changes and no tendency for tissue changes.
Intervention: An ideal cure. Watch for Hering's law of cure.

Q. 27. The Modus operandi of homeopathic medicines is explained in Organon of Medicine, in which §? (UPSC-2004)
  (a) § 26
  (b) § 25
  (c) § 29
  (d) § 39

Ans. (c)
Note
The Modus operandi of homeopathic medicines is explained in Organon of Medicine, in § '29'.
Also see
Following are the text of above aphorisms.
§ 26
This depends on the following homeopathic law of nature which was sometimes, indeed, vaguely surmised but not hitherto fully recognized, and to which is due every real cure that has ever taken place:
A weaker dynamic affection is permanently extinguished in the living organism by a stronger one, if the latter (whilst differing in kind) is very similar to the former in its manifestations.
§ 25
Now, however, in all careful trials, pure experience, the sole and infallible oracle of he healing art, teaches us that actually that medicine which, in its action on the healthy human body, has demonstrated its power of producing the greatest number of symptoms *similar* to those observable in the case of disease under treatment, does also , in doses of suitable potency and attenuation, rapidly, radically and permanently remove the totality of the symptoms of this morbid state, that is to say (§ 6 - 16), the whole disease present, and change it into health; and that all medicines cure, without exception, those diseases whose symptoms most nearly resemble their own, and leave none of them uncured.
§ 29
As every disease (not strictly belonging to the domain of surgery) depends only on a peculiar morbid derangement of our vital force in sensations and functions, when a homeopathic cure of the vital force deranged by natural disease is accomplished by the administration of a medicinal agent selected on account of an accurate similarity of symptoms a somewhat stronger, similar, artificial morbid affection is brought into contact with and, as it were pushed into the place of the weaker similar, natural morbid irritation, against which the instinctive vital force, now merely (through in a stronger degree) medicinally diseased, is then compelled to direct an increase amount of energy, but, on account of the shorter duration of the action of the medicinal agent that now morbid affects it, the vital force soon overcomes this, and as it was in the first instance relieved from the natural morbid affection, so it is now at last freed from the substituted artificial (medicinal) one, and hence, is enabled again to carry on healthily the vital operations of the organism (a). This highly probable explanation of the process rests on the following axioms.
§ 39 (in brief)
It is just in this way that violent treatment with allopathic drugs does not cure a chronic disease, but suppresses it only as long as the action of the powerful medicines, which are unable to excite any symptoms similar to the disease, lasts; after that, the chronic disease makes its appearance as bad or worse than before.
Ref: Organon By B.K. Sarkar

Q. 28. Which one of the following does not belong to "Causa Occasionalis"? (UPSC-04)
    (a)   Strong smelling flowers causes syncope
    (b)   Imperforated anus of infants
    (c)   Dyspnea from dust exposure
    (d)   Pthisis after chest injury

Ans. (d)
Note
From above (d) 'Pthisis after chest injury' do not belong to 'Causa Occasionalis'.
Also see
§ 7. Now, as in a disease, from which no manifest exciting or maintaining cause *(Causa Occasionalis)* has to be removed . We can perceive nothing but morbid symptoms, it must (regard being has to the possibility of a miasm, and attention paid to the accessory circumstances § 5) be symptoms along by which the disease demands and points to the remedy suited to relieve it – and moreover, the totality of these symptoms, *of this outwardly reflected picture of the internal essence of the disease, that is of the affection of the vital force, (a)* must be the principal, or the sole means where by the disease make known what remedy it requires – the only thing that can determine the choice of the most appropriate remedy – and thus, in a word, the totality of the symptoms must be the principal, indeed the only thing the physician has to take note of in every case of disease and to *remove* by means of his art, in order that it shall be cured and transformed into health. *(a)*
Ref: Organon By B.K. Sarkar

Q. 29. Mental diseases are (UPSC-04)
    (a)   Psoric in origin
    (b)   Pseudo-psoric in origin
    (c)   Syphilitic in origin
    (d)   Pseudo-syphilitic in origin

Ans. (a)
Note
Mental diseases are 'Psoric in origin'.
Also see
§ 210
Of psoric origin are almost all those diseases that I have above termed one-sided, which appear to be more difficult to cure in consequence of this one-sidedness, all their other morbid symptoms disappearing, as it were, before the single, great, prominent symptom. Of this character are what are termed *mental diseases*. They do not, however, constitute a class of disease the condition of the disposition and mind is always altered; and in all cases of disease we are called on to cure the state of the patient's disposition is to be particularly noted, along with the totality of the symptoms, if we would trace an accurate picture of the disease, we will be able to treat it homeopathically with success.
Ref: Organon By B.K. Sarkar

Q. 30. If psychotherapy is initially administered to the psychosomatic patient, it will cause (UPSC-04)
    (a)   Aggravation
    (b)   Homeopathic aggravation
    (c)   Amelioration
    (d)   Amelioration followed by aggravation

Ans. (c)
Note
If psychotherapy is initially administered to the psychosomatic patient, it will cause 'Amelioration'.
Also see
§ 226
It is only such emotional as these, which were first engendered and subsequently kept up by the mind, itself, that, *while they are yet recent and before they have made very great inroads on the corporeal state*, may , by means of psychical remedies, such as display of confidence, friendly exhortations, sensible advice, and often by as well disguised deception, be rapidly changed into a healthy state of the mind (and with appropriate diet and regimen, seemingly into a healthy state of the body also).
Ref: Organon By B.K. Sarkar

Brief of above aphorism is:
§ 226
These, if treated early, may be cured by psychical methods, gentle kind admonition, appeal to reason, skilful deception, or carefully regulated habits.
Ref: Organon of art of healing by Baldwin

Q. 31. Match List I (Topics) with List II (Aphorisms of the Fifth Edition of Organon of Medicine) and select the correct answer using the codes given below the lists (UPSC-04)

List -I	List -II
A. Idiosyncrasies	1. § 27 - 28
B. Kind of symptoms for choice of remedy	2. § 210 -230
C. Mental Diseases	3. §153
D. Therapeutic law of Nature	4. § 116 -117

Code

	A	B	C	D
(a)	4	3	2	1
(b)	2	3	4	1
(c)	4	1	2	3
(d)	2	1	4	3

Ans. (a)
Note
The correct match is as under

List -I	List -II
A. Idiosyncrasies	4. § 116 -117
B. Kind of symptoms for choice of remedy	3. §153
C. Mental Diseases	2. § 210 -230
D. Therapeutic law of Nature	1. § 27 - 28

Q. 32. Which one of the following causes pseudo chronic diseases (UPSC-04)
    (a) Maintaining cause
    (b) Fundamental cause
    (c) Sycosis
    (d) Syphilis

Ans. (a)
Note
From choice given above the 'Maintaining cause' belongs to 'Pseudo Chronic Diseases'.
Also see
§77
Those disease are inappropriately named chronic, which persons incur who expose themselves continually to avoidable noxious influences, who are in the habit of indulging in injurious liquors or ailments, are addicted to dissipation of many kinds which undermine the health, who undergo prolonged abstinence from things that are necessary for the support of life, who reside in unhealthy localities, especially marshy districts, who

are housed in cellars or other confined dwellings, who are deprived to exercise or of open air, who ruin their health by over exertion of body or mind, who live in a constant state of worry, etc. These states of ill-health, which persons bring upon themselves disappear spontaneously, provided no chronic miasm lurks in the body, under an improved mode of living, and they cannot be called chronic diseases.
Ref: Organon By B.K. Sarkar

Q. 33. First edition of Organon of medicine was published in (KPSC/Lect/Rep-04)
    (a)   1805
    (b)   1810
    (c)   1817
    (d)   1828

Ans. (b)
Note
The First edition of Organon was published in 1810. When Dr. Hahnemann was residing at 'Torgau' and it was published by the famous publisher 'Arnold of Dresden'.

Q. 34. Dr. Samuel Hahnemann has given idea about case taking in the § no (KPSC/Lect/Rep-04)
    (a)   § 1- 70
    (b)   § 71- 82
    (c)   § 83- 104
    (d)   §105- 145

Ans. (c)
Note
Dr. Hahnemann gives reference to case taking in 'Organon of Medicine' in § 83-104.

Also see
Refer: §84 - §104. Taking the case in brief is as under
§ 84
The patient and attendant narrates history of sickness and describes sensations, symptoms and behaviour, the physician observes with sight, hearing, touch and smell and allows story to be finished; only not allowing digressions.
§ 85
Write down each statement in a separate sentence one below the other.
§ 86
After the statement is voluntarily ended, review it, get each statement definitely restated. Get the exact location of each pain, the character of the pain, whether lasting or interrupted or shifting, time of each pain, position of aggravation or amelioration or how it responds to heat, cold, air, rest, motion, posture, contact, touch or pressure. Get a complete description of each attack.
§ 87
Don't ask direct question, or question that can be answered by yes or no.
§ 88
Don't ask leading question or questions that suggest an answer.
§ 84-99
Instructions to the physician for investigating and tracing the picture of the disease.
§ 100-102
Investigation of the epidemic diseases in particular.
§ 103
In like manner must the fundamental cause of (non-syphilitic) chronic diseases be investigated and the great entire picture of psora is displayed.
§ 104
Utility of noting down in writing the picture of the disease, for the purpose of curing, and in the progress of the treatment.
Ref: Organon By B.K. Sarkar, & Organon of art of healing by Baldwin

Q. 35. Number of § in fifth edition of Organon is: (KPSC/Lect/Rep-04)
    (a)   320
    (b)   294
    (c)   291
    (d)   318
Ans. (b)
Note
The number of Aphorisms in 5th Edition is 294.

Q. 36. Who gave the idea of complete symptom? (KPSC/Lect/Rep-04)
    (a)   Dr. S. Hahnemann
    (b)   Dr. Boenninghausen
    (c)   Dr. J.T. Kent
    (d)   Dr. Stuart Close
Ans. (b)
Note
The idea of complete symptom was given by 'Dr. Boenninghausen'.
Also see
Complete symptom according to Boenninghausen has following components: Location, Sensation, Modality and Concomitant.
Boenninghausen has given seven points to segregate the symptoms for a practical assessment. The points are represented in the forms of maxims. They are as under:
    a.   **Quis** - Peculiar constitution & temperament
    b.   **Quid** - Nature of disease
    c.   **Ubi** - Seat of disease
    d.   **Qiubis axillus** - Concomitants
    e.   **Cur** - Cause of the disease
    f.   **Quomodo** - Modalities of circumstances
    g.   **Quando** - Time modalities

Q. 37. General symptoms are those symptoms (KUPSC-Rep-04)
    (a)   Which refer to the person as a whole
    (b)   Which are uncommon in nature
    (c)   Which are common in nature
    (d)   All of the above
Ans. (a)
Note
General symptoms are those symptoms 'which refer to the person as a whole'.
Also see
The general symptoms or sensations that the patient predicts to himself or uses the first personal pronoun are general symptoms i.e., I am weak, or I am thirsty.
The generals are the expression of the whole person at a physical and mental level. When a certain symptoms run through all the particulars, it becomes generals. Generals can be:
    (a)   Physical general
    (b)   Mental general

Q. 38. Concomitant symptoms (KPSC/Lect/Rep-04)
    (a)   Have no value for disease diagnosis.
    (b)   Very important for individualizing the patient.
    (c)   Important for homeopathic therapeutic diagnosis.
    (d)   All of the above.
Ans. (d)
Note
Concomitant symptoms have all above characteristics.

MCQ's in Organon

Also see
Concomitant symptoms are those, which accompany the chief complaints, yet they don't have any pathological relationship with chief complaint.
Value
These symptoms thus represent the individuality of the patient and hence assume an important place in the construction of totality.

Q. 39. What is 'Causa occasionalis'? (KPSC-Rep-04)
 (a) Exciting cause
 (b) Maintaining cause
 (c) Both
 (d) None of the above

Ans. (c)
Note
'Causa occasionalis' refers to both exciting cause and maintaining cause.
Also see
§ 7
Now, as in a disease, from which no manifest exciting or maintaining cause *(Causa Occasinalis)* has to be removed. We can perceive nothing but morbid symptoms, it must (regard being has to the possibility of a miasm, and attention paid to the accessory circumstances § 5) be symptoms along by which the disease demands and points to the remedy suited to relieve it – and moreover, the totality of these symptoms, *of this outwardly reflected picture of the internal essence of the disease, that is of the affection of the vital force*, *(a)* must be the principal, or the sole means where by the disease make known what remedy it requires – the only thing that can determine the choice of the most appropriate remedy – and thus, in a word, the **totality of the symptoms** must be the principal, indeed the only thing the physician has to take note of in every case of disease and to *remove* by means of his art, in order that it shall be cured and transformed into health. *(a)*

Foot note to § 7
It is necessary to say that every intelligent physician would first remove this where it exists; the indisposition thereupon generally ceases spontaneously.
He will remove from the room strong smelling flowers, which have a tendency to cause syncope and hysterical sufferings; extract from the cornea the foreign body that excites inflammation of the eye; loosen the over-tight bandage on a wounded limb that threatens to cause mortification, and apply a more suitable one; lay bare and put a ligature on the wounded artery that produces fainting; endeavor to promote the expulsion by vomiting of belladonna berries, etc. that may have been swallowed; extract foreign substances that may have got into the orifices of the body (the nose, gullet, ears, urethra, rectum, vagina); crush the vesical calculus; open the imperforate anus of the new-born infant, etc.
Ref: Organon – By B.K. Sarkar

Q. 40. What is the main objective of Homeopathic case taking? (KPSC/Lect/Rep-04)
 (a) Diagnosis
 (b) Individualization
 (c) Prognosis
 (d) All of the above

Ans. (b)
Note
The main objective of homeopathic case taking is to 'individualization'.
Also see
§ 83 Each case demands individualization and faithful recording with unbiased judgement and sound sense. The 'Primary object' of homeopathic case taking is 'individualize the patient' and secondary object is to reach for diagnosis, prognosis. This individualization in core essence involves knowing him spiritually, emotionally, mentally, physically and sociologically etc.

Extended information
Advantage of individualization:
Advantage 1. Individualization of treatment – treatment directed to the patient himself, through symptoms, rather than at the disease as a name. (He may not have the disease suspected.)

Advantage 2. All drugs recommended have had extensive human experiment. We do not depend on guinea pigs, frogs, rabbits, etc., to outline the scope of medicine. (Drug proving.)

Advantage 3. By the homeopathic method of using symptoms (the "totality" which is the third principle of homeopathy) we can use symptoms as a guide, curatively, to eradicate the complex (disease) and not just palliatively in the sense that one takes aspirin for a headache or codeine for a cough or bicarbonate for a sour stomach.

Q. 41. What is the prognosis of third observation of Kent? (KPSC/Lect/Rep-04)
    (a)   Good
    (b)   Bad
    (c)   Very good
    (d)   Very bad

Ans. (c)
Note
The prognosis of the third observation of Kent is 'Very good'.
Also see
The 3rd observation of Kent
Aggravation is quick, short and strong with rapid improvement of the patient.
Interpretation
Remedy and potency both correct.
Comment

No irreversible or any structural changes in vital organs.
Intervention
Stop the medicine and observe till improvement takes place.

Q. 42. A full time amelioration of the symptoms, yet no special relief to the patient's is of Kent's which observation? (KPSC/Lect/Rep-04)
    (a)   Fifth
    (b)   Sixth
    (c)   Seventh
    (d)   Ninth

Ans. (c)
Note
A full time amelioration of the symptoms, yet no special relief to the patient's is of Kent's 7th Observation.
Also see
The 7th observation of Kent is
Rapid amelioration of the symptoms, yet no special relief of the patient.
Interpretation
Excellent palliative action.
Comment
    a.   If drug is similimum; case is incurable, having latent advanced organic changes.
    b.   If drug is partially similimum; acting as palliative.
Intervention
Watch the change in sign & symptoms, consider using low dilution.

Q. 43. The action of the medicine upon prover is the ─────── observation of Kent. (KPSC/Lect/Rep-04)
    (a)   Tenth
    (b)   Ninth
    (c)   Seventh
    (d)   Sixth

Ans. (b)
Note
Action of the medicine upon prover is the ninth observation of Kent.

Also see
Kent's ninth observation
New symptoms appear without appearance of old symptoms.
Interpretation
Action of medicine on healthy provers.
Comment
    a.   If symptoms belong to drug pathogenesis; correct remedy.
    b.   New symptom do not belong to drug pathogenesis, the drug symptoms may be missed while proving.
Intervention
No medication. Subject is sensitive to homeopathic drugs and can be a good prover.

Q. 44. In which year Dr. Hahnemann wrote the book on 'Medicine of Experience'? (KPSC/Lect/Rep-04)
    (a)   1803
    (b)   1805
    (c)   1810
    (d)   1819

Ans. (b)
Note
In the year '1805' Dr. Hahnemann wrote the book on 'Medicine of Experience'
Also see
The 'Medicine of Experience' was published in 1805, which was in every respect a forerunner of his Organon.

Q. 45. The word 'Homeopathy' is derived from (KPSC/Lect/Rep-04)
    (a)   German
    (b)   Latin
    (c)   French
    (d)   Greek

Ans. (d)
Note
The word Homeopathy is derived from the Greek homoi = similar, plus Pathos = suffering.

Q. 46. The word Organon is a derivation from (KPSC/Lect/Rep-04)
    (a)   Latin
    (b)   Greek
    (c)   German
    (d)   None of the above

Ans. (b)
Note
The word 'Organon' is a Greek derivation of the word 'Organum' which has following meanings
    a.   Literary work
    b.   A scientific investigation
    c.   Instrument of thought, system or logic
The word was first used by Greek Philosopher Aristotle (384- 312 BC) in his various treatises on logic were summed up under the common title 'Organon'.

Q. 47. 'Novum Organum' was written by (KPSC/Lect/Rep-04)
    (a)   Hahnemann
    (b)   Huges
    (c)   Lord Francis Bacon
    (d)   None of the above

Ans. (c)
Note
Lord Francis Bacon (1561- 1626 AD) wrote a book on Logic in Latin named 'Novum Organum'.

Q. 48. 'Aude Sapere' has originated from (KPSC/Lect/Rep-04)
    (a)   Greek
    (b)   German
    (c)   Latin
    (d)   None of the above

Ans. (c)
Note
'Aude' has originated from the Latin word 'Audhere' which means 'to dare', 'Sapere' means 'to be wise'. So 'Aude Sapere' means 'dare to be wise'. This quotation ('Aude Sapere') of Horace was used for the first time by Hahnemann as the concluding words of his 'Medicine of Experience' in 1805.

Q. 49. Idea about Hydrogenoid, Carbogenoid and Oxygenoid constitution was given by (KPSC/Lect/Rep-04)
    (a)   Dr. Grauvogl
    (b)   Dr. Adolph Lippe
    (c)   Dr. Roger Morrison
    (d)   Dr. Pierce Smith

Ans. (a)
Note
Idea about above constitutions was given by Dr. Grauvogl.
Also see
Von Grauvogl's classification of contitution: Von Grauvogl's arranged the morbid constitutions according to excess or deficiency of certain elements in the tissues and blood.
    a)   *The Carbo-nitrogenoid constitution:* An excess of carbon and nitrogen characterizes it. The carbo-nitrogenoid constitution is Hahnemann's psoric miasm.
    b)   *The Hydrogenoid constitution:* It is characterised by an excess of hydrogen and consequently of water in the blood and tissues. The hydrogenoid constitution corresponds closely with Hahnemann's sycotic miasm.
    c)   *The Oxygenoid constitution:* It is characterized by an excess of oxygen, or, at least, by an exaggerated influence of oxygen on the organism. The oxygenoid constitution corresponds to Hahnemann's syphilis miasm.

Q. 50. Who has worked on the chapter 'relationship of remedies'? (KPSC/Lect/Rep-04)
    (a)   Dr. R. Gibson Miller
    (b)   Dr. J.T. Kent
    (c)   Dr. William Boericke
    (d)   None of the above

Ans. (a)
Note
Dr. R. Gibson Miller has worked on the 'relationship of remedies'.
Also see
A vast amount of work on the relationship of remedies to each other, rather than to symptoms, has been done by such men as Boenninghausen, Hering, Clarke, Gibson Miller, Allens, Kent, Guernsey, and Lippe. Most of this work has been along one main line, that of complementary remedies. The best source for this are - Gibson Miller's little pamphlet, the 'Relationship of Remedies', printed in London.
Ref: 'Brief Study Course in Homeopathy', Remedy relationship by Wright, Elizabeth

Q. 51. The cause of disease action is from (KPSC/Lect/Rep-04)
    (a)   Center to circumference
    (b)   Circumference to center
    (c)   Below upwards
    (d)   None of the above

Ans. (a)
Note
The cause of disease action is from centre to circumference.

Also see
Everything that flows from a center must be considered in connection with that center. Man in his healthy state is the result of the normal activities of a unit, and he must be considered as a unit. In other words, his healthy vital force is the result of action from center.

Disease products are comparatively harmless were it not for the fact that they contain an innermost and it is the innermost itself that is causative. The bacteria are the result of conditions within, they are, as it were, evolved by a spontaneous generation-literally, that is what it is. Every virus is capable of assuming forms and shapes in ultimates. The causes of ultimate are not from without but the immaterial invisible center. Those things that appear to man's eye are evolved, just as man himself is formed from a center which has the power of evolving, an endowment from the Creator,. operating under fixed general laws.
Ref: Kent Lectures – Vital Force.

'There are miasms in the universe, acute and chronic. The chronic which have no tendency toward recovery, are three, psora, syphilis and sycosis; we shall study these later. Outside of acute and chronic miasms there are only the results of disease to be considered. The miasms are contagious; they flow from the innermost to the outer most and while they exist in organs yet they are imperceptible , for they cannot exist in man unless they exist in form subtle enough to operate upon the innermost of man's physical nature. The correspondence of this innermost cannot be discovered by man's eye, by his fingers, or by any of his senses, neither can any disease cause be found with the microscope. Disease can only be perceived by its results, and it flows from within out, from centre to circumferences, from the seat of government to the outermost. Hence cure must be from within out.'
Ref: Kent's Lectures.

In health and disease it is the same, both being essentially merely conditions of the life in the living organism, convertible each into the other. In each condition the modifying agent or factor acts primarily upon the internal life principle, which is the living substance of the organism. This reacts and produces external phenomena through the medium of the brain and nervous system which extends to every part of the body. Food or poison, toxins or antitoxins, therapeutic agents or pathogenic micro-organisms, all acts upon and by virtue of the existence of the reacting life principle or living substance of the organism.

Cure of disease or the restoration of health, likewise begins at the center and spreads outwardly, the symptoms disappearing from within outward, from above downward and in the reverse order of their appearance.
Ref: Stuart – Health and Disease.

Q. 52. Objective symptoms are the symptoms (KPSC/Lect/Rep-04)
    (a)   Noted by relatives
    (b)   Noted by friends
    (c)   Noted by physician
    (d)   All of the above
Ans. (d)
Note
Objective symptoms are the symptoms which are 'noted by; relatives, friends and physician' i.e. all of above.
Also see
Objective symptoms are also known as signs; they include those symptoms which are observed by the attendants, relatives of the patient and by the physician himself.
§ 6
He notices only the deviations from the former healthy state of the now disease individual, which are felt by the patient himself, remarked by those around him, and observed by the physician. All these perceptible signs represent the disease in its whole extent, that is, together they form the true and only conceivable portrait of the disease. *(a)*
Ref: Organon By B.K. Sarkar

Q. 53. Subjective symptoms are the symptoms, which are noted by (KPSC/Lect/Rep-04)
    (a)   Patient
    (b)   Friends of patient
    (c)   Relatives of patient
    (d)   Physician
Ans. (a)

Note
Subjective symptoms are the symptoms, which are noted by 'Patient' himself.
Also see
Subjective symptoms are those symptoms which are felt by the patient himself, without any external indications.
These include sensations, desire and aversions, dreams and modalities etc.
Value
According to homeopathic philosophy these are of utmost importance as:
- a. Hahnemann gave these symptoms a central role in analysis of a case. He found them to be the expressions of the interior states of the organism and mainly mental state.
- b. They represent the earliest deviation from the state of health.
- c. They help in individualizing the case.

Q. 54. Rare symptoms are the symptoms (KPSC/Lect/Rep-04)
    (a) Which appear in every prover
    (b) Appear on maximum prover
    (c) Appear only on few prover
    (d) Appear on fifty percent prover

Ans. (c)
Note
Rare symptoms are the symptoms 'appear only on few provers'.
Also see
The rare symptoms are the characteristic symptoms, which help in individualization. They may be mental, physical or particular generals.
Determinative symptoms whether encountered in disease or a drug proving are alike and usually consist of:
1. Modalities
2. Mental symptoms
3. Qualified basic or absolute symptoms
4. "Strange, rare, or particular symptoms" as mentioned by Hahnemann.

According to Boger
The peculiar strange rare symptoms are concomitants. Their presence cannot be explained by pathology, however, they accompany with the main complaint.
When a marked peculiar symptom belonging to the disease proper, makes the choice of remedy difficult, a concomitant will decidedly indicate the drug.

Q. 55. Most difficult task in a case recording is to obtain (KPSC/Lect/Rep-04)
    (a) Common symptoms
    (b) Mental symptoms
    (c) Physical symptoms
    (d) Individualizing characteristic symptoms.

Ans. (d)
Note
The most difficult job is to ascertain the 'Individualizing characteristic' symptoms and it may belong to the mental, physical or particular general.
Also see
Kent comments
"I do not say this to throw a cloud upon diagnosis, but to show that the study of diagnosis is not for the purpose of making a prescription. The more you dwell upon diagnostic symptoms, the more you will cloud the ideas entering the mind that lead towards a prescription. You might go into the room and work an hour individualizing a case".
Dr. Hahnemann tells us to individualize each particular individual case of chronic sickness under § 83. Each case demands individualization and faithful recording with unbiased judgement and sound sense.

MCQ's in Organon

Q. 56. Object of a homeopathic case taking is (KPSC/Lect/Rep-04)
    (a)   To get idea about common symptoms
    (b)   To get idea about mental symptoms
    (c)   To get idea about symptoms of body
    (d)   To obtain individual picture of the disease

Ans. (d)
Note
Object of a homeopathic case taking is to 'obtain individual picture of the disease'.

Also see
Prime object of the case taking is to collect the data, for selection of a remedy, for each individual picture of a person with disease, based on the homeopathic philosophy.
The pre-requisite for this is the background knowledge especially in the principles of homeopathy, basic medical sciences, clinical subjects and the ability to form a doctor patient relationship.

Extended information
§ 98
…the investigation of the true, complete picture and its peculiarities demands especial circumspection, tact, knowledge of human nature, caution in conducting the inquiry and patience in an eminent degree.
Ref: Organon By B.K. Sarkar

Q. 57. In which §, Dr. Samuel Hahnemann has given idea about homeopathic specific remedy?
(KPSC/Lect/Rep-04)
    (a)   § No. 18
    (b)   § No. 70
    (c)   § No. 71
    (d)   § No. 147

Ans. (d)
Note
The Dr. Hahnemann has given idea about homeopahtic 'specific remedy' in § 147.

Also see
§ 147
Which ever of these medicines that have been investigated as to their power of altering man's health we find to contain in the symptoms observed from its use the greatest similarity to the totality to the symptoms of a given natural disease, this medicine will and must be the most suitable the most certain homeopathic remedy for the disease; in it is found the specific remedy of this case of disease.
Ref: Organon By B.K. Sarkar

Q. 58. Who amongst the following brought the analogy of complete symptom with location, sensation, concomitant and Modality? (KPSC/Lect/Rep-04)
    (a)   Dr. J.T. Kent
    (b)   Dr. Boenninghausen
    (c)   H.A. Roberts
    (d)   Dr. Knerr

Ans. (b)
Note
Amongst above Dr. Boenninghausen brought the analogy of complete symptom with location, sensation, concomitant and modality.

Also see
Boenninghausen perceived and observed, in Materia Medica and patients that the manifestations in different localities showed a tendency to resemble each other rather than otherwise. He interpreted conjointly on grounds of analogy and postulated that whenever observations were missing in a particular area, they could validly be inferred from the characteristics expressions (Sensations or Modalities) in other areas. Thereby, it makes it possible for a physician to build up a workable totality for prescribing similimum. His idea was, "what is true of the part is true of the whole".

For Boenninghausen the individual symptoms are not important but groups are more important. According to Boenninghausen the patients symptoms are to be considered from the group aspect of:
- Location
- Sensation
- Modality
- Concomitants

Q. 59. Outwardly reflected picture of the internal essence of the diseases are (KPSC/Lect/Rep-04)
    (a)   Objective symptoms
    (b)   Subjective symptoms
    (c)   Totality of symptoms
    (d)   None of the above
Ans. (c)
Note
Outwardly reflected picture of the internal essence of the diseases are 'Totality of symptoms'.

Also see
§ 7 - ... and, moreover, the totality of these its symptoms, *of this outwardly reflected picture of the internal essence of the disease, that is, of the affection of the vital force*, must be the principal, or the sole means, whereby the disease can make known what remedy it requires-the only thing that can determine the choice of the most appropriate remedy-and thus, in a word, the totality of the symptoms must be the principal, indeed the only thing the physician has to take note of in every case of disease and to *remove* by means of his art, in order that it shall be cured and transformed into health.
Ref: Organon By B.K. Sarkar

Q. 60. The condition which affect or modify a symptom is called (KPSC/Lect/Rep-04)
    (a)   Aggravation
    (b)   Amelioration
    (c)   Causa occasionalis
    (d)   Modality
Ans. (d)
Note
The condition which affect or modify a symptom is called 'Modality'.

Also see
The condition that modify the symptom is called 'Modality' and it includes; (a) Cause (b) Prodrome, onset, pace, sequence, duration (c) Character, location, laterality, extension and radiation of pain or sensation (d) Concomitants and alternations (e) Aggravation or amelioration – time, temperature and weather, bath, rest, motion, position, external stimulus, eating, thirst, sleep, sweat, discharges, sexual, emotions.
Ref: A brief study course in homeopathy, by Elizabeth Wright

Q. 61. Totality of symptom was introduced in § (KPSC/Lect/Rep-04)
    (a)   § 2
    (b)   § 5
    (c)   § 7
    (d)   § 20
Ans. (c)
Note
Totality of symptom was introduced in § 7.

Also see
The totality of symptom was introduced in § 7.
See the note at Q No: 39 and 59.

Q. 62. Cure is effected by (KPSC/Lect/Org-05)
    (a)   Primary action of similar medicine
    (b)   Secondary action of similar medicine
    (c)   Both primary and secondary action of similar medicine
    (d)   Conjoint action
Ans. (b)

Note
Cure is affected by 'Secondary action of similar medicine'

Also see
Primary action of medicine:
It is the first action of medicine on the vital force. It can be defined as the first phase of the biphasic action of the medicine.

Secondary action of medicine:
It is automatic defensive reaction of the vital force against the primary action of the medicine which is called the secondary action. It is the second phase of biphasic action of the medicine.

Q. 63. Surrogates are (KPSC/Lect/Org-05) –Repeat Q. no-80
    (a)   Homeopathic medicines
    (b)   Substitutive medicines
    (c)   Allopathic medicines
    (d)   Antipathic medicines

Ans. (b)
Note
Surrogates are 'substitutive medicines'.

Also see
Foot note of §119
Any one who has a thorough knowledge of and can appreciate the remarkable difference of, effects on the health of man of every single substance from those of every other, will readily perceive that among them there can be, in a medical point of view, no equivalent remedies whatever, no *surrogates*. Only those who do not know the pure, positive effects of the different medicines can be so foolish as to try to persuade us that one can serve in the stead of the other and can in the same disease prove just as serviceable as the other. Thus do ignorant children confound the most essentially different things, because they scarcely know their external appearances, far less their real value, their true importance and their very dissimilar inherent properties.
Ref: Organon By B.K. Sarkar

Inference
As the action of every medicine differs from that of every other, therefore, in the true sense there can be no such things as surrogates.

Q. 64. Artificial chronic diseases are (KPSC/Lect/Org-05)
    (a)   Drug diseases
    (b)   Drug plus miasmatic diseases
    (c)   Miasmatic diseases
    (d)   None of the above

Ans. (a)
Note
Artificial chronic diseases are 'drug diseases'.

Also see
Following is the brief of the relevant aphorisms:

§ 74
The worst kinds of chronic diseases are those produced by the unskilfulness of allopathic physicians.

§ 75
These are the most incurable.

§ 76
It is only when the vital force is still sufficiently powerful, that the injury can then be repaired, often only after a long time, if the original disease be at the same time homeopathically eradicated.
Ref: Organon By B.K. Sarkar

Q. 65. Psora is the cause of (KPSC/Lect/Org-05)
    (a)   Non-veneral chronic diseases
    (b)   Veneral chronic diseases
    (c)   Both non-veneral and venereal chronic diseases
    (d)   All acute and chronic diseases

Ans. (a)
Note
Psora is the cause of 'Non-veneral chronic diseases'.
Also see
The relevant aphorisms from Organon are as under:
§ 80
Incalculably greater and more important than the two chronic miasms just, named, however, is the chronic miasm of psora, which, whilst those two reveal their specific internal dyscrasia, the one by the venereal chancre, the other by the cauliflower-like growths, does also, after the completion of the internal infection of the whole organism, announce by a peculiar cutaneous eruption, sometimes consisting only of a few vesicles accompanied by intolerable voluptuous tickling itching (and a peculiar odour), the monstrous internal chronic miasm – the psora, the only real *fundamental cause* and producer of all the other numerous, I may say innumerable, forms of disease, which under the name of nervous debility, hysteria, hypochondriasis, mania, melancholia, imbecility, madness, epilepsy and convulsions of all sorts softening of the bones (*rachitis*), scoliosis and kyphosis, caries, cancer, fungus, haematodes, neoplasms, gout, hemorrhoids, jaundice, cyanosis, dropsy, amenorrhoea, haemorrhages from the stomach, nose, lungs, bladder and womb, of asthma and ulceration of lungs, of impotence and barrenness, of megrim, deafness, cataract, amaurosis, urinary calculus, paralysis, defects of the senses and pains of thousands of kinds; etc. figure in systematic works on pathology as peculiar, independent diseases.

§ 81
The fact that this extremely ancient infecting agent has gradually passed, in some hundreds of generations, through many millions of human organisms and has thus attained an incredible developments, renders it in some measure conceivable how it can now display such innumerable morbid forms in the great family of mankind, particularly when we consider what a number of circumstances contribute to the production of these great varieties of chronic diseases (secondary symptoms of psora), besides the indescribable diversity of men in respect of their congenital corporeal constitutions, so that it is no wonder if such a variety of injurious agencies acting from within and from without and sometimes continually, on such a variety of organism permeated with the psoric miasm, should produce an innumerable variety of defects, injuries, derangements and sufferings, which have hitherto been treated of in the old pathological works, under a number of special *names*, as diseases of an independent character.
The brief of the relevant aphorisms is as under:
§73

Acute diseases are due to transient explosion of latent psora. Natural acute sickness due to natural causes are; 1. Epidemic 2. Endemic 3. Sporadic 4. Contagious 5. Infectious.
§ 80, 81
Psora; it is the mother of all true chronic diseases except the syphilitic and sycotic.
Ref: Organon By B.K. Sarkar

Q. 66. Primary action of medicine is (KPSC/Lect/Org-05)
    (a)   Actions of both medicine and vital principle
    (b)   Action of medicine
    (c)   Action of vital principle
    (d)   Reaction of vital principle

Ans. (a)
Note
Primary action of medicine is action of both 'medicine and vital principle'.
Also see
§ 63
Every agent that acts upon the vitality, every medicine, deranges more or less the vital force, and causes a certain alteration in the vital force, and causes a certain alteration in the health of the individual for a longer or

shorter period. This is termed *primary action*. Although a product of the medicinal and vital powers conjointly, it is principally due to the former power. To this action our vital force endeavours to oppose its own energy. This resistant action is a property, is indeed an automatic action of our life-preserving power, which goes by the name of *secondary action of counteraction*.
Ref: Organon By B.K. Sarkar
Brief of the other relevant aphorisms is as under:
§ 63
Every drug has two effects : 1st, primary drug effect; 2nd, secondary vital reaction just as does every other influence affecting the vitality, whether drug or morbific influence.
§ 64
The vitality passively receives the primary drug effects, and then actively by a secondary counter effect, curative crises, neutralizes the primary effects, if they are not so violent as to destroy the life of the individual.
§ 112
"Primary action (§63) is the proper action of the medicine on the vital force, and the reaction of the vital force of the organism, is secondary action (§ 62-67).
Ref: Organon of Art of Healing by Baldwin

Q. 67. Symptomatic treatment is (KPSC/Lect/Org-05)
    (a) Antipathic treatment
    (b) Allopathic treatment
    (c) Isopathic treatment
    (d) Homeopathic treatment
Ans. (a)
Note
Symptomatic treatment is 'Antipathic treatment'.
Also see
Foot note of § 7
In all times, the old school physicians, not knowing how else to give relief, have sought to combat and if possible to suppress by medicines, here and there, a *single* symptoms from among a number in diseases – a *one sided* procedure which under the name of *symptomatic treatment* has justly excited universal contempt, because by it, not only was nothing gained, but much harm was inflicted. A single one of the symptoms present is no more the disease itself than a single foot is the man himself.
Ref: Organon By B.K. Sarkar

Q. 68. A medicine may be called homeopathic, if it is (KPSC/Lect/Org-05)
    (a) Included in Homeopathic Materia Medica
    (b) Used in potensied form
    (c) Prepared according to Homeopathic pharmacopoeia
    (d) Based on the basis of similia
Ans. (d)
Note
A medicine may be called Homeopathic, if it is 'based on the basis of similia'.
Also see
What is medicine?
Medicine is a substance supposed to contain an element or elements having a definite relation to the symptoms of a disease, either that of suppressing the symptoms or relieving or "curing" them.

What is Homeopathy?
Homeopathy is a system of internal medicine or medicinal therapeutic, based on the principle "similia similibus curantur"- like cures like.

When a medicine may be called Homeopathic medicine?
It means that a medicine or a remedy to be curative to a disease, or a state of ill health, must be similar in medicinal nature and therapeutic range of action to the disease, as it is manifested in the patient by the symptoms present. In other words, the medicine in its proving on well people must have brought out or produced symptoms similar to those of which the patient complains. This includes all the symptoms, both the objective

and subjective; but from the standpoint of prescribing the correct remedy, the subjective symptoms are more important because they represent the individual reaction of the disease process within the body.

Q. 69. Vaccination against small pox was an imitation of (KPSC/Lect/Org-05)
    (a)   Homeopathy
    (b)   Antipathy
    (c)   Isopathy
    (d)   Allopathy

Ans. (a)
Note
Disease products, as in vaccination, to protect against a like disease. Hahnemann claimed this for what it is, HOMEOPROPHYLAXIS.

Also see
Disease products for the cure of the same disease? Again, unconscious homeopathy; and again, dating from Hahnemann. He discussed them - were they homeopathy or isopathy? "The cure in such cases," he asserts, "is homeopathy. It is the application of absolute simillimum to simillimum, the administration of a highly potentized and altered miasm to a patient." (By miasm, Hahnemann means germ-disease.)

Hahnemann says that homeopathic prescribing "is the only correct, direct means of cure, as it is only possible to draw one straight line between two given points".
It is true that, in medical conceptions, and even practice, the two schools are slowly, yet surely, converging. Yet the straight line remains straight, and the approach is all on the other side.
Ref: Isopathy - Besweir – Science and art?

Q. 70. Two dissimilar diseases, when both are of chronic character and of equal strength meeting together in the human being will cause (KPSC/Lect/Org-05)
    (a)   New one will be repelled by old one
    (b)   Old one to be suspended by new one
    (c)   A complex disease
    (d)   Neutralization by each other

Ans. (c)
Note
Two dissimilar diseases, when both are of chronic character and of equal strength meeting together in the human being will cause 'a complex disease'.

Also see
Brief of the relevant aphorism is as under:
§ 40
III. Or the new disease, after having long acted on the organism, at length, joins the old one that is dissimilar to it, and then arises a double (complex) disease; neither of these two dissimilar diseases removes the other.
Ref: Organon By B.K. Sarkar

Q. 71. Totality of symptoms includes (KPSC/Lect/Org-05)
    (a)   Only signs
    (b)   Only symptoms
    (c)   Both signs and symptoms
    (d)   Only keynote symptoms

Ans. Use your discretion
Note
Totality of symptoms includes 'both sign and symptoms' which of course includes the keynote symptoms also.
Also see
The related aphorisms are as under:
§ 6
The unprejudiced observer-well aware of the futility of transcendental speculations which can receive on confirmation from experience – be his powers of penetration ever so great, takes note of nothing in every individual disease except the changes in the health of the body and of the (*morbid phenomena, accidents,*

symptoms) which can be perceived externally by means of the senses; that is to say, the notices only deviations from the former healthy state of the now diseased individual, which are felt by the patient himself, remarked by those around him and observed by the physician. All these perceptible signs represent the disease in its whole extent that is together they form the true and only conceivable portrait of the disease.

§ 7

Now, as in a disease, from which no manifest exciting or maintaining cause (*causa occasionalis*) has to be removed. We can perceive nothing but morbid symptoms, it must (regard being had to the possibility of a miasm, and attention paid to the accessory circumstances § 5) be the symptoms alone by which the disease demands and points to the remedy suited to relieve it – and, moreover, the totality of these symptoms, *of this outwardly reflected picture of the internal essence of the disease, that is, of the affection of the vital force*, (a) must be the principal, or the sole means, whereby the disease makes known what remedy it requires – the only thing that can determine the choice of the most appropriate remedy – and thus, in a word, the totality of the symptoms must be the principal, indeed that only thing the physician has to take note of in every case of disease and to *remove* by means of his art, in order that it shall be cured and transformed into health.*(a)*

Ref: Organon By B.K. Sarkar

Q. 72. The doctrine of drug Dynamisation of the Organon of medicine was first introduced by Hahnemann in its (KPSC/Lect/Org-05)
   (a) 1st Edition
   (b) 2nd Edition
   (c) 3rd Edition
   (d) 5th Edition

Ans. (d)

Note
The doctrine of drug Dynamisation of the Organon of medicine was first introduced by Hahnemann in its '5th edition'.

Also see
The Doctrine of Vital force and Drug Dynamisation were introduced for the first time in 5th edition.
§ 269-271
The mode of preparing crude medicinal substances peculiar to homeopathy, so as to develop their curative powers to the utmost.
Ref: Organon By B.K. Sarkar

Q. 73. A homeopath may use medicines (KPSC/Lect/Org-05)
   (a) Only homeopathic
   (b) Both homeopathic and Antipathic
   (c) Homeopathic and Isopathic
   (d) All Homeopathic and Isopathic

Ans. Use your own discretion. (a)

Note
The homeopath may use medicine which is based on homeopathic law, and these are as stipulated in Organon of medicine'.

Also see
The choice is suggested is (a)
   - Only homeopathic; it is according to the fixed principals of homeopathic practice.
   - Both homeopathic and antipathic; not acceptable.
   - Homeopathic and isopathic; isopathic is also not acceptable as per the homeopathic laws.
   - All homeopathic and isopathic. Not acceptable.

Q. 74. Hahnemann wrote in (KPSC/Lect/Org-05)
   (a) Only German language
   (b) Both German and Latin
   (c) German, English and Latin
   (d) German, French and Latin

Ans. (b)

Note
Hahnemann wrote in both German and Latin.
Ref. Richard Haehl

Q. 75. Psora is the cause of (KPSC/Lect/Org-05). Similar to Q. 65. page 34
    (a) All diseases, acute and chronic
    (b) Only chronic diseases
    (c) Only non-veneral chronic diseases
    (d) Only veneral diseases

Ans. (c)
Note
Psora is the cause of 'Non veneral chronic disease'.
Also see
Psora is the fundamental (Primary) cause of all the diseases whether acute or chronic, and even secondary miasms like sycosis and syphilis.
Ref; Q. No. 65 for relevant notes.

Q. 76. The phrase "Aude sapere' was coined by (KPSC/Lect/Org-05) Similar to Q. 3.
    (a) Hippocrates
    (b) Horace
    (c) Hahnemann
    (d) Homer

Ans. (b)
Note
The phrase "Aude sapere' was coined by 'Horace'.
Also see
'Aude' has originated from Latin word, 'Audthere' which means 'to dare'; 'Sapere' means 'to be wise'. So 'Aude Sapere' means 'dare to be wise'. This quotation of Horace was used by Hahnemann for his 'Medicine of Experience' (1805).

Q. 77. Hahnemann died in the city of (KPSC/Lect/Org-05)
    (a) Meissen
    (b) Leipzig
    (c) Paris
    (d) Koethen

Ans. (c)
Note
Hahnemann died in the city of 'Paris'.
Also see
Hahnemann came to France in June 1835. By a Royal decree of August 12th 1836 Hahnemann was granted to practice Medicine in Paris. On 2nd July of 1843 at 5 am Hahnemann breathed his last at the age of 88 years.
Ref: A Treatise of Organon of Medicine Part –I, By A. K. Das.

Q. 78. Surrogates are (KPSC-Lect/Org/2005) Similar to Q. No 64.
    (a) Allopathic medicines
    (b) Antipathic medicines
    (c) Homeopathic medicines
    (d) Substitutive medicines

Ans. (d)
Note
Refer Q. No 63 for note.

Q. 79. Hahnemann mentioned about the law of similia for the first time in (KPSC/Lect/Org-05)
    (a)   1796 BC
    (b)   1790 AD
    (c)   1796 AD
    (d)   1805 BC

Ans. (c)

Note
Hahnemann mentioned about the law of similia for the first time in '1796 AD'.

Also see
Hahnemann in 1790, whilst translating Cullen's Materia Medica, came upon the therapeutic indications of Peruvian bark, where Cullen has attributed its success in the treatment of intermittent fever to the fact it was bitter. However, Hahnemann was not convinced and he experimented by taking 'twice a day, four drams of good china', and soon developed symptoms very similar to ague or malaria fever. This led Hahnemann to conclude that medicines cure diseases because they can produce similar diseases in healthy individuals.

In the year 1796, the discovery was brought to light in his essay titled "An essay on a New Principle for ascertaining the curative powers of Drugs and some Examinations of the previous principles". It was published in Hufeland's journal Vol. II Parts 3 and 4, pages 391 – 439 and 456 – 561. He put forward his new doctrine of "Similia Similibus Curantur" [Like cures like] in contrast to the age old "Contraria Contraris Curantur" [Opposite cures opposite]. Richard Haehl, Hahnemann's autobiographer tells us,"1796 is the year of birth of Homeopathy."
Ref: A Treatise of Organon of Medicine Part –I, By A. K. Das.

Q. 80. The 'Chronic Diseases' contains (KPSC/Lect/Org-05)
    (a)   Only provings of drugs
    (b)   Provings of drugs and nature of chronic diseases
    (c)   Proving, nature of chronic diseases and their effective treatment
    (d)   Nature of chronic diseases

Ans. (c)

Note
Chronic diseases contain 'Proving, nature of chronic diseases and their effective treatment.'

Q. 81. The fourth edition of Hahnemann's Organon contained sections numbering (KPSC/Lect/Org-05)
    (a)   318
    (b)   259
    (c)   315
    (d)   292

Ans. (d)

Note
The fourth edition of Hahnemann's Organon contained sections numbering '292'.

Also see
Following are the editions and number of aphorisms they contained:
First Edition – Contained § - 271
Second Edition – Contained § - 318
Third Edition – Contained § - 320
Fourth Edition – Contained § - 292
Fifth Edition – Contained § - 294
Sixth Edition - Contained § - 291

Q. 82. Pain in the head is a (KPSC/Lect/Org-05)
    (a)   Symptom
    (b)   Sign
    (c)   Characteristic
    (d)   Characteristic sign

Ans. (a)

Note
Pain in the head is a 'symptom'.

Also see
Any deviation from health is disease or ill health. Ill health consists primarily in a change or alteration of the normal functional activity of an organ or part of the body. This condition is usually expressed in signs and symptoms; of these the signs or objective symptoms can bee seen or detected, while the subjective ones are felt by the patient, and may consist of pain or a sensation of discomfort of an organ or any part of the body.

Q. 83. Tolle causam means (KPSC/Lect/Org-05)
  (a) Remove the diseases
  (b) Remove the maintaining cause
  (c) Remove the cause
  (d) Remove the fundamental cause

Ans. (c)
Note

Tolle causam means 'remove the cause'.

Also see
Sixth Edition of Organon in its Introduction by James Krauss, M.D. Boston September 30, 1921, translated by Dr. William Boericke, writes about 'Tolle Causam' (remove the cause) – in fifth paragraph – it is impossible to know all the antecedents' causative of disease consequents. 'Tolle causam' is easier said than done. How, then, shall we remove or palliate these effects by medical substances? Here, Hahnemann steps in to say, for the first time in all history, "remove the effects and you remove the disease, the cause of the effects. Cessat effectus cessat causa".
Ref: Organon of Medicine, Commentary by B.K. Sarkar, page 476.

Q. 84. Among all chronic diseases the most deplorable, incurable diseases are (KPSC/Lect/Org-05)
  (a) Pseudo-chronic diseases
  (b) Artificial chronic diseases
  (c) True natural chronic diseases
  (d) None of the above

Ans. (b)
Note
Among all chronic diseases the most deplorable, incurable diseases are 'artificial chronic diseases'.

Also see
Pseudo chronic diseases
§ 77
Those diseases are inappropriately named chronic, which persons incur who expose themselves continually to *avoidable* noxious influences, who are in the habit of indulging in injurious liquors or ailments, are addicted to dissipation of many kinds which undermine the health, who undergo prolonged abstinence from things that are necessary for the support of life, who reside in unhealthy localities, especially marshy districts, who are housed in cellars or other confined dwellings, who are deprived or exercise or of open air, who ruin their health by observation of body and mind, who live in constant state of worry, etc. These states of ill-health, which person brings upon themselves, disappear spontaneously, provided no chronic miasm lurks in the body, under an improved mode of living, and they cannot be called chronic diseases.

Brief of above
These are the one which are caused by persons themselves due to continuous exposure to some avoidable noxious influences i.e., addiction to liquor, overexertion of mind and body, residing in unhealthy localities.

Artificial chronic diseases
Brief of relevant aphorisms.
§ 41
Much more frequently than in the course of nature, an artificial disease caused by the long-continued employment of powerful, in-appropriated (allopathic) medicine in ordinary practice, associates itself with the

old natural disease, which is dissimilar to (and therefore not curable by) the former, and the chronic patient now becomes doubly diseased.
§ 74

The worse kinds of chronic diseases are those produced by the unskilfulness of allopathic physicians.
§ 75
These are the most in-curable.
Brief of above
These are the ones which are produced artificially by the allopathic non-healing art, due to prolonged use of violent heroic medicines in large and ever increasing doses.

The true natural chronic diseases
§ 78
True chronic diseases proper; they will arise from chronic miasms.
§ 79
Syphilis and sycosis.
§ 80, 81
Psora, it is the mother of all true chronic diseases except the syphilitic and sycotic.
Ref: Organon By B.K. Sarkar

Q. 85. Hahnemannian concept of general symptoms refers to (KPSC/Lect/Org-05)
    (a)   Common symptoms
    (b)   Uncommon symptoms
    (c)   Characteristic symptoms
    (d)   None of the above

Ans. (a)
Note
Hahnemannian concept of general symptoms refers to 'common symptoms'
Also see
The Hahnemann's concept of general symptoms is equivalent to Kentian concept of common symptoms.

Q. 86. Kentian concept of general symptoms refers to (KPSC/Lect/Org-05)
    (a)   Common symptoms
    (b)   Uncommon symptoms
    (c)   Symptoms related to the patient as a whole, which may be common or uncommon
    (d)   None of the above

Ans. (c)
Note
Kentian concept of general symptoms refers to 'symptoms related to the patient as a whole, which may be common or uncommon'
Also see
Kent divided the symptoms in to
        General
        Particular
        Common

General symptoms
- The general symptoms or sensations that the patient predicts to himself or uses the first personal pronoun are general symptoms i.e., I am weak, or I am thirsty.
- The generals are the expression of the whole person at a physical and mental level. When a certain symptoms run through all the particulars, it becomes generals. Generals can be;
    (a)   Physical general
    (b)   Mental general

These general symptoms may be common or uncommon.

Q. 87. In chronic case the most minute peculiarities must be attended because they (KPSC/Lect/Org-05)
    (a)   Are most characteristic
    (b)   Help in the choice of the remedy
    (c)   Have connection with principal remedy
    (d)   All of the above

Ans. (d)
Note
In chronic case the most minute peculiarities must be attended because they 'all of above are important'.
Also see
§ 95 (in brief)
Chronic cases need to be taken carefully. All trivial and obscure symptoms must not be overlooked. Each symptom objective and subjective, helps to complete the totality, and provide a basis for making a homeopathic prescription.
Ref: Organon of Art of Healing by Baldwin

Q. 88. Homeopathic specific remedy relates to (KPSC/Lect/Org-05)
    (a)   A medicine related to a particular disease
    (b)   A medicine in relation to a particular person
    (c)   A medicine related to a particular group of characteristic symptoms
    (d)   A medicine related to a particular group of symptoms

Ans. (c)
Note
Homeopathic specific remedy relates to 'a particular group of characteristic symptoms'.
Also see
§ 153
In this search for homeopathic specific remedy, that is to say, in this comparison of the collective symptoms of the natural disease with the list of symptoms of known medicines, in order to find among these an artificial morbific agent corresponding by similarity to the disease to be cured, the *more striking, singular, uncommon and peculiar* (Characteristic) signs and symptoms of the case of disease are chiefly and most solely to be kept in view; for it is *more particularly these that very similar ones in the list of symptoms of the selected medicine; must correspond to*, in order to constitute it the most suitable for affecting the cure.
Ref: Organon By B.K. Sarkar

Q. 89. Theoretic medicine is a (KPSC/Lect/Org-05)
    (a)   Substitutive medicine
    (b)   A palliative medicine
    (c)   Concept in relation to the development of diseases and their treatment
    (d)   A curative medicine

Ans. (c)
Note
Theoretic medicine is a 'concept in relation to the development of diseases and their treatment'.
Also see
§ 1
The physician's, high and only mission is to restore the sick to health, to cure, as it is termed.
Foot note to § 1

His mission is not, however, to construct so-called systems, by inter-weaving empty speculations and hypotheses concerning the internal essential nature of the vital processes and the mode in which diseases originate in the invisible interior of the organism, (whereon so many physicians have hitherto ambitiously wasted their talents and their time); nor is it to attempt to give countless explanations regarding the phenomena in diseases and their proximate cause (which must ever remain concealed), wrapped in unintelligible words and an inflated abstract mode of expression, which should sound very learned in order to astonish the ignorant-whilst sick humanity sighs in vain for aid. Of such learned reveries (to which the name of theoretic medicine is given, and for which special professorships are instituted) we have had quite enough, and it is now high time that

all who call themselves physicians should at length cease to deceive suffering mankind with mere talk, and begin now, instead, for once to act, that is, really to help and to cure.
Ref: Organon By B.K. Sarkar

Q. 90. In sec. 110 of Organon of Medicine (5th Edition) Dr. Hahnemann criticized the concept of "Doctrine of Signature" (KPSC/Lect/Org-05)
- (a) Yes
- (b) No
- (c) No reference of this concept
- (d) None of the above

Ans. (a)

Note
In section 110 of the Organon of Medicine (5th Edition) Dr. Hahnemann criticized the concept of 'Doctrine of Signature'.

Also see
§ 110
......Peculiar powers of medicines available for the cure of disease are to be learned neither by any ingenious *a priori* speculations, nor by the smell, taste or appearance of the drugs, nor by their chemical analysis, nor yet by the employment of several of them at one time in a mixture (prescription) in diseases..... .
Ref: Organon By B.K. Sarkar

Q. 91. According to Stuart Close constitution of an individual develops as a result of the following (KPSC/Lect/Org-05)
- (a) Interaction between hereditary and environmental factors
- (b) Interaction between simple substance and medicine
- (c) Interaction between simple substance and disease
- (d) None of the above

Ans. (a)

Note
According to Stuart Close constitution of an individual develops as a result of the 'Interaction between hereditary and environmental factors'.

Also see
According to Stuart Close – "constitution is that aggregate of hereditary characters influenced more or less by environment, which determines the individual's reaction successful or unsuccessful to the stress of environment".

Q. 92. Totality of symptoms (KPSC/Lect/Org-05)
- (a) Quantitative
- (b) Qualitative
- (c) Quantitative and qualitative
- (d) Not related to either quantity or quality

Ans. (b)

Note
Totality of symptoms is 'qualitative'.

Also see
Totality of symptom no doubt includes all the manifestation of internally deranged vital force, however the dependable totality is qualitative one and it includes those peculiar, uncommon singular and is distinguishing (characteristic) symptoms.
The suitable aphorism in this respect is as under
§ 154
If the antitype constructed from the list of symptoms of the suitable medicine contain those peculiar, uncommon, singular and distinguishing (characteristic) symptoms, which are to be met with in the disease to be cured in the greatest number and in the greatest similarity this medicine in the most appropriate homeopathic specific remedy for this morbid state; the disease, if it be not one of very long standing, will generally be removed and extinguished by the first dose of it, without any considerable disturbance.

Ref: Organon By B.K. Sarkar
Discussion
After a most thorough investigation, and guided by the most conspicuous and peculiar symptoms, a remedy in accordance with the strict similitude of symptoms should then be selected, anti-psoric, anti-syphilitic, anti-sycotic, as the case demands by its totality. Here the most conspicuous and peculiar / characteristic symptom refers to 'Qualitative one'.

Q. 93. In section 153 of Organon of Medicine (5th edition) Hahnemann actually evaluated the symptoms. (KPSC/Lect/Org-05)
(a) Yes
(b) No
(c) This section is not at all related to symptom classification
(d) This section is related to miasmatic diagnosis

Ans. (a)
Note
In section 153 of Organon of Medicine (5th edition) Hahnemann actually evaluated the symptoms.
Also see
§ 153 (Fifth Edition)
In this search for a homeopathic specific remedy, that is to say, in this comparison of the collective symptoms of the natural disease with the list of symptoms of known medicines, in order to find among these an artificial morbific agent corresponding by similarity to the disease to be cured, *the more striking, singular, uncommon and peculiar (characteristic) signs and symptoms of the case of disease are chiefly and most solely to be kept in view*; for it is more particularly these that very similar ones in the list of symptoms of the selected medicine must correspond to, *in order to constitute it the most suitable for effecting the cure.* The *more general and undefined symptoms: loss of appetite, headache, debility, restless sleep, discomfort, and so forth, demand but little attention* when of that vague and indefinite character, if they cannot be more accurately described, as symptoms of such a general nature are observed in almost every disease and from almost every drug.
Ref: Organon By B.K. Sarkar

Q. 94. The objective(s) of homeopathic case taking is (are) (KPSC/Lect/Org-05)
(a) Diagnosis of the disease
(b) Individualization
(c) Anamnesis
(d) All of the above

Ans. (d)
Note
The objective(s) of homeopathic case taking is (are); all of above.
Also see
The objectives of the case taking are multidimensional and according to the descending order of significance they are as under:

a. *Individualization*
   It is important as homeopathy believes in holistic concept that the person in question is sick and not his organs, therefore every case of sickness needs to be individualized.

b. *Anamnesis*
   It includes the following
   Whether the symptoms are complete or not; i.e., location, sensation, modality, extension?
   Whether they fall in the category of general or particular?
   What grade the symptom belongs to?
   Whether it is keynote symptom? What value one should attach to it?
   Whether it is symptom which can be used as eliminating symptom while deciding the repertorial analysis?

c. *Diagnosis*
   It includes the nosological nomenclature of the disease according to the current medical practice as adopted in accordance with ICD 10 and DSM IV. These are important from the legal and investigative point of view.

All the above aspects have a significant role in individual case management and includes nosological diagnosis, homeopathic drug diagnosis, prognosis, investigations from homeopathic point (miasm involve) and modern pathological ones, (when required) which is an integral aspect as a legal accountability of a concerned physician as well professional up-manship.

Q. 95. The importance of diagnosis of disease in the selection of homeopathic remedy is as follows: (KPSC/Lect/Org-05)
- (a) Nothing
- (b) Least
- (c) Highly
- (d) None of the above

Ans. (b)
Note
The importance of diagnosis of disease in the selection of homeopathic remedy is as follows 'least'
Also see
Selection of similimum / drug diagnosis is primary goal of any homeopath however the secondary goal is to go for nosological diagnosis by which we know the prognosis and general management in a given case.

Q. 96. According to __, "sycosis is contagious disease which results from suppression of chronic gonorrhoea. (KPSC/Lect/Org-05)
- (a) Hahnemann
- (b) J.T. Kent
- (c) J.H. Allen
- (d) Stuart Close

Ans. (a)
Note
Dr. Hahnemann has discussed the miasmatic theory of chronic sickness in his Book 'Chronic Diseases' following is brief note about sycosis:
The sycotic miasmatic dyscrasia is a direct result of suppressed or partly cured episode of acute gonorrhea. This condition is often expressed by the body in form of warty growths, moles or tumours, or as arthritic affections; and in one sided disease in the mental sphere there is a marked tendency to suicide.

Q. 97 Accessory miasm is related to (KPSC/Lect/Org-05)
- (a) Rabies vaccine
- (b) Cowpox vaccine
- (c) Smallpox vaccine
- (d) Measles vaccine

Ans. (b)
Note
Accessory miasm is related to 'Cowpox vaccine'.
Also see
§ 46
......The inoculated cow-pox, I say, after it has taken cures perfectly and permanently, in a homeopathic manner, by the similarity of this accessory miasm, analogous cutaneuous eruptions of children, often of very long standing and of a very troublesome character, as a number of observers assert.
Ref: Organon By B.K. Sarkar

Q. 98. Similar diseases can (KPSC/Lect/Org-05)
- (a) Co-exist in patient
- (b) Cannot co-exist in a patient
- (c) Can palliate a disease
- (d) Can suppress a disease

Ans. (b)
Note
Similar diseases 'can not co-exist in a pateint'

Also see

§ 44

The diseases *similar* to each other can either (as is asserted of dissimilar diseases in I [§ 36]) repel one another nor (as has been shown of dissimilar diseases in II [§ 38]) suspend one another, so that the old one shall return after the new one has run its course; and just as little can two *similar* diseases (as has been demonstrated in III [§ 40] respecting affections) *exist beside each other* in the same organism, or together form a double complex disease.

Brief of § 44

Two similar diseases cannot, like two dissimilar diseases; 1st, repel each other; 2nd, suspend each other, or, 3rd, complicate each other.

Ref: Organon By B.K. Sarkar

§ 45

On the contrary, two diseases differing in kind, similar in symptoms, when appearing in the same individual, the stronger will permanently overcome the weaker, which being a dynamic power without substance, i.e. a condition not a thing, ceases to exert an influence. By virtue of this principle, a successful vaccination with pure cow-pox will provide increased resistance to its most similar natural sickness, small-pox.

Ref: Organon of Art of Healing by Baldwin

Q. 99. Vital force exists in (KPSC/Lect/Org-05)
    (a)   The curative medicine
    (b)   The patient
    (c)   Both in medicine and the patient
    (d)   The palliative medicine

Ans. (b)

Note

Vital force exists in 'the patient'.

Also see

§ 9 (a)

In the healthy condition of man, the spiritual vital force (autocracy), the dynamics that animates the material body (organism) rules with unbounded sway, and retains all the parts of the organism in admirable harmonious, vital operation, as regards both sensations and functions, so that our indwelling, reason-gifted mind can freely employ this living, healthy instrument for the highest purposes of our existence.

Ref: Organon By B.K. Sarkar

§ 10

The material organism, without the vital force, is without conscious state or feeling and is dead. There is no reason in the attempt to divorce the psychic from the physical. The two are essential and indissoluble, in this life, forming the perfect unit. Consciousness is a manifestation of life not life of consciousness.

Ref: Organs of art of healing by Baldwin

Q. 100. A second disease when dissimilar to the first disease (KPSC/Lect/Org-05)
    (a)   Always cures
    (b)   Never cures
    (c)   Always palliates
    (d)   Never palliates

Ans. (b)

Note

A second disease when dissimilar to the first disease 'Never cures'.

Also see

The related aphorisms in brief are as follows:

§ 36

I. *The older disease existing in the body, if it be equally as strong or stronger, keeps away from the patient a new dissimilar disease.*

Therefore, suggested answer is (b).

However take note of the following:

§ 38
II. Or a new, stronger disease, attacking an individual already ill, suppresses only, as long it lasts, the old disease that is dissimilar to it, already present in the body, but never removes it.
Dissimilar diseases, of equal intensity, never unequal, may coexist in the same body.

§ 40
III. Or the new disease, after having long acted on the body, joins the old one that is dissimilar to it, and then arises a double (complex) disease; neither of these two dissimilar diseases removes the other.

§ 41
Much more frequently than in the course of nature, an artificial disease caused by the long – continued employment of powerful, inappropriate (Allopathic) medicine in ordinary practice, associates itself with the old natural disease, which is dissimilar to (and therefore not curable by) the former, and the chronic patient now becomes doubly diseased.

§ 42
These diseases that thus complicate one another take, on account of their dissimilarity, each the place in the organism suited for it.
Ref: Organon By B.K. Sarkar

Q. 101. Organon of medicine was first published in (KPSC/Lect/Org-05)
  (a) 1810 A.D
  (b) 1710 A.D
  (c) 1810 B.C
  (d) 1710 B.C

Ans. (a)
Note
The Organon of medicine was first published in 1810 A.D.

Q. 102. Hahnemann (KPSC/Lect/Org-05)
  (a) Invented Law of similars
  (b) Discovered Law of similars
  (c) Invented Law of contraria
  (d) None of the above

Ans. (b)
Note
Hahnemann discovered the 'law of similars'.

Also see
The natural law of cure is based on different natural experiments and observations. Hahnemann by his fine observations and inductive method of reasoning became convinced on the law of cure, *SIMILIA SIMILIBUS CURANTUR*. He embraced it and declared it to be universal, and a basic law of therapeutics. He did not invent the law of similars but he discovered its practical application to the art of healing.

Q. 103. Chronic diseases have (KPSC/Lect/Org-05)
  (a) Very rapid course and very abrupt onset
  (b) Very lingering course and very slow onset
  (c) Very rapid course and very slow onset
  (d) Very lingering course and very abrupt onset

Ans. (b)
Note
Chronic diseases have 'very lingering course and very slow onset'.

Also see
Brief of §72
Chronic diseases
The chronic diseases tend to have a chronic course. It's start is insidious, the continuation sustained, the outcome hopeless. According to Dr. Hahnemann, it is caused due to some internal dyscrasia called the miasm.

Q. 104. Nature's law of cure is found in (KPSC/Lect/Org-05)
    (a)   Allopathy
    (b)   Homeopathy
    (c)   Isopathy
    (d)   Enantiopathy

Ans. (b)
Note
Nature's law of cure is found in 'Homeopathy'.
Also see
§ 26 (a)
This depends on the following homeopathic law of nature which was sometimes, indeed vaguely surmised but not hitherto fully recognized, and to which is due every real cure that has ever taken place:
A weaker dynamic affection is permanently extinguished in the living organism by a stronger one, if the latter (whilst differing in kind) is very similar to the former in its manifestations.
Ref: Organon By B.K. Sarkar

Q. 105. A homeopathic physician may use medicines according to the (KPSC/Lect/Org-05)
    (a)   Law of similia only
    (b)   Laws of similia and contraries
    (c)   Laws of similia, contrariia and dissimilia
    (d)   Laws of similia and isopathia

Ans. (a)
Note
A homeopathic physician may use medicines according to the 'Laws of similia only'.
Also see
What is homeopathy?
Refer § 26 (a)
Homeopathy is a system of internal medicine or medicinal therapeutic, based on the principle "similia similibus curantur"- like cures like.
What is isopathy?
Refer foot note § 56

It is the use of disease products for the cure of the same disease? Again, unconscious homeopathy; and again, dating from Hahnemann. He discussed them - were they homeopathy or isopathy? "The cure in such cases," he asserts, "is homeopathy the application of absolute simillimum to simillimum the administration of a highly potentized and altered miasm to a patient." (By miasm, Hahnemann means germ-disease.)

Q. 106. In the western recorded history the law of simila was first mentioned by (KPSC/Lect/Org-05)
    (a)   Hahnemann
    (b)   Hippocrates
    (c)   Galen
    (d)   Aristotle

Ans. (b)
Note
In the western recorded history the law of simila was first mentioned by 'Hippocrates'.
Also see
"This recognition of law underlying cure is of ancient origin; no one knows when the first recognition of this law crept into use, but ancient Hindu manuscripts recorded its application. Certainly Aristotle recognized it, and *Hippocrates sensed the possibilities of this law and applied it in some recorded cases.* From time to time all through medical history this hypothesis was enunciated or demonstrated in greater or less degree. Hahnemann later demonstrated this law to be universal and not an occasional circumstance. He called the science and art of healing which naturally followed, homeopathy, but the thought was not a new one; it was age-old before a science of healing was based solely on this law".
Ref: Robert

Q. 107. The following is written by one of the below doctors: 'Biological development: Function creates and develops the organs. Of disease development: Functional symptoms are produced by the vital force in exact proportion to the profundity of the disturbance. Functional symptoms precede structural change'. (KPSC/Org/RE-05)
(a) Dr. Kent
(b) Dr. H.A. Roberts
(c) Dr. Stuart Close
(d) Dr. Hahnemann

Ans. (b)
Note
The above note is from 'Introduction to the study of Homeopathy' - by Dr. H. A. Roberts.

Q. 108. Of the below who said "A rational knowledge of anatomy is important. No homeopath ever discouraged the true study of anatomy and physiology"? (KPSC/Org/Re exam-05)
(a) Stuart Close
(b) Kent
(c) H.A. Roberts
(d) Hering

Ans. (b)
Note
A rational knowledge of anatomy is important. No homeopath ever discouraged the true study of anatomy and physiology. It is important not only to know the superficial but the real, profound character, to enable you to recognize one symptom-image from another.
Ref: Kent Lectures - The Examination of the Patient

Q. 109. By which method Hahnemann got the idea similia similibus curentur? (KPSC/Org/RE-05)
(a) Deduction
(b) Induction
(c) Generalization
(d) Individualization

Ans. (b)
Note
Dr. Hahnemann got the idea of 'similia similibus curentur' by method of Induction.
Also see
Experimentation is for one of two purposes, observation for induction, or verification of inductions. Experimentation is analysis, deduction, analytic deduction. We deduce from objects of nature, man or drug, properties in contrast with other properties. We observe by contrast. Observation is comparison, weighing, judging of contrasts. We compare for correspondence. We classify by resemblance. Classification is synthesis, induction, synthetic induction. We classify, conceive for reflection, thought, judgment. We think for expression. We formulate our propositions for verification. We verify by experimentation, by analytic deduction, the formulated propositions of science, of scientific inductions.
Inductive method is the scientific method that proceeds by induction that is by drawing universal conclusions from particular premise.

Q. 110. Of the below who said "We often hear patients classified on snap judgment as a Pulsatilla patient, a Nux vomica patient or perhaps a Phosphorous patient. Because of the general build and colouring associated with these remedies many mistakes have been made in prescribing on this so called type method"?(KPSC/Org/Re exam/2005)
(a) H.A. Roberts
(b) Kent
(c) Stuart Close
(d) Hahnemann

Ans. (a)

Note
The above passage is form the writings of 'Dr. H.A. Roberts'.
Also see

We often hear patients classified on snap judgments as a Pulsatilla patient, Nux vomica patient, or perhaps Phosphorus patient, because of the general build and colouring associated with these remedies. Many mistakes have been made in prescribing on this so-called type method. Let us analyses the reasons we have for considering a phlegmatic blonde woman as a Pulsatilla patient. Do we mean that this colouring always indicates Pulsatilla? Do we mean that a woman of this type never requires Nux vomica? If we do, we have based our conclusions on a half-truth. What we really mean is that the stout young woman with blue eyes, fair hair and pale skin has developed more, and more clearly cut symptoms under the proving than people of other colouring or stature. On the other hand, the best provers of Nux vomica were wiry dark men. This means that the natural physical makeup of certain people predisposing them to certain reactions under certain circumstances makes them particularly susceptible to certain disease influences, whether these disease influences are natural (created by themselves or their environment) or artificial (created by homeopathic provings). In other words, the temperament as cast in the beginning of their existence predisposes to certain morbific reactions, and, if not controlled, they will develop these reactions under certain circumstances. Ref: Robert – Temperament

Q. 111. Of these which is belonging to the individual? (KPSC/Org/RE-05)
    (a)   Peculiar symptoms
    (b)   General symptoms
    (c)   Local symptoms
    (d)   Past symptoms

Ans. (a)
Note
From above 'Peculiar symptoms' belong to the individual.
Also see
Peculiar symptoms are those symptoms which are strange or bizarre and may appear in any sphere whatsoever. They may be encountered in terms of - location, sensation, modalities, or connected with physical or mental generals etc. They are unique in themselves, which, makes them prominent as individual morbid expressions.

Q. 112. Of these which is acting more powerfully than others? (KPSC/Org/RE-05)
    (a)   Medicines act more powerfully
    (b)   Infections act more powerfully
    (c)   Telluric influences act more powerfully
    (d)   Meteoric influences act more powerfully

Ans. (a)
Note
From above the 'Medicines act more powerfully' than others.
Also see
§ 30
The human body appears to admit of being much more powerfully affected in its healthy medicines (partly because we have the regulation of the dose in our own power) than by natural morbid stimuli-for natural diseases are cured and overcome by suitable medicines.
Ref: Organon By B.K. Sarkar

Q. 113. Of the below which one complicates the chronic malady? (KPSC/Org/RE-05)
    (a)   Allopathic method
    (b)   Homeopathic method
    (c)   Two dissimilar affections
    (d)   Continuation of maintaining causes

Ans. (a)
Note
From above 'Allopathic method' is the one which complicates the chronic malady.

Also see
§ 41
Much more frequent than the natural disease associating with and complicating one another in the same body are the morbid complications resulting from the art of the ordinary practitioner, which the inappropriate medical treatment (the allopathic method) is apt to produce by the long-continued employment of unsuitable drugs. To the natural disease, which it is proposed to cure, there are then added, by the constant repetition of the unsuitable medicinal agent, the new, often very tedious, morbid conditions which might be anticipated from the peculiar powers of the drug; these gradually coalesce with and complicate the chronic malady which is dissimilar to them (which they were unable to cure by similarity of action, that is, homeopathically), adding to the old disease a new, dissimilar, artificial malady of a chronic nature, and thus give the patient a double in place of a single disease, that is to say, render him much worse and more difficult to cure, often quite uncurable.......
Ref: Organon By B.K. Sarkar

Q. 114. Who taught the palliative method? (KPSC/Org/RE-05)
    (a)   Galen's Teaching
    (b)   Plato's teaching
    (c)   Asclepias teaching
    (d)   Cullen's teaching

Ans. (a)
Note
Galen's Teaching taught the palliative method.

Also see
§ 56 (Sixth Edition of Organon)

By means of this palliative (antipathic, enantipathic) method, introduced according to Galen's teaching "Contraria contratris" for seventeen centuries, the physicians hitherto could hope to win confidence while they deluded with almost instantaneous amelioration. But how fundamentally unhelpful and hurtful this method of treatment is (in diseases not running a rapid curse) we shall see in what follows. It is certainly the only one of the modes of treatment adopted by the allopaths that had any manifest relation to a portion of the sufferings caused by the natural disease; but what kind of relation? Of a truth the very one (the exact contrary of the right one) that ought carefully to be avoided if we would not delude and make a mockery of the patient affected with a chronic disease.

Q. 115. Of the below in which palliative method is done? (KPSC/Org/RE-05)
    (a)   Natural disease
    (b)   Sudden accidents
    (c)   Incurable diseases
    (d)   Acute diseases

Ans. (b)
Note
From the choice given above in 'sudden accidents' calls for palliative method.

Also see
a.   For *natural diseases*
Only curative treatment is, homeopathic.
b.   For *sudden accidents:* (See foot note 1 of § 67)
Only in the most urgent cases where danger to life and imminent death allow no time for the action of homeopathic remedy- not hours, sometimes not even quarter-hours, and scarcely minutes- in sudden accidents occurring to previously healthy individuals- for example in asphyxia and suspended animation from lightning, from suffocation, freezing, drowning etc. - is it admissible and judicious, at all events as a preliminary measure, to stimulate the irritability and sensibility (the physical life) with a palliative....
Ref: Organon By B.K. Sarkar
c.   For *Incurable diseases:* the simillimum could act only as palliative.
    (Kent's –5th Observation)
d.   For *Acute diseases:* since these are self limiting and at the best can be managed with homeopathic medicines.

Q. 116. Of the below through which the medicine acts? (KPSC/Org/RE-05)
(a) Acts through blood vessels
(b) Acts through the tongue
(c) Acts through the nose
(d) Acts through the sentient nerves

Ans. (d)
Note
The medicines act 'through the sentient nerves'.
Also see
§ 16
Medicines acting upon our spirit-like vital force, which preserves them through the medium of the sentient faculty of the nerves everywhere present in the organism.
Ref: Organon By B.K. Sarkar

Q. 117. Of these which is deducted according to logic? (KPSC/Org/RE-05)
(a) Law of totality of symptoms
(b) Law of nature to cure diseases
(c) Law of modalities
(d) Law of generals

Ans. (b)
Note
From the choice given above 'Law of nature to cure diseases' is deducted according to logic.
Also see
Dr. Hahnemann had a great scientific approach in observation of nature (inductive logic) and he applied those findings in healing the sick through logical application (deductive logic) of the natural laws. Hahnemann followed the steps as under:

a. **The Exact observation of the law of nature**
§46 Examples illustrating the natural phenomena: 1, Smallpox has cured opthalmia; 2, Blindness, caused by suppressed eruption has been cured by smallpox; 3, Smallpox has cured deafness; 4, Smallpox has cured swelling of the testicles; 5, Cow-pox lessens the intensity of smallpox; 6, Vaccination with cow-pox is a recognized preventive of smallpox.
Through the unbiased observation in nature he formulated the following:
§45 Two diseases differing in kind, similar in symptoms, when appearing in the same individual, the stronger will permanently overcome the weaker.

b. **Correct interpretation and rational explanation:**
While translating the Cullen's Materia Medica the use of cinchona bark for intermittent fever attracted his attention. His interest thus aroused and his experiments with medicinal substances began.
The correct interpretation of the phenomenon produced by experiments or proving of the drugs thus provided similar results on him and his friends. It proved that cinchona is not curative in intermittent fever due to its bitter taste but because of its ability of producing symptoms similar to intermittent fever (inductive logic).

c. **Use of nature's law of cure as based on observed facts:**
Thus, Hahnemann insisted on the importance of this premise (similia similibus curentur) in treating the patients, as he was the first to test medical substance and apply the results with this purpose in mind by the rational explanation (inductive logic) of the whole phenomenon .

d. **The scientific construction:**
With the above facts in hand he applied the facts to resolve the certain medical problems with application of similia and to his anticipation he found the laws of nature of 'similia similibus curanture' as a 'true law of cure in nature' (deductive logic i.e. drawing a particular conclusion from a universal premise).

MCQ's in Organon

Q. 118. Of the below which eradicates permanently the other one? (KPSC/Org/RE-05)
    (a)   Two dissimilar diseases meet together
    (b)   Two similar diseases meet together
    (c)   Two mechanical injuries occur together
    (d)   Two poisonous stings occur together

Ans. (b)
Note
From above when 'two similar diseases meet together' the stronger one eradicates permanently the other.
Also see
§ 45
Two diseases differing in kind, similar in symptoms, when appearing in the same individual, the stronger will permanently overcome the weaker.
Ref: Organon of art of healing by Baldwin

Q. 119. Of the below which is the fixed miasm? (KPSC/Org/RE-05)
    (a)   Small pox
    (b)   Mechanical injury
    (c)   Surgical disease
    (d)   Congenital corporeal constitution

Ans. (a)
Note
The small pox belong to the category of 'fixed miasm'.
Also see
§ 73
Acute miasms which recur in the same manner (hence known by by some traditional name), *which either attack persons but once in a lifetime, as the smallpox, measles, whooping cough, the ancient smooth, bright red scarlet fever of Sydenham the mumps,* etc.
The above acute disease is referred to as fixed miasmatic ones as they affect the persons once in a life time.
Ref; Organon by B.K. Sarkar Clinical classification of diseases according to Hahnemann. Pg-336.

Q. 120. Of the below which is the curative action? (KPSC/Org/RE-05)
    (a)   Every medicine deranges the vital force
    (b)   Resistant action by the vital force
    (c)   Alternating action
    (d)   Action of miasms

Ans. (b)
Note
From above 'resistant action by the vital force' is the curative action.
Also see
Explanation of primary and secondary action.
§ 64 (in brief)
The vitality passively receives the primary drug effects, then actively by a secondary counter effect, curative crises, neutralizes the primary effects, if they are not so violent as to destroy the life of the individual.
Ref: Organon of art of healing by Baldwin

Q. 121. In which of the below it should not be treated immediately by antipsoric? (KPSC/Org/RE-05)
    (a)   Mental diseases resulting from corporeal maladies
    (b)   Schizophrenia
    (c)   Insanity caused by fright, vexation abuse of intoxicants
    (d)   Psychosomatic disorders

Ans. (c)
Note
From above the 'insanity caused by fright, vexation abuse of intoxicants' should not be treated immediately by antipsoric.

Also see
Abstracts of relevant aphorisms are as under:
§ 221
Insanity excited by fright, vexation, alcoholism, although resting on a substratum of psora, can be treated as an acute disease with bell., acon., stram., hyos., nux-v., merc., etc., and the psora returned to its latent state and appear to be cured.
§ 222

Although a patient is relieved of an acute mental disorder by means of non anti-psoric medicine, he should not be considered entirely cured.
Ref: Organon of art of healing by Baldwin

Q. 122. Of the below which is the correct method? (KPSC/Org/RE-05)
    (a)   In no case it is requisite to administer more than one single, simple medicinal substance at one time
    (b)   Combination of mother tinctures
    (c)   Combination of various triturations
    (d)   Combinations of mother tinctures and triturations

Ans. (a)
Note
From above the correct method is 'in no case it is requisite to administer more than one single, simple medicinal substance at one time'.
Also see
§ 272
In the treatment of disease only one simple medicinal substance should be used at a time in any single prescription.
§ 273
A mixture of medicines is irrational.
§ 274

It is unnecessary to apply a multiplicity of means where simplicity will accomplish the end.
Too many remedies, administered in a single prescription, confuse the vital force, neutralize medicinal effects, disorder the state of sickness, make obscure the true picture of sickness, teaches the physician nothing, creates within his mind a spirit of infidelity in medicine, cultivates a slovenly habit of prescribing and brings discredit upon the profession of medicine.
Ref: Art of healing

Q. 123. Of the below which type of pass diminishes the excessive restlessness and sleeplessness? (KPSC/Org/RE-05)
    (a)   By making a very rapid motion of the flat extended hand
    (b)   A gentle less rapid negative pass
    (c)   By touching from head to foot
    (d)   By touching from foot to head

Ans. (b)
Note
From the above 'a gentle less rapid negative pass' diminishes the excessive restlessness and sleeplessness.
Also see
§ 294 (last three lines)
In the manner, a gentle, less rapid, negative pass diminishes the excessive restlessness and sleeplessness accompanied with anxiety sometimes produced in very irritable persons by a too powerful positive pass, etc.
Ref: Organon By B.K. Sarkar.

Q. 124. Of the below which aphorism helped Kent to construct the mental generals? (KPSC/Org/RE/2005)
    (a)   § 211
    (b)   § 210
    (c)   § 209
    (d)   § 208

Ans. (a)

MCQ's in Organon

Note
From above '§ 211' helped Kent to construct the mental generals.
Also see
§ 211
This holds good to such an extent, that the state of the disposition of the patient often chiefly determines the selection of the homeopathic remedy, as being a decidedly characteristic symptom which can least of all remain concealed from the accurately observing physician.
Ref: Organon by B.K. Sarkar.
In brief:
The state of the patient's mind and temperament, least of all, should escape the physician's acute observation.
Ref: Organs of art of healing by Baldwin

Q. 125. Of the below which constitutes intermittent diseases? (KPSC/Org/RE-05)
    (a)   Sporadically appear
    (b)   Epidemically appear
    (c)   Complicated with sycosis
    (d)   Psoric complicated with syphilis

Ans. (d)
Note
From above given choice 'psoric complicated with syphilis' constitutes intermittent disease.
Also see
§ 232
These latter, alternating, diseases, are also very numerous, but all belong to the class of chronic diseases; they are generally a manifestation of developed psora alone sometimes, but seldom complicated with a syphilitic miasm, and therefore in the former case may be cured by antipsoric medicines in the latter however in alternating with anti-syphilitic as taught in my work on the Chronic Disease.

§ 233
The typical intermittent diseases are those where a morbid state of unvarying character returns at a tolerably fixed period whilst the patient is apparently in good health, and takes its departure at an equally fixed period; this is observed in those apparently non-febrile morbid states that come and go in a periodical manner (at certain times), as well as in those of a febrile character, to wit, the numerous varieties of intermittent fevers.

§ 234
Those apparently non-febrile, typical, periodically recurring morbid states just alluded to observed in one single patient at a time (they do not usually appear sporadically or epidemically) always belong to the chronic diseases, mostly to those that are purely psoric, but seldom complicated with syphilis, and are successfully treated by the same means; yet it is sometimes necessary to employ as an intermediate remedy a small dose of a potentized solution of cinchona bark, in order to extinguish completely their intermittent type.
Ref: Organon By By B.K. Sarkar Pg-231-232.

Q. 126. In which of the below the patient suffers all the more from the excessive medicinal disease and from the useless exhaustion of his strength? (KPSC/Org/RE-05)
    (a)   Antipathic treatment
    (b)   Small frequent doses
    (c)   Larger the dose with greater homeopathicity and the higher potency
    (d)   Large doses of allopathic medicine

Ans. (d)
Note
From above given choice 'large doses of allopathic medicine' causes patient to suffer all the more from excessive medicinal disease and useless exhaustion of his strength.

Also see
The relevant aphorisms are as under:
§ 74
Many disease conditions, which do not terminate cannot be classed with chronic diseases, but are the direct result of allopathic treatment, and the direct result of the continued use of violent, heroic medicines in large and increasing doses. Drug sickness is induced by abuse of calomel, corrosive sublimate, mercury and mercurial ointment, nitrate of silver, iodine ointments, and other ointments capable of suppressing eruptions, opium, valerian, quinine, coal tar products, synthetic pain killers, digitalis, ergot sulphur ointment, purgatives, salts, compound cathartic pills, patent and proprietary drug mixtures dispensed, with surprising profits, to a credulous and easily exploited public. Add to this vast army of persons suffering from disordered sickness and rendered incurable or difficulty curable by the indiscriminate use of drugs, the host of narcotic addicts, and it is easy to believe that medicine has been a curse, not a blessing to mankind. Medicine is here left open to attack by new healing cuts and suffers the reverse it deserves.
§ 75
Drugs may and have ruined health.
§ 76
Homeopathy cures all natural diseases, but cannot correct all drug diseases which are induced by indiscriminate and persistent use of drugs through a long period of time.
Ref: Organon of Art of Healing by Baldwin
Ref: Organon by B.K. Sarkar

Q. 127. Of the below which is recovery according to Stuart Close? (KPSC/Org/RE/2005)
(a) By the treatment which is not directly and specifically curative in nature
(b) By the administration of suitable antipsoric medicines
(c) By the administration of single high potency drug
(d) By the administration of single lower potency drug

Ans. (a)
Note
From the choice given above - recovery according to Stuart Close is 'by the treatment which is not directly and specifically curative in nature'.
Also see
Distinction between cure and recovery:

The favorable outcome of medical treatment may be either a cure or a recovery. To realize the ideal of cure, it is necessary to know the exact meaning of these terms and to be able to discriminate between them.

'A cure' - is always a result of art and is never brought about by nature'. Nature, however, aided or unaided, often brings about a recovery, under the operation of natural laws. Fortunate indeed is it for humanity that this is true.

Definition of recovery. - Recovery is the spontaneous return of the patient to health after the removal, disappearance or cessation of the exciting causes and occasion of disease, or as a result of treatment which is not directly and specifically curative in its nature.
Ref; Stuart, Cure and Recovery.

Q. 128. Of the below which is the correct one? (KPSC/Org/RE/2005)
(a) Theory of vital force and drug dynamisation was elaborated first in fifth edition of Organon
(b) Theory of vital force and drug dynamisation was elaborated first in fourth edition of Organon
(c) Theory of vital force and drug dynamisation was elaborated in third edition of Organon
(d) Theory of vital force and drug dynamisation was elaborated in second edition of Organon

Ans. (a)
Note
From the above choice the correct one is '(a)'
Also see
During his lifetime Hahnemann published five editions of Organon. The fifth one is the most popular. The sixth edition was published long after his death [1921]

The doctrine of vital force and drug dynamisation were introduced for the first time in 5th Edition of Organon.

Different editions of Organon at a glance

Edition	Name of book	Publication Year	Total No. of §	Important additions made
1st	Organon of Rational Art of Healing	1810	259	NA
2nd	Organon of Healing Art	1819	318 [315]	NA
3rd	do	1824	320 [317]	NA
4th	do	1829	292	Theory of chronic disease was introduced for the first time in this edition.
5th	do	1833	294	The doctrine of vital force and drug Dynamisation were introduced for the first time in this edition.
6th	Organon of Medicine	1921	291	Discussed in 'A Treatise on Organon of Medicine' Part III.

Q. 129. Of the below persons who introduced the clinical observation? (KPSC/Org/RE-05)
(a) Hippocrates
(b) Hahnemann
(c) Galen
(d) Paracelsus

Ans. (a)
Note
Hippocrates introduced the clinical observation.
Also see
Hippocrates (460-377BC)
Greatest physician of antiquity, regarded as the father of medicine. Approximately 70 works ascribed to him, and this Hippocratic collection reminds us, his teachings, sense of detachment, and ability to make direct, clinical observations.

Q. 130. Of the below who wrote the introduction to the sixth edition of Organon translated by Dr. William Boericke? (KPSC/Org/RE-05)
(a) Dr. William Boericke
(b) Dr. Hale
(c) Dr. Boger
(d) Dr. James Kraus

Ans. (d)
Note
Dr. James Kraus wrote the introduction to the sixth edition of Organon translated by Dr. William Boericke.

Q. 131. In which § the preserver of health is mentioned? (KPSC/Org/RE-05)
(a) 3rd §
(b) 4th §
(c) 7th §
(d) 9th §

Ans. (b)

Note
Preserver of health is mentioned in the 4th § of Organon.

Also see
§ 4
He is likewise a preserver of health, if he knows the things that derange health and cause disease, and how to remove them from persons in health.
Ref: Organon by B.K. Sarkar

Q. 132. Of these which term is used in sixth edition of Organon? (KPSC/Org/RE-05)
(a) Vital force
(b) Vital principle
(c) Dynamic power
(d) Dynamic energy

Ans. (b)
Note
From the choice given above 'vital principle' is the term used in sixth edition of Organon.

Also see
§ 29
Here in the sixth edition of Organon, Hahnemann substitutes "Vital energy (of the principle of life)" from "Vital force" (5th Edition).

Q. 133. Of the below periods in which period the manuscript of the sixth edition of Organon was in danger of being lost? (KPSC/Org/RE-05)
(a) Year 1870 to 1871 and years 1914 to 1918
(b) Year 1872 to 1873 and years 1919 to 1923
(c) Year 1874 to 1875 and years 1924 to 1928
(d) Year 1876 to 1877 and years 1929 to 1933

Ans. (a)
Note
The 'year 1870 to 1871 and 1914 to 1918' was the period the manuscript of sixth edition of Organon was in danger of being lost.

Q. 134. Of the below four persons by whom "Cessat-Effectus Cessat Causa" was declared? (KPSC/Org/RE-05)
(a) Galen
(b) Hippocrates
(c) Paracelsus
(d) Hahnemann

Ans. (d)
Note
From above given choices the 'Hahnemann' declared 'Cessat-Effectus Cessat Causa'.

Also see

The motto of the medical profession is still Tolle Causam (remove the cause), find the cause, and to-day there are many who consider that germ are the only cause of disease and are working to discover the specific germ or virus for well known clinical entities. Tolle causam (remove the cause) so often mentioned in the books of the allopaths.

Louis Pasteur, will for ever be remembered as the founder of the science of bacteriology. It was he who first isolated and identified a specific germ and related to a definite clinical entity (disease). Following upon his discoveries, medical science concentrated on the laboratory technique for the isolation and identification of a specific germ for each known disease, and the Koch postulates were accepted as the standard for declaring any germ capable of pathogenesis-of having power to cause disease.

It must now be accepted as scientific fact that specific germs, in many cases of disease, can be isolated and identified, but is it a true conclusion that the specific germ is always the cause of the disease?

MCQ's in Organon

In nature, where there is balance, there is no disease and the germ, in this case the E. Coli in the intestinal tract, performs a useful function. Where the intestinal mucosa is healthy the E. Coli a non-pathogenic. Any change in the host which affects the intestinal mucosa will upset the balance and will be followed by a change in the habit and the bio-chemistry of the E. Coli, which way then be said to become pathogenic, but is should be noted that the primary change, the disease originated in the host, which compelled the bacillus to modify its habit in order to survive.

Tolle causam is easier said than done. How, then, shall we remove or palliate these effects by medical substances? Here, Hahnemann steps in to say, for the first time in all history: Remove the effects and you remove the disease, the cause of the effects. Cessat effectus cessat causa.

Aetiology is of as much importance to the homeopathic prescriber as to the non-homeopathic. Where a cause is definite and operative, tolle causam is the motto of both of them. If a patient's sufferings are due to a vesicle calculus or to an intestinal volvulus, though a drug homeopathic or other, may relieve suffering or improve resisting power, may relieve suffering or improve resisting power, the actual mechanical cause must obviously be removed by appropriate means and with becoming speed.

Ref: Organon by Sarkar.
Ref: Organon 6th Edition Translated by Boericke, Introduction by James Krauss.

Q. 135. Of the below which method is palliative? (KPSC/Org/RE-05)
    (a)   Homeopathy
    (b)   Allopathy
    (c)   Isopathy
    (d)   Antipathy

Ans. (d)
Note
From the choice given above the 'antipathy' is palliative.

Also see
According to § 56 (Sixth Edition of Organon) this palliative (antipathic, enantipathic) method, introduced according to Galen's teaching "Contraria contratris" for seventeen centuries, the physicians hitherto could hope to win confidence while they deluded with almost instantaneous amelioration.

Q. 136. Of the below in which Aphorism "causes are mentioned"? (KPSC/Org/RE-05)
    (a)   5th §
    (b)   6th §
    (c)   7th §
    (d)   8th §

Ans. (a)
Note
From the choice given above 'causes are mentioned' in the 5th §.

Also see
§ 5
Useful to the physician in assisting him to cure are the particulars of the most probable *exciting cause* of acute disease as also the most significant points in the whole history of chronic disease to enable him to discover its *fundamental cause,* which is generally due to a chronic miasm. In these investigations the ascertainable physical constitution of the patient (especially when the disease is chronic), his moral, and intellectual character, his occupation, mode of living and habits, his social and domestic relations, his age, sexual function, etc., are to be taken into consideration. *(a)*
Ref: Organon by B.K. Sarkar

Q. 137. Of the below which is peculiar symptom? (KPSC/Org/RE-05)
    (a)   Single symptom
    (b)   Local symptom
    (c)   Multiple symptoms
    (d)   Singular symptom

Ans. (d)

Note
Out of above 'Singular symptom' is peculiar symptom.

Also see
§ 153
In this search for a homeopathic specific remedy, that is to say, in this comparison of the collective symptoms of the natural disease with the list of symptoms of known medicines in order to find among these an artificial morbific agent corresponding by similarity to the disease to be cured, the *more striking, singular, uncommon and peculiar* (characteristic) signs and symptoms of the case of disease are chiefly and most solely to be kept in view.
Ref: Organon by B.K. Sarkar

Q.138. Of the below which is homeopathic aggravation? (KPSC/Org/RE-05)
- (a) Appearance of old symptoms
- (b) Appearance of new symptoms
- (c) Secondary action
- (d) Primary action

Ans. (d)
Note
Out of above 'primary action' is homeopathic aggravation.

Also see
Homeopathic aggravation is an essential phenomenon in the process of homeopathic cure. It is produced by artificial disease which exhibits its dominancy over the natural disease.
§ 161
When I here limit the so-called homeopathic aggravation, or rather the primary action of the homeopathic medicine that seems to increase somewhat the symptoms of the original disease, to the first or few first hours, this is certainly true with respect to diseases of a more acute character and of recent origin; but where medicines of long action have to combat a malady of considerable or of very long standing, where no such apparent increase of the original disease ought to appear during treatment and it doses not so appear if the accurately chosen medicine was given in proper small, gradually higher doses, each somewhat modified with renewed Dynamisation (247) Such increase of the original symptoms of a chronic disease can appear only at the end of treatment when the cure is almost or quite finished.
Ref: Organon 6th Edition.

Q. 139. In which condition of the below it is said as accessory symptoms? (KPSC/Org/RE-05)
- (a) Indisposition
- (b) Distinctive symptoms
- (c) Vaguely described symptoms
- (d) New symptoms appear

Ans. (d)
Note
From listed above 'new symptoms appear' are said to be the accessory symptoms.

Also see
The new symptoms which appear after administration of a medicine is an '*accessory symptoms*'.

Discussion
The accessory symptoms may belong to following two areas:
(a) *Accessory Symptoms of Disease* are those symptoms from which the patient suffers for a considerable time, so that he becomes used to their long suffering and he pays little attention to them; and considers them as a part of his usual self.
(b) *Accessory Symptoms of Medicine*: After administration of a partially similar medicine some new symptoms appear which were not previously observed in the patient. These new symptoms are the accessory symptoms of the medicine.
Ref: A Treatise on Organon of Medicine, By A. K. Das

Q. 140. In which of the below imperfect selection of the medicine is inevitable? (KPSC/Org/RE-05)
    (a)   Psoric cases
    (b)   Syphilitic cases
    (c)   Present one or two severe violent symptoms
    (d)   Sycotic cases

Ans. (c)
Note
From above imperfect selection of the medicine is inevitable if one bases the prescription on 'one or two severe violent symptoms'.

Also see
§ 6.
The physician should understand that the observable morbid signs and symptoms represent the changes from normal in each individual disease, and that these observable signs, symptoms and sensations, taken together in their totality, represent the disease in its full extent. And the physician should understand that only with these changes in the sensorial condition of the body and mind, discernible through the senses, should he concern himself as an observer of individual cases of sickness. In the examination of any particular case the physician should not speculate or generalize and should not be biased by any previous observations. The unbiased observer observes, he does not speculate. He understands the futility of transcendental speculation unsupported by experience.

§ 7.
In disease, presenting no manifest exciting cause for removal, the totality of symptoms is the outward image of the inner disease, of the suffering vital force, related as cause and effect. These symptoms alone must constitute the medium through which the disease demands and points out its curative agent. In each case of disease only this totality of symptoms is to be recognized and removed, by the art of healing, that it may be cured and converted into health.
Ref: Organon of Art of Healing By Baldwin

Extended information
Whenever the medicine is selected on one or two severe violent symptoms the chances of imperfect selection of medicine is very much inevitable.
It has nothing to do with the miasmatic preponderance of the case in question whether it is psoric, sycotic or having a syphilitic background. The 'totality of symptom' needs to be considered for the selection of homeopathic simillimum.
Most of psoric patients who come with the complaints, which on scrutiny points to be of 'functional domain', may insist and influence the physician to give more significance to the certain symptoms, which every physician should avoid and must not give in such dictates.

Q. 141. Which of the below do not constitute sharply separated from all others? (KPSC/Org/RE-05)
    (a)   Psora
    (b)   Syphilis
    (c)   Mental diseases
    (d)   Sycosis

Ans. (a)
Note
Out of above 'psora' do not constitute sharply separated from all others.

Also see
Psora being the fundamental cause remains behind or facilitates the secondary miasms to take hold of the human organism. Therefore, sycosis and syphilitic miasms do not have an independent hold on the system. The mental diseases according to Dr. Hahnemann belong to psora so they are also not independent.
The individual presentations of chronic miasms i.e., psora, sycosis, and syphilis can be identified from their onset, clinical presentation and progression to the terminal stage and from each other. The mental diseases as such are the one sided diseases and according to Organon these belong to psoric.

Q. 142. Of the below which symptoms of the drug acts? (KPSC/Org/RE-05)
    (a)   All the symptoms of the drug
    (b)   Homeopathic symptoms
    (c)   Common symptoms of the drug
    (d)   Pathological symptoms

Ans. (a)
Note
Of the above 'all symptoms of the drug' act.
Also see
§ 18
Hence, the totality of symptoms, being the only visible aspect of the phenomena of sickness, is the only guide to the remedy.
§ 19
Therefore the curative power of medicines must rest alone on their power of altering the sensorial condition of the body, thus demonstrating their power of affecting the spirit-like dynamis.
§ 20
Drug effects cannot be determined by reason or conjecture, but only by proving. A curative remedy does not have anything to do with causes attacking man from without. That is purely a problem of sound hygiene.
§ 21
Therefore a drug's capacity for curing sickness will be determined by its capacity for producing symptoms on the healthy human being.
§ 22
Disease is manifest in its totality of symptoms. Drug action is manifest in its totality of symptomatology. Drugs must be applied, as remedies, to similar or contrary symptoms of disease as experience dictates.
Ref: Organon of Art of Healing By Baldwin
Also see
All the symptoms of drug which were produced on proving and subsequently recorded are suitable for the selection of medicine on the basis of totality of symptoms which are matched on 'similia'. All symptoms of drug so recorded can be taken for indication on the basis of similia and they will act according to the therapeutic law of nature. There is no entity as homeopathic symptom, or allopathic symptom.

Q. 143. Of the below which is advocated by Hahnemann in posthumous edition? (KPSC/Org/RE-05)
    (a)   Administration of one dose alone
    (b)   Gradually higher doses
    (c)   Only below 30th centesimal potency
    (d)   Only higher potency

Ans. (b)
Note
Of the above 'gradually higher doses' were advocated by Hahnemann in posthumous edition.
Also see
§ 246 (Sixth edition):
Every perceptibly progressive and strikingly increasing amelioration during treatment is a condition which, as long as it lasts, completely precludes every repetition of the administration of any medicine whatsoever, because all the good the medicine taken continues to effect is now hastening towards its completion. This is not infrequently the case in acute diseases, but in more chronic diseases, on the other hand, a single doses an appropriately selected homeopathic remedy will at times complete even with but slowly progressive improvement and give the help which such a remedy in such a case can accomplish naturally within 40, 50, 60, 100, days . This is, however, but rarely the case; and besides, it must be a matter of great importance to the physician, as well as to the patient that were it possible, this period should be diminished to one-half, one-quarter, and even still less, so that a much more rapid cure might be obtained. And this may be very happily affected, as recent and oft-repeated observations have taught me under the following conditions; firstly, if the medicine selected with the utmost care was perfectly homeopathic; secondly, if it is highly potentized, dissolved in water and given in proper small dose that experience has taught as the most suitable in definite intervals for the quickest accomplishment of the cure but with the precaution, that the degree of every dose deviate somewhat from the preceding and following in order that the vital principle which is to be altered to

a similar medicinal disease be not aroused to untoward reactions and revolt as is always the case {132 What I said in the fifth edition of the Organon, in a long note to this paragraph in order to prevent these undesirable reactions of the vital energy, was all that the experience I then had justified. But during the last four or five years, however, all these difficulties are wholly solved by my new altered but perfected method. The same carefully selected medicine may now be given daily and for months, if necessary in this way, namely, after the lower degree of potency has been used for one or two weeks in the treatment of chronic disease , advance is made in the same way to higher degrees, (beginning according to the new dynamization method, taught herewith the use of the lowest degrees). 132 with unmodified and especially rapidly repeated doses.
Ref: Organon 6th edition

Q. 144. In which condition of the below several anti psoric remedies are given in succession? (KPSC/Org/RE-05)
    (a)   Diseases of varying nature due to congenital corporeal constitution
    (b)   Indisposition
    (c)   Syphilitic miasm
    (d)   Sycotic miasm

Ans. (a)
Note
Of above 'diseases of varying nature due to congenital corporeal constitution' need several anti psoric remedies in succession.
Also see
In brief
§ 81
Diseases of varying nature due to congenital corporeal constitution are due to psora.
§ 171
In non-venereal chronic diseases it is often necessary to employ several antipsoric prescriptions in succession or repeated doses, in order to establish reaction and excite a curative crisis.
Ref: Organon of art of healing by Baldwin

Q. 145. In which of the below the local affection increases gradually? (KPSC/Org/RE-05)
    (a)   A part of the general disease
    (b)   By repeated application of antipathic drugs
    (c)   Mechanical irritation
    (d)   Sudden poisonings

Ans. (c)
Note
Of the above local affection increases gradually in 'mechanical irritation'.
Also see
One is the history of the development of malignant formation as the result of the frequent mechanical irritation of a simple mole on the face.
Irritation local or otherwise, affecting the tissue, may cause abnormal epithelial growths, which rising above the general level, may produce a wart.
Ref: Homoeopathic Treatment or 'Fifty Reasons, For Being A Homoeopath' By J. Compton Burnett M.D.

Q. 146. By whom law of similars was noted before Hahnemann? (KPSC/Org/RE-05)
    (a)   Law of similars is the original discovery of Hahnemann as Art-Science
    (b)   Law of similars was noted by Hippocrates before Hahnemann
    (c)   Law of similars was noted by Asclepias before Hahnemann
    (d)   Law of similars was noted by Cullen before Hahnemann

Ans. (b)
Note
'Law of similars' before Hahnemann. Aristotle recognized it, and *Hippocrates sensed the possibilities of this law and applied it in some recorded cases.*
Ref: Roberts.

Q. 147. Of the below statements which is correct? (KPSC/Org/RE-05)
    (a)   Asclepias in the balance written by Aristotle
    (b)   Asclepias in the balance written by Cullen
    (c)   Asclepias in the balance written by Plato
    (d)   Asclepias in the balance written by Hahnemann

Ans. (d)
Note
Hahnemann in 1805 has written - 'Asclepias in the Balance'.

Q. 148. Of the below in which edition the theory of chronic disease appeared first? (KPSC/Org/RE-05)
    (a)   Theory of chronic disease appeared first in the second edition of Organon
    (b)   Theory of chronic diseases appeared first in the third edition of Organon
    (c)   Theory of chronic diseases appeared first in the fourth edition of Organon
    (d)   Theory of chronic diseases first appeared in the fifth edition of Organon

Ans. (c)
Note
Theory of chronic diseases appeared first in the fourth edition of Organon.

Q. 149. Of the below which is a correct one. (KPSC/Org/RE-05)
    (a)   Every medicine acts on all parts of the body
    (b)   Every medicine acts in a determinate manner
    (c)   Every medicine either depresses or excites
    (d)   Every medicine acts as a tonic

Ans. (b)
Note
Of the above 'every medicine acts in a determinate manner' is correct.
Also see
§ 119
Each of these substances produces alterations in the health of human being in a peculiar, different, yet determinate manner, so as to preclude the possibility of confounding one with another. *(a)*
Ref: Organon by B.K. Sarkar

Q. 150. Of the below which is the suitable medicine? (KPSC/Org/RE-05)
    (a)   The medicine which has the greatest similarity to the totality of symptoms
    (b)   The medicine which has previously cured the same type of disease
    (c)   The medicine which has developed the same type of lesions in animal experimentation
    (d)   Medicines belonging to the same family of plant kingdom or animal kingdom when the indicated drug is not available

Ans. (a)
Note
Of the above 'the medicine which has the greatest similarity to the totality of symptoms' is the suitable medicine.
Also see
§147 Whichever of these medicines that have been investigated as to their power of altering man's health we find to contain in the symptoms observed from its use the greatest similarity to the totality of the symptoms of a given natural disease; this medicine will and must be the most suitable, the most certain Homeopathic remedy for the disease; in it is found the specific remedy of this case of disease.
Ref: Organon of Medicine 6th Edition.

Extended information
The most suitable medicine has the greatest similarity to the totality of symptoms.
Similarity of symptoms is, therefore, the natural guide to the curative remedy, as well as to the true diagnosis of the disease, and comparison of symptoms is the process by which the conclusion is reached.
Ref: Stuart – Pathology of Homeopathy.

MCQ's in Organon

Q. 151. Of the below which requires change in diet regulations? (KPSC/Org/RE-05)
    (a)   Indisposition
    (b)   Allopathic bungling
    (c)   Chronic disease
    (d)   Surgical disease

Ans. (a)
Note
Of the above 'indisposition' requires change in diet regulations.
Also see
§ 150 (Brief)

Indispositions require only change in diet or habits of living.
Ref: Organon of Art of Healing by Baldwin

In persons otherwise healthy, due to non-specific causes, such as indiscretions in diet or regimen, mechanical injuries, undue exertions or

Indulgences, emotional excesses, etc. Such conditions are not true diseases, but mere indispositions, which disappear of themselves under ordinary circumstances when the cause is removed, or yield easily to corrective hygienic, dietetic, moral or mechanical measures. They ordinarily require no medicine.
Ref: Stuart – Pathology of Homeopathy

Q. 152. In which § of the below Hahnemann has said that he opened the path of great truth homeopathy for the blessings of humanity? (KPSC/Org/RE-05)
    (a)   § 109
    (b)   § 110
    (c)   § 111
    (d)   § 112

Ans. (a)
Note
In § 109 Hahnemann has said that he opened the path of great truth homeopathy for the blessings of humanity.
Also see
§ 109
I was the first that opened up this path, which I have pursued with a perseverance that could only arise and be kept up by a perfect conviction of the truth, fraught with such blessings to humanity, that it is only by the homeopathic employment of medicines that the certain cure of human maladies is possible.
Ref: Organon 5th Edition

Q. 153. Of the below by which the correct data regarding the drug action can be obtained? (KPSC/Org/RE-05)
    (a)   All the alterations can be studied from a single prover.
    (b)   All the alterations can be ascertained at once in the same experiment.
    (c)   All the alterations can be ascertained by several experiments on several persons.
    (d)   All the alterations can be ascertained by the study on laboratory animals.

Ans. (c)
Note
The correct data regarding the drug action can be obtained 'all the alterations can be ascertained by several experiments on several persons.
Also see
§ 135
The whole of the elements of disease a medicine is capable of producing can only be brought to anything like completeness by numerous observations on suitable persons of both sexes and of various constitutions.
Ref: Organon by B.K. Sarkar

Q. 154. In which of the below that nothing can be accurately observed during proving? (KPSC/Org/RE-05)
    (a)   When large doses taken
    (b)   When more moderate doses taken
    (c)   When small doses taken
    (d)   When minute doses taken

Ans. (a)
Note
When large doses taken than nothing can be accurately observed during proving.

Also see
According to the Arndt-Schultz law, small drug doses stimulate cell activity, larger doses hinder it, still larger destroy it.
This has been recently demonstrated in a beautiful manner by Sir Jagadis Bose. According to Schultz, when drugs are administered to healthy persons the symptoms they elicit are a revelation as to the cells and tissues they affect. Drugs that derange, damage or destroy certain cells in medium to large doses will stimulate the same cells if given in small doses.
Disease symptoms are the expression of disordered cell and tissue activity, and their symptoms indicate the cells in need of stimulation. The ideal remedy will be the one which has produced similar symptoms on the healthy, so proving its power over precisely those cells affected by disease. On them, in minimal dose, it will act as a stimulus. And, as disease has made those particular cells abnormally sensitive, the stimulating dose must be very small indeed.
Ref: Homeopathy An Explanation of its Principles By Besweir

Q. 155. Of the below which type is cured by homeopathy in a few days? (KPSC/Org/RE-05)
    (a)   Acute disease
    (b)   Some what longer standing
    (c)   Complicated cases
    (d)   Allopathic bungling

Ans. (b)
Note
Some what longer standing type is cured by Homeopathy in a few days.

Also see
§ 149

When the suitable homeopathic remedy has been thus selected and rightly employed the acute disease we wish to cure, even though it be of a grave character and attended by many sufferings, subsides insensibly, in a few hours if it be of recent date, in a few days if it be a somewhat longer standing, along with all traces of indisposition, and nothing or almost nothing more of the artificial medicinal disease is perceived; there occurs, by rapid, imperceptible transitions, nothing but restore health, recovery. Diseases if long standing (and especially such as are of a complicated character) require for their cure a proportionately longer time. More especially do the chronic medicinal dyscrasia so often produced by allopathic bungling, along with the natural disease left uncured by it, require a much longer time for their recovery; often, indeed, are they, incurable, in consequence of the shameful robbery of the patient's strength and juices, the principal feat performed by allopathy in its so –called methods of treatment.
Ref: Organon by B.K. Sarkar

Q. 156. Of the below in which numerous striking symptoms are present? (KPSC/Org/RE-05)
    (a)   Indisposition
    (b)   Chronic diseases
    (c)   Acute diseases
    (d)   Poisoning cases

Ans. (c)
Note
Of above in 'acute diseases' numerous striking symptoms are present.

Also see
§ 152
The worse of the acute disease is, of so much the more numerous and striking symptoms is it generally composed.
Ref: Organon by B.K. Sarkar

Q. 157. Of the below which is the suitable method to obtain the pathogenetic power of the drugs? (KPSC/Org/RE-05)
    (a) Animal experiment
    (b) Experiment on plants
    (c) Experiment on diseased person
    (d) Experiment by the doctors taking the medicine internally

Ans. (d)
Note
Of the above 'experiment by the doctors taking the medicine internally' is the suitable method to obtain the pathogenetic power of the drugs.

Also see
As Hahnemann did and said:
§ 141 (In Brief) The healthy unprejudiced physician of fine perception makes the best prover. Every homeopathic physician should take an active part in proving some drugs as a part of the preparation for the practice of his art.
Ref: Organon of Art of Healing by Baldwin

Q. 158. Of the below who is fit to be a homeopathic physician? (KPSC/Org/RE-05)
    (a) Doctor framing questions so as to get answer yes or no
    (b) Doctor framing general expressions regarding the parts, mind
    (c) Doctor who writes prescriptions by seeing the report
    (d) Doctor who prescribes by simply seeing the patient

Ans. (b)
Note
Of the above 'doctor framing general expressions regarding the parts, mind' fit to be a homeopathic physician.

§ 6
The physician should understand that the observable morbid signs and symptoms represent the changes from normal in each individual disease, and that these observable signs, symptoms and sensations, taken together in their totality, represent the disease in its full extent. And the physician should understand that only with these changes in the sensorial condition of the body and mind, discernible through the senses, should he concern himself as an observer of individual cases of sickness. In the examination of any particular case the physician should not speculate or generalize and should not be biased by any previous observations. The unbiased observer observes, he does not speculate. He understands the futility of transcendental speculation unsupported by experience.
Ref: Organon of Art of Healing by Baldwin.

Q. 159. Of these which symptoms merit for prescription? (KPSC/Org/RE-05)
    (a) Symptoms gathered while taking the medicine
    (b) Symptoms expressed in vague terms
    (c) Symptoms pursued carefully and circumstantially
    (d) Symptoms obtain from the friends and relatives

Ans. (c)
Note
Of above 'symptoms pursued carefully and circumstantially' merit for prescription.
Also see
§ 95
In chronic diseases the investigation of the signs of disease above mentioned, and of all others, must be pursued as carefully and circumstantially as possible, and the most minute peculiarities must be attended to , partly

because in these diseases they are the most characteristic and least resemble those of acute diseases, and if a cure is to be affected they cannot be too accurately noted; partly because the patients become so used to their long sufferings that they pay litter or no need to the lesser accessory symptoms which are often very pregnant with meaning (characteristic)- often very useful in determining the choice of the remedy...
Ref: Organon of Medicine Sarkar

Q. 160. Of these which is required for the physician to prescribe the correct remedy? (KPSC/Org/RE-05)
(a) Knowledge of pathogenetic powers of few medicines
(b) Knowledge of pathogenetic effects of several drugs
(c) Knowledge of therapeutic hints
(d) Knowledge of previous experience treating the same type of disease

Ans. Use your discretion. (b)
Note
Of above 'knowledge of 'pathogenetic effects of several drugs' is required for the physician to prescribe the correct remedy?

Also see
The following points are of much more value in prescribing the correct remedy. Broadly speaking the physician should understand:
1st   What is curable in disease in general and in each individual case in particular?
2nd   What is curative in drugs in general and in each individual drug in particular?
3rd   How to apply, with distinct reason, what is curative in drugs to what is curable in diseases, i.e.
    a. How to match the proper remedy to the sickness?
    b. How properly to administer the proper dose?
    c. How properly to repeat the dose?
4th   And how to recognize and remove obstacles in the way of recovery. The physician should be able to recognize and remove causes of sickness from the healthy. Sanitation and Hygiene.
Ref: Organon of Art of Healing by Baldwin. § 2, 3, 4.

Extended information
Keeping in touch with above however, one should be very sure about the drugs which are used as medicine in a given case:
Original Provings and Sources of the Materia Medica - The first work embodying such record is that of Hahnemann, entitled, "Fragmenta de Viribus Medicamentorum Positivis.' It is a Latin work, and published in Leipsic in 1805. Twenty-seven drugs are treated of, containing symptoms Hahnemann himself had observed as effects of poisoning or from excessive dosing, and of provings on himself. " I have instituted experiments," he says in the preface, " in chief part on my own person, but also on some others whom I knew to be perfectly healthy and free from all perceptible disease.

In 1828, Hahnemann published his " Chronic Diseases," containing the symptomatology of a completely new series of medicines, a series of deeply acting drugs, like Calcarea, Sulphur, etc., the so-called antipsoric remedies. The symptomatology of these remedies was not wholly pathogenetic, but included observations at the bedside, so-called clinical symptoms.

A second edition greatly enlarged and now containing the symptomatology of twenty-five remedies, besides the twenty-two of the first edition, appeared between 1834 and 1838. A peculiar feature of the provings in this work is that the bulk of them must have been obtained with the thirtieth potency, and often are observations when given to the sick, differing entirely, therefore, from the *pathogenetic effects* of the Materia Medica Pura.
Ref: Foundations of Homeopathy - Hompath

"A true materia medica", he says, "will consist of the genuine, pure, and undeceptive effects of simple drugs"; and again, "Every such materia medica should exclude every supposition - every mere assertion and fiction - and its entire contents should be the language of nature, uttered in response to careful and faithful enquiry."

Many remedies, since Hahnemann's day, have been added to our armoury against disease; but all subsequent work has been done on his lines. It has never been found necessary to eliminate, or to alter. Recorded in the simple language of nature, free from theory, safe from the transient language of succeeding generations, they stand for all time, complete and true; while science, in discovering new truths, has never been able to touch Hahnemann's premises - except to confirm - since they are based on Law.
Ref: Homeopathy An Explanation of its Principles

Q. 161. Of the below small pox, measles whooping cough belong to which type? (KPSC/Org/RE-05)
    (a)   Acute diseases attacking individually
    (b)   Acute diseases attacking several persons
    (c)   Acute diseases attacking many persons by the same cause
    (d)   Acute diseases affecting once in a life time

Ans. (d)
Note
Of the above small pox, measles whooping cough belong to 'acute diseases affecting once in a life time'.
Also see
Small pox, measles, whooping cough fulfills the following:
    a.   All belong to category of acute diseases
    b.   All belong to the class of infectious diseases
    c.   On recovery from acute attack all provide lifelong immunity
However the peculiar to these from the miasmatic point of view is that they belong to type of fixed miasm and therefore on recovery from each one of above provides lifelong immunity.

Q. 162. Of these which is of indescribable diversity? (KPSC/Org/RE-05)
    (a)   Syphilis
    (b)   Psora
    (c)   Sycosis
    (d)   Drug diseases

Ans. (b)
Note
Of these 'psora' is of indescribable diversity.
Also see
§ 80 Psora, hydra-headed, is directly responsible for a host of so-called diseases which afflict the race.
§ 81 Here is presented a long list of presumably distinct diseases which have developed, through countless generations, and many million human organisms, with every variety of constitution and circumstance of living through the effect of the psora miasm. The race has been unable to escape from the chronic miasm, psora, by reason of the persistent and indiscriminate suppression of every manner of skin eruption, by the habitual use of ointments and astringent washes, by doctors and granny women, through countless generations.

Extended information
Of Hahnemann's three named Chronic Diseases, his PSORA was for him," the hydra-headed, most wide-reaching and difficult of all the chronic parasitic microbic diseases." He calls it "the oldest, most universal and most pernicious chronic parasitical disease, an ancient, smouldering contagion, of incomparably greater significance than either of the above named chronic miasms" (Syphilis and Gonorrhea).
The three chronic miasms, psora , syphilis and sycosis, are all contagious. In each instance there is something prior to the manifestations which we call disease. We speak of the signs and symptoms of a disease, we speak of the outcropping of the symptoms when we speak of syphilis, but remember there is a state prior to syphilis or syphilis would not exist. It could not come upon man except for a condition suitable to its development. In like manner psora could not exist except for a condition in mankind suitable for its development.
Psora being the first and the two coming later, it is proper for us to inquire into that state of the human race that would be suitable for the development of psora.
Ref: Kent Lectures

Q. 163. Of these which symptoms are pure symptoms? (KPSC/Org/RE-05)
    (a)   Symptoms before the use of medicine
    (b)   Symptoms while taking the medicine
    (c)   Symptoms while taking tranquillizers
    (d)   Symptoms after operation

Ans. (a)
Note
Of above 'symptoms before the use of medicine' are pure symptoms.

Also see
§ 91
The symptoms and feelings of the patient during a previous course of medicine do not furnish the pure picture of the disease; but, on the other hand, those symptoms and ailments which he suffered from *before the use of the medicines or after they had been discontinued for several days,* give the true fundamental idea of the original form of the disease, and these especially the physician must take note of. When the disease is of a chronic character, and the patient has been taking medicine up to the time he is seen, the physician may with advantage leave him some days quite without medicine, or in the meantime administer something of an unmedicinal nature and defer to a subsequent period the more precise scrutiny of the morbid symptoms, in order to be above to grasp in their purity the permanent uncontaminated symptoms of the old affection and to form a faithful picture of the disease.
Ref; Organon- B.K. Sarkar P172.

Q. 164. Of the below which is the correct one? (KPSC/Org/RE-05)
    (a)   Characteristic of an epidemic is obtained from the knowledge of previous epidemics
    (b)   Characteristics of an epidemic is obtained from the knowledge of study of several patient
    (c)   Characteristics of an epidemic is obtained by studying one patient
    (d)   Characteristics of an epidemic is obtained by the book knowledge

Ans. (b)
Note
Of the below 'Characteristics of an epidemic is obtained from the knowledge of study of several patient' is the correct one.
Also see
§102 (Brief)

The distinguishing characteristic of any epidemic sickness will be secured in the composite image of the totality of symptoms of several patients of different bodily constitution. This composite picture of the epidemic sickness will reveal the remedy for that epidemic. That remedy will master the epidemic, reduce the death rate, rob epidemics of their horror, and dedicate physicians to the mission of genuine public service.
Ref: Organon of art of healing by Baldwin

Q. 165. In which § "Homeopathic specific remedy" is given in the 5th edition of Organon of Medicine? (KPSC-Lect / Physio & Bioch - 05)
    (a)   § 241
    (b)   § 204
    (c)   § 246
    (d)   § 240

Ans. (a)
Note
In § 241 "Homeopathic specific remedy" is given in the 5th edition of Organon of Medicine.
Also see
§ 241
Epidemics of intermittent fever, in situations where none are endemic, are of the nature of chronic diseases, composed of single acute paroxysms; each single epidemic is of a peculiar, uniform character common to all the individuals attacked, and when this character is found in the totality of the symptoms common to all, it guides us to the discovery of the homeopathic (specific) remedy suitable for all the cases, which is almost universally serviceable in those patients who enjoyed tolerable health before the occurrence of the epidemic, that is to say, who were not chronic sufferers from developed psora.
Ref: Organon of Medicine 5th edition

Q. 166. No aggravation of the patient with recovery of the patient is (KPSC-Lect / Physio & Bioch-05)
    (a)   5th Observation
    (b)   2nd Observation
    (c)   3rd Observation
    (d)   6th Observation

Ans. Use your discretion

Note
No aggravation of the patient with recovery of the patient is given in '4th' Observation of Kent's. However, in the given choice it does not figure.

Also see
The 4th observation of Kent is
    -No aggravation, but steady improvement
Interpretation
    -Assessment and potency selection is extremely well
Comment
    -No tissue changes and no tendency for tissue changes.
Intervention/Observation
    -An ideal cure. Watch for Hering's law of cure.

Q. 167. How many aphorisms are present in the 4th edition of Organon of Medicine? (KPSC-Lect / Physio & Bioch-05)
    (a)   292
    (b)   320
    (c)   259
    (d)   318

Ans. (a)
Note
Fourth Edition – Contained 292 aphorisms.

Q. 168. Accessory symptom of the medicine is given in the § (KPSC-Lect / Physio & Bioch -05)
    (a)   § 179
    (b)   § 163
    (c)   § 170
    (d)   § 173

Ans. (b)
Note
Accessory symptom of the medicine is given in the §: 163.

Also see
§ 163
In this case we cannot indeed expect from this medicine a complete, untroubled cure; for during its use some symptoms appear which were not previously observable in the disease, accessory symptoms of the not perfectly appropriate remedy. This does by no means prevent a considerable part of the disease (the symptoms of the disease that resemble those of the medicine) from being eradicated by this medicine, thereby establishing a fair commencement of the cure, but still this does not take place without those accessory symptoms, which are, however, always moderate when the dose of the medicine is sufficiently minute.
Ref: Organon- By B.K. Sarkar

Q. 169. The Homeopathic law of nature and a provisional explanation of it (Kerala MD (Hom) Ent Paper-2 -01)
    (a)   § 26 – 35
    (b)   § 36 – 40
    (c)   § 99 - 104
    (d)   § 52 - 55

Ans. (a)
Note
The Homeopathic law of nature and a provisional explanation of it is given in
§ 26 – 35 of Organon.

Also see
The § 26 – 35 are as under:
§ 26
This is dependent on the therapeutic law of nature that a weaker dynamic affection in the living organism is permanently extinguished by one that is very similar to and stronger than it, only differing from it in kind.
NOTE - This applies both to physical affections and moral maladies.
§ 27
The curative power of medicines, therefore, depends on the symptoms they have similar to the disease.
§ 28-29
Attempt to explain this therapeutic law of nature.
§ 30-33
The human body is much more disposed to let its state of health be altered by medicinal forces than by natural disease.
§ 34-35
The correctness of the homeopathic therapeutic law is shown in the want of success attending every unhomeopathic treatment of a long-standing disease, and in this also, that two natural diseases meeting together in the body, if they be dissimilar to each other, do not remove or cure one another.
Ref: Organon – By B.K. Sarkar Pg.21-22

Q. 170. Clinical varieties of Acute Diseases (Kerala MD (Hom) Ent Paper-2 -01)
  (a) § 73
  (b) § 153
  (c) § 118
  (d) § 150

Ans. (a)
Note
Clinical varieties of Acute Diseases are given in § 73.
Also see
§ 73
As regards acute diseases, they are either of such a kind as attack human being individually, the exciting cause being injurious influences to which they were particularly exposed. Excesses in food, or an insufficient supply of it, severe physical impressions, chills, overheatings, dissipation, strains, etc., or physical irritations, mental emotions, and the like, are exciting causes of such acute febrile affections; in reality, however, they are generally only a transient explosion of latent psora, which spontaneously returns to its dormant state if the acute disease were not of too violent a character and were soon quelled. Or they are of such a kind as attack several persons at the same time, here and there (sporadically), by means of meteoric or telluric influences and injurious agents, the susceptibility for being morbidly affected by which is possessed by only a few persons at one time. Allied to these are those disease in which many persons are attacked with very similar sufferings from the same cause (epidemically); these disease generally become infectious (contagious) when they prevail among thickly congregated masses of human beings.
Ref: Organon – By B.K. Sarkar

Q. 171. Where the aggravation is quick, short and strong with rapid improvement of the patient (Kerala MD (Hom) Ent Paper-2 -01)
  (a) 1st observation of Kent
  (b) 5th observation of Kent
  (c) 3rd observation of Kent
  (d) 12th observation of Kent

Ans. (c)
Note
In Kent's 3rd observation 'aggravation is quick, short and strong with rapid improvement of the patient'.
Also see
3rd Observation of Kent
Aggravation is quick, short and strong with rapid improvement of the patient.
Interpretation

Remedy and potency both correct.
Comment
No irreversible or any structural changes in vital organs.
Intervention
Stop the medicine and observe till improvement takes place.

Q. 172. At the present day advanced thinkers are speaking of the fourth state of matter which is immaterial substance, who said this? (Kerala MD (Hom) Ent Paper-2 -01)
    (a) Boger
    (b) Robert
    (c) Dunham
    (d) J. T. Kent

Ans. (d)
Note
At the present day advanced thinkers are speaking of the fourth state of matter which is immaterial substance. We now say the solids, liquids and gases and the radiant form of matter. Substance in simple form is just as positively substance as matter in concrete form. The question then comes up for consideration and study. What is the vital force?
Ref: Kent Lectures – On Simple Substance.

Q. 173. "The removal of the totality of symptoms means removal of the cause", is the statement of (Kerala MD (Hom) Ent Paper-2 -01)
    (a) Hahnemann
    (b) Close
    (c) Dudgeon
    (d) J.T.Kent

Ans. (a)
Note
"The removal of the totality of symptoms means removal of the cause", is the statement of 'Hahnemann'.
Also see
§ 17

Now, as in the cure effected by the removal of the whole of the perceptible signs and symptoms of the disease the internal alteration of the vital principle to which the disease is due- consequently the whole of the disease - is at the same time removed, {A warning dream, a superstitious fancy, or a solemn prediction that death would occur at a certain day or at a certain hour, has not infrequently produced all the signs of commencing and increasing disease, of approaching death and death itself at the hour announced, which could not happen without the simultaneous production of the inward change (corresponding to the state observed externally); and hence in such cases all the morbid signs indicative of approaching death have frequently been dissipated by an identical cause, by some cunning deception or persuasion to a belief in the contrary, and health suddenly restored, which could not have happened without the removal, by means of this moral remedy, of the internal and external morbid change that threatened death.} it follows that the physician has only to remove the whole of the symptoms in order, at the same time, to abrogate and annihilate the internal change, that is to say, the morbid derangement of the
vital force-consequently the totality of the disease, the disease itself.
Ref: Organon – By B.K. Sarkar

Q. 174. The "Friend of Health" was written by (Kerala MD (Hom) Ent Paper-2 -01)
    (a) Hahnemann
    (b) Kent
    (c) J E Park
    (d) Socrates

Ans. (a)
Note
The "Friend of Health" was written by Dr. Hahnemann.

Q. 175. "Psora - It is the mother of all true chronic diseases except the syphilitic and sycotic"
(Kerala MD (Hom) Ent Paper-2 -01)
   (a)   § 70 – 71
   (b)   § 120 - 121
   (c)   § 80 - 82
   (d)   § 76 - 77

Ans. (c)
Note
"Psora - It is the mother of all true chronic diseases except the syphilitic and sycotic" is in § 80 -82.
Also see
§ 70 – 71
§ 70 and § 71: Recapitulation of all that proceeds and summary of all that follows:
   a)   Sickness reveals itself in no other way than symptoms, perceptible to the senses. Nothing else is to be removed; there is no other guide to the remedy.
   b)   No substance or drug can be used as a curative remedy that cannot change or alter the state of health of the healthy.
   c)   Diseases cannot be cured by drugs that produce dissimilar symptoms in the healthy, but only by that drug that has the power to produce an artificial condition most similar to that of the natural disease.
   d)   Experience teaches that medicines with opposite symptoms produce only transient relief of sickness. Medicines never cure which cannot aggravate the symptoms of the disease. Hence allopathy is not applicable to the cure of chronic serious sickness.
   e)   The homeopathic remedy is salutary, capable of creating similar symptoms where-by, when properly administered in the proper dose properly repeated, it is capable of establishing a healing crisis, what nature in accidental cures by similar diseases has demonstrated is necessary.

§71. Three questions answered in the next 222 paragraphs:
   a)   How does the physician gain the knowledge of disease necessary for the accomplishment of its cure?
   b)   How does the physician gain knowledge of drugs, as remedies, necessary for the cure of diseases?
   c)   How does the physician apply drugs effectively in the cure of disease?

§ 120 – 121
§ 120. Each remedy must be separately proved and tested.
§ 121. Strong drugs should be given in small doses, mild drugs in larger.

§ 80, 81, 82

§ 80. Psora, hydraheaded, is directly responsible for a host of so-called diseases which afflict the race. For an extended discussion of the chronic diseases psora, syphilis, sycosis (see Hahnemann's Chronic Diseases).

§ 81. Here is presented a long list of presumably distinct diseases which have developed, through countless generations, and many million human organisms, with every variety of constitution and circumstance of living through the effect of the psoric miasm. The race has been unable to escape from the chronic miasm, psora, by reason of the persistent and indiscriminate suppression of every manner of skin eruption, by the habitual use of ointments and astringent washes, by doctors and granny women, through countless generations.

§ 82.(in brief) Among the more specific remedies discovered for these chronic miasms, especially for psora, the selection of those for the cure of each individual case of chronic disease is to be conducted all the more carefully.

Ref: Organon By B.K. Sarkar Pg.25

§ 76-77

§ 76. Homeopathy cures all natural diseases, but cannot correct all drug diseases which are induced by indiscriminate and persistent use of drugs through a long period of time.

§ 77. True chronic sickness is due to infectious miasm and not to unhygienic living unless cured by the proper remedy.
Ref: Art of healing Hompoth

MCQ's in Organon

Q. 176. Inappropriately called chronic diseases (Kerala MD (Hom) Ent Paper-2 -01)
    (a) § 69 – 70
    (b) § 40 – 42
    (c) § 74 - 75
    (d) § 77

Ans. (d)
Note
Inappropriately called chronic diseases are delt in § 77.
Also see
§ 77
Those diseases are inappropriately named chronic, which persons incur who expose themselves continually to avoidable noxious influences, who are in the habit of indulging in injurious liquors or ailments, are addicted to dissipation of many kinds which undermine the health, who undergo prolonged abstinence from things that are necessary for the support of life, who reside in unhealthy localities, especially marshy districts, who are housed in cellars or other confined dwellings, who are deprived to exercise or of open air, who ruin their health by over exertion of body or mind, who live in a constant state of worry, etc. These states of ill-health, which persons bring upon themselves disappear spontaneously, provided no chronic miasm lurks in the body, under an improved mode of living, and they cannot be called chronic diseases.
Ref: Organon By B.K. Sarkar

Q. 177. "The Friend of Health" was published at Frankjoet in the year (Kerala MD (Hom) Ent Paper-2 -01)
    (a) 1792
    (b) 1790
    (c) 1796
    (d) 1810

Ans. (a)
Note
"The Friend of Health" was published at Frankjoet in the year 1792.

Q. 178. "The Medicine of experience' was written by (Kerala MD (Hom) Ent Paper-2 -01)
    (a) Jahr
    (b) Boenninghausen
    (c) Kent
    (d) Hahnemann

Ans. (d)
Note
The Medicine of experience' was written by Dr. Hahnemann.

Q. 179. "The subjects of Anatomy, Physiology are not life, but only results of life" is said by (Kerala MD (Hom) Ent Paper-2 -01)
    (a) Dunham
    (b) Close
    (c) Kent
    (d) Hahnemann

Ans. (c)

Q. 180. The 6th edition of Organon consists of (Kerala MD (Hom) Ent Paper-2 -01)
    (a) § 291
    (b) § 294
    (c) § 292
    (d) § 293

Ans. (a)
Note
The 6th Edition of Organon consists of 291 §.

Q. 181. Animal magnetism, mesmerism are in which § of 6th Edition (Kerala MD (Hom) Ent Paper-2 -01)
    (a)   § 288, 289
    (b)   § 278, 279
    (c)   § 281, 282
    (d)   § 286, 287

Ans. (a)
Note
§ 288, 289 in 6th edition of Organon contain instructions about Animal magnetism, mesmerism.

Q. 182. Massage in ___ (Kerala MD (Hom) Ent Paper-2 -01)
    (a)   § 280
    (b)   § 270
    (c)   § 260
    (d)   § 290

Ans. (d)
Note
Massage is discussed in § 290.
Also see
§ 290
Here belongs also the so-called massage of a vigorous good-natured person given to a chronic invalid, who, though cured, still suffers from loss of flesh, weakness of digestion and lack of sleep due to slow convalescence. The muscles of the limbs, breast and back, separately grasped and moderately pressed and kneaded arouse the life principle to reach and restore the tone of the muscles and blood and lymph vessels. The mesmeric influence of this procedure is the chief feature and it must not be used to excess in patients still hypersensitive.
Ref: Organon of Medicine 6th edition

Q. 183. Diet in acute diseases — (Kerala MD (Hom) Ent Paper-2 -01)
    (a)   § 259 – 261
    (b)   § 267 – 268
    (c)   § 142 – 143
    (d)   § 262 - 263

Ans. (d)
Note
Diet in acute diseases § 262 – 263

§ 262
In acute disease, on the other hand – except in cases of mental alienation – the subtle, unerring internal sense of awakened life-preserving faculty determines so clearly and precisely, that the physician only requires to counsel the friends and attendants to put no obstacles in the way of this voice of nature by refusing anything the patient urgently desires in the way of food, or by trying to persuade him to partake of anything injurious.

Ref: 5th Edition of Organon of Medicine, Commentary By B.K. Sarkar Pg-249

§ 263
The desire of the patient affected by an acute disease with regard to food and drink is certainly chiefly for things that give palliative relief; they are, however, not strictly speaking of a medicinal character, and merely supply a sort of want. The slight hindrances that the gratification of this desire, *within moderate bounds*, could oppose to the radical removal of the disease will be amply counteracted and overcome by the power of homeopathically suited medicine and the vital force set free by it, as also by the refreshment that follows from taking what has been so ardently longed for in like manner, in acute disease the temperature of room and the heat or coolness of the bed-coverings must also be arranged entirely in conformity with the patient's wish. He must be kept free from all over exertion of mind and exciting emotions. *(a)*
Ref: 5th Edition of Organon of Medicine, Commentary By B.K. Sarkar Pg-249

Q. 184. The manuscript of 6th Edition was left ready by our master 'Hahnemann' in the year (Kerala MD (Hom) Ent Paper-2 -01)
- (a) 1846
- (b) 1842
- (c) 1921
- (d) 1890

Ans. (b)

Note
According to Dr. Haehl, the biographer of Hahnemann, the date of confirmation is February, 1842, according to a manuscript copy made by Madame Hahnemann.
Ref: B.K. Sarkar, Orgnon of Medicine Pg-270.

Q. 185. The Homeopathic law of nature and a provisional explanation of is given under which section:
- (a) § 26 – 35
- (b) § 36 – 40
- (c) § 99 – 104
- (d) § 52 – 55

Ans. (a)

Note
The Homeopathic law of nature and a provisional explanation of is given under which section § 26 – 35

Also see
§ 26
This is dependent on the therapeutic law of nature that a weaker dynamic affection in the living organism is permanently extinguished by one that is very similar to and stronger than it, only differing from it in kind.
NOTE - This applies both to physical affections and moral maladies.
§ 27
The curative power of medicines, therefore, depends on the symptoms they have similar to the disease.
§ 28 – 29
Attempt to explain this therapeutic law of nature.
§ 30 – 33
The human body is much more disposed to let its state of health be altered by medicinal forces than by natural disease.
§ 34 – 35
The correctness of the homeopathic therapeutic law is shown in the want of success attending every unhomeopathic treatment of a long-standing disease, and in this also, that two natural diseases meeting together in the body, if they be dissimilar to each other, do not remove or cure one another.

Q. 186. In a case of 50 Millesimal potency, the method of repetition of doses in long lasting disease is: (UPSC-06)
- (a) Daily or every second day
- (b) Every 2, 3, 4 or 6 hours
- (c) Every hour
- (d) Every half hour

Ans. (a)

Note
In a case of 50 Millesimal potency, the method of repetition of doses in long lasting disease is 'on every second day'.

Also see
§ 248
The globule of the high potency is best crushed in a few grains of sugar of milk which the patient can put in the vial and be dissolved in the requisite quantity of water. (with perhaps 8, 10, 12, succussions) from which we give the patient one or (increasingly) several teaspoonful doses, in *long lasting diseases daily or every second day*, in acute diseases every two six hours and in very urgent cases every hour or oftener. Thus in chronic

diseases, every correctly chosen homeopathic medicine, even those whose action is of long duration, may be repeated daily for months with ever increasing success. If the solution is used up (in seven to fifteen days) it is necessary to add to the next solution of the same medicine if still indicated one or (though rarely) several pellets of a higher potency with which we continue so long as the patient experiences continued improvement without encountering one or another complaint that he never had before in his life.
Ref Organon 6th Edition.

Also see (brief)
To prescribe 50 Millesimal potency in a long lasting disease (chronic disease), the best choice is to prescribe daily, it will not cause any aggravation when favourable result (amelioration) appears then one can stop the medication. Very frequent repetition is suitable in acute case.

Q. 187. In case of intermittent fever, where the pyrexia stage is very short, the medicine should be administered during: (UPSC-06)
    (a)   Lucid interval
    (b)   Sweat state
    (c)   Declining period of paroxysm
    (d)   Heat stage

Ans. (c)
Note
In case of intermittent fever, where the pyrexia stage is very short, the medicine should be administered during 'declining period of paroxysm'.

Also see
§ 237
But if the stage of apyrexia be very short as happens in some very bad fevers, or if it be disturbed by some of the after sufferings of the previous paroxysms, the dose of the homeopathic medicine should be administered when the perspiration begins to abate or the other subsequent phenomena of the expiring paroxysms begin to diminish.
Ref Organon of Medicine (5th Edition), Commentary by B.K. Sarkar

Q. 188. Alternating disease belong to the domain of (UPSC-06)
    (a)   Psora
    (b)   Sycosis
    (c)   Chronic disease
    (d)   Sycosis, Syphilis

Ans. (a)
Note
Alternating disease belong to the domain of Psora.

Also see
§ 232
The later, *alternating* diseases, are also very numerous, but all belong to the class of chronic diseases, they are generally a manifestation of developed psora alone, sometimes, but *seldom, complicated with the syphilitic miasm* and therefore in the former case may be cured by antipsoric medicine, in the latter, however, in alteration with antisyphilitic as taught in my work on the *Chronic Diseases*.
Ref Organon By B.K. Sarkar Pg-231-232.

Q. 189. Psychotherapy is indicated in which type of the following mental diseases? (UPSC-06)
    (a)   Mental diseases originating from corporeal disease.
    (b)   Mental diseases or recent origin arising from psychogenic causes.
    (c)   Sudden outbursts of insanity.
    (d)   Mental diseases having physical or mental causes which are difficult to be ascertained.

Ans. (b)
Note
Psychotherapy is indicated in 'Mental diseases arising from psychogenic causes'.

Also see
§ 225 If the malady is the result of grief, mortification, vexation, insult, fear or fright it may profoundly affect the physical health.
§- 226 These, if treated early, may be cured by psychical methods, gentle kind admonition, appeal to reason, skilful deception, or carefully regulated habits.
Ref: Organon of art of healing by Baldwin

Q. 190. Assertion (A) (UPSC-06)
Suppression of eczemas by local applications has been known to produce colitis, asthma and bronchitis.
Reason (R)
Psora is the mother of all chronic diseases.
Code:
(a) Both A and R are individually true and R is the correct explanation of A.
(b) Both A and R are individually true but R is not the correct explanation of A.
(c) A is true but R is false.
(d) A is false but R is true.

Ans. (b)
Note
Both A and R are individually true but R is *not* the correct explanation of A.

Q. 191. Match List I with List II and select the correct answer using the code given below the lists: (UPSC-06)

List- I (Miasm)	List-II (Symptom)
A. Sycotic	1. Impatient
B. Syphilitic	2. Dyspnea worse in rainy season
C. Psoric	3. Intolerance to heat
D. Tubercular	4. Fastidious

Code:

	A	B	C	D
(a)	2	1	3	4
(b)	4	3	1	2
(c)	2	3	1	4
(d)	4	1	3	2

Ans. (c)
Note
The correct match is as under

List- I (Miasm)	List-II (Symptom)
A. Sycotic	2. Dyspnea worse in rainy season
B. Syphilitic	3. Intolerance to heat
C. Psoric	1. Impatient
D. Tubercular	4. Fastidious

Q. 192. Match List I with List II and select the correct answer using the code given below the lists: (UPSC-06)

List- I (Author)	List-II (Books)
A. E. A. Farrignton	1. The Genius of Homeopathy
B. R. E. Dudgeon	2. Clincial Materia Medica
C. Stuart Close	3. Lesser Writings of Hahnemann
D. Herbert A Roberts	4. Comparison of Chronic Miasms
E. Phyllis Speight	5. The Principle and Art of Cure by Homeopathy

Code

	A	B	C	D	E
(a)	2	5	1	3	4
(b)	4	3	2	5	1
(c)	2	3	1	5	4
(d)	4	5	2	3	1

Ans. (c)
Note
The correct match is as under:

List- I (Author)	List-II (Books)
A. E. A. Farrignton	2. Clincial Materia Medica
B. R. E. Dudgeon	3. Lesser Writings of Hahnemann
C. Stuart Close	1. The Genius of Homeopathy
D. Herbert A Roberts	5. The Principle and Art of Cure by Homeopathy
E. Phyllis Speight	4. Comparison of Chronic Miasms

Q. 193. Match List I with List II and select the correct answer using the code given below the lists (UPSC-06)

List- I (Aphorism)	List-II (Content)
A. Aphorism 1	1. Physician's Qualification
B. Aphorism 2	2. Physician is likewise preserver of health if he knows the things that derange health, cause disease, and their removal from persons in health.
C. Aphorism 3	3. Mission of Physician
D. Aphorism 4	4. Highest Ideal of Cure

Code

	A	B	C	D
(a)	2	4	1	3
(b)	3	4	1	2
(c)	2	1	4	3
(d)	3	1	4	3

Ans. (b)

MCQ's in Organon

Note
The correct match is as under:

List- I (Aphorism)	List-II (Content)
A. Aphorism 1	3. Mission of Physician
B. Aphorism 2	4. Highest Ideal of Cure
C. Aphorism 3	1. Physician's Qualification
D. Aphorism 4	2. Physician is likewise preserver of health if he knows the things that derange health, cause disease, and their removal from persons in health.

Q. 194. Consider the following: (UPSC-06)
1. Patient is intelligent and oversensitive.
2. Silent type of patient who goes out and commits suicide.
3. Sensitive to noise, to light and to odour.
4. All complaints are aggravated in winters.

Which of the above symptoms are related to 'Psoric Miasm'?
  (a) 1, 2 and 3
  (b) 1, 2 and 4
  (c) 1, 3 and 4
  (d) 2, 3 and 4

Ans. (c)
Note
The psoric patient is
 -Intelligent
 -Oversensitive to external impression – light, noise
 -Intolerance to cold – therefore worse in winters

Q. 195. Logic of Homeopathy is based on (UPSC-06)
  (a) Inductive method only
  (b) Both inductive and deductive method
  (c) Deductive method only
  (d) Aristotle's writing

Ans. (b)
Note
The logic can be defined as 'Science of Reasoning'.
Logic (Greek logos "word," "speech," "reason"), science dealing with the principles of valid reasoning and argument.
According to Bacon there are two scientific ways by which an inference can be tested;
  a. Inductive logic
  b. Deductive logic
The Inductive Logic
The Inductive method of logic proceeds by 'induction' by drawing an universal conclusion from a particular premise / inference.
 -The laws of homeopathy are based on inductive logic.
The deductive logic
In deductive logic we do the opposite and infer what will happen in consequences of law. Here a particular conclusion is drawn from a universal premise. Inference is drawn from general to particular.
The application of these laws are based on deductive logic.
Therefore the logic or Homeopathy is based on both.
Ref: Organon by B.K. Sarkar
Ref: A Treatise on Organon of Medicine Part III, By A. K. Das

Q. 196. In case of intermittent fever, the guidelines for prescription are given in which §? (UPSC-06)
    (a)   § 236
    (b)   § 36
    (c)   § 136
    (d)   § 286

Ans.   **(a)**

Note
In case of intermittent fever, the guidelines for prescription are given in § 236.

Also see
§ 236
The most appropriate and efficacious time for administering the medicine in these cases is immediately or very soon after the termination of the paroxysm, as soon as the patient has in some degree recovered from its effects; it has then time to effect all the changes in the organism requisite for the restoration of health, without any great disturbance or violent commotion; whereas the action of a medicine, be it ever so specifically appropriate, if given immediately before the paroxysm, coincides with the natural recurrence of the disease and causes such a reaction in the organism, such a violent contention, that an attack of that nature produces a the very least a great loss of strength, if it do not endanger life[2]. But if the medicine be given immediately after the termination of the fit, that is to say, at the period when the apyretic interval has commenced and a long time before are any preparations for the next paroxysm, then the vital force of the organism is in the best possible condition to allow itself to be quietly altered by the remedy, and thus restored to the healthy state.
Ref: Organon By B.K. Sarkar.

Q. 197. Only one wart on left index finger is a/an (UPSC-06)
    (a)   Internal one sided disease
    (b)   External one sided disease
    (c)   Artificial chroni c disease
    (d)   False chronic disease

Ans.   **(b)**

Note
Only one wart on left index finger is an 'External one sided disease'.

Also see
§ 173
The only diseases that seem to have but few symptoms, and on that account to be less amenable to cure, are those which may be termed one-sided, because they display only one or two principal symptoms which obscure almost all the others. They belong chiefly to the class of chronic diseases.

§ 174
Their principal symptom may be either an internal complaint (e.g. a headache of a many years' duration, a diarrhea of long standing, an ancient cardialgia, etc.), or it may be an affection more of an external kind. Diseases of the latter character are generally distinguished by the name of *local maladies*.
Ref: Organon of Medicine, Commentary by B.K. Sarkar

Extended information
Diseases with few symptoms
One-sided disease
1.   Diseases with only mental symptoms.
2.   Diseases with only physical symptoms.
These are further divided as
    a.   Internal physical symptoms (i.e., headache)
    b.   External physical symptoms
        i.   Surgical diseases:
            The treatment of such diseases is relegated to surgery, as the affected parts need mechanical aid, whereby the pathology is an obstruction to cure, and may be removed by mechanical aid.
        ii.   Non-Surgical diseases:
            Dynamic diseases, which appear on the external parts of the body i.e. wart.

Conclusion
From above it becomes clear that the wart on the finger is a example of external one sided dynamic disease.

Q. 198. Repertory part of the book 'Fragmenta De…..Observatis' is mentioned in the _____ (MD/NIH/98)
(a) First part
(b) Second part
(c) Both of above
(d) None of above

Ans. (b)

Note
Repertory part of the book 'Fragmenta De…..Observatis' is mentioned in the second part.

Also see
FRAGMENTA DE VIRIBUS
The First Materia Medica and Repertory of the Homoeopathy
(Fragmentary observations relative to the positive powers of medicine on the human body)
Fragmenta de viribus, as it is most popularly called was one of the first attempts made by Dr Samuel Hahnemann in the direction of a proper materia medica. This work was merely a glimpse of what was to come. It contained the accounts of his first provings of homoeopathic medicines. It was the precursor, the fore-runner of homoeopathic materia medica.

It was written in Latin language and was published in 1805. Publishers were M/s Sumpter Joan Ambrose Barthii of Leipzig.
It was published in two volumes:
(1) The first volume was published in 1805. It was called PARS PRIMA. It had 277 pages comprising of an 'Introduction' and the 'Main Text' of the book.
(2) The second volume was the 'Repertory' or 'Index.' It was called PARS SECUNDA. It had 476 pages comprising of 'Preface' and a 'Repertory' of 460 pages.

In the later editions, the two parts were combined in one volume. In 1834, Dr F.F. Quin, the erstwhile father of British homoeopathy, called for this book and published it in one volume from London.
Ref: http://www.homeorizon.com/mainpagegeneral.asp?t=fragmenta.htm#page%20top

Fragmenta ... Fragmenta de Viribus Medicamentorum Positivis Sive in Sano Humanis Corpore Observatis, 2 parts, 269 and 470 pages, J.A. Barth, Leipzig, 1805, by Hahnemann:

First Repertory

Abstract
The form of the repertory as we know it for the most part has its antecedents in Bönninghausen's *Systematic Alphabetic Repertory of Homoeopathic Medicines*. Our own research in this area has provided some insight into the process of *repertography* developed by Bönninghausen, and the ramifications on our modern day repertorial derivatives whose lineage[1] is traced to this original work.

From the Beginning
It was Hahnemann who first realised the need for some form of index for recalling the symptoms of our ever increasing provings, data, appending an *alphabetical index* to his *Fragmenta*[2] of 1805, and undertaking two further compilations which however were never published.[3] There followed a number of *indices* by various authors,[4] each listing a single remedy alongside a single symptom, more or less as it appeared[5] in the record.[6] These were not *repertories* as such, but rather, a re-organised[7] listing (for easier reference) of symptoms.[8]

The First Repertory
Bönninghausen's own life-saving experience of homoeopathy in 1828,[9] and his subsequent failure to induce any of the allopathic physicians around him to take up it's study,[10] moved him to pursue the study of this therapeutic method himself. His sharp mind being already trained in taxonomic definition was perfectly suited to this study,[11] and he quickly realised[12] the necessity of an accurate ready reference to our provings data, compiling a succession of precursors[13] before publishing his *Systematic Alphabetic Repertory of Homoeopathic Medicines [in two parts, antipsoric* (SRA) and non-antipsoric (SRN] medicines). This was *the first repertory*[14] as we know it, wherein provings were, for the first time, *represented* via rubrics,[15] *graded*

according to clinical verification,[16] arranged systematically,[17] and alphabetically, and thereby allowing ready access[18] to our materia medica.

Repeatedly urged by Hahnemann,[19] Bönninghausen set bout to bring out a single volume, combined edition of this work,[20] but ceased when he realised a different model of repertory (TT).[21] SRA/SRN have since remained largely unserviceable to the homoeopathic profession; only the SRA had been translated into English, whilst the more voluminous SRN had not.[22] Yet SRA/SRN, to which we now refer jointly as The First Repertory (TFR),[23] both conceptually and structurally, represents Bönninghausen's first method of repertory, and forms the very model of our modern repertories;[24] descended firstly through Jahr in his Handbuch (JHR),[25] the second edition of which was translated into English and published as the first English language repertory (1838).[26] This then found it's way via C.Lippe (LRMC), to E.J.Lee (LRC),[27] and on to J.T.Kent, being incorporated into his Repertory (KR),[28] whose basic structure was consistent with that of its predecessors.[29] Thus, it may be seen that Kent's Repertory, and its emulates,[30] wholly in structure and initially in content,[31] itself derives from the systematicalphabetic model of TFR[32]
Ref: http://www.vithoulkas.com/files/pdf/The_First_Repertory.pdf

Extended information
Organon § 109
I was the first that opened up this path, which I have pursued with a perseverance that could only arise and be kept up by a perfect conviction of the great truth, fraught with such blessings to humanity, that it is only by the homoeopathic employment of medicines[1] that the certain cure of human maladies is possible.[2]

1. It is impossible that there can be another true, best method of curing dynamic diseases (i.e., all diseases not strictly surgical) besides homoeopathy, just as it is impossible to draw more than one straight line betwixt two given points. He who imagines that there are other modes of curing diseases besides it could not have appreciated homoeopathy fundamentally nor practised it with sufficient care, nor could he ever have seen or read cases of properly performed homoeopathic cures; nor, on the other hand, could he have discerned the baselessness of all allopathic modes of treating diseases and their bad or even dreadful effects, if, with such lax indifference, he places the only true healing art on an equality with those hurtful methods of treatment, or alleges the latter to be auxiliaries to homoeopathy which it could not do without! My true, conscientious followers, the pure homoeopathists, with their successful, almost never-failing treatment, might teach these persons better.

2. The first fruits of these labors, as perfect as they could be at that time, I recorded in the Fragmenta de viribus medicamentorum positivis, sive in sano corpore humano observatis, pts. I, ii, Lipsiae, 8, 1805, ap. J. A. Barth; the more mature fruits in the Reine Arzneimittellebre, I Th., dritte Ausg.; II Th., dritte Ausg., 1833; III Th., zweite Ausg., 1825; IV Th., zw. Ausg., 1827 (English translation, Materia Medica Pura, vols I and ii); and in the second, third, and fourth parts of Die chronischen Krankheiten, 1828, 1830, Dresden bei Arnold (2nd edit., with a fifth part, Dusseldorf bei Schaub, 1835, 1839).

Q. 199. Diseases can be cured by a medicine which is _____ (MD/NIH/98/WB) Organon
    (a) Simillimum
    (b) Similar
    (c) Dissimilar
    (d) Same as the disease state

Ans. (a)
Note
Diseases can be cured by a medicine which is it's simillimum.
Also see
Aphorism 104
The image constructed by case taking as detailed above, is the basis for the selection of the remedy which has a strikingly similar pathogenesis. The remedy so selected is the similimum. The labor of making this selection constitutes the important item in the technique of homoeopathic prescribing. The well arranged repertory and the well stated materia medica facilitates the selection and lightens the labor. A preparation for

this labor involves the task of making acquaintance of a good repertory and mastering as far as is possible the peculiar genius of the best proved drugs. This latter achievement is no slight task and can be contemplated with equinimity only by feeling that the effort will be recompensed by a service to the sick, unequalled in curative merits by any other therapeutic modality known to the science of internal medicine. When the patient has received the similimum and all obstacles in the way of recovery have been removed the most has been done that can be done to insure a speedy, gentle, permanent cure.
Ref: Organon, aphorism 104.

Q. 200. All diseases are under the acute miasm except, _____ (MD/NIH/2000)
    (a)   Epidemic
    (b)   Sporadic
    (c)   Individual
    (d)   Venereal

Ans. (d)
Note
All diseases are under the acute miasm except, venereal diseases.

Also see
Aphorism 72
…The diseases to which man is liable are either rapid morbid processes of the abnormally deranged vital force, which have a tendency to finish their course more or less quickly, but always in a moderate time—these are termed acute diseases…
Clinical classification of diseases according to Hahnemann (according to aphorism 73):
Acute diseases include:
    (a)   Individual diseases: Diseases attacking 'individually'; these are the instances of transient explosions of latent psora due to:
        (i)   Excess in food.
        (ii)   Insufficient supply of food.
        (iii)   Severe physical impression for example, chill, overheating, dissipation, strains – mental or emotional, etc.
    (b)   Sporadic diseases: Diseases attacked 'sporadically'; for example, diseases that attack several persons at the same time here and there.
    (c)   Epidemic diseases: Or disease due to some general climatic conditions war, famine, etc. overpowering the resistance of a mass of people in some locality; or due to infection with some violent fixed miasms.
    Ref: Organon, page 337.

Q. 201. The role of vital force was first introduced in _____ edition of Orgnaon (MD/ACHMC/97)
    (a)   Third edition
    (b)   Fourth edition
    (c)   Fifth edition
    (d)   Sixth edition

Ans. (b)
Note
The role of vital force was first introduced in the fifth edition of Organon of Medicine.

Also see
The fifth edition of Organon of Medicine appeared in 1833. This edition since has been accepted as a standard textbook in homeopathic institution of the world. This was also the last edition published during the lifetime of Dr Hahnemann. This edition introduced two new doctrine viz., doctrine of vital force and doctrine of drug dynamization. By this time he had a clear conception of vital force and its working. The material living body serves as an instrument through which the vital force effects its working. The living body being the base and vital force, the source. Similarly, each medicinal substance possess a qualitative force which works in and through the physical material substance. Thus, by drug dynamization, the qualitative force of drug is released

which is capable of acting qualitatively on the dynamic vital force of living being.
In the sixth edition of Organon of Medicine, published after the death of Dr Hahnemann in 1921, another term, 'life principle' was introduced in preference to 'vital force.' Another change appeared in the sixth edition regarding a new method of potentizing medicines and their repetition. This new method of preparing potentised medicine is known as 50 millesimal scale as the material quantity of the medicine is decreased 50,000 times in each degree of dynamization. This method was introduced by him to avoid any homeopathic aggravation even if the medicine is repeated frequently to expediate cure in chronic diseases.
Ref: Organon of Medicine at a Glane, by A.C. Gupta, page 8.

Q. 202. Sycosis is _____ (PSC/WB/91)
(a) Inco-ordination of growth
(b) Ulcerative in nature
(c) Degenerative in nature
(d) Malignant in nature

Ans. (a)

Note
Sycosis is incoordination of growth.

Also see
Sycosis or the venereal wart disease, is the least frequently observed chronic miasm. Venereal warts, as primary lesions, complicate a certain type of gonorrhoea. The suppression of these primary warts is followed by a secondary stage that has not been carefully described. One pathology noted is the contraction of the tendons of the palms of the hands. The warts and moles that appear so frequently without apparent cause may be but mute evidence of the hereditary taint acquired from an immediate or remote ancestor. The genius of sycosis is to stack up redundant cell growth. It produces the hydrogenoid constitution which signifies excess of water and by virtue of this trait of stimulating or originating foci of proliferating cells is the substratum of those diseases characterized by exaggerated cell or tissue growth of which cancer is typical.
Ref: Organs of Art of Healing, by Baldwin – Hompath Archives.

Please Note
The inco ordination of growth is a character marker of cancer. Therefore both the features given in the choice as above are confusing in nature. Hoewever, the best choice is (a).

Q. 203. Which is the symptom of psora _____ (MD/NIH/98/RSC08)
(a) < daytime
(b) > warmth
(c) > movement
(d) < eating

Ans. Use your discretion

Note
Psora is covering two symptoms from the above and these are (a) and (b).

Also see
Psora, the internal itch miasm is the most universal and destructine of the three miasms. It is the oldest and most hydra-headed of all the chronic miasmatic diseases.

Psora	Sycosis	Syphilis
It is the outcome of evil thought.	It is the outcome of evil action.	It is the outcome of evil action.
Psoric mind is overactive.	The sycotic mind is mal-active.	Syphilitic mind is under active.
Psora is quick.	Sycotic is bad.	Syphilitic is slow.
Psora is intelligent.	Sycotic is mischievous.	Syphilitic is idiotic.
Psora manifests most strongly functional symptoms.	Sycosis has features of infiltration and overgrowth of tissues.	Syphilis has his hallmark ulceration and destruction of tissues.

Psora is over-sensitive both physically and mentally.	Sycotics are sensitive like a barometer.	Syphilitics have blunted sensitivity.
Psoric complaints are worse from sunrise to sunset.	Sycotic complaints are worse during twilight state.	Syphilitic complaints are worse from sunset to sunrise.
Wants warmth – both internally and externally. Aggravation from cold and during sleep.	Aggravation from rest, damp cold, moist cold, during thunderstorms and from heat.	Aggravation from natural discharges that is, perspiration, from extremes of temperature, at the seaside and from sea voyages, from thunderstorms, movements during summer, from warmth and from the warmth of the bed.

Ref: Homoeopathy – The Scientific Medicine, by E. Balkrishnan.
Ref: Miasmatic Diagnosis, by Subrata Kumar Banerjea, page 99, revised edition 2003.

Q. 204. A sycotic patient desires (MD/NIH/98/RSC/08)
  (a) Sweet
  (b) Narcotics
  (c) Beer
  (d) Cold food

Ans. (c)

Note
A sycotic patient desires beer.
Ref: Miasmatic Diagnosis, by Dr Subrata Kumar Banerjea, page 116, revised edition, 2004.

Also see
Psoric desires
Sweets, sugar, candies and syrup, hot food, acids, sour things, unusual things during pregnancy.
Sycotic desires
Craves beer, wine aggravates.
Syphilitic desires
Likes cold foods.
Ref: Perceving Crucial Symptoms, by S.M. Gunavante, page 116.
Ref: Miasmatic Diagnosis, by Subrata Kumar Banerjea, page 116, revised edition, 2003.

Q. 205. Hahnemann used the word miasm in sense of _____ (PSC/WB/91)
  (a) Infection
  (b) Influence
  (c) Pollution
  (d) Chronic syndrome

Ans. (c)

Note
Hahnemann used the word miasm in sense of 'pollution.'

Also see
The word 'miasm' comes from the Greek word 'miasma' which means taint, stain, pollution.
Haehl, the biographer of Hahnemann, also remarks that psora, as an expression, widely known in Hahnemann's time was the general germ for a whole series of skin troubles of the most varied kinds, welll known from the every earliest times. It was in this wider sense that his contemporaries used the word generally at the end of the eighteenth and in the first three decades of the nineteenth century, although at the same time they applied it in the narrower sense to itch proper. Hahnemann did not, therefore, coin this expression, but rather by his use of it showed his association with his contemporaries.
Ref: Organon, by Dr B.K. Sarkar, page 349.

Q. 206. Totality of symptoms comprises of _____ (PSC/WB/93)
    (a)   Sum total of all symptoms
    (b)   Symptoms which help in individualization
    (c)   Sum total of subjective symptoms
    (d)   Sum total of objective symptoms

Ans. (b)

Note
Totality of symptoms comprises of 'symptoms which help in individualization.'

Also see
The true 'totality' is more than the mere numerical totality or whole number of the symptoms. It may even exclude some of the particular symptoms if they cannot, at the time, be logically related to the case. Such symptoms are called 'accidental symptoms', and are not allowed to influence the choice of the remedy. The 'totality' is that concrete form which the symptoms take when they are logically related to each other and stand forth as an individuality, recognizable by anyone who is familiar with the symptomatic forms and lineaments of drugs and diseases.

Ref: Roberts
Ref: Essentials to Repertorization, Erecting a Totality, by S.K. Tiwari, page 39.

Q. 207. At the end of the treatment, the anti miasmatic medicine required is _____ (MD/NIH/98/RPSC/08)
    (a)   Anti-syphilitic
    (b)   Anti-sycotic
    (c)   Anti-psoric
    (d)   Anti-pseudopsoric

Ans. (c)

Note
At the end of treatment, the anti-miasmatic medicine required is anti-psoric.

Also see
Aphorism 195
In order to effect a radical cure in such cases, which are by no means rare, after the acute state has pretty well subsided, an appropriate antipsoric treatment (as is taught in my work on Chronic Diseases) must then be directed against the symptoms that still remain and the morbid state of health to which the patient was previously subject. In chronic local maladies that are not obviously venereal, the antipsoric internal treatment is, moreover, alone requisite.
Ref: Organon, by Sarkar, page 215, ninth revised edition, Birla Publication.

Q. 208. Prognosis of the patient after the administration of a medicine, was mentioned by_____ (MD/NIH/98)
    (a)   Hahnemann
    (b)   Hering
    (c)   Kent
    (d)   A.V. Haller

Ans. (c)

Note
Prognosis of the patient after the administration of medicine, was mentioned by Dr J.T. Kent.

Also see
Prognosis of the patient after the administration of a medicine, was mentioned by Dr Kent and this is known as Twelve Observations.
Ref: Philosophy, by Dr J. T. Kent, page 224.

Q. 209. 'Tolle Causam' means ----- (Similar /MD/Ent/NHMC/08)
(a) Remove the cause
(b) Total cause of disease
(c) Totality of symptoms
(d) Proximate cause

Ans. (a)

Note
'Tolle Causam' means remove the cause.

Also see
Introduction
The partisans of the old school of medicine flattered themselves that they could justly claim for it alone the title of 'rational medicine,' because they alone sought for and strove to remove the cause of disease, and followed the method employed by nature in diseases.

Tolle causam! they cried incessantly. But they went no further than this empty exclamation. They only fancied that they could discover the cause of disease; they did not discover it, however, as it is not perceptible and not discoverable. For as far the greatest number of diseases are of dynamic (spiritual) origin and dynamic (spiritual) nature, their cause is therefore not perceptible to the senses; so they exerted themselves to imagine one, and from a survey of the parts of the normal, inanimate human body (anatomy), compared with the visible changes of the same internal parts in persons who had died of diseases (pathological anatomy), as also from what they could deduce from a comparison of the phenomena and functions in healthy life (physiology) with their endless alterations in the innumerable morbid states (pathology, semeiotics), to draw conclusions relative to the invisible process whereby the changes which take place in the inward being of man in diseases are affected a dim picture of the imagination, which theoretical medicine regarded as its prima causa morbi,[1] and thus it was at one and the same time the proximate cause of the disease, and the internal essence of the disease, the disease itself – although, as sound human reason teaches us, the cause of a thing or of an event, can never be at the same time the thing or the event itself. How could they then, without deceiving themselves, consider this imperceptible internal essence as the object to be treated, and prescribe for it medicines whose curative powers were likewise generally unknown to them, and even give several such unknown medicines mixed together in what are termed prescriptions?

Ref: Organon of Medicine, translated from the fifth edition with an Appendix by R. E. Dudgeon MD, with additions and alterations as per the sixth edition translated by William Boericke, MD and an Introduciton by James Krauss MD.

It is impossible to know all the antecedents causative of disease consequents. Tolle causam is easier said than done. How, then, shall we remove or palliate these effects by medical substances? Here, Hahnemann steps in to say, for the first time in all history: Remove the effects and you remove the disease, the cause of the effects. Cessat effectus cessat causa.

Ref: Introduction to Dr Boericke's translation of the sixth edition of Hahnemann's 'Organon', by Dudgeon and Boericke.

Q. 210. Artificial chronic diseases are_____ (PSC/WB/91)
(a) Most difficult to treat
(b) Not at all curable
(c) Most difficult to cure
(d) Easily curable

Ans. (c)

Note
Artificial chronic disease is most difficult to cure.

Also see
Non-miasmatic expression of disease refers to chronic indisposition; artificial diseases (drug induced aphorism 74) or pseudo-chronic diseases (aphorism 77). In this category are included cases that resolve following changes in diet and lifestyle, correction of bad habits, or removal of offending drugs or environmental influences.

Aphorism 74, Fifth Edition
Among chronic diseases we must still, alas!, reckon those so commonly met with, artificially produced in allopathic treatment by the prolonged use of violent heroic medicines in large and increasing doses, by the abuse of calomel, corrosive sublimate, mercurial ointment, nitrate of silver, iodine and its ointments, opium, valerian, cinchona bark and quinine, foxglove, prussic acid, sulphur and sulphuric acid, perennial purgatives, venesections, leeches, issues, setons, etc., whereby the vital force is sometimes weakened to an unmerciful extent, sometimes, if it do not succumb, gradually abnormally deranged (by each substance in a peculiar manner) in such a way that, in order to maintain life against these inimical and destructive attacks, it must produce a revolution in the organism, and either deprive some part of its irritability and sensibility, or exalt these to an excessive degree, cause dilatation or contraction, relaxation or induration or even total destruction of certain parts, and develop faulty organic alterations here and there in the interior or the exterior[1] (cripple the body internally or externally), in order to preserve the organism from complete destruction of the life by the ever-renewed, hostile assaults of such destructive forces.

1. If the patient succumbs, the practiser of such a treatment is in the habit of pointing out to the sorrowing relatives, at the post-mortem examination, these internal organic disfigurements, which are due to his pseudo-art, but which he artfully maintains to be the original incurable disease (see my book, *Die Allöopathie, ein Wort deh Warnung an Kranke jeder Art*, Leipzig, bei Baumgärtner (translated in Lesser Writings)). Those deceitful records, the illustrated works on pathological anatomy, exhibit the products of such lamentable bungling.

Please Note
Organon mentions three classifications of long lasting diseases:
1. 'Those caused by continuing stress factors (disorders upheld by maintaining causes which by their nature are not necessarily true chronic disorders, §73).
2. Those caused by drug toxicity and faulty treatment (physician caused/drug induced, §74.),
3. And those caused by infectious miasms (naturally caused, §78).'

In modern times, the diseases produced by man-made toxins include the thousands of potential harmful chemicals released into our environment. As well as environmental degradation caused by massive industrialization, practice of compulsory immunization, and great numbers of new medicines produced by the pharmaceutical industry, and its ruthless use has resulted in tremendous growth of second category of chronic disease. These artificial chronic diseases are most difficult to cure.
Ref: What are Miasms?, by David Little.
http://www.wholehealthnow.com/homeopathy_pro/dl-miasms-03.html

Q. 211. Smallest possible dose can only be made with_____ (PSC/WB/91)
    (a)   Globules
    (b)   Purified H2O
    (c)   Cones
    (d)   Tabloid

Ans. (a)

Note
Smallest possible dose can only be made with 'globules'.

Also see
Aphorism 246, Fifth Edition
.......But the vital force shows the greatest resistance to the salutary action upon itself of the strongly indicated sulphur, and even exhibits manifest aggravation of the chronic disease, though the sulphur be given in the very smallest dose, though only a globule of the size of a mustard seed moistened with tinct. sulph X° be smelt, if the sulphur have formerly (it may be years since) been improperly given allopathically in large doses. This is one lamentable circumstance that renders the best medical treatment of chronic disease almost impossible among the many that the ordinary bungling treatment of chronic diseases by the old school would leave us nothing to do but to deplore, were there not some mode of getting over the difficulty.

In such cases we have only to let the patient smell a single time strongly at a globule the size of a mustard seed moistened with mercur metall. X, and allow this olfaction to act for about nine days, in order to make the vital

force again disposed to permit the sulphur (at least the olfaction of tinct. sulph. X°) to exercise a beneficial influence on itself – a discovery for which we are indepted to Dr Griesselich, of Carlsruhe.
Ref: Organon of Medicine.

Q. 212. In which edition of Organon did Hahnemann mention repetition (MD/Hydrabad)
    (a)   Fourth edition
    (b)   Fifth edition
    (c)   Sixth edition
    (d)   None of the above

Ans. (c)

Note
Hahnemann mentioned repetition in the sixth edition of Organon.

Also see
Hahnemann initially was against repetition but with constant experimentation he mentions repetition of doses more lucidly in the sixth editon.

The idea of repetition is a gradual one and has taken a long time to develop along with his experimentation and refinements as seen in different editions of Organon as under:

In the sixth edition of the Organon, Hahnemann recommended repetition (aphorism 246 and 248) 'at intervals that experience has shown to be the most distinctly appropriate for the best possible acceleration of treatment'; in chronic diseases of slow pace, this might be daily or every second day; in acute diseases, it might be every 6, 4, 3 or 2 hrs; in urgent cases, it could be hourly or even more frequently.

Ref: The Development of Approaches to the Repetition of Dose. in Hahnemann's Homoeopathy by Will Taylor, MD.
http://www.bringhealth.com/history_homeopathic_remedies_repetition_of_dose.html

Extended information
It was in 1829 that Hahnemann proposed the standardized use of the thirtieth centesimal potency, and this was his preferred preparation when he wrote Part 1 of Chronic Diseases in 1828. His posology in treating chronic disease is detailed on page 119-129, and page 137 (in the Jain edition). The carefully chosen dose and potency (most usually a single 30C pellet, dry or moistened) was allowed to act until the dose had exhausted its favourable action, with no other prescription to be considered so long as the improvement continued. Repetition or change of remedy was considered only when the old symptoms, which had been eradicated or very much diminished by the previous dose, commenced to rise again for a few days; discernment of the time to consider a second prescription required experience and careful observation.

The fourth edition of Organon, published the following year (1829), similarly advised that a 'single dose of a well-selected homeopathic medicine should always be allowed first fully to expend its action before a new medicine is given or the same one repeated.'

Constantine Hering left Germany for Surinam in 1827, and was shipwrecked off Martha's Vineyard on his attempt to return home in 1833. He settled in Philadelphia, well practiced in the methods of the fourth edition of Organon and the first edition of *Chronic Diseases*, and rooted the development of homeopathy in North America strongly with this 'wait and watch' methodology. Kent later provided perhaps the most eloquent and detailed description of this approach in his Lecture on the Second Prescription, read before the (AQ) International Hahnemannian Association at Niagara Falls in 1888.

When Hahnemann published the fifth edition of the *Organon* in 1833, he introduced an option he felt preferable to this 'wait and watch' approach, suggesting that a more rapid cure could be had by repeating a dose at 'suitable intervals which experience has proved to be best adapted' , guided by the 'nature of the medicinal substance, the corporeal constitution of the patient, and the magnitude of the disease.' He suggested repeating dry or moistened 30C globules (in Hahnemann's notation, X, referring to the decillionth dilution) at an unaltered dose and potency. Dosing frequency might range from every 7 to 14 days in a chronic illness of slow pace, to every five minutes in an acute illness of rapid pace, guided by clinical experience and observation of the progress of the case. This approach often required that an "intercurrent" remedy be given after several doses; a precaution that was reversed with the later introduction of gradual ascending potencies.

He modified the preparation of his centesimal potencies when intended to be used in this manner, reducing the number of successions at each dilution step from 10 to 2.

In 1838, Hahnemann developed his new potencies, his 'medicaments au globule' (the LM or Q or 50 millesimal potencies), which were intended to optimize the medicinal solution dosing approach described above. He shared his experience with these only with Boenninghausen, and first wrote about them in the sixth edition of Organon, the year prior to his death (1842), but which was only made available to the homeopathic community 80 years later, in 1921. Directions for the preparation of LMs are provided in the sixth edition of the Organon, in aphorism 270; and for their use in aphorisms 245-248 and 280-282. (also refer to Choudhury's book *Fifty Millesimal Potency - Theory and Practice*)

Ref: The Development of Approaches to the Repetition of Dose in Hahnemann's Homoeopathy by Will Taylor, MD.

http://www.bringhealth.com/history_homeopathic_remedies_repetition_of_dose.html

Q. 213. Surgical removal of an organ causes_____ (MD/NIH/98)
(a) Palliation
(b) Suppression
(c) Temperory relief
(d) Cure

Ans. (a)

Surgical removal of an organ causes 'suppression'.

Note
Suppression
A frequent form of suppression in modern days is the removal of disturbing organs by surgical means, again forbidding the expression of the vital force through its chosen organs, where it has expressed itself in a diseased state of the tonsils, the teeth, the sinuses, or any other part of the economy. The particular disturbance is shown by the symptom picture of the patient. In removing the tonsils, the teeth, or other organs by surgical operation we are dealing with the end product and not with the vital energy. We are cutting off the manifestation of disease and are doing nothing to set in order the vital energy or to prevent further disease manifestations. These diseased conditions have developed as an expression of the inward turmoil and distress under which the whole individual suffers.

Ref: The Principles and Art of Cure by Homoeopathy, by H.A. Robert, page 160.

Also see
Suppression
The 'suppressed' case always 'goes bad.' As an example of metastasis frequently observed and verified, take the surgical obliteration of a rectal fistula resulting from an ischio-rectal abscess in a tubercular patient, without having previously submitted the patient to a successful course of curative medical and hygienic treatment. What happens in such a case? The local, visible rectal symptoms are removed, the fistula is gone, but what about the patient? Presently the interior systemic disease which up to the time of the operation may be said to have been tentatively expressing itself in the rectal lesion, to the temporary relief of the organism and protection of vital organs, now breaks out in the lungs and hastens the patient to an untimely grave. A possibly curable case has been rendered incurable and a patient's life sacrificed because the physician or surgeon has failed to recognize the true indications in the case. The abscess and fistula act as if they were the 'Vent' or 'Exhaust' of the disease, affording temporary safety to vital organs. Close the exhaust and explosion follows.

Ref: Health and Disease, by Stuart.

Q. 214. Mental Disease is due to _____. (MD/NIH/98) -Organon
(a) Psora
(b) Pseudo-psora
(c) Sycosis
(d) Syphilis

Ans. (a)

Note
Mental disease is due to 'psora'.

Also see
Aphorism 210
Of psoric origin are almost all those diseases that I have above termed one-sided, which appear to be more difficult to cure in consequence of this one-sidedness, all their other morbid symptoms disappearing, as it were, before the single, great, **prominent symptom**. Of this character are what are termed mental diseases....
Ref: Organon of Medicine.

Q. 215. Subjective symptoms are_____ (PSC/WB/91)
    (a)   Narrated by the patient
    (b)   Narrated by the relatives
    (c)   Narrated by the patient in respect of his feelings
    (d)   Observed by attendants

Ans. (a)

Note
Subjective symptoms are narrated by the patient.

Also see
All the signs of disease expressed externally we find by observation of the so-called objective symptoms. Disease expresses itself also subjectively, the so-called subjective symptoms, which must be obtained from the patient. This is often very difficult. All too often the homeopath expects to be guided chiefly by the subjective signs, almost entirely neglecting the objective signs.
Ref: The Language of Disease (chapter 5).

According to Aphorism 95
Chronic cases cannot be taken too carefully. Trivial and obscure symptoms must not be overlooked. Each symptom, objective and subjective, helps to complete the totality, and provide a basis for making a homeopathic prescription.
Ref: Organon – Art Of Healing, by Baldwin.

Extended information
Subjective symptoms
A pure subjective symptom is one that the patient alone can feel and express, one that the doctor can neither see, hear, etc.
Ref: Handy Book of Reference, by Dr G. Royal.
Ref: http://www.homoeopathicdoctor.com/data.htm

Subjective symptoms are narrated by the patient. In addition to objective vital signs, clinicians need 'soft' data—subjective perceptions of symptoms and overall health and well-being, to manage their patients' health.

For example, to evaluate night-time dyspnoea, a clinician might select one or more of the following questions:
1. Have you experienced shortness of breath in bed?
2. Did you use extra pillows or sleep in a recliner?
3. Did breathing difficulty wake you up?
4. Did you sleep well last night?

Although self-reported symptoms may be less reliable than objective, machine-reported vital signs, they provide a sensitive diagnostic tool.
Ref: http://www.llmi.com/services/telemonitoring/subjective_symptoms.htm

Q. 216. In bad type of intermittent fever where the stage of apyrexia is very short, the medicine is to be applied_____ (PSC/WB/91)
    (a)   When chill is continuing
    (b)   When heat is continuing
    (c)   When sweat is continuing
    (d)   When perspiration begins to abate

Ans. (d)

Note
In bad type of intermittent fever where the stage of apyrexia is very short, the medicine is to be applied when perspiration begins to abate.

Also see
Aphorism 237
But if the stage of apyrexia be very short, as happens in some very bad fevers, or if it be disturbed by some of the after sufferings of the previous paroxysm, the dose of the homoeopathic medicine should be administered when the perspiration begins to abate, or the other subsequent phenomena of the expiring paroxysm begin to diminish.

Q. 217. Cure can take place by _____ (MD/NIH/98)
    (a) Primary action
    (b) Secondary action
    (c) Secondary counter action
    (d) Secondary curative action

Ans. (d)
Note
Cure takes place by Secondary curative action.

Also see
Primary and secondary action of the remedy from the Practical Part of Medicine, Organon of Medicine, by B.K. Sarkar, page 388.

Further reading:
The primary action of the homoeopathic remedy replaces the natural disease with a stronger but temporary medicinal disorder. The homoeopathic 'disease' is dependant of the duration of the remedy actions, which unlike chronic disease, is only temporary. In this way, a temporary medicinal disease removes a permanent chronic disease and a secondary curative action of the vital force 'directs its whole energy' against the remedy-disease 'which it soon overcomes.'
Ref: First Comments on the Vital Force, Primary and Secondary Actions, by David Little.
http://homepage.ntlworld.com/homeopathy_advice/Resources/ARCHIVE/vitalforce_davidlittle.html

Q. 218. 'Third prescription' is _____ (MD/NIH/98)
    (a) There is no third prescription
    (b) Any prescription made after the second prescription
    (c) A prescription made during the third visit
    (d) None of the above

Ans. (a)
Note
There is no third prescription.

Q. 219. 'By Miasm, Hahnemann means germ diseases' such a comment was made by _____ (MD/NIH/98)
    (a) Sir John Weir
    (b) M.L. Tyler
    (c) R. Hughes
    (d) Kent

Ans. (a)
Note
'By miasm, Hahnemann means germ diseases' – such a comment was made by Sir Hohn Weir.

Also see
Sir John Weir
Remarks in his book 'Science and Art of Homoeopathy'-"By miasm, Hahnemann means germ of diseases."
-The Science and Art of Homeopathy, British Homoeopathic Journal (1925).

Weir received his medical education first at Glasgow University MB, ChB 1907, and then was on a sabbatical year in Chicago, under the tutelage of Dr James Tyler Kent of Hering Medical College during 1908-9, along with Harold Fergie Woods and Douglas Morris Borland.

Weir reputedly first learned of homeopathy through his contact with Dr Robert Gibson Miller (1862-1919), head of the Glasgow Homeopathic Hospital, who had an important influence on the future Physician Royal, who he treated for boils and converted to homeopathy. "It was Dr Robert Gibson Miller who advised Sir John Weir to go to the USA."

Ref: http://homeopathy.wildfalcon.com/archives/2008/06/21/john-weir-and-homeopathy/

Extended information
DEFINITIONS

Hahnemann
Defines 'miasm as a morbific agent, which is inimical to life.' (aphorism 11)

Kent
Defines 'miasm as poisons on the dynamic plane.'

J.H. Allen
Miasm is the negative force linked to the vital force. Existence of a miasm is the true concept of chronic disease.

H.A. Roberts
'A miasm is defined as polluting exhalations or malarial poisons.'

Shakespeare
'Miasms are the maggots that are born within the brain.'

Dr P.S.Ortega
'This source or germ of suffering and death is positive, demonstrable and perfectly recognizable.'

A. J. Gross
'When we say miasms, we mean causes, the aetiology of acute and chronic diseases.'

George Vithoulkas
'Miasm is a predisposing weakness of the defense mechanism caused due to three factors such as hereditary infections, strong infectious diseases, and previous treatment.'

Foster
Defines 'miasm as a morbific emanation, which affects individuals directly, and not through the medium of another individual.'

Ref: Research on Efficacy of Homoeopathic Constitutional Medicine in Benign Hypertrophy of Prostate, Dr Joby Johny BHMS, MD (Hom), Trivandrum, Kerala, email : drjobyjohny@yahoo.com
Ref: http://www.similima.com/thesis46.html

Sir John Weir

Sir John Weir, GCVO, Royal Victorian Chain (19 October 1879 – 17 April 1971), MB ChB Glasgow, 1907, FFHom 1943, Physician Royal to several twentieth century monarchs.

Born in Paisley, Renfrewshire Scotland, Dr Weir was to become Physician Royal to King George V (reigned from 1910-36; Weir was his physician from 1918), King Edward VIII (reigned in 1936), King George VI (reigned from 1936-52), Queen Elizabeth II (physician to her from 1952-68), and King Haakon VII (from 1872-1957) of Norway, whose wife Maud (1869-1938) was the youngest daughter of King Edward VII (1841-1910).

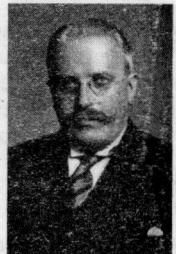

Sir John Weir, K.C.V.O. London, England President, I. H. A

Weir received his medical education first at Glasgow University, MB ChB, 1907, and then was on a sabbatical year in Chicago under the tutelage of Dr James Tyler Kent of Hering Medical College during 1908-9, along with Drs Harold Fergie Woods (1883-1961) and Douglas Borland (1885-1961).

Weir returned to the London Homeopathic Hospital as a consultant physician in 1910, and was appointed the **Compton-Burnett Professor of Materia Medica in 1911.** He rose to become President of the Faculty of **Homeopathy in 1923.**

Weir reputedly first learned of homeopathy through his contact with Dr Robert Gibson Miller (1862-1919), head of the Glasgow Homeopathic Hospital, who had an important influence on the future Physician Royal, who he treated for boils and converted to homeopathy (Bodman, 1971). "It was Dr Gibson Miller who advised Sir John Weir to go to the USA." (Stewart, 1967, page 260) This influence tended to get passed on: Dr Douglas Gibson (1888-1977) "became interested in homeopathy in 1936 through a meeting with Sir John Weir," (Gibson obit, 1977, 225).

Weir spoke on homeopathy before the Royal Society of Medicine in 1932, and was knighted by King George V that same year. The renovated Manchester Homoeopathic Institute and Dispensary was opened in Oxford Street by Sir John Weir in May 1939. Weir said in an address: homeopathy…is no religion, no sect, no fad, no humbug…remedies do not act directly on disease; they merely stimulate the vital reactions of the patient, and this causes him to cure himself. (Sir John Weir, 1931, 200-201) Having advanced through all levels of the Royal Victorian Order he was, as a rare distinction, awarded the Royal Victorian chain in 1947, possibly as a mark of the medical care he gave to the ailing King George VI.
Ref: http://en.wikipedia.org/wiki/John_Weir

Q. 220. 'Reine arzneimittellehre' indicates _____ (MD/NIH/98)
    (a) Medicine of Experience
    (b) Materia Medica Pura
    (c) Chronic Diseases
    (d) Organon of Medicine

Ans. (b)
Note
'Reine arzneimittellehre' indicates, Materia Medica Pura.

Also see
Aphorism 109 (Footnote)

.... Reine Arzneimittellebre, I Th., dritte Ausg.; II Th., dritte Ausg., 1833; III Th., zweite Ausg., 1825; IV Th., zw. Ausg., 1827 (English translation, Materia Medica Pura, volumes I and II); and in the second, third, and fourth parts of Die Chronischen Krankheiten, 1828, 1830, Dresden bei Arnold (second edition, with a fifth part, Dusseldorf bei Schaub, 1835, 1839).
Ref: Organon of Medicine.

...*Organon der rationellen Heilkunst* (1810; 'Organon of Rational Medicine'), contains an exposition of his system, which he called *Homöopathie*, or homeopathy. His Reine *Arzneimittellehre*, sixth volume. (1811; 'Pure Pharmacology'), detailed the symptoms produced by "proving" a large number of drugs—that is, by systematically...
Discussed in biography (in Hahnemann, Samuel)
Ref: http://www.britannica.com/EBchecked/topic/496589/Reine-Arzneimittellehre

Q. 221. Best time for giving an antipsoric medicine is ____(MD/NIH/98)
    (a) **During pregnancy**
    (b) **Before menses**
    (c) **After menses**
    (d) **During menses**

Ans. (a)
Note
Best time for giving antipsoric medicine is during pregnancy.

Also see
Aphorism 284, sixth edition (Footnote)
1. The power of medicines acting upon the infant through the milk of the mother or wet nurse is wonderfully helpful. Every disease in a child yields to the rightly chosen homoeopathic medicines given in moderate doses to the nursing mother and so administered, is more easily and certainly utilized by these new world-citizens than is possible in later years. Since most infants usually have imparted to them psora through the milk of the nurse, if they do not already possess it through heredity from the mother, they may be at the same time protected antipsorically by means of the milk of the nurse rendered medicinally in this manner. But the case of mothers in their (first) pregnancy by means of a mild antipsoric treatment, especially with sulphur dynamizations prepared according to the directions in this edition (§ 270), is indispensable in order to destroy the psora – that producer of most chronic diseases – which is given to them hereditarily; destroy it both within themselves and in the foetus, thereby protecting posterity in advance. This is true of pregnant women thus treated; they have given birth to children usually more healthy and stronger, to the astonishment of everybody. A new confirmation of the great truth of the psora theory discovered by me.
Ref: Organon of Medicine.

Where antipsoric treatment is properly conducted, the strength of the patient increases from the start and this increase in strength continues during the whole treatment until the organism unfolds its regenerated life.

The best time for taking an antipsoric is in the morning, before breakfast and the patient ought then to wait about an hour before eating or drinking anything.

Antipsorics should neither be taken immediately before, nor during menstruation. If menses appear too soon, too abundant, and last too long, she may smell on the fourth day of a globule of a high potency of Nux vomica, and several days after the antiposric may be taken. Nux restores the harmony of the nerves functions and calms the irritability which inhibits the action of the antipsoric.

Pregnancy offers a brilliant sphere of action to antipsoric remedies, but only the highest potencies ought to be employed. Nurslings ought to get their medicine through the milk of the mother or wet nurse.

Ref: A Compend of the Principles of Homoeopathy as Taught by Hahnemann and Verified by a Century of Clinical Application, by Dr William Boericke.

Ref: http://books.google.co.in/books?pg=PA151andlpg=PA151anddq=Best+time+for+giving+antipsoric+medicineandsig=L2Ky4-zyWRIg38x52_vYNphEn28andei=XIWOSbqrDIiO6gOouey9Cgandct=resultandid=KI27WZcVVXICandots=52_lJi9_t2andoutput=html

Q. 222. Homeopathic cure described in aphorism _____ (MD/Hydrabad/99)
    (a) 29
    (b) 39
    (c) 30
    (d) 147

Ans. (a)
Note
Homeopathic cure is described in aphorism 29.

Also see
Aphorism 29, sixth edition
As every disease (not entirely surgical) consists only in a special, morbid, dynamic alteration of our vital energy (of the principle of life) manifested in sensation and motion, so in every homeopathic cure this principle of life dynamically altered by natural disease is seized through the administration of a medicinal potency selected exactly according to symptom-similarity by a somewhat stronger, similar artificial disease-manifestation. By this the feeling of the natural (weaker) dynamic disease-manifestation ceases and disappears. This disease-manifestation no longer exists for the principle of life which is now occupied and governed merely by the stronger, artificial disease-manifestation. This artificial disease-manifestation has soon spent its force and leaves the patient free from disease, cured. The dynamis, thus freed, can now continue to carry life on in health. This most highly probable process rests upon the following propositions.

Ref: Organon of Medicine.

Q. 223. In homeopathic aggravation____ (MD/Hydrabad/ 99)
    (a) Medicine is correct
    (b) This < wished to (AQ)
    (c) Occurs in primary action
    (d) All of the above

Ans. (d)

Note

Homeopathic aggravation is a term used to describe a temporary intensification of symptoms before a condition improves.

Aggravation is a sign that the remedy is correct or is the simillmum, and this aggravation is due to the 'primary action' of the drug on the vital force. With this, the secondary action of the vital force will initiate the curative secondary curative action.

It is best to wait and watch unless the aggravation is very severe, which will require to be antidoted.

Aphorism 158

This slight homoeopathic aggravation during the first hours – a very good prognostic that the acute disease will most probably yield to the first dose – is quite as it ought to be, as the medicinal disease must naturally be somewhat stronger than the malady to be cured if it is to overpower and extinguish the latter, just as a natural disease can remove and annihilate another one similar to it only when it is stronger than the latter (§43 - 48).

Aphorism 160

But as the dose of a homoeopathic remedy can scarcely ever be made so small that it shall not be able to relieve, overpower, indeed completely cure and annihilate the uncomplicated natural disease of not long standing that is analogous to it (§ 249, note), we can understand why a does of an appropriate homoeopathic medicine, not the very smallest possible, does always, during the first hour after it's ingestion, produce a perceptible homoeopathic aggravation of this kind.

Aphorism 161, sixth edition

When I here limit the so-called homoeopathic aggravation, or rather the primary action of the homoeopathic medicine that seems to increase somewhat the symptoms of the original disease, to the first or few first hours, this is certainly true with respect to diseases of a more acute character and of recent origin, but where medicines of long action have to combat a malady of, considerable or of very long standing, where no such apparent increase of the original disease ought to appear during treatment and it does not so appear if the accurately chosen medicine was given in proper small, gradually higher doses, each somewhat modified with renewed dynamization (§ 247). Such increase of the original symptoms of a chronic disease can appear only at the end of treatment when the cure is almost or quite finished.

Aphorism 282, fifth edition

The smallest possible dose of homoeopathic medicine capable of producing only the very slightest homoeopathic aggravation, will, because it has the power of exciting symptoms bearing the greatest possible resemblance to the original disease (but yet stronger even in the minute dose), attack principally and almost solely the parts in the organism that are already affected, ...
Ref: Organon of Medicine.

Q. 224. Amelioration of all complaints by unnatural discharge is _____ miasm (MD/Hydrabad/99)
    (a) Sycotic
    (b) Syphilitic
    (c) Tubercular
    (d) Psoric

Ans. (a)

Note

Ameliorated from motion, unnatural discharges (which are generally greenish/yellow in colour) and unnatural eliminations through the mucous surfaces, for example, leucorrhoea, nasal discharge, etc. Physiological eliminations do not ameliorate.

Ref: Miasmatics Interpretation in Homoeopathic Prescribing, by Dr Subrata Kumar Banerjea.
http://homeopatia.edu.pl/index.asp?idm=2andidp=13andide=42

Q. 225. Hahnemann got his MD in the year ___ (MD/NIH/98)
(a) 1778
(b) 1779
(c) 1780
(d) 1781

Ans. (b)

Note

Hahnemann got his MD in 1779.

Also see

Hahnemann's thesis in 1779 – A Consideration of Etiology and Therapeutics of Spasmodic Affections. He got MD at the age of 24 on 10 April, 1779.

Ref: Repertory – Last Moment Revision, by Dr K.R. Mansoor Ali.

Q. 226. 'Aude sapere' was introduced for first time in ____ edition of Organon (MD/NIH/98)
(a) First
(b) Second
(c) Third
(d) Fourth

Ans. (b)

Note

'Aude sapere' was introduced for the first time in 'the second edition' of Organon of Medicine.

Also see

Sapere aude is a Latin phrase meaning 'dare to know.' It was originally used by Horace. It is a common motto for universities and other institutions, after becoming closely associated with 'The Enlightenment' by Immanuel Kant in his seminal essay, 'What is Enlightenment?'
Ref: http://en.wikipedia.org/wiki/Sapere_aude

In the Organon, it has been called the 'Bible of Homoeopathy.' It contains a complete and exhaustive exposition of Hahnemann's discoveries, experiments and opinions, concerning the healing of the sick.

The title page of the first edition bears the following motto from the poet Gellert :
'The truth we mortals need
Us blest to make and keep,
The All-wise slightly covered o'er,
But did not bury deep.'
This motto is changed in the other editions to the words 'Aude sapere'; and the title itself becomes : 'Organon der Heilkunst.'

He says in the Preface:
'The results of my convictions are set forth in this book. It remains to be seen, whether physicians, who mean to act honestly by their conscience and by their fellow creatures, will continue to stick to the pernicious tissue of conjectures and caprice, or can open their eyes to the salutary truth.

I must warn the reader that indolence, love of ease and obstinacy preclude effective service at the altar of truth, and only freedom from prejudice and untiring zeal qualify for the most sacred of all human occupations, the practice of the true system of medicine.

The physician who enters on his work in this spirit becomes directly assimilated to the Divine Creator of the world, whose human creatures he helps to preserve, and whose approval renders him thrice blessed.'

The book consists of two parts: The Introduction and the Organon proper. The introduction is first devoted to an analysis of the imperfect and erroneous method, distinguishing the old school of medicine.
Ref: http://www.homeoint.org/books4/bradford/chapter20.htm

Q. 227. Cure is possible in which dose (MD/NIH/98)
    (a)   Sub-physiological dose
    (b)   Sub-lethal dose
    (c)   Infinite dose
    (d)   Too frequent small dose

Ans. (c)

Note
Cure is possible in an infinite dose.

Also see
Homoeopathy achieves its ends and accomplishes its purposes by the use of single, simple, pure drugs; refined and deprived of the injurious properties and enhanced in curative power by the pharmacodynamical processes of mechanical communication, trituration, solution and dilution according to scale; in minimum or infinitesimal doses, administered by the mouth; the remedy having been selected by comparsion of the symptoms of the sick with symptoms of drugs produced by tests in healthy human subjects; under the principle of symptom- similarity, as enunciated in the maxims, 'Similia, Similibus Curantur.- Simplex Simile, Minimum.'
Ref: Development in Philosophy, by Stuart.

According to aphorism 16
The spirit-like dynamis, when disordered, is affected only by spirit-like morbid agencies. Hence the dynamic action of remedial agencies must be used for the purpose of cure. Life is the chemistry of the infinitesimal, the infinitesimal only can alter its processes or correct its disorder.

According to aphorism 269
The medicinal power of a crude substance is developed to an unparalleled degree by potentization. This process especially develops the medicinal powers of crude drugs, which in their crude state have no medicinal effect on the human body……. Homoeopathy potentizes the inert element, by a mathematical progression, to liberate its spirit-like dynamis that it may be employed to correct disorders of cell chemistry. Cell chemistry is the chemistry of the infinitesimal, the potentized crude element. Thus Hahnemann, by his carefully devised process of potentization has stolen from nature her secret means of initiating life and correcting its defects.

However it is interesting to know:
I am not without enemies in my own profession, they have been sent me from above for the purification of my heart, but I conquer them by silence and frequent remarkable cures with medicines which have neither smell nor taste, but usually help in a permanent manner without causing much discomfort. On those occasions I see that I am not lacking the necessaries of life, and have the sweet assurance that I have, taking all things into consideration, made unhappy people happy.
Ref: To Councillor Becker, by Hahnemann (in response to attacks on Hahnemann), Torgau, June 11, 1806.

Q. 228. Drug proving on healthy persons was thought of for the first time by _____ (PSC/WB/93)
    (a)   Hippocrates
    (b)   Von Haller
    (c)   Parcelsus
    (d)   Hahnemann

Ans. (b)

Note
Drug proving on healthy persons was thought of for the first time by 'Albrecht Von Haller.'

Also see
Aphorism 108
There is, therefore , no other possible way in which the peculiar effects of medicines on the health of individuals can be accurately ascertained – there is no sure, no more natural way of accomplishing this object,

than to administer the several medicines experimentally, in moderate doses, to healthy persons, in order to ascertain what changes, symptoms and signs of their influence each individually produces on the health of the body and of the mind; that is to say, what disease elements they are able and tend to produce[1], since, as has been demonstrated (§24-27), all the curative power of medicines lies in this power they possess of changing the state of man's health and is reveled by observation of the latter.

Footnote

1. Not one single physician, as far as I know, during the previous two thousand five hundred years, thought of this so natural, so absolutely necessary and only genuine mode of testing medicines for their pure and peculiar effects in deranging the health of man, in order to learn what morbid state each medicine is capable of curing, except the great and immortal Albrecht von Haller. He alone, besides myself, saw the necessity of this (vide the Preface to the Pharmacopoeia Helvet., Basil,1771, fol., p.12): Nempe primum in corpore sano medela tentanda est, sine peregrina ulla miscela; odoreque et sapore ejus exploratis, exiguaillius dosis ingerenda et ad omnes, quae inde contingunt, affectiones, quis pulsus, qui calor, quae respiratio, quaenam excretiones, pulsus, qui calor, quae respiratio, quaenam excretiones, attendendum. Inde ad ductum phaenomenorum, in sano obviorum, transeas ad experimenta in corpore aegroto," etc. But no one, not a single physician, attended to or followed up this invaluable hint.

Ref: Organon, by Sarkar, page 180, 181, Birla Publication.

Q. 229. Homeopathic drugs cause cure because _____ (PSC/WB/93)
- (a) Similarity of symptoms
- (b) Minuteness of dose
- (c) Potentization of drugs
- (d) Infrequent repetition of drug

Ans. (a)

Note

Homeopathic drugs cause cure because of similarity of symptoms.

Also see

Aphorism 29, sixth edition

As every disease (not entirely surgical) consists only in a special, morbid, dynamic alteration of our vital energy (of the principle of life) manifested in sensation and motion, so in every homoeopathic cure this principle of life dynamically altered by natural disease is seized through the administration of medicinal potency selected exactly according to symptom-similarity by a somewhat stronger, similar artificial disease-manifestation. By this the feeling of the natural (weaker) dynamic disease-manifestation ceases and disappears. This disease-manifestation no longer exists for the principle of life which is now occupied and governed merely by the stronger, artificial disease-manifestation. This artificial disease-manifestation has soon spent its force and leaves the patient free from disease, cured. The dynamis, thus freed, can now continue to carry life on in health. This most highly probable process rests upon the following propositions.

Ref: Organon of Medicine.

Or

Homeopathic treatment involves giving extremely small doses of substances that produce characteristic symptoms of illness in healthy people when given in larger doses. This approach is called 'like cures like.' The word homeopathy is a Greek derivation where 'homeos' means 'similar' and 'pathos' means 'suffering.' It is founded on a law – 'Similia Similibus Curantur' which means 'like cures like', the choice of the medicine is fundamentally based on the principle that the medicine must have the capability of producing most similar symptoms of the disease to be cured in a healthy person. So homeopathy may be defined as the therapeutic method of symptom similarity.

Q. 230. A simillimum medicine is given to a morbid patient in ____ potency (MD/NIH/98)
- (a) High
- (b) Medium
- (c) Low
- (d) Highest

Ans. (c)

Note
A simillimum medicine is given to a morbid patient in 'low' potency.

Also see
A medicine which when given by itself in a sufficiently large dose to a healthy individual produces a definite effect, that is, a number of its own peculiar symptoms, preserving its own tendencies, will be able to produce them even in the smallest dose . . . for curative purposes incredibly small doses are sufficient. . . if instead of smaller and smaller doses, increasingly large ones were given, then (after the original disease, has disappeared) there arise merely medicinal symptoms, a kind of artificial and unnecessary disease. . . How much the sensitiveness of the body towards medicinal stimuli increases, the illness can only be appreciated by the accurate observer. Especially when the disease has become very serious, this surpasses all belief. . . On the other hand, it is just as true as it is remarkable that even the most robust people, who are suffering from a chronic disease, notwithstanding their abundant physical strength, as soon as they are given the medicine positively helpful in their chronic disease, experienced just as great an impression from the smallest possible dose, as if they were suckling babes.'
Ref: Hompath.

Administer a low potency when a simillimum medicine is given to a morbid patient as this is based on the principle 'Similars cure similars.' The vital force is hypersensitive and susceptible to a similar remedy in a small dose of a potency.
Ref: http://homepage.ntlworld.com/homeopathy_advice/Resources/ARCHIVE/vitalforce_davidlittle.html

Q. 231. Diseases having few symptoms are called____(MD/NIH/98)
    (a) One-sided
    (b) Local disease
    (c) Partial disease
    (d) Mental malady

Ans. (a)
Note
Diseases having few symptoms are called one-sided disease.

Also see
Aphorism 173
The only diseases that seem to have but few symptoms, and on that account to be less amenable to cure, are those which may be termed one-sided, because they display only one or two principal symptoms which obscure almost all the others. They belong chiefly to the class of chronic diseases.
Ref: Organon of Medicine.

Q. 232. Best time for administration of medicine in intermittent fever____ (MD/NIH/98)
    (a) During the apyrexial state
    (b) During pyrexia
    (c) At the declining phase of pyrexia
    (d) At the onset of pyrexia

Ans. (a)
Note
Best time for administration of medicine in intermittent fever is during the apyrexial state.

Also see
Aphorism 236
The most appropriate and efficacious time for administering the medicine in these cases is immediately or very soon after the termination of the paroxysm, as soon as the patient has in some degree recovered from its effects; it has then time to effect all the changes in the organism requisite for the restoration of health, without any great disturbance or violent commotion; whereas the action of a medicine, be it ever so specifically appropriate, if given immediately before the paroxysm, coincides with the natural recurrence of the disease and causes such a reaction in the organism, such a violent contention, that an attack of that nature produces at the very least a great loss of strength, if it do not endanger life. But if the medicine be given immediately after

the termination of the fit, that is to say, at the period when the apyretic interval has commenced and a long time before there are any preparations for the next paroxysm, then the vital force of the organism is in the best possible condition to allow itself to be quietly altered by the remedy, and thus restored to the healthy state.
Ref: Organon of Medicine.

Q. 233. 'Prophylaxis' is a _____ (MD/NIH/98)
(a) Preventive therapy
(b) Curative therapy
(c) Palliative therapy
(d) Suppressive therapy

Ans. (a)

Note
Prophylaxis is a preventive threapy.

Also see
After working in an epidemic for a few weeks, you will find, perhaps that half-a-dozen remedies are indicated daily and one of these in a large number of cases than any other. This one remedy seems to be best suited to the general nature of the sickness. Now you will find that for prophylaxis there is required a less degree of similitude than is necessary for curing. A remedy will not have to be so similar to prevent disease as to cure it, and these remedies in daily use will enable you to prevent a large number of people from becoming sick. We must look to homeopathy for our protection as well as for our cure.
Ref: Kent Lecture – Idiosyncrasies.

Q. 234. Susceptibility means_____ (MD/NIH/98)
(a) Capabilities of man, both inherent and acquired
(b) General quality of a living organism of receiving impressions
(c) One of the fundamental attributes of life
(d) All of the above

Ans. (d)
Susceptibility means all of the above.

Note
General pathology of homeopathy (pathology of homeopathy)
…..By idiosyncrasy we mean a habit or quality of the organism peculiar to the individual. It is a peculiarity of the constitution, inherited or acquired, which makes the individual morbidly susceptible to some agent or influence which would not so affect others…..
Ref: By Stuart.

Susceptibility reaction and immunity (Immunity):
By susceptibility we mean the general quality or capability of the living organism of receiving impressions; the power to react to stimuli. Susceptibility is one of the fundamental attributes of life. Upon it depends all functioning, all vital processes, physiological and pathological. Digestion, assimilation, nutrition, repair, secretion, excretion, metabolism and katabolism, as well as all disease processes arising from infection or contagion depend upon the power of the organism to react to specific stimuli.
Ref: By Stuart.

Q. 235. > by pressure belongs to _____ miasm (MD/Hyderabad/98
(a) Psoric
(b) Syphilitic
(c) Sycotic
(d) Tubercular

Ans. (c)
Amelioration by pressure belongs to sycotic miasm.

Note

The colic of sycosis is better by bending double, by motion or hard pressure; this it not so of psora; we often find the worst forms of constipation or inactivity of the bowels in psoric or pseudo-psoric patients. Sometimes in disease states of the abdomen, the patient is very sensitive to motion. In psora we often have a beating or throbbing as of a pulse in the abdomen, while in tubercular patients, you can often feel the beating of the carotids through the abdominal walls.

Ref: The Chronic Miasms: Sycosis, Psora and Pseudopsora, by J.H. Allen.

Q. 236. In case of local disease, _____ procedure will be most effective for quick and radical cure (PSC/WB/91)
- (a) Internal and external administration of the same medicine which is found most homeopathically selected under the circumstances
- (b) Only internal administration of the well selected medicine
- (c) External administration of constitutional medicine
- (d) None of the above

Ans. (b)

In case of local disease, only internal administration of a well selected medicine will be most effective for a quick and radial cure.

Note
Aphorism 191

This is confirmed in the most unambiguous manner by experience, which shows in all cases that every powerful internal medicine immediately after its ingestion causes important changes in the general health of such a patient, and particularly in the affected external parts (which the ordinary medical school regards as quite isolated), even in a so-called local disease of the most external parts of the body, and the change it produces is most salutary, being the restoration to health of the entire body, along with the disappearance of the external affection (without the aid of any external remedy), provided the internal remedy directed towards the whole state was suitable chosen in a homoeopathic sense.

Ref: Organon of Medicine.

Also see

The treatment of local affections by the external employment of medicine is inadmissible for the following reasons:
- (a) All local affections, whether acute or chronic are only an inseparable part of the whole disease.
- (b) If a case of prominent local affection, recovers more rapidly with local applications than the internal disease, it often leads to the deceptive impression that a complete cure has been affected.
- (c) For the same reason, the medicine, homeopathically indicated for the whole case, should not be used exclusively as a topical application to the local symptoms of chronic miasmatic disease. With the disappearance of the chief local symptom, the residual picture of the whole disease remains in a mutilated and vague form, thus depriving the physician to get hold of individualizing symptoms for the selection of a simillimum.

Ref: Organon, by Sarkar, page 410, section 194-200.

Q. 237. 'Chronischen Krankheiten' means _____ (MD/NIH/98)
- (a) Chronic disease
- (b) Chronic miasm
- (c) Deep acting drugs
- (d) Crude drugs

Ans. (a)

Note
Chronischen Krankheiten (German) = *Chronic Diseases*

Also see
Chronic Disease was published by Hahnemann in 1828.

Ref:
Hahnemann's Die Chronischen Krankheiten
4 volumes.
1, 2, 3 volumes – published in 1828.
4th volume - published in 1830.
First Volume – Theory of chronic diseases.
Second, third and fourth volumes – Pathogenesis of medicines, new to Materia Medica Pura or to any materia medica.
17 new remedies + 2 old remedies.
Total of 22 remedies.
Second and third volumes – 15 remedies.
Fourth volume – 7 remedies [5 old (Con.,Carb.v.,Carb.-an., Caust. and Sulph.) of materia medica pura + 2 new (Nat.-mur. and Kali.-c.].
Symptoms drawn from action of medicine on sick.
No acknowledgement of fellow observers.
Potency 18 – 30 (Centesimal).
Magnesia muriatica – 6 potency.
Natrium carbonicum – 12 potency.
Violent effect from using 6, 9 and 12 potencies.
Sepia officinalis and Carbo vegetabilis for itch in 3 potency.
Violent effects of 2 – 12 potencies experienced by the sick from the bulk of symptoms.
Natrum muriaticum was proved on healthy people in 30 potency.

Hahnemann's second edition of Die Chronischen Krankheiten
5 volumes.
First and second volumes – published in 1835.
Third volume – published in 1837.
Fourth volume – published in 1838.
Fifth volume – published in 1839.
22 medicines of First edition + 25 remedies (13 new + 12 old in Materia Medica Pura)
Total of 47 remedies.
Pathogenesis in a continuous list.
Those already appeared have more additions.
He has acknowledged the contributions of fellow provers.
27 provers.
Hahnemann included -
(a) The works of Hartlaub and Trinks (Arzneimittellehre of their own)
(b) Independent provings of Stapf.
(c) Stapf (Archiv - A Journal).
(d) Prof. Jorg's provings on himself and his students.
Hughes says Hahnemann added the collateral effect of drugs with 30 potency in chronic patients.
30 potency in Centesimal.
Hughes says that the enormity of symptoms is due to the provings on sick.
On reproving less number of symptoms were got on healthy.
Hughes says that the bulk of symptoms cannot be relied upon unlike in Materia Medica Pura.
Note: Provings on healthy individuals was conducted by Haller, Stoerck and Alexander before Hahnemann.
English translation of Materia Medica Pura and Chronic Diseases by Hempel fell short of original.
In Materia Medica Pura of Hempel, medicines were arranged in Latin alphabetical order.
All names of authorities omitted.
Here there was no separation between symptoms of Hahnemann and others.
In Bryonia alba, symptoms of Hahnemann follow others and symptoms of Hahnemann are enclosed in brackets.
In Argentum metallicum and Camphora officinalis, symptoms are thrown together without distinction.
Symptoms are printed continuously without being divided into separate paragraphs and into section with headings.

The second volume of Materia Medica Pura was translated in 1824 and not in 1833.
Ferrum mettalicum and Verbascum Thapsus were omitted.
Medicines in Chronic Diseases were omitted from Materia Medica Pura.
Wholesome omission and careless rendering of symptoms and also of introductions and notes.
New English translation is of Hughes and Dudgeon of Materia Medica Pura.
Chronic Diseases is translated by Hughes and Louis. H. Tafel.
Ref: http://www.similima.com/mm2.html

Sources of Homeopathy Materia Medica
Dr K.R. Mansoor Ali, BHMS, MD (Hom)
Govt. Homeopathic Medical College, Calicut, Kerala
Approved practitioner, Ministry of Health, UAE.

Email : info@similima.com

Q. 238. Mental diseases are due to_____ (MD/NIH/98/WB)
 (a) Psora
 (b) Pseudopsora
 (c) Sycosis
 (d) Syphilis

Ans. (a)

Note
Mental diseases are due to Psora.

Also see
Aphorism 210
Of psoric origin are almost all those disease that I have above termed one-sided, which appear to be more difficult to cure in consequence of this one-sidedness, all their other morbid symptoms disappearing, as it were, before the single, great, prominent symptom. Of this character are what are termed mental diseases. They do not, however, constitute a class of disease sharply separated from all others, since in all other so-called corporeal diseases the condition of the disposition and mind is always altered.[1]
Ref: Organon of Medicine.

Q. 239. Idiosyncrasy is helpful in _____ (PSC/WB/93)
 (a) Assessment of prognosis
 (b) Drug proving
 (c) Management of cases
 (d) Case taking

Ans. (b)

Note
Idiosyncrasy is helpful in drug proving.

Also see
There is another reaction that we find in some patients, and that is purely hysterical. They seem to prove any remedy you may give them and get an aggravation from it. This may be because of an idiosyncrasy for the remedy or because of too sensitive a reaction of the vital energy. It may be almost impossible to do anything with them in a curative way, but it may be of inestimable help in proving a remedy.
Ref: Remedy Reaction, by Roberts.

Aphorism 117
To the latter category belong the so-called idiosyncrasies, by which are meant peculiar corporeal constitutions which, although otherwise healthy, possess a disposition to be brought into a more or less morbid state by certain things which seem to produce no impression and no change in many other individuals.[1] But this inability to make an impression on every one is only apparent. For as two things are required for the production of these as well as all other morbid alterations in the health of man – to wit., the inherent power of the influencing substance, and the capability of the vital force that animates the organism to be influenced by it – the obvious derangements of health in the so-called idiosyncrasies cannot be laid to the account

of these peculiar constitutions alone, but they must also be ascribed to these things that produce them, in which must lie the power of making the same impressions on all human bodies, yet in such a manner that but a small number of healthy constitutions have a tendency to allow themselves to be brought into such an obvious morbid condition by them. That these agents do actually make this impression on every healthy body is shown by this, that when employed as remedies they render effectual homoeopathic service to all sick persons for morbid symptoms similar to those they seem to be only capable of producing in so-called idiosyncratic individuals.

Q. 240. Repetition of first prescription is required _____ (PSC/WB/93)
    (a)   When symptoms have aggravated
    (b)   When symptoms have returned
    (c)   When order of symptoms have changed
    (d)   When original symptoms have returned

Ans. (d)

Note

Repetition of first prescription is required when the original symptoms return.

Also see

The second prescription presupposes that the first one has been a correct one, that it has acted, and that it has been let alone. If the first prescription has not acted curatively, or has not been permitted to act the full time, it is impossible to get a second observation. The second observation is made when the case comes to a standstill, for after the first prescription has been made, changes occur; there is a coming and going of symptoms, and while these changes are occurring no rational observation can be made of the case; if a second prescription is made during this time, it will most likely spoil the whole case. If the patient is not given perfect rest, if medicines are not kept out of the case, we will have no opportunity to make a rational second prescription. But if these precautions are observed, then we can really make an observation upon the return of the original symptoms, which is the first thing to be considered. Perhaps they are not so marked, but that is always the first thing to be looked for, the return of the original symptoms. While the confusion is going on after the administration of the remedy, while an internal order is being established in the economy, we do not have the return of the original symptoms...... If, after an interval of two or more months, the original symptoms return, we need very little information beyond this to know that the first prescription was a good one. In such a case, when the symptoms return, when the patient has the same general and particulars as formerly, it means that the first prescription was a good one, that the case is curable, and that the second prescription must be a repetition of the former.

Ref: Kent's Lectures; second Prescription.

Q. 241. 'What the pathologists of today call gonorrhoeal infection is what we term sycosis' – who made this comment (MD/NIH/98)
    (a)   J.H. Allen
    (b)   H.A. Roberts
    (c)   H. Farrington
    (d)   Richard Haehl

Ans. (a)

Note

'What the pathologists of today call gonorrhoeal infection is what we term sycosis' was commented by Dr J.H. Allen

Also see

Sycosis:

Sycosis is not a new name for gonorrhoea, neither is it gonorrhoea in any sense of the word. The well known specific urethritis, presents only in its initial stage, similar phenomena to that of sycosis, the history of the two diseases differs widely in their constitutional developments and progress. Gonorrhoea simplex is not a basic miasm, while sycosis comprises one of the chronic miasms of Hahnemann, and next to psora it is the most persistent of the great triune (AQ) of the subversive forces, syphilis, sycosis and psora. Sycosis, implanted on a rich pseudo-psoric soil, develops into one of the most formidable enemies of the race, whose destructive power and depth of action upon the organism cannot be expressed by any combination

of words. What the pathologists of today call gonorrhoeal infection, is what we term sycosis. But it is not an infection from a supposed gonorrhoeal catarrh, for gonorrhoea simplex does not affect the organism as does gonorrhoeal sycosis.
Ref: The Chronic Miasms, Volume II, Chapter-Sycosis, page 13, by J.H. Allen.

Q. 242. Too short a relief of symptoms after the application of deep acting remedies means_____ (PSC/WB/91)
    (a)   The remedy is to be repeated
    (b)   The remedy is to be applied in a higher potency
    (c)   There is a structural change in the patient
    (d)   The patient is of low susceptibility

Ans. (c)
Too short a relief of symptoms after the application of deep acting remedy means there is a structural change in the patient.

Note
Kent's sixth observation:

Too short a relief of symptoms.
When a high and right potency acts in curable case – the remedy acts at once and establishes a condition of order, after which there is no need of giving more medicine. This order may continue for a considerable length of time, sometimes several months. The patient gets along without any medicine. But, the patient may come back at the end of the first, second and third week and say he has done well, that he has been improving all the time, but at the end of the fourth week he returns with suffering.

- This could be due to some obstacle – something that has spoiled the action of the medicine. This condition is an unfavorable one.
- If relief after the constitutional remedy does not last long enough, it is because of some condition that interferes with the action of the remedy; it may be unconscious on the part of the patient, or it may be intentional. A quick rebound means everything in the remedy, means that it is well chosen, that the vital economy is in a good state, and if everything goes well, recovery will take place.
- In acute cases, when there is too short an amelioration of the symptoms, the remedy has to be repeated. If it is too short an amelioration in acute cases, it is because high grade inflammatory action is present and that organs are threatened by the rapid processes going on.
- If it is too short an amelicration in chronic diseases, it means that there are structural changes and organs are destroyed or being destroyed.

Bibliography

Books
1. Organon of Medicine, Commentary - B.K. Sarkar – Birla Publications (P) Ltd., New Delhi.
2. Introduction to Study of Homeopathy – Roberts – B. Jain Publishers (P) Ltd., New Delhi.
3. Lectures on Homeopathic Philosophy – J.T. Kent – B. Jain Publishers (P) Ltd., New Delhi.
4. Organon of Art of Healing – Baldwin – B. Jain Publishers (P) Ltd., New Delhi.
5. A Brief Study Course in Homeopathy – Elizabeth Wright – B. Jain Publishers (P) Ltd., New Delhi.
6. Lectures by Besweir
7. Life and works of Hahnemann – Richard Haehl – B. Jain Publishers (P) Ltd., New Delhi.
8. Fifty Reasons for Being a Homoeopath – J.C. Burnett – B. Jain Publishers (P) Ltd., New Delhi.
9. A Treatise on Organon of Medicne - Ashok Kumar Das – Hahnemann Homoeo Publications, Calcutta.

Websites
www.similima.com

Softwares
RADAR

Chapter 2
MATERIA MEDICA

Q. 1. Semilateral headache with blurred vision or blindness preceding the attack – must lie down, aversion to light and noise, sight returns as headache increases, headache in small spot can be covered by tip of finger, indicate the remedy from the following (UPSC-02)
    (a)   Gelsemium sempervirens
    (b)   Kali-bichromicum
    (c)   Sanguinaria canadensis
    (d)   Spigelia

Ans. (b)
Note
Above features are indicative of 'Kali-bi'.
Also see
(a)   Gels
Headache: preceeded by blindness (Kali-bi.) > by profuse urination. Headache: beginning in the cervical spine; pains extend over the head, causing a bursting sensation in forehead and eyeballs [Sang., Sil., begins in same way, but semi-lateral]; < by mental exertion; from smoking; heat of sun; lying with head low. Sensation of band around the head above eyes (Carb-ac., Sulph.); scalp sore to touch.
Ref: Allen's Key Notes
(b)   Kali-bi.
Headache: *blurred vision or blindness precedes the attack [Gels., Lac-d.]; must lie down; aversion to light and noise; sight returns as headache increases* (Iris, Nat-m., Lac-d.). Pains: in small spots, can be covered with point of finger.
Ref: Allen's Key Notes
(c)   Sang
Headache; worse right side, sun headache. Periodical sick headache; pain begins in occiput, spreads upwards, and settles over eyes, especially right. Veins and temples are distended. Pain better lying down and sleep. Headaches return at climacteric; every seventh day. (Sulph., Sabad.) Pain in small spot over upper left parietal bone. Burning in eyes. Pain in the back of head "like a flash of lightning".
Ref: Boericke's materia medica
(d)   Spig.
Nervous headache; periodical, beginning in morning at base of brain, spreading over the head and locating in eye, orbit at temple of left side (right side, Sang., Sil.); pain pulsating, violent throbbing. Headache; at sunrise, at its height at noon, declines till sunset (Nat-m., Tab.).
Ref: Allen's Key Notes

Q. 2. It is slow, deep acting remedy, belongs to anti-psoric, anti-sycotic and anti-syphilitic family, there is a tendency of destruction of tissues, especially syphilitic complaints and bone disease. Patient is very hot. Which one of the following is the correct remedy? (UPSC-02)
    (a)   Carbolicum acidum
    (b)   Mercurius solubilis
    (c)   Fluoricum acidum
    (d)   Nitricum acidum

Ans. (c)
Note
Above features belong to 'Fluoricum Acidum.
Also see
Fluoricum acidum

It is a very deep-acting medicine and an antipsoric, antisyphilitic and anti-sycotic. It is an unusually hot-blooded remedy. Think of the remedy, then, in vicious bone diseases, in necrosis and caries.
Ref: Kent lectures-Materia Medica

Q. 3. Match a List – I (Symptoms triads) with the List II (Medicine) and select the correct answer using the codes given below the lists. (UPSC-02)

List I (Symptom Triad)	List II (Medicine)
A. Constriction, Contraction, Congestion	1. Argentum nitricum
B. Apprehension, anticipation, hurried	2. Cactus grandiflorus
C. Chilly, dirty, offensive	3. Cantharis vesicatoria
D. Sexual instinct, sexual thought, sexual frenzy	4. Psorinum

Code

	A	B	C	D
(a)	3	4	1	2
(b)	2	1	4	3
(c)	3	1	4	2
(d)	2	4	1	3

Ans. (b)

Note
Correct match is as under:

List I (Symptom Triad)	List II (Medicine)
A. Constriction, Contraction, Congestion	2. Cactus grandiflorus
B. Apprehension, anticipation, hurried	4. Psorinum
C. Chilly, dirty, offensive	1. Argentum nitricum
D. Sexual instinct, sexual thought, sexual frenzy	3. Cantharis Vesicatoria

Also see
Arg-n.
Apprehension when ready for church or opera, diarrhea sets in (Gels.). Time passes slowly (can-i); impulsive, wants to do things in a hurry; must walk fast; is always hurried; anxious, irritable, nervous (Aur., Lil-t.).
Ref: Allen's Key Notes
Cact.
Constrictions, contractions and congestions run through Cact.
Ref: Kent's Lectures- materia medica
Canth.
Acute mania, generally of a sexual type; amorous frenzy; fiery sexual desire.
Ref: Boericke's materia medica
Psor.
Great sensitiveness to cold air or change of weather; wears a fur cap, overcoat or shawl even in hottest summer weather.
The skin over the body, especially of the face, looks filthy, though it has been well washed. A dingy, dirty, foul look, as if covered with dirt.
The oozing is offensive like carrion or decomposed meat; nauseating odor from the oozing fluid.
Ref: Kent's Lectures- materia medica

Q. 4. Bad effects of anger, grief, or disappointed love, broods in solitude over imaginary troubles, persons mentally and physically exhausted by long concentrated grief. Which one of the following is the correct remedy for above symptom complex? (UPSC-2002)
(a) Agaricus muscarius
(b) Cuprum metallicum
(c) Hyoscyamus niger
(d) Ignatia amara

Ans. (d)
Note
Above features belong to 'Ign.'.
Also see
Ign.
Bad effects of anger, grief, or disappointed love (Calc-p., Hyos.); broods in solitude over imaginary trouble. Persons mentally and physically exhausted by long-concentrated grief.
Ref: Allen's Key Notes

Q. 5. Match List – I (Homeopathic medicines) with List-II (Time of aggravation) and select the correct answer using the codes given below: (UPSC-2002)

List I (Homeopathic Medicine)	List II (Time of Aggravation)
A. Arsenicum album	1. 10 or 11 AM
B. Syphilinum	2. 4 to 9 PM
C. Natrium muriaticum	3. Sunset to Sunrise
D. Colocynthis	4. 1 to 2 AM

Code

	A	B	C	D
(a)	4	3	1	2
(b)	1	1	4	3
(c)	4	2	1	3
(d)	1	3	4	4

Ans. (a)
Note
Correct match is as under:

List I (Homeopathic Medicine)	List II (Time of Aggravation)
A. Arsenicum album	4. 1 to 2 AM
B. Syphilinum	3. Sunset to Sunrise
C. Natrium muriaticum	1. 10 or 11 AM
D. Colocynthis	2. 4 to 9 PM

Also see
Ars.
Worse: Midnight; after. 2 A.M.
Ref: Phatak's materia medica

English Kent

GENERALS - NIGHT - midnight, - amel. - 1 a.m.
ARS.$_k$ caul.$_k$ cocc.$_k$ lachn.$_k$ mag-m.$_k$ mur-ac.$_k$ psor.$_k$
Syph.
Worse: at night, sundown to sunrise, seashore, in summer.
Ref: Boericke's materia medica
Nat-m.
Worse: At 10 or 11 A.M.; at the seashore or from sea air; heat of sun or stove; mental exertion, talking, writing, reading, lying down.
Ref: Allen's key Notes
Colo.

English Kent

GENERALS - AFTERNOON - 4 p.m.
alum.$_k$ anac.$_k$ arum-t.$_k$ calc-p.$_k$ carb-v.$_k$ *Caust.*$_k$ chel.$_k$ cob.$_k$ *Coloc.*$_k$ gels.$_k$ *Hell.*$_k$ kali-c.$_k$ lachn.$_k$ **LYC.**$_k$ mag-m.$_k$ mur-ac.$_k$ nat-s.$_k$ puls.$_k$ stront-c.$_k$

English Kent

GENERALS - AFTERNOON - 4 to 8 p.m.
alum.$_k$ bov.$_k$ *Hell.*$_k$ **LYC.**$_k$ mag-m.$_k$ nux-m.$_k$ sulph.$_k$

English Kent

GENERALS - AFTERNOON - 4 to 10 p.m.
alum.$_k$ chel.$_k$ plat.$_k$

Q. 6. Consider the following symptoms regarding hemorrhagic diathesis (UPSC-02)
    (I)   Hamamelis virginiana- Prostration out of proportion to the amount of blood loss.
    (II)   Secale cornutum - Continuous oozing of sanguineous liquid blood.
    (III) Lachesis mutus- Hemorrhage from left side of the body, bright red and coaguable.
    (IV) Cinchona officinalis - Aversion to sour things during hemorrhage.
Which of these statements is / are correct?
    (a)   (I) only
    (b)   (I) and (II)
    (c)   (II), (III), and (IV)
    (d)   (III) and (IV)
Ans. (a)
Note
From above correct statement is (I).
Also see
    (I)   Ham.: Prostration out of all proportion to amount of blood lost (Hydr.). Bad effects from loss of blood (Cinch.).
    (II)   Sec.: NA
    (III) Lach.: NA
    (IV) Chin.: Haemorrhages: of mouth, nose, bowels or uterus; long continued; longing for sour things.
Ref: Allen's Key Notes

Q. 7. A 7-year-old child with convulsions screams and has violent jerking of hands and feet. He has pinching colic in abdomen before passing stool with mucous like while pieces of popped corn; also grinds teeth at night. Choose the correct remedy from the following (UPSC-02)
    (a)   Belladonna
    (b)   Chamomilla
    (c)   Cicuta virosa
    (d)   Cina
Ans. (d)

Note
Above features point to remedy 'Cina'.
Also see
Cina
Convulsions, with screams and violent jerkings of the hands and feet. Stool: White mucous, like small pieces of popped corn, proceeded by pinching colic. Grits teeth during sleep.
Ref: Boericke's materia medica

Q. 8. Match List – I (Medicines) with List-II (Symptoms in a case of prolapse uterus) and select the correct answer using the codes given below in the lists

List I (Homeopathic Medicine)	List II (Symptoms in case of prolapsed uterus)
A. Stannum metallicum	1. Worse during stool
B. Belladona	2. Better standing and sitting erect
C. Sepia	3. Better supporting vulva with hands
D. Lilium tigrinum	4. Better by sitting close

Code

	A	B	C	D
(a)	1	2	4	3
(b)	2	3	4	1
(c)	3	4	1	2
(d)	4	1	2	3

Ans. (a)

Note
Correct match is as under (a):

List I (Homeopathic Medicine)	List II (Symptoms in case of prolapsed uterus)
A. Stannum metallicum	1. Worse during stool
B. Belladona	2. Better standing and sitting erect
C. Sepia	4. Better by sitting close
D. Lilium tigrinum	3. Better supporting vulva with hands

Also see
(a) *Stann.*
Prolapsus, worse during stool (with diarrhea, Pod.)
Ref: Allen's Key Notes
(b) *Bell.*
Sensitive forcing downwards, as if all the viscera would protrude at genitals. Better semi-erect.
Ref: Boericke's materia medica
(c) *Lil-t.*
Bearing-down sensation; in abdomen and pelvis, as though all organs would escape (Lac c., Murx, Sep.) < supporting vulva with hand.
Ref: Allen's Key Notes

(d) *Sep.*
Prolapsus of uterus and vagina; pressure and bearing down as if every thing would protrude from pelvis; must cross limbs tightly or "sit close" to prevent it.

Ref: Allen's Key notes

Q. 9. A 46 –year old woman consults you for painful swelling of the throat for about 12 days. The complaints started with fever (mild) with chilliness followed by painful swelling. Associated with suffocation and attacks of palpitations. No cough. Wants to keep feet in cool place. Very hungry. All complaints are better by eating. Thirst is excessive. On examination; thyroid is enlarged. Which one of the following will you choose in this case? (UPSC-02)
   (a) Iodium
   (b) Phosphorus
   (c) Spongia
   (d) Sulphur

Ans. (a)

Note
The remedy for above clinical presentation is 'Iodium'.

Also see
The case appears to be of acute thyroiditis. The onset is sudden and initial symptoms i.e., fever and chilliness belongs to common symptoms of fever due to any cause. The painful swelling at neck is goiter painful (Ref: Kent Repertory-Chapter-External throat- Rubric; Goiter painful- 3:Iod, 2:Plat, 1:Spong). Hungry with much thirst. Better after eating are prominent symptoms of 'Iod.'. Palpitation is due to tachycardia is also covered by 'Iod'. Therefore the most appropriate choice appears to be 'Iod.'.

Q. 10. Regarding simple hypertrophy of heart, consider the following symptoms and remedies mentioned against them (UPSC-02)
   (I)   Chronic hypertrophy without valvular lesions – Naja tripudians
   (II) Hypertrophy with vascular lesions and cardiac dropsy - Adonis vernalis
   (III) Hypertrophy without vascular lesion and extreme dyspnea on least exertion- Crataegus
   (IV) Atheroma without weakness of heart – Cactus grandiflorus

Which of these are correct?
   (a) I and II
   (b) II and III
   (c) III only
   (d) I, II, III and IV

Ans. Use your discretion.

Note
Naja
Simple hypertrophy of heart. For restoring a heart damaged by acute inflammation or from relief of *sufferings of chronic hypertrophy and valvular lesions.*
Ref: Allen's Key Notes
Comment; not applicable as the heart complaint is with valvular lesions.

Adonis vernalis
Mitral and aortic regurgitation. Chronic aortitis. Fatty heart pericarditis. Rheumatic endocarditis (kalmia). Precordial pain, palpitation and dyspnea. Marked venous engorgement. Cardiac asthma. (quebracho), fatty heart. Myocarditis, irregular cardiac action, constriction and vertigo. Pulse rapid, irregular.
Ref: Boreicke's materia medica
Comment: The hypertrophy is without vascular lesions – i.e., arterio-venous fistulae, or hypertension. Of course it could be due to valvular lesions like aortic and mitral regurgitation.

Crataegus
Cardiac dropsy. Fatty degeneration. Aortic disease. Extreme dyspnea on least exertion, without much increase of pulse. Pain in region of heart and under left clavicle. Heart muscles seem flabby, worn out. Heart dilated; first sound weak. Pulse accelerated, irregular, feeble, and intermittent. Valvular murmurs, angina pectoris. Cutaneous chilliness, blueness of fingers and toes; all aggravated by exertion or excitement. Sustains heart in infectious diseases.
Ref: Boericke's materia medica

Cactus grandiflorus
Heart feels as if clasped and unclasped rapidly by an iron hand; as if bound, "had no room to beat".
Ref: Allen's Key Notes
Comment: Without atheroma there cannot be angina.

Q. 11. A nine-year-old child is brought to you with complaints of moderate fever and sore throat for 2 days. There is sore aching bruised feeling all over the body. On examination, head is hot and limbs are cold. Tonsils are red with white patches. He also feels as if a hot coal were present in his throat. Which one of the following will you chose for him? (UPSC-02)
   (a)   Belladonna
   (b)   Arnica montana
   (c)   Mercurius cynapium
   (d)   Phytolacca decandra

Ans. (d)

Note
The boy is suffering from tonsillitis.

Also see
Bell.
Dry, as if glazed; angry-looking congestion; red worse on right side. Tonsils enlarged; Throat feels constricted, difficult deglutition; worse, liquids.

Arn.
It has sore bruised feeling all over but it is more in tune with typhoid.

Merc cyn.
Feels raw and sore. Mucous membranes broken down, ulcerated. Looks raw in spots, especially in public speakers. Hoarseness and talking is painful. Necrotic distruction of soft parts of palate and fauces. Intense redness of fauces. Swallowing very difficult. Dark blood from nose.
Ref: Boericke's materia medica

Phyt.
Aching, soreness, restlessness, prostration, are general symptoms guiding to Phyt. Pre-eminently a glandular remedy. Glandular swellings with heat and inflammation. Has a typical sensation of great pain at root of tongue when swallowing burning as from a coal of fire or a red-hot iron is typical of Phyt.
Ref: Boericke's materia medica

Q. 12. A female of 45 years of age has sciatica of right side which always aggravates in night during sleep and is better when not lying on right side. She has gnawing pains in stomach but feels better by eating. Throat is painful on swallowing which becomes worse after taking warm liquids. She requires (UPSC-02)
   (a)   Lycopodium clavatum
   (b)   Phytolacca decandra
   (c)   Lachesis mutus
   (d)   Mercurius iodatus flavus

Ans. (c)

Note
She requires 'Lachesis'.

Also see
Lachesis
- Lach. is for females in climacteric period.
- Right sided sciatica (can be left) with oversensitiveness to touch.
- Stomach; gnawing pressure made better by eating.
- Pain throat < hot drinks.

Ref: Boericke's materia medica

Q. 13. Consider the following drugs (UPSC-02)
    (I)   Rhus toxicodendron
    (II)   Conium maculatum
    (III) Nux vomica
    (IV) Ranunculus bulbosus

Which of the above are obtained from poisonous plants?
    (a)   (I),(II), (III) & (IV)
    (b)   (II), (III) & (IV)
    (c)   (I), (II), & (III)
    (d)   (I) & (IV)

Ans. (a)

Note
All of above are obtained from poisonous plants.

Also see
Rhus-t.
The poison ivy grows in thickets and low grounds in North America, flowering in June. It was introduced into England as a plant in 1640. In 1798 Dufresnoy of Valenciennes first used it as a medicine. It was brought to his notice by the cure of a young man of a herpetic eruption (dartre) of six years duration, through his being accidentally poisoned with the plant. Dufresnoy used it successfully in eruptive diseases, paralysis, rheumatism, and amaurosis. The milky juice, which turns black on exposure, is used as a marking ink (like Anac.) and as an ingredient of varnishes for finishing boots. The tincture contains rhoitannic acid ($C_{18}H_{28}O_{13}$) and toxicodendric acid, a poisonous, volatile principle.
Ref: Clarke.

Con.
Con. or poison hemlock is a native Europe. The active principle is Conia, a yellowish, oily, transparent fluid, lighter than water, of an acrid, nauseous, tobacco-like taste. It is very volatile; slightly soluble in water; its combinations with acids do not easily crystallize, and are very soluble and poisonous. It was known in ancient times, but not used until recently as an internal medicine. It was employed in the execution of political offenders, and was the means of Socrates' death.
Ref: Hering.

Nux-v.
Nux-v. or poison nut. Nux Vomica seeds contain strychnine and nearly the allied alkaloid brucine, for action, principle being strychnine $C_{21}H_{22}H_2O_2$. Strychnine has a powerful stimulant action on the CNS especially on the spinal cord. First there is a feeling of stiffness in the muscles of the neck, face. Reflex action is so much increased that a slight touch evokes a sudden and violent movement. This increased movement is accompanied by restlessness. Tremors and involuntary movements are noticed. At the beginning of the convulsion the muscles are tonically contracted, hard and firm. But soon tremors develop and the muscles go into relaxation, soon a second convulsion ensues. As a rule, after a few convulsion death ensue, from asphyxia due to respiratory

failure. Strychnine causes flow of saliva and increased appetite. It is absorbed from intestines and increases the movements of the bowels.
Ref: Pharmacy Chapter 15 Hompath

Ran-b.
The juice or sap of this plant is excessively irritating to skin. When applied locally, it produces erythema followed later by an eruption which is at first vesicular in character and attended with burning, smarting and itching. If the symptoms continue, even the gangrene of part may follow.
Ref: Farrignton's Lectures.

Q. 14. A patient cannot walk with eyes closed, trembles with general debility, has paralysis with mental and abdominal symptoms, has rigidity of calves with debility, walks and stands unsteady especially when unobserved. Has numbness in arms and post diphtheric paralysis. Remedy suitable for this patient is (UPSC-02)
    (a)   Gelsemium sempervirens
    (b)   Causticum
    (c)   Chamomilla
    (d)   Argentum nitricum

Ans. (d)

Note
Remedy suitable for this patient is 'Arg-n'.

Also see
Arg-n.
Cannot walk with eyes closed. Trembling, with general debility. Paralysis, with mental and abdominal symptoms. Rigidity of calves. Debility in calves especially. Walks and stands unsteadily, especially when unobserved. Numbness of arms. Post-diphtheritic paralysis after Gels.
Ref: Boericke's materia medica.

Q. 15. Match the list –I (Medicine) with List –II (Disease) and select the correct answer using the codes given below the lists (UPSC-02)

List I (Homeopathic Medicine)	List II (Diseases)
A. Parotidinum	1. Quinsy
B. Pertussinum	2. Puerperal fever
C. Pyrogenium	3. Whooping cough
D. Baryta carbonicum	4. Mumps

Code

(a)	A	B	C	D
	4	3	2	1
(b)	A	B	C	D
	4	3	1	2
(c)	A	B	C	D
	3	4	2	1
(d)	A	B	C	D
	3	4	1	2

Ans. (a)

Note
The correct codes are as under (a)

List I (Homeopathic Medicine)	List II (Diseases)
A. Parotidinum	4. Mumps
B. Pertussinum	3. Whooping cough
C. Pyrogenium	2. Puerperal fever
D. Baryta carbonicum	1. Quinsy

Also see
Parotidinum
It is a nosode of mumps. It is used as a prophylactic against mumps.
Ref: Boericke's materia medica Augmented Editioin, Pg-1172
Pertussinum
Taken from the glairy and stringy mucous containing the virus of whooping cough. Introduced by John H. Clarke for the treatment of whooping cough and other spasmodic coughs.
Ref: Boericke's materia medica Augmented Editioin, Pg-1488
Pyrogenium
This remedy was introduced by English homeopaths, prepared from decomposed lean beef allowed to stand in the sun for two weeks and then potentized. Pyrogen is a great remedy for septic states, with intense restlessness.
Ref: Boericke's materia medica Augmented Editioin, Pg-523
Baryta carbonicum
This medicine is especially indicated in infancy and old age. Quinsy.
Ref: Boericke's materia medica Augmented Editioin, Pg-106-107
After Bar-c., Psor. Will often eradicate the constitutional tendency to quinsy.
Ref: Allen's Key Notes

Q. 16. Which of the following is the correct order that matches with the sequential order of "desire for sweets", "aversion to sweets" and "aggravation from sweets"? (UPSC-02)
(a) Arg-n. Chin., Graph.
(b) Chin., Arg-n. Graph.
(c) Graph., Arg-n., Chin.
(d) Chin., Graph., Arg-n.

Ans. (d)
Note
The correct order that matches with the sequential order of "desire for sweets", "aversion to sweets" and "aggravation from sweets" is (d).

Also see
Desire for sweets
STOMACH - DESIRES - sweets
Am-c. arg-met. **ARG-N.** ars. bar-c. *Bry.* bufo *Calc-s. Calc. Carb-v.* **CHIN.** chinin-ar. *Elaps Ip.* kali-ar. *Kali-c.* kali-p. *Kali-s.* **LYC.** *Mag-m. Med.* merc. nat-act. *Nat-c.* nat-m. nux-v. op. petr. *Plb. Rheum Rhus-t Sabad. Sec. Sep.* **SULPH.** *Tub.*

Aversion to sweets
STOMACH - AVERSION to - sweets
Ars. bar-c. *Caust.* **GRAPH.** hipp. lac-c. *Merc.* nit-ac. *Phos. Sin-n. Sulph. Zinc.*

Aggravation from sweets
GENERALS - FOOD, - sweets agg.
acon. am-c. *Ant-c.* ARG-N. calc. *Cham.* fl-ac. *Graph.* **IGN.** *Merc.* nat-c. ox-ac. phos. *Sel.* spig. *Sulph.* thuj. zinc.

Ref: Kent's Repertory of Homeopathic Mateia Medica

MCQ's in Materia Medica

Q. 17. Consider the following medicines and symptoms regarding abdominal colic (UPSC-02)
- (I) Colocynthis; Pain in abdomen with restlessness and better by hard pressure and bending double.
- (II) Platina; Pain in abdomen with restlessness and better by hard pressure and warmth application.
- (III) Magnesium phosphoricum; Pain in abdomen better by passing stool.
- (IV) Chamomilla; Pain in abdomen with irritability.

Which of these statements is / are correct?
- (a) (I), (II), & (III)
- (b) (I) & (IV)
- (c) (II) & (III)
- (d) (IV) Only

Ans. (b)

Note
Correct statement for above symptoms is (b).

Also see
- (I) Colocynthis: Agonizing pain in abdomen causing patient to bend double, with restlessness, twisting and turning to obtain relief >, by hard pressure (>. by heat, Mag.-p.).
  Ref: Allen's Key Notes
- (II) Platina: The pains increase gradually and as gradually decrease [Stann.]; are attended with numbness of parts (Cham.).
  Ref: Allen's Key Notes
- (III) Mag-p.: Pains: sharp, cutting, stabbing; shooting, stitching; lightning-like in coming and going (Bell.); intermittent paroxysm becoming almost unbearable, driving patient to frenzy; rapidly changing place (Lac c., Puls.), with a constricting sensation (Cac., Iod., Sulph.), cramping, in neuralgia affections of stomach, abdomen and pelvis (Caul. > bending double; heat; warmth; pressure (burning pain >. by heat, Ars.)
  Ref: Allen's Key Notes
- (IV) Cham: Peevish, irritable, oversensitive to pain, driven to despair (Coff.); snappish, cannot return a civil answer. Child exceedingly irritable, fretful; quiet only when carried; impatient, wants this or that and becomes angry when refused, or when offered, petulantly rejects it.
  Ref: Allen's Key Notes.
  Considering the above symptoms choice of (b); (I) and (IV) is most appropriate.

Q. 18. Over sensitiveness of nerves, scratching of linen or silk, crackling of papers is unbearable' is a characteristic symptom of (UPSC 2002)
- (a) Antimonium crudum
- (b) Staphysagria
- (c) Asarum europaeum
- (d) Ptelea

Ans. (c)

Note
Above symptopm is characteristic of 'Asarum europaeum'.

Also see
Asarum europaeum:
Oversensitiveness of nerves, scratching of linen or silk, crackling of paper is unbearable (Fer., Tar.).
Ref: Allen's Key Notes

Q. 19. From amongst the remedies (anti-miasmatic) given below, pick up the "Grand Anti –sycotic" remedies (UPSC-02)
    (a)   Arg-n., Med., Nat-s., Sep.
    (b)   Ars-i, Kali-i, Merc-c., Med.
    (c)   Nat-s., Sep., Aur-m-n., Kali-i.
    (d)   Merc-c., Kali-i., Aur-m-n., Ars-i.

Ans. (a)

Note
Amongst the above grand antisycotic remedies include 'Arg-n, Med, Nat-s, Sep'.

Also see

English Kent

GENERALS - SYCOSIS
$Agar._k$ $alumn._k$ $alum._k$ $anac._k$ $ant-c._k$ $ant-t._k$ $Apis_k$ $aran._k$ **ARG-MET.**$_k$ **ARG-N.**$_k$ $Aster._k$ $aur._k$ $Aur-m._k$ $Bar-c._k$ $bry._k$ $Calc._k$ $carb-an._k$ $carbn-s._k$ $carb-v._k$ $Caust._k$ $cham._k$ $cinnb._k$ $con._k$ $Dulc._k$ $euphr._k$ $Ferr._k$ $Fl-ac._k$ $Graph._k$ $hep._k$ $Iod._k$ $kali-c._k$ **KALI-S.**$_k$ $Lach._k$ $Lyc._k$ $Mang._k$ **MED.**$_k$ $merc._k$ $Mez._k$ **NAT-S.**$_k$ **NIT-AC.**$_k$ $amyg-p._k$ $Phyt._k$ $puls._k$ $sabin._k$ $Sars._k$ $Sec._k$ $Sel._k$ **SEP.**$_k$ $Sil._k$ **STAPH.**$_k$ $Sulph._k$ **THUJ.**$_k$

Ref: Kent's Repertory of Homeopathic Mateia Medica (RADAR 10)

Q. 20. Patient is fat, chilly with delayed menstrual history. Nails are deformed, crumbling and brittle, sore and painful. The remedy is (UPSC-02)
    (a)   Calarea carbonicum
    (b)   Mercurius solubilis
    (c)   Sulphur
    (d)   Graphites

Ans. (d)

Note
Above symptoms point to 'Graphites'.

Also see
Graphites
Suited to women, inclined to obesity, who suffer from habitual constipation; with a history of delayed menstruation. The nails brittle, rumbling, deformed (Ant. c); painful, sore, as if ulcerated; thick and crippled, and takes cole easily.
Ref: Allen's Key notes

Q. 21. Consider the following medicines (UPSC-02)
    (I)   Mercurius solubilis
    (II)   Coffea cruda
    (III)   Plantago
    (IV)   Bismuth

Which of the above medicine are applicable in the case of toothache amelioration by holding ice cold water inside the mouth? (UPSC 2002)
    (a)   (I) & (II)
    (b)   (III) Only
    (c)   (I) & (IV)
    (d)   (II), (III) & (IV)

Ans. Use your discretion

Note
The choice given above is covered by two drugs; Coff. and Bism. their features are given below.

Also see
Merc sol
Toothache: pulsating, tearing, lacerating, shooting into face or ears; < in damp weather or evening air, warmth of bed, from cold or warm things; > from rubbing the cheek. Crowns of teeth decay, roots remain (crowns intact, roots decay, Mez.).
Ref: Allen's Key Notes
Coffea cruda
Toothache: intermittent, jerking, relieved by holding ice-water in the mouth, but returns when water becomes warm (Bis., Bry., Puls., Caust., Sep., Nat-s.).
Ref: Allen's Key Notes
Plantago
Toothache, better while eating.
Ref: Boericke's materia medica
Bismuth
Toothache; better, cold water in mouth (Coff.)
Ref: Boericke's materia medica
From above the correct choice is (II and IV). However, this choice is not given.

Directions
The following 'six 'items consists of two statements, one labeled as "Assertion A" and the other labeled as "Reason R". You are to examine these two statements carefully and decide if the Assertion (A) and the Reason (R) are individually true and if so, whether the Reason is a correct explanation of the Assertion. Select your answers to these items using the codes given below and mark your answer sheet accordingly: (UPSC-02)

Answer Code:
- (a) Both A and R is true and R is the correct explanation of A.
- (b) Both A and R is true but R is not a correct explanation of A.
- (c) A is true but R is false.
- (d) A is false but R is true.

Q. 22. **Assertion (A): Magnesium phosphoricum is preferred to Belladonna in spasmodic pains.**
Reason (R): In Belladonna congestion is marked and pain appears and disappears suddenly.

Answer Code:
- (a) Both A and R is true and R is the correct explanation of A.
- (b) Both A and R is true but R is not a correct explanation of A.
- (c) A is true but R is false.
- (d) A is false but R is true.

Ans. (b)

Q. 23. **Assertion (A): Alumina is 'the Aconite of chronic disease".**
Reason (R): The treatment of all the chronic diseases can be initiated with Alumina without considering the symptom totality or any other criterion whatsoever.

Answer Code:
- (a) Both A and R is true and R is the correct explanation of A
- (b) Both A and R is true but R is not a correct explanation of A
- (c) A is true but R is false
- (d) A is false but R is true

Ans. (c)

Q. 24. Assertion (A): Typhoid fever ————
Reason (R): Baptisia in low dilutions produced a form of antibodies to the bacterial typhus.

Answer Code:
    (a)   Both A and R is true and R is the correct explanation of A
    (b)   Both A and R is true but R is not a correct explanation of A
    (c)   A is true but R is false
    (d)   A is false but R is true

Ans. (d)

Q. 25. A assertion (A): Sulphur is a great Antipsoric remedy.
Reason (R): Sulphur often has a great use in beginning the treatment of the psoric cases.

Answer Code:
    (a)   Both A and R is true and R is the correct explanation of A
    (b)   Both A and R is true but R is not a correct explanation of A
    (c)   A is true but R is false
    (d)   A is false but R is true

Ans. (b)

Q. 26. Assertion (A): It seems probable that Ars-i., there is a remedy most closely allied to the manifestations of tuberculosis.
Reason (R): Clinically it is advisable in tuberculosis to begin the treatment with Ars-i.

Answer Code:
    (a)   Both A and R is true and R is the correct explanation of A
    (b)   Both A and R is true but R is not a correct explanation of A
    (c)   A is true but R is false
    (d)   A is false but R is true

Ans. (c)

Q. 27. Assertion: (A): Ars. alb. is a sheep remedy, Ant-c. is Horse's remedy and Puls. is a pig's remedy.
Reason (R): According to tests ars. acts best vegetable eating animals than carnivore; have power to wished with nervous restlessness. Anti-c. has tendency to grow fat; and Puls. tends to get frightened with dullness of intelligence.

Answer Code:
    (a)   Both A and R is true and R is the correct explanation of A
    (b)   Both A and R is true but R is not a correct explanation of A
    (c)   A is true but R is false
    (d)   A is false but R is true

Ans. (d)
Note
The reason is correct but the assertion is wrong.

Q. 28. During difficult dentition, children are unable to digest milk. This is a characteristic symptom of (UPSC-02)
    (a)   Magnesium muriaticum
    (b)   Natrium muriaticum
    (c)   Arsenic album
    (d)   Rhus toxicodendron

Ans. (a)
Note
Above symptom is characteristic of 'Mag-m'.

MCQ's in Materia Medica

Also see

English Kent

STOMACH - INDIGESTION (Includes Complaints After Substances Not Otherwise Described) - milk, after
AETH.$_k$ ambr.$_k$ *Ant-c.*$_k$ *Calc.*$_k$ **CHIN.**$_k$ *Iris*$_k$ *Mag-c.*$_k$ **MAG-M.**$_k$ **NIT-AC.**$_k$ *Nux-v.*$_k$ **SULPH.**$_k$
Ref: Kent's Repertory of Homeopathic Mateia Medica (RADAR 10)

Mag-m.

Children who cannot digest milk. Constipation of infants during dentition; only passing small quantity; stools knotty, like sheep's dung, crumbling at verge of anus.

Ref: Boericke's materia medica.

Nat-m.

Hungry, yet loose flesh. (Iod.) Heartburn, with palpitation. Unquenchable thirst. Sweats while eating. Craving for salt. Aversion to bread, to anything slimy, like oysters; fats. Throbbing in pit. Sticking sensation in cardiac orifice.

Ref: Boricke's materia medica.

Ars.-alb

Cannot bear the sight or smell of food. Great thirst; drinks much, but little at a time. Nausea, retching, vomiting, after eating or drinking. Ill effects of vegetable diet, melons, and watery fruits generally. Craves milk.

Ref: Boericke's materia medica.

Rhus-t.

Want of appetite for any kind of food, with unquenchable thirst. bitter taste. (cupr.) nausea, vertigo, and bloated abdomen after eating. Desire for milk. Great thirst, with dry mouth and throat. Pressure as from a stone. (bry., ars.) Drowsy after eating.

Ref: Boericke's materia medica.

Q. 29. Match list–I (Medicines) with List II (Disease) and select the correct answer using the codes given below the lists (UPSC 2002)

List I (Homeopathic Medicine)	List II (Time of Aggravation)
A. Urtica urens	1. Eye injury
B. Secale cornutum	2. Superficial burn
C. Kalium bichromicum	3. Gangrene
D. Symphytum	4. Full thickness burn

Code

	A	B	C	D
(a)	4	1	2	3
(b)	2	3	4	1
(c)	4	3	2	1
(d)	2	1	4	3

Ans. **(b)**

Note
Correct match is as under:

List I (Homeopathic Medicine)	List II (Time of Aggravation)
A. Urtica urens	2. Superficial burn
B. Secale cornutum	3. Gangrene
C. Kalium bichromicum	4. Full thickness burn
D. Symphytum	1. Eye injury

Q. 30. Consider the following medicines (UPSC-02)
  I. Causticum
  II. Lachesis
  III. Colocynthis
  IV. Magnesium phosphoricum

Which of the above mentioned medicines are applicable in case of left sided sciatica pain?
  (a) I and III
  (b) II and IV
  (c) II and III
  (d) II and IV

Ans. (a)

Note
The choice for
  I. Causticum: *Left-sided sciatica*, with numbness.
      Ref: Boericke's materia medica
  II. Lachesis: Sciatica, right side, better lying down.
      Ref: Boericke's materia medica
  III. Colocynthis: *Sciatic pain, left side*, drawing, tearing; better, pressure and heat; worse, gentle touch.
      Ref: Boericke's materia medica
  IV. Magnesium Phosphoricum: Sciatica; feet very tender. Darting pains. Modality: Worse, right side, cold, touch, night. Better, warmth, bending double, pressure, friction.
      Ref: Boericke's materia medica

Q. 31. Match list – I (Symptoms) with List – II (Medicines) and select the correct answer using the codes given below the lists; (UPSC-02)

List I (Symptoms)	List II (Medicine)
A. Children aversion to	1. Sepia officinalis
B. Cannot look at blood	2. Platinum metallicum
C. Business aversion to	3. Alumina
D. Talks of business	4. Bryonia alba

Code

	A	B	C	D
(a)	2	3	1	4
(b)	1	4	2	3
(c)	2	4	1	3
(d)	1	3	2	4

Ans. (a)

MCQ's in Materia Medica

Note
The correct match is as under:

List I (Symptoms)	List II (Medicine)
A. Children aversion to	2. Platinum metallicum
B. Cannot look at blood	3. Alumina
C. Business aversion to	1. Sepia officinalis
D. Talks of business	4. Bryonia alba

Also see
Platinum metallicum
Repertory Kent-Mind-Children; Aversion to- 1: Plat.
Alumina
Repertory Kent-Mind-Blood, cannot look at, or a knife: 3:Alum.
Sepia officinalis
Repertory Kent-Mind-Business; Averse to: 2:Brom., 2:Con., 2:Lach., 2: Phyt., 2:Puls., 3:Sep., 2:Sul.
Bryonia alba
Repertory Kent-Mind-Business: Talks of: 3:Bry., 2:Hyos.

Q. 32. In the controlled and blind trial of drugs in the Homeopathic drug proving protocols, who is/are kept blind about the nature of the drug? (UPSC-02)
    (a) Prover
    (b) Proving master
    (c) Prover and the proving master both
    (d) Neither the prover nor the proving master

Ans. (a)
Note
In Drug proving Protocols, 'prover' is kept blind about the nature of the drug.

Also see
Randomised controlled clinical trials (RCCT's)
These are under taken to elicitation of new clinical symptoms. Proving master designs the trial and selects the medicine and different potencies to be proved. He directs the research assistant / researcher to conduct the proving on selected subjects which are known as provers. RCCT involves:

Single Blinded Trial
Group A
- Patient knows he is getting medicine, but researcher thinks it might be medicine or placebo.
Group B
- Patient is told he might get either medicine or placebo, but the researcher knows that medicine or placebo is given.

Double Blinded Trial
Group A
- Patient is given medicine, but neither he nor the researcher knows whether medicine or placebo is given.
Group B
- Patient is given placebo, but neither he nor the researcher knows whether medicine or placebo is given.
In both the conditions proving master knows the medicine given but patient are kept blind about the medicine in single blind trial and in case of double blind trial both researcher and patient do not know about the medicine.
Ref: Preliminary Guidelines for Research in Homeopathy By Dr. V.K. Chauhan and Dr. Meeta Gupta

Q. 33. Dr. Hahnemann while proving the Peruvian bark, took (UPSC-02)
    (a) Four drams of China twice a day
    (b) One dram of China three times a day
    (c) Two drams of China once a day
    (d) Four drams of China once a day

Ans. (d)

Note
Hahnemann took 'four drams of china once a day'.

Also see
Hahnemann was, in all essentials, a flawless experimenter. He took four drachms of china once a day. He had paroxysms of chill and fever.

Ref: Introduciton to Hahnemann's Organon of Medicine 6th Edition (Boericke's translation) By James Krausss MD Boston, Sept 30 1930

Q. 34. The first nosode proved by Dr. C.F.S. Hahnemann was (UPSC-02)
- (a) Medorrhinum
- (b) Parotidinum
- (c) Psorinum
- (d) Bacillinum

Ans. (c)

Note
The first nosode proved by Dr. C.F.S. Hahnemann was 'Psorinum'.

Also see
Psorinum; the nosode of psora. (The seropurulent matter of a scabies vesicle was used by Hahnemann.
Ref; Clark.
Direction:

The following 8 (eight) items consist of two statement; one labeled as the 'Assertion (A)'and the other as 'Reason (R)'. You are to examine these two statements carefully and select the answers to these items using the codes given below: (UPSC-04)
Codes:
- (a) Both A and R are individually true and R is the correct explanation of A
- (b) Both A and R are individually true but R is not correct explanation of A
- (c) A is true but R is false
- (d) A is false but R is true

Q. 35. Assertion (A): Thuja is the king of antisycotic remedies.
Reason (R): Thuja can cure each and every kind of warts at each and every location. (UPSC-04)

Ans. (c)

Q. 36. Assertion (a): The object of Materia Medica is to formulate the symptom register.
Reason(R): In the process of cure, a physician tries to analyse the data from the symptoms register to match the portrait of disease with that of drug. (UPSC-04)

Ans. (b)

Q. 37. Assertion (A): Toxicological cases can be successfully treated by Homeopathic medicine.
Reason(R): Toxicological action is more of a chemical action than a dynamic action. (UPSC-04)

Ans. (d)

Q. 38. Assertion (A): Belladonna is a proven prophylactic against Japanese Encephalitis.
Reason(R): Belladonna is a viricidal agent and kills the J.E. virus. (UPSC-04)

Ans. (c)

Q. 39. Assertion (A): Belladona is a medicine for inflammation.
Reason(R): Atropine being the active principle of Belladona can act as a surrogate.(UPSC-04)

Ans. (c)

Q. 40. Assertion (A): The most common cause of female sterility is failure to ovulate.
Reason (R): The female sterility can result from salpingitis which in the past was common outcome of gonococcal infection.(UPSC-04)

Ans. (b)

Q. 41. Assertion (A): Staphysagria is a frequently indicated remedy for honeymoon cystitis.
Reason (R): Staphysagria alters the pH value of urine. (UPSC-04)

Ans. (c)

Q. 42. Assertion (A): Hamamelis and Millefolium belong to same family.
Reason (R): Hamamelis and Millefolium are antihaemorrhagic medicines. (UPSC-04)

Ans. (d)

Q. 43. Match List-I (Medicine) with List-II (keynote) and select the correct answer using the codes given below the lists (UPSC-04)

List – I Medicine	List – II (Keynote)
A. Camphora officinalis	1. Leucorrhea preventing pregnancy
B. Caulophyllum	2. Sequelae of measles
C. Thuja occidentalis	3. Coition prevented by extreme sensitiveness of vagina
D. Lycopodium clavatum	4. Coition prevented by extreme dryness of vagina

Answer Codes

(a)	A	B	C	D
	2	1	3	4
(b)	A	B	C	D
	2	1	4	3
(c)	A	B	C	D
	1	2	4	3
(d)	A	B	C	D
	4	3	1	2

Ans. (a)

Note
The correct match is as under

List – I Medicine	List – II (Keynote)
A. Camphora officinalis	2. Sequelae of measles
B. Caulophyllum	1. Leucorrhea preventing pregnancy
C. Thuja occidentalis	3. Coition prevented by extreme sensitiveness of vagina
D. Lycopodium clavatum	4. Coition prevented by extreme dryness of vagina

Also see
Camphora
All sequelae of measles.
Ref: Allen's Key Notes

Caulophyllum
Leucorrhoea: acrid, exhausting; upper eyelids heavy, has to raise them with fingers (Gels.); with "moth spots" on forehead (Sep.); in little girls (Calc.); preventing pregnancy.
Ref: Allen's Key Notes

Thuja
Coition prevented by extreme sensitiveness of the vagina (Plat. - by dryness, Lyc., Lys., Nat-m.).
Ref: Allen's Key Notes

Lycopodium
Dryness of vagina; burning in, during and after coition (Lys.).
Ref: Allen's Key Notes

Q. 44. Match List-I (Symptoms) with List-II (medicine) and select the correct answer using the codes given below the lists- (UPSC-04)

List – I (Symptoms)	List – II (Medicines)
A. Hemorrhage of black blood from all the outlets of body	1. Cinchona officinalis
B. Hemorrhage long continued; longing for sour things	2. Crocus sativus
C. Hemorrhage after extraction of teeth	3. Bovista
D. Hemorrhage from any part black blood viscid clotted forming into long black sting hanging from the bleeding surface	4. Sulphuricum acidum

Answer Codes

	A	B	C	D
(a)	1	2	3	4
(b)	2	1	4	3
(c)	3	2	1	4
(d)	4	1	3	2

Ans. (d)

Note
The correct match is as under:

List – I (Symptoms)	List – II (Medicines)
A. Hemorrhage of black blood from all the outlets of body	4. Sulphuricum acidum
B. Hemorrhage long continued; longing for sour things	1. Cinchona officinalis
C. Hemorrhage after extraction of teeth	3. Bovista
D. Hemorrhage from any part black blood viscid clotted forming into long black sting hanging from the bleeding surface	2. Crocus sativus

Also see
Cinchona
Hemorrhages: of mouth, nose, bowels or uterus; long continued; longing for sour things.
Ref: Allen's Key Notes.
Crocus sativus
Hemorrhage from any part, blood black, viscid, clotted, forming into long black strings, and hanging from bleeding surface (Elaps).
Ref: Allen's Key Notes.
Bovista
Hemorrhage: after extraction of teeth (Ham.); from wounds; epistaxis.
Ref: Allen's Key Notes.
Sulphuricum acidum
Hemorrhage of black blood from all the outlets of the body (Crot., Mur-ac., Nit-ac., Ter.).
Ref: Allen's Key Notes.

Q. 45. Consider the following symptoms (UPSC-04)
1. Stool, partly expelled, recedes.
2. Much urging, but inability to expel.
3. Stool lies in rectum without urging until there is a large accumulation.
4. Stool hard as stone.

Which of these are the guiding symptoms of Sanicula constipation?

Answer code
    (a)   2 and 3
    (b)   1 and 3
    (c)   1,2,3 and 4
    (d)   1 only

Ans. (b)
Note
The guiding symptoms of 'sanicula constipation is 1 and 3.
Also see
Sanicula
Constipation; no desire until a large accumulation; after great straining stool partially expelled, recedes; large evacuation of small dry, gray balls, must be removed mechanically. Stool; hard, impossible to evacuate, of grayish-white balls, like burnt lime, crumbling from verge of anus; with odor or limburger cheese.
Ref: Allen's Key Notes
Sanicula
Stools large, heavy and painful. Pain in whole perineum. No desire until a large accumulation. After great straining only partially expelled; recedes, crumbles at verge of anus.
Ref: Boericke's materia medica

Q. 46. Marasmus of Abrotanum is characterised by (UPSC-04)
    (a)   Marasmus of Neck
    (b)   Marasmus of lower extremities
    (c)   Marasmus of breast
    (d)   Marasmus of whole body

Ans. (b)
Note
Marasmus of Abrotanum is characterized by 'Marasmus of lower extremities'.
Also see
Abrotanum
Marasmus of children with marked emaciation, especially of legs (Iod. Sanic. , Tub.); the skin is flabby and hangs loose in folds (of neck, Nat-m., Sanic.)
Ref: Allen's Key Notes

Q. 47. Inordinate craving for meat in children of tuberculous is parentage is characteristic of (UPSC-04)
    (a)   Magnesium carbonicum
    (b)   Magnesium muriaticum
    (c)   Antimonium crudum
    (d)   Sulphur

Ans. (a)
Note
Mag-c.
Inordinate craving for meat in children of tuberculous parentage.
Ref: Allen's Key Notes

Q. 48. Traumatic chronic neuritis, neuralgia of stump after amputation, burning and stinging pain are characteristics of (UPSC-04)
    (a)   Ledum palustre
    (b)   Staphysagria
    (c)   Allium cepa
    (d)   Hypericum perforatum

Ans. (c)

Note
Allium cepa
Neuralgic pains like a long thread; in face, head, neck, and chest. Traumatic chronic neuritis; neuralgia of stump after amputation; burning and stinging pains.

Ref: Allen's Key Notes

Q. 49. Pain at conclusion of urination is a characteristic of (UPSC-04)
    (a)   Berberis vulgaris
    (b)   Cantharis
    (c)   Sarsaparilla
    (d)   Lycopodium clavatum

Ans. (c)

Note
Sarsaparilla
Severe, almost unbearable pain at conclusion of urination (Berb., Equis., Med., Thuj.). Passage of gravel or small calculi; renal colic; stone in bladder; bloody urine.

Ref: Allen's Key notes and also Boericke's materia medica

Q. 50. Which one of the following statements is not correct? (UPSC-04)
    (a)   Agaricus muscarius affects left shoulder and right hip joint.
    (b)   Hammamelis is the aconite of arterial capillary system.
    (c)   Abrotanum can cure marasmus of lower limbs.
    (d)   In epilepsy indicating Cuprum metallicum, aura begins in the knees and ascends.

Ans. (b)

Note
Hamamelis
It is adapted to venous hemorrhage from every orifice of the body; nose, lungs, bowels, uterus, bladder. Venous congestion: passive, of skin and mucous membranes; phlebitis, varicose veins; ulcers, varicose, with stinging, pricking pain; hemorrhoids.

Ref: Allen's Key Notes

Q. 51. Which one of the following does not belong to the pathogenesis of Mezerium? (UPSC-04)
    (a)   Aggravation of complaints at night.
    (b)   Ulcers with thick whitish yellow scab.
    (c)   Teeth decay specially at the edges of the gums.
    (d)   Bad effects of vaccination.

Ans. (c)

Note
All of the above belong to Mezerium except teeth decay (Caries), decayed, hollow; gums at the edge of: 1:Calc., 1:Syph., 2:Thuj.

Ref: Kent's Repertory

Q. 52. Profuse perspiration after acute disease with relief of all sufferings is the peculiar symptoms of (UPSC-04)
    (a)   Mercurius sulubilis
    (b)   Psorinum
    (c)   Sulphur
    (d)   Syphilinum

Ans. (b)

Note
Psorinum
Profuse perspiration after acute diseases, with relief of all suffering (Calad., Nat-m.).

Ref: Allen's Key Notes

Q. 53. Decided aversion to coition (both sexes) is found in (UPSC-04)
    (a)   Sepia officinalis
    (b)   Lycopodium clavatum
    (c)   Graphites
    (d)   Selenium

Ans. (c)
Note
Decided aversion to coition in both sexes is found in 'Graphites'
Also see
FEMALE GENITALIA - COITION, - aversion to
agar. *Agn.* alum. am-c. arund. bov. cann-s. carb-an. carbn-s. *Caust. Clem.* coff. cub. ferr-ma. ferr-p. fl-ac. *Graph.* hell. ign. *Kali-br.* kali-c. kali-n. kali-p. kali-s. *Lach.* lyc. mag-c. *Med.* **NAT-M.** onos. op. *Petr. Phos.* plat. plb. *Psor.* ran-s. *Rhod.* **SEP.** stann. staph. stram. sul-ac. sulph. tarent. ther. thuj.

MALE GENITALIA - COITION, - aversion to
agar. agn. astac. borx. bufo cann-s. caust. chlor. clem. **GRAPH.** kali-c. **LYC.** nat-m. petr. phos. *Psor. Rhod.*

Graphites
Decided aversion to coition (both sexes).
Ref: Allen's Key Notes
Graphites
Female
Decided aversion to coition.
Male
Sexual debility, with increased desire; aversion to coition; too early or no ejaculation.
Ref: Boericke's materia medica

Q. 54. Great indignation about things done by oneself or by others is a characteristic of (UPSC-04)
    (a)   Aurum metallicum
    (b)   Staphysagria
    (c)   Lycopodium clavatum
    (d)   Gelsemium sempervirens

Ans. (b)
Note
Staphysagria
Very sensitive to slightest mental impressions; least action or harmless word offends (Ign.). Great indignation about things done by others or by himself; grieves about consequences.
Ref: Allen's Key Notes

Q. 55. Which one of the following drugs is required by a girl in her teens with nervous exhaustion, who suffers from incessant and violent fidgety feeling in feet or lower extremities and moves them constantly? (UPSC-04)
    (a)   Helleborus niger
    (b)   Kalium bromaticum
    (c)   Sulphur
    (d)   Zincum metallicum

Ans. (d)
Note
Zincum metallicum
Incessant and violent fidgety feeling in feet or lower extremities; must move them constantly. Always feels better every way as soon as the menses begin to flow; it relieves all her sufferings; but they return again as soon after the flow ceases.
Ref: Allen's Key Notes

Q. 56. Which one of the following is not a symptom of Euphrasia in respect of menses? (UPSC-04)
    (a)   Early
    (b)   Scanty
    (c)   Short duration
    (d)   Painful

Ans. (a)
Note
Euphrasia
Menses: painful, regular, now lasting only one hour; or late, scanty, short, lasting only one day (Bar.).
Ref: Allen's Key Notes

Q. 57. A child suffering from acute tonsillitis is presented with the symptom of throat pain associated with pain in ears which got aggravated by warm drinks and better by cold drinks. Which one of the following is likely remedy? (UPSC-04)
    (a)   Mercurius solubilis
    (b)   Belladonna
    (c)   Arsenicum album
    (d)   Phytolacca decandra

Ans. (d)
Note
Phytolacca decandra
Then ulceration of mouth and throat: follicular sore throat: patches in throat: even diphtheria with these symptoms, i.e. the blueness, the dryness, the pain (root of tongue and throat) shooting into ears: the worse for hot drinks. All worse for cold, except the throat symptoms, which are worse for hot drinks. Ref: Tyler

Q. 58. Abdominal colic of colocynthis is ameliorated by (UPSC-04)
    (a)   Bending double
    (b)   Bending backward
    (c)   Bending sidewise
    (d)   Standing erect

Ans. (a)
Note
Colocynthis
Agonizing pain in abdomen causing patient to bend double, with restlessness, twisting and turning to obtain relief > by hard pressure (> by heat, Mag-p.). Pains: are worse after eating or drinking; compel patient to bend double (Mag-p. - <by bending double, Dios.).
Ref: Allen's Key Notes

Q. 59. Which one of the following is the correct order that matches with the sequential order of 'amelioration from coffee', 'aggravation from coffee' and 'desire for coffee'? (UPSC-04)
    (a)   Ignatia, Angustura, Chamomilla
    (b)   Angustura, Ignatia, Chamomilla
    (c)   Ignatia, Chamomilla, Angustura
    (d)   Chamomilla, Ignatia, Angustura

Ans. (d)
Note
Correct sequential order of amelioration from coffee, aggravation from coffee' and desire for coffee' is 'Cham., Ign., and Ang.'.
Also see

English Kent

GENERALS - FOOD, - coffee - amel.
acon.$_k$ agar.$_k$ arg-met.$_k$ *Ars*.$_k$ cann-i.$_k$ canth.$_k$ **CHAM.**$_k$ *Coloc.*$_k$ eucal.$_k$ euphr.$_k$ hyos.$_k$ lach.$_k$ op.$_k$ phos.$_k$

English Kent

GENERALS - FOOD, - coffee - agg.
Aeth.$_k$ all-c.$_k$ ars.$_k$ arum-t.$_k$ aster.$_k$ bell.$_k$ bov.$_k$ bry.$_k$ *Cact.*$_k$ calc.$_k$ *Calc-p.*$_k$ **CANTH.**$_k$ *Caps.*$_k$ carb-v.$_k$ **CAUST.**$_k$ **CHAM.**$_k$ cist.$_k$ *Cocc.*$_k$ colch.$_k$ cycl.$_k$ fl-ac.$_k$ form.$_k$ glon.$_k$ grat.$_k$ *Hep.*$_k$ **IGN.**$_k$ *Ip.*$_k$ kali-bi.$_k$ kali-n.$_k$ *Lyc.*$_k$ mag-c.$_k$ mang.$_k$ *Merc.*$_k$ nat-m.$_k$ *Nat-s.*$_k$ nit-ac.$_k$ **NUX-V.**$_k$ ox-ac.$_k$ *Ph-ac.*$_k$ plat.$_k$ *Puls.*$_k$ rhus-t.$_k$ sep.$_k$ stram.$_k$ sulph.$_k$ sul-ac.$_k$ *Thuj.*$_k$ vinc.$_k$

English Kent

STOMACH - DESIRES - coffee
Alum.$_k$ **ANG.**$_k$ arg-met.$_k$ arg-n.$_k$ *Ars.*$_k$ aster.$_k$ *Aur.*$_k$ *Bry.*$_k$ calc-p.$_k$ *Caps.*$_k$ *Carb-v.*$_k$ cham.$_k$ chel.$_k$ *Chin.*$_k$ colch.$_k$ *Con.*$_k$ gran.$_k$ lach.$_k$ lec.$_k$ lob.$_k$ *Mez.*$_k$ mosch.$_k$ nat-m.$_k$ *Nux-m.*$_k$ nux-v.$_k$ ph-ac.$_k$ sabin.$_k$ *Sel.*$_k$ sol-t-ae.$_k$ sulph.$_k$
Ref: Kent's repertory (RADAR 10)

Q. 60. Consider the following symptom (UPSC-04)
1. Bad effect from loss of sleep.
2. Nausea, vomiting from riding in carriage.
3. Gall stones with pain under right shoulder blade.
4. Excessive prostration at menstrual sinus.

Which of these are the guiding symptoms of cocculus indicus?
 (a) 1,3 and 4
 (b) 2,3 and 4
 (c) 1,2 and 4
 (d) 1,2 and 3

Ans. (c)
Note
The guiding symptom of cocculus indicus are options 1, 2 and 4.
Also see
Cocculus indicus
1. Bad effects: from loss of sleep, mental excitement and night watching; feel weak if they lose but one hour's sleep; convulsions after loss of sleep; of anger and grief.
2. Nausea or vomiting from riding in carriage, boat or railroad car (Arn., Nux-m.), or even looking at a boat in motion; sea-sickness; car-sickness.
3. NA.
4. During the effort to menstruate she is so weak she is scarcely able to stand from weakness of lower limbs (Alum., Carb-an.).
Ref: Allen's Key Notes.

Q. 61. Consider the following symptom (UPSC-04)
1. Rheumatism and dysentery alternate
2. Sexual desire absent in thin people
3. Headache preceded by blindness
4. Round ulcers of stomach

Which of the above features is/are found in Kali-bi.?
 (a) 1 and 2
 (b) 1 only
 (c) 1,3 and 4
 (d) 2 and 4

Ans. (c)
Note
The features found in Kali-bi. are options 1, 3 and 4.

Also see
Kali-bi.
1. Rheumatism alternating with gastric symptoms, one appearing in the fall and the other in the spring; rheumatism and dysentery alternate (Abrot.).
2. Sexual desire absent in *fleshy* people.
3. Headache: blurred vision or blindness precedes the attack (Gels., Lac-d.); must lie down; aversion to light and noise; sight returns as headache increases (Iris, Nat-m., Lac-d.).
4. Gastric complaints: bad effects of beer; loss of appetite; weight in pit of stomach; flatulence; <. Soon after eating; vomiting of ropy mucous and blood; round ulcer of stomach (Gym.).

Ref; Allen's Key Notes.

Q. 62. Which of the symptom given below is / are helpful for confirmation of Phosphorus as remedy? (UPSC-04)
1. Anxiety for health of
2. Desires salt, ice-cream, chocolates
3. Fair, fat, flabby
4. Sleeps on right side.

Select the correct answer from the codes given below:
(a) 3 only
(b) 1, 2 and 4
(c) 1 and 3
(d) None

Ans. (b)

Note
Symptoms given above as options for confirmation of Phosphorus as remedy are 1, 2 and 4.

Also see
1. **Anxiety for health**

> English Kent

MIND - ANXIETY - health, about
acet-ac.$_k$ acon.$_k$ alum.$_k$ *Arg-met.*$_k$ arg-n.$_k$ arn.$_k$ ars.$_k$ bry.$_k$ calad.$_k$ *Calc.*$_k$ calc-s.$_k$ cocc.$_k$ grat.$_k$ ign.$_k$ **KALI-AR.**$_k$ kali-c.$_k$ kali-p.$_k$ lac-c.$_k$ lach.$_k$ mag-m.$_k$ nat-c.$_k$ nat-p.$_k$ **NIT-AC.**$_k$ nux-m.$_k$ nux-v.$_k$ ph-ac.$_k$ Phos.$_k$ psor.$_k$ puls.$_k$ *Sep.*$_k$ sil.$_k$ staph.$_k$ sulph.$_k$

2. **Desires salt, ice cream, chocolates**

> English Kent

STOMACH - DESIRES - ice cream
Calc.$_k$ Eup-per.$_k$ **PHOS.**$_k$ tub.$_k$ verat.$_k$
Kent: Stomach; Desires: Chocolate- 1: Lepi, 1: Lyss

> English Kent

STOMACH - DESIRES - salt things
Aloe$_k$ **ARG-N.**$_k$ atro.$_k$ *Calc.*$_k$ *Calc-p.*$_k$ calc-s.$_k$ **CARB-V.**$_k$ *Caust.*$_k$ cocc.$_k$ *Con.*$_k$ *Cor-r.*$_k$ **LAC-C.**$_k$ Lyss.$_k$ Manc.$_k$ Med.$_k$ meph.$_k$ merc-i-f.$_k$ merc-i-r.$_k$ **NAT-M.**$_k$ *Nit-ac.*$_k$ **PHOS.**$_k$ Plb.$_k$ Sanic.$_k$ sel.$_k$ sulph.$_k$ Tarent.$_k$ teucr.$_k$ thuj.$_k$ tub.$_k$ **VERAT.**$_k$

3. **Fair, fat, flabby**
Phos has physical constitution as under:
Adapted to tall slender persons of sanguine temperament, fair skin, eyelashes, fine blond, or red hair, quick perceptions, and very sensitive nature. Young people who grow too rapidly are inclined to stoop (to walk stooped, Sulph.]; who are chlorotic or anemic; old people, with morning diarrhea. Nervous, weak; desires to be magnetized (Sil.).
Ref: Allen's Key Notes

GENERALS - OBESITY

agar.k ambr.k *Am-m.*k *Ant-c.*k asaf.k *Aur.*k bar-c.k borx.k bry.k **CALC.**k *Calc-ar.*k camph.k canth.k **CAPS.**k chin.k cocc.k con.k *Cupr.*k euph.k **FERR.**k **GRAPH.**k guaj.k iod.k ip.k *Kali-bi.*k *Kali-c.*k *Lac-d.*k lach.k laur.k *Lyc.*k mag-c.k merc.k mur-ac.k nat-c.k nux-m.k olnd.k op.k plat.k plb.k *Puls.*k sabad.k sars.k seneg.k sep.k sil.k spig.k spong.k *Sulph.*k thuj.k verat.k

4. Sleeps on right side
   Phos patient is aggravated: Evening, before midnight (Puls., Rhus-t.); lying on left or painful side; during a thunderstorm; weather changes.
   Ref: Allen's Key Notes.

Q. 63. Match List-I (Medicine) with List-II (Guiding Mental Attributes) and select the correct answer using the codes given below the lists (UPSC-04)

List-I (Medicine)	Ist-II (Guiding Mental Attributes)
A. Tuberculinum	1. Sympathetic
B. Lycopodium clavatum	2. Melancholic
C. Causticum	3. Cosmopolitan
D. Aurum metallicum	4. Greedy

Codes

	A	B	C	D
(a)	1	4	3	2
(b)	3	4	1	2
(c)	2	3	4	1
(d)	1	3	2	4

Ans. (b)
Note
The correct match is as under:

List-I (Medicine)	Ist-II (Guiding Mental Attributes)
A. Tuberculinum	3. Cosmopolitan
B. Lycopodium clavatum	4. Greedy
C. Causticum	1. Sympathetic
D. Aurum metallicum	2. Melancholic

Q. 64. Dulcamara is incompatible before or after administering which one of the following drug? (UPSC-04)
   (a) Aceticum acidum
   (b) Aceticum acidum and Belladonna
   (c) Aceticum acidum, Belladonna and Lachesis
   (d) Aceticum acidum, Lachesis and Natrium sulphuricum

Ans. (c)
Note
Dulcamara is incompatible with, Acet-ac. Bell., Lach. Should not be used before or after.
Ref: Allen's Key Notes

Q. 65. Consider the following statement: (UPSC-04)
   1. Hahnemann Materia Medica Pura as left by him had six volumes.
   2. Synthetic repertory by Barthel and Klunker has three volumes.
   3. Allen's encyclopedia has 12 volumes.
   4. Hering's guiding symptoms has 10 volumes.

Which of the statement given above are correct?
(a) 1,2,3 and 4
(b) 1 and 4
(c) 2,3 and 4
(d) 1,2 and 3

Ans. (a)
Note
Statements given at 1, 2, 3, 4 all are correct.

Q. 66. Which one of the following is the correct remedy for caries of fibula? (UPSC-04)
(a) Acidum fluoricum
(b) Silicea
(c) Hepar sulphuricum
(d) Calendula officinalis

Ans. (b)
Note
Remedy for caries of fibula is Silicea.
Also see
Caries of bone; Fibula: 3:SIL.
Ref: Repertory-Kent, Chapter- Extremities

Q. 67. Match List-I (symptoms) with List-II (medicine) and select the correct answer using the codes given below the lists (UPSC-04)

List-I (symptoms)	List-II (medicine)
A. Ardent	1. Mercurius solubilis
B. Hypocraisy	2. Ignatia amara
C. Inconstancy	3. Phosphorus
D. Precocity	4 Nux vomica

Codes

	A	B	C	D
(a)	2	3	4	1
(b)	4	1	2	3
(c)	2	1	4	3
(d)	4	3	2	1

Ans. (d)
Note
The correct match is as under:

List-I (symptoms)	List-II (medicine)
A. Ardent	4 Nux vomica
B. Hypocraisy	3. Phosphorus
C. Inconstency	2. Ignatia amara
D. Precocity	1. Mercurius solubilis

Also see
References from Kent's repertory

-Kent: Mind; Ardent- 1: Nux-v.
-Kent: Mind; Hypocraisy- 1: Phos.
-Kent: Mind; Inconstancy- 1: Act-sp, 1: Agar, 1: Ars, 1: Asaf, 1: Bism, 1: Canth, 1: Cimic, 1: Coff, 1: Dros, 3: Ign, 1: Lac-c, 1: Lach, 1: Led, 1: Nat-c, 1: Op, 1: Plan, 1: Sil, 1: Spig, 1: Thuja.
-Kent: Mind; Precocity- 1: Merc.

Reference from Synthesis:
Hypocrisy: 3: LYC. 2: Puls., 2:Sep., 2: Sulph. (Ref; Synthesis-Mind)
Ref: Synthesis:
Precocity: 2:Calc., 2: Merc., 3:VERAT. (Ref; Synthesis – Mind)

68. Pain as if bones were all torn to pieces is the particular of (KPSC/Lect/Rep-04)
    (a) Cimicifuga
    (b) Colocynthis
    (c) Ipecacuanha
    (d) Magnesium phosphoricum

Ans. (c)
Note
Pains as if bones were all torn to pieces is the particular of 'Ipec'.
Also see
Ipecacuanha
Pains as if bones were all torn to pieces as if broken, (Eup.).
Ref: Allen's Key Note

Q. 69. Nit-ac. is complementary to (KPSC/Lect/Rep-04)
    (a) Arsenicum album
    (b) Caladium
    (c) Both
    (d) None of the above

Ans. (c)
Note
Nit-ac. is complementary to 'Ars and Caladium'.
Also see
Relationship
Complementary: *Ars.; Calad.; Lac-c.; Sep..*
Inimical: *Lach.*
Compare: *Merc. Kali-c.; Thuj.; Hep.; Calc.*
Ref: Boericke's materia medica

Q. 70. "Pains are drawing, tearing, erratic rapidly shifting from one part to another' is in (KPSC/Lect/Rep-04)
    (a) Kalium bichromicum
    (b) Lac caninum
    (c) Pulsatilla nigricans
    (d) All of the above

Ans. (d)
Note
"Pains are drawing, tearing, erratic rapidly shifting from one part to another' is in all of the above – Kali-bi., Lac-c. and Puls.
Also see
Repertory reference:
Extremities-Pain: Wandering, shifting: 3:AM.M., 2:Arn., 2:Cal-p., 3:CARBN-S., 2:Caul., 2:Caust., 2:Kali-Bi., 3:KALI-S., 2:Kalm., 3:LAC-C., 2:Lyc., 2:Mag-p., 2:Med., 2:Nux-v., 2:Phyt., 2:Plb., 3:PULS., 2:Rhod., 2:Still., 2:Terent., 2:Tub., 2:Verat-v.
Ref: Kent's Repertory
Lac-c.

Symptoms erratic, pains constantly flying from one part to another (Kali Bi., Puls.); changing from side to side every few hours or days.
Ref: Allen's Key Notes

Q. 71. 'Kali-bi.' is antidote to (KPSC/Lect/Rep-04)
    (a)   Arsenicum album
    (b)   Lachesis mutus
    (c)   Pulsatilla nigricans
    (d)   All of the above

Ans. (d)
Note
Kali-bi. is antidote to Ars, Lach and Puls.
Also see
Kali-bi.
Relationship - Antidotes: *Ars, Lach.*
Ref: Boericke's's materia medica
Kali-bi. antidotes – Ars, Lach, Puls.
Ref: Relationship of remedies - Gibson miller

Q. 72. 'Acridity and putridity' of all the discharges from mucous membrane is the keynote symptom of (KPSC/Lect/Rep-04)
    (a)   Kreosotum
    (b)   Lachesis mutus
    (c)   Nitricum acidum
    (d)   All of the above

Ans. (a)
Note
'Acridity and putridity' of all the discharges from mucous membrane is the keynote symptom of 'Kreosotum'.

Also see
Kreosote
Corrosive, fetid, ichorous discharges from mucous membranes.
Ref: Allen's Key Notes
Excoriating, burning, and offensive discharges.
Ref: Boericke's materia medica
Repertory Reference:
Generals- Acridity, excoriations, etc: 3:ARS, 2Brom, 2:Caust, 2:Graph, 2:Iod, 2:Kreos, 3:MERC, 2:Nit-ac, 2:Rhus-t., 2:Sep., 2:Sil., 3:SULPH.
Ref: Synthesis

Q. 73. Perspiration, smelling like honey is the characteristic of (KPSC/Lect/Rep-04)
    (a)   Calcarea carbonicum
    (b)   Thuja occidentalis
    (c)   Both
    (d)   None of the above

Ans. (b)
Note
Perspiration, smelling like honey is the characteristic of 'Thuja'.
Also see
Thuj.
Sweat; only uncovered parts; or all over, except the head (rev.of Sil.); when he sleeps, stops when he wakes (rev. of Samb.); profuse, sour smelling, fetid, at night. Perspiration, smelling like honey, on the genitals.
Ref: Allen's Key Notes

Q. 74. 'Lecture on Homeopathic philosophy' by Dr. J.T. Kent was published in the year: (KPSC/Lect/Rep-04)
    (a) 1870
    (b) 1897
    (c) 1900
    (d) 1921

Ans. (c)

Note
'Lecture on Homeopathic philosophy' by Dr. J.T. Kent was published in the year '1900'.

Also see
Contributions of Dr. J.T. Kent:
-Repertory of the Homeopathic Materia Medica (1877) - Initially compiled by him for his own use. Other homeopaths began asking for their own copies. Revised by his widow Clara (and others) up to 1961. Forms the basis of many of the more recent repertories.
-What the Doctor Needs to Know in Order to Make a Successful Prescription (1900)
-Lectures on Homeopathic Philosophy (1900)
-Lectures on Homeopathic Materia Medica (1904). Drawn from his lectures on remedies from Hering's Guiding Symptoms of our Materia Medica.
-New Remedies, Clinical Cases, Lesser Writings, Aphorisms and Precepts (1926).
-High potency prescription (200C and above for chronic cases)
-Single remedy prescribing
-Emphasis on "Mentals" and "Generals"
-"Wait and Watch" methodology from the 4th Edition Organon (the dry dose medicine was not repeated until all improvement from the previous dose had ceased)

Q. 75. 'An essay on a new principle for ascertaining the curative powers of Drugs' was written in the year (KPSC/Lect/Rep/04)
    (a) 1790
    (b) 1796
    (c) 1803
    (d) 1810

Ans. (b)

Note
'An essay on a new principle for ascertaining the curative powers of Drugs' was written in the year '1796'.

Hahnemann's most important works:
    -*Essay on a New Principle [1796]*
    -Are the Obstacles to Medical Practice Insurmountable? [1797]
    -Cure & Prevention of Scarlet Fever [1801]
    -On the Power of Small Doses [1801]
    -Aesculapius in the Balance [1805]
    -Fragmenta de viribus medicamentorum positivis [1805]
    -The Medicine of Experience [1805]
    -On the Value of the Speculative Systems of Medicine [1808]
    -Observations on the Three Modes of Medical Practice [1809]
    -Hellebore thesis [1812]
    -Sources of the Materia Medica [1817]
    -Contrast of Old and New Medical Systems [1825]
    -Four essays on Cholera [1831]
    -All these essays can all be read in his Lesser Writings edited by Dudgeon, some of which are viewable online at:
Ref: http://www.minutus.org/lesser.htm

Q. 76. The following symptoms are observed on patients, but not on prover (KPSC/Lect/Rep/04)
    (a) Pathological
    (b) Toxicological
    (c) Clinical
    (d) None of the above

Ans. (c)

Note
From above 'Clinical' symptoms are observed on patients, but not on prover.
Also see

Homeopathic proving is carried on healthy humans. The medicines are not given till the tissue changes occur. The change is noticed in the subjective sphere.

However, in case of a patient the objective symptoms are certain changes in organ systems which can be examined at bed side and are included in clinical signs.

Q. 77. What is the common name of Apocynum? (KPSC/Lect/Rep-04)
    (a) Honey bee
    (b) Indian hemp
    (c) Indian turnip
    (d) None of the above
Ans. (b)
Note
The common name of Apocynum is 'Indian Hemp', it belong to Apocynaceae family.
Ref: Allen's Key Notes.

Q. 78. Great pain throat, burning as if from coal of fire or a red-hot iron with dryness is in: (KPSC/Lect/Rep-04)
    (a) Nitricum acidum
    (b) Lachesis mutus
    (c) Phytolacca decandra
    (d) Belladonna
Ans. (c)
Note
Great pain throat, burning as if from coal of fire or a red-hot iron with dryness is in 'Phyt.'.
Also see
Nit-ac.
Throat; Dry. Pain into ears. Hawks mucous constantly. White patches and sharp points, as from splinters, on swallowing.
Ref: Boericke's materia medica
Lach.
Diphtheria and tonsillitis, beginning on the left and extending to right side (Lac c., Sabad.); dark purple appearance (Naja); < by hot drinks, after sleep; liquids more painful than solids when swallowing (Bell., Bry., Ign.); prostration out of all proportion to appearance of throat.
Ref: Allen's Key Notes
Phyt.
Diphtheria: pains shoot from throat into ears on swallowing; great pain at root of tongue when swallowing burning as from a coal of fire or a red-hot iron; dryness.
Ref: Allen's Key Notes
Bell.
Thaoat; dry, as if glazed; angry-looking congestion (Gins.); red worse on right side. Tonsils enlarged; throat feels constricted, difficult deglutition; worse, liquids. Sensation of a lump. Esophagus dry; feels contracted. Spasms in throat. Continual inclination to swallow. Scraping sensation. Muscles of deglutition very sensitive. Hypertrophy of mucous membrane.
Ref; Boericke's materia medica.

Q. 79. 'Chelidonium majus' belongs to the family of (KPSC/Lect/Rep-04)
    (a) Cucurbitaceae
    (b) Liliaceae
    (c) Loganiaceae
    (d) Papaveraceae
Ans. (d)

Note
Chelidonium majus belongs to the family of Papaveraceae.
Ref: Allen's Key Notes.

Q. 80. 'Worm Seed' is the common name of (KPSC/Lect/Rep-04)
    (a)   Chamomilla.
    (b)   Cina
    (c)   Cinchona officinalis
    (d)   Drosera

Ans. (b)
Note
'Worm Seed' is the common name of 'Cina'.
Also see
The common names are as:
    a.   Chamomilla – Matricaria chamomilla.
    b.   Cina- Worm Seed
    c.   Cinchona officinalis - Peruvian Bark
    d.   Drosera - Sundew
Ref: Allen's Key Notes

Q. 81. 'Vertigo on seeing the flowing water' is the characteristic of (KPSC/Lect/Rep-04)
    (a)   Theridion
    (b)   Conium maculatum
    (c)   Ferrum metallicum
    (d)   All of the above

Ans. (c)
Note
'Vertigo on seeing the flowing water' is the characteristic of 'Ferr.'.
Also see
Theridion
Vertigo: on closing the eyes (Lach., Thuj. - on opening them, Tab.; on looking upward, Puls., Sil.); from any, even least, noise; aural or labyrinthine (Meniere's disease).
Ref: Allen's Key Notes
Conium
Vertigo: especially when lying down or turning in bed; moving the head slightly, or even the eyes; must keep head perfectly still; in turning the head to the left (Col.); of old people; with ovarian and uterine complaints.
Ref: Allen's Key Notes
Ferrum metallicum
Vertigo: With balancing sensation, as if on water; on seeing flowing water; when walking over water, as when crossing a bridge (Lys.); on descending (Borx., Sanic.).
Ref: Allen's Key Notes

Q. 82. Nose bleeding when washing the face is marked feature of (KPSC/Lect/Rep-04)
    (a)   Hamamelis
    (b)   Belladonna
    (c)   Phosphorus
    (d)   Ammonium carbonicum

Ans. (d)
Note
Nose bleeding when washing the face is marked feature of 'Ammonium carbonicum'.
Also see
Ammonium carbonicum
Nosebleed: when washing the face (Arn, Mag-c.) and hands in the morning, from left nostril; after eating.
Ref: Allen's Key Notes

Q. 83. Vertigo when ascending is the marked feature of (KPSC/Lect/Rep-04)
- (a) Belladonna
- (b) Bryonia alba
- (c) Arsenicum album
- (d) Calcarea carbonicum

Ans. (d)
Note
Vertigo when ascending is the marked feature of 'Calc c'.
Also see
Calc.
Vertigo on ascending, and when turning head.
Ref: Boericke's materia medica

Q. 84. Toothache ameliorated by holding cold water in the mouth is marked in: (KPSC/Lect/Rep-04)
- (a) Coffea crudum
- (b) Belladonna
- (c) Aconite napellus
- (d) None of the above

Ans. (a)
Note
Toothache ameliorated by holding cold water in the mouth is marked in 'Coffea'.
Also see
Coffea
Toothache: intermittent, jerking, relieved by holding ice-water in the mouth, but returns when water becomes warm
(Bis., Bry., Puls., Caust., Sep., Nat-s.).
Ref: Allen's Key Notes

Q. 85. Palpitation from least exertion is the marked feature of (KPSC/Lect/Rep-04)
- (a) Natrium muriaticum
- (b) Lycopodium clavatum
- (c) Argentum nitricum
- (d) Iodium

Ans. (d)
Note
Palpitation from least exertion is the marked feature of 'Iodium'.
Also see
Iod
Palpitation, worse from least exertion (compare Dig. - from least mental exertion, Calc-ar.).
Ref: Allen's Key Notes
Extended information
Iod
Heart feels squeezed. Myocarditis, painful compression around heart. Feels as if squeezed by an iron hand (Cact.) followed by great weakness and faintness. Palpitation from least exertion. Tachycardia.
Ref: Boericke's materia medica
Lyco
Aneurysm (Bar-c.) Aortic disease. Palpitation at night. Cannot lie on left side.
Ref: Boericke's materia medica
Nat-m.
Tachycardia. Sensation of coldness of heart. Heart and chest feel constricted. Fluttering, palpitating; intermittent pulse. Heart's pulsations shake body. Intermits on lying down.
Ref: Boericke's materia medica

MCQ's in Materia Medica

Q. 86. Constipation even soft stool requires great straining is the marked feature of (KPSC/Lect/Rep/04)
    (a) Alumina
    (b) Bryonia
    (c) Sulphur
    (d) Natrium muriaticum

Ans. (a)
Note
Constipation even soft stool requires great straining is the marked feature of 'Alumina'.
Also see
Alum.
Tendency to paretic muscular states. Old people, with lack of vital heat, or prematurely old, with debility. Rectum sore, dry, inflamed, bleeding. Itching and burning at anus. Even a soft stool is passed with difficulty. Great straining. Constipation of infants (Coll.; Psor.; Paraf.) and old people from inactive rectum, and in women of very sedentary habit.
Ref: Boericke's materia medica

Q. 87. Leucorrhea like white of egg especially after every urination is marked feature of (KPSC/Lect/Rep-04)
    (a) Ammonium muriaticum
    (b) Sepia officinalis
    (c) Alumina
    (d) Kreosotum

Ans. (a)
Note
Leucorrhea like white of egg especially after every urination is marked feature of 'Am-m.'.
Also see
Ammonium muriaticum
Leucorrhea: like white of egg, preceded by griping pain about the navel; brown, slimy, painless, after every urination.
Ref: Allen's Key Notes

Q. 88. Irresistible desire to talk in rhymes is the marked feature of (KPSC/Lect/Rep-04)
    (a) Thuja occidentalis
    (b) Stramonium
    (c) Lachesis mutus
    (d) Antimonium crudum

Ans. (d)
Note
Irresistible desire to talk in rhymes is the marked feature of 'Antimonium crudum'.
Also see
Ant-c.
Great sadness, with weeping. Loathing life. Anxious lachrymose mood, the slightest thing effects her (Puls.); object despair, suicide by drowning. Irresistible desire to talk in rhymes or repeat verses. Sentimental mood in the moonlight, especially ecstatic love; bad effects of disappointed affection. (Calc.-p.).
Ref: Allen's Key Notes

Q. 89. Hardness of hearing, relieved by riding in a carriage or train (KPSC/Lect/Rep-04)
    (a) Pulsatilla nigricans
    (b) Nitricum acidum
    (c) Thuja occidentalis
    (d) Capsicum annum

Ans. (b)

Note
Hardness of hearing, relieved by riding in a carriage or train is a feature of 'Nit-ac'.
Also see
Nit-ac.
Difficult hearing; better by riding in carriage or train. Very sensitive to noise, as the rattle of wagons over pavements.
Ref: Boericke's materia medica

Q. 90. Corns on soles of feet, which are very sensitive and painful (KPSC/Lect/Rep-04)
    (a)   Ranunculus bulbosus
    (b)   Sulphur
    (c)   Thuja occidentalis
    (d)   Natrium muriaticum

Ans. (a)
Note
Corns on soles of feet, which are very sensitive and painful is a feature of 'Ranunculus bulbosus'.
Also see
Ran-b.: Corns sensitive.
Ref: Boericke's materia medica

Q. 91. Rashes on the body before menses is in (KPSC/Lect/Rep-04)
    (a)   Colocynthis
    (b)   Bryonia alba
    (c)   Aconitum napellus
    (d)   Dulcamara

Ans. (d)
Note
Rashes on the body before menses is a featue of 'Dulcamara'.
Also see
Dulcamara
Before appearance of menses, a rash appears on skin, or sexual excitement.
Ref: Boericke's materia medica

Q. 92. Mental symptom "feels that life is constant burden for him" is in (KPSC/Lect/Rep/04)
    (a)   Veratrum album
    (b)   Thuja occidentalis
    (c)   Aurum metallicum
    (d)   Sulphur

Ans. (c)
Note
Mental symptom "feels that life is constant burden for him" is found in 'Aur. met'.
Also see
Aur.
Constantly dwelling on suicide (Naja - but is afraid to die, Nux-v). Profound melancholy: feels hateful and quarrelsome; desire to commit suicide; *life is a constant burden*; after abuse of mercury; with nearly all complaints.
Ref: Allen's Key Notes

Q. 93. Podophyllum has fever paroxysm usually at (KPSC/Lect/Mat-Med-04)
    (a)   3.00 p.m.
    (b)   12.00 at midnight
    (c)   11.00 a.m.
    (d)   7.00 a.m.

Ans. (d)

Note
Podophyllum has fever paroxysm usually at '7.00 am.'
Also see
Podophyllum
Fever; Chills at 7 a.m., with pain in hypochondria, and knees, ankles, wrists. Great loquacity during fever. Profuse sweat.
Ref: Boericke's materia medica

Q. 94. Complementary relationship is found in (KPSC/Lect/Mat-Med-04)
    (a)   Aconitum napellus - Sulphur
    (b)   Mercurius solubilis – Silicea
    (c)   Causticum - Phosphorus
    (d)   Nux vomica – Camphora

Ans. (a)
Note
a. *Acon.*
    Complementary; Coff.; Sulph. Sulphur may be considered a chronic Aconite. Often completes a cure begun with Acon..
    Ref: Boericke's materia medica
b. *Merc.*
    Complementry: Bad.
    Ref: Boericke's materia medica
c. *Caust.*
    Complementary; Carb.; Petros.
    Ref: Boericke's materia medica
d. *Nux-v.*
    Complementry: Sulph. in nearly all diseases.
    Ref: Allen's Key Notes

Q. 95. "Coition prevented by extreme sensitiveness of vagina" is a symptom of (KPSC/Lect/Mat-Med/04)
    (a)   Thuja occidentalis only
    (b)   Platina only
    (c)   Both Thuja occidentalis and Platina
    (d)   Neither Thuja occidentalis nor Platina

Ans. (c)
Note
"Coition prevented by extreme sensitiveness of vagina" is a symptom of 'Thuj. and Plat.'.
Also see
Thuj.
Coition prevented by extreme sensitiveness of the vagina (Plat. - by dryness, Lyc, Lys., Nat-m).
Ref: Allen's Key Notes
Plat.
Sexual organs exceedingly sensitive; cannot bear the napkin to touch her; will go into spasms from an examination; vulva painfully sensitive during coitus; will faint during, or cannot endure, coitus.
Ref: Allen's Key Notes.

Q. 96. Thuja is indicated in diarrhea resulting from (KPSC/Lect/Mat-Med-04)
    (a)   Coffee only
    (b)   Onion only
    (c)   Vaccination only
    (d)   All of the above

Ans. (d)
Note
Thuj. is indicated in diarrhea resulting from all of above.

Also see
Thuj.
Diarrhea: early morning; expelled forcibly with much flatus (Aloe); gurgling, as water from a bunghole; < after breakfast, coffee, fat food, vaccination, onions.
Ref: Allen's Key Notes

Q. 97. "Sensation of something alive in the abdomen" is found in (KPSC/Lect/Mat-Med-04)
    (a) Nux-moschata only
    (b) Sulphur only
    (c) Crocus sativus only
    (d) Nux moschata, Sulphur and Crocus sativus

Ans. Use your discretion.
Note
"Sensation of something alive in the abdomen" is found in 'Sulph. and Croc.' only and not in Nux-m. The options given above are inconsistent.
Also see

English Kent

ABDOMEN - ALIVE, sensation of something
calc-p.$_k$ cann-s.$_k$ conv.$_k$ **CROC.**$_k$ cur.$_k$ *Cycl.*$_k$ hyos.$_k$ ign.$_k$ kali-i.$_k$ lyc.$_k$ merc.$_k$ nux-v.$_k$ sabad.$_k$ sabin.$_k$ sang.$_k$ sep.$_k$ stram.$_k$ stront-c.$_k$ sulph.$_k$ **THUJ.**$_k$
(See movements)
Ref: Kent's Repertory (RADAR 10)
Abdomen –Alive sensation of something: CROC, sulph, THUJ..
Ref: Synthesis

Extended information
Sulph
Movement in abdomen as of a child (Croc., Thuj.).
Ref: Allen's Key Notes
Croc.
Sensation as if something alive were moving in the stomach, abdomen, uterus, arms or other parts of the body (Sab., Thuj., Sulph.).
Ref: Allen's Key Notes

Q. 98. "Patient perspires when he sleeps but stops when he wakes up" may require (KPSC/Lect/Mat-Med-04)
    (a) Thuja occidentalis
    (b) Sambucus nigra
    (c) Thuja occidentalis and Sambucus nigra
    (d) Neither Thuja occidentalis nor Sambucus nigra

Ans. (a)
Note
"Patient perspires when he sleeps but stops when he wakes up" may require 'Thuj.'.
Also see
Thuj.
Sweat: only uncovered parts; or all over except the head (rev.of Sil.); when he sleeps, stops when he wakes [rev. of Samb.]; profuse, sour smelling, fetid, at night. Perspiration, smelling like honey, on the genitals.
Ref: Allen's Key Notes

Q. 99. "Time passes too quickly" is a feature of (KPSC/Lect/Mat-Med-04)
    (a) Argentum nitricum
    (b) Theridion
    (c) Cannabis indica
    (d) Nux moschata

Ans. (b)

Note
Theridion
Mind: Restless; finds pleasure in nothing. Time passes too quickly.
Ref: Boericke's materia medica

Q. 100. "Vertigo on closing the eyes" belongs to the portrait of (KPSC/Lect/Mat-Med-04)
  (a) Lachesis only
  (b) Lachesis and Theridion only
  (c) Theridion and Thuja occidentalis only
  (d) Lachesis, Thuja occidentalis and Theridion

Ans. **(d)**
Note
Thuj.
Vertigo, when closing the eyes (Lach., Ther.).
Ref: Allen's Key Notes

Q.101. "Palpitation violent when lying on left side, goes off when turning to the right" belongs to the pathogenesis of (KPSC/Lect/Mat-Med-04)
  (a) Gelsemium sempervirens
  (b) Tabacum
  (c) Thuja occidentalis
  (d) Cactus grandiflorus

Ans. (b)
Note
"Palpitation violent when lying on left side goes off when turning to the right" belongs to the pathogenesis 'Tabacum'.
Also see
Tabacum
Palpitation: violent when lying on left side; goes off when turning to the right. Pulse: quick, full large; small, intermittent, exceedingly slow; feeble, irregular, almost imperceptible. Hands icy cold, body warm.
Ref: Allen's Key Notes

Q. 102. Which of the following is not correct in respect of the bad effects of Tobacco? (KPSC/Lect/Mat-Med-04)
  (a) Phosphorus for tobacco heart
  (b) Ignatia amara for hiccough
  (c) Nux vomica for occipital headache and vertigo
  (d) Sepia for right sided facial neuralgia

Ans. (c)
Note
From the options given above 'Nux-v. for occipital headache and vertigo' is not correct in respect of the bad effects of Tobacco.
Also see
Tobacco; Relations with above drugs:
Phos.
Palpitation, tobacco heart, sexual weakness.
Ign.
For annoying hiccough from tobacco chewing.
Nux-v.
For the gastric symptoms next morning after smoking.
Sep
Neuralgic affections of right side of face; dyspepsia; chronic nervousness, especially in sedentary occupations.
Ref: Allen's Key Notes

Q. 103. "Aversion to alcohol" is not found in (KPSC/Lect/Mat-Med-04)
- (a) Psorinum only
- (b) Tuberculinum only
- (c) Sulphur only
- (d) All of these drugs

Ans. (d)
Note
"Aversion to alcohol" is not found in 'all of the above options'.
Also see
STOMACH - AVERSION to - alcoholic stimulants
ant-t. ars. bell. *Hyos.* ign. manc. merc. nux-v. ph-ac. *Rhus-t.* stram.
Ref: Kent's repertory.

Q. 104. According to Dr. H.C. Allen, when Nux vom and Sulphur improved, but fail to cure piles, which of the following drugs is useful: (KPSC/Lect/Mat-Med-04)
- (a) Psorinum
- (b) Aesculus hippocastanum
- (c) Acidum nitricum
- (d) Ratanhia

Ans. (b)
Note
According to Dr. H.C. Allen, when Nux-v. and Sulph. improved, but fail to cure piles, the 'Aesc.' is useful.
Also see
Aesculus hipocastanum
Relations:
Aesc. often cures. Useful after Nux-v. and Sulph. have improved, but failed to cure piles.
Ref: Allen's Key Notes

Q. 105. "Child unable to hold up the head" is a feature of (KPSC/Lect/Mat-Med-04)
- (a) Aethusa cynapium only
- (b) Abrotanum only
- (c) Both Aethusa cynapium and Abrotanum
- (d) Neither Aethusa cynapium nor Abrotanum

Ans. (c)
Note
"Child unable to hold up the head" is a feature of both 'Aethusa and Abrotanum'.
Also see
Aethusa cynapium
Especially for children during dentition in hot summer weather; children who cannot bear milk. Great weakness: children cannot stand; unable to hold up the head (Abrot.); prostration with sleepiness.
Ref: Allen's Key Notes

Abrotanum
Marasmus of children with marked emaciation, especially of legs (Iod., Sanic. , Tub.); the skin is flabby and hangs loose in folds (of neck, Nat-m., Sanic.). In marasmus, head weak, cannot hold it up. (Aeth.) Marasmus of lower extremities only.
Ref: Allen's Key Notes

Q. 106. "Complaints appear diagonally; upper right and lower left" is found in (KPSC/Lect/Mat-Med-04)
- (a) Ambra grisea only
- (b) Bromium only
- (c) Medorrhinum only
- (d) All of these medicines

Ans. (d)

Note
"Complaints appear diagonally; upper right and lower left" is found in 'all of above'.
Also seet
Complaints appear diagonally; upper right and lower left; Ambr., Brom., Med, Phos., Sul-ac.
Ref: Repertory Boericke – Chapter- Generalities.

Q. 107. "Imaginary odour before the nose, as of herring or musk" is a symptom of (KPSC/Lect/Mat-Med-04)
    (a)   Agnus castus
    (b)   Lycopodium clavatum
    (c)   Kalium bichromicum
    (d)   Platina

Ans. (a)
Note
"Imaginary odour before the nose, as of herring or musk" is a symptom of 'Agnus castus'.
Also see
Agnus castus
Complaints of imaginary odor before the nose, as of herring or musk.
Ref: Allen's Key Notes

Q. 108. "Colicky pain in abdomen after eating cucumber" can be cured by (KPSC/Lect/Mat-Med-04)
    (a)   China officinalis
    (b)   Allium cepa
    (c)   Colocynthis
    (d)   Pulsatilla nigricans

Ans. (b)
Note
"Colicky pain in abdomen after eating cucumber" can be cured by 'Allium cepa'.
Also see
All-c.
Colic : from cold by getting feet wet; overeating; from cucumbers; salads.
Ref: Allen's Key Notes.
Colic, pain; cause and nature; eating cucumber salad from: All-c.
Ref: Repertory- Boericke – Chapter- Abdomen

Q. 109. Which of the following features is common to Aloe, Psorinum, Rumex and Sulphur? (KPSC/Lect/Mat-Med-04)
    (a)   Headache < in winter.
    (b)   Itching of the skin, < from cold, > by warmth.
    (c)   Early morning diarrhea driving the patient out from bed.
    (d)   When passing flatus, sensation as if stool would pass with it.

Ans. (c)
Note
"Early morning diarrhea driving the patient out from bed" of above is a feature common to Aloe, Psorinum, Rumex and Sulphur.
Also see
Aloe
Diarrhea: has to hurry to closet immediately after eating and drinking (Crot-t.); with want of confidence in sphincter ani; driving out of bed early in the morning (Psor., Rumx., Sulph.). When passing flatus, sensation as if stool would pass with it (Olnd., Mur-ac., Nat-m.).
Ref: Allen's Key Notes

Q. 110. Which of the following medicines is called as "Aconite of chronic diseases"? (KPSC/Lect/Mat-Med-04)
    (a)   Hamamelis
    (b)   Sulphur
    (c)   Hepar sulphuricum
    (d)   Alumina

Ans. (d)
Note
"Alumina" from above medicines is called as "Aconite of chronic diseases".
Also see
Alumina
Adapted to persons who suffer from chronic diseases; "the Aconite of chronic diseases."Constitutions deficient in animal heat (Calc., Sil.).
Ref: Allen's Key Notes

Q. 111. "Even soft stool requires great straining" is a symptom of (KPSC/Lect/Mat-Med-04)
    (a)   Alumina only
    (b)   Anacardium orientalis and Platina only
    (c)   Alumina and Platina only
    (d)   Alumina, Anacardium orientalis and Platina

Ans. (d)
Note
From options given above "Even soft stool requires great straining" is a symptom of 'Alumina, Anacardium and Platina'.
Also see
Alumina
Constipation : no desire for and no ability to pass stool until there is a large accumulation (Meli.); great straining, must grasp the seat of closet tightly; stool hard, knotty, like laurel berries, covered with mucous; or soft, clayey, adhering to parts (Plat.) Inactivity of rectum, even soft stool requires great straining (Anac., Plat., Sil., Verat.). Constipation: of nursing children, from artificial food; bottle-fed babies; of old people (Lyc., Op.) of pregnancy, from inactive rectum (Sep.).
Ref: Allen's Key Notes

Q. 112. "Presence of others, even the nurse is unbearable during stool" is a symptom of (KPSC/Lect/Mat-Med-04)
    (a)   Ignatia amara
    (b)   Calcarea carbonicum
    (c)   Ambra grisea
    (d)   Natrium muriaticum

Ans. (c)
Note
From the options given above "Presence of others, even the nurse is unbearable during stool" is a symptom of 'Ambra grisea'.
Also see
Ambra grisea
One thing running through this remedy is that the presence of other persons aggravates the symptoms; also the marked aggravation from conversation. A woman, when attended by a nurse, *is unable to have a stool without sending the nurse into another room*. In spite of much straining she can do nothing unless alone. It is said that in Natrium muriaticum the patient cannot urinate in the presence of other persons. The urine will not start when anyone is around. That is a sort of general feature of this remedy. Confusion of mind and embarrassment in the presence of other persons. Embarrassment in company.
Ref: Kent materia medica

Q. 113. "Diarrhea before menses" is a feature of (KPSC/Lect/Mat-Med-04)
    (a)   Ammonium carbonicum
    (b)   Podophyllum
    (c)   Pulsatilla
    (d)   Arsenicum album

Ans. (a)
Note
"Diarrhea before menses" is a feature of 'Ammonium carbonicum'.
Also see
Ammonium carbonicum
Cholera-like symptoms at the commencement of menstruation (Bov, Verat).
Ref: Allen's Key Notes

Q. 114. "Menstrual bleeding worse at night" is found in (KPSC/Lect/Mat-Med-04)
    (a)   Bovista only
    (b)   Ammonium muriaticum only
    (c)   Both (a) and (b).
    (d)   Neither (a) not (b)

Ans. (b)
Note
"Menstrual bleeding worse at night" is found in 'Am-m. only'.
Also see
Bovista
Menses: flow only at night; not in the daytime.
Ref: Allen's Key Notes
Ammonium muriaticum
Menses too early, too free, dark, clotted; flow more at night.
Ref: Boericke's materia medica

Q. 115. Which of the following symptom is common to Anacardium, Lac caninum and Lilium tigrinum (KPSC/Lect/Mat-Med-04)
    (a)   Forgets recent things, but remembers remote things.
    (b)   Aggravation in empty stomach.
    (c)   Irresistible desire to curse and swear.
    (d)   Lack of confidence in himself and others.

Ans. (c)
Note
'Irresistible desire to cures and swear' of the above symptom is common to Anac., Lac-c. and Lil-t.
Also see
Anacardium
Disposed to be malicious, seems bent on wickedness. Irresistible desire to curse and swear (Lac-c., Lil-t., Nit-ac. wants to pray continually, Stram.). Lack of confidence in himself and others.
Ref: Allen's Key Notes

Q. 116. Which of the following symptoms is not peculiar to Antimonium crudum? (KPSC/Lect/Mat-Med-04)
    (a)   Loss of voice from becoming over-heated
    (b)   Craving for cold bathing
    (c)   Constant discharge of flatus up and down, for years ; belching tasting of ingesta
    (d)   Irresistible desire to talk in rhymes

Ans. (b)
Note
'Craving for cold bathing' of the above symptoms is not peculiar to Ant-c.

Also see
Antimonium crudum
Aversion to cold bathing; child cries when washed or bathed with cold water; cold bathing causes violent headache; causes suppressed menses; colds from swimming or falling into water (Rhus).
Ref: Allen's Key Notes

Q. 117. "Extraordinary craving for apples" is found in (KPSC/Lect/Mat-Med-04)
    (a) Aloe only
    (b) Antimonium tartaricum only
    (c) Aloe and Antimonium tartaricum
    (d) Antimonium tartaricum and Antimonium crudum

Ans. (c)
Note
"Extraordinary craving for apples" is found in 'Aloe and Ant-t.'.
Also see
Desires; Apples: 1:Aloe., 1:Ant-t., 2:Guaj., 1:Tell.
Ref: Repertory-Kent-Chapter-Stomach

Q. 118. "Vomiting in any position except lying on right side" is a characteristic feature of (KPSC/Lect/Mat-Med-04)
    (a) Arsenicum album
    (b) Ipecacuanha
    (c) Bismuth
    (d) None of these drugs

Ans. (d)
Note
"Vomiting in any position except lying on right side" is a characteristic feature of 'None of these drugs'.
Also see
Vomiting-retching: concomitants with: Relief of symptoms from: Lying on right side: 2:Ant-t.
Ref: Repertory –Boericke- Chapter –Stomach
Ant-t.
Vomiting: in any position except lying on right side; until he faints; followed by drowsiness and prostration.
Ref: Allen's Key Notes

Q. 119. Which of the following symptoms is common to Kalium bichromicum, Apis mellifica and Lac caninum? (KPSC/Lect/Mat-Med-04)
    (a) Shifting nature of pain
    (b) Thirstlessness with dry tongue
    (c) Obsessiveness with forgetfulness
    (d) Delayed, scanty, painful menses with increased sexual desire and weeping disposition

Ans. (a)
Note
'Shifting nature of pain' of the above symptoms is common to Kali-bi, Apis and Lac-c.
Also see
Apis
Pain: burning, stinging, sore; suddenly migrating from one part to another (Kali-bi., Lac-c., Puls.).
Ref: Allen's Key Notes
Kali-bi.
Pains: in small spots, can be covered with point of finger (Ign.); shift rapidly from one part to another (Kali S., Lac-c., Puls.); appear and disappear suddenly (Bell., Ign., Mag.-p.).
Ref: Allen's Key Notes
Lac-c.
Symptoms erratic, pains constantly flying from one part to another (Kali-bi., Puls.); changing from side to side every few hours or days.
Ref: Allen's Key Notes

MCQ's in Materia Medica

Q. 120. "Vicarious menstruation" is a common feature of (KPSC/Lect/Mat-Med-04)
    (a)   Bryonia alba and Phosphorus
    (b)   Phosphorus and Sabina
    (c)   Bryonia alba and Sabina
    (d)   Bryonia alba, Sabina and Phosphorus

Ans. (a)
Note
"Vicarious menstruation" is a common feature of 'Bryonia and Phosphorus'.
Also see
Bryonia
Vicarious menstruation; nosebleed when menses should appear (Phos.); blood spitting, or haemoptysis.
Ref: Allen's Key Notes

Q. 121. "Craving for salt" is a common feature of (KPSC/Lect/Mat-Med-04)
    (a)   Natrium muriaticum and Sepia officinalis
    (b)   Natrium muriaticum and Graphites
    (c)   Phosphorus and Graphites
    (d)   Phosphorus and Argentum nitricum

Ans. (d)
Note
"Craving for salt" is a common feature of Arg –n., Nat-m. and Phos. However, Sepia and Graphite has aversion to salt. Therefore, the correct choice is (d).
Also see

▶ **English Kent**

STOMACH - DESIRES - salt things
Aloe. **ARG-N.**k atro.k *Calc.*k *Calc-p.*k calc-s.k **CARB-V.**k *Caust.*k cocc.k *Con.*k *Cor-r.*k **LAC-C.**k Lyss.k Manc.k *Med.*k meph.k merc-i-f.k merc-i-r.k **NAT-M.**k *Nit-ac.*k **PHOS.**k *Plb.*k Sanic.k sel.k sulph.k Tarent.k teucr.k thuj.k tub.k **VERAT.**k

▶ **English Kent**

STOMACH - AVERSION to - salt food
acet-ac.k carb-v.k card-m.k **COR-R.**k **GRAPH.**k *Nat-m.*k *Sel.*k *Sep.*k sil.k
Ref: Kent's Repertory (RADAR 10)
Natrium muriaticum
Craving for salt (Calc., Caust.).
Ref: Allen's Key Notes

Q. 122. "Craving for milk" is found in (KPSC/Lect/Mat-Med-04)
    (a)   Rhus toxicodendron and Aethusa cynapium
    (b)   Sabadilla and Natrium carbonicum
    (c)   Rhus toxicodendron and Sabadilla
    (d)   Rhus toxicodendron and Natrium carbonicum

Ans. (c)
Note
"Craving for milk" is found in 'Rhus toxicodendron and Sabadilla'.
Also see
Rhus-t.
Desire for milk.
Ref: Boericke's materia medica
Nat-c.
Averse to milk. Diarrhea from milk.
Ref: Boericke's materia medica

Aeth.
Especially for children who cannot bear milk. Intolerance of milk: cannot bear milk in any form; it is vomited in large curds as soon as taken.
Ref: Allen's Key Notes
Sabad.
Craves; hot things, sweets, milk.
Ref: Phatak

Extended information

English Kent

STOMACH - DESIRES - milk
anac.$_k$ *Apis.*$_k$ *Ars.*$_k$ *Aur.*$_k$ bapt.$_k$ borx.$_k$ bov.$_k$ *Bry.*$_k$ *Calc.*$_k$ *Chel.*$_k$ *Elaps*$_k$ kali-i.$_k$ *Lac-c.*$_k$ mag-c.$_k$ mang.$_k$ Merc.$_k$ Nat-m.$_k$ Nux-v.$_k$ phel.$_k$ *Ph-ac.*$_k$ **RHUS-T.**$_k$ *Sabad.*$_k$ sabin.$_k$ *Sil.*$_k$ Staph.$_k$ Stront-c.$_k$ sulph.$_k$
Ref: Kent's Repertory (RADAR 10)

Q. 123. Opium, Chelidonium and Plumbum metallicum, have the following characteristic symptom in common (KPSC/Lect/Mat-Med-04)
(a) 'Right sided' paralysis
(b) Black, ball like stool
(c) Sweat on the covered parts
(d) Dementia of the aged persons

Ans. (b)
Note
Opium, Chelidonium and Plumbum metallicum, have the abvoe characteristic symptom in common 'Black ball like stool'.

Also see
Opium
Constipation: of children; of corpulent, good - natured women (Graph.); from inaction or paresis, no desire; from lead poisoning; stool hard, round, black balls (Chel., Plumb., Thuj.); feces protrude and recede (Sil., Thuj.). Stool: involuntary, especially after fright (Gels.); black and offensive; from paralysis of sphincter.
Ref: Allen's Key Notes

Additional information
STOOL - BALLS,like - black
ALUMN. OP. *Plat.* **PLB.** *Pyrog. Verat.*

Please take not of the above list of drugs given in Kent's Reperotry mentions drug which is different in above reference to the Allen's key Notes.

Q. 124. Petroleum, Natrium carbonicum and Phosphorus manifest which the following symptoms, in common? (KPSC/Lect/Mat-Med-04)
(a) Aggravation from eating cabbage
(b) Diarrhea after taking milk
(c) Ailments from riding in a carriage
(d) Complaints worse before and during thunderstorm

Ans. (d)
Note
From above the symptom 'Complaints worse before and during thunderstorm' is common to Petroleum, Natrium carbonicum and Phosphorus.

Also see
Petroleum
Ailments which are worse before and during a thunderstorm (Nat-c., Phos., Psor.).
Ref: Allen's Key Note

MCQ's in Materia Medica

Q. 125. "Aversion to sweet" is found in (KPSC/Lect/Mat-Med-04)
    (a) Sepia
    (b) Tuberculinum
    (c) Staphysagria
    (d) Graphites

Ans. (d)
Note
"Aversion to sweet" is found in 'Graphites'.
Also see
Graph
Aversion to meat. Sweets nauseate.
Ref: Boericke's materia medica

Extended information
Aversion-Sweets; 2:Ars., 1:Bar-c., 2:Caust., 3:GRAPH., 1:Hipp., 1:Lac-c., 2:Merc., 1:Nit-ac., 2:Phos., 2:Sin-n., 2:Sulph., 2:Zinc.
Ref: Repertory –Kent -Chapter-Stomach.

Q. 126. The medicine (s) usually used in contused wound is/are (KPSC/Lect/Mat-Med-04)
    (a) Arnica montana only
    (b) Hamamelis only
    (c) Arnica montana and Hamamelis
    (d) Neither Arnica montana nor Hamamelis

Ans. (c)
Note
The medicine usually in contused wound is 'Arnica montana and Hamamelis'.
Also see
Hamamelis
"Bruised soreness of affected parts (Arn.); rheumatism, articular and muscular. Wounds: incised, lacerated, contused; injuries from falls; checks hemorrhage, removes pain and soreness (Arn.).
Ref: Allen's Key Notes

Extended information
Wounds (Injuries in general, falls, bruises, blows, contusions); Contused, crushed, blows, etc: Arn., Con., Euph., Hep., Petr., Puls., Ruta., Sul-ac.
Ref: Repertory Boenninghausen -Chapter Skin and exterior body.
Please note that the Hamamelis is missing in drug list of Kent above.

Q. 127. According to H.C. Allen, in "delirium": (KPSC/Lect/Mat-Med-04)
    (a) Belladonna occupies a place midway between Hyoscyamus niger and Stramonium
    (b) Hyoscyamus niger occupies a place midway between Belladonna and Stramonium
    (c) Stramonium occupies a place midway between Belladonna and Hyoscyamus niger
    (d) Stramonium can be prescribed when Belladonna and Hyoscyamus niger fail to relieve

Ans. (b)
Note
According to H.C. Allen, in "delirium" 'Hyoscyamus occupies a place midway between Belladonna and Stramonium'.
Also see
Hyoscyamus
In delirium, Hyoscyamus occupies a place midway between Belladonna and Stramonium; lacks the constant cerebral congestion of the former and the fierce rage and maniacal delirium of the latter.
Ref: Allen's Key Notes

Q. 128. In Hyoscyamus, cough is (KPSC/Lect/Mat-Med-04)
(a) < when lying down, at night, after drinking, talking and > by sitting up
(b) < while sitting up, during day time, after eating, > while lying down
(c) < While lying down, at night, > after eating and drinking
(d) < Talking, singing, > while lying down

Ans. (a)
Note
In Hyoscyamus, cough is 'Worse when lying down, at night, after drinking, talking and better by sitting up'.
Also see
Hyoscyamus
Cough: dry, nocturnal, spasmodic; < when lying down, relieved by sitting up (Dros.); < at night, after eating, drinking, talking, singing (Dros, Phos. > When lying down, Mang-m.).
Ref: Allen's Key Notes

Q. 129. "Thin, watery Leucorrhea" is commonly not found in (KPSC/Lect/Mat-Med-04)
(a) Sepia officinalis
(b) Alumina
(c) Syphilinum
(d) Hydrastis canadensis

Ans. (c)
Note
"Thin, watery leucorrhea" is commonly not found in 'Syphilinum'.
Also see
a. *Sepia*
Leucorrhea, yellow, greenish; with much itching.
Ref: Allen's Key Notes
b. *Alumina*
Leucorrhoea; acrid and profuse, running down to the heels (Syph.); worse during the daytime; > by cold bathing.
Ref: Allen's Key Notes
c. *Syphilinum*
Leucorrhea: profuse, soaking through the napkins and running down to the heels.
Ref: Allen's Key Notes
Leucorrhea Profuse, thin, watery, acrid, with sharp, knife-like pain in ovaries.
Ref: Boericke materia medica
d. *Hydrastis*
Leucorrhea: ropy, thick, viscid, yellow; hanging from os in long strings (Kali bi.); pruritus.
Ref: Allen's Key Notes

Q. 130. Find the correct order/sequence of medicines to be prescribed: (KPSC/Lect/Mat-Med-04)
(a) Sulphur → Calcarea carbonicum → Lycopodium clavatum
(b) Calcarea carbonicum → Sulphur → Lycopodium clavatum
(c) Lycopodium clavatum → Calcarea carbonicum → Sulphur
(d) Sulphur → Lycopodium clavatum → Calcarea carbonicum

Ans. (c)
Note
The correct order/sequence of medicines to be prescribed is Lyco → Calc → Sulph.
Also see
Lyco
Relationship
Follows well: after, Calc., Carbo-v., Lach., Sulph. It is rarely advisable to begin the treatment of a chronic disease with Lyc. unless clearly indicated; it is better to give first another antipsoric. Lyc. is a deep-seated, long-acting remedy, and should rarely be repeated after improvement begins.
Ref: Allen's Key Notes

Calc.
Complementary: Calcarea acts best: before, Lyc, Nux, Phos., Sil. It follows: Nit. Ac., Puls., Sulph.
Ref: Allen's Key Notes

Q. 131. Find the odd match (Drug - symptom) out (KPSC/Lect/Mat-Med-04)
   (a) Sepia - fond of company
   (b) Causticum – Sympathetic
   (c) Lachesis - loquacious
   (d) Natrium muriaticum – obsessive

Ans. (a)
Note
The odd match from the options given above is 'Sepia –fond of company'.
Also see
Company aversion to: Dreads being alone, yet: 2:Clem., 2:Nat-C, 2:Sep.
Ref: Repertory-Kent-Chapter Mind

Q. 132. Which of the following medicines is fastidious? (KPSC/Lect/Mat-Med-04)
   (a) Lycopodium clavatum
   (b) Aconitum napellus
   (c) Carcinosinum
   (d) Tuberculinum

Ans. (c)
Note
From options given above the 'Carcinosinum' is fastidious.
Also see

📖 English Kent

MIND - FASTIDIOUS
Ars.$_k$ *Nux-v.*$_k$

📖 Schroyens F., Synthesis Treasure Edition Vet ▸ Full Synthesis ▾

MIND - FASTIDIOUS
ALOE$_{sne}$ *Anac.*$_{st1,vh}$ **ARS.**$_{bg2,br1,k,mrr1,mtf33,ptk1,ptk2,tl1,vh/dg,vhx2}$ *Aur-m-n.*$_{wbt2}$ *Aur-s.*$_{wb}$ *Carc.*$_{c,gk6,mlr1,mrr1,mtf33,sk1,sp1,sst2,st1,vh/dg,vhx3}$ *Caust.*$_{mrr1}$ *Graph.*$_{bg2,mtf33,ptk1,st1,yh}$ *Kali-ar.*$_{gk}$ *Kali-c.*$_{gg,mtf33}$ **KALI-S.**$_{fd,fd4,de}$ *Nat-m.*$_{ckh1,k2,mrr1,mtf33,vh,vh/dg,vhx1,vh}$ **NAT-SIL.**$_{fd,fd3,de}$ *Nicc.*$_{stj1}$ *Nux-v.*

Ref: Repertory –Synthesis -Chapter; Mind (RADAR 10)

Q. 133. In which of the following medicines, "aversion to company" is found (KPSC/Lect/Mat-Med-04)
   (a) Natrium muriatium
   (b) Bismuth
   (c) Lac caninum
   (d) Kalium carbonicum

Ans. (a)
Note
The aversion to company is found in 'Natrium muriaticum'.
Also see

📖 English Kent

MIND - COMPANY, - aversion to
acon., *Aloe*, alum.$_k$ *Ambr.*$_k$ **ANAC.**$_k$ anan.$_k$ ant-c.$_k$ ant-t.$_k$ atro. *Aur.*$_k$ *Aur-s.*$_k$ **BAR-C.**$_k$ bar-m.$_k$ *Bell.*$_k$ *Bry.*$_k$ bufo-s.$_k$ bufo. *Cact.*$_k$ calc.$_k$ *Calc-p.*$_k$ calc-s.$_k$ cann-i.$_k$ **CARB-AN.**$_k$ carbn-s.$_k$ *Carb-v.*$_k$ cedr.$_k$ **CHAM.**$_k$ *Chin.*$_k$ **CIC.**$_k$ cimic.$_k$ cinnb.$_k$ clem.$_k$ coca.$_k$ *Coloc.*$_k$ *Con.*$_k$ cop.$_k$ *Cupr.*$_k$ cur.$_k$ *Cycl.*$_k$ dig.$_k$ dios.$_k$

elaps.k eug. *Ferr.*k ferr-i.k ferr-p.k fl-ac. **GELS.**k graph.k grat.k ham.k *Hell.*k helon. *Hep.*k *Hipp.*k hydr.k *Hyos.*k **IGN.**k *Iod.*k jug-c.k kali-bi.k kali-br.k kali-c.k kali-p.k kali-s.k *Lac-d.*k *Lach.*k *Led.*k *Lyc.*k mag-m.k mang. meny.k *Nat-c.*k **NAT-M.**k nat-p.k nicc.k **NUX-V.**k *Oxyt.*k petr.k phos.k pic-ac.k *Plat.*k psor.k ptel.k *Puls.*k *Rhus-t.*k sec.k *Sel.*k *Sep.*k *Stann.*k *Sulph.*k sul-ac.k tarent.k tep.k *Thuj.*k til.k ust.k verat.k
Company-aversion to; 3: NAT-M.

Ref: Repertory- Kent- Chapter- Mind -From the above group of drugs only one medicine is present in first grade.

Q.134. **Calcarea phosphoricum, Baryta carbonicum and Gelsemium have the following symptom, in common (KPSC/Lect/Mat-Med-04)**
(a) Amelioration of complaints when thinking of them
(b) Aggravation of symptoms when thinking of them
(c) Aggravation of symptoms when lying on the left side
(d) All symptoms are worse during menses mental labour and at night

Ans. (b)
Note
From options given above 'Aggravation of symptoms when thinking of them' is in common for Calc-p., Bar-c. and Gels.
Also see
Ref: Repertory: Kent -Chapter -Mind

Q. 135. **Complementary to Psorinum is (KPSC/Lect/Mat-Med-04)**
(a) Sulphur only
(b) Tuberculinum only
(c) Both Sulphur and Tuberculinum
(d) Neither Sulphur nor Tuberculinum

Ans. (a)
Note
Complementary to Psorinum is 'Sulphur'.
Also see
Psorinum
Relationship - Complementary: Sulphur.
Ref: Boericke's materia medica

Q. 136. **According to William Boericke, Psorinum patient does not improve while using (KPSC/Lect/Mat-Med-04)**
(a) Coffee
(b) Cigarette
(c) Tea
(d) Opium

Ans. (a)
Note
According to William Boericke, Psorinum patient does not improve while using 'Coffee'.
Also see
Psorinum
Modalities - Worse, coffee; Psorinum patient does not improve while using coffee.
Ref: Boericke's materia medica

Q. 137. **"Alternate Diarrhea and constipation" is not found in (KPSC/Lect/Mat-Med-04)**
(a) Abrotanum
(b) Croton tiglium
(c) Antimonium crudum
(d) Sulphur

Ans. (b)

MCQ's in Materia Medica

Note
"Alternate Diarrhea and constipation" is not found in 'Crot-t'.

Also see
Constipation: Alternating with Diarrhea: 2:Abrot., 3:ANT-C., 2:Arg-n., 2:Ars, 2:Aur., 2:Bry, 2:Carb-ac, 2:Card-m, 2:Cas, 3:CHEL, 2:Cimic, 2:Cob, 2:Coll, 2:Con, 2:Cupr, 2:Dig, 2:Ferr-I, 2:Hydr, 2:Ign, 2;Kali-C, 2:Lac-d., 2:Lach, 2:Lact, 2:Lec, 2:Mánc, 2:Mang, 2:Nat-m., 2:Nat-s., 3:Nit-ac, 2:Nux-m., 3:NUX-V, 3:OP, 2:Phos., 2:Plb., 3:PODO., 2:Ptel., 2:Puls., 2:Sulph, 2:Tub., 2:Zinc.
Ref: Repertory- Kent- Chapter- Rectum.

Extended information
Crot-t.
Affects mucous membrane of intestinal tract, producing transudations of watery portions of blood, a copious, watery Diarrhea (Verat.), and develops and acute eczema over whole body (Rhus-t.). The bowels are moved as if by spasmodic jerk, "coming out like a shot" (Gamb.); as soon as patient eats, drinks, or even while eating; yellow watery stool. Constant urging to stool followed by sudden evacuation, which is shot out of the rectum (Gamb., Grat., Pod.,Thuj.). Swashing sensation in intestines, as from water, before stool (rumbling before stool, Aloe).
Ref: Allen's Key Notes

Q. 138. "Bleeding from warts" is the characteristics symptom of (KPSC/Lect/Mat-Med-04)
    (a) Nitrium acidum
    (b) Calcarea carbonicum
    (c) Dulcamara
    (d) Natrium muriaticum

Ans. (a)
Note
"Bleeding from warts" is the characteristics symptom of 'Nit-ac'.

Also see
Warts: Bleeding; CAUST, Nit-ac., Rhus-t., THUJA.
Ref: Repertory- Synthesis- Chapter- Skin

Extended information
Skin; Warts, large jagged; bleed on washing. Ulcers bleed easily, sensitive; splinter-like pains; zigzag, irregular edges; base looks like raw flesh. Exuberant granulations.
Ref: Boericke materia medica.

Q. 139. "Urticaria after violent exercise" indicates (KPSC/Lect/Mat-Med-04)
    (a) Sepia officinalis
    (b) Natrium muriaticum
    (c) Rhus toxicodendron
    (d) Arnica montana

Ans. (b)
Note
"Urticaria after violent exercise" indicates 'Natrium muriaticum'.

Also see
Natrium muriaticum
Urticaria, acute or chronic; over whole body, especially after violent exercise (Apis, Calc., Hep., Sanic., Urt-u.).
Ref: Allen's Key Notes

Q. 140. "Itching without eruptions" belongs to the pathogenesis of (KPSC/Lect/Mat-Med-04)
    (a) Graphites
    (b) Dolichos
    (c) Natrium muriaticum
    (d) Sarsaparilla

Ans. (b)

Note
"Itching without eruptions" belongs to the pathogenesis of 'Dolichos'.

Also see
Dolichos
A right-sided medicine, with pronounced liver and skin symptoms. A general intense itching without eruption. Exalted nervous sensibility. Senile pruritus.
Ref: Boericke's materia medica

Q. 141. "Pain better while thinking of it" is a feature of (KPSC/Lect/Mat-Med-04)
- (a) Camphora only
- (b) Helleborus niger only
- (c) Both Camphora and Helleborus niger
- (d) Neither Camphora nor Helleborus niger

Ans. (a)

Note
"Pain better while thinking of it" is a feature of 'Camphor'.

Also see
Camphora
Pain better while thinking of it (Hell. - Worse, Calc-p., Helon, Ox-ac.).
Ref: Allen's Key Notes

Q. 142. During collapse, the body surface is cold to touch, yet the patient cannot bear covering. This is a symptom of (KPSC/Lect/Mat-Met-04)
- (a) Camphora only
- (b) Medorrhinum only
- (c) Secale cornutum only
- (d) Camphora, Medorrhinum and Secale cornutum

Ans. (d)

Note
During collapse, the body surface is cold to touch, yet the patient cannot bear covering. This is a symptom of 'Camphora, Medorrhinum and Secale cornutum'.

Also see
Camphora
Bad effects of shock from injury; surface of body cold, face pale, blue, lips livid; profound prostration. Surface cold to touch, yet cannot bear to be covered; throws off all coverings (Med., Sec.).
Ref: Allen's Key Notes

Q. 143. Find the symptom common to Alumina, Carbo animalis and Cocculus indicus. (KPSC/Lect/Mat-Med-04)
- (a) Vertigo while riding in a carriage
- (b) Physically and mentally too weak after menses
- (c) Aversion to open, dry, cold air
- (d) Time passes too quickly

Ans. (b)

Note
From above symptom common to Alumina, Carbo animalis and Cocculus indicus is 'Physically and mentally too weak after menses'.

Also see
Alumina
After menses: exhausted physically and mentally, scarcely able to speak (Carbo-an., Coc.).
Ref: Allen's Key Notes

MCQ's in Materia Medica

Q. 144. "Toothache during pregnancy and at night" is a symptom of (KPSC/Lect/Mat-Med-04)
  (a) Magnesium carbonicum
  (b) Thyroidinum
  (c) Plantago
  (d) Magnesium phosphoricum

Ans. (a)

Note
"Toothache during pregnancy and at night" is a symptom of 'Mag-c.'.

Also see
Mag-c.
Toothache, during pregnancy < at night.
Ref: Allen's Key Notes

Q. 145. The common feature of Lachesis, Llium tigrinum and Thuja occidentalis is (KPSC/Lect/Mat-Med-04)
  (a) Left sided complaints
  (b) Anti-sycotic background
  (c) Menses flow only when moving about
  (d) Indifference

Ans. (a)

Note
The common feature of Lach., Lil-t. and Thuj. is 'Left sided complaints'

Also see
Lil-t: Affects principally the left side of the body (Lach., Thuj.).
Ref: Allen's Key Notes

Q. 146. "Consolation aggravates" is found in (KPSC/Lect/Mat-Med-04)
  (a) Natrium muriaticum only
  (b) Lilium tigrinum only
  (c) Natrium muriaticum and Lilrium tigrinum
  (d) Neither Natrium muriaticum nor Lilium tigrinum

Ans. (c)

Note
"Consolation aggravates" is found in 'Nat-m. and Lil-t.'.

Also see
Consolation Agg; 2:Ars, 2:Bell., 2:Calc-p., 2:Hell, 3:IGN, 2:Lil-t., 3:NAT-M., 2:Plat., 3:SEP, 3:SIL.
Ref: Repertory-Kent –Chapter- Mind

Extended information
Natrium muriaticum
Marked disposition to weep; sad weeping mood, without cause Puls., but consolation from others < her troubles.
Ref: Allen's Key Notes

Lilium tigrinum
Tormented about her salvation [Lyc., Sulph., Ver.], with ovarian or uterine complaints; consolation <.
Ref: Allen's Key Notes

Q. 147. "Thyroidinum" is a (KPSC/Lect/Mat-Med-04)
  (a) Nosode
  (b) Sarcode
  (c) Imponderabilia
  (d) Plant product

Ans. (b)

Note
"Thyroidinum" is a 'Sarcode'.

Also see
Thyroidinum
Thyroid extract. A Sarcode.
Ref: Allen's Key Notes

Sarcodes are prepared from the secretion of healthy organism: Insulin - (B cells of the islets of Langerhans of the pancreas); Thyroidinum - (Thyroid gland).

Q. 148. The source of "Lobelia inflata" is (KPSC/Lect/Mat-Med-04)
    (a)   Plant
    (b)   Animal
    (c)   Mineral
    (d)   None of the above

Ans. (a)
Note
The source of "Lobelia inflata" is 'Plant'.

Also see
Lobelia Inflata is; Indian tobacco, Family; Lobeliaceae
Ref: Allen's Key Notes

Q. 149. In tonsillitis, "pain extending from left side of throat to right side" indicates (KPSC/Lect/Mat-Med-04)
    (a)   Lachesis and Sabadilla only
    (b)   Lachesis and Lac-caninum only
    (c)   Lac-caninum and Sabadilla only
    (d)   Lac-caninum, Lachesis and Sabadilla

Ans. (d)
Note
In tonsillitis, "pain extending from left side of throat to right side" indicates 'Lac-caninum, Lachesis, and Sabadilla.

Also see
Lachesis
Diphtheria and tonsillitis, beginning on the left and extending to right side (Lac-c., Sabad.); dark purple appearance (Naja); <. by hot drinks, after sleep; liquids more painful than solids when swallowing (Bell., Bry., Ign.);
Ref: Allen' Key Notes

Extended information
Pain: Sore: Left: Extending to right: 3:LACH, 1:Plb, 2:Sabad.
Ref: Repertory-Kent- Chapter-Throat

Q. 150. "Profuse sweat over entire body during waking hours" is a symptom of (KPSC/Lect/Mat-Med-04)
    (a)   Thuja
    (b)   Sambucus nigra
    (c)   China officinalis
    (d)   Conium maculatum

Ans. (b)
Note
"Profuse sweat over entire body during waking hours" is a symptom of 'Sambucus'.

Also see
Sambucus nigra

Profuse sweat over entire body during waking hours; on going to sleep, dry heat returns (Sweats as soon as he closes his eyes to sleep, Cinch., Con.)
Ref: Allen's Key Notes

Extended informaiton
Perspiration awake only, while: 3:Samb., 1:Sep.
Ref: Repertory – Kent – Chapter -Perspiration

Q. 151. "Stool crumbles at the verge of anus" is a characteristic symptom of (KPSC/Lect/Mat-Med-04)
- (a) Sanicula only
- (b) Magnesium muriatium only
- (c) Both Sanicula and Magnesium muriaticum
- (d) Neither Sanicula nor Magnesium muriaticum

Ans. (c)
Note
"Stool crumbles at the verge of anus" is a characteristic symptom of Saincula & Magnesium muriaticum both.
Also see
Sanicula
Constipation: No desire until a large accumulation; after great straining stool partially expelled, recedes (Sil., Thuj.); large evacuation of small dry, gray balls, must be removed mechanically (Sel.). Stool: hard, impossible to evacuate; of grayish-white balls, like burnt lime; crumbling from verge of anus (Mag-m.).; with the odor of limburger cheese.
Ref: Allen's Key Notes

Q. 152. Which of the following is not true in respect of Secale cornutum? (KPSC/Lect/Mat-Med-04)
- (a) Leucorrhea — green, brown, offensive
- (b) Boils - small, painful with green contents
- (c) Diarrhea - painless, involuntary, stood discharged with great force ; anus wide open
- (d) Gangrene - dry, senile, > from external heat

Ans. (d)
Note
'Gangreen –dry, senile > from external heat from above is not true in respect of Secale cornutum
Also see
Secale cornutum
Gangrene; Dry, senile, < from external heat.
Ref: Allen's Key Notes

Q. 153. Patient is very forgetful in business, but during sleep, dreams of what he had forgotten. He requires (KPSC/Lect/Mat-Med-04)
- (a) Selenium
- (b) Bryonia alba
- (c) Lachesis
- (d) Nux vomica

Ans. (a)
Note
Patient is very forgetful in business, but during sleep, dreams of what he had forgotten. He requires 'Selenium'.
Also see
Selenium
Adapted to light complexion; blondes; great emaciation of face, hands, legs, feet, or single parts. Very forgetful in business, but during sleep dreams of what he had forgotten.
Ref: Allen's Key Notes

Q. 154. "According to H.C. Allen, lack of vital heat in acute disease" is a feature of (KPSC/Lect/Mat-Med-04)
    (a)   Sepia
    (b)   Ledum palustre
    (c)   Calcarea carbonicum
    (d)   Secale cornutum

Ans. (b)
Note
"According to H.C. Allen, lack of vital heat in acute disease" is a feature of 'Sepia'.
Also see
Sep.
Particularly sensitive to cold air, "chills so easily"; lack of vital heat, especially in chronic diseases (in acute diseases, Led.).
Ref: Allen's Key Notes

Q. 155. Patient having "vertigo, on looking upwards" may need (KPSC/Lect/Mat-Med-04)
    (a)   Spigelia
    (b)   Phosphorus
    (c)   Kalmia
    (d)   Silicea

Ans. (d)
Note
Patient having "vertigo, on looking upwards" may need 'Silicea'.
Also see
Silicea
Vertigo: spinal ascending from the back of neck to head; as if one would fall forward, from looking up (Puls - looking down, Kalm., Spig.).
Ref: Allen's Key Notes

Q. 156. Cough worse from taking sweets and cold drinks may be cured by (KPSC/Lect/Mat-Med-04)
    (a)   Drosera rotundifolia
    (b)   Spongia tosta
    (c)   Rumex crisspus
    (d)   Corallium rubrum

Ans. (b)
Note
Cough worse from taking sweets and cold drinks may be cured by 'Spongia'.
Also see
Spongia
Cough: dry, sibilant, like a saw driven through a pine board; < sweets, cold drinks, smoking, lying with head low, dry cold winds; <reading, singing, talking, swallowing; > eating or drinking warm things.
Ref: Allen's Key Notes

Q. 157. Find the odd symptom out in respect of Stannum metallicum (KPSC/Lect/Mat-Med-04)
    (a)   Sad, feels like crying all the time, but crying makes her worse
    (b)   Faints especially when going upstairs
    (c)   Colic > by hard pressure
    (d)   Menses too early and too profuse

Ans. (b)
Note
The odd symptom out in respect of Stann. is 'Faints especially when going upstairs.'

Also see
Stannum metallicum
Sad, despondent, feels like crying all the time, but crying makes her worse (Nat-m., Puls. Sep.); faint and weak, especially when going down stairs; can go up well enough (Borx. - rev of, Calc.). Colic: > by hard pressure, or by laying abdomen across knee or shoulder (Col.); lumbrici; passes worms. Menses: too early, too profuse.
Ref: Allen's Key Notes

Q. 158. Which of the following drug (s) crave 'Sympathy from others' (KPSC/Lect/Mat-Med-04)
      (a)   Ignatia amara
      (b)   Natricum muriaticum
      (c)   Pulsatilla nigricans
      (d)   Arnica montana

Ans. (c)
Note
Pulsatilla from the above drug (s) crave 'Sympathy from others'
Also see
Puls.
Weeps easily. Timid, irresolute. Fears in evening to be alone, dark, ghosts. Likes sympathy. Children like fuss and caresses. Easily discouraged. Morbid dread of the opposite sex. Religious melancholy. Given to extremes of pleasure and pain. Highly emotional. Mentally, an April day.
Ref: Boericke's materia medica
Puls.
Mind: Mild, timid, emotional and tearful. Disgusted at everything. Discouraged. Easily offended. Whining. Craves sympathy. Children like fuss and caresses. Morbid dread of the opposite sex; marriage; thinks that sexual intercourse is a sinful act.
Ref: Phatak materia medica
Sympathy Craves; Phos., Puls.
Ref: Repertory – Boenninghhauen –Chapter -Mind

Q. 159. Headache of Arsenicum album gets relieved by (KPSC/Lect/Mat-Med-04)
      (a)   Cold application
      (b)   Warm application
      (c)   Both cold and warm application
      (d)   Neither cold nor warm application

Ans. (a)
Note
Headache of Ars-alb. gets relieved by cold applications.
Also see
Ars-alb
Headaches relieved by cold, other symptoms worse.
Ref: Boericke's materia medica

Q. 160. "Bed feels so hot, she cannot lie on it" indicates (KPSC/Lect/Mat-Med-04)
      (a)   Arnica montana
      (b)   Bryonia alba
      (c)   Pyrogenium
      (d)   Opium

Ans. (d)
Note
"Bed feels so hot, she cannot lie on it" indicates – Opium.
Also see
Opium
Bed feels so hot she cannot lie on it (bed feels hard, Arn., Bry, Pyrog.); moves often in search of a cool place; must be uncovered.
Ref: Allen's Key Notes

Q. 161. Which of the following features does not belong to the pathogenesis of Medorrhinum? (KPSC/Lect/Mat-Med-04)
  (a) State of collapse, skin cold, yet throws of the covers.
  (b) Cannot speak without weeping.
  (c) Extraordinary craving for alcohol.
  (d) During dyspnea, can exhale easily, but no power to inhale.

Ans. (d)
Note
'During dyspnea, can exhale easily, but no power to inhale' is the feature from above which does not belong to the pathogenesis of Medorrhinum.

Also see
Medorrhinum
Dyspnea and sense of constriction; can inhale with ease, but no power to exhale (Samb.).
Ref: Allen's Key Notes

Q. 162. Aggravation of complaints at night, ulcers with thick whitish yellow scab, bad effects of vaccination. and teeth decay at the roots are the symptoms found in (KPSC/Lect/Mat-Me-04)
  (a) Mercurius solubilis
  (b) Mezereum
  (c) Kreosotum
  (d) Syphilinum

Ans. (b)
Note
Mezereum
Aggravation; Cold air: cold washing; *at night*; touch or motion.
Ulcers with thick, yellowish-white scabs.
Eczema and itching eruptions after *vaccination*.
Toothache: in carious teeth (Kreos.); feels elongated, dull pain when biting on them and when touched with tongue, < at night; > with mouth open and drawing in air; *roots decay* (rev. of Mer.).
Ref: Allen's Key Notes

Q. 163. Which of the following medicines does not have craving for sweets? (KPSC/Lect/Mat-Med-04)
  (a) Graphites
  (b) Causticum
  (c) Both Graphites and Causticum
  (d) Neither Graphites not Causticum

Ans. (c)
Note
Caust
Stomach; Greasy taste. Aversion to sweets.
Ref: Boericke's materia medica
Graph
Stomach; Aversion to meat. Sweets nauseate.
Ref: Boericke's materia medica
Aversion: Sweets; 2: Ars, 2:Caust, 3: GRAPH, 2:Merc, 2:Phos, 2:Sin-n., 2:Sulph., 2:Zinc.
Ref: Repertory-Kent-Chapter-Stomach

Q. 164. "Extraordinary craving for alcohol" is found in (KPSC/Lect/Mat-Med-04)
  (a) Calcarea arsenicosa only
  (b) Sulphuricum acidum only
  (c) Asarum europaeum only
  (d) All of these medicines

Ans. (d)

Note
"Extraordinary craving for alcohol" is found in 'all of above medicine'
Also see
Calcarea arsenicosa
Complaints of drunkards, after abstaining; craving for alcohol (Asar., Sul-ac.).
Ref: Allen's Key Notes
Asarum europaeum
Unconquerable longing for alcohol; a popular remedy in Russia for drunkards.
Ref: Allen's Key Notes
Sulphuricum acidum
Water drunk causes coldness of the stomach unless mixed with alcoholic liquor.
Ref: Allen's Key Notes

Q. 165. Which of the following symptoms is/are common to the pathogenesis of Ammonium muriaticum, Magnesium muriaticum and Natrium muriaticum (KPSC/Lect/Mat-Med-4)
    (a)   Stool hard and crumbles at the verge of anus.
    (b)   Great sensitiveness to noise.
    (c)   Offensive foot sweat.
    (d)   Urticaria after violent exercise.
Ans. (a)
Note
'Stool hard and crumbles at the verge of anus' of the above symptoms is/are common to the pathogenesis of Am-m., Mag-m. and Nat-m.
Also see
Natrium muriaticum
Constipation: Stools dry, hard, difficult, crumbling (Am-c., Mag-m.).
Ref: Allen's Key Notes

Q. 166. 'Unbearable pain towards the end of urination" can be cured by (KPSC/Lect/Mat-Med-04)
    (a)   Sarsaparilla only
    (b)   Medorrhinum only
    (c)   Both Sarsaparilla and Medorrhinum
    (d)   Neither Sarsaparilla nor Medorrhinum
Ans. (c)
Note
'Unbearable pain towards the end of urination" can be cured by 'Both Sarsaparilla and Medorrhinum'
Also see
Sarsparilla
Severe, almost unbearable pain at conclusion (end) of urination (Berb., Equis., Med., Thuj.).
Ref: Allen's Key Notes

Q. 167. "Cough during day time only' is found in (KPSC/Lect/Mat-Med-04)
    (a)   Euphrasia only
    (b)   Ferrum metallicum only
    (c)   Natrium muriaticum only
    (d)   Both Euphrasia and Ferrum metallicum
Ans. (d)
Note
'Cough during day time only' is found in 'Ferr.'.
Also see
Ferr.
Cough only in the day time (Euphr.); relieved by lying down.
Ref: Allen's Key Notes

Q. 168. Which of the following is not usually a symptom of China officinalis? (KPSC/Lect/Mat-Med-04)
    (a) Gall stone colic < bending double.
    (b) Flatulence after eating fruits.
    (c) Headache after sexual excesses.
    (d) Has no desire to live, but lacks courage to commit suicide.

Ans. (a)
Note
From above 'Gall stone colic < bending double' is not usually a symptom of 'China.'

Also see
China
Colic: at a certain hour each day; periodical, from gall-stones (Card-m.); worse at night and after eating; better bending double (Coloc.).
Ref: Allen's Key Notes

Q. 169. Find the odd symptom out in respect of Ledum palustre (KPSC/Lect/Mat-Med-04)
    (a) Affects right shoulder and left hip joint.
    (b) Foots cold to touch, but not cold subjectively to patient.
    (c) Easy spraining of ankles and feet.
    (d) Ascending type of rheumatism.

Ans. (a)
Note
Led. has no such symptom as 'affects right shouldedr and left hip joint'.

Also see
Complaints appear; diagnonally, upper right, lower left side; 2: Ambr., 2: Brom., 2: Med., 2: Phos., 2: Sul-ac.
Ref: Repertory- Boericke- Chapter – Generalities

Q. 170. "Illusion of a mouse running from under the chair" is a symptom of (KPSC/Lect/Mat-Med-04)
    (a) Ignatia amara
    (b) Moschus
    (c) Actaea racemosa
    (d) Platina

Ans. (c)
Note
"Illusion of a mouse running from under the chair" is a symptom of 'Actaea racemosa'.

Also see
Actaea racemosa
Illusion of a mouse running from under her chair (Lac-c., Aeth.).
Ref: Allen's Key Notes

Q. 171. Find the odd symptom out (KPSC/Lect/Mat-Med-04)
    (a) Hamamelis is the Aconite of venous capillary system.
    (b) Abrotanum is indicated for marasmus of lower limbs.
    (c) In epilepsy indicating Cuprum metallicum, aura begins in the elbows and ascends.
    (d) Agaricus affects left shoulder and right hip joint.

Ans. (c)
Note
The odd symptom is 'In Epilepsy indicating Cupr. met, aura begins in the elbows and ascends

Also see
Cupr. met
Epilepsy: aura begins in knees and ascends.
Ref: Allen's Key Notes

MCQ's in Materia Medica

Q. 172. For "Humid asthma", which of the following medicines is commonly used? (KPSC/Lect/Mat-Med-04)
    (a)   Aconitum napellus
    (b)   Natrium sulphuricum
    (c)   Platina
    (d)   Glonoine

Ans. (b)
Note
For "Humid asthma", from above 'Nat-s.' is commonly used.
Also see
Nat-s.
Humid asthma in children; with every change to wet weather; with every fresh cold; always worse in damp, rainy weather; sputa green, greenish, copious (greenish gray, Cop.).
Ref: Allen's Key Notes

Q. 173. Which of the following features is/are not correct in respect of Dulcamara? (KPSC/Lect/Mat-Med-04)
    (a)   Urticaria < in cold air
    (b)   Fleshy, smooth warts
    (c)   Chyluria
    (d)   Rash before menses

Ans. (a)
Note
'Urticaria < in cold air' from above is not correct in respect of Dulcamara.
Also see
Dulcamara
Urticaria; every time patient takes cold or is long exposed to cold. Urticaria over whole body, no fever; itching burns after scratching; < in warmth, > in cold.
Warts, fleshy, large, smooth; on face or back of hands and fingers (Thuj.).
Catarrhal ischuria in grown-up children, with milky urine.
Rash before the menses (Con. - during profuse menses, Bell., Graph.).
Ref: Allen's Key Notes

Q. 174. "Menses scanty, painful and of short duration" is found in (KPSC/Lect/Mat-Med-04)
    (a)   Euphrasia
    (b)   Ferrum metallicum
    (c)   Platina
    (d)   Tuberculinum

Ans. (a)
Note
"Menses scanty, painful and of short duration" is found in 'Euphrasia'.
Euphrasia
Menses: painful, regular, now lasting only one hour; or late, scanty, short, lasting only one day (Bar-c.).
Ref: Allen's Key Notes

Q. 175. Find the odd one out in respect of Drug ~ Family relation (KPSC/Lect/Mat-Med-04)
    (a)   Cina - Compositae
    (b)   Belladonna – Ranunculaceae
    (c)   Croton tigrinum – Euphorbiaceae
    (d)   Nux vomica – Loganiaceae

Ans. (b)

Note

Drug	Family	Remark	Reference
a. Cina	Compositae	Correct	Ref: Allen's key Notes
b. Belladonna	Ranunculaceae	Incorrect	Solanaceae Ref: Allen's key Notes
c. Croton tigrinum	Euphorbiaceae	Correct.	Ref: Allen's key Notes
d. Nux vomica	Loganiaceae	Correct.	Ref: Allen's key Notes

Q. 176. Arnica montana belongs to the family (KPSC/Lect/Mat-Med-04)
    (a) Umbellitferae
    (b) Rubiaceae
    (c) Compositae
    (d) Scrophularaceae

Ans. (c)
Note
Arnica montana (Commmon name; Leopard's Bane) belongs to compositae family.
Ref: Allen's Key Notes

Q. 177. The common name of 'Aethusa cynapium" is (KPSC/Lect/Mat-Med-/04)
    (a) Horse chestnut
    (b) Wild hop
    (c) Witch hazel
    (d) Fool's Parsley

Ans. (d)
Note
The common name of 'Aethusa cynapium' is 'Fool's Parsley'.
Ref: Allen's Key Notes

Q. 178. Find the odd pair out (Drug-Common name) (KPSC/Lect/Mat-Med-04)
    (a) Calendula officinalis - Puffball
    (b) Baptisia - Wild indigo
    (c) Lycopodium clavatum - Wolf's foot
    (d) Nux moschata – Nutmeg

Ans. (a)
Note
Calendula is commonly known as Marigold.
Ref: Allen's Key Notes

Q. 179. Which of the following is not commonly found in the symptomatology of Tuberculinum? (KPSC/Lect/Mat-Med-04)
    (a) Early morning diarrhea.
    (b) Tubercular deposits begin in the lower lobe of the right lung.
    (c) Crops of boils containing green fetid pus, appear successively on nose.
    (d) Changeable temperament.

Ans. (b)
Note
Tuberculinum
(a) Diarrhea: *early morning, sudden*, imperative (Sulph); emaciating though eating well. – Correct
(b) *Tubercular deposit begins at apex of lungs, usually the left* [Phos., Sulph., Ther.] – Incorrect
(c) Crops of small boils, intensely painful, successively appear in the nose; green, fetid pus [Sec.]. – Correct
(d) Symptoms ever changing; Melancholy, despondent; morose, irritable, fretful, peevish; taciturn, sulky; naturally of a sweet disposition, now on the borderland of insanity.

Correct
All above are usually found under the symptomatology of Tuberculium; except the tubercular deposit begins at apex of the lungs, usually the left.
Ref: Allen's Key Notes

Q. 180. The relationship between Belladonna and Dulcamara is (KPSC/Lect/Mat-Med-04)
    (a)   Complementary
    (b)   Antidote
    (c)   Cordial
    (d)   Inimical

Ans. (b)
Note
Dulcamara
Relationship
Incompatible: with, Acet-ac., Bell. , Lach. Should not be used before or after.
Ref: Allen's Key Notes

Q. 181. Which of the following statements is not true? (KPSC/Lect/Mat-Med-04)
    (a)   Rhus-t. belongs to the family Anacardiaceae.
    (b)   Graphites has aversion to sweets.
    (c)   Abrotanum, Antimonium crudum and Alumina have alternate diarrhea and constipation.
    (d)   Sepia has craving for bitter things.

Ans. (c)
Note
The statement from above 'Abrotanum, Antimonium crudum and Alumina have alternate diarrhea and constipation' is not true.

Also see
a.   Rhus-t. belongs to the family Anacardaceae – Correct
    Ref: Allen's Key Notes
b.   Graphites has aversion to sweets- Correct.
    Aversion- Sweet- 2:Ars, 1: Bar-c, 2: Caust., 3:GRAPH, 1:Hipp., 1:Lac-c., 2:Merc, 1:Nit-ac, 2:Phos., 2:Sin-n., 2:Sulph., 2:Zinc.
    Ref: Kent Repertory: Stomach- Aversion- Sweet
c.   Abrotanum and Antimonium crudum have alternate diarrhea and constipation. However, alumina has only constipation. Therefore this statement appears to be inconsistent – *Incorrect*
    Ref: Allen's Key Notes
d.   Sepia has craving for bitter things - Correct.
    Ref: Synthesis
Bitter drinks: 1:Acon., 1:Dig., 2:Nat-m., 1:Ter.
Ref: Kent Repertory-Stomach
Desires Bitter food: 1:Dig., 2:Nat-m.
Ref: Kent Repertory-Stomach

Q. 182. Which of the following statements is/are correct? (KPSC/Lect/Mat-Med-04)
    (a)   All symptoms of Phosphorus are aggravated from cold and ameliorated from warmth in general except stomach complaints.
    (b)   All symptoms of Arsenicum album are worse from cold and better from warmth.
    (c)   All complaints of Actaea racemosa are worse from warmth and better from cold in general except headache.
    (d)   All ailments of Lycopodium are aggravated from warmth and better from cold.

Ans. (b)
Note
The statement from above 'All symptoms of Ars. are worse from cold and better from warmth' is not true

Also see
(a) *Phos.*
Worse:
Touch; physical or mental exertion; twilight; warm food or drink; change of weather, from getting wet in hot weather; evening; lying on left or painful side; during a thunder-storm; ascending stairs.
Better:
In dark, lying on right side, cold food; cold; open air; washing with cold water; sleep.
Ref: Boericke's materia medica.
(b) *Ars.*
Worse:
Wet weather, after midnight; from cold, cold drinks, or food. Seashore. Right side.
Better:
From heat; from head elevated; warm drinks.
Ref: Boericke's materia medica
(c) *Actaea racemosa (Cimic.)*
Worse:
Morning, cold (except headache), during menses; the more profuse the flow, the greater the suffering.
Better:
Warmth, eating.
Ref: Boericke's materia medica
(d) *Lyc.*
Worse:
Right side, from right to left, from above downward, 4 to 8 p.m.; from heat or warm room, hot air, bed. Warm applications, except throat and stomach which are better from warm drinks.
Better:
By motion, after midnight, from warm food and drink, on getting cold, from being uncovered.
Ref: Boericke's materia medica

Q. 183. Which of the following drugs belongs to carbonitrogenoid constitution? (KPSC/Lect/Mat-Med-04)
    (a) Natrium sulphuricum
    (b) Sulphur
    (c) Antimonium tartaricum
    (d) Syphilinum

Ans. (b)
Note
From above options 'Sulphur' belongs to carbonitrogenoid constitution.
Also see
Von Grauvogl had arranged the morbid constitutions according to excess or deficiency of certain elements in the tissues and blood. For every organ and every tissue breathes, and if the lungs are the gateway and the blood the carrier it is the tissues, which are the ultimate recipients of the oxygen that is inbreathed.
The Carbonitrogenoid constitution:
-An excess of carbon and nitrogen characterizes it.
-The *Carbonitrogenoid constitution* is *Hahnemann's Psoric miasm.*
-Important corresponding drugs are; Sulph., Psor., Graph.
Ref: Hompath; Philosophy Archives.

Q. 184. "Thuja" belongs to which of the following constitutions? (KPSC/Lect/Mat-Med-04)
    (a) Oxygenoid
    (b) Carbonitrogenoid
    (c) Hydrogenoid
    (d) Strumous

Ans. (c)
Note
"Thuja" belongs to hydrogenoid constitution.

Also see
The hydrogenoid constitution
It is characterized by an excess of hydrogen and consequently of water in the blood and tissues. It covers a much wider area and is not by any means confined to the acquired or inherited results of gonorrhoeal infection. The *hydrogenoid constitution* corresponds closely with *Hahnemann's Sycotic miasm*.
Important corresponding drugs are; Thuj., Ant-c.
Ref: Hompath; Philosophy Archives.

Q. 185. Find the odd pair out (KPSC/Lect/Mat-Med-04)
    (a)   Carcinosin - Cafe au lait
    (b)   Bromium – Brunette
    (c)   Sepia — Sallow complexion
    (d)   Natrium muriaticum — Cachectic

Ans. (b)
Note
The odd pair from above is 'Bromium – Burunette'.
Also see
(a) Carcinosin - Cafe au lait
    Skin: Dark, brownish complexion. CAFE-AU-LAIT spots.
    Ref : Radar key note.
(b) Bromium – Brunette
    It acts best, but not exclusively, on persons with light-blue eyes, flaxen hair, light eyebrows, fair, delicate skin; *blonde*, red-cheeked, scrofulous girls.
    Ref: Allen's Key Notes
(c) Sepia — Sallow complexion
    Adapted to persons of dark hair, rigid fibre, but mild and easy disposition (puls.). Yellowness: of the face; conjunctiva; yellow spots on the chest; a yellow saddle across the upper part of the cheeks and nose; a "tell tale face" of uterine ailments.
    Ref: Allen's Key Notes
(d) Nat-m. — Cachectic
    For the anemic and cachectic, whether from loss of vital fluids - profuse menses, seminal losses - or mental affections. Great emaciation; losing flesh while living well (Abrot., Iod.); throat and neck of children emaciate rapidly during summer complaint (Sanic.).
Ref: Allen's Key Notes

Q. 186. Find the odd pair out (KPSC/Lect/Mat-Med-04)
    (a)   Tuberculinum – Cosmopolitan
    (b)   Lycopodium clavat. – Greedy
    (c)   Causticum - Selfish
    (d)   Aurum metallicum. – Melancholic

Ans. (c)
Note
The odd pair from above is 'Causticum – Selfish'.
Also see
Cosmopolitan (See Traveling desire for): 3:Calc-p., 2:Car., 2:Hipp., 2:Ign., 2:Iod., 2: Merc., 3:TUB.
Ref: Synthesis
Greedy: Greed, cupidity: 2Ars, 2:Chin, 2:Hyos., 2:Lyc., 2:Merc., 2:Puls., 2:Sep.
Ref: Synthesis
Selfish: 2:Calc., 2:Med., 3:PLAT., 2:Puls, 2:Sulph., 2:Verat.
Ref: Synthesis
Melancholic: 3:AUR.
Ref: Synthesis

Q. 187. Natrium muriaticum is suitable to the persons of which temperament ? (KPSC/Lect/Mat-Med-04)
   (a) Fastidious
   (b) Obsessive
   (c) Hypochondriac
   (d) Hysterical

Ans. Use your discretion

Note
From the options given above 'Nat-m.' covers all above 'mental traits'.

Also see
Reference from Kent Repertory for rubrics is as:
a. **Mental General; Fastidious** – *Ars, Nux-v.*
b. **Obsessive**- (Cross reference- Anxiety, Cleanliness, excessive, delusions, Dwells on past disagreeable occurances, Fanaticism, Fears, Ideas; abundant, clearness of mind, same ides. Ideas; fixed, monomania, phobias, thoughts; persistent. Thoughts; repetition of. Washing; always, her hands. **Washing, cleanliness, mania for:** syph.
   Thought persistent: *Ambr., Arg-n., Ars., Calc.,* **CANN-I.,** *Chin., Graph., Ign., Iod.,* NAT-M., *Nux-v., Ph-ac., Psor., Puls., Rhus-t., Stram., Sulph., Thuj.*
c. Mental General; **Hypochondriacal Humour** –see **Sadness**, mental depression – **NAT –M**
d. Hysterical; Mental General; Hysteria; **NATRIUM MURIATICUM.**
   Reference from Synthesis 7.0 is as under:
a. Fastidious: -Chapter- Mind; Rubric- Fastidious *Anac,* **ARS***, Calc, Graph, Kali-ar, Kali-c., Nat – m. Nux-v.*
b. Obsessive: - Chapter- Mind; Rubric- Obsession- see 'hought – persistent –
   Ambr, Arg-n., Ars., Bell., **CANN-I.,** *Carb-v., Graph., Ign., Iod.,* **NAT-M.**, *Nux-v., Ph-ac., Psor., Rhus-t., Sabad., Sil., Staph., Stram., Sulph., Thuja.*
c. Hypochondriac: Chapter –Mind; Hypochondriasis – **NAT- M.**
d. Hysterical: Chapter- Mind; Hysteria – **NAT-M.**

Inference
There appears to be some difference in terms of drugs related to the rubric fastidious in both the repertories. However, use your discretion – as from the point of view of references from the Synthesis -
The Nat-m. is qualifying for (a), (c) and (d) options.

Q. 188. Which of the following pair is not correct? (KPSC/Lect/Mat-Med-04)
   (a) Rheumatic - Spigelia
   (b) Tubercular - Baryta carbonicum
   (c) Sycotic - Alumina
   (d) Haemorrhagic - Ammonium carbonicum

Ans. (c)

Note
The pair 'Sycotic - Alumina' is not correct.

Also see
Spigelia
Adapted to anemic debilitated subjects of *rheumatic diathesis*; to scrofulous children afflicted with ascarides and lumbrici [Cina, Stan.].
Ref: Allen's Key Notes
Baryta Carabonicum
Especially adapted to complaints to first and second childhood; the psoric or *tubercular*.
Alunina
Adapted to persons who suffer from chronic diseases; "the Aconite of chronic diseases."Constitutions deficient in animal heat [Calc., Sil.]. Spare, dry, thin subjects; dark complexion; mild, cheerful disposition; hypochondriacs; dry, tettery, itching eruption, worse in winter [Petr.]; intolerable, itching of whole body when getting warm in bed [Sulph.], scratches until bleeds, then becomes painful.

Ammonium carbonicum
Hemorrhagic diathesis, fluid blood and degeneration of red blood-corpuscles; ulcerations tend to gangrene. Stout, fleshy women with various trouble in consequence of leading a sedentary life; delicate women who must have the "smelling-bottle" continually at hand; readily catch cold in water. Children dislike washing [Ant- c., Sulph.].

Q. 189. Which of the following medicines cannot tolerate "tea"? (KPSC/Lect/Mat-Med-04)
(a) Arsenicum album
(b) Natrium carbonicum
(c) Argentum nitricum
(d) Nux vomica

Ans. (d)
Note
From options given above 'Nux-v.', cannot tolerate "tea".
Also see
Tea: Agg- 2:Aesc., 2:Chin., 1:Coff., 1:Dios., 2:Ferr., 1:Lach., 1:Rumx., 3:Sel., 2:Thuj., 1:Verat.
Ref: Repertory- Kent, Chapter-Generalities Food
Aggravaton; Tea: Abies-n., Cinch., Dros., Lob., Nux-v., Puls., Sel., Thuj.
Ref: Repertory-Boericke, Chapter: Modalities.
Tea effects of: Abies-n., Chin., Dios., Lob., Nux-v., Thuj.
Repertory-Clarke, Chapter-Clinical
Tea agg: 2: Abies-n., 2:Aesc., 2:Chin., 2:Ferr., 2:Nux-v., 2:Rhus-t., 3:SEL., 3:SEP., 2:Spig., 2:Thuj.
Ref: Reperoty-Synthesis- Chapter-Generals –Food and Drinks

Q. 190. Antimonium crudum patients cannot tolerate (KPSC/Lect/Mat-Med-04)
(a) Milk
(b) Pastries
(c) Coffee
(d) Sweet

Ans. (b)
Note
Ant-c. patients cannot tolerate 'Pastries'.
Also see
Ant-c.
Gastric and intestinal affections; from bread and pastry; acids, especially vinegar; sour or bad wine.
Ref: Allen's Key Notes

Extended information
Repertory reference:
Chapter-Generals – Food and Drinks -Pastry agg: 3:ANT-C., 2:Bry., 2:Kali-c., 2:Kali-chl, 2:Lyc., 2:Phos., 3:PULS., 2:Verat.
Ref: Repertory-Synthesis

GENERALS - FOOD, - pastry agg.
ant-c. arg-n. ars. carb-v. ip. *Kali-chl. Lyc. Phos.* **PULS.**
Ref: Kent Repertory.

Q. 191. Of these which drug is having longing for alcohol a popular remedy in Russia for drunkards? (KPSC/Lect/Org/RE-05)
(a) Nux vomica
(b) Quercus glandium spiritus
(c) Asarum europaeum
(d) Capsicum annum

Ans. (c)

Note
Asarum europaeum
Unconquerable longing for alcohol; a popular remedy in Russia for drunkards. "Horrible sensation" of pressing, digging in the stomach when waking in the morning (After a debauch). Great faintness and constant yawning.
Ref: Allen's Key Notes

Q. 192. Of these which symptoms are pure symptoms? (KPSC/Lect/Org/RE-05)
(a) Symptoms before the use of medicine
(b) Symptoms while taking the medicine
(c) Symptoms while taking tranquillizers
(d) Symptoms after operation

Ans. (a)
Note
Pure symptoms
These are the symptoms, which are present before taking any medicinal substance.

Q. 193. Of the below drugs which is used in kidney affections? (KPSC/Lect/Org/RE-05)
(a) Cephalandra indica
(b) Coleus aromaticus
(c) Calotropis gigantea
(d) Carica papaya

Ans. (b)
Note
Of the above 'Calotropis gingantea' is used in kidney affections.

Also see
    a. Cephalandra indica: Diabetes mellitus, and insipidus.
    b. Coelus aromaticus: Action genitourinary organs.
    c. Calotropis gigantea: Respiratory and GIT and rheumatic affections.
    d. Carica papaya: GIT affections.
Ref: Boericke's materia medica

Q. 194. Of the below which forms the Materia Medica Pura? (KPSC/Lect/Org/RE-05)
(a) Collection of real, pure, reliable modes of action of simple medicinal substances.
(b) Collection of details from the experience of physicians.
(c) Collection of details from poisonings.
(d) Collection of details from animal experimentation.

Ans. (a)
Note
Of the above 'Colleciton of real, pure, reliable modes of action of simple medicinal substances' forms the Materia Medica Pura

Also see
Guidelines for Collection of real, pure, reliable modes of action of simple medicinal substances are given in Organon as under:
§122. Drugs to be proven must not be mixed with other medicinal substance.
§123. The drug should be of unquestioned purity and full strength.
§124. Drugs must be taken pure and alone not alternated or mixed.
§125. Diet during proving should be plain, simple and free from spices or vegetables having any medicinal properties.
§126. During proving the prover should avoid distracting affairs that absorb the attention.
§127. Male and female should jointly participate in provings.
§128. The drug finely divided by potentization, trituration or succussion yields a greater wealth of symptoms than if taken crude or undivided.
§129. Prover should begin with small doses and increase dose as proving progresses, as susceptibility can not be predicted.

§130. A strong initial dose will more exactly exhibit the primary and the order of the appearance of its symptoms, but repeated experiments are necessary to acquire all this information.

§131. Too frequent repetition of the dose, to the prover, often confuses the symptoms, however, for some drugs several doses will be necessary before symptoms appear.

§132. However the order of the appearance of symptoms for mild drugs will be observed only after giving repeated small doses to a sensitive person.

§133. When symptoms begin to appear it is useful to observe effect of position, heat, cold, air, rest, motion, contact, eating, drinking, coughing, talking, sneezing, time of aggravation or amelioration of the pains, sensations or symptoms. These are the modalities of the drugs.

§134. No one prover will experience the whole possible pathogenesis of any one drug during one trial.

§135. Many provers of both sexes should participate in the proving of each drug in order to make a totality of pathogenesis available in one experiment.

§136. A drug so proven will be a remedy for sickness having symptoms most similar to its pathogenesis. The presence of such symptoms in sickness proves the susceptibility of the patient to the drug similar. This remedy is called the similimum. An aggravation must be expected if such remedy is administered in too large a dose or too frequently repeated. This explains the small dose of the homeopath and assigns sufficient reason for it.

§137. Provers should be intelligent, truthful, observing, in sympathy with the work, and feel that they are serving humanity. Care should be taken, too, that the dose is small enough to avoid violent reaction.

§138. Every alteration from normal should be observed and noted in plain simple terms with absolute regard for the truth. If any of the symptoms have ever been felt before they should be recorded for symptoms cannot come of themselves.

§139. Provers must make record of sensations while sensations are felt. Record must be made from day to day, through the whole course of the provings.

§140. If prover cannot keep record, some one skilled in observing, should keep a daily record, recounted by the prover. No guess, supposition or extorted statement should be allowed to enter into the record.

§141. The healthy unprejudiced physician of fine perception, makes the best prover. Every Homeopathic physician should take an active part in proving some drugs as a part of the preparation for the practice of his art.

Q. 195. "Cough with irritation in larynx as if some fluid had gone the wrong way" is feature of (KPSC/ Lect/Physio & Bioch-05)
    (a)   Drosera rotundifolia
    (b)   Ignatia amara
    (c)   Kalium carbonicum
    (d)   Lachesis mutus

Ans. (d)

Note
"Cough with irritation in larynx as if some fluid had gone the wrong way" is feature of 'Lachesis'.

Also see
Lachesis
Respiratory; suffocation and strangulation, on lying down; on dropping to sleep; must spring from bed and rush for open air window. Feels he must take deep breath. Air hunger. Tickling, choking cough worse touching neck or auditory canal; better retching out a little expectoration. Cough during sleep without being conscious of it. As of a skin hanging in or a valve in larynx. As of a plug moving up and down with cough. Larynx painful to touch. Last stage of pneumonia. Abscess of the lungs. Expectoration; frothy, purulent, difficult, bloody with excessive perspiration. Loss of voice; from paralysis of vocal cords, or Oedema. Cough as if some fluid has gone into wrong way; most during day.
Ref: Phatak.
Ref: Allen's Key notes – NA
Ref: Boericke's materia medica- NA

Extended information
Chapter-Cough-Irritation: Larynx in, from: as if some fluid had gone the wrong way: 3:Lach.
Ref: Kent Repertory

Q. 196. Indurations of glands after injuries is seen in (KPSC/Lect/Physio & Bioch-05)
  (a) Silicea
  (b) Carbo animalis
  (c) Conium maculatum
  (d) Iodium

Ans. (c)
Note
Indurations of glands after injuries is seen in 'Conium'.
Also see
Conium maculatum
Glandular induration of stony hardness; of mammae and testicles in persons of cancerous tendency; after bruises and injuries of glands [compare, Aster. Rub.].
Ref: Allen's Key Notes

Extended information
Chapter – Generalities - Indurations; Glands: Injury After: 3:Con.
Ref: Kent Repertory

Q. 197. Nux moschata was introduced to Homeopathic world by (KPSC/Lect/Physio & Bioch-05)
  (a) Dr. Hahnemann
  (b) Dr. Helbig
  (c) Dr. Hering
  (d) Dr. Bute

Ans. (b)
Note
Nux-m. was introduced by Dr. Helbig.
Ref: Hering materia medica.

Q. 198. In stomatitis, deep longitudinal cracks on tongue and excessive flow of saliva runs out of mouth when sleeping (KPSC/Lect/Practice of Med-2005)
  (a) Syphilinum
  (b) Mercurius solubilis
  (c) Nitricum acidum
  (d) Muriaticum acidum

Ans. (a)
Note
Syphilinum
Mouth: Teeth decay at gum; edges serrated, dwarfed. Tongue coated, teeth- indented; deep longitudinal cracks. Ulcers smart and burn. Excessive flow of saliva; it runs out of mouth when sleeping.
Ref: Boericke's materia medica.

Q. 199. In duodenal ulcer canine hunger and tendency to eat far beyond the capacity to digest (KPSC/Lect/Practice of Med-05)
  (a) Nux vomica
  (b) Abies canadensis
  (c) Abies nigra
  (d) Sulphur

Ans. (b)
Note
Abies canadensis
Great appetite, craving for meat, pickles, radishes, turnips, artichokes, coarse food. Tendency to eat far beyond capacity for digestion.
Ref: Boericke materia medica

MCQ's in Materia Medica

Q. 200. Best tonic for debility after exhausting diseases (KPSC/Lect/Practice of Med-05)
    (a)   China officinalis
    (b)   Selenium
    (c)   Avena sativa
    (d)   Psorinum

Ans. (c)
Note
Best tonic for debility after exhausting diseases is 'Avena sativa'.
Also see
Avena sativa
Has a selective action on brain and nervous system, favorably influencing their nutritive function. Nervous exhaustion, sexual debility, and the morphine habit call for this remedy in rather material dosage. Best tonic for debility after exhausting diseases.
Ref: Boericke's materia medica

Q. 201. In Hyperchlorhydria with aversion to milk and fat food (KPSC/Lect/Practice of Med-05)
    (a)   Pulsatilla
    (b)   Robinia
    (c)   Acidum sulphuricum
    (d)   Calcarea carbonicum

Ans. (d)
Note
Above featues are found in 'Calcarea carbonicum'.
Also see
Calcarea carbonicum
Stomach: Acidity and dislike of fat. Aversion to meat, boiled things. Milk disagrees. Frequent sour eructations; sour vomiting. Dislike of fat. Loss of appetite when overworked. Heartburn and loud belching. Thirst; longing for cold drinks. Aggravation while eating. Hyperchlorhydria (Phos.).
Ref: Boericke's materia medica

Q. 202. Dry hacking cough expelling an offensive breath from lungs (KPSC/Lect/Practice of Med-05)
    (a)   Pulsatilla nigricans
    (b)   Kalium iodatum
    (c)   Capsicum anum
    (d)   Nitricum acidum

Ans. (c)
Note
The above features are found in 'Capsicum'.
Also see
Capsicum
Respiratory: Constriction of chest; arrests breathing. Hoarseness. Pain at apex of heart or in rib region, worse touch. Dry, hacking cough, expelling an offensive breath from lungs. Dyspnea. Feels as if chest and head would fly to pieces. Explosive cough. Threatening gangrene of lung. Pain in distant parts on coughing—bladder, legs, ears, etc.
Ref: Boericke's materia medica

Q. 203. Gastralgia relieved with eating with hepatic symptoms (KPSC/Lect/Practice of Med-05)
    (a)   Podophyllum
    (b)   Chelidonium
    (c)   Anacardium orientalis
    (d)   Mercurius solubilis

Ans. (b)
Note
Gastralgia relieved with eating with hepatic symptoms is 'Chelidonium'.

Also see
Chelidonium
Stomach: Gastralgia. Eating relieves temporarily, especially when accompanied with hepatic symptoms.
Ref: Boericke's materia medica

Q. 204. Angina pectoris with sensation as if the heart ceased to beat then starts very suddenly (KPSC/Lect/Practice of Med-05)
    (a)   Cactus grandiflorus
    (b)   Digitalis purpura
    (c)   Lilium tigrinum
    (d)   Convallaria majalis

Ans. (d)
Note
Angina pectoris with sensation as if the heart ceased to beat then starts very suddenly is a feature of 'Convallaria majalis'.

Also see
Convallaria majalis
A heart remedy. Increases energy of heart's action, renders it more regular of use when the ventricles are overdistended and dilatation begins, and when there is an absence of compensatory hypertrophy, and when venous stasis is marked. Heart: sensation as if heart ceased beating, then starts very suddenly. Palpitation from the least exertion.
Ref: Boericke's materia medica

Q. 205. Painful cracks of the corner of the mouth with cancer of stomach (KPSC/Lect/Practice of Med-05)
    (a)   Nitricum acidum
    (b)   Bismuth
    (c)   Antimonium crudum
    (d)   Condurango

Ans. (d)
Note
Painful cracks of the corner of the mouth with cancer of stomach is a feature of 'Condurango'.

Also see
Condurango
Painful cracks in corner of mouth are a guiding symptom of this drug. Chronic gastric catarrh, syphilis, and cancer.
Ref: Boericke's materia medica

Q. 206. Renal colic with pain in small of back before micturation and ceases after flow (KPSC/Lect/Practice of Med-05)
    (a)   Berberis vulgaris
    (b)   Lycopodium clavatum
    (c)   Pulsatilla nigricans
    (d)   Nux vomica

Ans. (b)
Note
Renal colic with pain in small of back before micturation and ceases after flow is a feature of 'Lycopodium'.

Also see
Lycopodium
Urine: Pain in back before urinating; ceases after flow.
Ref: Boeircke's materia medica

Q. 207. Asthma in children as a constitutional remedy in sycotic subjects (KPSC/Lect/Practice of Med-05)
    (a)   Natrium sulphuricum
    (b)   Antimonium tartaricum
    (c)   Silicea
    (d)   Hepar sulphuricum

Ans. (a)
Note
Asthma in children as a constitutional remedy in sycotic subjects is 'Natrium sulphuricum'.

Also see
Natrium sulphuricum
Respiratory: Dyspnea, during damp weather. Must hold chest when coughing. Humid asthma; rattling in chest, at 4 and 5 a.m. Cough, with thick, ropy, greenish expectoration; chest feels all gone. Constant desire to take deep, long breath. Asthma in cildren, as a constitutional remedy. Delayed resolution in pneumonia.
Ref: Boericke's materia medica

Natrium sulphuricum
Respiratory; Dyspnea. Asthma, sycotic; in children as a constitutional remedy, worse early morning. Loose but violent cough; better sitting; must hold the chest or sides. Pain, piercing through lower left chest. Every fresh cold or any unusual exertion, brings on an attack of asthma. Breathing short while walking; constant desire to take deep, long breath. Asthma, with early morning diarrhea. Expectoration, greenish, copious.
Ref: Phatak materia medica

Q. 208. Rheumatism associated with urticarea like eruptions (KPSC/Lect/Practice of Med-05)
    (a)   Rhus toxiodendron
    (b)   Graphites
    (c)   Urtica urens
    (d)   Dulcamara

Ans. (c)
Note
Rheumatism associated with urticarea like eruptions is 'Uritica urens'.

Also see
Urtica urens
Skin: Itching blotches. Urticaria, burning heat, with formication; violent itching. Consequences of suppressed nettle-rash. Rheumatism alternates with nettle-rash.
Ref: Boericke's materia medica

Q. 209. In apoplexy (rupture of artery) with headache and sensation of a lump of ice on the vertex (KPSC/Lect/Practice of Med-05)
    (a)   Glonoine
    (b)   Belladonna
    (c)   Gelsemium
    (d)   Veratrum album

Ans. (d)
Note
In apoplexy (rupture of artery) with headache and sensation of a lump of ice on the vertex is 'Veratrum Album'.

Also see
Glonoine
Head- Throbbing headache.
Ref: Boericke's materia medica

Belladonna
Head - Palpitation reverberating in head with labored breathing. Pain; fullness, especially in forehead, also occiput, and temples. Headache from suppressed catarrhal flow. Sudden outcries. Pain worse light, noise, jar,

lying down and in afternoon, better by pressure and semi-erect posture.
Ref: Boericke's materia medica

Gelsemium
Head- Heaviness of head; band-feeling around and occipital headache.
Ref: Boericke's materia medica

Veratrum album
Head- Sensation of a lump of ice on vertex.
Ref: Boericke's materia medica

Q. 210. An important remedy for pericarditis is (KPSC/Lect/Practice of Med-05)
    (a)   Kalium carbonicum
    (b)   Apis mellifica
    (c)   Spigelia
    (d)   Bryonia alba

Ans. (c)
Note
Spigelia is an important remedy in pericarditis and other diseases of the heart, because the provings were conducted with the greatest regard for objective symptoms and the subjective symptoms are by innumerable confirmations proved to be correct.
Ref: C. Hering materia medica

Also see
Spigelia
Heart: Violent palpitation. Praecordial pain and great aggravation from movement. Frequent attacks of palpitation, especially with foul odor from mouth. Pulse weak and irregular. Pericarditis, with sticking pains, palpitation, dyspnea. Neuralgia extending to arm or both arms. Angina pectoris. Craving for hot water which relieves. Rheumatic carditis, trembling pulse; whole left side sore. Dyspnea; Must lie on right side with head high.
Ref: Boericke's materia medica

Q. 211. A medicine for post herpetic neuralgia (KPSC/Lect/Practice of Med-05)
    (a)   Mezereum
    (b)   Sulphur
    (c)   Bryonia alba
    (d)   Phosphorus

Ans. (a)
Note
Mezereum
Neuralgic burning pains after zona.
Ref: Allen's Key Notes

Q. 212. Rheumatism of the right wrist (KPSC/Lect/Practice of Med-05)
    (a)   Sulphur
    (b)   Viola odorata
    (c)   Bryonia alba
    (d)   Benzoic acidum

Ans. (b)
Note
Viola odorata
Extremities: Rheumatism of the deltoid muscle. Trembling of limbs. Pressing pain in right carpal and metacarpal joints.
Ref: Boericke's materia medica

Q. 213. In plica polonica (KPSC/Lect/Practice of Med-05)
    (a)   Mercurius solubilis
    (b)   Natrium muriaticum
    (c)   Vinca minor
    (d)   Sulphur

Ans. (c)
Note
In plica polonica medicine is 'Vinca minor'.
Also see
Vinca minor
General
A remedy for skin affections, eczema, and especially plica polonica; also for hemorrhages and diphtheria.
Head
Tearing pain in vertex, ringing and whistling in ears. Whirling vertigo, with flickering before eyes. Spots on scalp, oozing moisture, matting hair together. corrosive itching of scalp. Bald spots. Plica polonica. Irresistible desire to scratch.

Extended information
Ref: Repertory: Boericke –Chapter: Head – Symptom: Scalp; Eruption; Plica polonica; Ant-t., Bar-c., Bor x., Graph., **Lyc.**, Nat-m., Psor., Sars., Tub., **Vinc.**, Viol–t.

Q. 214. A medicine for rectal cancer (KPSC/Lect/Practice of Med-05)
    (a)   Ruta graveolens
    (b)   Sulphur
    (c)   Aloe socotrina
    (d)   Mercurius solubilis

Ans. (a)
Note
A medicine for rectal cancer is 'Ruta'.
Also see
Ruta
Rectum: Carcinoma affecting lower bowel.
Ref: Boericke's materia medica

Q. 215. Epistaxis painless with bright red blood (KPSC/Lect/Practice of Med-05)
    (a)   Nitricum acidum
    (b)   Sabina
    (c)   Millefolium
    (d)   Secale cornutum

Ans. (c)
Note
Epistaxis painless with Bright Red Blood 'Millefolium'.
Also see
Millefolium
Haemorrhages: Painless, without fever, bright red, fluid blood (Acon., Ip., Sabad.,); from lungs, bronchi, larynx, mouth, nose, stomach, bladder, rectum, uterus; of mechanical origin (Arn.); of wounds (Ham.).
Ref: Allen's Key Notes

Q. 216. Asthma during sexual contact is a feature of (KPSC/Obs-Gyn-05)
    (a)   Ambra grisea
    (b)   Natrium muriaticum
    (c)   Sepia officinalis
    (d)   Kreosotum

Ans. (a)

Note
Asthma during sexual contact is a feature of 'Ambra grisea'.

Also see
Ambra grisea
Asthmatic breathing; in old people; worse by coition.
Ref: Phatak materia medica

Extended information
Respiration- Asthmatic- Coition –During- 2:Aeth., 1:Ambr.
Ref: Kent's Repertory

Q. 217. Which medicine have inflammation of ovaries during childhood? (KPSC/Obs-Gyn-05)
    (a)   Aconitum napellus
    (b)   Apis mellifica
    (c)   Pulsatilla nigricans
    (d)   Rhus toxicodendron

Ans. (b)
Note
'Apis' is the most appropriate medicine for inflammation of ovaries during childhood.

Also see
Aconitum napellus
Constitution: It is generally indicated in acute or recent cases occurring in young persons, especially girls of a full, plethoric habit who lead a sedentary life; persons easily affected by atmospheric changes. Acute inflammation of ovaries from suppression of menses.
Ref: Allen's Key Notes

Apis
Constitution: Adapted to the strumous constitution; glands enlarged, indurated; scirrhous or open cancer. Women, especially widows; children and girls who, though generally careful, become awkward, and let things fall while handling them (Bov.). Bad effects of acute exanthema imperfectly developed or suppressed (Zinc.); measles, scarlatina, urticaria. Cyst right ovary, enlargement of dropsy of right ovary; right testicle.
Ref: Allen's Key Notes

Discussion
The common causes of inflammation of ovary are usually metastasis of mumps or measles which can cause ovaritis. Therefore, it is the most probable remedy for inflammation of ovary during childhood.

Pulsatilla nigricans
Constitution: Adapted to persons of indecisive, slow, phlegmatic temperament; sandy hair, blue eyes, pale face, easily moved to laughter or tears; affectionate, mild, gentle, timid, yielding disposition - the woman's remedy. Weeps easily: almost impossible to detail her ailments without weeping (weeps when thanked, Lyc.). Especially in diseases of women and children.
Ref: Allen's Key Notes

Rhus toxicodendron
Constitution: Adapted to persons of rheumatic diathesis; bad effects of getting wet, especially after being over-heated.
Ref: Allen's Key Notes

Q. 218. Leucorrhea like curds, white of an egg is a feature of (KPSC/Obs-Gyn-05)
    (a)   Mercurius solubilis
    (b)   Borax
    (c)   Calcarea carbonicum
    (d)   Sepia officinalis

Ans. (b)
Note
Leucorrhea like curds, white of an egg is a feature of 'Borax'.

Also see
Mercurius
Leucorrhea: acrid, burning, itching with rawness; always worse at night; pruritus, < from contact of urine which must be washed off (Sulph.).
Ref: Allen's Key Notes

Borax
Leucorrhea: profuse, albuminous, starchy, with sensation as if warm water were flowing down; for two weeks between the catamenia (compare, Bov., Con.).
Ref: Allen's Key Notes

Calcarea carbonicum
Leucorrhea: Milky (Sep.).
Ref: Boericke's materia medica

Sepia officinalis
Leucorrhoea: yellow, greenish; with much itching.
Ref: Boericke's materia medica

Q. 219. Atrophy of breast with absence of menses is a feature of (KPSC/Obs-Gyn-05)
- (a) Damiana
- (b) Pituitrinum
- (c) Iodium
- (d) Onosmodium

Ans. (c)

Note
Atrophy of breast with absence of menses is a feature of 'Iodium'.

Also see
Damiana
Said to be of use in sexual neurasthenia; impotency. Sexual debility from nervous prostration. Incontinence of old people. Chronic prostatic discharge. Renal and cystic catarrh; Frigidity of females. Aids the establishment of normal menstrual flow in young girls.
Ref: Boericke's materia medica

Pituitrinum
Pituitary exercises a superior control over the growth and development of the sexual organs, stimulates muscular activity and overcomes uterine inertia.
Ref: Boericke's materia medica

Iodium
Sterility from atrophy of ovaries and mammae.
Ref: Phatak's materia medica

Onosmodium
Severe uterine pains; bearing-down pains; old pains return sexual desire completely destroyed. Feels as if menses would appear. Aching in breasts. Nipples itch. Menses too early and too prolonged. Soreness in uterine region. Leucorrhoea, yellow, acrid, profuse.
Ref: Boericke's materia medica

Extended information
Also see

English Kent

CHEST - ATROPHY, - mammae
anan.$_k$ ars.$_k$ bar-c.$_k$ *Chim.*$_k$ **CON.**$_k$ **IOD.**$_k$ **KALI-I.**$_k$ *Kreos.*$_k$ lac-d.$_k$ *Nat-m.*$_k$ *Nit-ac.*$_k$ *Nux-m.*$_k$ plb.$_k$ sacch.$_k$ sars.$_k$ *Sec.*$_k$

English Kent

FEMALE GENITALIA - MENSES, - absent,amenorrhoea
Acon.k aesc.k agar.k agn.k alet.k Am-c.k am-m.k Ant-c.k Apis.k Apoc.k arg-n.k Ars.k Ars-i.k **AUR.**k Bar-c.k Bell.k benz-ac.k berb.k Borx.k Bry.k Calc.k calc-s.k canth.k **CARBN-S.**k carb-v.k card-m.k Caul.k Caust.k Cham.k chel.k Chin.k chinin-ar.k cic.k cimic.k cina Cocc.k colch.k Coll.k Coloc.k **CON.**k croc.k crot-t.k Cupr.k Cycl.k dig. Dros.k **DULC.**k euph.k **FERR.**k Ferr-ar.k **FERR-I.**k Ferr-p.k gels.k Goss.k **GRAPH.**k Guaj.k Ham.k Hell.k helon.k Hyos.k Ign.k Iod.k Kali-ar.k **KALI-C.**k kali-i.k Kali-n.k Kali-p.k kali-s.k Lach.k lil-t.k lob.k **LYC.**k Mag-c.k Mag-m.k Merc.k mill.k nat-c.k Nat-m.k nat-p.k Nux-m.k Nux-v.k ph-ac.k Phos.k Plat.k podo.k **PULS.**k Rhus-t.k Sabad.k sabin.k sang.k sec.k **SENEC.**k **SEP.**k **SIL.**k Staph.k stram.k **SULPH.**k **TUB.**k Valer.k verat.k verat-v.k xan.k Zinc.k
Above repertory references points to 'Iod' as the most possible choice.
Ref: Kent's Repertory (RADAR 10)

Q. 220. Absence of menses due to Jaundice is a features of (KPSC/Obs-Gyn-05)
    (a) Chelidonium majus
    (b) Chionanthus
    (c) Bryonia alba
    (d) Nux vomica

Ans. (b)
Note
Above feature is found in 'Chionanthus'.

Also see
Chionanthus
Hepatic derangement. Jaundice. Enlarged spleen. (Cean.) Jaundice, with arrest of menses. A prominent liver remedy.
Ref: Boericke's materia medica

Q. 221. Blood from vagina every time the child takes breast (KPSC/Obs-Gyn-05)
    (a) Pulsatilla nigricans
    (b) Silicea
    (c) Medorrhinum
    (d) Bryonia alba

Ans. (b)
Note
Above feature is found in 'Silicea'.

Also see
Silicea
Discharge of blood from vagina every time child is nursed.
Ref: Boericke's materia medica

Q. 222. Which medicine have abortion due to mental strain? (KPSC/Obs-Gyn-05)
    (a) Gelsemium sempervirens
    (b) Sabina
    (c) Secale cornutum
    (d) Aurum muriaticum

Ans. (a)
Note
'Gels' is the choice from above options for 'Abortion due to mental strain'.

Also see
Repertory-Kent-Chapter- Genitalia female – Abortion; Excitement-3:GELS.
Repertory-Kent-Chapter- Genitalia female – Abortion; Fright from- 2:Acon., 2:Gels., 2:Ign, 2:Op.
Repertory-Synthesis 7.0 Chapter-Gemale Genitalia-Abortion; excitement; from emotional -2:Bapt., 1: Cham, 3:GELS., 2:Helon., 2:Op.

Q. 223. Which medicine is good for sterility due to atrophy of ovaries? (KPSC/Obs-Gyn-05)
(a) Kalium bromatum
(b) Iodium
(c) Sepia officinalis
(d) Xanthoxylum

Ans. (b)

Note
Iodium
Sterility from atrophy of ovaries and mammae.
Ref: Phatak materia medica

Also see

> Boericke O., Repertory

FEMALE SEXUAL SYSTEM - Conception - Difficult
Agn.$_{bro1}$ alet.$_{bro1}$ am-c.$_{bro1}$ aur.$_{bro1}$ *Bar-m.*$_{bro1}$ *Borx.*$_{bro1}$ calc.$_{bro1}$ cann-i.$_{bro1}$ caul.$_{bro1}$ *Con.*$_{bro1}$ eup-pur.$_{bro1}$ goss.$_{bro1}$ *Graph.*$_{bro1}$ helon.$_{bro1}$ *Iod.*$_{bro1}$ lec.$_{bro1}$ *Med.*$_{bro1}$ nat-c.$_{bro1}$ *Nat-m.*$_{bro1}$ nat-p.$_{bro1}$ phos.$_{bro1}$ *Plat.*$_{bro1}$ *Sabal*$_{bro1}$

> English Kent

FEMALE SEXUAL SYSTEM - Ovaries - Atrophy
Iod.$_{bro1}$ orch.$_{bro1}$ ov.$_{bro1}$
Ref: Pocket manual of Hom. Mat. Med. and Repertory, Boericke (RADAR 10)

> English Kent

FEMALE GENITALIA - ATROPHY, ovaries
apis$_k$ *Bar-m.*$_k$ *Carbn-s.*$_k$ *Con.*$_k$ helon.$_k$ **IOD.**$_k$ plb.$_k$
Ref: (RADAR 10)

Q. 224. Menses bleeding only during day time (KPSC/Obs-Gyn/05)
(a) Magnesium carbonicum
(b) Bovista
(c) Bryonia alba
(d) Nux vomica

Ans. Use your discretion

Note
Chapter Genitalia Female Menses: Daytime only gives following medicines – 1: Cact, 2:Caust, 2:Coff, 3:Cycl, 1:Ham, 3:Puls.
Ref: Kent's Repertory

Also see
However, Menses night only has following drugs:
Genitalia female-Menses:Night only: 1:Borx., 3:Bov., 1:Coff., 1:Cycl., 1:Mag-c.
Ref: Kent's Repertory
Female genitalia / Sex: Menses-Daytime only: 1:Cact., 2: Caust., 1:Coff., 1:Cycl., 1:Ham., 1:Kali-c, 3:Puls.
Ref: Synthesis
No remedy suggested in the above rubric is represented in the choice. Use your discretion.

Q. 225. Which medicine shows delayed labour in second stage due to uterine inertia (KPSC/Obs-Gyn/05):
(a) Pituitrinum
(b) Caulophyllum
(c) Cuprum metallicum
(d) Pulsatilla nigricans

Ans. (a)

Note
From above options 'Pituitrinum' shows delayed labour in second stage due to uterine inertia.
Also see
Pituitrinum
Uterine inertia in second stage of labor where os is fully dilated.
Ref: Boericke's materia medica

Q. 226. Nipples cracked and ragged extreme sensitive cannot bear to touch this symptom peculiar to (KPSC/Obs-Gyn-05)
    (a)   Silicea
    (b)   Castor equi
    (c)   Sarasaparilla
    (d)   Graphites

Ans. (b)
Note
Nipples cracked and ragged extreme sensitive cannot bear to touch this symptom peculiar to 'Castor equi'.

Also see
Castor equi (Rudimentary Thumb-nail of the Horse)
Chest: Cracked, sore nipples, excessively tender.
Ref: Boericke's materia medica

Q. 227. Vomiting of pregnancy in women have the colour of dark olive green is a feature of (KPSC/Obs-Gyn-05)
    (a)   Carbolicum acidum
    (b)   Cerium oxalicum
    (c)   Sepia officinalis
    (d)   Symphoricarpus racemosa

Ans. (a)
Note
Vomiting of pregnancy in women have the colour of dark olive green is a feature of 'Carbolicum acidum'.
Also see
Carbolicum acidum
Stomach: Constant belching, nausea, vomiting, dark olive green.
Ref: Boericke's materia medica

Q. 228. Which medicine is more suitable for habitual abortion? (KPSC/Obs-Gyn-05)
    (a)   Sabina
    (b)   Viburnum opulus
    (c)   Sepia officinalis
    (d)   Pulsatilla nigricans

Ans. (b)
Note
Viburnum is more suitable for habitual abortion.

Choice of (b) appears to be most suitable answer, however, use your discretion.
Also see
Sabina
Tendency to miscarriage, especially at third month.
Ref: Boericke's materia medica
Viburnum
Frequent and very early miscarriage, causing seeming sterility.
Ref: Boericke's materia medica
Sepia
Tendency to abortion.
Ref: Boericke's materia medica

Pulsatilla
Miscarriage / abortion symptoms -NA.
Ref: Boericke's materia medica

Q. 229. Which medicine shows retention of urine with albuminuria? (KPSC/Obs-Gyn-05)
    (a)   Cantharis vesicatoria
    (b)   Terebinthiniae oleum
    (c)   Apis mellifica
    (d)   Helonias dioica

Ans. (b)
Note
'Ter. has the feature of retention of urine with albuminuria'.

Also see
Terebinthiniae
Violent burning and cutting in bladder; tenesmus; sensitive hypogastrium; cystitis and retention from atony of fundus. Albuminuria: acute, in early stages, when blood and albumin abound more than casts and epithelium.
Ref: Allen's Key Notes

Q. 230. Which medicine have aversion for bread during pregnancy? (KPSC/Obs-Gyn-05)
    (a)   Sepia officinalis
    (b)   Lycopodium clavatum
    (c)   Colchicum autumnale
    (d)   Arsenicum album

Ans. (a)
Note
'Sepia' has aversion for bread during pregnancy.

Also see
Generals-Food and Drinks-Aversion to bread during pregnancy; 1:Ant-t, 1:Laur., 2:Sep.
Ref: Synthesis

Q. 231. Reflex cough of pregnant women is a feature of (KPSC/Obs-Gyn-05)
    (a)   Kalium bromatum
    (b)   Kalium sulphuricum
    (c)   Causticum
    (d)   Conium maculatum

Ans. (a)
Note
Reflex cough of pregnant women is a feature of 'Kalium bromatum'.

Also see
Kali-br.
Nervous cough during pregnancy; dry, hard, almost incessant, threatening abortion (Con.).
Ref; Allen's Key Notes
Kali-br.
Spasmodic croup. Reflex cough during pregnancy. Dry, fatiguing, hacking cough at night.
Ref: Boericke materia medica
Kali-s.
Post-grippal cough especially in children. Bronchial asthma, with yellow expectoration. Cough; worse in evening and in hot atmosphere.
Caust
Cough with rawness and soreness in chest; with inability to expectorate. Ref: Allen's Key Notes
Con.
Cough: In spasmodic paroxysms caused by dry spot in larynx (in throat, Act.); with itching chest and throat (Iod.); worse at night, when lying down, and during pregnancy (Caust., Kali-bi.).
Ref: Allen's Key Notes

Extended information
Cough Pregnancy during: 2:Caust. 2:Con., 2:Nux-m., 3:Phos., 3:Sep.
Ref: Synthesis

Q. 232. Madness during pregnancy is found in one of the following medicine (KPSC/Obs-Gyn-05)
    (a)   Stramonium
    (b)   Nux moschata
    (c)   Cicuta virosa
    (d)   Actaea racemosa

Ans. Use your discretion as (a) and (d) both have the above symptom

Note
Stramonium
Puerperal mania, with characteristic mental symptoms and profuse sweatings.
Ref: Boericke materia medica
Nux moschata
Symptoms of mania / madness NA.
Ref: Allens Key Notes
Cicuta virosa
Puerperal convulsions.
Ref: Allen's Key Notes
Actaea racemosa
Puerperal mania; thinks she is going crazy (compare, Syph), tries to injure herself.
Ref: Allen's Key Notes

Extended information
Mania, madness: 3:Stram., 2:Nux-m. 3: Cimic. The medicine missing is Cicuta and Actaea racemosa.
Ref: Kent Repertory –Mania, madness

Q. 233. Toothache in pregnancy is relieved by keeping cold water (KPSC/Obs-Gyn/05)
    (a)   Coffea cruda
    (b)   Kreosotum
    (c)   Pulsatilla nigricans
    (d)   Chamomilla

Ans. Use your discretion

Note
Teeth-Pain, toothache in general: Pregnancy during: 1:Alum, 1:Apis, 2: Bell, 1:Bry, 2:Calc, 2:Cham, 2:Hyos, 3:Lyss, 2:Mag-c., 2:merc, 2:Nux-m, 1:Nux-v, 2:Puls, 2:Rat, 1:Rhus-t., 3:Sep, 2:Staph, 2:Tab.
Ref: Kent's Repertory

Also see
Coffea
Toothache: intermittent, jerking, relieved by holding ice-water in the mouth, but returns when water becomes warm (Bis., Bry., Puls., Caust., Sep., Nat-s.)
Ref: Allen's Key Notes

Coffea
Toothache, better by cold water.
Ref: Clarke's materia medica

Kreosote
Very rapid decay of teeth, with spongy, bleeding gums; teeth dark and crumbly. (Staph. Ant-c.)
Ref: Boericke's materia medica

Puls
Toothache: relieved by holding cold water in the mouth (Bry., Coff.);
worse from warm things and heat of room.
Ref: Allen's Key Notes

Chamomilla
Toothache if anything warm is taken into the mouth [Bis., Bry., Coff.]; on entering warm room; in bed; from coffee; during menses or pregnancy
Ref: Allen's Key Notes

Chamomilla
Odontalgia, most frequently semi-lateral, and chiefly at night, when warm in bed, with insupportable pains which almost induce despair, swelling, heat, and redness of the cheek, swelling, burning of the gums, and painful swelling of the sub-maxillary glands. The toothache recommences when entering a warm room. Toothache, after a cold and suppressed perspiration. Affects teeth on left lower side, under jaw. The pains are commonly drawing and pulling, or pulsative and shooting, or searching and gnawing, in the hollow teeth, appearing frequently after drinking or eating anything hot (or cold), and chiefly after taking coffee. Toothache better by dipping finger in cold water and applying it to affected part. Loosening of the teeth. Dentition, with convulsions.
Ref: Clarke's materia medica

Q. 234. Leucorrhea, profuse, watery, during pregnancy, at night (KPSC/Obs-Gyn/05)
    (a) Alumina
    (b) Syphillinum
    (c) Both (a) and (b)
    (d) None of the above

Ans. Not suggested

Note
Use your Discretion

Also see
Alumina
Leucorrhea : acrid and profuse, running down to the heels [Syph.]; worse during the daytime; > by cold bathing.
Ref: Allen's Key Notes

Alumina
Leucorrhea acrid, profuse, transparent, ropy, with burning; worse during daytime, and after menses. Relieved by washing with cold water.
Ref: Boericke's materia medica

Syphilinum
Leucorrhea: profuse, soaking through the napkins and running down to the heels [Alum.].
Ref: Allen's Key Notes

Extended information
Female genitalia; leucorrhea –Pregnancy; 3:Alum, 2:Cocc, 3:Kreos, 2:Puls, 3:Sep.
Female genitalia; leucorrhea-Night; 1:Alum, 2:Syph.
Female genitalia; leucorrhea- Copious; 2:Alum, 1:Puls, 3:Sep, 2:Syph.
Ref: Repertory- Synthesis

Q. 235. If vertigo and headache be very persistent or prostration be prolonged after Natrium Muriaticum, will relieve (Kerala MD(Hom)/Entr/Paper 2-01)
    (a) Gelsemium sempervirens
    (b) Apis mellifica
    (c) Glonoine
    (d) Nux vomica

Ans. (d)

Note
In above clinical situation after 'Natrium muriaticum' the follows well is 'Nux-v'.

Also see
Natrium muriaticum
Relationship:
If vertigo and headache be very persistent, or prostration be prolonged after Nat-m., Nux-v. will relieve.
Ref: Allen's Key note

Q. 236. Believes that she is going to die soon that she cannot be helped (Kerala MD(Hom)/Entr /Paper 2-01)
  (a) Aconitum napellus
  (b) Hydrastis canadensis
  (c) Agnus castus
  (d) Helleborus niger

Ans. (c)
Note
For the above clinical presentation suggested choice is 'Agn'.

Also see
Agn
Fear of death. SADNESS WITH IMPRESSION OF SPEEDY DEATH.
Ref: Boericke's materia medica

Extended information
Chapter- Mind-Death: Presentiment of: Believes that she will die soon and that she cannot be helped: 2:Agn.
Ref: Kent's Repertory

Q. 237. Irritable pains are accompanied by excitement (Kerala MD(Hom)/Entr/Paper 2-01)
  (a) Aconitum napellus
  (b) Cinchona officinalis
  (c) Coffea cruda
  (d) Causticum

Ans. (c)
Note
The above features of pain are represented by 'Coffea'.

Also see
Coffea
Extreme sensitiveness characterizes this remedy. Neuralgia in various parts; always with great nervous excitability and intolerance of pain, driving to despair.
Ref: Boericke's materia medica

Q. 238. Convulsions of single muscle (Kerala MD(Hom)/EP2/01)
  (a) Ignatia amara
  (b) Cuprum metallicum
  (c) Magnesium-phosphoricum
  (d) Bufo rana

Ans. NA
Note
Use your discretion.

Also see
Ignatia amara
Twitching, jerking, even spasms of single limbs or whole body, when falling asleep. Pain in small, circumscribed spots.
Ref: Allen's Key note
Cuprum metallicum

Convulsions, with blue face and clenched thumbs. Cramps in the extremities; pains, soles, calves with great weariness of limbs. Clonic spasms, beginning in fingers and toes, and spreading over entire body; during pregnancy; puerperal convulsions; after fright or vexation; from metastasis from other organs to brain (Zinc.).
Ref: Allen's Key note

Magnesium phosphorium
Cramps: of extremities; during pregnancy; of writers, piano or violin players.
Ref: Allen's Key note

Bufo rana
Of use in feeble-minded children. Prematurely senile. Epileptic symptoms. Convulsive seizures occur during sleep at night. More or less connected with derangements of the sexual sphere, seem to come within the range of this remedy. Injuries to fingers; pain runs in streaks up the arms.
Ref: Boericke's materia medica

Q. 239. Tension is the key-note of (Kerala MD(Hom)/EP2/01):
    (a)   Aconitum napellus
    (b)   Argentum nitricum
    (c)   Gelsenium sempervirens
    (d)   Oxalicum acidum

Ans. (a)
Note
Tension is key note of 'Aconite'.
Also see
Aconite
Dr. Hughes has acutely remarked that the condition to which acon. is Homeopathic is one of tension, and this word gives the best idea of the action and sphere of acon.
Ref: Clarke's materia medica

Q. 240. 4-8 P.M. aggravation in bowel nosodes (Kerala MD(Hom)/EP2/01)
    (a)   Morgan-Gaertner
    (b)   Morgan pure
    (c)   Proteus
    (d)   Bacillus-7

Ans. (a)
Note
The agg 4-8 pm is a feature of 'Morgan Gaertner'.
Also see
Morgan Gaertner (Paterson)
Most useful in acute inflammatory conditions as in renal colic and gallstone colic Aggravation at 4- 8 pm.

Q. 241. Morning diarrhea and evening constipation (Kerala MD(Hom)/EP2/01)
    (a)   Aloe socotrina
    (b)   Sulphur
    (c)   Bryonia alba
    (d)   Natrium muriaticum

Ans. NA
Note
-Use your discretion.
Also see
Aloe socotrina
Diarrhea driving out of bed very early in morning.
Ref: Allen's Key Notes

Sulphur
Diarrhea: after midnight; painless; driving out of bed early in the morning (Aloes, Psor); as if the bowels were too weak to retain their contents. Constipation: stools hard, knotty, dry, as if burnt (Bry.); large painful, child is afraid to have the stool on account of pain, or pain compels the child to desist on first effort; alternating with Diarrhea.
Ref: Allen's Key Notes

Bryonia alba
Constipation: inactive, no inclination; stool large, hard dark, dry, as if burnt; on going to sea (Plat.). Diarrhea: during a spell of hot weather; bilious, acrid with soreness of anus; like dirty water; of undigested food; from cold drinks when overheated, from fruit or sourkrout; < in morning, on moving, even a hand or foot.
Ref: Allen's Key Notes

Natrum muriaticum
Constipation: sensation of contraction of anus; torn, bleeding, smarting afterwards, stool dry, hard, difficult, crumbling [Am-c., Mag-m.]; stitches in rectum [Nit-ac.]; involuntary, knows not whether flatus or feces escape [Aloe, Iod., Mur-ac., Olnd., Pod.].
Ref: Allen's Key Notes

Extended information

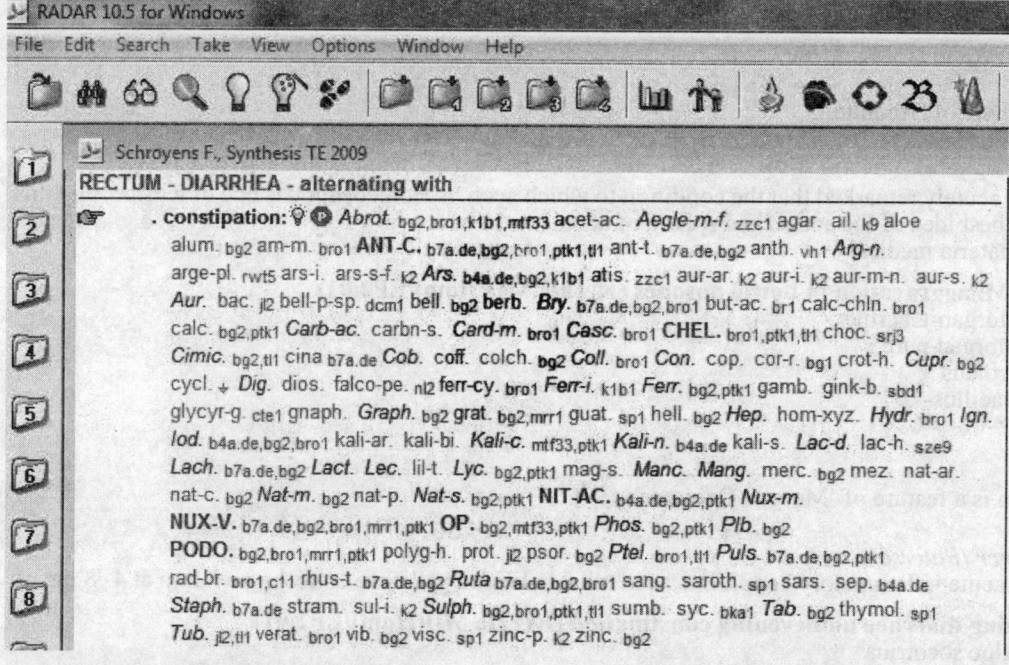

Temperaments - constipation - lymphatic persons disposed to, or to morning diarrhoea
sulph.c2
Ref: (RADAR 10)

Q. 242. Aversion to mother (Kerala MD(Hom)/EP2/01)
(a) Raphanus
(b) Silicea
(c) Causticum maculatum
(d) Thuja occidentalis

Ans. (d)
Note
The above feature belongs to 'Thuj.'.
Also see
Chapter – Mind – Aversion to Mother – 1: Thuj.
Ref: Repertory – Synthesis

Q. 243. Back-ache is relieved by lying on abdomen. One drug is aceticum acidum; another is (Kerala MD(Hom)/EP2/01)
    (a)   Natricum muraticum
    (b)   Medorrhinum
    (c)   Kalium carbonicum
    (d)   Tuberculinum

Ans. NA
Note
Use your discretion.
Also see

> English Kent

BACK - PAIN - lying, - abdomen,on - amel.
Acet-ac.$_k$ chel.$_k$ mag-c.$_k$ Nit-ac.$_k$ sel.$_k$

Aceticum acidum
Cannot sleep lying on the back (sleeps better on back Ars.); sensation of sinking in abdomen causing dyspnea; rests better lying on belly (Am-c.).
Ref: Allen's Key Notes
Discussion
The backache is better by lying on abdomen the reference from acet-ac. is am-c., however the choice is given in (c) is Kalium carbonicum which appears to be a typhographical mistake. Therefore, the choice given does not corroborate.

Q. 244. Slow in learning to walk and talk due to sluggish development of mind (Kerala MD(Hom)/EP2/01):
    (a)   Agaricus muscarius
    (b)   Calcarea carbonicum
    (c)   Aethusa cynapium
    (d)   Baryta carbonicum

Ans. NA
Note
Use your discretion.
Also see
Agaricus
Morose, self-willed, stubborn, slow in learning to walk and talk.
Ref: Clarke materia medica

Calcarea carbonicum
Psoric constitutions; pale, weak, timid, easily tird when walking. Disposed to grow fat, corpulent, and unwieldy. Children with red face, flabby muscles, who sweat easily and take cold readily in consequence. Large heads and abdomens; fontanelles and sutures open; bones soft, develop very slowly. Curvature of bones, especially spine and long bones; extremities crooked, deformed; bones irregularly developed. Diseases: arising from defective assimilation; imperfect ossification; difficulty in learning to walk or stand; children have no disposition to walk and will not try; suppressed sweat.
Ref: Allen's Key Notes

Aethusa
Children who cannot bear milk. Great weakness: children cannot stand; unable to hold up the head [Abort.]; prostration with sleepiness. Idiocy in children : incapacity to think; confused.
Ref: Allen's Key Notes

Baryta carbonicum
Especially adapted to complaints to first and second childhood; the psoric or tubercular. Memory deficient; forgetful, inattentive; child cannot be taught for it cannot remember; threatened idiocy. Scrofulous, dwarfish

children who do not grow [children who grow too rapidly, Calc.]; scrofulous ophthalmia, cornea opaque; abdomen swollen; frequent attacks of colic; face bloated; general emaciation. Children both physically and mentally weak. Dwarfish.
Ref: Allen's Key Notes

Extended information

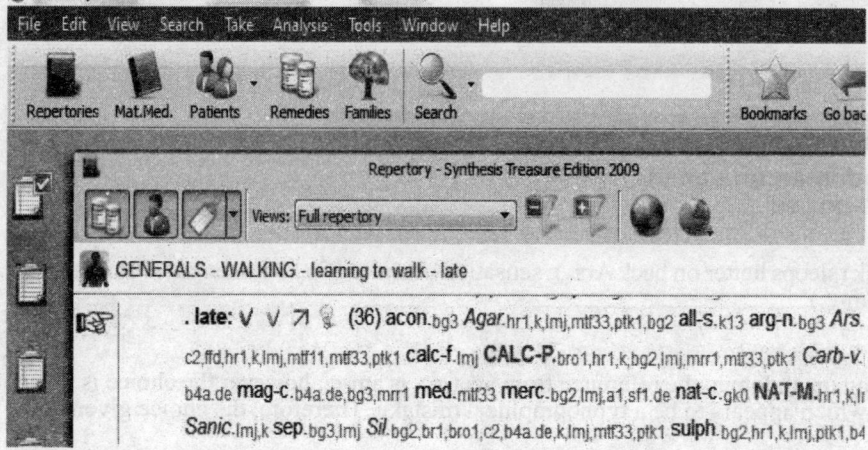

Ref: Synthesis / Radar 10

Q. 245. Marasmus with retracted abdomen (Kerala MD(Hom)/EP2/01)
    (a)   Abrotanum
    (b)   Natrium muriaticum
    (c)   Calcarea carbonicum
    (d)   Calcarea phosphoricum

Ans. (d)
Note
Above feature is in favour of Calc-p.

Also see
a. *Abrotanum*
Marasmus of children with marked emaciation, especially of legs (Iod. Sanic. , Tub.); the skin is flabby and hangs loose in folds (of neck, Nat-m., Sanic.). In marasmus, head weak, cannot hold it up (Aeth.). Marasmus of lower extremities only. Ravenous hunger; losing flesh while eating well (Iod., Nat-m., Sanic. , Tub.).
Ref: Allen's Key Notes

b. *Natrium muriaticum*
Great emaciation; losing flesh while living well (Abrot., Iod.); throat and neck of children emaciate rapidly during summer complaint (Sanic.).
Ref: Allen's Key Notes

c. *Calcarea carbonicum*
Disposed to grow fat, corpulent, unwieldy. Children with red face, flabby muscles, who sweat easily and take cold readily in consequence. Large heads and abdomens; fontanelles and sutures open; bones soft, develop very slowly.
Ref: Allen's Key Notes

d. *Calcarea phosphoricum*
Children: emaciated, unable to stand; slow in learning to walk (Calc., Sil.); sunken, flabby abdomen.
Ref: Allen's Key Notes

MCQ's in Materia Medica

Q. 246. Angry at trifles and perfectly harmless things, but is soon sorry for it (Kerala MD(Hom)/EP2/01)
- (a) Natrium muriaticum
- (b) Ignitia amara
- (c) Chamomilla
- (d) Mezereum

Ans. (d)

Note
Above features are in favour of 'Mezereum'.

Also see
Mezereum
Hypochondriacal and despondent; indifferent to everything and every one; angry at trifles and perfectly harmless things, but is soon sorry for it.
Ref: Allen's Key Notes

Q. 247. Asthma worse in foggy weather as per Boericke (Kerala MD(Hom)/EP2/01)
- (a) Natrium sulphuricum
- (b) Dulcamara
- (c) Rhus toxicodendron
- (d) Hypericum

Ans. (d)

Note
Above feature in found in 'Hypericum'.

Also see
Hypericum
Respiration: Asthma worse foggy weather and relieved by profuse perspiration.
Ref: Allen's Key Notes

Q. 248. Complaints from eating melons and drinking impure water as per Boericke (Kerala MD(Hom)/EP2/01)
- (a) Zingiber
- (b) Pyrogenium
- (c) Dulcamara
- (d) Natrium sulphuricum

Ans. (a)

Note
Above feature is found in 'Zingiber'.

Also see
Zingiber
Complains form eating melons and drinking impure water.
Ref: Boericke's materia medica

Q. 249. Calcarea carbonicum and Baryta carbonicum - Drug relation (Kerala MD(Hom)/EP2/01):
- (a) Concordant
- (b) Incompatible
- (c) Antidote
- (d) Complementary

Ans. (b)

Note
Baryta carbonicum
Incompatible: after Calc. in scrofulous affections.
Allen's Key Notes

Baryta carbonicum
Relationship: Incompatible: Calc.
Ref: Boericke's materia medica

Q. 250. All acid drugs are thirstless except (Kerala MD(Hom)/Entr/Paper 2-2001)
    (a)   Acidum picricum
    (b)   Lactis acidum
    (c)   Oxalicum acidum
    (d)   Aceticum acidum

Ans. NA
Note
Use your discretion
All acid drugs are thirstless except 'Aceticun acidum'.
Also see
Acidum picricum
Stomach; Bitter taste; with thirst. Aversion to food. Vomits suddenly, without warning; vomits bright yellow, bitter.
Phatak materia medica
Lactis acidum
This acid is found in buttermilk and is a valuable remedy for morning sickness, diabetes, rheumatic affections; breast troubles. It is suitable to anaemic, pale women. Nausea; on waking better by eating; in diabetes or pregnancy. Thirst.
Phatak materia medica
Oxalicum acidum
Mouth; Tongue swollen, sensitive, red, dry, burning, swollen, with thick, white coating. Tongue coated white, with nausea, thirst, and loss of taste. Sour taste in mouth. In mouth, pain, accumulation of saliva, water, or mucus.
Ref: Clarke's materia medica
Aceticum acidum
Thirst: intense, burning, insatiable even for large quantities in dropsy, diabetes, chronic diarrhea; but no thirst in fever.
Ref: Boericke's materia medica
Also see

English Kent

STOMACH - THIRSTLESS
acet-ac., *Aesc.*$_k$ agar.$_k$ *Agn.*$_k$ all-c.$_k$ ambr.$_k$ am-c.$_k$ *Am-m.*$_k$ *Ant-c.*$_k$ **ANT-T.**$_k$ **APIS**$_k$ *Arg-n.*$_k$ Ars.$_k$ Asaf.$_k$ Bell.$_k$ *Bov.*$_k$ brom.$_k$ bry.$_k$ bufo$_k$ calad.$_k$ *Camph.*$_k$ canth.$_k$ caps.$_k$ caust.$_k$ chel.$_k$ **CHIN**.$_k$ cimic.$_k$ cocc.$_k$ **COLCH**.$_k$ *Con.*$_k$ cor-r.$_k$ crot-t.$_k$ *Cycl.*$_k$ dios.$_k$ euph.$_k$ *Ferr.*$_k$ ferr-ar.$_k$ ferr-m.$_k$ gamb.$_k$ **GELS**.$_k$ ham.$_k$ **HELL**.$_k$ hep.$_k$ *Hydr-ac.*$_k$ ign.$_k$ indg.$_k$ *Ip.*$_k$ iris$_k$ kali-ar.$_k$ *Kali-c.*$_k$ kali-p.$_k$ led.$_k$ *Lyc.*$_k$ *Mang.*$_k$ **MENY**.$_k$ merc-c.$_k$ mez.$_k$ mur-ac.$_k$ nat-act.$_k$ nat-c.$_k$ nat-m.$_k$ nat-s.$_k$ nit-ac.$_k$ **NUX-M**.$_k$ nux-v.$_k$ *Olnd.*$_k$ onos.$_k$ *Op.*$_k$ ox-ac.$_k$ petr.$_k$ **PH-AC**.$_k$ phos.$_k$ plat.$_k$ ptel.$_k$ **PULS**.$_k$ **SABAD**.$_k$ *Samb.*$_k$ sars.$_k$ *Sep.*$_k$ spig.$_k$ *Staph.*$_k$ stram.$_k$ sulph.$_k$ tab.$_k$ thuj.$_k$ valer.$_k$ verat.$_k$
Ref: (RADAR 10)

Q. 251. 3 P.M. and 3 A.M. aggravation - drug is (Kerala MD(Hom)/Entr/Paper-2-01)
    (a)   Pulsatilla nigricans
    (b)   Apis mellifica
    (c)   Kalium carbonicum
    (d)   Thuja occidentalis

Ans. (d)
Note
Thuja
Aggravation: At night; from heat of bed; at 3 A. M. and 3 P. M.; from cold, damp air; narcotics.
Ref: Boericke's materia medica

Q. 252. Cough is better by lying down and aggravated in day time (Kerala MD(Hom)/Entr/Paper-2-01)
      (a)   Hyoscyamus niger
      (b)   Medorrhinum
      (c)   Pulsatilla nigricans
      (d)   Manganum aceticum

Ans. (d)

Note
The symptoms are in favour of 'Manganum'.

Also see
Hyos.
Cough: dry, nocturnal, spasmodic; < when lying down, relieved by sitting up [Dros.]; < at night, after eating, drinking, talking, singing [Dros., Phos. -> when lying down, Mang-m.].
Ref: Allen's Key Notes
Med.
Cough: dry, incessant, severe; painful, as if mucous membrane was torn from larynx; deep, hollow, like coughing in a barrel; < at night, from sweets, on lying down; > by lying on stomach.
Ref: Allen's Key Notes
Puls.
Dry cough in evening and at night; must sit up in bed to get relief; and loose cough in the morning; with copious mucous expectoration.
Ref: Boericke's materia medica
Mang.
There is one curious symptom they have in common: Cough better by lying down. If there is any difference, the Mang cough is more apt to be deep, and it is also worse in damp weather.
Ref: Clarke's materia medica

Extended information

English Kent

COUGH - DAYTIME - only
Am-c.$_k$ Arg-met.$_k$ brom.$_k$ *Calc.*$_k$ chin.$_k$ cic.$_k$ dulc.$_k$ **EUPHR.**$_k$ *Ferr.*$_k$ graph.$_k$ hep.$_k$ kali-n.$_k$ *Lach.*$_k$ laur.$_k$ lyc.$_k$ *Mang.*$_k$ merc.$_k$ nit-ac.$_k$ nux-m.$_k$ *Phos.*$_k$ *Rumx.*$_k$ sep.$_k$ sin-n.$_k$ stann.$_k$ *Staph.*$_k$ thuj.$_k$ viol-o.$_k$

English Kent

COUGH - DRY - lying,while - amel.
am-c.$_k$ **MANG.**$_k$ sep.$_k$ zinc.$_k$
Ref: Kent's repertory (RADAR 10)

Q. 253. The pains are tearing and aching - the seat of the disease is (Kerala MD(Hom)/Entr/Paper- 2-01)
      (a)   Serous membranes
      (b)   Mucous membrane
      (c)   Tendons
      (d)   Muscles

Ans. (d)

Note
For tearing and aching pain the seat of the disease is tendons.

Q. 254. A 52 year old man, senior executive with sedentary habits, fond of eating good food and drinking alcohol, complains of pain in back in lumbar region. The pain is felt more at night while lying in bed. He must sit up to turn over. What is the remedy? (UPSC-06)
      (a)   Nux vomica
      (b)   Rhus toxicodendron
      (c)   Staphysagria
      (d)   Sulphur

Ans. (a)

Note
The most suitable remedy in above case is 'Nux vomica'.

Also see
The patient characteristics here are in tune with Nux vomica. (However these features are precipitating factors to Coronary Artery Disease and Gouty arthritis. However, here these are pointing to the lifestyle of Nux vomica patient). The pain in the lumbar region and worse at night lying in bed and that he must sit up and turn over – in a way point to the Rhus Tox. However, this symptom is a distracter here.

Extended information
Back – Pain: Turning: in bed: Must sit up to turn over – two medicines come –1: Kali-p and 3: Nux-v.
Therefore, the answer is Nux-v.
Ref: Kent's Repertory

Q. 255. A very gentle and soft spoken lady tearfully complaints of wandering pain in both the extremities. Since her puberty she lived with chill feeling, thirstlessness and a sense of comfort in an open area outside the room. Which one of the following is the indicated remedy? (UPSC-06)
    (a)   Sepia
    (b)   Pulsatilla
    (c)   Platina
    (d)   Kalium bichromicum

Ans. (b)

Note
The above clinical presentation is in favour of 'Puls'.

Also see
Synthesis based on information given in the MCQ is as under:
The opening lines- 'A very gentle and soft spoken lady tearfully complaints' is strongly suggestive of the constitutional type of the pulsatilla lady. Then comes – 'complaint of wandering pains in both the extremities' – the pulsatilla complaints are always shifting and changing location. The further narration goes, since her puberty (it is the onset of her complaints which dates back to the onset of puberty – typical of Puls.) she lived with chill feeling, (Typically puls is a chilly patient) thirstlessness (once again the Puls. is a thirstless subject) and a sense of comfort in an open area outside the room (the Pulsatilla subject is better in open air – step by step the narration goes in favour of one and only drug the Pulsatilla.).

Extended information
Compare with the choice given above

Sepia
Adapted to persons of dark hair, rigid fiber, but mild and easy disposition (Puls.). Diseases of women; especially those occurring during pregnancy; childbed and lactation; or diseases attended with sudden prostration and sinking faintness (Murx., Nux-m.); "the washerwoman's remedy," complaints that are brought on by or aggravated after laundry work. Pains extend from other parts of the back (rev. of, Sab.); are attended with shuddering (with chilliness, Puls.). Particularly sensitive to cold air, "chills so easily"; lack of vital heat, especially in chronic diseases.
Ref: Allen's Key Notes

Comment
There are many similarities with Sepia but these are very superficial.

Platina
Adapted to women, dark hair, rigid fibre; thin of a sanguine temperament; who suffer from too early and too profuse menses. Sexual organs exceedingly sensitive; cannot bear the napkin to touch her; will go into spasms from an examination; vulva painfully sensitive during coitus; will faint during, or cannot endure, coitus (compare, Murx., Orig.). The pains increase gradually and as gradually decrease (Stann.); are attended with numbness of parts (Cham.). For hysterical patients, alternately gay and sad, who cry easily (Croc, Ign., Puls.); pale, easily fatigued. Arrogant, proud, contemptuous, and haughty; pitiful "looking down" upon people.
Ref: Allen's Key Notes

Comment
It differs from Pulsatilla in the temperament.

Kali-bi.
Fat, light-haired persons who suffer from catarrhal syphilitic or psoric affections. Fat, chubby, short-necked children disposed to croup and croupy affections. Affections of the mucous membranes - eyes, nose, mouth, throat, bronchi; gastro-intestinal and genito-urinary tracts - discharge of a tough, stringy mucous which adheres to the parts and can be drawn into long strings (compare, Hydr., Lys.). Complaints occurring in hot weather. Liability to take cold in open air. Rheumatism alternating with gastric symptoms, one appearing in the fall and the other in the spring; rheumatism and dysentery alternate (Abrot.). Pains: in small spots, can be covered with point of finger (Ign.); shift rapidly from one part to another (Kali-s., Lac-c., Puls.); appear and disappear suddenly (Bell., Ign., Mag-p.).
Ref: Allen's Key Notes

Comment
It is very much different from pulsatilla in the modality as well as the pains.

Q. 256. Women complaints of swollen painful breasts before the onset of menses. The pain gets better after the appearance of menstrual flow, but is worst least jar. She dreams of snakes, what is the remedy? (UPSC-06)
    (a)   Calcarea carbonicum
    (b)   Lac caninum
    (c)   Conium maculatum
    (d)   Mercurius solubilis

Ans. (b)
Note
The above presenting features are suggestive of 'Lac-c'.
Also see
The important remedies covering the symptom- "Swollen painful breast before the onset of menses" – include; Calc, Lac-c., Con. from the above list.
Reference from the Kent's repertory:
-Chest – Swelling: Mammae: Menses Before: 2: Calc, 1: Con, 1: Kali-c., 1: Kali-s., 2: Lac-c., 1: Murx. 2: Tub).
-Chest: Pain: Mammae: Menses Before: 3:Calc., 3:Con., 1: Kali-c., 2: Lac-c., 1: Nux-v., 1: Sang. 1: Spong.
Compare:
Calc
Hot swelling breasts. Breasts tender and swollen before menses. Agg: from exertion, mental or physical; ascending; cold in every form; water, washing, moist air, wet weather; during full moon; standing.
Ref: Boericke's materia medica

Lac-c.
Breasts swollen; painful before (Calc.; Con.; Puls.) and better on appearance of menses. Mastitis; Worse least jar. Sleep: Dreams of snakes.
Ref: Boericke's Materia Medica

Q. 257. "Over-sensitiveness of nerves, scratching of linen or silk, crackling of paper is unbearable" is a characteristic of which one of the following? (UPSC-06)
    (a)   Arnica montana
    (b)   Asarum europaeum
    (c)   Antimonium crudum
    (d)   Arum triphyllum

Ans. (b)
Note
The above clinical presentation is suggestive of 'Asar'.
Also see
Arnica montana
Nervous, cannot bear pain; whole body over-sensitive. Everything on which he lies seems too hard. It is especially suited to cases when any injury, however remote, seems to have caused the present trouble. Gout

and rheumatism, with great fear of being touched or struck by persons coming near him.
Ref: Allen's Key Notes

Asarum europaeum
A remedy for nervous affections, loss of energy, with excessive erethism. Scratching on silk or linen or paper unbearable.
Ref: Boericke's materia medica

Antimonium crudum
Excessive irritability and fretfulness, together with a thickly-coated white tongue, are true guiding symptoms to many forms of disease calling for this remedy. All the conditions are aggravated by heat and cold bathing. Cannot bear heat of sun. Tendency to grow fat. An absence of pain, where it could be expected, is noticeable.
Ref: Boericke's materia medica

Arum triphyllum
Inflammation of mucous surfaces and destruction of tissue. 'Acridity' is the keynote of Arum.
Ref: Boericke's materia medica

Q. 258. Which one of the following is true in respect of Abrotanum? (UPSC-06)
- (a) Marasmus of upper extremities only
- (b) Marasmus of lower extremities
- (c) Emaciation of neck
- (d) Emaciation of breast

Ans. (b)

Note
From the above true statement in respect of 'Abrotanum' is 'Marasmus of lower extremities'.

Also see
Abrotanum
A very useful remedy in marasmus, especially of lower extremities only, yet with good appetite.
Ref: Boericke's Materia Medica.

Extended information
Additional references from Repertory:
Emaciation of upper extremity: Repertory – Boenninghausen – Chapter: upper extremity – Symptom – Emaciation – Plb met.
Emaciation of Neck; Emaciation most notable in neck. – Nat-m.
Ref: Boericke's materia medica
Emaciation of Breast: Repertory –Allen – Mamma – Emaciation – Con., Frag., Hall, Iod, Kali-i, Kreos.

Q. 259. Match the List I with List II and select the correct answer using the code given below the lists (UPSC-06)

List- I (Symptom)	List-II (Medicine)
A. Insatiable thirst before and during chill and fever	1. Lilium tigrinum
B. Must keep busy to repress sexual desire	2. Bromium
C. Physometra	3. Bryonia alba
D. Vicarious menstruation	4. Eupatorium perfoliatum

Code

	A	B	C	D
(a)	3	2	1	4
(b)	4	1	2	3
(c)	3	1	2	4
(d)	4	2	1	3

Ans. (b)

Note
The correct match is as under:

List- I (Symptom)	List-II (Medicine)
A. Insatiable thirst before and during chill and fever	4. Eupatorium perfoliatum
B. Must keep busy to repress sexual desire	1. Lilium tigrinum
C. Physometra	2. Bromium
D. Vicarious menstruation	3. Bryonia alba

Also see
Lilium tigrinum
Disposed to curse, strike, to think obscene things (Anac., Lac-c.); alternates with uterine irritation. Listless, yet cannot sit still; restless, yet does not want to walk; must keep busy to repress sexual desire.
Ref: Allen's Key Notes

Bromium
Physometra; loud emission of flatus from the vagina (Lyc.); membranous dysmenorrhea (Lac-c.).
Ref: Allen's Key Notes

Bryonia
Vicarious menstruation; nosebleed when menses should appear (Phos.) blood spitting, or hemoptysis.
Ref: Allen's Key Notes

Eupatorium perfoliatum
Insatiable thirst before and during chill and fever; knows chill is coming because he cannot drink enough.
Ref: Allen's Key Notes

Q. 260. "Thirsty in dropsy, but thirstless in fever" is a symptom of which one of the following? (UPSC-06)
  (a) Aceticum acidum
  (b) Apis mellifica
  (c) China officinalis
  (d) Pulsatilla nigricans

Ans. (a)
Note
"Thirsty in dropsy, but thirstless in fever" is a symptom of 'Aceticum acidum'.
Also see
Aceticum acidum
Thirst: intense, burning, insatiable even for large quantities in dropsy, diabetes, chronic diarrhea; but no thirst in fever.
Ref: Allen's Key-Notes.

Apis mellifica
Thirst: Thirstlessness; in anasarca; ascites.
Ref: Allen's Key-Note.

China officinalis
Thirst: Intermittent, paroxysms anticipate; return every week. All stages well marked. Chill generally in forenoon, commencing in breast; thirst before chill, and little and often.
Ref: Boericke materia medica

Pulsatilla nigricans
Thirst: thirstlessness with nearly all complaints. Great dryness of mouth in morning, without thirst.
Ref: Allen's Key-Notes.

Q. 261. "Great sadness and weeping. Dread of being alone, of men, of meeting friends; with uterine troubles" is a symptom of which of the following? (UPSC-06)
    (a)   Sepia officinalis
    (b)   Pulsatilla nigricans
    (c)   Selenium
    (d)   Aconitum napellus

Ans. (a)

Note
The above symptoms are suggestive for 'Sepia'.

Also see
Sepia
Great sadness and weeping. Dread of being alone, of men; of meeting friends; with uterine troubles. Indifferent: even to one's family, to one's occupation (Fl-ac., Ph-ac.); to those whom she loves best.
Ref: Allen's Key Notes

Pulsatilla
Easily moved to laughter or tears; affectionate, mild, gentle, timid, yielding disposition. Weeps easily: almost impossible to detail her ailments without weeping (weeps when thanked, Lyc.).
Ref: Allen's Key Notes

Selenium
Very forgetful in business, but during sleep dreams of what he had forgotten.
Ref: Allen's Key Notes

Aconite
Great fear and anxiety of mind, with great nervous excitability; afraid to go out, to go into a crowd where there is any excitement or many people; to cross the street.
Ref: Allen's Key Notes

Q. 262. "Consolation aggravates" is not a symptom of which one of the following (UPSC-06)
    (a)   Sepia
    (b)   Lilium tigrinum
    (c)   Silicea
    (d)   Pulsatilla

Ans. (d)

Note
"Consolation aggravates" is not a symptom of 'Pulsatilla'.

Also see
Mind – Consolation Agg:
2:Ars, 2:Bell, 2:Calc-p., 2:Hell, 3:IGN, 2: Lil-t., 3:Nat-m., 2:Plat, 3:SIL.
Ref: Kent's Repertory
Mind – Consolation Ame:
2:Puls.
Ref: Kent's Repertory
Please take note of the language – 'Consolation aggravates' - The Pulsatilla is the one which is better by consolation. Others do not.

Sepia
It is a distracter here.

Lilium tigrinum
Worse by consolation.

Silicea
Worse by consolation.

Pulsatilla
Better by consolation.

Q. 263. Match List I with List II and select the correct answer using the code given below the lists (UPSC-06)

List-I (Desires)	List-II (Drugs)
A. Sweet	1. Hepar sulphuricum
B. Salt	2. Antimonium tartaricum
C. Sour	3. Argentum nitricum
D. Apple	4. Natrium muriaticum

Code:

	A	B	C	D
(a)	3	4	1	2
(b)	2	1	4	3
(c)	3	1	2	4
(d)	2	4	1	3

Ans. (a)

List-I (Desires)	List-II (Drugs)
A. Sweet	3. Argentum nitricum
B. Salt	4. Natruim muriaticum
C. Sour	1. Hepar sulphuricum
D. Apple	2. Antimonium tartaricum

Note
The correct code is as under:

Also see
Argentum nitricum
Craves sugar; child is fond of it, but diarrhea results from eating (craves salt or smoked meat, Calc-p.).
Ref: Allen's Key Notes
Natrium muriaticum
Craving for salt (Calc., Caust.); great aversion to bread.
Ref: Allen's Key Notes
Hepar sulphuricum
Desire for sour: Not given.
Ref: Allen's Key Notes
Longing acids, wine and strong testing food.
Ref: Boericke's materia medica
Antimonium tartaricum
Desire for apples, fruits, and acids generally.
Ref: Boericke's materia medica

Extended information

🔖 **English Kent**

STOMACH - DESIRES - sour,acids,etc.
alumn.ₖ alum.ₖ am-c.ₖ am-m.ₖ *Ant-c.*ₖ *Ant-t.*ₖ *Apis*ₖ arg-n.ₖ *Arn.*ₖ *Ars.*ₖ arund.ₖ bell.ₖ bol-la.ₖ *Borx.*ₖ *Brom.*ₖ *Bry.*ₖ *Calc.*ₖ calc-s.ₖ carb-an.ₖ carbn-s.ₖ *Carb-v.*ₖ *Cham.*ₖ chel.ₖ chin.ₖ chinin-ar.ₖ *Cist.*ₖ *Con.*ₖ conv.ₖ **COR-R.**ₖ corn.ₖ cub.ₖ cupr.ₖ dig.ₖ elapsₖ *Ferr.*ₖ ferr-ar.ₖ *Ferr-m.*ₖ ferr-p.ₖ *Fl-ac.*ₖ gran.ₖ **HEP.**ₖ

hipp., *Ign.*, *Kali-ar.*, kali-bi., *Kali-c.*, kali-p., kali-s., kreos., *Lach.*, *Mag-c.*, mang., *Med.*, merc-i-f., Nat-m., phel., *Phos.*, plb., *Podo.*, psor., ptel., *Puls.*, rhus-t., *Sabad.*, Sabin., Sec., Sep., Squil., Stram., *Sulph.*, Sul-i., thea, ther., thuj., ust., **VERAT.**, ziz.,
Ref: RADAR 10

Q. 264. The symptoms are "Mastitis after delivery, breasts very hard, like a cake, swollen hot and painful with fever. Every time the child nurses, the pains spread all over the body from nipples". What is the remedy? (UPSC-06)
   (a)   Belladonna
   (b)   Bryonia alba
   (c)   Conium maculatum
   (d)   Phytolacca

Ans. (d)
Note
The remedy for above symptoms syndrome is 'Phytolacca'.
Also see
Belladonna
Mastitis pain, throbbing, redness, streaks radiate from nipple. Breasts feel heavy; are hard and red.
Ref: Allen's Key-Notes.
Bryonia alba
Mammae heavy, of a stony hardness; pale but hard; hot and painful; must support the breasts (Phyt.).
Ref: Allen's Key-Notes.
Conium maculatum
Glandular induration of stony hardness; of mammae and testicles in persons of cancerous tendency; after bruises and injuries of glands (compare, Aster.). Breasts sore, hard and painful before and during menstruation (Lac-c., Kali-c.).
Ref: Allen's Key-Notes.
Phytolacca
Breast, shows an early tendency to cake; is full; stony, hard and painful, especially when suppuration is inevitable; when child nurses pain goes from nipple all over body (goes to back, Crot-t.; to uterus, Plus., Sil.).
Ref: Allen's Key Notes
Mastitis: mammae hard and very sensitive. Tumors of the breasts with enlarged axillary glands. Cancer of breast. Breast is hard, painful and of purple hue. Mammary abscess. When child nurses, pain goes from nipple all over body.
Ref: Boericke's materia medica

Q. 265. A 25 year old man comes with a complaint of dry cough for about two weeks. Cough is much aggravated at night, but he feels better by lying on the stomach with face down and with protruding tongue. Which is the remedy? (UPSC-06)
   (a)   Ammonium carbonicum
   (b)   Causticum
   (c)   Medorrhinum
   (d)   Phosphorus

Ans. (c)
Note
The above clinical presenatation is in favour of 'Medorrhinum'.
Also see
Ammonium carbonicum
Dyspnea with palpitation, worse by exertion or on ascending even a few steps; worse in a warm room. One of the best remedies in emphysema. Cough: dry, from tickling in throat as from dust every morning from 3 to 4 A. M.
Ref: Allen's Key-Notes.

Causticum
Cough: with rawness and soreness in chest; with inability to expectorate, sputa must be swallowed (Arn., Kali-c.); relieved by swallow of cold water; on expiration (Acon.); with pain in hips; remaining after pertussis; with expectoration chiefly at night.

Ref: Allen's Key-Notes.

Medorrhinum
Asthma: choking caused by a weakness of spasm of epiglottis; larynx stopped so that no air could enter, only > by lying on face and protruding tongue.

Ref: Allen's Key-Notes.

Phosphorus
Cough: going from warm to cold air (rev. of, Bry.); < from laughing, talking, reading, drinking, eating, lying on the left side (Dros., Stan.).

Ref: Allen's Key-Notes.

Q. 266. A patient suffering from painless diarrhea, coming out of bed early in the morning. Which one of the following is the indicated remedy? (UPSC-06)
    (a) Sulphur
    (b) Kalium sulphuricum
    (c) Podophyllum
    (d) Argentum nitricum

Ans. (a)

Note
In above cinical presentation 'Sulphur' is indicated remdy.

Also see
Sulphur
Diarrhea: after midnight; painless; driving out of bed early in the morning (Aloe, Psor.); as if the bowels were too weak to retain their contents. Constipation: stools hard, knotty, dry, as if burnt (Bry.); large painful, child is afraid to have the stool on account of pain, or pain compels the child to desist on first effort; alternating with diarrhea.

Ref: Allen's Key-Notes

Kalium sulphuricum
Colicky pains; abdomen feels cold to touch; tympanitic, tense. Yellow, slimy diarrhea.

Ref: Boericke's materia medica

Podophyllum
Diarrhea: of long standing; early in morning, continues through forenoon, followed by natural stool in evening (Aloe), and accompanied by sensation of weakness or sinking in abdomen or rectum. Diarrhea of children: during teething: after eating; while being bathed or washed; of dirty water soaking napkin through (Benz-ac); with gagging. Stool: green, watery, foetid, profuse (Calc.); gushing out (Gamb., Jat., Phos); chalk-like, jelly-like (Aloe) undigested (Cinch., Ferr); yellow meal- like sediment; prolapse of rectum before or with stool.

Ref: Allen's Key-Notes

Argentum nitricum
Diarrhea; green mucous, like chopped spinach in flakes; turning green after remaining on diaper; after drinking; after eating candy or sugar; masses of muco-lymph in shreddy strips or lumps (Asar); with much noisy flatus (Aloe). Diarrhea as soon as he drinks (Ars, Crot-t., Thro.).

Ref: Allen's Key-Notes.

Q. 267. 'Presence of others, even the nurse is unbearable during stool, with frequent, ineffectual desire which makes her anxious' is a characteristic feature of which one of the following? (UPSC-06)
    (a) Alumina
    (b) Aloe socotrina
    (c) Ambra grisea
    (d) Actaea racemosa

Ans. (c)

Note
The above presentation is a characteristic feature of 'Ambra grisea.

Also see
Ambra grisea
One thing running through this remedy is that the presence of other persons aggravates the symptoms; also the marked aggravation from conversation. A woman, when attended by a nurse, is unable to have a stool without sending the nurse into another room. In spite of much straining she can do nothing unless alone.
Ref: Kent's materia medica

Natrium muriaticum
It is said that in Natrium muriaticum; the patient cannot urinate in the presence of other persons. The urine will not start when anyone is around.
Ref: Kent's materia medica

Alumina
Diarrhea when she urinates. Has to strain at stool in order to urinate.
Ref: Allen's Key-Notes

Aloes
Diarrhea : has to hurry to closet immediately after eating and drinking (Crot-t.); with want of confidence in sphincter ani; driving out of bed early in the morning. When passing flatus, sensation as if stool would pass with it (Olean., Mur-ac., Nat-m.).
Ref: Allen's Key-Notes

Q. 268. A patient is suffering from tonsillitis with very offensive smell from the mouth. He can swallow liquid food, but solid food causes choking with no pain in throat. Which one of the following is the likely remedy? (UPSC-06)
    (a)   Phytolacca
    (b)   Mercurius solubilis
    (c)   Baptisia tinctoria
    (d)   Baryta carbonica

Ans. (c)

Note
The above features are in suggestive of 'Baptisia-tinctoria'.

Also see
Phytolacca
Sore throat; of a dark red color; uvula large, dropsical, almost translucent (Kali-bi., Rhus-t.). Diphtheria: pains shoot from throat into ears on swallowing; great pain at root of tongue when swallowing burning as from a coal of fire or a red-hot iron; dryness; difficult to swallow with trembling of the hands; sensation of a lump in the throat with continuous desire to swallow; tonsils, uvula and back part of the throat covered with ash-colored membrane; cannot drink hot fluids (Lach.). Carotid and submaxillary glands indurated after diphtheria.
Ref: Allen's Key-Note.

Mercurius solubilis
Tonsils enlarged. As if something rising in the throat, with desire to swallow it down. Offensive, putrid odour from mouth. Painful ragged, swollen, bleeding gums. Gumboil teeth; hollow, black; pain worse heat and cold, night; feel tender and elongated. Aphthae. Salive; increased; flows during sleep; yellow; bloody, bad tasting, offensive. Tongue; broad, flabby, yellow, Indented; needle pricks at tip. Furrow across upper portion of the tongue; with pricking. Sweetish, metallic taste.
Ref: Phatak's materia medica

Baptisia tinctoria
All exhalations and discharges fetid, especially in typhoid or other acute diseases; (Compare the tonsillitis with offensive breath). Can swallow liquids only (Bar-c); least solid food gags (can swallow liquids only, but has aversion to them, Sil). Painless sore throat; tonsils, soft palate and parotids dark red, swollen; putrid, offensive discharge (Diph).
Ref: Allen's Key-Note.

MCQ's in Materia Medica

Baryta carbonica
Persons subjects to quinsy, take cold easily, or with every, even the least, cold have an attack of tonsillitis, prone to suppuration (Hep., Psor.). Inability to swallow anything but liquids (Bap., Sil).
Ref: Allen's Key-Note.

Q. 269. An 18 year old girl, unmarried, complaints of having missed periods for about two months. Menstrual cycle has been irregular since menarche. She has increased frequency of urination, more at night. She gets frequent attacks of sore throat usually before menses. What is the remedy? (UPSC-06)
  (a) Kalium carbonicum
  (b) Natrium muriaticum
  (c) Pulsatilla nigricans
  (d) Sanicula

Ans. NA

Note
Use your discretion

Also see
The important components of above MCQ are as under:
An 18 year old girl, unmarried, complaints of having missed periods for about two months. Menstrual cycle has been irregular since menarche.

Suggestion for Pulsatilla
Especially in diseases of women and children. Women inclined to be fleshy, with scanty and protracted menstruation [Graph.]. The first serious impairment of health is referred to puberic age, have "never been well since"
Allen's Key Notes

Missed periods for about two months.

> English Kent

FEMALE GENITALIA - MENSES, - absent, amenorrhoea
Acon.$_k$ aesc.$_k$ agar.$_k$ agn.$_k$ alet.$_k$ *Am-c.*$_k$ am-m.$_k$ *Ant-c.*$_k$ *Apis*$_k$ *Apoc.*$_k$ arg-n.$_k$ *Ars.*$_k$ *Ars-i.*$_k$ **AUR.**$_k$ Bar-c.$_k$ *Bell.*$_k$ benz-ac.$_k$ berb.$_k$ *Borx.*$_k$ *Bry.*$_k$ *Calc.*$_k$ calc-s.$_k$ canth.$_k$ **CARBN-S.**$_k$ carb-v.$_k$ card-m.$_k$ *Caul.*$_k$ *Caust.*$_k$ *Cham.*$_k$ chel.$_k$ *Chin.*$_k$ chinin-ar.$_k$ cic.$_k$ cimic.$_k$ cina *Cocc.*$_k$ colch.$_k$ *Coll.*$_k$ *Coloc.*$_k$ **CON.**$_k$ croc.$_k$ crot-t.$_k$ *Cupr.*$_k$ *Cycl.*$_k$ dig.$_k$ *Dros.*$_k$ **DULC.**$_k$ euph.$_k$ **FERR.**$_k$ *Ferr-ar.*$_k$ **FERR-I.**$_k$ *Ferr-p.*$_k$ gels.$_k$ *Goss.*$_k$ **GRAPH.**$_k$ *Guaj.*$_k$ *Ham.*$_k$ *Hell.*$_k$ helon.$_k$ *Hyos.*$_k$ *Ign.*$_k$ *Iod.*$_k$ *Kali-ar.*$_k$ **KALI-C.**$_k$ kali-i.$_k$ *Kali-n.*$_k$ *Kali-p.*$_k$ kali-s.$_k$ *Lach.*$_k$ lil-t.$_k$ lob.$_k$ **LYC.**$_k$ *Mag-c.*$_k$ *Mag-m.*$_k$ *Merc.*$_k$ mill.$_k$ nat-c.$_k$ *Nat-m.*$_k$ nat-p.$_k$ *Nux-m.*$_k$ *Nux-v.*$_k$ ph-ac.$_k$ *Phos.*$_k$ *Plat.*$_k$ podo.$_k$ **PULS.**$_k$ *Rhus-t.*$_k$ *Sabad.*$_k$ sabin.$_k$ sang.$_k$ sec.$_k$ **SENEC.**$_k$ **SEP.**$_k$ **SIL.**$_k$ *Staph.*$_k$ stram.$_k$ **SULPH.**$_k$ **TUB.**$_k$ *Valer.*$_k$ verat.$_k$ verat-v.$_k$ xan.$_k$ *Zinc.*$_k$

Above is suggestive of : Puls., Sep.

Menstrual cycle has been irregular since menarche.

> English Kent

FEMALE GENITALIA - MENSES, - irregular
Apis$_k$ apoc.$_k$ aran.$_k$ *Arg-n.*$_k$ *Art-v.*$_k$ aur-m-n.$_k$ *Benz-ac.*$_k$ *Calc.*$_k$ calc-p.$_k$ calc-s.$_k$ *Carb-ac.*$_k$ carbn-s.$_k$ caul.$_k$ *Caust.*$_k$ chel.$_k$ *Cimic.*$_k$ *Cocc.*$_k$ *Con.*$_k$ cur.$_k$ cycl.$_k$ *Dig.*$_k$ ferr.$_k$ ferr-p.$_k$ ham.$_k$ hyos.$_k$ *Ign.*$_k$ *Iod.*$_k$ *Ip.*$_k$ *Iris*$_k$ kali-bi.$_k$ kali-p.$_k$ *Kreos.*$_k$ *Lac-d.*$_k$ *Lach.*$_k$ lil-t.$_k$ *Lyc.*$_k$ mag-c.$_k$ mag-m.$_k$ merc.$_k$ *Murx.*$_k$ *Nit-ac.*$_k$ **NUX-M.**$_k$ *Nux-v.*$_k$ oena.$_k$ op.$_k$ phos.$_k$ plb.$_k$ puls.$_k$ ruta$_k$ sabad.$_k$ **SEC.**$_k$ *Senec.*$_k$ *Sep.*$_k$ *Sil.*$_k$ *Staph.*$_k$ *Sulph.*$_k$ *Tub.*$_k$ ust.$_k$ verat.$_k$ vesp.$_k$ xan.$_k$

Above has important suggestions: Puls., Sep.

She has increased frequency of urination, more at night.

> English Kent

BLADDER-URINARY ORGANS - URGING to urinate (morbid desire) - night
agar.$_k$ *Alum.*$_k$ am-c.$_k$ anac.$_k$ ant-t.$_k$ apis$_k$ *Arn.*$_k$ *Ars.*$_k$ *Ars-i.*$_k$ *Aur-m.*$_k$ *Bell.*$_k$ *Borx.*$_k$ bry.$_k$ *Calc.*$_k$ carbn-s.$_k$

carb-v.$_k$ caust.$_k$ chim.$_k$ cina$_k$ clem.$_k$ *Con.*$_k$ croc.$_k$ cupr.$_k$ **DIG.**$_k$ equis-h.$_k$ *Ery-a.*$_k$ euphr.$_k$ *Graph.*$_k$ hep.$_k$ hyper.$_k$ iod.$_k$ kali-ar.$_k$ *Kali-bi.*$_k$ kali-c.$_k$ kali-p.$_k$ kali-s.$_k$ *Kreos.*$_k$ *Lach.*$_k$ **LYC.**$_k$ mag-c.$_k$ *Mag-m.*$_k$ med.$_k$ meph.$_k$ *Merc.*$_k$ mez.$_k$ mur-ac.$_k$ nat-act.$_k$ nat-c.$_k$ *Nat-m.*$_k$ nat-p.$_k$ nicc.$_k$ *Nit-ac.*$_k$ nux-m.$_k$ *Nux-v.*$_k$ petr.$_k$ ph-ac.$_k$ *Phos.*$_k$ puls.$_k$ *Rhus-t.*$_k$ sabin.$_k$ *Samb.*$_k$ sec.$_k$ sep.$_k$ **SIL.**$_k$ spig.$_k$ squil.$_k$ stram.$_k$ **SULPH.**$_k$ sul-ac.$_k$ syph.$_k$ tab.$_k$ *Thuj.*$_k$ zinc.$_k$

Suggestive of - Puls., Mag-c.

She gets frequent attacks of sore throat usually before menses.

THROAT INTERNAL - INFLAMMATION - menses, - before
Mag-c.$_k$

English Kent

THROAT INTERNAL - PAIN - menses, - before
lac-c.$_k$ *Mag-c.*$_k$

Suggestive of - Mag-c.

Repertory References are as under:
Kent-Genitalia female-Menses: absent, amenorrhea: 3:KALI-C, 2:Nat-m., 3:PULS.
Kent-Genitalia female-Menses: Irregular: 1:Puls.
Kent-Bladder-Urging to urinate (morbid desire): Night: 1:Kali-c., 2:Nat-m., 1:Puls,
Kent-Throat-Pain: Sore: Menses Before: 2:Lac-c., 2:Mag-c.

Comment:
-No single medicine is covering the all above symptoms therefore choice of correct medicine is difficult.

Q. 270. Match List I with List II and select the correct answer using the code given below the lists (UPSC-06)

List- I (Medicine)	List-II (Craving for Type of food)
A. Phosphorus	1. Bitter
B. Medorrhinum	2. Egg
C. Calcarea carbonicum	3. Sweet
D. Sepia	4. Salt

Code

	A	B	C	D
(a)	1	3	2	4
(b)	4	2	3	1
(c)	1	2	3	4
(d)	4	3	2	1

Ans. (d)

List- I (Medicine)	List-II (Craving for Type of food)
A. Phosphorus	4. Salt
B. Medorrhinum	3. Sweet
C. Calcarea carbonicum	2. Egg
D. Sepia	1. Bitter

Note
The correct match is as under:

Also see
Phosphorus
Desire for salt.
Ref: Allen's Key Notes

English Kent

STOMACH - DESIRES - salt things
Aloe.$_k$ **ARG-N.**$_k$ atro. Calc.$_k$ Calc-p.$_k$ calc-s. **CARB-V.**$_k$ Caust.$_k$ cocc. Con. Cor-r.$_k$ **LAC-C.**$_k$ Lyss.$_k$ Manc.$_k$ Med.$_k$ meph.$_k$ merc-i-f.$_k$ merc-i-r.$_k$ **NAT-M.**$_k$ Nit-ac.$_k$ **PHOS.**$_k$ Plb.$_k$ Sanic.$_k$ sel.$_k$ sulph.$_k$ Tarent.$_k$ teucr.$_k$ thuj.$_k$ tub.$_k$ **VERAT.**$_k$

Medorrhinum
Insatiate craving: for liquor, which before she hated (Asar.); for salt (Calc., Nat-m.); for sweets (Sulph.); for ale, ice, acids, oranges, green fruits.
Ref: Allen's Key Notes

English Kent

Am-c.$_k$ arg-met.$_k$ **ARG-N.**$_k$ ars.$_k$ bar-c.$_k$ Bry.$_k$ bufo$_k$ Calc.$_k$ Calc-s.$_k$ Carb-v.$_k$ **CHIN.**$_k$ chinin-ar.$_k$ Elaps$_k$ Ip.$_k$ kali-ar.$_k$ Kali-c.$_k$ kali-p.$_k$ Kali-s.$_k$ **LYC.**$_k$ Mag-m.$_k$ Med.$_k$ merc.$_k$ nat-act.$_k$ Nat-c.$_k$ nat-m.$_k$ nux-v.$_k$ op.$_k$ petr.$_k$ Plb.$_k$ Rheum.$_k$ Rhus-t.$_k$ Sabad.$_k$ Sec.$_k$ Sep.$_k$ **SULPH.**$_k$ Tub.$_k$

Calcarea carbonicum
During either sickness or convalescence, great longing for eggs; craves indigestible things (Alum.); aversion to meat.
Ref: Allen's Key Notes

Sepia
Desire for bitter.
Ref: Allen's Key Notes
Repertory –kent- Stomach- Desires; Bitter Drinks: 1Aon, 1:Dig, 2:Nat-m., 1:Ter
Repertory –kent- Stomach- Desires; Bitter Food: 1:Dig, 2:Nat-m.

Ref: RADAR 10

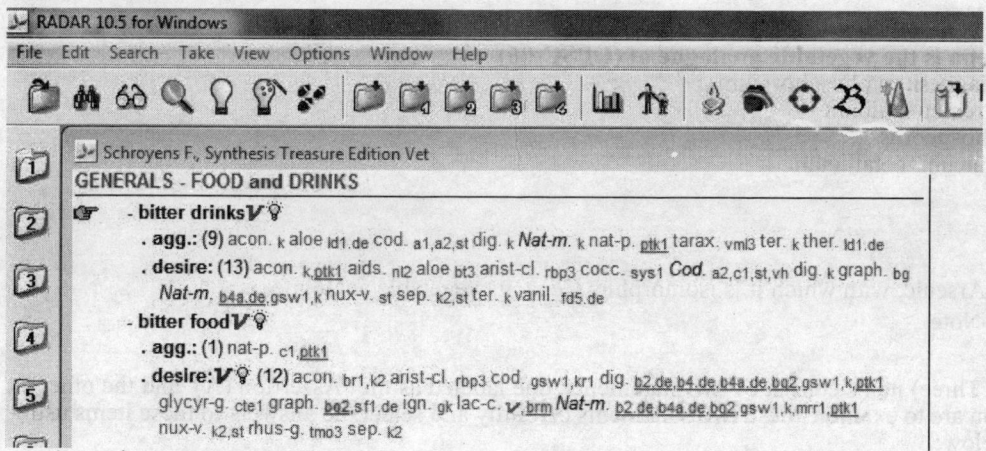

Q. 271. Mental calmnests is a contraindication for which one of the following medicine? (UPSC-06)
(a) Nux vomica
(b) Chamomilla
(c) Tarentula hispanica
(d) Rhus toxicodendron

Ans. (b)
Note
A disposition that is mild, calm and gentle; sluggish and constipated bowels contra-indicate chamomilla.
Ref: Boericke's Materia Medica.

Q. 272. The symptom is 'Twitching and jerking of single muscle with weakness and trembling of hands while writing'. What is the remedy? (UPSC-06)
    (a) Plumbum metallicum
    (b) Causticum
    (c) Argentum nitricum
    (d) Zincum metallicum

Ans. (d)
Note
The remedy is Zincum metallicum
Also see
Zincum
Twitching and jerking of single muscles (Agar., Ign.). Weakness and trembling of extremities; of hands while writing.
Ref: Allen's Key notes.

Q. 273. A 26 year old man has premature graying of hair. He remains under constant mental strain. Which one of the following is the likely remedy for him? (UPSC-06)
    (a) Calcarea fluoricum
    (b) Calcarea phosphoricum
    (c) Lycopodium clavatum
    (d) Calcarea sulphuricum

Ans. (c)
Note
The most likely remedy for above condition is 'Lycopodium'.
Also see
Lycopodium
Complexion pale, dirty; unhealthy; sallow, with deep furrows, looks older than he is.
Ref: Allen's Key-Note.

Q. 274. Allium cepa is the vegetable analogue of (UPSC-06)
    (a) Magnesium phosphoricum
    (b) Arenicum album
    (c) Phosphorus
    (d) Zincum metallicum

Ans. (c)
Note
Phosphorus
Complementary: Arsenic, with which it is isomorphic; Cepa, its vegetable analogue.
Ref: Allen's Key-Note.

Directions
The following 3 (Three) items consist of two statements: one labeled as the 'Assertion (A)' and the other as 'Reason (R)'. You are to examine these two statements carefully and select the answers to these items using the code given below:

Code
    (a) Both A and R are individually true and R is the correct explanation of A.
    (b) Both A and R are individually true but R is not the correct explanation of A
    (c) A is true but R is false
    (d) A is false but R is true

Q. 275. Assertion (A): Spongia is one of the best remedies for goiter.
Reason (R): Spongia has proven precursor of thyroxin. (UPSC-06)

Ans. (c)

Note

Ans. (c) Suggests
Assertion A: Spongia is one of the best remedies for goiter- is true.
Reason (R): Spongia has proven precursor of thyroxin. – is not true.

Discussion
Homeopathically speaking the spongia is made from spong which is rich in iodine. That way it is supposed to be the good medicine for iodine deficiency goiter. Yet there is no scientific basis to prove the above hypothesis.

Q. 276. The "Balm of Gilead" for diseases of old maids and women during and after climacteric; bad effects of suppressed sexual desire, or suppressed menses is (UPSC-06)
    (a) Conium maculatum
    (b) Sepia officinalis
    (c) Lachesis mutus
    (d) Causticum

Ans. (a)
Note
Conium maculatum
The "Balm of Gilead" for diseases of old maids and women during and after climacteric. Especially for diseases of old men; old maids. Bad effects: of suppressed sexual desire, or suppressed menses; non-gratification of sexual instinct, or from excessive indulgence.
Ref: Allen's Key-Note

Q. 277. "Threatened abortion especially at third month, prolonged bearing down forcing pains. During labour, pains irregular, too weak, feeble, everything seems loose and open, but no expulsive action, fainting". Which one of the following is a remedy for above condition? (UPSC-06)
    (a) Sabina
    (b) Secale cornutum
    (c) Magnesium carbonicum
    (d) Caulophyllum

Ans. (b)
Note
For the above clinical presentation most indicated remedy is 'Secale cornutum'.

Also see
Sabina
Has a special action on the uterus; also upon serous and fibrous membranes; hence its use in gout. Pain from sacrum to the pubis. Hemorrhages, where blood is fluid and clots together. Tendency to miscarriage, especially at third month. Violent pulsations; wants windows open.
Ref: Boericke's materia medica

Secale cornutum
Threatened abortion especially at the third month [Sab.]; prolonged, bearing down, forcing pains. During labor; pains irregular; too weak; feeble or ceasing; everything seems loose and open but no expulsive action; fainting. Ref: Allen's Key-Note.

Magnesium carbonicum
Sore throat before menses appears. Before menses, coryza and nasal stoppage. Menses too late and scanty, thick, dark, like pitch; mucous leucorrhea. Menses flow only in sleep; more profuse at night (Am-m.), or when lying down; cease when walking.
Ref: Boericke's materia medica

Caulophyllum
This is a woman's remedy. Want of tonicity of the womb. During labor, when the pains are deficient and the patient is exhausted and fretful. Extraordinary rigidity of os. (Bell, Gels, Verat-v.) Spasmodic and severe pains, which fly in all directions; shivering, without progress: false pains. Revives labor pains and furthers progress of labor. After pains. Habitual abortion from uterine debility.
Ref: Boericke's materia medica

Q. 278. Match List I with List II and select the correct answer using the code given below the lists (UPSC-06)

List- I (Symptoms)	List-II (Medicine)
A. Day time cough	1. Kreosotum
B. Nocturnal Enuresis	2. Apis mellifica
C. 3 p.m. chilliness	3. Podophyllum
D. 7 a.m. fever	4. Ferrum metallicum

Code:

	A	B	C	D
(a)	4	2	1	3
(b)	4	1	2	3
(c)	3	2	1	4
(d)	3	1	2	4

Ans. (b)
Note
The correct match is as under:

List- I (Symptoms)	List-II (Medicine)
A. Day time cough	4. Ferrum metallicum
B. Nocturnal Enuresis	1. Kreosotum
C. 3 p.m. chilliness	2. Apis mellifica
D. 7 a.m. fever	3. Podophyllum

Also see
Ferrum
Cough only in the day time (Euphr.); relieved by lying down; > by eating (Spong.).
Ref: Allen's Key-Notes
Kreosotum
Incontinence of urine; can only urinate when lying; copious, pale; urging, cannot get out of bed quick enough (Apis, Petros.); during first sleep (Sep.), from which child is roused with difficulty.
Ref: Allen's Key-Notes
Apis mellifica
Intermittent fever; chill 3 P. M., with thirst, always (Ign.); < warm room and from external heat (Thuj., 3 A.M. and at 3 P.M.).
Ref: Allen's Key-Notes.
Podophyllum
Fever paroxysm at 7 A.M. With great loquacity during chill and heat; sleep during perspiration.
Ref: Allen's Key-Notes

Q.279. Consider the following symptoms (UPSC-06)
1. Tendency to small, painful boils, one after another, extremely sore
2. Retention of urine or incontinence after labour
3. Ribbon like stool in females due to re-troverted uterus
4. Heat of the upper part of body, coldness of lower part.

Which of the above are the features pertaining to Arnica montana?
    (a) 2 and 3
    (b) 1 and 4
    (c) 2, 3 and 4
    (d) 1, 2, 3 and 4

Ans. (d)

Note
Features pertaining to Arnica montana are given at (d).
Also see
Arnica montana

Nervous women, sanguine plethoric persons, lively expression and very red face. For the bad effects resulting from mechanical injuries; even if received years ago. Especially adapted to those who remain long impressed by even slight mechanical injuries. Sore, lame, bruised feeling all through the body as if beaten; traumatic affections of muscles. Mechanical injuries, especially with stupor from concussion; involuntary feces and urine. After injuries with blunt instruments (Symph.). Compound fractures and their profuse suppuration (Calen.). Concussions and contusions, results of shock or injury; without laceration of soft parts; prevents suppuration and septic conditions and promotes absorption. Nervous, cannot bear pain; whole body oversensitive (Cham, Coff., Ign.). Everything on which he lies seems too hard; complains constantly of it and keeps moving from place to place in search of a soft spot [the parts rested upon feel sore and bruised, Bapt., Pyrog., must move continually to obtain relief from the pain, Rhus-t.]. *Heat of upper part of body; coldness of lower*. The face or head and face alone is hot, the body cool. Unconsciousness; when spoken to answers correctly, but unconsciousness and delirium at once return (falls asleep in the midst of a sentence, Bapt.). Says there is nothing the matter with him. Meningitis after mechanical or traumatic injuries; from falls, concussion of brain, etc. When suspecting exudation of blood, to facilitate absorption. Hydrocephalus; deathly coldness in forearm of children (in diarrhea, Brom.). Apoplexy; loss of consciousness, involuntary evacuation from bowels and bladder; in acute attack, controls hemorrhage and aids absorption; should be repeated and allowed to act for days or weeks unless symptoms call for another remedy. Conjunctival or retinal hemorrhage, with extravasation, from injuries or cough (Led, Nux-v.). Gout and rheumatism, with great fear of being touched or struck by persons coming near him. Cannot walk erect on account of a bruised sort of feeling in the pelvic region.(1) *Tendency to small, painful boils, one after extremely sore* (small boils in crops, Sulph.). Paralysis [left sided]; pulse full, strong; stertor, sighing, muttering. Belching; eructations; foul, putrid, like rotten eggs. Dysentery; with ischuria, fruitless urging; long interval between the stools. Constipation: rectum loaded, faeces will not come away; (3) ribbon-*like stools from enlarged prostate or retroverted uterus*. Soreness of parts after labor; prevents post-partum hemorrhage and puerperal complications. *(2) Retention or incontinence of urine after labor* (Op.).
Ref: Allen's Key-Notes

Q. 280. A patient is suffering from high temperature with thirst being very prominent especially before and during chill; bilious vomiting after drinking, heat stage characterised by severe bone pain which is relieved by sweat. What is the likely remedy? (UPSC-06)
    (a)   China officinalis
    (b)   Eupatorium perfoliatum
    (c)   Apis mellifica
    (d)   Natrium muriaticum

Ans. (b)
Note
The most likely remedy is Eupatorium perfoliatum.
Also see
China officinalis
Intermittent fever; paroxysm anticipates from two to three hours each attack [Chin-s.]; returns every seven or fourteen days; never at night; sweats profusely all over on being covered, or during sleep [Con.].
Ref: Allen's Key-Notes
Eupatorium perfoliatum
Fever: Chill to 9 A. M. one day, at noon the next day; bitter vomiting at close of chill; drinking hastens chill and causes vomiting; bone pains, before and during chill. Insatiable thirst before and during chill and fever; knows chill is coming because he cannot drink enough.
Ref: Allen's Key-Notes
Eupatorium perfoliatum
Great thirst. Vomiting and purging of bile, of green liquid several quarts at a time. Vomiting preceded by thirst.

Perspiration relieves all symptoms except headache. Chill between 7 and 9 a.m., preceded by thirst with great soreness and aching of bones. Nausea, vomiting of bile at close of chill or hot stage; throbbing headache. Knows chill is coming on because he cannot drink enough.
Ref: Boericke's materia medica
Apis mellifica
Intermittent fever; chill 3 P. M. , with thirst, always [Ign.]; < warm room and from external heat [Thuja, 3 A. M. and at 3 P. M.].

Ref: Allen's Key-Notes
Natrium muriaticum
Intermittent: Paroxysm at 10 or 11 A.M.; old chronic, badly treated cases, especially after suppression by quinine; headache, with unconsciousness during chill and heat; sweat > pains.

Extended information
Repertorial anamnesis from Radar 7.0
High temperature:
-Fever intense heat: ACON, *Apis,* ARN, ARS, BELL, *Bry,* CON, GELS, MEZ, NAT-M, PULS, PYROG, RHUS-T, SEC. (Ref: Radar-7.0)
Fever with thirst, before and during chill:
-Thirst in all stages of fever; acon, bry, Eup-per, Nat-m. (Ref: Radar-7.0)
Bilious vomiting after drinking:
-Vomiting bile cold water, after: Eup-p., Rhus-t.
Heat stage is characterized by sever bony pain > by sweat
-Extremities pain – bone: ASAF, EUP-PER, MERC, NIT-AC, NUX-V, PH-AC, PULS, PYROG, RUTA. (Radar: 7.0)
-Perspiration ameliorates: BRY, CUPR, Eup-per, GELS, NAT-M, RHUS-T.
Discussion:
The above remedies do have high fever and thirst. The Bone pains are a typical finding with fever and which is relieved is by sweat is only covered by Eup-per.

Q. 281. A 45 years old patient has been diagnosed as a case of cystitis. He is passing very offensive urine which is brown in colour, acidic in character with excess of uric acid. Which one of the following is the indicated remedy? (UPSC-06)
    (a)   Baptisia
    (b)   Benzoicum acidum
    (c)   Acidum nitricum
    (d)   Pyrogenium

Ans. (b)
Note
From the remedies above, indicated remedy is 'Benzoicum acidum'.
Also see
All above are highly offensive remedies. However, the – Benzoicum acidum and Acidum nitricum – have highly offensive urine. The Baptisia and Pyrogenium have general offensiveness of all the discharges. Therefore only two remedies are to be differentiated that is Nit-ac. and Benz-ac. The redline symptom 'offensive urine which is brown in colour, acidic in character with excess of uric acid" is a characteristic of Benz-ac. The Nit-ac. urine has – bloody, offensive and phosphatic'.

Q. 282. The symptom is: 'Cough with expectoration of much tough, ropy white mucous; associated with gagging and vomiting while brushing teeth in the morning'. What is the remedy? (UPSC-06)
    (a)   Coccus cacti
    (b)   Drosera rotundifolia
    (c)   Hydrastis canadensis
    (d)   Kalium bichronicum

Ans. (a)
Note
The 'stringy discharge' is covered by all the above drugs except 'Drosera'.
The morning aggravation and that too especially while brushing teeth is can be seen in Kent's Repertory as-

Cough – Brushing teeth – 1: Coc-c, 1: Staph. However, Staph is not included in the choice above.
The gagging and vomiting while brushing teeth in the morning can be further verified form Boericke Materia Medica
Therefore only drug which covers the symptom is Coc-c.

Q. 283. Consider the following statements (UPSC-06)
    1.   Graphites patient craves for sweets.
    2.   Sepia patient has aversion to bitter things.

Which of the statements given above is/ are correct
    (a)   1 Only
    (b)   2 Only
    (c)   Both 1 and 2
    (d)   Neither 1 nor 2

Ans. (d)

Note
The first statement 'Graphites' patient craves for sweet – is incorrect.
The second statement 'Sepia' patient has aversion to bitter things – is incorrect.

Also see
Sepia
Aversion to Fat and salt.
Desires – sweets, chocolate, vinegar, sour bread, salt stimulants and 'Bitter.'
References especially for 'desire for bitter' can be found at two places only – Synthesis and Murphy's Repertory.
Desire for sweet can be seen for sepia in Kent Repertory as under:

English Kent

STOMACH - DESIRES - sweets
Am-c.$_k$ arg-met.$_k$ **ARG-N.**$_k$ ars.$_k$ bar-c.$_k$ *Bry.*$_k$ bufo$_k$ *Calc.*$_k$ *Calc-s.*$_k$ *Carb-v.*$_k$ **CHIN.**$_k$ chinin-ar.$_k$ *Elaps*$_k$ *Ip.*$_k$ kali-ar.$_k$ *Kali-c.*$_k$ kali-p.$_k$ *Kali-s.*$_k$ **LYC.**$_k$ *Mag-m.*$_k$ *Med.*$_k$ merc.$_k$ nat-act.$_k$ *Nat-c.*$_k$ nat-m.$_k$ nux-v.$_k$ op.$_k$ petr.$_k$ *Plb.*$_k$ *Rheum*$_k$ *Rhus-t.*$_k$ *Sabad.*$_k$ *Sec.*$_k$ *Sep.*$_k$ **SULPH.**$_k$ *Tub.*$_k$

Discussion
In the reference of above - Both the statements 1 and 2 are incorrect.

Therefore, the answer suggested is – (d)

Q. 284. Match List I with List II and select the correct answer using the code given below the lists: (UPSC-06)

List- I (Symptoms)	List-II (Remedies)
A. Headache with blindness	1. Kalium bichromicum
B. Headache relieved by passing urine	2. Gelsemium sempervirens
C. Headache relieved by talking	3. Dulcamara
D. Headache relieved by eating	4. Anacardium orientalis

Code

	A	B	C	D
(a)	1	2	3	4
(b)	1	3	2	4
(c)	4	2	3	1
(d)	4	3	2	1

Ans. (a)

Note
The correct sequence is as under:

List- I (Symptoms)	List-II (Remedies)
A. Headache with blindness	1. Kalium bichromicum
B. Headache relieved by passing urine	2. Gelsemium sempervirens
C. Headache relieved by talking	3. Dulcamara
D. Headache relieved by eating	4. Anacardium orientalis

Also see
Kali-bi.
Headache: blurred vision or blindness precedes the attack (Gels. Lac-d.); must lie down; aversion to light and noise; sight returns as headache increases (Iris, Nat-m., Lac-d.).
Ref: Allen's Key Notes
Gelsemium
Headache: proceeded by blindness (Kali-bi.), >. by profuse urination.
Ref: Allen's Key Notes
Dulcamara
Headache relieved by talking; NA
Ref: Allen's Key Notes
Headache relieved by conversation.
Ref: Boericke's materia medica
Anacardium
Headache: relieved entirely when eating [Psor.]; when lying down in bed at night, and when about falling asleep; worse during motion and work.
Ref: Allen's Key Note

Q. 285. Match List I with List II and select the correct answer using the code given below the lists (UPSC-06)

List- I (Medicine)	List-II (Symptoms)
A. Conium maculatum	1. Sweats during waking hours
B. Thuja occidentalis	2. Sweats on the face only while walking
C. Sambucus nigra	3. Sweats as soon as one sleeps
D. Ignatia amara	4. Sweats only on uncovered parts

Code

	A	B	C	D
(a)	3	4	1	2
(b)	2	1	4	3
(c)	3	1	4	2
(d)	2	4	1	3

Ans. (a)
Note
The correct sequence is as under:

List- I (Medicine)	List-II (Symptoms)
A. Conium maculatum	3. Sweats as soon as one sleeps
B. Thuja occidentalis	4. Sweats only on uncovered parts
C. Sambucus nigra	1. Sweats during waking hours
D. Ignatia amara	2. Sweats on the face only while walking

Here the walking is to be replaced as no such symptom is there in Ingnatia, however, we find sweats on the face only while 'eating'.

Review
Reference for Conium:
Repertory Kent- Perspiration –Sleep; Even when closing the eyes: 1:Carb-an, 3:Con.
In reference to Thuja:
Repertory Kent- Perspiration –Uncovered Parts, on: 2:Puls., 1:Thuj.
In reference to Sambucus:
Repertory Kent – Perspiration: Daytime: Awake, while: 3:Samb.
In reference to Ignatia:
Repertory Kent –Face-Perspiration: Eating: While: 2:Ign, 2:Nat-m, 2:Sulph.
Repertory Kent –Face-Perspiration: Walking, While: 1: Valer.
Repertory Kent -Perspiration: Profuse: Walking while: 1:Bry, 1:Canth, 1:Chin-s, 1:Kali-c, 2:Merc, 3:Psor, 1:Sel, 2:Sel, 2:Sulph.

Comment:
It appears that in reference to Ignatia – in place of 'walking' it should have been 'Eating'.

Q. 286. Constitutional medicine for haemorrhoids of pregnant women is ____. (MD/ NIH/98)
    (a)   Collinsonia canadensis
    (b)   Lachesis mutus
    (c)   Sulphur
    (d)   Aloe socotrina

Ans. (a)

Note
From the choice given above, the constitutional medicine for haemorrhoids of pregnant women is Collinsonia canadensis.

Also see
Collinsonia canadensis
Pelvic and portal congestion resulting in dysmenorrhoea and haemorrhoids. Congestion of pelvic viscera, with haemorrhoids, especially in latter months of pregnancy. After heart is relieved, old piles reappear, or suppressed menses return. Chronic, painful, bleeding piles; sensation as if sticks, sand or gravel had lodged in rectum (Aesc.). Haemorrhoidal dysentery with tenesmus. Alternate constipation and diarrhoea; congestive inertia of lower bowel; stools sluggish and hard with pain and great flatulence. Constipation. Pruritus in pregnancy with haemorrhoids, unable to lie down.
Ref: Allen's Keynotes.

Lachesis mutus
Persons of a less melancholic temperament, dark eyes, and a disposition to low spirits and indolence. Women of choleric temperament, with freckles and red hair (Phos.). Better adapted to thin and emaciated than to fleshy persons; to those who have been changed, both mentally and physically, by their illness. Climacteric ailments: haemorrhoids, haemorrhages; hot flushes and hot perspiration; burning vertex headache, especially at or after menopause (Sang, Sulph.). Piles: with scanty menses; at climaxis; strangulated; with stitches shooting upward (Nit-ac.).
Ref: Allen's Keynotes.

Sulphur
Adapted to persons of a scrofulous diathesis, subject to venous congestion; especially of portal system. Haemorrhoids that have been treated with ointments.
Ref: Allen's Keynotes.

Aloe socotrina
Haemorrhoids: blue, like a bunch of grapes (Mur.-ac.); constant bearing down in rectum; bleeding, sore, tender, hot, relieved by cold water; intense itching. Itching and burning in anus, preventing sleep (Ind.).

Adapted to indolent, 'weary' persons; averse to either mental or physical labour; mental labour fatigues. Old people, especially women of relaxed, phlegmatic habit.
Ref: Allen's Keynotes.

Extended information
Following are the repertory references:
Ref: Kent's Repertory.

[kent] [Rectum]Haemorrhoids:Pregnancy,during:
Aesc,Am-m,Ant-c,Caps,Coll,Lach,Lyc,Nat-m,Nux-v,Sep,Sulph,

[knerr] [Stool and Rectum]Hemorrhoids:Pregnancy, during:
AESC,AM-M,ANT-C,CAPS,COLL,Crot-h,HYDR,LYC,NAT-M,Nux-v,SULPH,

[knerr] [Pregnancy, Parturition, Lactation]Pregnancy:Haemorrhoids:
AESC,AM-M,ANT-C,CAPS,COLL,Crot-h,HYDR,LYC,NAT-M,NUX-V,SULPH,ZINC,

Q. 287. Irritable, nervous fidgety, hard to please_____. (ACHMCH/98/WB) and (MD/ACMCH/BBSR/98)
    (a)   Apis mellifica
    (b)   Natrium muriaticum
    (c)   Silicea terra
    (d)   Helonias dioica

Ans. (a)
Note
Apis mellifica is irritable, nervous fidgety, and hard to please.

Also see
Apis mellifica
Adapted to the strumous constitution; glands enlarged, indurated; scirrhus or open cancer. Women, especially widows; children and girls who, though generally careful, become awkward, and let things fall while handling them (Bov.). Bad effects of acute exanthema imperfectly developed or suppressed (Zinc.); measles, scarlatina, urticaria. Ailments from jealousy, fright, rage, vexation and bad news. Irritable; nervous; fidgety; hard to please. Weeping disposition; cannot help crying; discouraged, despondent (Puls.).
Ref: Allen's Keynote.

Q. 288. Extreme hunger even when stomach is full of food_____. (DM/Hydrabad/99)
    (a)   Iodium
    (b)   China officinalis
    (c)   Staphysagria
    (d)   Calcarea carbonica

Ans. (c)
Note
Extreme hunger even when stomach is full – Staphysagria.

Also see
Staphysagria
Teeth turn black, show dark streaks through them; cannot be kept clean; crumble, decay on edges (at the roots, Mez., Thuj.); scorbutic cachexia. Craving for tobacco. Extreme hunger even when stomach is full of food. Sensation as if abdomen and stomach were hanging down relaxed (Agar., Ip., Tab.).
Ref: Allen's Keynotes.

Extended information
Ref: Gentry's Concordance Repertory.

[Gentry] [Stomach]Hunger:Extreme H., even when stomach is full of food:

1: Staph

3 Alternate canine H. and want of appetite:	3 Great H. after fever:
3 Canine H., even after eating:	3 H., with aversion to food:
3 Ravenous, canine H.:	3 H. soon after eating:
3 Loss of appetite or canine H.:	3 Sensation of H., but no appetite:
3 Excessive, ravenous, canine H.; must eat	3 Extreme H., even when stomach is full of
3 Canine H. alternating with loss of appetite	3 H., with headache
3 Canine H.; worse after vomiting:	3 H., with inability to swallow:
3 Appetite excited, even to canine H.:	3 H., with colic:
3 Canine H., with torpid fever:	3 H., with thirst:
3 Ravenous H., after a stool:	3 H., with yawning:
3 Vomiting, with H.:	3 Gnawing sensation in stomach, as from H
3 Ravenous H., with want of appetite:	3 H.; cannot satisfy it:
3 Ravenous morbid H.; cannot be satisfied:	3 H. soon satisfied:
3 Ravenous H., with weakness:	3 H., but a mouthful satisfies:
3 Ravenous H., with trembling from longing	3 Violent H. and appetite, yet a little food sa

Iodium
Empty eructations from morning to night, as if every particle of food was turned into air (Kali-c.). Suffers from hunger, must eat every few hours, anxious and worried if he does not eat (Cina, Sulph.); feels > while eating or after eating, when stomach is full. Itching: low down in the lungs, behind the sternum, causing cough; extends through bronchi to nasal cavity (Coc-c., Con., Phos.).

Q. 289. Menstruation only during daytime, ceases when lying down (MD/NIH/98)
  (a) Causticum annuum
  (b) Cactus grandiflorus
  (c) Magnesia carbonica
  (d) Lilium tigrinum

Ans. (a)
Note
Above symptom is covered by 'Causticum'.
Also see
Causticum annuum
Menses: too early; too feeble; only during the day; ceases on lying down.
Ref: Allen's Keynotes.

Magnesium carbonica
Menses preceded by sore throat (Lac-c.), labour-like pain, cutting colic, backache, weakness, chilliness; flows only at night or when lying, ceases when walking (Am.-m., Kreos. - reverse of Lil-t.).
Ref: Allen's Keynotes.

Lilium tigrinum
Menses early, scanty, dark, offensive; flow only when moving about; ceases to flow when she ceases to walk (Caust., – on lying down, Kreos., Mag-c.).
Ref: Allen's Keynotes.

Extended information
[kent] Genitalia, Female, Menses, daytime
FEMALE GENITALIA - MENSES, - daytime only
cact. *Caust.* coff. cycl. ham. **PULS.**

Ref: Kent's Repertory.

Q. 290. Sweat in axilla smells like onions _____. (PSC/WB/91)
    (a) Bovista lycoperdon
    (b) Thuja occidentalis
    (c) Sulphur
    (d) Sepia officinalis

Ans. (a)

Note
Sweat in axilla smells like onion is Bovista lycoperdon.

Also see
Bovista lycoperdon
Sweat in axilla, smells like onions.
Ref: Allen's Keynotes.

Thuja occidentalis
Sweat only on uncovered parts; or all over except the head (reverse of Sil.); when he sleeps, stops when he wakes (reverse of Samb.); profuse, sour smelling, foetid, at night. Perspiration, smelling like honey, on the genitals.
Ref: Boericke's Materia Medica.

Sulphur
Dry skin and great thirst. Night sweat, on nape and occiput. Perspiration of single parts. Disgusting sweats. Remittent type.
Ref: Boericke's Materia Medica.

Sepia officinalis
Sweat on feet, worse on toes; intolerable odour. Lentigo in young women. Ichthyosis with offensive odour of skin.
Ref: Boericke's Materia Medica.

Q. 291. _____ is indicated for vertigo after coition. (PSC/WB/91) (RSC/08)
    (a) Acidum phosphoricum
    (b) Conium maculatum
    (c) Sulphur
    (d) Gelsemium sempervirens

Ans. (a)

Note
From the choice given above, Acidum phosphoricum is indicated for vertigo after coition.

Also see

[kent] [Vertigo]Coition,after:

1: Ph-ac   1: Sep

Ref: Kent's Repertory.

Q. 292. Fluoricum acidum is complementary of _____. (PSC/WB/91)
    (a) Pulsatilla nigricans
    (b) Silicea terra
    (c) Hepar sulphuris
    (d) Mercurius solubilis

Ans. (b)

Note
Fluoricum acidum is complementary of Silicea terra.

Also see
Fluoricum acidum
Relations
Complementary: Coca, Sil. Follows well: after, Ars. in ascites of drunkards; after, Kali-c. in hip disease; after, Coff., Staph. in sensitive teeth; after, Ph.-ac. in diabetes; after Sil., Symph. in bone diseases; after, Spong in goitre.
Ref: Allen's Keynotes.

Q. 293. Sanguine, ruddy people_____. (MD/ACHMH/97)
    (a)   Aurum metallicum
    (b)   Arnica montana
    (c)   Ignatia amara
    (d)   Cactus grandiflorus

Ans. (a)

Q. 294. Prolapsus, post-climacteric, bearing down pain almost intolerable. Pain in left ovary, right hip.
    (a)   Sanicula aqua
    (b)   Agaricus muscarius
    (c)   Lilium tigrinum
    (d)   Lachesis mutus

Ans. (b)
Note
From the choice given above Agaricus muscarius is the remedy.
Also see
Agaricus Muscarius (Agar.)
Every motion, every turn of body, causes pain in spine. Single vertebra sensitive to touch. Prolapsus, post-climacteric; bearing down pain almost intolerable (compare, Lil-t., Murx., Sep.). Extremely sensitive to cold air (Calc., Kali-c., Psor.). Complaints appear diagonally; upper left and lower right side (Ant-t., Stram. upper right, lower left, Ambr. , Brom. , Med., Phos. , Sul-ac.).
Ref: Allen's Keynotes.

Q. 295. Rash before menses_____. (MD/NIH/98) Rept (RSC/08)
    (a)   Dulcamara
    (b)   Natrium muriaticum
    (c)   Belladonna
    (d)   Graphites

Ans. (a)
Note
Rash before menses is Dulcamara.
Also see
Dulcamara
Catarrhal ischuria in grown-up children, with milky urine; from walking with bare feet in cold water; involuntary. Rash before menses (Cocc- During profuse menses, Bell. , Graph.). Urticaria over whole body, no fever; itching burns after scratching; < in warmth, >. in cold. Thick brown-yellow crusts on scalp, face, forehead, temples, chin; with reddish borders, bleeding when scratched. Warts, fleshy, large, smooth; on face or back of hands and fingers (Thuja).
Ref: Allen's Keynotes.

Q. 296. 'Bed feels hard'_____. (MD/NIH/98/RSC/08)
    (a)   Pyrogenium
    (b)   Baptisia tinctoria
    (c)   Arnica montana
    (d)   Opium

Ans. (a)

Note
From the choice given above, Pyrogenium is the most suitable answer.

Also see

Pyrogenium
The bed feels hard (Arn.); parts lain on feel sore and bruised (Bapt.); rapid decubitus (Carb-ac.). Great restlessness; must move constantly to > the soreness of parts (Arn., Eup).
Ref: Allen's Keynotes.

Baptisia tinctoria
In whatever position the patient lies, the parts rested upon feel sore and bruised (Pyrog. – compare, Arn., Pyrog.). Decubitus in typhoid (Arn, Mur-ac., Pyrog.).
Ref: Allen's Keynotes.

Arnica montana
Nervous, cannot bear pain; whole body over-sensitive (Cham., Coff., Ign.). Everything on which he lies seems too hard; complains constantly of it and keeps moving from place to place in search of a soft spot (the parts rested upon feel sore and bruised, Bapt., Pyrog., must move continually to obtain relief from the pain, Rhus-t.).
Ref: Allen's Keynotes.

Opium
Sleeplessness with acuteness of hearing, clock striking and cocks crowing at a great distance keep her awake. Loss of breath on falling asleep (Grind., Lach.). Bed feels so hot she cannot lie on it (bed feels hard, Arn., Bry., Pyrog.); moves often in search of a cool place; must be uncovered.
Ref: Allen's Keynotes.

GENERALS - HARD bed, sensation of

  HARD bed, sensation of: (37) acon. agar. **ARN.** *Ars. Bapt.* bar-c. bry. caust. con. dros. *Ferr. Ferr-p.* graph. ip. kali-c. lyc. mag-c. mag-m. manc. merc. nux-m. nux-v. op. phos. plat. puls. *Pyrog. Rhus-t. Ruta* sabad. **SIL.** spong. stann. sulph. tarax. thuj. verat.

Also see
On consulting Kent's Repertory for the above condition, we find that – Pyrogenium, Baptisia tinctoria, Arnica montana and Opium are all covered the same.

Q. 297. Headache preceeded by blindness, ameliorated by the process of urination (PSC/WB/91)
    (a) Natrium muriaticum
    (b) Gelsemium sempervirens
    (c) Thuja occidentalis
    (d) Belladonna

Ans. (b)

Note
Headache preceeded by blindness, ameliorated by the process of urination is Gelsemium sempervirens.

Also see

Gelsemium sempervirens
Headache preceeded by blindness (Kali-bi.), > by profuse urination. Lack of muscular co-ordination; confused; muscles refuse to obey the will. Headache beginning in the cervical spine; pains extend over the head, causing a bursting sensation in forehead and eyeballs (Sang., Sil., begins in same way, but semi-lateral); < by mental exertion; from smoking; heat of sun; lying with head low.
Ref: Allen's Keynotes.

Q. 298. Mapped tongue, with involuntary urination when coughing, walking and laughing___ (MD/NIH/99)
    (a) Causticum
    (b) Natrium muriaticum
    (c) Taraxacum officinale
    (d) Squilla maritima

Ans. (b)

Note
Mapped tongue, with involuntary urination while coughing, walking, laughing is Natrium muriaticum.

Also see
Natrium muriaticum
Tongue: mapped, with red insular patches; like ringworm on sides (Ars., Lach., Merc., Nit.-ac., Tarax.); heavy, difficult speech, children slow in learning to walk. Constipationsensation of contraction of anus; torn, bleeding, smarting afterwards, stool dry, hard, difficult, crumbling (Am-c., Mag-m.); stitches in rectum (Nit.-ac.); involuntary, knows not whether flatus or faeces escape (Aloe, Iod., Mur.-ac., Oldn., Podo.). Urine: involuntary when walking, coughing, laughing (Caust., Puls., Squil.); has to wait a long time for urine to pass, if others are present (Hep., Mur-ac.); cutting in urethra after (Sars.).
Ref: Allen's Keynotes.

Q. 299. Delirium with desire of light and company_____ (MD/NIH/98)
    (a)   Belladonna
    (b)   Stramonium
    (c)   Hyoscyamus niger
    (d)   Bismuthum

Ans. (b)

Note
Delirium with a desire for light and company is Stramonium.

Also see
Stramonium
Disposed to talk continually (Cic., Lach.); incessant and incoherent talking and laughing; praying, beseeching, entreating; with suppressed menses. Desires light and company; cannot bear to be alone (Bism.); worse in the dark and solitude; cannot walk in a dark room. Awakens with a shrinking look, as if afraid of the first object seen. Hallucinations which terrify the patient. Desire to escape, in delirium (Bell., Bry., Op.,) Rhus-t.
Ref: Allen's Keynotes.

Q. 300. Avarice in BTPB is found in chapter_____ (MD/NIH/97)
    (a)   Mind
    (b)   Intellect
    (c)   Internal head
    (d)   Vision

Ans. (a)

Note
Avarice in BTPB is found in chapter 'Mind.'

Also see
Avarice in BTPB is found under chapter 'Mind'. It contains the following drugs: ARS, Calc-c., Lyc., Nat-c., PULS., Sep.

Extended information
There are a total of 18 rubrics in the 'Mind' section.
Ref: BTPB, page 18, reprint edition 1990, B. Jain Publishers.

Q. 301. Urticaria aggravated in warmth but better in cold ____ (PSC/WB/91)
    (a)   Thuja occidentalis
    (b)   Dulcamara
    (c)   Rhus toxicodendron
    (d)   Sulphur

Ans. (b)

Note
From the variable provided above for urticaria aggravated in warmth but better in cold is best covered by Dulcamara.

Also see
Dulcamara
Urticaria over whole body, no fever; itching burns after scratching; < in warmth, > in cold.
Ref: Allen's Keynotes.

Q. 302. Vicarious menstruation_____ (PSC/WB/91)
    (a)   Pulsatilla pratensis
    (b)   Arnica montana
    (c)   Bryonia alba
    (d)   Causticum annuum

Ans. (c)
From the above given choice, the most appropriate choice is Bryonia alba.

Also see
Bryonia alba
Excessive dryness of mucous membranes of entire body; lips and tongue dry, parched, cracked; stool, dry as if burnt; cough, dry, hard, racking, with scanty expectoration; urine, dark and scanty; great thirst. Vicarious menstruation; nosebleed when menses should appear (Phos.); blood spitting, or heamoptysis.
Ref: Allen's Keynotes.

Q. 303. Which of the medicines is indicated for 'Excoriated lips from acrid saliva' (PSC/WB/91)
    (a)   Kreosotum
    (b)   Petroleum
    (c)   Acidum nitricum
    (d)   Silicea terra

Ans. (c)
Note
From the choice given above 'Acidum Nitricum' covers the symptom 'excoriated lips from acrid saliva'.

Also see

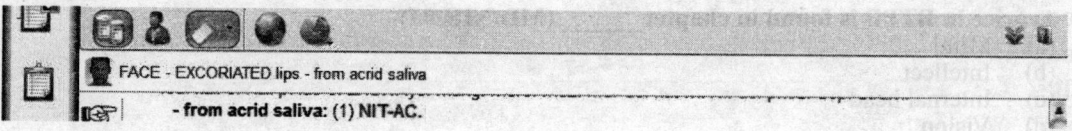

Q. 304. Indication of China officinalis in intermittent fever is warranted where there is _____ (PSC/WB/93)
    (a)   Thirst during heat
    (b)   Thirst at the onset of chill and heat stages
    (c)   Thirst during heat
    (d)   Thirst before chill

Ans. (d)
The indication of China officinalis in intermittent fever is warranted where there is 'thirst before chill'.
Note
China officinalis
Paroxysms every 7 or 14 days, with thirst before the chill begins, which ceases as chill increases. General shaking chill over whole body increases the chill.
Ref: Comparative Materia Medica by Ernest Albert Farrington, page 456.
Ref: Kent's Lectures on Materia Madica, page 789.
Ref: Boericke's Materia Medica, page 204.

Q. 305. A child appears to be intelligent but delayed in learning to talk. Which of the following medicines is applicable (PSC/WB/93)
    (a)   Baryta carbonica
    (b)   Natrium muriaticum

(c) Calcarea carbonica
(d) Sulphur

Ans. (b)

Note
Mind; talking, slow learning to talk; NATRIUM MURIATICUM.

Also see

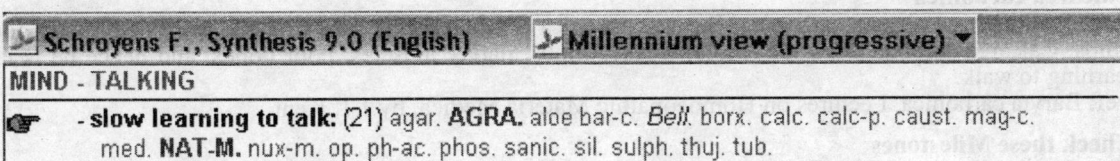

Ref.: (AQ)

Talk:	
Symptoms Covered by Drugs	**Nat-m**
2 Talk:	
3 Indisposed to, desire to be silent, taciturn:	2:Nat-m
4 Forenoon:	1:Nat-m
4 Afternoon:	1:Nat-m
3 Slow learning, to:	**3:Nat-m**
2 Talking:	
3 Pleasure in his own talking:	1:Nat-m
3 Sleep, in:	2:Nat-m
2 Talks:	
3 Dead people, with:	1:Nat-m
2 Thinking:	
3 Aversion to:	1:Nat-m
3 Complaints, of:	
4 Agg:	1:Nat-m
2 Thoughts:	
Symptom Count/Total Weightage:	**433/695**

kent->Mind Repertory

Also see late learning to walk:
Among the choice given above 'Calcarea carbonica' is the most suitable choice for a child who is intelligent but delayed in learning to walk.

Extended information
Baryta carbonica
'Late learning to walk' is Baryta carbonica. Baryta carbonica has great bearing over the development of the young and is expressed as 'dwarfishness'. Children are late coming into usefulness; or activity; late with their studies; late learning to talk; late learning to read; late learning to make the combinations that enter into

life; late learning to take in images, and form perceptions; to take on their activities; to do their work. Baryta carbonica has late learning how to walk, even with pretty good limbs.

Natrium muriaticum
'Late learning to walk' is Baryta carbonica, Borax veneta and Natrium muriaticum. All three of these medicines have a peculiar kind of tardiness in the development of the brain, so that they are late learning to do things; late in developing. But Baryta carbonica leads them all in this late coming into the activities and uses of life.

Calcarea carbonica
'Late walking' is Calcarea carbonica. Baryta carbonica is late learning how to walk, even with pretty good limbs. Calcarea carbonica has miserable, weakly limbs, flabby muscles, poor bones, and hence he is late learning to walk.
Ref: Baryta carbonica, Lectures on Homoeopathic Materia Medica, by J.T. Kent.

Check these Milestones
Here is a set of milestones which, if not met by any child in time, should make one look for medical help:
1. Not rolling over by six months.
2. Having head lag when pulled to a sitting position after six months.
3. Not sitting by himself/herself without support by eight months.
4. Not crawling by twelve months.
5. Not walking by fifteen months.
6. Not speaking a single word (mamma, dadda) by fifteen months.
7. Not pointing to named objects (dog, nose) between twelve to twenty four months.
8. Not initiating speech sounds by twelve months.
9. Not adding more words every month.
Ref: From the web.

Q. 306. _____ is indicated for tough and greasy stools. ((PSC/WB/93)
    (a) Antimonium tartaricum
    (b) Causticum
    (c) Ledum palustre
    (d) Hydrastis canadensis

Ans. (b)

Note
Causticum is indicated for tough and greasy stools.

Also see
Causticum
Constipation frequent, ineffectual desire (Nux-v.); stool passes better when person is standing; impeded by haemorrhoids; tough and shining, like grease; in children with nocturnal enuresis.
Ref: Allen's Keynotes.
Ref: Boericke's Materia Medica.

Extended information
Antimonium tartaricum
Cholera morbus. Diarrhoea in eruptive diseases.
Ref: Boericke's Materia Medica.

Ledum palustre
ANAL FISSURES. Haemorrhoidal pain.
Ref: Boericke's Materia Medica.

Hydrastis canadensis
Prolapsed; anus fissured. CONSTIPATION, with sinking feeling in stomach and dull headache. During stool, smarting pain in rectum. After stool, long lasting pain (Nit-ac.) Haemorrhoids; even a light flow exhausts. Contraction and spasm.
Ref: Boericke's Materia Medica.

MCQ's in Materia Medica

Q. 307. Intense sympathy for the suffering of others___ (PSC/WB/93)
    (a) Causticum
    (b) Ignatia amara
    (c) Pulsatilla pratensis
    (d) Arnica montana

Ans. (a)

Note
Intense sympathy for the suffering of others is Causticum.

Also see
Causticum
Melancholic mood: sad, hopeless; from care, grief, sorrow; with weeping, 'The least thing makes the child cry.' Intense sympathy for the sufferings of others. Ailments from long lasting grief and sorrow (Ph.-ac.); from loss of sleep, night watching (Cocc., Ign.); from sudden emotions, fear, fright, joy (Coff., Gels.); from anger or vexation; from suppressed eruptions.
Ref: Allen's Keynotes.

Extended information

[kent] [Mind]Sympathetic:
Carl,*Caust*,*Cic*,Croc,*Ign*,Iod,Lyc,Manc,*Nat-c*,*Nat-m*,*Nit-ac*,Nuph,*Nux-v*,**PHOS**,Puls,

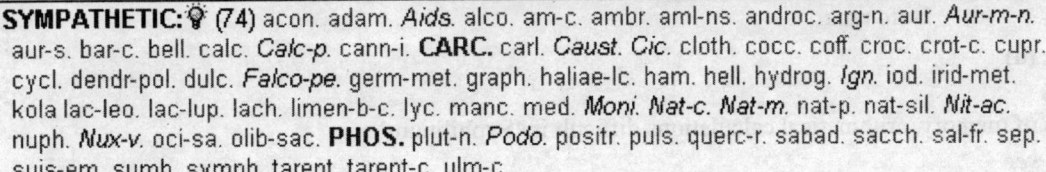

Q. 308. Number of medicines mentioned in the Boericke's Materia Medica (MD/ NIH/ 98)
    (a) 1214
    (b) 1412
    (c) 1414
    (d) 1428

Ans. (c)

Note
Number of medicines mentioned in Boericke's Materia Medica are 1414.

Also see
The repertory has a total number of 1409 medicines. The index provides a list of 1414 medicines but 5 medicines appear twice because of their dual names.
Ref: Essentials of Repertorization, by S.K. Tiwari, page 523, third revised enlarged edition.

Q. 309. Menses at regular time, too short, scanty; pains all relieved by flow (MD/ Hydrabad-99)
    (a)   Zincum metallicum
    (b)   Lachesis mutus
    (c)   Lyssinum
    (d)   Allium cepa

Ans. (b)

Note
Menses at regular time, too short, scanty; pains all relieved by flow is covered by 'Lachesis mutus' from the above given choices.

Also see
Lachesis mutus
Menses at regular time; too short, scanty, feeble; pains all relieved by the flow; always better during menses (Zinc.).
Ref: Allen's Keynote.

Q. 310. Loss of memory, arithmetical calculations difficult_____ (MD/BBSR/98)
    (a)   Syphilinum
    (b)   Medorrhinum
    (c)   Arsenicum album
    (d)   Bufo rana

Ans. (a)

Note
Loss of memory, arithmetical calculations difficult is 'Syphilinum'.

Also see
Syphilinum
Heart, lancinating pains from base to apex, at night (from apex to base, Med.; from base to clavicle, or shoulder, Spig.). Loss of memory; cannot remember names of books, persons or places; arithmetical calculation difficult. Sensation as if going insane, as if about to be paralyzed; of apathy and indifference.
Ref: Allen's Keynotes.

Q. 311. All female symptoms are associated with restlessness, especially of the feet; coldness, depression, and spinal tenderness ameliorated during menstrual flow; which one of the following medicines is indicated in such patients (PSC/WB/98)
    (a)   Sepia officinalis
    (b)   Zincum metallicum
    (c)   Lachesis mutus
    (d)   Secale Cornutum

Ans. (b)

Note
Zincum metallicum is the indicated medicine for the above mentioned symptoms.

Also see
Zincum metallicum
Persons suffering from cerebral and nervous exhaustion; defective vitality; brain or nerve power wanting; too weak to develop exanthemata or menstrual function, to expectorate, to urinate; to comprehend, to memorize. Incessant and violent fidgety feeling in feet or lower extremities; must move them constantly. Always feels

better every way as soon as the menses begin to flow; it relieves all her sufferings; but they return again as soon after the flow ceases.
Ref: Allen's Keynotes.

Female: ovarian pain, ESPECIALLY LEFT; CAN'T KEEP STIL. (VIB.) Nymphomania of lying-in women. Menses too late, suppressed; lochia suppressed (Puls.). Breasts painful. Nipples sore. Menses flow more at night (Bov.). Complaints all better during menstrual flow (Eupi., Lach.). All the female symptoms are associated with restlessness, depression, coldness, spinal tenderness and restless feet. Dry cough before and during menses.
Ref: Boericke's Materia Medica.

Q. 312. Fluent discharge acrid from the nose but bland from the eyes_____ better in open air and worse in a warm room, neuralgia of stump after amputation. Which one of the following medicines is indicated in such a patient (PSC/WB/93)
(a) Arsenicosum iodatum
(b) Allium cepa
(c) Staphysagria
(d) Euphrasia officinalis

Ans. (b)

Note
The indicated medicine from above is Allium cepa.

Also see
Allium cepa
Eyes burning, biting, smarting as if from smoke, must rub them; watery and suffused; capillaries injected and there in excessive lachrymation. Coryza profuse, watery and acrid nasal discharge, with profuse, bland lachrymation (profuse, full of acrid tears, bland and fluent coryza, Euphr.). Acrid, watery discharge dropping from tip of nose (Ars., Ars-iod.). Spring coryza: after damp north-easterly winds; discharge burns and corrodes nose and upper lip.

Traumatic chronic neuritis; neuralgia of stump after amputation; burning and stinging pains. Panaritia: with red streaks up the arm; pains drive to despair; in child-bed.
Ref: Allum cepa, Allen's Keynotes.

Q. 313. Hemiopia; sees only the lower half_____ (MD/NIH/98)
(a) Aurum metallicum
(b) Lycopodium clavatum
(c) Syphilinum
(d) Lithium carbonicum

Ans. (a)

Note
Hemiopia; sees only the lower half is 'Aurum metallicum'.

Also see
Aurum metallicum
Hemiopia; sees only the lower half (sees only the left half, Lith.-c., Lyc.).
Ref: Allen's Keynotes.

Extended Information

[kent] [Vision]Hemiopia:Upper lost:
Ars,AUR, Camph, Dig, Gels,
Ref: Kent's Repertory.

Q. 314. Toothache from coffee drinking____ (MD/NIH/98)
(a) Apis mellifica
(b) Nux vomica
(c) Coffea cruda
(d) Mezereum

Ans. (b)

Note
From the choice given above for toothache from coffee drinking is Nux vomica.

Also see

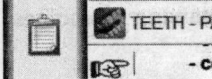

TEETH - PAIN, - coffee,from

- **coffee,from:** (13) anan. *Bell. Camph.* carb-v. **CHAM.** cocc. *Ign.* lachn. merc. *Nux-v. Puls.* rhus-t. sil.

Ref: Kent's Repertory.

Q. 315. Child cries whole night but remains quiet during daytime. Which of the following medicines should be applicable (PSC/WB/91)
(a) Lycopodium clavatum
(b) Chamomilla
(c) Belladonna
(d) Jalapa

Ans. (d)

Note
Child cries whole night but remains quiet during daytime is Jalapa.

Also see
Jalapa
General:
Causes and cures colic and diarrhoea. The child is good all day, but screams and is restless and troublesome at night.
Ref: Boericke's Materia Medica.

Q. 316. Which of the following medicines is applicable in case of eruptions severely itching but ameliorated by warm application (PSC/WB/91)
(a) Sulphur
(b) Mercurius solubilis
(c) Croton tiglium
(d) Rumex crispus

Ans. (d)
Note
From the choice given above Rumex crispus is the remedy which covers the above symptom.

Also see:
Sulphur
Skin itching, voluptuous; scratching causes burning; < from heat of bed (Merc.); soreness in folds (Lyc.).
Ref: Allen's Keynotes.

Mercurius solubilis
ITCHING; worse from warmth of bed.
Ref: Allen's Keynotes.

Croton tiglium
Intense itching of skin, but so tender is unable to scratch; > by gently rubbing; eczema over whole body. Intense itching of genitals in both sexes (Rhus-t.); vesicular eruption on male; so sensitive and sore is unable to scratch.
Aggravation: diarrhoea; every motion; after drinking; while eating or nursing (Arg-n., Ars.); during summer; from fruit and sweetmeats (Gamb.); the least food or drink.

Rumex crispus
Intense itching of skin, especially of lower extremities; worse, exposure to cold air and when undressing.
Ref: Boericke's Materia Medica.

Skin itching of various parts; < by cold, > by warmth; when undressing, uncovering or exposing to cold air (Hep., Nat-s., Olnd.).
Ref: Allen's Keynotes.

Q. 317. Sensation of great dryness without real thirst____ (MD/BBSR/99)
    (a)   Pulsatilla pratensis
    (b)   Nux moschata
    (c)   Bryonia alba
    (d)   Gelsemium sempervirens

Ans. (b)
Note
From the choice given above Nux moschata covers the above symptom.
Also see
Nux moschata
Great dryness of mouth (Apis, Lach.); tongue so dry it adheres to roof of mouth; saliva seems like cotton; throat dry, stiffened, no thirst (Puls.). Sensation of great dryness without real thirst and without actual dryness of the tongue.
Ref: Allen's Keynotes.

Q. 318. A lady was very thirsty in her normal condition but developed complete aversion to drinking water; even the sight of water induced vomiting. Which of the following medicines may be applicable? (PSC/WB/93)
    (a)   Apis mellifica
    (b)   Bryonia alba
    (c)   Natrium muriaticum
    (d)   Phosphorus

Ans. (d)
Note
From the choice given above Phosphorus covers the above symptom.
Also see
Phosphorus
During pregnancy; unable to drink water; sight of it causes vomiting; must close her eyes while bathing (Lyss.).
Ref: Allen's Keynotes.

Q. 319. Sensation as if a thread was hanging down the throat____ (MD/NIH/98)
    (a)   Sabadilla
    (b)   Drosera rotundifolia
    (c)   Hyoscyamus niger
    (d)   Valeriana officinalis

Ans. (d)
Note
Sensation as if a thread was hanging down the throat is Valeriana officinalis.
Also see
Valeriana officinalis
Sensation as if a thread was hanging down the throat (on tongue, Nat-m., Sil.).
Ref: Allen's Keynotes.

Q. 320. Gunshot diarrhoea is seen in ____ (MD/NIH/98)
(a) Antimonium crudum
(b) Podophyllum peltatum
(c) Croton tiglium
(d) Phosphoricum acidum

Ans. (c)

Note
From the choice given above 'Croton tiglium' covers the above symptom.

Also see
Croton tiglium
The bowels are moved as if by spasmodic jerk, 'coming out like a shot' (Gamb.); as soon as patient eats, drinks, or even while eating; yellow watery stool. Constant urging to stool followed by sudden evacuation, which is shot out of the rectum (Gamb., Grat., Podo., Thuj.). Swashing sensation in intestines, as from water, before stool (rumbling before stool, Aloe).
Ref: Allen's Keynotes.

Q. 321. Drawing pain through chest from breast to scapula of same side everytime the child nurses, nipple very sore____ (PSC/WB/91)
(a) Croton tiglium
(b) Graphites
(c) Silicea terra
(d) Phytolacca decandra

Ans. (a)

Note
From the choice given above 'Croton tiglium' covers the above symptom.

Also see
Croton tiglium
Drawing pain through the chest from breast to scapula, of same side every time the child nurses; nipple very sore. Intense itching of skin, but so tender is unable to scratch; > by gently rubbing; eczema over whole body.
Ref: Allen's Keynotes.

Q. 322. Nitricum acidum covers _____ miasm (MD/NIH/2000)
(a) Psora
(b) Sycosis
(c) Psora, Syphilis
(d) Psora, Sycosis, Syphilis

Ans. (d)

Note Nitricum acidum covers all three miasms – psora, sycosis and syphilis.

Also see
Nitricum acidum
'Phthisis,' 'syphilis,' and 'warty growths' represent Hahnemann's three miasms, psora, syphilis and sycosis. Nit-ac. belongs almost equally to all three. But in addition to its miasm relationship. Nit-ac. has drug relationships of great importance. It is one of the chief antidotes of Mercurius, and it is in cases of syphilis that have been overdosed with Mercurium that its action is most brilliant.
Ref: Clarke's Materia Medica.
Ref: Chronic Diseases, page 271-272.

Q. 323. Cancerous degeneration of the cervix; cutting pain in abdomen and haemorrhage at every stool (MD/NIH/98)
(a) Conium maculatum
(b) Mercurius solubilis
(c) Iodium
(d) Collinsonia canadensis

Ans. (c)

Note
Above symptom is covered by Iodium.

Also see
Iodium
Leucorrhoea: acrid, corrosive, straining and corroding the linen; most abundant at times of menses. Cancerous degeneration of the cervix; cutting pains in abdomen and haemorrhage at every stool. Constipation, with ineffectual urging, > by drinking cold milk. Croup: membranous, hoarse, dry cough, worse in warm, wet weather; with wheezing and swaying respiration (Spong.). Child grasps the larynx (All-c.); face pale and cold especially in fleshy children.
Ref: Allen's Keynotes.

Q. 324. Which of the following medicines is more applicable for crops of tiny boils mostly appearing on the face behind the ears, etc. in summers (PSC/WB/91)
    (a) Hepar sulphuris
    (b) Mercurius solubilis
    (c) Calcarea sulphurica
    (d) Arnica montana

Ans. (c)

Q. 325. Toothache relieved by holding cold water in the mouth____(PSC/WB/93)
    (a) Thuja occidentalis
    (b) Ignatia amara
    (c) Natrium sulphuricum
    (d) Nux vomica

Ans. (c)

Note
Toothache in general relieved by cold water in the mouth is Natrium sulphuricum.

Also see
Thuja occidentalis
Teeth decay next to gums; very sensitive; gums retract.
Ref: Boericke's Materia Medica.

Ignatia amara
Toothache; worse after drinking coffee and smoking.
Ref: Boericke's Materia Medica.

Natrium sulphuricum
Nosebleed during menses (instead of menses, Bry., Puls.).Toothache > by cold water, cool air (Coff., Puls.). Dirty, greenish-grey or brown coating on tongue.
Ref: Allen's Keynotes.

Nux vomica
Teeth ache; worse, cold things. Gums swollen, white and bleeding.
Ref: Boericke's Materia Medica.

Extended information

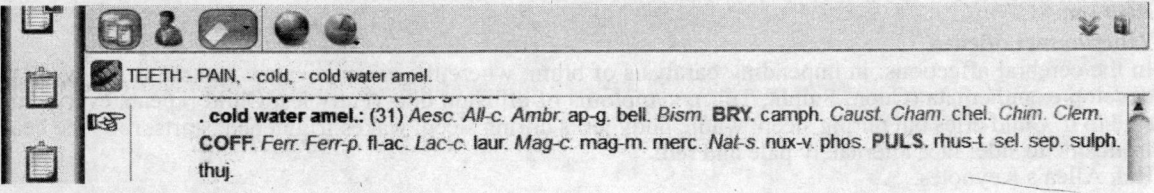

Ref: Kent's Repertory.

Q. 326. Flapping of alae nasi. All are true except___ (MD/NIH/98)
    (a) Lycopodium clavatum
    (b) Antimonium tartaricum
    (c) Bromium
    (d) Silicea terra

Ans. (d)

Note
Choice given above are all true for 'flapping of alae nasi' except 'Silicea terra.'

Also see

Bromium
It acts best, but not exclusively, on persons with *light blue eyes, flaxen hair, light eyebrows, fair, delicate skin; blonde, red cheeked, scrofulous girls*. Sensation of cobweb on the face (Bar-c, Borx., Graph.). Fan-like motion of the alae nasi (Ant-t., Lyc.). Sailors suffer with asthma 'on shore.' Stony, hard, scrofulous or tuberculous swelling of glands, especially on lower jaw and throat (thyroid, submaxillary, parotid, testes).
Ref: Allen's Keynotes.

Q. 327. Mercury's vegetable analogue is ___ (MD/NIH/2000)
    (a) Podophyllum peltatum
    (b) Mezereum
    (c) Silicea terra
    (d) Phytolacca decandra

Ans. (b)

Note
Mercury's vegetable analogue is Mezereum.

Also see

Mercurius solubilis
Relations
Follows well: after, Bell, Hep., Lach., Sulph., but should not be given before or after Sil. If given in low (weak) potencies hastens rather than aborts suppuration. The bad effects of Merc. are antidoted by Aur., Hep., Lach., Mez., Nit-ac., Sulph., and by a strong (high) potency of Merc, when the symptoms correspond. Compare: Mezereum, it's vegetable analogue for bad effects of large doses or of too frequent repetition. Mercury is < by heat of, but > by rest in, bed. Arsenicum is > by heat of, but < by rest in, bed.
Ref: Allen's Keynotes.

Q. 328. Child repeats everything said to it___ (MD/Hydrabad/99)
    (a) Agaricus muscarius
    (b) Helleborus niger
    (c) Zincum metallicum
    (d) Graphites

Ans. (c)

Note
Child repeats everything said to it is Zincum metallicum.

Also see

Zincum metallicum
In the cerebral affections: in impending paralysis of brain; where the vis medicatrix naturae is too weak to develop exanthemata (Cupr., Sulph., Tub.); symptoms of effusion into ventricles. Child repeats everything said to it. Child cries out during sleep; whole body jerks during sleep; wakes frightened, starts, rolls the head from side to side; face alternately pale and red.
Ref: Allen's Keynotes.

MCQ's in Materia Medica

Q. 329. Which of these is indicated for contradictory and alternating states of symptoms (PSC/WB/93)
    (a) Ignatia amara
    (b) Sulphur
    (c) Sepia officinalis
    (d) Natrium sulphuricum

Ans. (a)

Note
Ignatia amara is indicated for contradictory and alternating states of symptoms.

Also see
Ignatia amara
Especially suited to nervous temperament; women of a sensitive, easily excited nature; dark hair and skin but mild disposition, quick to perceive, rapid in execution. In striking contrast with the fair complexion, yielding, lachrymose, but slow and indecisive Pulsatilla. Remedy of great contradictions: the roaring in ears > by music; the piles > when walking; sore throat feels > when swallowing; empty feeling in stomach not > by eating; cough < the more he coughs; cough on standing still during a walk (Astac.); spasmodic laughter from grief; sexual desire with impotency; thirst during a chill, no thirst in the fever; the colour changes in the face when at rest.
Ref: Allen's Keynotes.

Q. 330. ____ is indicated for changeable stool (PSC/WB/91)
    (a) Pulsatilla pratensis
    (b) Nux vomica
    (c) Mercurius solubilis
    (d) Argentum nitricum

Ans. (a)

Note
Pulsatilla pratensis is indicated for changeable stool.

Also see
Pusatilla pratensis
Great dryness of mouth in the morning, without thirst (Nux-m. – mouth moist, intense thirst, Merc.). Mumps; metastasis to mammae or testicles. 'All-gone' sensation in stomach, in tea drinkers especially. Diarrhoea: only, or usually at night, watery, greenish-yellow, very changeable; as soon as they eat; from fruit, cold food or drinks, ice cream (Ars., Bry.; eating pears, Verat., Chin; onions, Thuj.); oysters, Brom., Lyc.; milk, Calc., Nat.-c., Nicc., Sulph.; drinking impure water, Cramp., (AQ) Zing.).
Ref: Allen's Keynotes.

Q. 331. Which has prominent properties of the syphilitic miasm (PSC/WB/91)
    (a) Pulsatilla nigricans
    (b) Phytolacca decandra
    (c) Selenium metallicum
    (d) Secale cornutum

Ans. (b)

Note
From the choice given above, Phytolacca decandra has the prominent properties of syphilitic miasm.

Also see
The syphilitic miasmatic skeletal complaints are consistent with:
Necrosis leading to crippling deformities of joints (primary degenerative osteoarthropathy, dental caries before teeth erupt; bone and periosteal pain at night, relieved by cold applications and movement, skeletal deformities, etc.

Phytolacca decandra

You will notice the resemblance of this drug to Mercury, and it is an antidote to mercury. In those lingering mercurial bone pains, where the patient has been salivated; the pains come on at night from the warmth of the bed; the body aches; a chronic, sore, bruised state; soreness of the periosteum where the flesh is thin, over the tibia; joints; soreness of the muscles; drawing and cramping; drawing in the muscles of the back; backache, worse at night; worse from the warmth of the bed.

...Phytolacca ought to be called 'vegetable Mercury' because it is so full of symptoms analogous to Mercury.

Ref: Lectures on Materia Medica, by J.T. Kent.

Miasmatic Preponderance for Phytolacca decandra

Medicine	Psora	Sycosis	Syphilis
Pulsatilla nigricans	++	+++	+
Phytolacca decandra	++	++	+++
Selenium metallicum	+	+++	+
Secale cornutum	++	++	+

Ref: Miasmatic Diagnosis, by Dr Banerjee.

Q. 332. In the early months of pregnancy, the lady can lie comfortably only on the abdomen. ____ medicine is applicable (PSC/WB/91)
(a) Medorrhinum
(b) Cina maritima
(c) Stannum metallicum
(d) Podophyllum peltatum

Ans. (d)

Note
From the given choices above, Podophyllum peltatum is the most suitable remedy for the above mentioned symptomatology.

Also see

Podophyllum peltatum
In early months of pregnancy, can lie comfortably only on stomach (Acet-ac.). Patient is constantly rubbing and shaking the region of liver with his and. Fever paroxysm at 7 am with great loquacity during chill and heat; sleep during perspiration.
Ref: Allen's Keynotes.

Q. 333. Cough deep, dry, precedes fever paroxysm____ (MD/NIH/2000)
(a) Sambucus nigra
(b) Hepar sulphuris
(c) Aconitum napellus
(d) Sabadilla

Ans. (a)

Note
From the choices given above, Sambucus nigra is the most appropriate choice.

Also see

Sambucus nigra
Cough: suffocative, with crying children; worse about midnight; hollow, deep, whooping, with spasm of chest; with regular inhalations but sighing exhalations. Cough deep, dry, precedes the fever paroxysm. Fever: dry heat while he sleeps; on falling asleep; after lying down; without thirst, dreads uncovering (must be covered in every stage, Nux-v.).
Ref: Allen's Keynotes.

Q. 334. Rarely repeated during active pulmonary tuberculosis____ (MD/NIH/98)
    (a)   Acalypha indica
    (b)   Arsenicum iodatum
    (c)   Ferrum phosphoricum
    (d)   Bacillinum

Ans. (d)

Note
Among the choices given above, Bacillinum is rarely repeated during active pulmonary tuberculosis.

Bacillinum
Has been employed successfully in the treatment of tuberculosis; its good effects are seen in the change of sputum, which reduces in quantity and becomes more aerated and less purulent. Many forms of chronic non-tubercular diseases are influenced favourably by Bacillinum, especially when bronchorrhoea and dyspnoea are present.

Doses
The dose is important. It should not be given below the thirtieth, and not repeated frequently. One dose a week is often sufficient to bring about a reaction. It is rapid in action, and good results are ought to be seen soon, otherwise there is no need of repetition.
Ref: Boericke's Materia Medica.

Also see
Acalypha indica
It is indicated in incipient phthisis, with hard, racking cough, bloody expectoration, arterial haemorrhage, but no febrile disturbance. Very weak in the morning, gains strength during the day. Progressive emaciation. All pathological haemorrhages having a notably morning aggravation.
Ref: Boericke's Materia Medica.

Arsenicum iodatum
Arsenicum iodatum, we have a remedy most closely allied to manifestations of tuberculosis. In the early stages of tuberculosis, even though there is an afternoon rise in temperature, Arsenicum iodatum is very effective. It will be indicated by profound prostration, rapid irritable pulse, recurring fever and sweats, emaciation and a tendency to diarrhoea. Chronic pneumonia, with abscess in the lung. Hectic debility; night sweats. This remedy is also to be remembered in phthisis with a hoarse, racking cough and profuse expectoration of a purulent nature, and attended with cardiac weakness, emaciation and general debility.
Ref: Boericke's Materia Medica.

Ferrum phosphoricum
In acute exacerbation of tuberculosis, a fine palliative of wonderful power. Corresponds to Grauvogl's oxygenoid constitution – the inflammatory, febrile, emaciating, wasting consumptive.
Ref: Boericke's Materia Medica.

Q. 335. Baseless fear of impending poverty, talks of his business in delirium, likes to lie listlessly. Which medicine is helpful to this patient____ (PSC/WB/91)
    (a)   Gelsemium sempervirens
    (b)   Bryonia alba
    (c)   Acidum phosphoricum
    (d)   Arnica montana

Ans. (b)

Note
From the choice given above, Bryonia alba has the feature of 'baseless fear of impending poverty, talks of his business in delirium.'

Also see
Bryonia alba
Delirium: talks constantly about his business; desire to get out of bed and go home (Cimic,, Hyos.).
Ref: Allen's Keynotes.

....Business concerns occupy their subconscious mind; as a consequence, they often **talk about business** while in a **delirium**. ......a sense of financial insecurity dwells, and the primary expression of this insecurity in Bryonia alba patients is a fear of poverty. They are afraid of being poor one day, irrespective of the degree of their bank balance or business success.....
Ref: Bryonia - The Essential Homeopathic Features and Generalities.
http://www.vithoulkas.com/content/view/104/9/lang,en/\

Q. 336. Fever returning annually; paroxysm every spring (PSC/WB/93)
    (a) Rhus toxicodendron
    (b) Belladonna
    (c) Lachesis mutus
    (d) Aconitum napellus

Ans. (c)
Note
From the choice given above, 'fever usually returning annually; paroxysm every spring' is a feature in Lachesis mutus.
Also see
Lachesis mutus
Sensation as of a ball rolling in the bladder. Fever annually returning; paroxysm every spring (Carb-v., Sulph.), after suppression by quinine the previous autumn.
Ref: Allen's Keynotes.

Q. 337. All are complementary except_____ (MD/NIH/2000)
    (a) Ignatia amara – Natrium muriaticum
    (b) Mercurius solubilis – Silicea terra
    (c) Belladonna – Calcarea carbonica
    (d) Apis mellifica – Natrium muriaticum

Ans. (b)
Note
All are complementary except Mercurius solubilis–Silicea terra.
Also see
Complementary:
    (a) Ignatia amara and Natrium muriaticum – Nat-m is chronic of Ignatia amara, which is it's vegetable analog. This is followed by Sepia officinalis and Thuja occidentalis.
    (b) Mercurius solubilis should not be given before or after Silicea terra.
    (c) Apis mellifica and Natrium muriaticum.
    (d) Belladonna – Calcarea carbonica
Ref: Allen's Keynotes.

Q. 338. The symptoms of Staphysagria include _____ (MD/NIH/2000)
    (a) Craving for tobacco
    (b) Bad effects of onanism
    (c) Cough only during daytime
    (d) All of the above

Ans. (d)
Note
All the above mentioned the symptoms belong to Staphysagria.
Also see
Staphysagria
Toothache: during menses; sound as well as decayed teeth; painful to the touch of food or drink; but not from biting or chewing; < drawing cold air into the mouth; < from cold drinks and after eating. Teeth turn black, show dark streaks through them; cannot be kept clean; crumble; decay on edges (at the roots, Mez., Thuja); scorbutic cachexia. Craving for tobacco. Extreme hunger even when stomach is full of food. Sensation as if

stomach and abdomen were hanging down relaxed (Agar., Ip., Tab.). Onanism; persistently dwelling on sexual subjects; constantly thinking of sexual pleasures. Spermatorrhoea: with sunken features; guilty, abashed look; emission followed by headache, weakness; prostration and relaxation or atrophy of sexual organs. Cough: only in the daytime, or only after dinner, worse after eating meat; after vexation or indignation; excited by cleaning the teeth.

Aggravation
Mental affections; from anger, indignation, grief, mortification; loss of fluids; tobacco; onanism; sexual excesses; from the least touch on affected parts.
Ref: Allen's Keynotes.

Q. 339. Heat and cold on vertex___ (MD/NHI/98)
    (a)   Sanguinaria canadensis
    (b)   Veratrum album
    (c)   Sepia officinalis
    (d)   Sulphur

Ans. (b)

Note
From the sensation given above, Veratrum Album covers it.

Also see

Veratrum album
Sensation of a lump of ice on vertex, with chilliness (Sep.); as of heat and cold at same time on scalp; as if brain were torn to pieces.
Ref: Allen's Keynotes.

Q. 340. Shingles; vesicles may have a bluish appearance (MD/NIH/98)
    (a)   Tarantula hispanica
    (b)   Ranunculus bulbosus
    (c)   Lachesis mutus
    (d)   Ledum palustre

Ans. (b)

Note
Shingles; vesicles may have a bluish appearance is Ranunculus bulbosus.

Also see

Ranunculus bulbosus
Intercostal rheumatism; chest sore, bruised, < from touch, motion or turning the body (Bry.); in wet, stormy weather (Rhus-t.). Shingles: preceded or followed by intercostal neuralgia (Mez.); vesicles may have a bluish appearance.
Ref: Allen's Keynotes.

Q. 341. Menorrhagia with scanty, black, acrid and indelible bloody discharge. Which one is the indicated medicine (PSC/WB/91)
    (a)   Medorrhinum
    (b)   Secale cornutum
    (c)   Ustilago maydis
    (d)   Kreosotum

Ans. (c)

Note

Medorrhinum
Metrorrhagia: at climacteric; profuse for weeks, flow dark, clotted, offensive; in gushes, on moving with malignant disease of uterus. Intense menstrual colic, with drawing up of knees and terrible bearing down labor-like pains; must press feet against support, as in labor. Intense
pruritus of labia and vagina, < by thinking of it. Breasts and nipples sore and sensitive to touch.

Scale Cornutum
Menses: irregular; copious, dark fluid; with pressing, labor-like pains in abdomen, continuous discharge of watery blood until next period. Threatened abortion, especially at the third month (Sabin.); prolonged, bearing down, forcing pains. During labor – pains irregular; too weak; feeble or ceasing; everything seems loose and open but no expulsive action; fainting. After pains: too long; too painful; hour-glass contractions.

Ustiligo maydis
Menorrhagia, with displaced uterus. Flabby, relaxed condition of pelvic organs, atonic condition of uterus; a state of weakness, relaxation and atony. Flushes of heat and disturbances of circulation similar to those occurring at climaxis, or from premature suppression of menses; ovaries inflamed, irritable, sensitive and swollen; burning distress in both ovaries.

Kreosotum
Menses: too early, profuse, protracted; pain during, but < after it; flow on lying down, ceases on sitting or walking about; cold drinks relieve menstrual pains; flow intermits, at times almost ceasing, then commencing again (Sulph.). Incontinence of urine; can only urinate when lying; copious, pale; urging, cannot get out of bed quick enough (Apis, Petros.); during first sleep (Sep.), from which child is roused with difficulty.

Q. 342. Hears better when in a noise (PSC/WB/98)
    (a)   Aconitum napellus
    (b)   Thuja occidentalis
    (c)   Graphites
    (d)   Belladonna

Ans. (c)

Note
Hears better when in a noise is **Graphites**.

Also see
Graphites
…..Suffering parts emaciate. Hears better when in a noise; when riding in a carriage or car, when there is a rumbling sound (Nit-ac.).
Ref: Allen's Keynotes.

Q. 343. Every stool is followed by thirst and every drink by shuddering ___ (PSC/WB/93)
    (a)   Aloe socotrina
    (b)   Cantharis vesicatoria
    (c)   Capsicum annuum
    (d)   Nux vomica

Ans. (c)

Note
Every stool is followed by thirst and every drink by shuddering is Capsicum annuium.

Also see
Capsicum annuum
Every stool is followed by thirst and every drink by shuddering. As the coldness of the body increases, so also does the ill-humour.
Ref: Allen's Keynotes.

Q. 344. ___ is indicated after Arnica montana in traumatic affections of the ovaries (PSC/WB/99)
    (a)   Psorinum
    (b)   Bellis perennis
    (c)   Ruta graveolens
    (d)   Hypericum perforatum

Ans. (a)

Note
Psorinum is indicated after Arnica montana in traumatic affections of the ovaries.

MCQ's in Materia Medica 235

Also see
Psorinum
Relations
Sulphur and Tuberculinum. Is followed well: by, Alum., Borx., Hep., Sulph., Tub. After: Lac-ac., in vomiting of pregnancy. After: Arn. in traumatic affections of ovaries. Sulphur follows Psorinum well in mammary cancer. Whether derived from purest gold or purest filth, our gratitude for its excellent service, forbids us to enquire or care. – J. B. Bell.
Ref: Allen's Keynotes.

Q. 345. Bad effects; from loss of sleep, mental excitement and night watching, feel weak if they lose but one hour's sleep, convulsions after loss of sleep, of anger and grief (PSC/WB/91)
    (a)   Cocculus indicus
    (b)   Nitricum acidum
    (c)   Nux vomica
    (d)   Zincum sulphuricum

Ans. (a)
Note
Bad effects from the above mentioned causes are covered by Cocculus indicus.

Also see
Cocculus indicus
Loss of appetite, with metallic taste (Merc.). Time passes too quickly (too slowly, Arg-n., Cann-i.). Great lassitude of the whole body; it requires exertion to stand firmly; feels too weak to talk loudly. Bad effects: from loss of sleep, mental excitement and night watching; feels weak if they lose but one hour's sleep; convulsions after loss of sleep; of anger and grief. Trembling of arms and legs; from excitement, exertion or pain.
Ref: Allen's Keynotes.

Q. 346. After overaction, from repeated doses of Belladonna in whooping cough___ (MD/NIH/98)
    (a)   Stramonium
    (b)   Drosera rotundifolia
    (c)   Belladonna
    (d)   Sulphur

Ans. (a)
Note
After overaction, from repeated doses of Belladonna in whooping cough, Stramonium is indicated.

Also see
Stramonium
Relations
Stramonium often follows: Bell, Cupr, Hyos, Lyss. In metrorrhagia from retained placenta with characteristic delirium, Sec. often acts promptly when Stram. has failed (with fever and septic tendency, Pyrog.). After overaction, from repeated doses of Bell., in whooping cough.
Ref: Allen's Keynotes.

Q. 347. In the treatment of psoric cases, Hahnemann has recommended Sulphur with one of the following as an intercurent remedy (PSC/WB/91)
    (a)   Lycopodium clavatum
    (b)   Sepia officinalis
    (c)   Calcarea carbonica
    (d)   Psorinum

Ans. (a)
Note
In the treatment of psoric cases, Hahnemann has recommended Sulphur with Lycopodium clavatum as an intercurent remedy.

Also see
Relations
Complementary: Iodine. Bad effects: of onions, bread; wine, spiritous liquors; tabacco smoking and chewing (Ars.). Follows well: after, Calc., Carb-v., Lach., Sulph. It is rarely advisable to begin the treatment of a chronic disease with Lyc. unless it is clearly indicated; it is better to first give another antipsoric. Lyc. is a deep seated, long acting remedy, and should rarely be repeated after improvement begins.
Ref: In reference to Lycopodium, Boericke's Materia Medica.

Q. 348. Cannot bear the smell or sight of food (PSC/WB/93)
    (a)   Arsenicum album
    (b)   Ammonium carbonicum
    (c)   Calcarea carbonica
    (d)   Aethusa cynapium

Ans. (a)

Note
Cannot bear the smell or sight of food is Arsenicum album.

Also see
Arsenicum album
Burning thirst without a special desire to drink; the stomach does not seem to tolerate, because it cannot assimilate cold water; lies like a stone in the stomach. It is wanted, but he cannot or dare not drink it. Cannot bear the smell or sight of food (Colch., Sep.). Great thirst for cold water; drinks often, but little at a time; eats seldom, but much. Gastric derangements; after cold fruits; ice cream; ice water; sour beer; bad sausage; alcoholic drinks; strong cheese. Teething children are pale, weak, fretful, and want to be carried rapidly.
Ref: Allen's Keynotes.

Q. 349. Cold sensation in larynx on inspiration, > shaving is a symptom of ___ (MD/NIH/2000)
    (a)   Conium maculatum
    (b)   Sulphur
    (c)   Bromium
    (d)   Carbo animalis

Ans. (b)

Note
Cold sensation in larynx on inspirations > shaving is a symptom of Bromium.

Also see
Bromium
Physometra; loud emission of flatus from the vagina (Lyc.); membranous dysmenorrhoea (Lac-c.). Cold sensation in larynx on inspiration (Rhus-t. Sulph.); > after shaving (< after shaving, Carb-an.).
Ref: Allen's Keynotes.

Q. 350. Violently irritable, prays with folded hands, incessant talking, irrelevant laughing, rapid change from joy to sadness, lewd nature. _____ medicine is indicated (PSC/WB/91)
    (a)   Stramonium
    (b)   Hyoscyamus niger
    (c)   Platinum metallicum
    (d)   Lachesis mutus

Ans. (a)

Note
From the choice of drugs above, the most suitable one is Stramonium.

Also see
Stramonium
Mind: devout, earnest, beseeching and ceaseless talking. Loquacious, garrulous, laughing, singing, swearing, praying, rhyming. Sees ghosts, hears voices, talks with spirits. Rapid changes from joy to sadness. Violent and lewd. Delusions about his identity; thinks himself tall, double, a part missing. Religious mania. Cannot bear solitude or darkness; must have light and company. Sight of water or anything glittering brings on

spasms. Delirium, with a desire to escape (Bell.; Bry.; Rhus-t.)
Ref: Boericke's Materia Medica.

Hyoscyamus niger
Mind: very suspicious. Talkative, obscene, lascivious mania, uncovers body; jealous, foolish. Great hilarity; inclined to laugh at everything. Delirium, with an attempt to run away. Low, muttering speech; constant carphologia, deep stupor.
Ref: Boericke's Materia Medica.

Platinum metallicum
Mind: irresistible impulse to kill. Self-exaltation; contempt for others. Arrogant, proud. Weary of everything. Everything seems changed. Mental troubles, associated with suppressed menses. Physical symptoms disappear as mental symptoms develop.
Ref: Boericke's Materia Medica.

Lachesis mutus
Mind: great loquacity. Amative. Sad in the morning; no desire to mix with the world. Restless and uneasy; does not wish to attend to business; wants to be off somewhere all the time. Jealous. (Hyos.) Mental labour best performed at night. Euthanasia. Suspicious; nocturnal delusion of fire. Religious insanity. (Verat.; Stram.) Derangement of the sense of time.
Ref: Boericke's Materia Medica.

Q. 351. Menses only during the day, cease on lying down___ (PSC/WB/91)
    (a) Causticum
    (b) Pulsatilla nigricans
    (c) Sepia officinalis
    (d) Bovista lycoperdon

Ans. (a)

Note
From the choice given above, Causticum covers the above symptom.

Also see
Causticum
'Menses: too early; too feeble; only during the day; cease on lying down'.
Ref: Allen's Keynotes.

Pulsatilla nigricans
Derangements at puberty; menses, suppressed from getting the feet wet; too late, scanty, slimy, painful, irregular, intermittent flow, with evening chilliness; with intense pain; great restlessness and tossing about (Mag-p.); flows more during the day (on lying down, Kreos.). Delayed first menstruation.
Ref: Allen's Keynotes.

Sepia officinalis
Irregular menses of nearly every form – early, late, scanty, profuse, amenorrhoea or menorrhagia.
Ref: Allen's Keynotes.

Bovista lycoperdon
Menses: flow only at night; not during daytime (Mag-c. – only in the day, ceases on lying, Cact., Caust., Lil-t.); every two weeks, dark and clotted; with painful bearing down (Sep.).
Ref: Allen's Keynotes.

Q. 352. Tickling, constant cough < by talking, entry of air through mouth or nose. So the patient avoids talking and tries to cover mouth and nose often with a piece of cloth Which medicine is indicated (PSC/WB/91)
    (a) Ipecacuanha
    (b) Squilla maritima
    (c) Spongia tosta
    (d) Rumex crispus

Ans. (c)

From the choice given above, Rumex crispus covers the above listed symptom.

Note

Rumex crispus
Tickling in throat pit, causing dry, teasing cough. Dry, incessant, fatiguing cough; worse from changing air or room (Phos., Spong.); evening after lying down; touching or pressing the throat pit; lying on left side (Phos.); from slightest inhalation of cold air; covers head with bedclothes to make air warmer; little or no expectoration. The cough is < in cool air or by anything which increases the volume or rapidity of inspired air......
Ref: Allen's Keynotes.

Q. 353. Eczema mainly in genitalia spreading to perianal region; severely itching and followed by severe soreness so that the patient cannot touch the area in spite of the desire to scratch. Which medicine is indicated? (PSC/WB/91)
(a) Sulphur
(b) Mercurius solubilis
(c) Croton tiglium
(d) Graphites

Ans. (c)
For the above symptom, Croton tiglium is the suitable choice.

Note

Croton tiglium
Intense itching of skin, but so tender is unable to scratch; > by gently rubbing; eczema over whole body. Intense itching of genitals of both sexes (Rhus-t.); vesicular eruption on males; so sensitive and sore is unable to scratch.
Ref: Allen's Keynotes.

Q. 354. Bed feels hard____ (MD/NIH/98)
(a) Pyrogenium
(b) Baptisia tinctoria
(c) Arnica montana
(d) Opium

Ans. (a)
From the choice given above, Pyrogenium is the most appropriate remedy for the mentioned symptom.

Note
From the choice given above, both Arnica montana and Pyrogenium have a hard bed sensation. However, under the repertory reference of Kent, Arnica montana has more intensity than Pyrogenium.

Also see

Opium
Sleep: heavy, stupid; with stetorous breathing, red, face, eyes, half closed, blood shot; skin covered with hot sweat; after convulsions. Sleepy, but cannot sleep (Bell., Cham.), sleeplessness with acuteness of hearing, clock striking and cocks crowing at great distance keep her awake. Loss of breath on falling asleep (Grind., Lach.). Bed feels so hot she cannot lie on it (bed feels hard, Arn., Bry., Pyrog.); moves often in search of a cool place; must be uncovered.
Ref: Allen's Keynotes.

Extended information
Kent repertory reference:

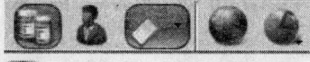

 GENERALS - HARD bed, sensation of

HARD bed, sensation of: (37) acon. agar. **ARN**. *Ars*. *Bapt*. bar-c. bry. caust. con. dros. *Ferr*. *Ferr-p*. graph. ip. kali-c. lyc. mag-c. mag-m. manc. merc. nux-m. nux-v. op. phos. plat. puls. *Pyrog*. *Rhus-t*. *Ruta* sabad. **SIL**. spong. stann. sulph. tarax. thuj. verat.

MCQ's in Materia Medica

Q. 355. Vicarious menstruation_____ (PSC/WB/91)
(a) Pulsatilla nigricans
(b) Arnica montana
(c) Bryonia alba
(d) Causticum annuum

Ans. (c)
Note
Vicarious menstruation is 'Bry'.

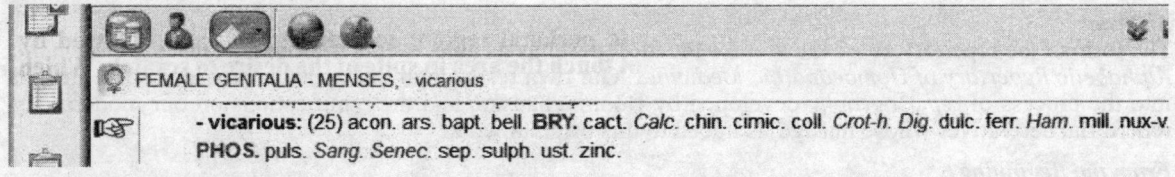

Ref: Kent's Repertory

Q. 356. Teeth decay at edges _____ (MD/NIH/98)
(a) Staphysagria
(b) Thuja occidentalis
(c) Kreosotum
(d) Magnesia carbonica

Ans. (a)
From the choice of drugs given above, 'staphysagria' has the feature 'teeth decay at edges.'

Note
Staphysagria
Teeth turn black, show dark streaks through them; cannot be kept clean; crumble, decay on edges (at the roots, Mez., Thuj.); scorbutic cachexia. Craving for tobacco.
Ref: Allen's Keynotes.

Q. 357. Repertory part of the book 'Fragmenta De…..Observatis' is mentioned in the _____ (MD/NIH/98)
(a) First part
(b) Second part
(c) Both of above
(d) None of above

Ans. (b)
Note
Repertory part of the book 'Fragmenta De…..Observatis' is mentioned in the second part.

Also see
FRAGMENTA DE VIRIBUS
The First Materia Medica and Repertory of the Homoeopathy
(Fragmentary observations relative to the positive powers of medicine on the human body)
Fragmenta de viribus, as it is most popularly called was one of the first attempts made by Dr Samuel Hahnemann in the direction of a proper materia medica. This work was merely a glimpse of what was to come. It contained the accounts of his first provings of homoeopathic medicines. It was the precursor, the fore-runner of homoeopathic materia medica.

It was written in Latin language and was published in 1805. Publishers were M/s Sumpter Joan Ambrose Barthii of Leipzig.
It was published in two volumes:

(1) The first volume was published in 1805. It was called PARS PRIMA. It had 277 pages comprising of an 'Introduction' and the 'Main Text' of the book.

(2) The second volume was the 'Repertory' or 'Index.' It was called PARS SECUNDA. It had 476 pages comprising of 'Preface' and a 'Repertory' of 460 pages.

In the later editions, the two parts were combined in one volume. In 1834, Dr F.F. Quin, the erstwhile father of British homoeopathy, called for this book and published it in one volume from London.
Ref: http://www.homeorizon.com/mainpagegeneral.asp?t=fragmenta.htm#page%20top

Fragmenta ... Fragmenta de Viribus Medicamentorum Positivis Sive in Sano Humanis Corpore Observatis, 2 parts, 269 and 470 pages, J.A. Barth, Leipzig, 1805, by Hahnemann:

First Repertory

Abstract
The form of the repertory as we know it for the most part has its antecedents in Bönninghausen's *Systematic Alphabetic Repertory of Homoeopathic Medicines*. Our own research in this area has provided some insight into the process of *repertography* developed by Bönninghausen, and the ramifications on our modern day repertorial derivatives whose lineage$_1$ is traced to this original work.

From the Beginning
It was Hahnemann who first realised the need for some form of index for recalling the symptoms of our ever increasing provings, data, appending an *alphabetical index* to his *Fragmenta*$_2$ of 1805, and undertaking two further compilations which however were never published.$_3$ There followed a number of *indices* by various authors,$_4$ each listing a single remedy alongside a single symptom, more or less as it appeared[5] in the record.$_6$ These were not *repertories* as such, but rather, a re-organised$_7$ listing (for easier reference) of symptoms.$_8$

The First Repertory
Bönninghausen's own life-saving experience of homoeopathy in 1828,$_9$ and his subsequent failure to induce any of the allopathic physicians around him to take up it's study,$_{10}$ moved him to pursue the study of this therapeutic method himself. His sharp mind being already trained in taxonomic definition was perfectly suited to this study,$_{11}$ and he quickly realised$_{12}$ the necessity of an accurate ready reference to our provings data, compiling a succession of precursors,$_{13}$ before publishing his *Systematic Alphabetic Repertory of Homoeopathic Medicines [in two parts, antipsoric* (SRA) *and non-antipsoric* (SRN] *medicines*). This was *the first repertory*$_{14}$ as we know it, wherein provings were, for the first time, *represented* via *rubrics*,$_{15}$ graded according to clinical verification,$_{16}$ arranged systematically,$_{17}$ and alphabetically, and thereby allowing ready access$_{18}$ to our materia medica.

Repeatedly urged by Hahnemann,$_{19}$ Bönninghausen set bout to bring out a single volume, combined edition of this work,$_{20}$ but ceased when he realised a different model of repertory (TT).$_{21}$ SRA/SRN have since remained largely unserviceable to the homoeopathic profession; only the SRA had been translated into English, whilst the more voluminous SRN had not.$_{22}$ Yet SRA/SRN, to which we now refer jointly as The First Repertory (TFR),$_{23}$ both conceptually and structurally, represents Bönninghausen's first method of repertory, and forms the very model of our modern repertories;$_{24}$ descended firstly through Jahr in his Handbuch (JHR),$_{25}$ the second edition of which was translated into English and published as the first English language repertory (1838).$_{26}$ This then found it's way via C.Lippe (LRMC), to E.J.Lee (LRC),$_{27}$ and on to J.T.Kent, being incorporated into his Repertory (KR),$_{28}$ whose basic structure was consistent with that of its predecessors.$_{29}$ Thus, it may be seen that Kent's Repertory, and its emulates,$_{30}$ wholly in structure and initially in content,$_{31}$ itself derives from the systematicalphabetic model of TFR$_{32}$
Ref: http://www.vithoulkas.com/files/pdf/The_First_Repertory.pdf

Extended information
Organon § 109
I was the first that opened up this path, which I have pursued with a perseverance that could only arise and be kept up by a perfect conviction of the great truth, fraught with such blessings to humanity, that it is only by the homoeopathic employment of medicines[1] that the certain cure of human maladies is possible.[2]

1. It is impossible that there can be another true, best method of curing dynamic diseases (i.e., all diseases not strictly surgical) besides homoeopathy, just as it is impossible to draw more than one straight line betwixt two given points. He who imagines that there are other modes of curing diseases besides it could not have appreciated homoeopathy fundamentally nor practised it with sufficient care, nor could he ever have seen or read cases of properly performed homoeopathic cures; nor, on the other hand, could he have discerned the baselessness of all allopathic modes of

treating diseases and their bad or even dreadful effects, if, with such lax indifference, he places the only true healing art on an equality with those hurtful methods of treatment, or alleges the latter to be auxiliaries to homoeopathy which it could not do without! My true, conscientious followers, the pure homoeopathists, with their successful, almost never-failing treatment, might teach these persons better.

2. The first fruits of these labors, as perfect as they could be at that time, I recorded in the Fragmenta de viribus medicamentorum positivis, sive in sano corpore humano observatis, pts. I, ii, Lipsiae, 8, 1805, ap. J. A. Barth; the more mature fruits in the Reine Arzneimittellebre, I Th., dritte Ausg.; II Th., dritte Ausg., 1833; III Th., zweite Ausg., 1825; IV Th., zw. Ausg., 1827 (English translation, Materia Medica Pura, vols I and ii); and in the second, third, and fourth parts of Die chronischen Krankheiten, 1828, 1830, Dresden bei Arnold (2nd edit., with a fifth part, Dusseldorf bei Schaub, 1835, 1839).

Q. 358. A patient feels too hot, cannot tolerate least exposure to sun's ray, dislikes covering even in winter, very eager to have cold bath. Which one of the following medicines is strongly indicated (PSC/WB/91)
   (a) Natrium muriaticum
   (b) Carbo vegetabilis
   (c) Acidum fluoricum
   (d) Carbo animalis

Ans. (c)

Q. 359. Bitter taste, nausea, gall bladder swollen and tender, stool bright yellow, hard, knotty sometimes alternates with diarrhoea, stitching pain in lower right ribs with jaundice, urine golden yellow colour. Which is the indicated medicine (PSC/WB/93)
   (a) Carduus mariannus
   (b) Ipecacuanha
   (c) Chelidonium majus
   (d) Nux vomica

Ans. (c)

Note
The medicine is 'Chelidonium majus.'

Also see
Chelidonium majus

Stomach:
Tongue yellow, with imprint of teeth; large and flabby. (Merc.; Hydr.) **Taste bitter**, pasty. Bad odour from mouth. PREFERS HOT FOOD AND DRINK. **Nausea**, vomiting; BETTER, VERY HOT WATER. **Pain through stomach to back and right shoulder blade**. Gastralgia. EATING RELIEVES TEMPORARILY, especially when accompanied with hepatic symptoms.

Abdomen:
Jaundice due to hepatic and gall bladder obstruction. Gall colic. Distention. Fermentation and sluggish bowels. Constriction across, as by a string. Liver enlarged. Gall stones. (Berb.)

Urine:
Profuse, foaming, **yellow urine, like beer**. (Chen.) Dark, turbid.

Stool:
Constipation; **stools hard, round balls**, like sheep's dung, bright yellow, pasty; clay coloured, stools float in water; ALTERNATION OF DIARRHOEA AND CONSTIPATION. Burning and itching of anus (Rat. Sulph.).

Ref: Boericke's Materia Medica.

Q. 360. When treating a case of non – febrile intermittent disease, Hahnemann has recommended an intercurrent drug. Which one of the following is correct (PSC/WB/91)
  (a) Arsenicum album
  (b) Sulphur
  (c) China officinalis
  (d) Ipecacuanha

Ans. (c)

Note
Hahnemann has recommended the intercurrent drug China officinalis.

Q. 361. Ravenous appetite; hungry soon after eating
  (a) Cina maritima
  (b) Lycopodium clavatum
  (c) Iodium
  (d) All of the above

Ans. (d)

Note
Ravenous appetite; hungry soon ofter eating includes all the above remedies.

Also see

[Kent] [STOMACH] - APPETITE, - ravenous,canine,excessive - eating - after,soon
acon. agar. *Arg-met.* asc-c. bov. *Calc.* CHININ-S. *Cic.* CINA coc-c. com. fago. grat. IOD. kali-p. lach. LYC. *Med. Merc.* myric. PHOS. phyt. plb. *Psor.* sarr. *Staph.* stront-c. *Sulph.* zinc.

Q. 362. Appetite, ravenous / canine, excessive; emaciation with
  (a) Calcarea carbonica
  (b) Ignatia amara
  (c) Natrium muriaticum and Petroleum
  (d) All of the above

Ans. (d)

Note
Ravenous / canine, excessive, emaciation with, includes all the above mentioned medicines.

Also see

[Kent] [STOMACH] - APPETITE, - ravenous,canine,excessive - emaciation,with
Abrot. CALC. IOD. NAT-M. PETR. *Phos.* psor. *Sulph. Tub.*

Q. 363. Aversion to fish
  (a) Graphites
  (b) Nux vomica
  (c) Lycopodium clavatum
  (d) Thuja occidentalis

Ans. (a)

Note
Aversion to fish is Graphites.

Also see

[Kent] [STOMACH] - AVERSION to - fish
Colch. GRAPH. guare. nat-m. *Phos.* sulph. *Zinc.*

Q. 364. **Aversion to hot food:**
(a) Nux vomica
(b) China officinalis
(c) Lycopodium clavatum
(d) Argentum nitricum

Ans. (a)

Note
Aversion to hot food is China officinalis.

Also see

[Kent] [STOMACH] - AVERSION to - food - hot
CHIN. ferr. kali-s. merc-c. petr.

Q. 365. **Aversion to warm food**
(a) Sulphur
(b) Carbo vegetabilis
(c) Natrium muriaticum
(d) Graphites

Ans. (d)

Note
Aversion to warm food is Graphites.

Also see

[Kent] [STOMACH] - AVERSION to - food - warm
Bell. Calc. Chin. cupr. **GRAPH.** guare. *Ign. Lach. Lyc.* mag-c. mag-s. *Merc-c.* merc. petr. **PHOS.** psor. **PULS.** *Sil. Verat.* zinc.

Bibliography

Books
- Allen's Key Notes – B. Jain Publishers (P) Ltd., New Delhi
- Pocket Manual of Homeopathic Materia Medica & Repertory – B. Jain Publishers (P) Ltd., New Delhi
- Relationship of Remedies and Sides of the Body – R.Gibson Miller – B. Jain Publishers (P) Ltd., New Delhi
- Homeopathic Drug Pictures – M.L. Tyler – B. Jain Publishers (P) Ltd., New Delhi
- Lectures on Homeopathic Materia Medica – By Kent – B. Jain Publishers (P) Ltd., New Delhi
- Repertory of the Homeopathic Materia Medica – Dr. Kent – B. Jain Publishers (P) Ltd., New Delhi
- Hering's Guiding Symptoms of Materia Medica – C. Hering – B. Jain Publishers (P) Ltd., New Delhi
- Dictionary of Practical Materia Medica – J.H.Clarke – B. Jain Publishers (P) Ltd., New Delhi
- Materia Medica of Hom. Medicine – S.R. Phatak, B. Jain Publishers (P) Ltd., New Delhi
- Lotus Materia Medica – Robin Murphy – B. Jain Publishers (P) Ltd., New Delhi
- Synthesis Repertory – Version-9.1 – B. Jain Publishers (P) Ltd., New Delhi

Websites
www.similima.com

Softwares
RADAR
HOMPATH

Chapter 3
ANATOMY

Q. 1. The median cubital vein is the vein of choice for intravenous injection for withdrawing blood from donors and for catheterization because it is (UPSC-02)
    (a)   A long vein
    (b)   Does not slip while drawing the blood
    (c)   Is an accessory vein
    (d)   Is a deep vein

Ans. (b)
Note
The median cubital vein is the vein of choice for intravenous injection, for withdrawing blood from donors, and for cardiac catheterization, because it is fixed by the perforators and does not slip away during piercing. When the median cubital vein is absent, the basilica or median basilica vein is preferred over the cephalic because the former is a more efficient channel.
Ref: Human Anatomy Vol-I, By B. D. Chaurasia 3rd Ed Pg-64

Q. 2. The most important part of levator ani is (UPSC-02)
    (a)   Iliococcygeus
    (b)   Ischiococcygeus
    (c)   Pubococcygeus
    (d)   Ischiopubic part of coccygeus

Ans. (c)
Note
Levator ani muscle
Levator ani is the main muscle of the pelvic floor. It forms a funnel-shaped diaphragm in the pelvis between the lateral hip walls, the pubis anteriorly and the coccyx posteriorly.
Often, levator ani is considered as several separate muscle parts:
    (a)   Pubovaginalis
    (b)   Coccygeus
    (c)   Iliococcygeus
    (d)   Pubococcygeus
    (e)   Puborectalis
However they have common features:
Origin:
From a tendinous arch between the pubis and ischial spine on the internal surface of the pelvis.
Insertion:
    (a)   Perineal body
    (b)   External wall of anal canal
    (c)   Anococcygeal ligament
    (d)   Coccyx
Therefore the main part of levator ani is *pubococcygeus part* as it has a crucial role in the maintenance of continence.
The Pubococcygeus
a.   Anterior fibers of this part arises from the medial part of the pelvic surface of the body of the pubis. In the males these fibers closely surround the prostate and constitute the levator prostatae. In females these fibres surround the vagina and form the sphincter vaginae. Both in the male and female the anterior fibres are inserted into the perineal body.
b.   Posterior fibres of pubococcygeus arise from the lateral part of the pelvic surface of the body of the pubis; and from the anterior half of the white line on the obturator fascia. They partly form loop or a sling around

the anorectal junction; and are partly continuous with the longitudinal muscle coat of the rectum. These middle fibres constitute the puborectalis.

During coughing, sneezing, lifting and other muscular efforts, the pubococcygeus part of levator ani and coccygei counteract and help to maintain continence of bladder and rectum.

In micturition, defecation and parturition a particular pelvic outlet is open, but contraction of fibers around other openings resists increased intra-abdominal pressure and prevents any prolapse through the pelvic floor.

The coccygei pull forwards and support the coccyx, after it has been pressed backwards during defecation or parturition.

Ref: Human Anatomy Vol-II, By B. D. Chaurasia Ed 3rd Pg-346

Q. 3. Disease of hip may produce referred pain in knee because of (UPSC-02)
    (a)   Femoral and Sciatic nerve
    (b)   Femoral and Obturator nerve
    (c)   Obturator and Sciatic nerve
    (d)   Only Sciatic nerve

Ans. (b)

Note
Diseases of hip like tuberculosis may cause referred pain in the knee because of the common nerve supply of the two joints.

The hip joint is supplied by:
    (i)   Femoral nerve
    (ii)   Ant. division of obturator nerve

The knee joint is supplied by:
    (iii)   Femoral and
    (iv)   Obturator nerve (Post. division of obturator nerve supplies both to hip and knee joint)

Ref: Human Anatomy Vol-II, By B. D. Chaurasia 3rd Ed Pg-122 & 129
Ref: Snell's 7th Ed Pg Pg 639

Q. 4. The submucosa of which one of the following GIT organs is completely filled with Brunner's glands? (UPSC-02)
    (a)   Appendix
    (b)   Colon
    (c)   Duodenum
    (d)   Oesophagus

Ans. (c)

Note
Brunner's glands are submucosal glands located throughout the duodenum. The main function of these glands is to produce an alkaline secretion (containing bicarbonate) in order to:
    (i)   Protect the duodenum from the acidic content of chyme (which is introduced into the duodenum from the stomach).
    (ii)   Provide an alkaline condition for the intestinal enzymes to be active.
    (iii)   Lubricate the intestinal walls.

Ref: Human Anatomy Vol-II, By B. D. Chaurasia 3rd Ed. Pg-212

Q. 5. Arch of aorta lies behind the (UPSC 2002)
    (a)   Lower half of manubrium sterni
    (b)   Xiphoid process of sternum
    (c)   Middle one third of manubrium sterni
    (d)   Jugular notch

Ans. (a)

Note
The arch or aorta is present in superior mediastinum behind the lower half of the manubrium sterni.
Ref: Human Anatomy Vol-I, By B. D. Chaurasia 3rd Ed. Pg-234

Q. 6. Which rib of our body is more oblique? (UPSC-02)
    (a)   1st Rib
    (b)   2nd Rib
    (c)   9th Rib
    (d)   10th Rib

Ans. (c)
Note
Most Oblique rib in the body is 9th rib.
Ref: B.D. Chaurasia Vol I 2nd Ed. Pg-127

Q. 7. Consider the following: (UPSC 2002)
    I.   Pacinian corpuscle
    II.   Krause's corpuscle
    III.   Meissner's Corpscle
    IV.   Ruffin's corpuscle
Which one of the above are nerve endings?
    (a)   1, 2 and 4
    (b)   2, 3 and 4
    (c)   1, 2 and 3
    (d)   1, 3 and 4

Ans. (d)
Note
Pacinian corpuscle → Deep pressure
Krause's corpuscle → Cold
Meissner's corpuscle → Touch
Ruffiani's corpuscle → Warmth
Ref: B.D. Chaurasia Vol III 2nd Ed. Pg-294
Ref: Human Physiology By C.C. Chatterjee Vol II Pg- 5.67

Q. 8. Which one is called musician's nerve? (UPSC-02)
    (a)   Radial Nerve
    (b)   Ulnar Nerve
    (c)   Median Nerve
    (d)   Sciatic Nerve

Ans. (b)
Note
The ulnar nerve is also known as 'Musician's nerve' because it supplies the muscles producing the fine moments of the fingers.
Ref: Human Anatomy Vol-I, By B. D. Chaurasia 3rd Ed. Pg-106

Q. 9. The Spinal cord in an adult ends at the level of (UPSC-04)
    (a)   Lumbar – 1
    (b)   Lumbar – 4
    (c)   Lumbar – 5
    (d)   Sacral – 1

Ans. (a)
Note
In the fetus the spinal cord is up to sacrum and after birth due to growth of vertebral column its recessation takes place. In the adults it ends at the level of lower border of L1.
Ref: Human Anatomy Vol-III, By B. D. Chaurasia 3rd Ed. Pg-247

Q. 10. Angle of Louis is (UPSC 2004)
    (a)   Used in measuring genu valgus.
    (b)   The angle between the neck and shaft of femur.

(c) The angle of femoral triangle.
(d) Used in counting ribs.

Ans. (d)

Note
Sternal angle (Angle of louis): It marks the manubrio-sternal joint, and lies at the level of the second costal cartilage anteriorly, and the disc between the 4th and 5th thoracic vertebrae posteriorly. It is situated 5 cm below the suprasternal notch. It is an important landmark and from this point the ribs can be counted downwards.
Ref: Human Anatomy Vol-I, By B. D. Chaurasia 3rd Ed. Pg-162

Q. 11. How many fontanelles are present in a foetus? (KPSC / Lect/ Organon /Re-Exam -05)
(a) Four fontanelles
(b) Three fontanelles
(c) Two fontanelles
(d) Five fontanelles

Ans. Use your discretion

Note
However, the unossified membranous intervals, termed fontanelles, are seen at the angles of the parietal bones; these fontanelles are six in number: two, an anterior and a posterior, are situated in the middle line, and two, an antero-lateral and a postero-lateral, on either side.
Ref: Gray's Anatomy.
Fontanelles are 6.
Ref: Dutta Obstetrics 5th Ed. Pg- 91

Q. 12. Which artery is obliterated after the birth of the infant? (KPSC / Lect/ Organon /RE-05)
(a) Obliteration of the hypogastric arteries
(b) Obliteration of epigastric arteries
(c) Obliteration of the renal artery
(d) Obliteration of the brachial artery

Ans. (a)

Note
The hypogastric arteries in fetus become the umbilical artery at umbilicus. However, after birth of the infant the hypogastric artery obliterates / closes. Functional closure is almost instantaneous preventing even slight amount of the foetal blood to drain out. Actual obliteration takes about 2 – 3 months. The distal part forms the lateral umbilical ligament and the proximal part remains open as superior vesical artery.
Ref: Textbook of Obstetrics by D. C. Dutta 5th Ed. Pg- 44.

Q. 13. Anatomical capacity of human urinary bladder (in ml) is (KPSC / Lect/ Organon /RE-05)
(a) 500
(b) 1000
(c) 1500
(d) 2000

Ans. (a)

Note
The capacity of adult male urinary bladder is 500 ml.
Ref; Snell's Clinical Anatomy 6th Ed. Pg- 862
The capacity of adult male urinary bladder is 120 – 320 ml.
Ref: Human Anatomy Vol-II, By B. D. Chaurasia 3rd Ed. Pg- 306

Q. 14. Motor speech area is (KPSC / Lect/ Organon /RE-05)
(a) Wernicke's area
(b) Angular gyms
(c) Arcuate fasciculus
(d) Broca's area

Ans. (d)

Note
Motor speech area is called as 'Broca's area' and is situated in the inferior frontal gyrus of the left cerebral hemisphere in the right handed person.
Injury to this area results in inability to speak (aphasia).
Ref: Human Anatomy Vol-III, By B. D. Chaurasia 3rd Ed. Pg-274

Q. 15. Deep branch of ulnar nerve supplies the following muscles except (KPSC/Lect/Organon/RE-05)
(a) Adductor pollicis
(b) First lumbricals
(c) First dorsal interosseous
(d) Third lumbricals

Ans. (b)
Note
The first lumbrical is supplied by median nerve.
(However for information sack- First and Second lumbricals both are being supplied by median nerve.)
Ref: Human Anatomy Vol-I, By B. D. Chaurasia 3rd Ed. Pg- 118

Q. 16. Superior cerebral vein drains into (KPSC/Lect/Organon/RE-05)
(a) Great cerebral vein
(b) Vein of Galen
(c) Superior sagittal sinus
(d) Inferior sagittal sinus

Ans. (c)
Note
The superior cerebral vein terminates into superior sagittal sinus. (The superior cerebral veins are six to twelve in number. They drain superolateral surface of the hemisphere. They terminate into superior sagittal sinus)
Ref: Human Anatomy Vol-III, By B. D. Chaurasia 3rd Ed Pg 303

Q. 17. 53. AV node is located in the (KPSC/Lect/Organon/RE-05)
(a) Inter atrial septum
(b) Moderator band
(c) Muscular part of inter ventricular septum
(d) Membranous part of inter ventricular septum

Ans. (a)
Note
A.V. node is situated in the lower and dorsal part of inter-atrial septum above the opening of coronary sinus just above attachment of septal cusp of tricuspid valve.
Ref: Human Anatomy Vol-I, By B. D. Chaurasia 3rd Ed. Pg-225
Ref: Snell's 7th Ed Pg 116

Q. 18. The vein into which the external jugular vein usually drains is (KPSC/Lect/Organon /RE-05)
(a) Internal jugular
(b) Subclavin
(c) Branchiocephalic
(d) Azygous

Ans. (b)
Note
The external jugular vein drains into subclavian vein and then subclavian vein drains into internal jugular vein.
Ref: Human Anatomy Vol-II, By B. D. Chaurasia 3rd Ed. Pg-148

Q. 19. Ossification center appearing just before birth is (KPSC/Lect/Organon/RE-05)
  (a) Upper end of humerus
  (b) Lower end of tibia
  (c) Lower end of femur
  (d) Scaphoid.

Ans. (c)
Note
The femur ossifies from one primary and four secondary centres. The primary centre for the shaft appears in the 7th week of intra-uterine life. *The secondary centres appear one for the lower end at the end of 9th month of Intra Uterine Life* immediately before birth. One for the head during the first 6 months of life.
Ref: Human Anatomy Vol-II, By B. D. Chaurasia 3rd Ed. Pg-17

Q. 20. Nerve supply of larynx are all of the following, except (MD (Hom) EP-1/01)
  (a) Superior laryngeal nerve
  (b) Recurrent laryngeal nerve
  (c) Ext. branch of superior laryngeal nerve
  (d) Ansa cervicalis nerve

Ans. (d)
Note
Ansa cervicalis is formed by a superior and an inferior root. The superior root is the continuation of the descending branch of hypoglossal nerve. Its fibers are derived from C1, this root descends the internal carotid artery and the common carotid artery. The inferior root descending cervical nerve is derived from spinal nerves C2, 3 and it supplies; the infrahyoid muscles.
Ref: Human Anatomy Vol-III, By B. D. Chaurasia 3rd Ed. Pg-105

Q. 21. Primary motor area of the brain (MD (Hom) Q. EP-1/01)
  (a) Superior temporal gyri
  (b) Post central gyri
  (c) Pre central gyri
  (d) Inferior frontal gyri

Ans. (c)
Note
The motor area is located in the precentral gyrus on the superolateal surface of the hemisphere, and in the anterior part of the paracentral lobule. Stimulation of this area results in the movement in the opposite half of the body. The body is represented upside down in this area.
Ref: Human Anatomy Vol-III, By B. D. Chaurasia 3rd Ed. Pg-274

Q. 22. Adductor pollicis muscle is supplied by nerve (MD (Hom) EP-1/01)
  (a) Radial nerve
  (b) Median nerve
  (c) Deep branch of peroneal nerve
  (d) Deep branch of ulnar nerve

Ans. (d)
Note
Adductor pollicis muscle is supplied by the deep branch of ulnar nerve (C8T1)
Ref: Human Anatomy Vol-I, By B. D. Chaurasia Ed. Pg-111

Q. 23. Posterior inferior cerebellar artery is a branch of (MD (Hom) EP-1/01)
  (a) Vertebral artery
  (b) Posterior cerebellar artery
  (c) Basilar artery
  (d) Internal carotid artery

Ans. (a)

Note
The posterior cerebellar artery is the largest cranial branch of verterbral artery. It supplies parts of medulla, pons and cerebellum.
Ref: Human Anatomy Vol-III, By B. D. Chaurasia 3rd Ed. Pg-171

Q. 24. One of the boundary of inguinal triangle is (MD (Hom) EP-1/01)
  (a) Conjoint tendon
  (b) Pectineal line
  (c) Linea semilunaris
  (d) Inferior epigastric artery

Ans. (d)
Note
The Inguinal triangle or Hesselbach's triangle is formed by:
  (a) Lateral border of rectus abdominus, medially.
  (b) Inferior epigastric artery, laterally.
  (c) Inguinal Ligament, inferiorly.
Ref: Human Anatomy Vol-II, By B. D. Chaurasia 3rd Ed. Pg-180

Q. 25. All of the following structures pass through cavernous sinus except (MD (Hom) EP -1/01)
  (a) Internal carotid artery
  (b) Occulomotor nerve
  (c) Abducent nerve
  (d) Mandibular branch of trigeminal nerve

Ans. (d)
Note
All the above structures pass through the cavernous sinus except mandibular branch of trigeminal nerve.
Ref: Human Anatomy Vol-III, By B. D. Chaurasia 3rd Ed. Pg-73

Q. 26. Gluteus maximus muscle is inserted into (MD (Hom) EP-1/01)
  (a) Greater tronchanter
  (b) Shaft of femur
  (c) Gluteal tuberosity and iliotibial tract
  (d) Ilio-tibial tract

Ans. (c)
Note
Gluteus maximus muscle is inserted into Gluteal tubersoity of the femur and ilio-tibial tract.
Ref: Human Anatomy Vol-II, By B. D. Chaurasia 3rd Ed. Pg-61*

Q. 27. Inferior epigastric artery is a branch of (MD (Hom) EP-1/01)
  (a) Femoral artery
  (b) Ext. iliac artery
  (c) Internal iliac artery
  (d) Lateral circumflex artery

Ans. (b)
Note
Inferior epigastric artery is derived from external iliac artery near its lower end, immediately above, inguinal ligament lower and medial part.
Ref: Human Anatomy Vol-II, By B. D. Chaurasia 3rd Ed. Pg-174

Q. 28. Muscle attached to ulnar tuberosity (MD (Hom) EP-1/01)
  (a) Supinator
  (b) Biceps brachi
  (c) Brachialis
  (d) Flexor-carpi ulnaris

Ans. (c)

Note
The muscle attached to ulnar tuberosity and roughed depression on anterior surface of coronoid process is Brachialis.
Ref: Human Anatomy Vol-I, By B. D. Chaurasia 3rd Ed. Pg-79

Q. 29. Anterior fold of axilla is formed by (MD (Hom) EP-1/01)
- (a) Pectoralis major + minor
- (b) Pectoralis major + serratus anterior
- (c) Pectoralis major + clavi pectoral fascia
- (d) Pectoralis major + subscapularis

Ans. (c)
Note
Anterior wall of axilla is formed by pectoralis major in front and clavi-pectoral fascia enclosing the pectoralis minor and the subclavius, all deep to pectoralis major.
Ref: Human Anatomy Vol-II, By B. D. Chaurasia 3rd Ed. Pg-306

Q. 30. Attachment of semi membranous include (MD (Hom) EP-1/01)
- (a) Ischial tuberosity + medial tibial condyle
- (b) Ischial tuberosity + tibial shaft
- (c) Ischial tuberosity + fibular head
- (d) Ischial tuberosity + lateral condyle of tibia

Ans. (a)
Note
Origin of semimembranous is from suprolateral impression on the upper part of ischial tuberosity and it is inserted into groove on the posterior surface of the medial condyle of tibia.
Ref: Human Anatomy Vol-II, By B. D. Chaurasia 3rd Ed. Pg-74*

Q. 31. Uterine artery is a branch of (MD (Hom) EP-1/01)
- (a) Common iliac artery
- (b) Internal iliac artery
- (c) External iliac artery
- (d) Lateral sacral artery

Ans. (b)
Note
Uterine artery is a branch of anterior division of internal iliac artery.
Ref: Human Anatomy Vol-II, By B. D. Chaurasia 3rd Ed. Pg-319

Q. 32. Duodenal ulcer bleeds from (MD (Hom) EP-1/01)
- (a) Left gastric artery
- (b) Gastro duodenal artery
- (c) Gastric artery
- (d) Superior pancreatico duodenal artery

Ans. (b)
Note
Duodenal ulcer bleeds from gastro-duodenal artery.
Ref: Human Anatomy Vol-II, By B. D. Chaurasia 3rd Ed. Pg-306

Q. 33. Neck pulsation felt inferiorly at medial border of sternocleidomastoid muscle is (MD (Hom) EP-1/01)
- (a) Vertebral
- (b) Brachial
- (c) Subclavian
- (d) Internal jugular

Ans. (c)

Note
Neck pulsations are felt inferiorly at medial border of sternocleidomastoid muscle is of subclavian artery.
Ref: Human Anatomy Vol-III, By B. D. Chaurasia 3rd Ed. Fig 3.9 Pg-57
The surface marking of subclavian artery:
It is marked by a broad curved line, convex upwards, by joining the following two points:
    a.   A point on the sternoclavicular joint.
    b.   A second point at the middle of the lower border of the clavicle.
The artery rises about 2 cm above the clavicle.
The thoracic part of left subclavian artery is marked by a broad vertical line along the left border of manubrium a little to left of the left common carotid artery.
Ref: Human Anatomy Vol-III, By B. D. Chaurasia 3rd Ed. Surface marking at Pg- 235-b.

Q. 34. Mandibular nerve lesion at its origin involves all of following muscles except (MD (Hom) EP-1/01)
    (a)   Buccinator
    (b)   Masseter
    (c)   Lateral pterigoid
    (d)   Tensor tympani

Ans. (a)
Mandibular nerve lesion at its origin involves all of the following muscles except buccinator which is supplied by facial nerve.
Ref: Human Anatomy Vol-III, By B. D. Chaurasia 3rd Ed. Pg-125

Q. 35. Following have lymphatics except (MD (Hom) EP-1/01)
    (a)   Brain
    (b)   Dermis
    (c)   Eye
    (d)   Internal ear

Ans. (a)
Note
CSF replaces lymph in the CNS (Brain).
Ref: Human Anatomy Vol-III, By B. D. Chaurasia 3rd Ed. Pg- 245

Q. 36. Trachea bifurcates at the level of (during deep inspiration) (MD (Hom) EP-1/01)
    (a)   T6-7
    (b)   T3-4
    (c)   T 5-6
    (d)   T4-5

Ans. (a)
Note
Trachea bifurcates at the level of T6-7 during deep inspiration.

Q. 37. Oesophagus and duodenum share (MD (Hom) EP-1/01)
    (a)   Submucous glands
    (b)   Mucous cells
    (c)   Pseudo-stratified columnar epithelium
    (d)   All of the above

Ans. (a)
Note
Oesophagus and duodenum share submucous glands.
Ref: Human Anatomy Vol-III, By B. D. Chaurasia 3rd Ed. Pg-125

MCQ's in Anatomy

Q. 38. Ovarian artery is a branch of (MD (Hom) EP-1/01)
    (a) Internal iliac
    (b) External iliac artery
    (c) Common iliac artery
    (d) Aorta

Ans. (d)
Note
Ovarian (Gonadal) arteries are the branches of aorta. These are small arteries (two in number) that arise from the front of aorta a little below the origin of renal arteries.
Ref: Human Anatomy Vol-III, By B. D. Chaurasia 3rd Ed. Pg-273

Q. 39. Phrenic nerve receives the branches from roots of (MD (Hom) EP-1/01)
    (a) C 2, 3
    (b) C 1, 2, 3
    (c) C 3, 4, 5
    (d) C 4, 5, 6

Ans. (c)
Note
The phrenic nerve on both sides originates from the ventral rami of the third to fifth cervical nerves.
Phrenic nerve:
It is a mixed nerve carrying motor fibers to the diaphragm and sensory fibers from the diaphragm, the pleura, the pericardium, and part of the peritoneum.
Origin:
It arises from the 4th cervical nerve but receives contributions from C3 and C5. The contribution from C5 may come directly from the root or indirectly through the nerve to the subclavius. In the latter case the contribution is known as the *accessory phrenic nerve.*
Ref: Human Anatomy Vol-III, By B. D. Chaurasia 3rd Ed. Pg-159

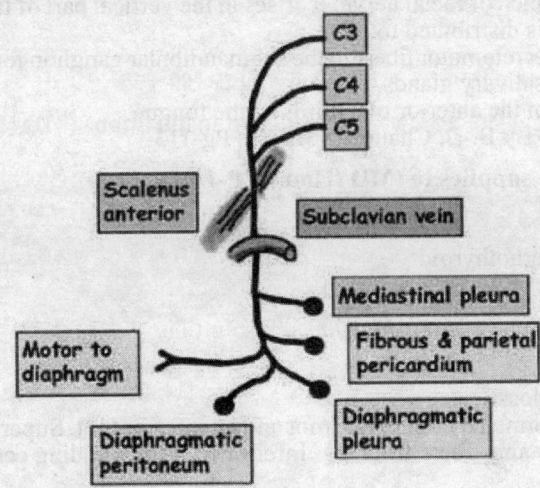

Q. 40. Deep peroneal nerve supplies to (MD (Hom) EP-1/01)
    (a) Lateral group of muscles of leg
    (b) Peroneous longus + Extensor digitorum braves
    (c) Lateral group of muscles of leg + extensor digitorum braves
    (d) Posterior muscles of leg

Ans. NA

Note
Deep peroneal (Anterior Tibial) nerve: Muscular branches:
a. Muscles of the anterior compartment of the leg; (all are dorsiflexors of the foot)-(1) Tibialis anterior, (2) Extensor digitorum longus, (3) Extensor Halucis longus (4) Peroneous tertius.
b. The extensor digitorum brevis (on the dorsum of the foot
c. First and second dorsal interossei
Ref: Human Anatomy Vol-II, By B. D. Chaurasia 3rd Ed. Pg-83

Q. 41. Thoracic duct ends at (MD (Hom) EP-1/01)
(a) Junction of left subclavian and internal jugular veins
(b) Left jugular vein
(c) Left subclavian vein
(d) Right jugular vein

Ans. (a)
Note
Thoracic duct (Largest lymphatic vessel in body – 18 inches long):
Origin: upper end of cisterna chyli at lower border of 12th thoracic vertebrae.
Course: crosses posterior and superior part of mediastinum.
Ends: By opening into the angle of junction of between the left subclavian and left internal jugular veins.
Ref: Human Anatomy Vol-I, By B. D. Chaurasia 3rd Ed. Fig. 20.6 Pg-242

Q. 42. Chorda tympani nerve is a branch of (MD (Hom) EP-1/01)
(a) Trigeminal
(b) Facial nerve
(c) Glossopharyngeal
(d) Vagus

Ans. (b)
Note
Chorda tympani nerve is a branch of facial nerve. It arises in the vertical part of facial canal about 6 mm above the stylomastoid foramen. It is distributed to:
a. Preganglionic secretomotor fibers to the submandibular ganglion for supply of the submandibular and sublingual salivary glands.
b. Taste fibers form the anterior two thirds of the tongue.
Ref: Human Anatomy Vol-II, By B. D. Chaurasia 3rd Ed. Pg-113

Q. 43. Ansa cervicalis nerve supplies to (MD (Hom) EP-1/01)
(a) Sternohyoid
(b) Thyrohyoid
(c) Omohyoid + Sternothyroid
(d) All of the above

Ans. (d)
Note

Ansa cervicalis (Ansa Hypoglossi)
It is a thin nerve loop that is formed by a superior root and an inferior root. Superior root is descending branch of hypoglossal nerve and contains fibers from C1. Inferior root (descending cervical nerve) is derived from spinal nerves C2, C3.
Distribution
a. Superior root; to superior belly of omohyoid.

b. *Ansa cervicalis; to sternohyoid, the sternothyroid and inferior belly of omohyoid.*

Note that the thyrohyoid and geniohyoid are supplied by separate branches from the first cervical nerve through the hypoglossal nerve.
Ref: Human Anatomy Vol-II, By B. D. Chaurasia 3rd Ed. Pg-105

Q. 44. Nerve supply of extraocular muscles (MD (Hom) EP-1/01)
    (a)   Occulomotor
    (b)   Abducent
    (c)   Trochlear
    (d)   All of the above

Ans. (d)
Note
Nerve supply of extraocular muscles:
    a.   The superior oblique is supplied by the 4th cranial (Trochlear) nerve.
    b.   The lateral rectus is supplied by the 6th cranial (Abducent) nerve.
    c.   The remaining extraocular muscles; superior, inferior and medial recti, inferior oblique and levator palpebrae superioris are all supplied by 3rd cranial (Oculomotor) nerve.
Ref: Human Anatomy Vol-III, By B. D. Chaurasia 3rd Ed. Pg-85

Q. 45. The sphenoid air sinus opens into (MD (Hom) EP-1/01)
    (a)   Middle meatus
    (b)   Spheno-ethmoidal recess
    (c)   Inferior meatus
    (d)   Bulla ethmoid

Ans. (b)
Note
The spheno-ethmoidal recess is a triangular fossa just above the superior concha. It receives the opening of sphenoidal air sinus. Sphenoidal air sinus lies within the body of sphenoid bone.
Ref: Human Anatomy Vol-III, By B. D. Chaurasia 3rd Ed. Pg-197

Q. 46. Medial side of great toe is supplied by nerve (MD (Hom) EP-1/01)
    (a)   Saphenous
    (b)   Tibial posterior
    (c)   Anterior tibial
    (d)   Deep peroneal

Ans. (a)
Note
Saphenous nerve is a branch of posterior division of femoral nerve. It pierces the deep fascia on the medial side of the knee between the Sartorius and Gracilis, and runs downwards in front of the great saphenous vein. It supplies the skin of the medial side of leg and the medial border of foot upto the ball of the great toe
Ref: Human Anatomy Vol-III, By B. D. Chaurasia 3rd Ed. Pg-81

Q. 47. Pisiform bone gives attachment to (MD (Hom) EP-1/01)
    (a)   Pisohamate ligament
    (b)   Abductor pollicis
    (c)   Extensor carpi ulnaris
    (d)   Flexor pollicis

Ans. (a)
Note
Pisiform bone gives attachments to:
    a.   Flexor carpi ulnaris
    b.   Flexor retinaculum
    c.   Abductor digiti minimi
    d.   Extensor retinaculum
    e.   Pisohamate ligament
Muscular attachments are given, but pisohamate ligament is not mentioned by Chaurasia. Since both the bones are present together on the lateral side these are connected together to by pisohamate ligament.
Ref: Human Anatomy Vol-I, By B. D. Chaurasia 3rd Ed. Pg-23 Fig. 2.10.

Q. 48. Internal pudendal artery is a branch of (MD (Hom) EP-1/01)
(a) Superior iliac
(b) Common peroneal
(c) Internal iliac
(d) Abdominal aorta

Ans. (c)
Note
Internal pudendal artery is a branch of internal iliac artery. It enters the gluteal region through the greater sciatic foramen. It leaves the gluteal region by passing into the lesser sciatic foramen through which it reaches the ischiorectal fossa.
Ref: Human Anatomy Vol-III, By B. D. Chaurasia 3rd Ed. Pg-66

Q. 49. Narrowest part of male urethra is at (MD (Hom) EP-1/01)
(a) Fossa navicularis
(b) Bulbar urethra
(c) External meatus
(d) Prostatic urethra

Ans. (c)
Note
The membranous part of the male urethra is the narrowest and least dilatable part of the urethra. With the exception of urethral orifice (External meatus),
Ref: Human Anatomy Vol-III, By B. D. Chaurasia 3rd Ed. Pg-293

Q. 50. Double nerve supply is received by (MD (Hom) EP-1/01)
(a) Adductor magnus
(b) Abductor longus
(c) Abductor bravis
(d) Gracilis

Ans. (a)
Note
The Adductor magnus has dual nerve supply:
  a. Adductor part (Origin- inferior ramus of pubis, ramus of ischium. Insertion- linea aspera of femur) is supplied by posterior division of obtruator nerve
  b. Hamstring / Extensor part (Origin- ischial tuberosity. Insertion- Adductor tubercle of femur) is supplied by tibial part of sciatic nerve.
Ref: Dorland's Pocket Medical Dictionary 21st Ed. Pg- 394

Q. 51. Superior rectal vein drains into (MD (Hom) EP-1/01)
(a) Portal vein
(b) Internal iliac vein
(c) Renal vein
(d) Inferior vena cava

Ans. (a)
Note
Superior rectal vein
The tributaries of this vein begin from the internal rectal venous plexus, they pass upwards in the rectal submucosa, pierce the muscular coat about 7.5 cm above the anus and unite to form the superior rectal vein which continues upwards as the inferior mesenteric vein (Pg-334). It opens into the splenic vein or sometimes into its junction with the superior mesenteric vein- forming Portal vein (Pg-233).
Ref: Human Anatomy Vol-II, By B. D. Chaurasia 3rd Ed. Pg-334 & 233

Q. 52. Dentate nucleus is a part of (MD (Hom) EP-1/01)
  (a) Mid brain
  (b) Pons
  (c) Medulla
  (d) Cerebellum

Ans. (d)
Note
The gray matter of cerebellum consists of:
  a. Dentate nucleus (It is a part of neo-cerebellum).
  b. Nucleus globosus (It is the part of paleo-cerebellum).
  c. Nucleus emboliformis (it is also a part of paleo-cerebellum).
  d. Nucleus fastigii (It is the part of archi cerebellum).
Ref: Human Anatomy Vol-III, By B. D. Chaurasia 3rd Ed. Pg-265

Q. 53. Duct of wirsung opens at (MD (Hom) Ent / Paper -1 /2001)
  (a) Minor papilla
  (b) Major papilla
  (c) Upper 2nd Molar
  (d) Side of the frenulum of tongue

Ans. (b)
Note
Wirsung's duct (The excretory duct of the pancreas into the duodenum.)
Ref: Dorland's Pocket Medical Dictionary 21st Ed.. Pg-200
Also known as: Duct of Wirsung / Ductus pancreaticus Wirsungi / Ductus Wirsungianus Wirsung's canal. It is named on the person: Johann George Wirsung
The Pancreatic duct opens into major papillae and the accessory pancreatic duct opens into the minor papilla.
Ref: Human Anatomy Vol-II, By B. D. Chaurasia 3rd Ed. Pg-249

Q. 54. Surface ectoderm gives rise to all of the following structures except (AIIMS/May-03)
  (a) Lens
  (b) Corneal epithelium
  (c) Conjunctival epithelium
  (d) Anterior layers of iris

Ans. (d)
Note
Surface ectoderm gives rise to (a) Lens, (b) Corneal epithelium (c) Conjunctival epithelium, except (d) Anterior layers of iris.

Q. 55. All of the following ligaments contribute to the stability of ankle (talocrural) joint except (AIIMS/May-03)
  (a) Calcaneonavicular (spring)
  (b) Deltoid
  (c) Lateral
  (d) Posterior tibiofibular

Ans. (a)
Note
Calcaneonavicular (Spring Ligament); it is the ligament which maintains the median longitudinal arch of the foot. It is attached posteriorly to the anterior margin of the sustentaculus tali, and anteriorly to the plantar surface of the navicular bone (Pg-137).
Ligaments which contribute to the stability of ankle joint are:
Deltoid (Medial) ligament: Consists of a. Tibionavicular, b. Tibiocalcaneal and Tibiotalar.
Lateral ligament (On lateral side) consist of a. Ant. Talofibular, b. Post. Talofibular, c. Calcaneofibular.
Ref: Human Anatomy Vol-II, By B. D. Chaurasia 3rd Ed. Pg-133

Q. 56. In dislocation of the jaw, displacement of the articular disc beyond the articular tubercle of the temporo-mandibular joint results from spasm or excessive contraction of the following muscle? (AIIMS/May-03)
- (a) Buccinator
- (b) Lateral pterygoid
- (c) Masseter
- (d) Temporalis

Ans. (b)
Note
Dislocation of temporo-mandibular joint occurs when the mandible is depressed. During this movement head of mandible and articular disc both move forwards until they reach the summit of the articular tubercle. In this position the joint is unstable, and sudden contraction of lateral pterygoid muscles, (as in yawning) is sufficient to pull the disc forward beyond the summit.
Ref; Snell's Clinical Anatomy. 7th Ed, Pg-783

Q. 57. Following surgical removal of a firm nodular cancer swelling in the right breast and exploration of the right axilla, on examination the patient was found to have a winged right scapula. Most likely this could have occurred due to injury to the (AIIMS/May-03)
- (a) Subscapular muscle
- (b) Coracoid process of scapula
- (c) Long thoracic nerve
- (d) Circumflex scapular artery

Ans. (c)
Note
The long thoracic nerve (C 5, 6 and 7) is well known to get injured during the surgical procedure of radical mastectomy.
Ref; Snell's Clinical Anatomy. 7th Ed, Pg-577

Q. 58. A 50 year old man suffering from carcinoma of prostate showed areas of sclerosis and collapse of T10 and T11 vertebrae in X-ray. The spread of this cancer to the above vertebrae was most probably through (AIIMS/May-03)
- (a) Sacral canal
- (b) Lymphatic vessels
- (c) Internal vertebral plexus of veins
- (d) Superior rectal veins

Ans. (c)
Note
There are many connections between prostatic venous plexus and vertebral veins; while coughing and straining intrabdominal pressure is raised. It leads to reverse flow of blood which enters the vertebral veins. This explains the frequent occurrence of skeletal metastasis in the lower vertebral column.
Ref: Snell's Clinical Anatomy. 7th Ed, Pg-939-940

Q. 59. The Pronator quadratus has the same innervation as one of the following muscles (AIIMS / Nov-03)
- (a) Flexor digitorum superficialis
- (b) Palmaris longus
- (c) Flexor pollicis longus
- (d) Flexor digitorum profundus of middle finger

Ans. (c)
Note
Pronator quadratus is supplied by anterior interosseous nerve and same imervation is for Flexor pollicis longus.
Ref: Human Anatomy Vol-I, By B. D. Chaurasia 3rd Ed. Pg-98

MCQ's in Anatomy

Q. 60. All of the following are pneumatic bones except (AIIMS /Nov-03)
- (a) Maxilla
- (b) Parietal
- (c) Ethmoid
- (d) Mastoid

Ans. (b)
Note
The air filled spaces present within some of the skull bones, especially which are situated around the nasal cavity. These are collectively called as paranasal sinuses. The sinuses (pneumatic spaces in bones contain large air spaces to make the skull light in weight, and help in resonance of voice) are present in (a) Maxilla, (c) Ethmoid, and (d) Mastoid, however, (b) the Parietal bones of skull do not contain any such air cavity.
Ref: Human Anatomy Vol-III, By B. D. Chaurasia 3rd Ed. Pg-198

Q. 61. The kinetic energy of the body is least in one of the following phases of walking cycle (AIIMS /Nov-03)
- (a) Heel strike
- (b) Mid-stance
- (c) Double support
- (d) Toe-off

Ans. (b)
Note
The kinetic energy of the body is least in Mid-stance.
Ref: Gray's Anatomy 38th Ed. Pg-898, 899.

Q. 62. When a heavy object in hand is lowered, the extension at the elbow is brought about by (AIIMS /Nov-03)
- (a) Active shortening of the extensors
- (b) Passive shortening of the extensors
- (c) Active lengthening of the flexors
- (d) Active shortening of the flexors

Ans. (c)
Note
When a heavy object in hand is lowered, the extension at the elbow is brought about by active lengthening of the flexors.
Ref; Gray's Anatomy 38th Ed. Pg-843

Q. 63. A 40 year old tailor complains of pain, numbness and weakness of the right hand for the last three months. On examination, there is hypoaesthesia and atrophy of thenar eminence. Which one of the following nerves is likely to be involved? (AIIMS /Nov-03)
- (a) Ulnar
- (b) Radial
- (c) Axillary
- (d) Median

Ans. (d)
Note
The hypoaesthesia and atrophy of thenar eminence corresponds to the motor and sensory distribution of 'Median nerve'.
The Median nerve in the hand supplies the following muscles:
- (1) Abductor pollicis brevis
- (2) Superficial head of Flexor pollicis brevis
- (3) Opponens pollicis (shared with the ulnar nerve) and
- (4) First and second lumbrical muscles. Along with palmar skin over the middle and distal phalanges of the lateral and half fingers.

Ref: Human Anatomy Vol-I, By B. D. Chaurasia 3rd Ed. Pg-118

Q. 64. Meiosis occurs in human males in (AIIMS /May-04)
    (a)   Epididymis
    (b)   Seminiferous tubules
    (c)   Vas deferens
    (d)   Seminal vesicles

Ans. (b)
Note
The spermatogenesis occurs in the seminiferous tubules. Therefore the meiotic division also takes place in seminferous tubules. The primary spermatocyte has 46 chromosomes and after meiosis it becomes secondary sperpmatocyte which contains 23 chromosomes.

Q. 65. The right lobe of liver consists of which of the following segments (AIIMS /May-04)
    (a)   V, VI, VII and VIII
    (b)   IV, V, VI, VII and VIII
    (c)   I, V, VI,VII and VIII
    (d)   I, IV, V, VI, VII and VIII

Ans. (a)
Note
Right lobe of liver consists of (a) V, VI, VII and VIII, surgical segments.

Q. 66. A young boy who was driving motorcycle at a high speed collided with a tree & was thrown on his right shoulder. Though there was no fracture, his right arm was medially rotated and forearm pronated. The following facts concerning this patient are correct, except (AIIMS /May-04)
    (a)   The injury was at Erb's point.
    (b)   A lesion of C5 and C6 was present.
    (c)   The median and ulnar nerves were affected.
    (d)   Supraspinatus, infraspinatus, subclavius & biceps brachii were paralyzed.

Ans. (c)
Note
All the facts regarding this patient are correct i.e., (a), (b), and (d), except (c).
It is a injury resulted from excessive displacement of head to the opposite side and depression of the shoulder on the same side causing injury to upper part of brachial plexus. Therefore it is consistent with the features of Erb's paralysis. It involves C5 and C6 roots. The suprascapular nerve, the nerve to the subclavius, and the musculocutaneous and axillary nerve all possess the fibers derived from C5 and C6 roots and therefore become functionless. The muscles paralysed are; (a) Supraspinatus (abductor of the shoulder), (b) the subclavius (Depresses the clavicle), (c) Biceps brachii (Supinator of the forearm, flexor of the elbow, weak flexor of shoulder) and (d) Deltoid; abductor of the shoulder joint. Teres minor (lateral rotator of shoulder joint). Thus the limb hangs by the side, medially rotated and forearm pronated.
Ref: Human Anatomy Vol-I, By B. D. Chaurasia 3rd Ed. Pg-44

Chapter 4
PHYSIOLOGY

Q. 1. Which one of the following enzymes is antagonistic to insulin? (UPSC-02)
    (a) Glucagon
    (b) Pepsin
    (c) Serotonin
    (d) Trypsin

Ans. (a)
Note
Glucagon acts mostly on the liver and adipose tissue where it antagonizes the action of insulin. Glucagon increases the breakdown of liver glycogen to glucose, producing a rapid rise in blood glucose within few minutes.
Ref: Textbook of Physiology by Prof. A.K.Jain, Volume II, Unit IX, Endocrine System, Ch.7, Pancreas, Pg -720

Q. 2. Adrenocorticotrophic hormone (ACTH) principally controls the secretion of (UPSC-02)
    (a) Thyroid hormones
    (b) Cortisol
    (c) Follicle-stimulating hormone
    (d) Luteinizing hormone

Ans. (b)
Note
Regulation of glucocorticoids (Cortisol) secretion is brought about by regulation of ACTH. Both basal secretion of GC and increased secretion provoked by stress are dependent upon ACTH from anterior pituitary.
Ref: Textbook of Physiology by Prof. A. K. Jain, Volume II, Unit IX, Endocrine System, Ch.5, The Adrenal Cortex, Pg-692

Q. 3. Which of the following is/are due to the closure of 'Semilunar Valves' and mark(s) the onset of ventricular diastole? (UPSC-02)
    (a) First Heart Sound
    (b) Second Heart Sound
    (c) Both First and Second Heart Sound
    (d) Third and Fourth Heart Sound

Ans. (b)
Note
At end of ventricular systole, ventricular pressure drops more rapidly. During this phase, the arterial pressure is better sustained due to elastic recoil of the vessel wall and immediately the arterial pressure exceeds that in the ventricle. This results in closure of semilunar valves, causing sharp second heart sound. After that there is isovolumetric ventricular relaxation i.e. initial part of ventricular diastole, which begins after closure of semilunar valves.
Ref: Textbook of Physiology by Prof. A.K.Jain, Volume I, Unit V, Cardiovascular System, Ch. 3,The Cardiac Cycle, Pg- 283

Q. 4. The breakdown of haemoglobin takes place mainly in (UPSC-04)
    (a) Liver cells
    (b) Kidney tubules
    (c) Erythrocytes
    (d) Reticulo-endothelial system

Ans. (a)

Note
Red blood cells that have reached the end of their lives are engulfed by phagocytic cells called 'Kupffer cells' which line the sinusoids.

Q. 5. The Hepatic triad constitutes (UPSC-04)
  (a) Interlobular branches of portal vein, branch of hepatic artery and bile duct
  (b) Central vein, bile duct and branch of hepatic artery
  (c) Central vein, lymphatics and bile duct
  (d) Interlobular branches of portal vein, branch of hepatic artery and lymphatics

Ans. (a)

Note
Liver structure: Hepatic triad—composed of portal vein, hepatic artery, & bile duct. Liver allows very close contact between blood & hepatocytes.

Q. 6. Cancer cells derive their energy primarily from (UPSC-04)
  (a) Aerobic glycolysis
  (b) Anaerobic glycolysis
  (c) Utilisation of nitrogen
  (d) Utilisation of carbohydrates

Ans. (b)

Note
The 1931 Nobel laureate in medicine, German Otto Warburg, PhD, first discovered that cancer cells have a fundamentally different energy metabolism compared to healthy cells. The crux of his Nobel thesis was that malignant tumours frequently exhibit an increase in anaerobic glycolysis - a process whereby glucose is used as a fuel by cancer cells with lactic acid as an anaerobic by product - compared to normal tissues. The large amount of lactic acid produced by this fermentation of glucose from cancer cells is then transported to the liver. This conversion of glucose to lactate generates a lower, more acidic pH in cancerous tissues as well as overall physical fatigue from lactic acid build-up Thus, larger tumours tend to exhibit a more acidic pH.

Q. 7. In infants, defecation often follows a meal due to (UPSC-04)
  (a) Gastro-ileal reflex
  (b) Gastro-colic reflex
  (c) Entero-gastric reflex
  (d) Increased levels of circulating CCK

Ans. (b)

Note
Gastro-colic reflex: A mass movement of the contents of the colon, often preceded by a similar movement in the small intestine that sometimes occurs immediately after food enters the stomach.

Q. 8. Specific gravity of blood rises: (UPSC-04)
  (a) When excessive water is lost from the body.
  (b) In the event of severe hemorrhage.
  (c) After injection of saline into the veins.
  (d) When large quantity of water is taken.

Ans. (a)

Note
The specific gravity of blood rises; when excessive water is lost from the body, causing hemoconcentration.

Q. 9. Which is the sensory tract? (KPSC- RE/Organon-05)
  (a) Rubro spinal tract
  (b) Tecto spinal tract
  (c) Olivo spinal tract
  (d) Tract of Burdach

Ans. (d)

Note
The Tract of Burdach (Fasciculus Cuneatus) is sensory tract.
The fasciculus cuneatus (tract of Burdach) is triangular on transverse section, and lies between the fasciculus gracilis and the posterior column, its base corresponding with the surface of the medulla spinalis. Its fibers, larger than those of the fasciculus gracilis, are mostly derived from the same source, viz, the posterior nerve roots. Some ascend for only a short distance in the tract, and, entering the gray matter, come into close relationship with the cells of the dorsal nucleus; while others can be traced as far as the medulla oblongata, where they end in the gracilis and cuneate nuclei.

Q. 10. Which is responsible to maintain 85% colloidal osmotic pressure? (KPSC- RE/Organon-05)
    (a)   Albumin
    (b)   Fibrinogen
    (c)   Prothrombin
    (d)   Globulin

Ans. (a)

Note
Colloidal osmotic pressure is inversely proportional to the molecular size and shape, and is directly related to the concentration of molecules. Therefore, 80% of COP is due to albumin because of least molecular weight (i.e. molecular size) and maximum concentration.
Ref: Textbook of Physiology by Prof. A.K. Jain, Volume I, Unit II, Blood, Ch. 2,The Plasma Proteins, Pg- 47

Q. 11. Which is responsible for the second sound of the heart? (KPSC- RE/Organon-05)
    (a)   Sudden closure of AV valves
    (b)   Closure of the semilunar valves
    (c)   Opening of the AV valves
    (d)   Opening of the semilunar valves

Ans. (b)

Note
At end of ventricular systole, ventricular pressure drops more rapidly. During this phase, the arterial pressure is better sustained due to elastic recoil of the vessel wall and immediately the arterial pressure exceeds that in the ventricle. This results in closure of semilunar valves, causing a sharp second heart sound.
Ref: Textbook of Physiology by Prof. A.K.Jain, Volume I, Unit V, Cardiovascular System, Ch. 3,The Cardiac Cycle, Pg-283

Q. 12 Which group is the universal donor of blood? (KPSC- RE/Organon-05)
    (a)   A Group
    (b)   B Group
    (c)   AB Group
    (d)   O Group

Ans. (d)

Note
Universal donor; a person who has group O blood and is therefore able to serve as a donor to a person of any other blood group in the ABO system.
Persons of Group O contain no agglutinogen and can be given to anyone; therefore, its RBCs are not agglutinated by the members of group, called Universal Donors.
Ref: Textbook of Physiology by Prof. A.K. Jain, Volume I, Unit II, Blood, Ch. 9 the Blood Groups, Pg- 102

Q. 13. Astigmatism is corrected by using _____ lens. (KPSC/Lect/Phy & Bioch-05)
    (a)   Concave
    (b)   Convex
    (c)   Cylindrical
    (d)   None of the above

Ans. (c)

Note
Astigmatism is an error of vision in which the light rays are not brought to a point focus on the retina. This is most commonly due to a difference in horizontal and vertical curvature of cornea. Astigmatism can be corrected with cylindrical lens placed in such a way so that the refraction from all the meridians becomes equal.
Ref: Textbook of Physiology by Prof. A.K. Jain, Volume II, Unit XII, The Special Senses, Ch.4, The Eye, Pg-1088

Q. 14. Which of the following is present in pancreatic secretion (KPSC/Lect/Phy & Bioch-05)
    (a)   Pepsin
    (b)   Renin
    (c)   Trypsin
    (d)   Enteropeptidase
Ans. (c)

Note
Trypsin is the most powerful proteolytic enzyme of the pancreatic juice. It hydrolyses proteins by splitting bonds in the protein molecule. Therefore; proteins are digested mainly to small polypeptides.
Ref: Textbook of Physiology by Prof. A. K. Jain, Volume I, Unit IV, Digestive System, Ch.5, Pancreas, Pg- 224

Q. 15. Which of the following is a dietary fiber (KPSC/Lect/Phy & Bioch-05)
    (a)   Collagen
    (b)   Pectin
    (c)   Keratin
    (d)   Elastin
Ans. (b)

Note
The carbohydrates (e.g. pectin, cellulose, and hemicellulose) and some non-carbohydrate substances (e.g. lignin) are collectively called dietary fiber. It resists digestion and is found in vegetables, fruits and grains.
Ref: Textbook of Physiology by Prof. A. K. Jain, Volume II, Unit VIII, Metabolism and Nutrition, Ch.5, Food and Nutrition, Pg- 606

Q. 16. Which is a function of albumin (KPSC/Lect/Phy & Bioch-05)
    (a)   Maintain plasma osmotic pressure
    (b)   Maintain plasma hydrostatic pressure
    (c)   Coagulation of blood
    (d)   Immunity
Ans. (a)

Note
The functions of albumin are:
    a.   Controls colloidal osmotic pressure.
    b.   Helps in transport of anions, cations, dyes, drugs, hormones, fatty acids, metals, amino acids, enzymes and bilirubin.
Ref: Textbook of Physiology by Prof. A.K. Jain, Volume I, Unit II, Blood, Ch. 2, The Plasma Proteins, Pg- 44

Q. 17. All the following can be measured by simple spirometry except (KPSC/Lect/Phy & Bioch-05)
    (a)   Inspiratory reserve volume
    (b)   Expiratory reserve volume
    (c)   Residual volume
    (d)   Tidal volume
Ans. (c)

Note
a.   Inspiratory reserve volume
    The maximal volume of air that can be inhaled after a normal inspiration also called complemental air.

b. Expiratory reserve volume
The maximal volume of air, usually about 1000 milliliters, that can be expelled from the lungs after normal expiration also called reserve air, supplemental air.
c. Residual volume
The volume of air remaining in the lungs after a maximal expiratory effort also called residual air, residual capacity.
d. Tidal volume
The volume of air inhaled and exhaled at each breath.

Q. 18. In athletes bradycardia is because of (KPSC/Lect/Phy & Bioch-05)
(a) Decreased sympathetic tone
(b) Increased vagal tone
(c) Decreased vagal tone
(d) Increased sympathetic tone

Ans. (b)
Note
Adaptive effects of endurance training on autonomic function in athlets indicated that vagal activities enhances, which contributes to the resting bradycardia.
Ref: Medicine & Science in Sports & Exercise. 29(11):1482-1490, November 1997. *SHIN, KUNSOO; MINAMITANI, HARUYUKI; ONISHI, SHOHEI; YAMAZAKI, HAJIME; LEE, MYOUNGHO*

Q. 19. Testes does not produce (KPSC/Lect/Phy & Bioch-05)
(a) Estradiol
(b) Testosterone
(c) Fructose
(d) Inhibin

Ans. (c)
Note
The testis secretes principal male sex hormone, the 'testesterone'; it also secretes 'oestrogen' in small amounts. Some unidentified testicular factor, inhibin is derived from the seminiferous tubules (Sertoli cells).
Ref: Textbook of Physiology by Prof. A. K. Jain, Volume II, Unit X, Reproductive System, Ch. 2, Male Reproductive System, Pg- 769, 771

Q. 20. Osmolality of plasma in a normal adult (in mOsm/L) is (KPSC/Lect/Phy & Bioch-05)
(a) 250 - 270
(b) 270 - 290
(c) 300 - 320
(d) 320 - 340

Ans. (b)
Note
Osmolality is the number of osmoles per kilogram of the solvent. The osmolality of normal human plasma is 290 msOm/ L.
Ref: Textbook of Physiology by Prof. A.K .Jain, Volume I, Unit I, The General Physiology, Ch. 2, Transport Across Cell Membranes, Pg-12

Q. 21. Normal level of creatinine in serum (in mg %) is (KPSC/Lect/Phy & Bioch-05)
(a) 0.6—1.2
(b) 1.2—2
(c) 2 —2.6
(d) 2.6—3.2

Ans. (a)
Note
Normal creatinine levels in blood: 0.6 – 1.2 mg%
Ref: Textbook of Physiology by Prof. A. K. Jain, Volume I, Unit II, Blood, Ch. 1, Composition and Functions of Blood, Pg- 42

Q. 22. Maximum enzyme activity is observed at (KPSC/Lect/Phy & Bioch-05)
  (a) Acidic pH
  (b) Optimum pH
  (c) Alkaline pH
  (d) None of the above

Ans. (b)
Note
Effects of pH
Enzymes are affected by changes in pH. The most favorable pH value - the point where the enzyme is most active - is known as the optimum pH.

Q. 23. All of the following are examples for ketogenic amino acid, except (KPSC/Lect/Phy & Bioch-05)
  (a) Leucine
  (b) Isoleucine
  (c) Phenyl alanine
  (d) Valine

Ans. (d)
Note
The ketogenic amino acids are amino acids that can be converted into ketone bodies through ketogenesis. Important amino acids in this group are; Isoleucin, leucine, lysine, phenylalanine, threonine, tryptophan, tyrosine.
Ref: http://en.wikipedia.org/wiki/Category:Ketogenic_amino_acids

Q. 24. Active site of enzyme (KPSC/Lect/Phy & Bioch-05)
  (a) Have a rigid shape
  (b) Bind the substrate
  (c) Are preserved even after denaturation
  (d) Decided by primary structure alone

Ans. (b)
Note
The active site of an enzyme is the binding site where catalysis occurs the structure and chemical properties of the active site allow the recognition and binding of the substrate.

Q. 25. "Fats" are chemically (KPSC/Lect/Phy & Bioch-05)
  (a) Lipoproteins
  (b) Prostaglandins
  (c) Triglycerides
  (d) Phospholipids

Ans. (a)
Note
a. Lipoproteins
   Lipoproteins are compounds of protein that carry fats and fat-like substances such as cholesterol in the blood.
b. Prostaglandins
   Any of a group of hormone like substances produced in various tissues that are derived from amino acids and mediate a range of physiological functions, such as metabolism and nerve transmission.
c. Triglycerides
   Ester formed from glycerol and one to three fatty acids, fats and oils are triglycerides. In a simple triglyceride such as palmitin or stearin, all three fatty-acid groups are identical. In a mixed triglyceride, two or even three different fatty-acid groups are present; most fats and oils contain mixed triglycerides.
d. Phospholipids
   Any of various phosphorous-containing lipids that are composed mainly of fatty acids, a phosphate group, and a simple organic molecule, they are also called phosphatide.

Q. 26. Hypoalbuminemia may be a feature of the following conditions except (KPSC/Lect/Phy & Bioch-05)
    (a)   Cirrhosis of liver
    (b)   Nephrotic syndrome
    (c)   Malnutrition
    (d)   Hyperlipoproteinemia

Ans. (d)

Note
Hypoalbuminemia is not a feature of hyperlipoprotenemia.

Q. 27. Urea is the catabolic product of (KPSC/Lect/Phy & Bioch-05)
    (a)   Proteins
    (b)   Lipids
    (c)   Purines
    (d)   Carbohydrates

Ans. (a)

Note
Urea is a water-soluble compound that is the major nitrogenous end product of protein metabolism and is the chief nitrogenous component of the urine in mammals and other organisms. Also called carbamide.

Also see
Proteins are complex molecules built mainly from amino acids linked together in chains. Amino acids which are not used as such undergo 'oxidative deamination', primarily in the liver. The overall reaction is the transformation of an amino acid to the corresponding keto acid. This involves an oxidation to give amino acid, followed by hydrolysis liberating ammonia. The ammonia thus formed is then used up in the synthesis of other amino acids or excreted as urea.
Ref: Textbook of Physiology by Prof. A. K. Jain, Volume II, Unit VIII, Metabolism and Nutrition, Ch. 4, Protein Metabolism, Pg- 596

Q. 28. Scurvy is due to deficiency of (KPSC/Lect/Phy & Bioch-05)
    (a)   Thiamin
    (b)   Vitamin C
    (c)   Riboflavin
    (d)   Folic acid

Ans. (b)

Note
Vitamin C deficiency causes scurvy which is characterized by painful swelling of gums and joints, multiple hemorrhages and anemia.
Ref: Textbook of Physiology by Prof. A.K. Jain , Volume II , Unit VIII, Metabolism and Nutrition, Ch.5, Food and Nutrition, Pg- 609

Q. 29. Which of the following is a lipotropic factor? (KPSC/Lect/Phy & Bioch-05)
    (a)   Proline
    (b)   Inositol
    (c)   Cardiolipin
    (d)   Choline

Ans. (d)

Note
A substance which reduces the amount of liver fat is called a lipotropin (lipotropic factor). The lipotropins are effective because they contain choline or because they promote choline synthesis.
Ref: Textbook of Physiology by Prof. A. K. Jain, Volume II, Unit VIII, Metabolism and Nutrition, Ch.3, Fat Metabolism, Pg- 589

Q. 30. Number of ATP produced during anaerobic glycolysis is (KPSC/Lect/Phy & Bioch-05)
    (a)   12
    (b)   8
    (c)   38
    (d)   2

Ans. (d)
Note
During aerobic glycolysis, the net production of ATP is 19 times as great as the 2 ATPs formed under anaerobic conditions.
Ref: Textbook of Physiology by Prof. A. K. Jain, Volume II, Unit VIII, Metabolism and Nutrition, Ch.2, Carbohydrate Metabolism, Pg-582

Q. 31. Which test is used to detect urine sugar? (KPSC/Lect/Phy & Bioch-05)
    (a)   Biuret test
    (b)   Hay's test
    (c)   Molisch's test
    (d)   Benedict's test

Ans. (d)
Note
Benedict's test is used to detect urine sugar.

Q. 32. Specific gravity of urine is increased in (KPSC/Lect/Phy & Bioch-05)
    (a)   Diabetes mellitus
    (b)   Steatorrhea
    (c)   Diabetes insipidus
    (d)   Chronic nephritis

Ans. (a)
Note
Normal specific gravity: 1005-1030
Increase in specific gravity of urine is seen in:
-Low water intake
-Diabetes mellitus due to presence of glucose
-Albuminuria
-Acute nephritis
Ref: Textbook of Physiology by Prof. A. K. Jain, Volume I, Unit VII, Excretory System, Ch. 7, Kidney Function Tests, Pg- 550

Q. 33. Normal potassium level is (KPSC/Lect/Phy & Bioch-05)
    (a)   35—50 mEq/L
    (b)   13.5—14.5 mEq/L
    (c)   3.5 —5.0 mEq/L
    (d)   05 —15 mEq/L

Ans. (c)
Note
Normal potassium (s) levels are 3.5- 5.0 mEq/L.
Ref: Textbook of Physiology by Prof. A.K.Jain , Volume I , Appendix II, Ranges of Normal Values in Human Whole Blood, Plasma or Serum, Pg- vii

Q. 34. An example for sulphur containing amino-acid is (KPSC/Lect/Phy & Bioch-05)
    (a)   Alanine
    (b)   Glutamic acid
    (c)   Histidine
    (d)   Methionine

Ans. (d)
Note
Neutral amino acids- one of the type is sulphur containing amino acids: cysteine, cystine, methionine.

Ref: Textbook of Physiology by Prof. A. K. Jain, Volume II, Unit VIII, Metabolism and Nutrition, Ch.4, Protein Metabolism, Pg- 595

Q. 35. Negative N₃ balance is observed in (KPSC/Lect/Phy & Bioch-05)
    (a)   Pregnancy
    (b)   Chronic illness
    (c)   Growth period
    (d)   Convalescence

Ans. (b)
Note
A subject whose intake of nitrogen is smaller than the output (e.g. in starvation, forced immobilization) is said to have a negative nitrogen balance.
Ref: Textbook of Physiology by Prof. A. K. Jain, Volume II, Unit VIII, Metabolism and Nutrition, Ch.4, Protein Metabolism, Pg- 596

Q. 36. In a healthy adult the upper limit of serum creatinine is (KPSC/Lect/Phy & Bioch-05)
    (a)   0.75 mg/dl
    (b)   1.20 mg/dl
    (c)   1.60 mg/dl
    (d)   2.00 mg/dl

Ans. (b)
Note
Normal creatinine levels in blood: 0.6 – 1.2 mg/dl
Ref: Textbook of Physiology by Prof. A. K. Jain, Volume I, Unit II, Blood, Ch. 1, Composition and Functions of Blood, Pg- 42

Q. 37. Biological value of egg is (KPSC/Lect/Phy & Bioch-05)
    (a)   100
    (b)   90
    (c)   80
    (d)   50

Ans. (b)
Note
The Biological Value (BV) of a protein is a value that measures how well the body can absorb and utilize a protein. The higher the Biological Value of the protein you use, the more nitrogen your body can absorb, use, and retain as a result, proteins with the highest BV promote the most lean muscle gains.

Q. 38. The major cation of intracellular fluid is (KPSC/Lect/Phy & Bioch-05)
    (a)   Ca and Mg
    (b)   Ca and K
    (c)   K and Mg
    (d)   K and Na

Ans. (c)
Note
Sodium, calcium, chloride and bicarbonate are largely extracellular, whereas potassium, magnesium, organic phosphates and proteins are predominantly present in intracellular fluid.
Ref: Textbook of Physiology by Prof. A. K. Jain, Volume I, Unit I, The General Physiology, Ch. 3, Body Water and Body Fluids, Pg- 21

Q. 39. The normal pH of blood plasma is (KPSC/Lect/Phy & Bioch-05)
    (a)   7.0
    (b)   7.2
    (c)   7.4
    (d)   7.6

Ans. (c)

Note
Blood pH always refers to plasma pH (7.4). Optimal pH range for blood at which human body functions properly is 7.35 to 7.45. Clinically blood pH < 7.35, referred as acidosis and blood pH > 7.45, referred as alkalosis.
Ref: Textbook of Physiology by Prof. A.K.Jain, Volume I, Unit I, The General Physiology, Ch. 3, Body Water and Body Fluids, Pg- 23

Q. 40. Which of the following is not a ketone body? (KPSC/Lect/Phy & Bioch-05)
    (a)   Acetone
    (b)   Acetoacetate
    (c)   Pyruvate
    (d)   Beta-Hydroxybutyrate

Ans. (c)

Note
The ketone bodies or acetone bodies are substances, which form a metabolically related group, e.g. acetoacetic acid, beta hydroxybutyric acid and acetone.
Ref: Textbook of Physiology by Prof. A. K. Jain, Volume II, Unit VIII, Metabolism and Nutrition, Ch.3, Fat Metabolism, Pg- 590

Q. 41. Which of the following human tissues contains the greatest amount of body glycogen? (KPSC/Lect/Phy & Bioch-05)
    (a)   Liver
    (b)   Pancreas
    (c)   Kidney
    (d)   Skeletal muscle

Ans. (a)

Note
Glycogen is the body's main source of stored energy. Made from glucose (from excess carbs), glycogen is stored primarily in liver and muscle cells. It is stored with water, in the ratio 1 gram of carbohydrates to 3 grams of water.
Most glycogen is found in the liver (comprising about 10 percent of the liver); with muscles containing a relatively smaller amount. Liver-glycogen is more readily available for energy and blood glucose maintenance, while muscle-glycogen is used primarily for muscle-energy.

Also see
Glucose is converted into glycogen in most tissues of the body, especially in liver and muscle. Liver content of glycogen is 60gm (4% by weight of liver) which increases to 5% after a high carbohydrate meal and decreases with fasting. The glycogen content in resting muscle is 150gm (0.7 to 1 % by weight of muscles)
Ref: Textbook of Physiology by Prof. A. K. Jain, Volume II, Unit VIII, Metabolism and Nutrition, Ch.2, Carbohydrate Metabolism, Pg- 577

Q. 42. The major role of glucocorticoids in carbohydrate metabolism is (KPSC/Lect/Phy & Bioch-05)
    (a)   Stimulates glycogenesis in muscle
    (b)   Stimulates glycolysis in muscle
    (c)   Stimulates gluconeogenesis in liver
    (d)   Increased uptake of glucose by extrahepatic tissues

Ans. (c)

Note
Glucocorticoids have the following action on carbohydrate metabolism:
1. It increases liver glucose-6-phosphatase activity to increase glucose formation and prevents peripheral utilization of glucose. Thus increases blood glucose.
2. Increases glycogen synthesis by increasing glycogen synthetase and indirect inhibition of glycolysis in the liver

Ref: Textbook of Physiology by Prof. A. K. Jain, Volume II, Unit IX, Endocrine System, Ch.5, The Adrenal Cortex, Pg-695

Q. 43. Which of the following is absorbed in the colon (KPSC/Lect/Phy & Bioch-05)
  (a) Iron
  (b) Protein
  (c) Bile salt
  (d) Sodium

Ans. (d)
Note
Some sodium diffuses into or out of small intestine 'passively' depending on concentration gradient. In addition, sodium is actively transported out of the lumen into the small intestine and colon by sodium- potassium pumps.
Ref: Textbook of Physiology by Prof. A. K. Jain, Volume I, Unit IV, Digestive System, Ch.9, Digestion and Absorption in GIT, Pg- 264

Q. 44. Pacinian corpuscles are major receptors for (KPSC/Lect/Phy & Bioch-05)
  (a) Pressure
  (b) Pain
  (c) Touch
  (d) Temperature

Ans. (a)
Note
Pacinian corpuscles- These are nerve terminals of Aβ fibres mainly and concerned with perception of pressure (or sustained touch).
Ref: Textbook of Physiology by Prof. A. K. Jain, Volume II, Unit XI, The Nervous System, Ch. 3, Receptors, Pg- 844

Q. 45. Organ of corti is concerned with (KPSC/Lect/Phy & Bioch-05)
  (a) Hearing
  (b) Vision
  (c) Smell
  (d) Taste

Ans. (a)
Note
The primary receptor of hearing is the organ of corti which is located on the basilar membrane extending from the apex to the base of cochlea.
Ref: Textbook of Physiology by Prof. A. K. Jain, Volume II, Unit XII, The Special Senses, Ch. 3, The Ear, Pg- 1046

Q. 46. Under resting condition, the cardiac output (in L/minute) is (KPSC/Lect/Phy & Bioch-05)
  (a) 2
  (b) 4
  (c) 5
  (d) 9

Ans. (c)
Note
The amount of blood pumped out by each ventricle into the circulation per minute is called cardiac output. Cardiac output can be calculated as heart rate X stroke volume. Normally it is 5-6 L/min (average: 5.5 L/min).
Ref: Textbook of Physiology by Prof. A.K. Jain, Volume I, Unit V, CVS, Ch.8, The Cardiac Output, Pg-334

Q. 47. Plateau phase of action potential curve of cardiac tissue is due to (KPSC/Lect/Phy & Bioch-05)
  (a) Opening of sodium channels
  (b) Opening of potassium channels
  (c) Opening of calcium channels
  (d) Closing of sodium channels

Ans. (c)

Note
A plateau phase in which the membrane potential falls slowly only to -40mV due to inactivation of sodium influx which starts appearing at zero potential and calcium influx and potassium efflux continue at a slow rate.
Ref: Textbook of Physiology by Prof. A. K. Jain, Volume I , Unit III , Nerve Muscle Physiology, Ch. 7 , Cardiac Muscle, Pg- 165

Q. 48. Swallowing centre is located in (KPSC/Lect/Phy & Bioch-05)
(a) Mid brain
(b) Pons
(c) Medulla
(d) Cerebellum

Ans. (c)
Note
Swallowing is a reflex response controlled via vagus nerve and its centre is located in the medulla oblongata.
Ref: Textbook of Physiology by Prof. A.K. Jain, Volume I, Unit IV, Digestive System ,Ch.3 , Mouth and Oesophagus, Pg-199

Q. 49. Calcitonin is produced by (KPSC/Lect/Phy & Bioch-05)
(a) Adrenal cortex
(b) Adrenal medulla
(c) Parathyroid
(d) Thyroid

Ans. (d)
Note
Thyroid hormones are:
1. Thyroxine
2. Tri-iodo-thyronine
3. Calcitonin

Calcitonin is secreted by parfollicular cells or C cells which lie in between the follicular cells.
Ref: Textbook of Physiology by Prof. A. K. Jain, Volume II, Unit IX, Endocrine System, Ch.3, The Thyroid Gland, Pg-652

Q. 50. The normal life span of RBC (in days) is (KPSC/Lect/Phy & Bioch-05)
(a) 30
(b) 120
(c) 150
(d) 180

Ans. (b)
Note
Life span of RBC is 120 days
Ref: Textbook of Physiology by Prof. A. K. Jain , Volume I, Unit II, Blood, Ch. 4 , Erythrocyte-RBC, Pg- 56

Q. 51. Oxygen dissociation curve is shifted to the right in all except (KPSC/Lect/Phy & Bioch-05)
(a) Fall in pH
(b) Rise in temperature
(c) Increase of 2, 3, DPG
(d) HbF

Ans. (d)
Note
Causes of oxygen haemoglobin dissociation curve shift to right:
a. Fall in blood pH
b. Increase in body temperature
c. Increase in concentration of 2,3, diphosphoglyceric acid

Ref: Textbook of Physiology by Prof. A. K. Jain, Volume I, Unit VI, The Respiratory System, Ch.3, Transport of Gases

Q. 52. Which is metabolised like xenobiotics? (MD/Hom/Ent-1/01)
- (a) Myoglobulin
- (b) Biliverdin
- (c) Hemoglobin
- (d) Bilirubin

Ans. (d)
Note
A xenobiotic (from the Greek words xenos: stranger/foreign and bios: life) is a chemical which is found in an organism but which is not normally produced or expected to be present in it.
Specifically, drugs such as antibiotics are xenobiotics in humans as human body cannot produce them itself and they are not expected to be present as part of a normal diet. The term is also used in the context of pollutants such as dioxins and polychlorinated biphenyls and their effect on the biota.
The body removes xenobiotics by xenobiotic metabolism. This consists of the deactivation and the secretion of xenobiotics, and happens mostly in the liver. Secretion routes are urine, feces, breath, and sweat.
Ref: http://en.wikipedia.org/wiki/Xenobiotic

Q. 53. Gastrin is secreted from (MD/Hom/Ent-1/01)
- (a) Duodenum
- (b) Pyloric antrum
- (c) Lesser curvature
- (d) Cardiac

Ans. (b)
Note
Gastrin is secreted by G-cells from deeper portion of pyloric (antral) glands in the gastric mucosa.
Ref: Textbook of Physiology by Prof. A. K. Jain , Volume I, Unit IV, Digestive System ,Ch.4, The Stomach, Pg-205

Q. 54. Pulse pressure varies as blood flows to the extremities due to (MD/Hom/Ent-1/01)
- (a) Change in velocity
- (b) Change in viscosity
- (c) Cross sectional area
- (d) Change in vessel wall

Ans. (d)
Note
Pulse pressure is difference of SBP and DBP. It determines the pulse volume and high PP is indicative of systolic hypertension and indirectly determines decrease in elasticity of blood vessels.
Ref: Textbook of Physiology by Prof. A.K. Jain , Volume I , Unit V, CVS ,Ch. 9 , The Arterial Blood Pressure, Pg- 343

Q. 55. Plateaue phase of action potential is seen in (MD/Hom/Ent-1/01)
- (a) A V Node
- (b) S A Node
- (c) Atrial fibres
- (d) Ventricular fibres

Ans. (d)
Note
This "plateau" phase of the cardiac action potential is sustained by a balance between inward movement of Ca^{2+} (ICa) through L-type calcium channels and outward movement of K^+ through the slow delayed rectifier potassium channels, IKs. The sodium-calcium exchanger current, INa,Ca and the sodium/potassium pump current, INa,K also play minor roles during phase 2 and occus in ventricular fibers.
Ref: http://en.wikipedia.org/wiki/Cardiac_action_potential

Q. 56. Which gas is not responsible for green house effect? (MD/Hom/Ent-1/01)
    (a)   Ozone
    (b)   Nitrogen
    (c)   Nitrous oxide
    (d)   Carbon-dioxide

Ans. (b)
Note
The earth's "greenhouse effect" is what makes this planet suitable for life as we know it. The earth's atmosphere contains trace gases, some of which absorb heat. These gases (water vapor, carbon dioxide, methane, ozone, and nitrous oxide) are referred to as "greenhouse gases."
Ref: http://www.ucar.edu/learn/1_3_1.htm
Nitrous oxide (N_2O), a colorless gas with a sweetish taste and odor. A major use of nitrous oxide is in anesthesia, e.g., in dentistry. It is commonly called laughing gas since it produces euphoria and mirth when inhaled in small amounts. It is also used in making certain canned pressurized foods, e.g., instant whipped cream. It was discovered (1772) by Joseph Priestley.

Q. 57. Sperm motility is caused by (MD/Hom/Ent-1/01)
    (a)   Epididymis
    (b)   Testis
    (c)   Vas-deferens
    (d)   Prostatic secretion

Ans. (a)
Note
Spermatozoa (sperms) in the semeniferous tubular lumen are moved along the tubules to the Ductuli Efferentes which lead to the epididymis. The spermatozoa are then stored in the tail of epididymis, where they can remain viable for a month.
Ref: Textbook of Physiology by Prof. A.K.Jain, Volume II, Unit X, Reproductive System, Ch. 2, Male Reproductive System, Pg- 767

Q. 58. Normal mitral valve area in adults is (MD/Hom/Ent-1/01)
    (a)   05 - 2cm
    (b)   1-4 cm
    (c)   4-6 cm
    (d)   6-8 cm

Ans. (c)
Note
Symptoms of mitral stenosis generally develop when the area of the valve is reduced to less than 50% of its normal size (normal valve area: 4 to 6 cm2). In most cases, symptoms do not occur at rest until the valve becomes at least moderately stenotic (valve area: 1 to 1.5 cm2). Severe mitral stenosis (valve area: < 1 cm2) is almost always symptomatic.
Ref: http://www.clevelandclinicmeded.com/medicalpubs/diseasemanagement/cardiology/mitralvalve/mitralvalve.htm

Q. 59. Daily loss of water from skin in absence of visible sweating is (MD/Hom/Ent-1/01)
    (a)   1.5 liters
    (b)   1 liter
    (c)   500 - 700 ml
    (d)   200 - 300 ml

Ans. (b)
Note
Water is lost from the body as urine, in feces and by evaporation from the skin and lungs (the latter two make up what is called "insensible water loss"). More water is lost from the skin and lungs in high temperatures, at high altitude and when the air is dry. Even in the absence of visible perspiration, approximately half of water loss occurs through the lungs and skin. Water loss through the skin is usually about 800-1000ml per day.

MCQ's in Physiology

Also see
Table : WHO recommendations for daily requirements of drinking water

	Average conditions	Manual labour in high temperatures	Total needs in pregnancy/lactation
Female adults	2.2 litres	4.5 litres	4.8 litres (pregnancy) 5.5 litres (lactation)
Male adults	2.9 litres	4.5 litres	-

Table : Example of water balance in the body in a temperate climate

Source	Water intake (ml/day)	Source	Water loss (ml/day)
Food	1120	Urine	1300
Drink	1180	Lungs	300
Oxidation of nutrients (metabolic water	280	Skin	920
	258	Faeces	60
Total	2580	Total	2580

Ref: http://www.water.org.uk/home/water-for-health/medical-facts/adults

Q. 60. Iron absorption is increased by (MD/Hom/Ent-1/01)
   (a)   Fiber diet
   (b)   Vit-C
   (c)   Phosphates
   (d)   Phytic Acid

Ans. (d)
Note
Phytic acid (found in cereals), phosphates, oxalates, pancreatic juice react with iron to form insoluble compounds in the intestine and thereby decreases iron absorption.
Ref: Textbook of Physiology by Prof. A.K. Jain , Volume I , Unit IV, Digestive System ,Ch.9, Digestion and Absorption in GIT, Pg- 265

Q. 61. Pulse blood pressure is (MD/Hom/Ent-1/01)
   (a)   Diastolic + 1/3 systolic
   (b)   Diastolic × systolic
   (c)   1/3 diastolic ÷ systolic
   (d)   (Systolic - Diastolic)

Ans. (d)
Note
Pulse pressure is difference of SBP and DBP. It determines the pulse volume and high PP is indicative of systolic hypertension and indirectly determines decrease in elasticity of blood vessels.
Ref: Textbook of Physiology by Prof. A.K.Jain , Volume I , Unit V, CVS ,Ch. 9 , The Arterial Blood Pressure, Pg- 343

Q. 62. Renal artery constriction is associated with (MD/Hom/Ent-1/01)
   (a)   Heart disease
   (b)   Carotid artery stenosis
   (c)   Azotemia
   (d)   Hypertension

Ans. (d)
Note
Renal artery constriction is associated with hypertension.

Q. 63. Sodium is maximum in (MD/Hom/Ent-1/01)
 (a) Extra cellular spaces
 (b) Intra cellular spaces
 (c) Interstitial spaces
 (d) Bone

Ans. (a)
Note
Sodium, calcium, chloride and bicarbonate are largely extracellular, whereas potassium, magnesium, organic phosphates and proteins are predominantly present in intracellular fluid.
Ref: Textbook of Physiology by Prof. A. K. Jain, Volume I, Unit I, The General Physiology, Ch. 3, Body Water and Body Fluids, Pg- 21

Q. 64. Normal glucose level present in CSF is (MD/Hom/Ent-1/01)
 (a) 50 mg to 80 mg
 (b) 80 mg to 120 mg
 (c) 120 mg to 180 mg
 (d) Not present

Ans. (a)
Note
Glucose composition (mg %) in CSF is 64 (50- 85).
Ref: Textbook of Physiology by Prof. A. K. Jain , Volume I, Unit V, CVS , Ch. 10, The Regional Circulation, Pg- 368

Q. 65. Normal daily secretion of gastric intestinal tract is (MD/Hom/Ent-1/01)
 (a) 2000 cc
 (b) 3000 cc
 (c) 5500 cc
 (d) 8000 cc

Ans. (b)
Note
Daily secretion of gastric juice is 2.5 – 3 litres/day, "isotonic" with plasma.
Ref: Textbook of Physiology by Prof. A. K. Jain, Volume I, Unit IV, Digestive System ,Ch. 4, The Stomach, Pg- 207

Q. 66. Beta-Endorphins are released from (MD/Hom/Ent-1/01)
 (a) Adrenal cortex
 (b) Anterior and intermediate lobe of pituitary
 (c) Posterior lobe of pituitary
 (d) Thyroid

Ans. (b)
Note
Beta-endorphins (β-endorphins) are the most powerful endorphins in the body. They are usually found in the hypothalamus and pituitary gland. More endorphins are released in the pituitary gland during times of pain or stress. Exercise increases the endorphin release too. For the same reason, exercise results in a better mood. Beta-endorphin is an endogenous opioid, secreted by the anterior pituitary, that is more powerfully analgesic
http://simple.wikipedia.org/wiki/Endorphin

Q. 67. Glomerular filtration is most dependent on (MD/Hom/Ent-1/01)
 (a) Renal blood flow
 (b) Pressure in bowman's capsule
 (c) Glomerular capillary pressure
 (d) Plasma membrane pressure

Ans. (c)

Note
The mechanism of glomerular filtration across the glomerular capillaries is the same as the mechanism governing the filtration across all other body capillaries i.e. the hydrostatic pressure gradient across the capillary wall, the osmotic pressure gradient across the capillary wall, the permeability of capillaries and size of capillary bed.
Ref: Textbook of Physiology by Prof. A. K. Jain, Volume I, Unit VII, Excretory System, Ch. 2, Mechanism of Formation of Urine, Pg- 503

Q. 68. During action potential permeability of following increases (MD/Hom/Ent-1/01)

-**Ans. (b)**
Note
During action potential, in Phase 0, there is rapid depolarization and potential reaches +20 to +30 mV. This is due to 100 fold increase in sodium permeability resulting in sodium influx and marked increase in calcium permeability causing calcium influx.
Ref: Textbook of Physiology by Prof. A. K. Jain, Volume I, Unit III, Nerve Muscle Physiology, Ch. 7, Cardiac Muscle, Pg- 165

Q. 69. Auditory impulses relay to (MD/Hom/Ent-1/01)
    (a) Sup colliculus
    (b) Medial leminiscus
    (c) Inferior geniculate
    (d) Medial geniculate body

Ans. (d)
Note
Auditory pathways- From the inferior colliculi many fibres project and relay in the medial geniculate bodies; medial geniculate body neurons finally project to the primary auditory cortex.
Ref: Textbook of Physiology by Prof. A. K. Jain, Volume II, Unit XII, The Special Senses, Ch. 3, The Ear, Pg- 1047

Q. 70. Iron (Fe) absorption decreases by following except (MD/Hom/Ent-1/01)
    (a) Phytates
    (b) Phosphate
    (c) Vit-C
    (d) Taurine

Ans. (c)
Note
Phytic acid (found in cereals), phosphates, oxalates, pancreatic juice react with iron to form insoluble compounds in the intestine and thereby decreases iron absorption.
Ref: Textbook of Physiology by Prof. A. K. Jain, Volume I, Unit IV, Digestive System, Ch.9, Digestion and Absorption in GIT, Pg-265

Q. 71. Thirst center is situated in (MD/Hom/Ent-1/01)
    (a) Hypothalamus
    (b) Cerebellum
    (c) Medulla Oblongata
    (d) Cerebrum

Ans. (a)
Note
The hypothalamus is involved in the maintenance of fluid balance by participating in the control of water intake as well as in the control of water loss by the body. Though hypothalamus is primarily involved in the control of drinking, other areas such as septal nuclei, amygdale and hippocampus can influence water intake.
Ref: Textbook of Physiology by Prof. A. K. Jain, Volume II, Unit XI, The Nervous System, Ch. 16, The Hypothalamus, Pg- 984

Q. 72. Most accurate measurement of extracellular fluid volume (ECF) can be done by using (AIIMS/May-03)
(a) Sucrose
(b) Mannitol
(c) Inulin
(d) Aminopyrine

Ans. (c)
Note
Most accurate method to measure extracellular fluid volume is by using inulin. Radio-active inulin levels are easily determined by counting the samples with suitable radiation detectors.
Ref: Textbook of Physiology by Prof. A. K. Jain, Volume I, Unit I, The General Physiology, Ch. 3, Body Water and Body Fluids, Pg- 20

Q. 73. A shift of posture from supine to upright posture is associated with cardiovasucular adjustments. Which of the following is not true in this context? (AIIMS/May-03)
(a) Rise in central venous pressure
(b) Rise in heart rate
(c) Decrease in cardiac output
(d) Decrease in stroke volume

Ans. (a)
On assumption of erect posture, the force of gravity causes pooling of blood in lower extremities, leading to decrease return through inferior vena cava and it causes decrease in central venous pressure.

Q. 74. There is a mid-cycle shift in the basal body temperature (BBT) after ovulation in women This is caused by (AIIMS/May-03)
(a) FSH peak
(b) LH peak
(c) Estradiol
(d) Progesterone

Ans. (d)
Note
Ovulation is the release of the ovum from the ovary at fairly fixed intervals. It can be determined by recording the basal body temperature i.e. recording the body temperature, before getting up in the morning. In the preovulatory phase the oral BBT is 36.3-36.8 degree Celsius, which increases by 0.3 to 0.5 degee Celsius. It is probably due to the increase in progesterone secretion, since progesterone is thermogenic.
Ref: Textbook of Physiology by Prof. A.K. Jain, Volume II, Unit X, Reproductive System, Ch. 3, Female Reproductive System, Pg- 781

Q. 75. A 55-year-old male accident victim in casualty urgently needs blood. Blood bank is unable to determine his ABO group, as his red cell group and plasma group do not match. Emergency transfusion of patient should be with (AIIMS/May-03)
(a) RBC corresponding to his red cell group and colloids/crystalloid
(b) Whole blood corresponding to his plasma group
(c) O positive RBC and colloids/crystalloid
(d) AB negative whole blood

Ans. (c)
Note
If time does not permit the grouping and cross-matching of the recipient, 'O' Rh negative blood should be used. In case of extreme emergency like war casualties, train accidents etc., 'O' Rh positive blood should be given (in case if 'O' Rh negative blood is not available).
Ref: Textbook of Physiology by Prof. A. K. Jain, Volume I, Unit II, Blood, Ch. 9, Blood Groups, Pg- 103

Q. 76. All are correct about potassium balance except (AIIMS/May-03)
(a) Most of potassium is intracellular.
(b) Three quarter of the total body potassium is found in skeletal muscle.

(c) Intracellular potassium is released into extra-cellular space in response to severe injury or surgical stress.
(d) Acidosis leads to movement of potassium from extracellular to intracellular fluid compartment.

Ans. (d)

All of above are correct about potassium balance except; (d) that acidosis leads to movement of potassium from extracellular to intracellular fluid compartment. However, the opposite takes place – to maintain electronutrality of the plasma the K+ from the cells comes out causing increased K+ concentration in plasma.

Q. 77. In angina pectoris, the pain radiating down the left arm is mediated by increased activity in afferent (sensory) fibers contained in the (AIIMS/May-03)
(a) Carotid branch of the glossopharyngeal nerve
(b) Phrenic nerve
(c) Vagus nerve and recurrent laryngeal nerve
(d) Thoracic splanchnic nerve

Ans. (d)
Note
The referred pain is felt at the dermatome which corresponds to the viscerotome of the pain producing viscus. Therefore, the pain is felt at an area where the viscus was situated in the embryonic stage. As the heart originated in the neck as well as the arms therefore both of these structures receive pain nerve fibers from the same spinal segment. The afferent sympathetic nerve carrying pain sensation from the heart ends in upper thoracic segment. Upper thoracic splanchnic nerve originating in sympathetic trunks (T1-4) carries pain sensation from heart and lungs.

Q. 78. Osteoclast has specific receptor for (AIIMS/May-03)
(a) Parathyroid hormone
(b) Calcitonin
(c) Thyroxine
(d) Vitamin D3

Ans. (b)
Note
Osteoclast has specific receptors for calcitonin.

Q. 79. Hypocalcemia is characterized by all except
(a) Numbness and tingling of circumoral region
(b) Hyperactive tendon reflexes and positive Chvostek's sign
(c) Shortening of Q-T interval in ECG
(d) Carpopedal spasm

Ans. (c)
Note
In hypoparathyroidism, as calcium exerts a stabilizing effect on the cell membranes of excitable tissues, therefore hypocalcaemia increases the excitability of muscle and nerve membranes, which get potentiated by ischemia. Features-
1. Numbness, tingling of extremeties and feeling of stiffness with cramps in extremeties.
2. Facial irritability- Chvostek's sign.
3. Carpopedal spasm.
4. ECG changes- ST segment is prolonged with abnormal T wave.

Ref: Textbook of Physiology by Prof. A. K. Jain, Volume II, Unit IX, Endocrine System, Ch. 4, Parathyroids, Calcitonin and Vitamin D, Pg- 684

Q. 80. The mechanism that protects normal pancreas from autodigestion is
(a) Secretion of bicarbonate
(b) Protease inhibitors present in plasma
(c) Proteolytic enzymes secreted in inactive form
(d) The resistance of pancreatic cells

Ans. (c)

Note
Proteolytic enzymes secreted in inactive form are responsible for protecting normal pancreas from autodigestion.

Q. 81. Although more than 400 blood groups have been identified, the ABO blood group system remains the most important in clinical medicine because:
    (a)   It was the first blood group system to be discovered.
    (b)   It has four different blood groups A, B, AB, O (H).
    (c)   ABO (H) antigens are present in most body tissues and fluids.
    (d)   ABO (H) antibodies are invariably present in plasma when a person's RBC lacks the corresponding antigen.

Ans. (d)
Note
Although more than 400 blood groups have been identified, the ABO blood group system remains the most important in clinical medicine because ABO (H) antibodies are invariably present in plasma when a person's RBC lacks the corresponding antigen.

Q. 82. Father to son inheritance is never seen in case of
    (a)   Autosomal dominant inheritance
    (b)   Autosomal recessive inheritance
    (c)   X- linked recessive inheritance
    (d)   Multifactorial inheritance

Ans. (c)
Note
Father to son inheritance is never seen in case of X- linked recessive inheritance.

Q. 83. The hormone associated with cold adaptation is
    (a)   Growth hormone
    (b)   Thyroxine
    (c)   Insulin
    (d)   Melanocyte stimulating hormone

Ans. (b)
Note
Thyroxine is the hormone associated with cold adaptation.
Ref: http://www.thieme-connect.com/ejournals/abstract/hmr/doi/10.1055/s-2005-870420

Q. 84. Brain lipid binding proteins are expressed by which of the following
    (a)   Mature astrocytes
    (b)   Oligodendrocytes
    (c)   Purkinje cells
    (d)   Pyramidal neurons

Ans. (a)
Note
Astrocytes are found throughout the brain joining to the blood vessels and investing synaptic structures, neuronal bodies and neuronal processes. Function is support, transport, inflammatory and repairative reactions and helps forming the blood brain barrier. They also help in maintaining optimal concentration of ions and neurotransmitters in the brain neurons.
Ref: Textbook of Physiology by Prof. A.K. Jain, Volume I, Unit III, Nerve Muscle Physiology, Ch.1, Structure and Function of Nervous Tissues, Pg- 132

Q. 85. Several hormones regulate the tubular reabsorption of water and electrolytes at different sites in the nephron. Which of the following combination is correct? (AIIMS/Nov-03)
    (a)   Angiotensin in distal tubule
    (b)   Aldosterone in collecting ducts
    (c)   ADH in proximal tubule
    (d)   ANP in loop of Henle

Ans. (b)

Note
Aldosterone causes retention of sodium from the kidney and increased urinary excretion of potassium. It acts on the distal collecting tubule and collecting tubules to increase sodium reabsorption in exchange for potassium and hydrogen which are then excreted in the urine.
Ref: Textbook of Physiology by Prof. A. K. Jain, Volume II, Unit IX, Endocrine System, Ch. 5, The Adrenal Cortex, Pg- 700

Q. 86. Relative colour and luminosity of photoreceptive input under changing light conditions are regulated and maintained by (AIIMS/Nov-03)
- (a) Muller cells
- (b) Amacrine cells
- (c) Ganglion cells
- (d) Retinal astrocytes

Ans. (c)
Note
Ganglion cells discharge can be increased or decreased by shining light on a small circular region of the retina (receptive field). Some ganglion cells respond to steady illumination: others respond only to changes in illumination.
Ref: Textbook of Physiology by Prof. A. K. Jain, Volume II, Unit XII, The Special Senses, Ch. 4, The Eye, Pg- 1095

Q. 87. Exposure to darkness leads to increased melatonin secretion. It is brought about by (AIIMS/Nov-03)
- (a) Decreasing the activity of suprachiasmatic nuclei
- (b) Increasing the serotonin N-acetyl transferase
- (c) Decreasing the hydroxy-indole-O-methyl transferase activity
- (d) Blocking the release of norepinephrine from sympathetic nerve terminals

Ans. (b)
Note
Melatonin secretion are increased during the dark period of the day and maintained at a low level during daylight hours.
5HT
N-acetyltransferase and acetyl CoA
N-acetyl 5HT
Hydroxy indole-O-methyl transferase
N-Acetyl-5-methoxy-tryptamine or melatonin
Ref: Textbook of Physiology by Prof. A. K. Jain, Volume II, Unit IX, Endocrine System, Ch. 9, The Pineal Gland, Pg- 739

Q. 88. Which one of the following clearly states the role of cerebellum in motor performance (AIIMS/May-04)
- (a) Planning and programming of movement
- (b) Convert abstract thought into voluntary action
- (c) Initiation of skilled voluntary action
- (d) Smoothens and coordinates ongoing movements

Ans. (d)
Note
The cerebellum does not initiate movements; rather it coordinates movements that are initiated in the motor system. Coordination of movements is the result of appropriate regulation of time, rate, range force and direction of muscular activity.
Ref: Textbook of Physiology by Prof. A. K. Jain, Volume II, Unit XI, The Nervous System, Ch. 12, The Cerebellum, Pg- 946

Q. 89. Which of the following phrase adequately describes Pacinian corpuscles (AIIMS/May-04)
- (a) A type of pain receptors
- (b) Slowly adapting touch receptors

(c) Rapidly adapting touch receptors
(d) Located in the joints

Ans. (c)
Note
Pacinian corpuscles- These are nerve terminals of Aβ fibres mainly and concerned with perception of pressure (or sustained touch). They respond to deformation caused by firm pressure and are quickly adapting.
Ref: Textbook of Physiology by Prof. A. K. Jain, Volume II, Unit XI, The Nervous System, Ch. 3, Receptors, Pg- 844

Q. 90. Ovulation is associated with sudden rise in (AIIMS/May-04)
(a) Prolactin
(b) Testosterone
(c) LH
(d) Oxytocin

Ans. (c)
Note
Ovulation occurs about 9 hours after the 'LH surge'. Therefore LH is also called "Ovulating Hormone".
Ref: Textbook of Physiology by Prof. A. K. Jain, Volume II, Unit X, Reproductive System, Ch. 3, Female Reproductive System, Pg- 784

Q. 91. The normal adult human electroencephalogram (EEG) (AIIMS/May-04)
(a) Will not show high frequency waves during stage 3 sleep
(b) Shows alpha rhythm when a person is awake but inattentive
(c) Has lower frequency waves during mental activity
(d) Is predominated by large amplitude waves during REM sleep

Ans. (a)
Note
In non- rapid eye movement (NREM) sleep or slow wave sleep, stage 3 , EEG shows sleep spindles superimposed on a background of waves of delta type (frequency 1-2 Hz).
Ref: Textbook of Physiology by Prof. A.K. Jain , Volume II , Unit XI, The Nervous System, Ch. 14, The Electroencephalogram and Sleep , Pg- 964

Q. 92. The afferent fibers which are most sensitive to local anesthetic belong to group (AIIMS/May-04)
(a) A
(b) B
(c) C
(d) D

Ans. (c)
Note
Mammalian nerve fibres are having three type; A, B and C. The 'A' and 'B' type of fibres are myelinated and the 'C' fibers are unmyelinated.
The 'C' group is most susceptible to local anaesthetics, whereas 'B' is intermediate, and 'A' is least susceptible.

Q. 93. Lower esophageal sphincter (AIIMS/May-04)
(a) Has no tonic activity
(b) Has a tone which is provided by the sympathetic system
(c) Relaxes on increasing abdominal pressure
(d) Relaxes ahead of the peristaltic wave

Ans. (d)
Note
Lower esophageal sphincter – The last 2.5cm of esophagus is sphincteric in action. At rest it is in a state of tone and its walls are tightly in apposition. Swallowing or distension of esophagus with food causes reflex relaxation of sphincter. When peristaltic contractions reach this region the sphincter closes and may undergo a strong and prolonged after contraction, thereby preventing regurgitation of food, gastric juice and air.

Ref: Textbook of Physiology by Prof. A. K. Jain, Volume I, Unit IV, Digestive System ,Ch.3 , Mouth and Oesophagus, Pg- 201

Q. 94. When information memorized afterwards is interfered by the information learnt earlier, it is called (AIIMS/May-04)
  (a) Retroactive inhibition
  (b) Proactive inhibition
  (c) Simple inhibition
  (d) Inhibition

Ans. (b)
Note
Inhibition:
 -Inhibition is imposition of restraint or arrest of a process.
Retroactive inhibition:
 -When learning one thing inhibits the retention of something that was learned earlier.
Proactive inhibition:
 -When the things learned earlier interfere with the things learned latter.

Q. 95. Wedged hepatic venous pressure represents pressure in (AIIMS/May-04)
  (a) Main portal vein
  (b) Main hepatic vein
  (c) Sinusoids
  (d) Central vein radicles

Ans. (c)
Note
Wedged hepatic venous pressure: it is recorded by a catheter wedged in a hepatic vein, however it reflects the portal venous pressure via hepatic sinusoids.

Also see
The mean pressure of the hepatic artery that converges on the hepatic sinusoids is 90mmHg. Both arterial and hepatic blood flow join to produce a sinusoidal pressure called the hepatic venous pressure of 6.8mmHg.
Ref: Textbook of physiology by A. K. Jain, 2nd edition, Vol 1, unit V, Ch. 10, pg 379, 380

Q. 96. The pressure-volume curve is shifted to the left in (AIIMS/May-04)
  (a) Mitral regurgitation
  (b) Aortic regurgitation
  (c) Mitral stenosis
  (d) Aortic stenosis

Ans. (d)
Note
The pressure volume curve is shifted to the left in case of aortic stenosis.
Volume overload, as observed in chronic aortic and/or mitral valvular regurgitant disease, shifts the entire diastolic pressure-volume curve to the right, indicating increased chamber stiffness.
Pressure overload that leads to concentric LV hypertrophy (as occurs in aortic stenosis, hypertension, and hypertrophic cardiomyopathy) shifts the diastolic pressure-volume curve to the left along its volume axis so that at any diastolic volume ventricular diastolic pressure is abnormally elevated, although chamber stiffness may or may not be altered.
Ref: http://www.emedicine.com/med/topic3552.htm

Q. 97. The intrafusal fibers of the striated skeletal muscles are innervated by one of the following types of motor neurons (AIIMS/May-04)
  (a) Alpha
  (b) Beta
  (c) Gamma
  (d) Delta

Ans. (c)

Note
The intrafusal fibers of the striated skeletal muscles are innervated by gamma neurons.

Q. 98. The inhibitory neurotransmitter in CNS neurons is (AIIMS/May-04)
- (a) Glutamate
- (b) Aspartate
- (c) Gamma-amino butyric acid
- (d) Taurine

Ans. (c)
Note
The inhibitory neurotransmitter in CNS is:
a. Glutamate or glutamic acid is an important excitatory neurotransmitter in dorsal root afferents and at other sites in the CNS.
b. Aspartate its role as an excitatory neurotransmitter is less certain though it is known to act as one.
c. GABA: It is an inhibitory transmitter in spinal cord and to the cells of the cerebral cortex. In spinal cord it is responsible for presynaptic inhibition.
Ref: Textbook of physiology by A.K. Jain, 2nd edition, Vol 2, unit XI, Ch. 20, pg 1025

Q. 99. The correct sequence of cell cycle is (AIIMS/May-04)
- (a) G0-G1-S-G2-M
- (b) G0-G1-G2-S-M
- (c) G0-M-G2-S-G1
- (d) G0-G1-S-M-G2

Ans. (a)
Note
The cell cycle is the phase between two consecutive divisions. There are four sequential phases:
1. G_1 or Gap 1 in this phase the messenger RNA for proteins and the proteins required for DNA synthesis are synthesized.
2. S phase: Replication of nuclear DNA takes place.
3. G_2 phase or short gap phase is the stage when messenger RNA for mitosis is synthesized.
4. M phase: In which process of mitosis to form 2 daughter cells is completed.

Ref: Textbook of pathology by Harsh Mohan, Ch 2, Pg 17

Q. 100. Which of the following is the best-known metabolic function of the lung? (AIIMS/Nov-04)
- (a) Inactivation of serotonin
- (b) Conversion of angiotensin-I to angiotensin-II
- (c) Inactivation of bradykinin
- (d) Metabolism of basic drugs by cytochrome P-450 system

Ans. (b)
Note
The metabolic and endocrine functions of lungs are:
1. Surfactant production
2. Substances synthesized by the lung:
   - PGE_2 and PGF_2
   - Histamine is released from the mast cells in the lung inresponse to pulmonary embolism
   - Kallikrein
3. Substances removed from the blood by the lungs:
   - Bradykinin
   - Adenine derivatives
   - Serotonin
   - Norepinephrine
   - Acetylcholine
   - Prostaglandins
4. Substances activated in lung:
   Angiotensin I (inactive form) Angiotensin 2 (active form)

5. Vasoactive hormones that pass through the lungs: epinephrine, dopamine, oxytocin, vasopressin
6. Storage of hormones such as VIP, substance P, CCK-PZ and somatostatin, etc.
7. Contain fibrinolytic system that lyses clot in the pulmonary vessels.

Ref: Textbook of physiology by A. K. Jain, 2nd edition, Vol 1, unit VI, Ch. 1, pg 405, 406

Q. 101. When the aviator is subjected to negative G (AIIMS/Nov-04)
(a) The hydrostatic pressure in veins of lower limb increases.
(b) The cardiac output decreases.
(c) Black out occurs.
(d) The cerebral arterial pressure rises.

Ans. (d)
Note
When the aviator is subjected to negative G, the blood gets centrifuged to the head and therefore the cerebral arterial pressure rises.

Also see
During acceleration downwards force acts toward the head (negative 'G') increases arterial pressure at head level, the intracranial pressure also rises.(this is the reason why the vessels do not rupture)
During acceleration upwards (positive 'G') blood moves towards the feet and arterial pressure as well as the venous pressure decreases.
Ref: -Textbook of physiology by A. K. Jain, 2nd edition, Vol 1, unit V, Ch. 10, pg 365

Q. 102. Which combination of the following statements is correct with reference to hypoxia? (AIIMS/Nov-04)
a When it is severe, causes stimulation of the sympathetic nervous system.
b It leads to the accumulation of hydrogen and lactate ions.
c It causes decrease in cerebral blood flow.
d If it is chronic, causes rightward shift of oxygen Hb curve.

Answer Code
(a) All of the above statements are correct
(b) b and c
(c) a, b and d
(d) b, c and d

Ans. (c)
Note
The following statements are correct with reference to hypoxia:
i. When it is severe, causes stimulation of the sympathetic nervous system.
ii. It leads to accumulation of hydrogen and lactate ions.
iii. If it is chronic, causes rightward shift of oxygen Hb curve
The options (c) a, b and d is the most appropriate choice.

Q. 103. Which one of the following acts to increase the release of Ca^{2+} from endoplasmic reticulum? (AIIMS/Nov-04)
(a) Inositol triphosphate
(b) Parathyroid hormone
(c) 1, 25-dihydroxy cholecalciferol
(d) Diacyglycerol

Ans: (a)
Note
Inositol triphosphate activates the IP3 receptor, which is a membrane glycoprotein complex and activates Ca^{2+} channel.
Ref: http://en.wikipedia.org/wiki/Inositol_triphosphate_receptor

Q. 104. Erythropoiesis is promoted by all of the following except (AIIMS/Nov-04)
(a) ACTH
(b) Thyroxine

(c) Estrogen
(d) Prolactin

Ans: (c)

Note

Erythropoiesis is controlled by erythropoietin. Factors increasing erythropoietin synthesis are:
- Hypoxia due to haemorrhage, high altitude, cardio-respiratory disturbances
- Vasoconstrictor agents
- Nucleotides
- Haemolysis
- Hormones such as thyroxine, androgens, anterior pituitary hormones

Factors decreasing erythropoiesis are:
- Estrogens: it decreases hepatic synthesis of globulin and decreases erythropoietin response hypoxia.

Ref: Textbook of physiology by A. K. Jain, 2nd edition, Vol 1, unit II , Ch. 4, pg 63,64

Q. 105. Trendelenberg position produces decrease in all of the following except (AIIMS/Nov-04)
(a) Vital capacity
(b) Functional residual capacity
(c) Compliance
(d) Respiratory rate

Ans. (d)

Note

Trendelenburg's position; where a patient I splaced in such a position that his head is lower than the feet.

Also see

a. In such a position there would be a decrease in the vital capacity because: The venous return would increase and secondly the diaphragm would move up. (Page 412)

b. Functional residual capacity is the volume of air contained in the lung at end expiratory position. There would be a decrease in functional residual volume because, there would be increased congestion of blood in the lung and consequently the volume of air that can be contained in the lung at end of expiration should decrease. (Pg 412)

c. Compliance is the measurement of distensibility of the lungs and the chest wall.

The lung compliance will also decrease because of increased venous return to the heart and consequently to the pulmonary capillaries. (Pg. 418-420)

Ref: Textbook of physiology by A. K. Jain, 2nd edition, Vol 1, unit VI, Ch. 2

Q. 106. Which one of the following phenomena is closely associated with slow wave sleep (AIIMS/Nov-04)
(a) Dreaming
(b) Atonia
(c) Sleep walking
(d) Irregular heart rate

Ans. (c)

Note

Slow wave sleep is also called as Non-REM sleep. Dreaming is a feature of REM sleep. REM sleep is a light sleep and is characterized by: muscular atony, increased PR, RR and BP and movements of small muscle groups occurring intermittently.

NREM sleep is deep sleep. Sleep disorders occurring during NREM sleep are: sleep walking, night terrors, bedwetting, bruxism, sleep talking.

Ref: A short textbook of psychiatry by Neeraj Ahuja, 6th sdition, Ch. 11, page 146-154.

Q. 107. If a single spinal nerve is cut, the area of tactile loss is always greater than the area of loss of painful sensations, because (AIIMS/Nov-04)
(a) Tactile information is carried by myelinated fast conducting fires
(b) Tactile receptors adapt quickly
(c) Degree of overlap of fibres carrying tactile sensation is much less
(d) In the primary sensory cortex tactile sensation is represented on a larger area

Ans. (c)

Note
If a single spinal nerve is cut the area of tactile (sensory) loss is always less than its anatomical distribution, as the adjacent nerve fibers overlap the area.

Q. 108. Massage and the application of liniments to painful areas in the body relieves pain due to (AIIMS/Nov-04)
  (a) Simultaneous inhibition of endogenous analgesic system
  (b) Release of endorphins by the first order neurons in the brain stem
  (c) Release of glutamate and substance P in the spinal cord
  (d) Inhibition by large myelinated afferent fibres

Ans. (d)
Note
Massage and application of liniments causes stimulation of a large number of A and B both myelinated sensory fibers from the peripheral tactile receptors which in-turn depress the transmission of pain signals.

Also see
Touching or shaking an injured area decreases the pain of injury because such stimulation produces a profound reduction of pain by inhibiting pain pathways. Two main pathways are involved:
1. Segmental inhibition: stimulation of nerves in the same segment in which pain is felt can relieve such a pain.
2. Supra spinal inhibition: a descending inhibitory pathway from the brainstem to the rexed laminae I and V can also produce analgesia.

Ref: Textbook of physiology by A.K. Jain, 2nd edition, Vol 2, unit II, Ch. 5, pg 878

Q. 109. Which of the following produces the least damage to blood elements? (AIIMS/Nov-04)
  (a) Disc oxygenator
  (b) Membrane oxygenator
  (c) Bubble oxygenator
  (d) Screen oxygenator

Ans. (b)
Note
The oxygenator is designed to transfer oxygen to infused blood and remove carbon dioxide from the venous blood. Cardiac surgery was made possible by CPB using bubble oxygenators, but membrane oxygenators have supplanted bubble oxygenators since the 1980s.
Bubble oxygenators have no intervening barrier between blood and oxygen; these are called 'direct contact' oxygenators.
Membrane oxygenators introduce a gas-permeable membrane between blood and oxygen that decreases the blood trauma of direct-contact oxygenators.
Another type of oxygenator gaining favor recently is the heparin-coated blood oxygenator which is believed to produce less systemic inflammation and decrease the propensity for blood to clot in the CPB circuit.
Ref: http://en.wikipedia.org/wiki/Heart-lung_machine

Q. 110. In a fetus the insulin secretion begins by (AIIMS/May-05)
  (a) 3rd month
  (b) 5th month
  (c) 7th month
  (d) 9th month

Ans. (a)
Note
In a foetus the insulin secretion begins by 3rd month.
Ref: Textbook of Obstetrics By Dutta, 5th Edition Pg-43

Q. 111. Which of the following hormones is an example of a peptide hormone? (AIIMS/May-05)
  (a) Parathormone
  (b) Adrenaline
  (c) Cortisol
  (d) Thyroxine

Ans. (a)

Note
Parathormone (PTH) is a polypeptide with MW 9500, its primary function is to keep the calcium concentration in ECF and ICF constant. This is brought about by its action on both bone and kidney via activation of adenyl cyclase which increases formation of cAMP. It increases plasma Ca^{2+} and decreases Plasma PO_4^{3-}
Ref: -Textbook of physiology by A. K. Jain, 2nd edition, Vol 2, unit IX, Ch. 4, pg 680

Q. 112. The intrapleural pressure is negative both during inspiration and expiration because (AIIMS/May-05)
(a) Intrapulmonary pressure is always negative
(b) Thoracic cage and lungs are elastic structures
(c) Transpulmonary pressure determines the negativity
(d) Surfacant prevents the lungs to collapse

Ans. (b)
Note
The lungs and the chest wall are elastic structures. At the end of expiratory position the tendency for the lungs to recoil from the chest wall is just balanced by the tendency of the chest wall to recoil in opposite direction. This causes a subatmospheric pressure to develop say of 2mmHg between the two layers of pleura at the start of inspiration called as intrapleural pressure or intrathoracic pressure. It is directly proportional to the thoracic expansion. Therefore the lungs are pulled into a more expanded position causing the intrapleural pressure to decrease to about -6mmHg.
Ref: Textbook of physiology by A.K. Jain, 2nd edition, Vol 1, unit VI, Ch. 2, pg 409

Q. 113. Synaptic potentials can be recorded by (AIIMS/May-05)
(a) Patch clamp technique
(b) Voltage clamp technique
(c) Microelectrode
(d) EEG

Ans. (c)
Note
The events occurring at various synapses in the nervous system are similar to those occurring at the spinal synapses. The synaptic activity is studied by inserting a microelectrode into the soma of a motor neuron.
Ref: Textbook of physiology by A.K. Jain, 2nd edition, Vol 1, unit II, Ch. 2, pg 831

Q. 114. The ECG of a 40-year-old male was recorded using standard bipolar limb leads. The sum of voltages of the three standard leads was found to be 5 millivolts. This indicates (AIIMS/May-05)
(a) A normal heart
(b) Right ventricular hypertrophy
(c) Left ventricular hypertrophy
(d) Increased cardiac muscle mass

Ans. (d)
Note
The voltage in the three standard bipolar limb leads, as measured from the peak of the R wave to the botton of the S wave, vary between 0.5 to 2.0 millivolts, with lead III usually recording the lowest voltage and lead II the highest. When the sum of the voltage of all the QRS complexes of the three standard leads is greater than 4 millivolts the patient is considered to have a high voltage ECG and the common cause of high voltage QRS complexes is due to increased muscle mass of the heart.
Ref: Textbook of Medial Physiology, Guyton 10th Edition Pg-127

Q. 115. The velocity of blood is maximum in the (AIIMS/May-05)
(a) Large veins
(b) Small veins
(c) Venules
(d) Capillaries

Ans. (a)

Note
An increase in total cross sectional area of blood vessels decreases the linear mean velocity of blood flow.

	Total cross sectional area	Linear mean velocity
Aorta	$4 cm^2$	22.5 cm/sec
Small arteries	$63 cm^2$	1.4 cm/sec
Capillaries	$2800 cm^2$	0.3 mm/sec
Venules	$400 cm^2$	1-2 cm/sec
Small veins	$80 cm^2$	1-2 cm/sec
IVC and SVC (large veins)	$6 cm^2$	7-8 cm/sec

Ref: Textbook of physiology by A.K. Jain, 2nd edition, Vol 1, unit V, Ch. 5, pg 309

Q. 116. Which of the following methods is not used for measurement of body fluid volumes? (AIIMS/May-05)
- (a) Antipyrine for total body water.
- (b) Inulin for extracellular fluid.
- (c) Evens blue for plasma volume.
- (d) 125I-albumin for blood volume.

Ans. (d)
Note
Use of radioactive inulin is the most useful method to measure CEFV. Other methods are: Radioactive isotopes of Cl^-, Br, SO_4^{3-} etc.
Plasma volume is measured by employing certain substances that never leave the vascular system nor penetrate the RBCs. E.g.
- Evans blue dye (T-1824) that binds to plasma proteins.
- Radio-iodinated human serum albumin (RISA).
- Radio-iodinated gamma globulin and fibrinogen.

Ref: Textbook of physiology by A.K. Jain, 2nd edition, Vol 1, unit I, Ch. 3, pg 20,21

Q. 117. Group A nerve fibers are most susceptible to (AIIMS/May-05)
- (a) Pressure
- (b) Hypoxia
- (c) Local anaesthetics
- (d) Temperature

Ans. (a)
Note
Nerve fibres are classified according to physio clinical basis depending on their sensitivity to hypoxia, pressure and anaesthetic agents.
-Hypoxia: Pre-ganglionic autonomic 'B' fibres are most susceptible to it.
-Pressure: Group A fibres; these fibres are responsible for touch, pressure, pain, temp, proprioception etc.
-Local anaethetics: group C fibres (they include post ganglionic sympathetic fibres and fibres carrying pain, touch and temperature) are most sensitive to local anaesthetics.

Ref: Textbook of physiology by A. K. Jain, 2nd edition, Vol 1, unit III, Ch. 3, pg 137,138

Q. 118. Phantom limb sensations are best described by (AIIMS/May-05)
- (a) Weber Fechner law
- (b) Power law
- (c) Bell-magendie law
- (d) Law of projection

Ans. (d)
Note
The law of projection states that no matter where a particular sensory pathway is stimulated along its course to the cortex, the conscious sensation produced is referred to the location of the receptor.
For e.g., A limb that has been lost by amputation, the patient usually experiences intolerable pain and proprioceptive sensations in the limb that is no longer there is called as the phantom limb. These sensations

are due to irritation of the damaged receptive and proprioceptive afferents at the stump of the removed limb. This generates impulses in nerve fibres that previously came from the receptors in the removed limb, and the sensations produced are projected to where the receptors used to be located.
Ref: Textbook of physiology by A.K. Jain, 2nd edition, Vol 2, unit XI, Ch. 3, pg 849

Q. 119. The following statements are true regarding the SA node except (AIIMS/May-05)
  (a) Is located at the right border of the ascending aorta.
  (b) It contains specialized nodal cardiac muscle.
  (c) It is supplied by the atrial branches of the right coronary artery.
  (d) It initiates cardiac conduction.

Ans. (a)
Note
SA Node is located on the posterior aspect of the heart at the junction of the superior vena cava with the right atrium. It consists of thin elongated muscle fibres rich in glycogen and mitochondria. It is innervated by the right vagus nerve.
It is supplied by the right coronary artery which also supplies the whole of the right atrium, greater part of the rt. ventricle, a small part of the left ventricle, posterior part of the interventricular septum and most of the conducting system.
Ref: Textbook of physiology by A.K. Jain, 2nd edition, Vol 1, unit V, Ch. 1 and 10, pg 277, 354

Q. 120. The type of hemoglobin that has least affinity for 2,3-diphosphoglycerate (2,3-DPG) or (2,3-BPG) is (ALL INDIA/ 05)
  (a) Hb A
  (b) Hb F
  (c) Hb B
  (d) Hb A2

Ans. (b)
Note
Hb F is fetal haemoglobin and has greater affinity for O_2 as compared to Hb A, because of poor binding to 2,3 DPG, therefore it binds with Oxygen at a much lower Pressure than Hb A. Thus it causes the oxygen dissociation curve to shift to the left.
Hb A2 produces as such no abnormality and is regarded as normal Hb. Approximately 2.5 % of total Hb A is Hb A2.
Ref: Textbook of physiology by A.K. Jain, 2nd edition, Vol 1, unit II,VI Ch. 3, pg 54,434

Q. 121. Cellular and flagellar movement is carried out by all of the following except (ALL INDIA/ 05)
  (a) Intermediate filaments
  (b) Actin
  (c) Tubulin
  (d) Myosin

Ans. (d)
Note
Intermediate filaments provide flexible scaffolding for the cells that organizes the cytoplasm and helps in resisting external pressure. These include keratins, neuro-filaments, desmin, viamentin, glial cells and they are in no way involved in cellular or flagellar movements.
Actin and myosin are microfilments, which help in leucocyte movements and phagocytosis.
Tubulin are microtubules composed of slender tubes made up of protein. These are essential for leucocyte migration and phagocytosis.

Q. 122. Heme is converted into bilirubin mainly in (ALL INDIA/ 05)
  (a) Kidney
  (b) Liver
  (c) Spleen
  (d) Bone marrow

Ans. (c)

MCQ's in Physiology

Note
Most suitable answer is (c) however, note the following also.
RBCs are ingested and destroyed by in the tissue macrophage system or RES and form and release bilirubin. They include:
- Littoral cells of the blood sinuses in the bone marrow
- Kuppfer cells which lie along the vascular capillaries of the liver
- Reticulum cells: Found in both white and red pulp of the spleen
- L.N. (Lymph Nodes)
- Osteoclasts in the bone
- Microglia in the brain
- Pulmonary alveolar macrophages
- Subcutaneous tissue

Ref: Ref: Textbook of physiology by A.K. Jain, 2nd edition, Vol 1, unit II, Ch. 10, pg 106

Q. 123. Normal CSF glucose level in a normoglycemic adult is (ALL INDIA/ 05)
(a) 20-40 mg/dl
(b) 40-70 mg/dl
(c) 70-90 mg/dl
(d) 90-110 mg/dl

Ans. (b)
Note
Composition of CSF is:
- Na^+ 147 meq/l
- K^+ 2.9 meq/ml
- Ca^{2+} 2.3 meq/ml
- Cl^- 113 meq/ml
- HCO_3^- 25.1 meq/ml
- Proteins 25mg%
- Glucose 64mg%
- pH 7.33

Ref: Textbook of physiology by A.K. Jain, 2nd edition, Vol 1, unit V, Ch. 10, pg 368

Q. 124. Which one of the following molecules is used for cell signaling? (ALL INDIA/ 05)
(a) CO_2
(b) O_2
(c) NO
(d) N_2

Ans. (c)
Note
NO (Nitric Oxide) is a gas which acts as a neurotransmitter, neuromodulator in nervous system of mammals.
Ref: Ganong

Q. 125. Osteoclasts are inhibited by (ALL INDIA/ 05)
(a) Parathyroid hormone
(b) Calcitonin
(c) 1,25-dihydroxycholecalciferol
(d) Tumor necrosis factor

Ans. (b)
Note
Osteoclasts are large multinuclear giant cells containing numerous lysosomes. They erode and reabsorb previously formed bone. Osteoclastic activity is inhibited by calcitonin. It also lowers serum Ca levels and decreases renal formation of 1,25 DHCC.
Ref: Textbook of physiology by A. K. Jain, 2nd edition, Vol 2, unit IX, Ch. 2, pg 682

Q. 126. CO_2 is majorly transported in the arterial blood as (ALL INDIA/ 05)
    (a) Dissolved CO_2
    (b) Carbonic acid
    (c) Carbamino-hemoglobin
    (d) Bicarbonate

Ans. (d)
Note
CO_2 is carried in plasma and RBC in three forms:
    -In dissolved form (0.3 ml%)
    -As carbamino compound (0.7 ml%)
    -As bicarbonate (3 ml%)
Ref: Textbook of physiology by A.K. Jain, 2nd edition, Vol 1, unit VI, Ch. 3, pg 437

Q. 127. Both vitamin K and C are involved in (ALL INDIA/ 05)
    (a) The synthesis of clotting factors
    (b) Post translational modifications
    (c) Antioxidant mechanisms
    (d) The microsomal hydroxylation reactions

Ans. (b)
Note
The major function of the K vitamins is in the maintenance of normal levels of the blood clotting proteins, factors II, VII, IX, X and protein C and protein S, which are synthesized in the liver as inactive precursor proteins. Conversion from inactive to active clotting factor requires a posttranslational modification of specific glutamate (E) residues. This modification is a carboxylation and the enzyme responsible requires vitamin K as a cofactor.
Deficiency in vitamin C leads to the disease scurvy due to the role of the vitamin in the post-translational modification of collagens.
Ref: http://web.indstate.edu/thcme/mwking/vitamins.html#c

Q. 128. The main site of bicarbonate reabsorption is (ALL INDIA/ 05)
    (a) Proximal convoluted tubule
    (b) Distal convoluted tubule
    (c) Cortical collecting duct
    (d) Medullary collecting duct

Ans. (a)
Note
HCO_3^- reabsorption occurs throughout the nephron except in descending limb of loop of henle. Approximately 90% of the filtered HCO_3^- is reabsorbed into the proximal convoluted tubule (PCT) by secondary active transport. Remaining 10-15% of filtered HCO_3^- is reabsorbed into DCT and CT
Ref: Textbook of physiology by A. K. Jain, 2nd edition, Vol 1, unit VII, Ch. 2, pg 513, 514

Q. 129. The membrane protein, clathrin is involved in (ALL INDIA/ 05)
    (a) Cell motility
    (b) Receptor-mediated endocytosis
    (c) Exocytosis
    (d) Cell shape

Ans. (b)
Note
Endocytosis is a process whereby cells absorb material (molecules such as proteins) from the outside by engulfing it with their cell membrane. There are three types of endocytosis: namely, macropinocytosis, clathrin-mediated endocytosis, and caveolar endocytosis.
Clathrin-mediated endocytosis is the specific uptake of large extracellular molecules such as proteins, membrane localized receptors and ion-channels. These receptors are associated with the cytosolic protein clathrin which initiates the formation of a vesicle by forming a crystalline coat on the inner surface of the cell's membrane.
Ref: http://en.wikipedia.org/wiki/Endocytosis

Q. 130. The parvocellular pathway from lateral geniculate nucleus to visual cortex is most sensitive for the stimulus of (ALL INDIA/ 05)
(a) Color contrast
(b) Luminance contrast
(c) Temporal frequency
(d) Saccadic eye movements

Ans. (a)
Note
Parvocellular pathway carries signals for color vision, texture shape and fine details to visual cortex, from 3, 4, 5 and 6 layers of lateral geniculate nucleus.

Q. 131. The fibers from the contralateral nasal hemiretina project to the following layers of the lateral geniculate nucleus (ALL INDIA/ 05)
(a) Layers 2, 3 & 5
(b) Layers 1, 2 & 6
(c) Layers 1, 4 & 6
(d) Layers 4, 5 & 6

Ans. (c)
Note
The fibres from contralateral nasal hemiretina project to the 1, 4 and 6 layer of the lateral geniculate nucleus.

Also see
The grey matter of Lateral Geniculate body shows 6 clear cut layers numbered from 1 to 6. The fibers from the retina to the contralateral side end in layers 1, 4 and 6.
The fibers from the ipsilateral retina end in layers 2, 3 and 5.
Ref: Textbook of physiology by A. K. Jain, 2nd edition, Vol 2, unit XII, Ch. 4, pg 1072

Q. 132. All endothelial cells produce thrombomodulin except for those found in (ALL INDIA/ 05)
(a) Hepatic circulation
(b) Cutaneous circulation
(c) Cerebral microcirculation
(d) Renal circulation

Ans. (c)
Note
All endothelial cells except for those of cerebral microcirculation produce thrombomodulin, a thrombin binding protein that converts thrombin to protein C activator. This activates protein C, a naturally occurring anticoagulant protein that inactivates Factors V and VII and inactivates tissue plasminogen activator, thus increasing fibrinolysis and preventing formation of a clot in cerebral circulation.
Ref: Textbook of physiology by A. K. Jain, 2nd edition, Vol 1, unit II, Ch. 8, pg 92

Q. 133. SA node acts as a pacemaker of the heart because of the fact that it (ALL INDIA/ 05)
(a) Is capable of generating impulses spontaneously
(b) Has rich sympathetic innervations
(c) Has poor cholinergic innervations
(d) Generates impulses at the highest rate

Ans. (d)
Note
SA node is located on the posterior aspect of heart at the Junction of SVC with right atrium. It normally generates and discharges impulses more rapidly than any other pace maker tissue and their rate of discharge determines the rate at which the heart beats. That is why SA node is also called as the pace maker of the heart.
Ref: Textbook of physiology by A. K. Jain, 2nd edition, Vol 1, unit V, Ch. 1, pg 277

Q. 134. The first physiological response to high environmental temperature is (ALL INDIA/ 05)
(a) Sweating
(b) Vasodilatation

(c) Decreased heat production
(d) Non-shivering thermogenesis

Ans. (b)

Note
On Exposure to heat the thermoregulatory mechanism is called into action which includes:
1. Increased heat loss: By cutaneous vasodilatation, sweating and increase in respiratory rate. (It is the first physiological response for thermoregulation)
2. Decreased heat production: This is achieved by:
   -Anorexia
   -Decreased sympathetic activity
   -Apathy and inertia
   -Decreased TSH secretion from anterior pituitary.

Ref: Textbook of physiology by A.K. Jain, 2nd edition, Vol 1, unit VII, Ch. 9, pg 567

Q. 135. All of the following factors normally increase the length of the ventricular cardiac muscle fibres except (ALL INDIA/ 05)
(a) Increased venous tone
(b) Increased total blood volume
(c) Increased negative intrathoracic pressure
(d) Lying-to-standing change in posture

Ans. (d)

Note
Factors that normally increase the length of the ventricular cardiac muscle fibres are:
  -increased venous tone
  -increase total blood volume
  -increased negative intrathoracic pressure
  -strong atrial contractions
Whereas the factors which normally decrease the length of ventricular cardiac muscle fibres are:
  -lying-to-standing change in posture
  -standing
  -increased pericardial pressure
  -decreased ventricular compliance

Ref: Ganong

Q. 136. The vasodilatation produced by carbon dioxide is maximum in one of the following (ALL INDIA/ 05)
(a) Kidney
(b) Brain
(c) Liver
(d) Heart

Ans. (b)

Note
The most pronounced vasodilatation produced by carbon dioxide is in the skin and brain. As the skin is not given as a choice, therefore the option brain is the most suitable choice.

Also see
Metabolic changes that produce vasodilatation include:
1. Decreased arterial pO_2 or hypoxia
2. Decreased blood pH
3. Increased arterial pCO_2 : it is a direct dilator and its action is most pronounced on the skin and brain
4. Increased blood osmolality
5. Increased body temperature
6. Lactic acid accumulation

Ref: Textbook of physiology by A. K. Jain, 2nd edition, Vol 1, unit V, Ch. 6, pg 316

Q. 137. Which one of the following statements is true regarding water reabsorption in the tubules? (ALL INDIA/ 05)
    (a)   The bulk of water reabsorption occurs secondary to Na+ reabsorption
    (b)   Majority of facultative reabsorption occurs in proximal tubule
    (c)   Obligatory reabsorption is ADH dependent
    (d)   20% of water is always reabsorbed irrespective of water balance

Ans. (a)

Note
Passive reabsorption of water in proximal convoluted tubule (PCT) secondary to active reabsorption of Na^+ is called as obligatory reabsorption of water.
Reabsorption of water under the influence of ADH is called as facultative reabsorption of water.
Water is mainly absorbed passively along the osmotic gradient established by reabsorption of Na^+ and Cl^-
Ref: Textbook of physiology by A. K. Jain, 2nd edition, Vol 1, unit VII, Ch. 2, pg 517

Q. 138. Urinary concentrating ability of the kidney is increased by (ALL INDIA/ 05)
    (a)   ECF volume contraction
    (b)   Increase in RBF
    (c)   Reduction of medullary hyperosmolarity
    (d)   Increase in CFR

Ans. (a)

Note
ECF volume contraction is a decrease in extra cellular fluid volume caused by loss of water and total body Na^+ content. Causes include vomiting, sweating, diarrhoea, burns, diuretic use, and renal failure. Clinical features include diminished skin turgor, dry mucous membranes, tachycardia, and orthostatic hypotension. During ECF volume depletion, normally functioning kidneys conserve Na^+. Thus, the urine Na^+ concentration is usually < 15 mEq/L; the fractional excretion of Na^+ is usually < 1%; also, urine osmolality is often > 450 mOsm/kg.
Ref: http://www.merck.com/mmpe/sec12/ch156/ch156c.html#sec12-ch156-ch156c-676

Q. 139. Distribution of blood flow is mainly regulated by the (ALL INDIA/ 05)
    (a)   Arteries
    (b)   Arterioles
    (c)   Capillaries
    (d)   Venules

Ans. (b)

Note
Arterioles offer maximum resistance to the blood flow towards the capillaries and thus are the main sites for peripheral resistance; therefore the blood flow to the different body organs is regulated by small changes in the caliber of the arterioles.
Ref: Textbook of physiology by A. K. Jain, 2nd edition, Vol 1, unit I, Ch. 5, pg 306

Q. 140. In which of the following a reduction in arterial oxygen tension occurs? (ALL INDIA/ 05)
    (a)   Anaemia
    (b)   CO poisoning
    (c)   Moderate exercise
    (d)   Hypoventilation

Ans. (d)

Note
In hyperventilation there is wash out of CO_2, pCO_2 also decreases but alveolar pO_2 increases.
Hypoventilation is a state contrary to this, thus we can draw the conclusion that in hypoventilation pO_2 would decrease and pCO_2 will increase.
Ref: Textbook of physiology by A. K. Jain, 2nd edition, Vol 1, unit VI, Ch. 4, pg 458, 459

Q. 141. With which one of the following, lower motor neuron lesions are associated? (ALL INDIA/ 05)
   (a)   Flaccid paralysis
   (b)   Hyperactive stretch reflex
   (c)   Spasticity
   (d)   Muscular incoordination

Ans. (a)
Note
Lower motor neuron lesion occurs when the lesion is at the spinal and cranial motor neurons that directly innervates the muscle spindle. Muscle becomes 'completely flaccid' due to complete loss of muscle tone which depends on the integrity of the reflex arc.
Other features are:
   -disuse atrophy
   -absent reflexes
   -muscle twitching
Ref: Textbook of physiology by A. K. Jain, 2nd edition, Vol 2, unit XI, Ch. 6, pg 892

Q. 142. Which of the following statements can be regarded as primary action of inhibin? (ALL INDIA/ 05)
   (a)   It inhibits secretion of prolactin.
   (b)   It stimulates synthesis of estradiol.
   (c)   It stimulates secretion of TSH.
   (d)   It inhibits secretion of FSH.

Ans. (d)
Note
Inhibin is an unidentified testicular factor derived from the seminiferous tubules. It provides a negative feedback to the secretion of FSH.
This has been proven by the fact that patients having atrophy of seminiferous tubules show elevated plasma FSH levels with normal testosterone and LH.
Ref: Textbook of physiology by A. K. Jain, 2nd edition, Vol 2, unit X, Ch. 2, pg 772

Q. 143. To which of the following family of chemical mediators of inflammation, the Lipoxins belong? (ALL INDIA/ 04)
   (a)   Kinin system
   (b)   Cytokines
   (c)   Chemokines
   (d)   Arachidonic acid metabolites

Ans. (d)
Note
Arachidonic acid metabolites are cell derived mediators of inflammation. They are of types:
1.   Metabolites via cyclo-oxygenase pathway
2.   Metabolites via lipo-oxygenase pathway
Arachidonic acid generates substances called **lipoxins** that work to stop inflammatory activity. In the lungs and respiratory passages, another type of arachidonic acid-derived eicosanoid, **leukotrienes,** constrict the airway muscles making breathing more difficult.
Ref: Textbook of Pathology, Harsh mohan, Ch. 5, page 121
http://www.fatsoflife.com/fatsoflife/inflammation-and-the-immune-system.asp

Q. 144. The main excitatory neurotransmitter in the CNS is (ALL INDIA/ 04)
   (a)   Glycine
   (b)   Acetylcholine
   (c)   Aspartate
   (d)   Glutamate

Ans. (d)

Note
Glutamic acid is an important excitatory neurotransmitter in dorsal root afferents and at other sites in the CNS.
The role of aspartate as an excitatory neurotransmitter is less certain.
Inhibitory neurotransmitters are: GABA and Glycine
Ref: Textbook of physiology by A. K. Jain, 2nd edition, Vol 2, unit XI, Ch. 20, pg 1024, 1025

Q. 145. During the cardiac cycle the opening of the aortic valve takes place at the (ALL INDIA/ 04)
    (a)   Beginning of systole
    (b)   End of isovolumetric contraction
    (c)   End of diastole
    (d)   End of diastasis

Ans. (b)
Note
The period of isovolumetric contraction is when ventricle contracts as a closed chamber with both of the atrio-ventricular (Semilunar) valves are closed.
According to Ganong opening of the aortic valve occurs at the end of isovolumetric contraction.
Ref: Ganong 20th Edition Pg- 54

Q. 146. The patients having acute cardiac failure do not show oedema, because (ALL INDIA/ 04)
    (a)   The plasma osmatic pressure is high.
    (b)   There is renal compensation.
    (c)   Increased cardiac output.
    (d)   There is a fall in the systemic capillary hydrostatic pressure.

Ans. (d)
Note
Oedema in chronic heart disease is caused by increased capillary hydrostatic pressure to a level more than plasma osmatic pressure resulting in minimal or no reabsorption of fluid at the venular end resulting in oedema.
In acute cardiac failure there is sudden systemic hypotension (leading to a fall in hydrostatic pressure) preventing peripheral oedema.
Ref: Textbook of pathology, Harsh Mohan, 4th Edition
Pg- 80, 281

Q. 147. During acclimatization to high altitude all of the following take place, except (ALL INDIA/ 04)
    (a)   Increase in minute ventilation
    (b)   Increase in the sensitivity of central chemoreceptors
    (c)   Increase in the sensitivity of carotid body to hypoxia
    (d)   Shift in the oxygen dissociation curve to the left

Ans. (d)
Note
Within a few hours of exposure to hypoxia at high altitude, there is increase in the amount of 2, 3 DPg in RBCs. This shifts the O_2 – Hb dissociation curve to shift to the right releasing more oxygen from Hb.
Ref: Textbook of physiology by A. K. Jain, 2nd edition, Vol 1, unit VI, Ch. 6, pg 473

Q. 148. Duchenne muscular dystrophy is a disease of (ALL INDIA/ 04)
    (a)   Neuromuscular junction
    (b)   Sarcolemmal proteins
    (c)   Muscle contractile proteins
    (d)   Disuse atrophy due to muscle weakness

Ans. (b)
Note
DMD is a type of muscular dystrophy due to defect in dystrophin- glycoprotein complex. This is a large protein complex that connects the thin filaments to the transmembranous proteins in the sarcolemma and thus provides support and strength to the myofibrils.
Ref: Textbook of physiology by A. K. Jain, 2nd edition, Vol 1, unit III, Ch. 6, pg 162

Q. 149. Sertoli cells have receptors for (ALL INDIA/ 04)
   (a) Inhibin
   (b) Luteinising hormone
   (c) Follicle stimulating hormone
   (d) Melatonin

Ans (c)
Note
FSH acts on the sertoli cells and facilitate the last stage of spermatid maturation.
LH stimulates leydig cells to cause testosterone secretion.
Ref: Textbook of physiology by A. K. Jain, 2nd edition, Vol 2, unit X, Ch. 2, pg 766

Q. 150. Before the onset of puberty the GnRH neurons are under the inhibitory control of (ALL INDIA/ 04)
   (a) Glycine
   (b) Glutamate
   (c) Gamma amino butyric acid (GABA)
   (d) Beta-endorphin

Ans. (c)
Note
GnRH stimulates the release of FSH and LH, which in turn determine the changes occurring at puberty. GnRH neurosecretion has been shown to be under the control of many neurotransmitters and neuropeptides. Among the latter, two aminoacids have a predominant action: glutamate which has an excitatory effect and whose levels increase before puberty, and gamma aminobutyric acid (GABA) which exerts an important inhibitory action on GnRH secretion and whose concentrations diminish at puberty.
Ref: http://www.endotext.org/pediatrics/pediatrics13/pediatrics13.htm

Q. 151. The enzyme associated with the conversion of androgen to oestrogen in the growing ovarian follicle is (ALL INDIA/ 04)
   (a) Desmolase
   (b) Isomerase
   (c) Aromatase
   (d) Hydroxylase

Ans. (c)
Note
Aromatase is an enzyme of the cytochrome P450 group (EC 1.14.14.1), whose function is to mediate the aromatization of androgens (that is, to selectively increase their aromaticity), producing estrogens.
Ref: http://en.wikipedia.org/wiki/Aromatase

Q. 152. Which of the following is a membrane-bound enzyme that catalyzes the formation of cyclic AMP from ATP ? (ALL INDIA/ 04)
   (a) Tyrosine kinase
   (b) Polymerase
   (c) ATP synthase
   (d) Adenylate cyclase

Ans. (d)
Note
Conversion of ATP to cAMP occurs during glycogenolysis in presence of enzyme – Adenylate cyclase.
In this cycle glycogen gets converted to glucose in the liver.
Ref: Textbook of physiology by A.K. Jain, 2nd edition, Vol 2, unit VII, Ch. 2, pg 578,579, Fig 8.2.1

Q. 153. The transmembrane region of a protein is likely to have (ALL INDIA/ 04)
   (a) A stretch of hydrophilic amino acids
   (b) A stretch of hydrophobic amino acids
   (c) A disulphide loop
   (d) Alternating hydrophilic and hydrophobic amino acids

Ans. (b)

Note
Chemically a biomembrane consists of lipids (20-40%) and proteins (60-70%) and carbohydrates (1-5%). The lipids and proteins contain both polar (hydrophillic) and non polar (hydrophobic) ends. The hydrophobic ends of proteins are either kept folded or used to establish connections with hydrophobic part of lipids.
Ref: Truman's Elementary Biology, Vol 1, Unit 2, cp- 8, pg 91

Q. 154. In which of the following forms the antidiuretic hormone (ADH) is circulated in plasma (ALL INDIA/ 04)
(a) Bound to neurophysin-I
(b) Bound to neurophysin-II
(c) Bound to plasma albumin
(d) Free form

Ans. (d)
Note
ADH is a hypothalamic hormone synthesised in the cells of the supraoptic nucleus. The hormones then pass down the axons bound to carrier protein Neurophysin II. This is only a physiological carrier protein for intraneuronal transport of ADH and are released in the circulation with the neurosecretory products without being bound to the hormones.
Ref: Textbook of physiology by A.K. Jain, 2nd edition, Vol 2, unit IX, Ch. 2, pg 645

BIOCHEMISTRY

Q. 155. The most abundant glycoprotein present in basement membrane is
(a) Laminin
(b) Fibronectin
(c) Collagen type 4
(d) Heparan sulphate

Ans. (a)
Note
Basement membranes are positive amorphous structures (PAS) that lie underneath epithelia of different organs and endothelial cells. They consist of collagen type IV protein and laminin.
Ref: Textbook of pathology, Harsh Mohan, 4th edition, Ch. 5, page 157

Q. 156. An enzyme that makes a double stranded DNA copy from a single stranded RNA template molecule is known as
(a) DNA polymerase
(b) RNA polymerase
(c) Reverse transcriptase
(d) Phosphokinase

Ans. (c)
Note
Retroviruses exhibit a unique replicative strategy. Their single stranded RNA is converted into RNA:DNA hybrid by the viral reverse transcriptase enzyme, it is a RNA directed DNA polymerase. The ds DNA is then synthesized from the RNA DNA hybrid. The ds DNA from the virus is then integrated with the host DNA, which causes transformation of cell and neoplasia.
Ref: Textbook of microbiology, R. Ananthanarayan, Ch. 48, page 404

Q. 157. A person on a fat free carbohydrate rich diet continues to grow obese. Which of the following lipoproteins is likely to be elevated in his blood?
(a) Chylomicrons
(b) VLDL
(c) LDL
(d) DHDL

Ans. (b)

Note
Diets rich in cholesterol or saturated fats tend to raise blood LDL cholesterol, while high carbohydrate intake or excessive alcohol consumption may increase plasma VLDL. Thus any diet aimed at reducing cholesterol must not only restrict fats but also carbohydrates.
Ref: Principles and practice of medicine, Davidsons, 19th edition, Ch. 10, page 310

Q. 158. A genetic disorder renders fructose 1,6- bisphosphatase in liver less sensitive to regulation by fructose 2,6-bisphosphate. All of the following metabolic changes are observed in this disorder, except
    (a)   Level of fructose 1,6-bisphosphate is higher than normal
    (b)   Level of fructose 1,6-bisphosphate is lower than normal
    (c)   Less pyruvate is formed
    (d)   Less ATP is generated

Ans. (b)
Note
Fructose-1,6- biphosphatase regulates conversion of fructose-6-phosphate to fructose-1,6-biphosphate. If the enzyme is defective and less sensitive to fructose-6-phosphate then it is no longer converted to fructose-1,6-biphosphate and its level in blood falls.
Ref: Textbook of physiology by A.K. Jain, 2nd edition, Vol 2, unit VIII, Ch. 2, pg 580, fig 8.2.2

Q. 159. Xeroderma pigmentosum is produced as a result of a defect in
    (a)   DNA polymerase II
    (b)   DNA polymerase I
    (c)   DNA exonuclease
    (d)   DNA ligase

Ans. (c)
Note
Damage to DNA in epidermal cells occurs during exposure to UV-C light. The absorption of the high energy light leads to the formation of pyrimidine dimers, namely CPDs (Cyclobutane-Pyrimidine-Dimers) and 6-4PP (pyrimidine-6-4-pyrimidone photoproducts). The pathway, using multiple enzymes which repair the UV-damage in healthy cells, is called nucleotide excision repair. The damage is excised by exonucleases, then the gap is filled by a DNA polymerase and sealed by a ligase. The most common defect in xeroderma pigmentosum is a genetic defect whereby nucleotide excision repair (NER) enzymes are mutated, leading to less or no repair of UV-lesions.
Ref: http://en.wikipedia.org/wiki/Xeroderma_pigmentosum

Q. 160. Radio isotopes are used in the following techniques, except
    (a)   Mass spectroscopy
    (b)   RIA
    (c)   ELISA
    (d)   Sequencing of nucleic acid

Ans. (c)
Note
ELISA (Enzyme Linked Immunoabsorbent Assay) is so named because it involves the use of an immunosorbent, and it does not use radioactive isotopes.
RIA (Radioimmunoassay), Mass spectroscopy, Sequencing of nucleic acid, all these procedures involved use of radioisotopes.
Ref: Textbook of microbiology, R. Ananthanarayan, Ch. 13, page 100

Q. 161. Alpha helix and beta pleated sheet are examples of
    (a)   Primary structure
    (b)   Secondary structure
    (c)   Tertiary structure
    (d)   Quaternary structure

Ans. (b)

Note
A protein can have up to 4 levels of organization:
a. Primary: It is the description of the basic structure of the proteins.
b. Secondary: They are of three types:
    - α helix-Polypeptide chain is coiled spirally in right handed manner.
    - β pleated-2 or more polypeptide chains are connected by hydrogen bonds.
    - Collagen helix: 3 strands of Polypeptide chains are coiled around each other.
c. Tertiary: Bending and folding of various types to form spheres, rods etc.
d. Quaternary structure: Is the arrangement of multiple folded protein molecules in a multi-subunit complex.

Ref: Truman's Elementary Biology, unit 2, Ch. 6, page 57, 58

Q. 162. Which of the following substances acts to increase the release of Ca^{2+} from endoplasmic reticulum?
    (a) Inositol triphosphate
    (b) Parathyroid hormone
    (c) 1,25-dihydroxy cholecalciferol
    (d) Diacyl glycerol

Ans. (a)
Note
a. Inositol triphosphate triggers the release of Ca^{2+} into the cytoplasm from the endoplasmic reticulum.
b. Parathyroid hormone increases blood calcium.
c. 1,25-dihydroxy cholecalciferol maintains blood calcium level and is needed for mineralisation.
d. Diacyl glycerol activates Protien C.

Ref: http://www.targetpg.com/exams/aipg/2004/2004aipgphys.doc

Q. 163. Which of the following elements is known to influence the body's ability to handle oxidative stress?
    (a) Calcium
    (b) Iron
    (c) Potassium
    (d) Selenium

Ans. (d)
Note
Selenium is part of the enzyme glutathione peroxidase which helps prevent free radical damage to cells. Thus selenium helps in preventing free radical damage.
Selenium is also part of the enzyme responsible for the conversion of thyroxine to triiodothyronine. Its deficiency has been reported to cause cardiomyopathy in children.

Ref: Davidson's principles and practice of medicine, 19th edition, Ch. 10, page 325

Q. 164. In which of the following conditions the level of creatinine kinase-1 increases?
    (a) Myocardial ischemia
    (b) Brain ischemia
    (c) Kidney damage
    (d) Electrical cardioversion

Ans. (b)
Note
Creatinine Kinase (CK, CPK) is an enzyme found primarily in the heart and skeletal muscles, and to a lesser extent in the brain.
There are 3 forms of CK:
CPK-1 or CPK-BB: found in brain and lungs.
CPK-2-or CPK-MB: found in the cardiac muscles.
CPK-3 or CPK-MM: found in skeletal muscle.
Significant injury to any of these structures will lead to a measurable increase in CK levels.
    -Once elevated, CK remains elevated for several days, if the injury is acute.

-If there is on-going injury, the CK will remain elevated indefinitely.
Ref: Textbook of Pathology, Harsh Mohan, 4th edition, Ch. 11, Page 295

Q. 165. Proteins targeted for destruction in eukaryotes are covalently linked to
    (a)   Clathrin
    (b)   Pepsin
    (c)   Laminin
    (d)   Ubiquitin

Ans. (d)
Note
Ubiquitin is a small protein which is present in eukaryotic cells. It targets many intracellular proteins for degradation which include newly produced abnormal proteins and aged normal proteins.
The 'C' terminal residue of ubiquitin becomes covalently attached to lysine residue of proteins that are then degraded.
Ref: Ganong

Q. 166. Which of the following groups of proteins assist in the folding of other proteins?
    (a)   Proteases
    (b)   Proteosomes
    (c)   Templates
    (d)   Chaperone

Ans. (d)
Note
Chaperones are proteins whose function is to assist other proteins in achieving proper folding. Many chaperones are heat shock proteins, that is, proteins expressed in response to elevated temperatures or other cellular stresses. The reason for this behaviour is that protein folding is severely affected by heat and, therefore, some chaperones act to repair the potential damage caused by misfolding.
Ref: http://en.wikipedia.org/wiki/Chaperone

Q. 167. An increase in which of the following parameters will shift the O_2 dissociation curve to the left? (ALL INDIA/03)
    (a)   Temperature
    (b)   Partial pressure of CO_2
    (c)   2,3 DPG concentration
    (d)   Oxygen affinity of haemoglobin

Ans. (d)
Note
The curve relating %O_2 saturation of Hb to the pO_2 is called as oxygen-hemoglobin dissociation curve. It is sigmoid in shape.
Shift to the right: at any pO_2 the oxygen content that can be held by the blood decreases causing unloading of O_2
Causes
    a.   Fall in blood pH due to increased pCO_2.
    b.   Increased body temperature.
    c.   Increased concentration of 2,3 DPG (DPG competes with O_2 for binding sites on the hemoglobin molecule therefore the percentage saturation of Hb with O_2 will be reduced in presence of 2,3 DPG).
Shift to the left: i.e. affinity of hemoglobin to combine with O_2 increases causing less release of oxygen to the tissues.
Causes
    a.   CO
    b.   HbF
    c.   Myoglobin
    d.   Decreased body temperature

Ref: Textbook of physiology by A.K. Jain, 2nd edition, Vol 1, unit VI, Ch. 3, pg 433,434

Q. 168. A lesion of ventrolateral part of spinal cord (below the level of lesion) will lead to loss of (ALL INDIA/03)
  (a) Pain sensation on the ipsilateral side
  (b) Proprioception on the contralateral side
  (c) Pain sensation on the contralateral side
  (d) Proprioception on the ipsilateral side

Ans. (c)

Note
The lateral white column of spinal cord carries the following tracts:
  -Lateral spinothalamic tract: It carries pain, temperature impulses of the opposite side
  -Anterior and posterior spinocerebellar tracts: are responsible for maintenance of posture, thus if this tract is affected then there is disturbance in posture.
Proprioception, tactile localization, fine touch, kinesthetic sensations are carried in the dorsal column. Which are unaffected in ventro-lateral lesions of the spinal cord.
Ref: Textbook of physiology by A.K. Jain, 2nd edition, Vol 2, unit XI, Ch. 5, pg 866-869

Q. 169. As a part of space-research program, a physiologist was asked to investigate the effect of flight-induced stress on blood pressure. Accordingly the blood pressure of the cosmonauts were to be measured twice: once before the take-off, and once after the spacecraft entered the designated orbit around the earth. For a proper comparison, the preflight blood pressure should be recorded in (ALL INDIA/03)
  (a) The lying down position
  (b) The sitting position
  (c) The standing position
  (d) Any position, as long as the post-flight recording is made in the same position

Ans. (a)

Note
The pressure in any vessel below the level of heart is increased and a vessel above the level of heart is decreased by the effect of gravity. The magnitude of gravity at normal density of blood is 0.77mmHg.
Ref: Textbook of physiology by A.K. Jain, 2nd edition, Vol 1, unit V, Ch. 9, pg 344
Since the pressure has to be measured in space where the element of gravity is eliminated therefore on ground also the BP should be measured with the patient in lying down position.

Q. 170. The renal plasma flow (RPF) of a patient was to be estimated through the measurement of Para Amino Hippuric acid (PAH) clearance. The technician observed the procedure correctly but due to an error in the weighing, inadvertently used thrice the recommended dose of PAH The RPF estimated is likely to be (ALL INDIA/03)
  (a) False-high
  (b) False-low
  (c) False-high or false-low depending on the GFR
  (d) Correct and is unaffected by the PAG overdose

Ans. (b)

Note
Para Amino Hippuric acid (PAH) is used to measure renal plasma flow according to the following formula:
RPF = amount of PAH excreted in urine/ min X V

$A_{PAH} - V_{PAH}$
Where V is Rate of urine flow
A_{PAH} or V_{PAH} concentration of PAH in renal Artery and renal Vein respectively
If the dose of PAH given is more than the concentration of PAH in renal Artery consequently urinary concentration of PAH is also more. Therefore it shouldn't affect the RPF value.
Ref: Textbook of physiology by A.K. Jain, 2nd edition, Vol 1, unit VII, Ch. 3, pg 522

Q. 171. Which of the following statements is true for excitatory postsynaptic potentials? (EPSP) (ALL INDIA/03)
(a) Are self propagating
(b) Show all or none response
(c) Are proportional to the amount of transmitter released by the presynaptic neuron
(d) Are inhibitory at presynaptic terminal

Ans. (c)

Note
Excitation post synaptic potentials are proportional to the amount of transmitter released by the presynaptic neuron. Excitation post synaptic potentials are small depolarization of the post-synaptic membrane due to discharge of chemical transmitter by a few pre-synaptic knobs in response to small stimuli. These depolarization's are small and do not result in genesis of an action potential in the post-synaptic membrane. However, these small depolarization can add up to reach the threshold level in which case an action potential is then generated. The excitation post synaptic potentials are directly proportional to the strength of initial stimuli.

Also see
The initial depolarizing impulse produced by a single stimulus to the sensory nerve begins about 0.5 msec after the impulse enters the spinal cord; if it is not sufficient to produce a depolarization then it declines. During this potential the excitability of the neuron to other stimuli is increased, therefore the potential is called an excitatory post-synaptic potential. It is also called as Graded potential.
EPSP due to activity in one synaptic knob is small, but EPSP produced by each of the active knobs summate. This can occur by two mechanisms:
1. Spatial summation
2. Temporal summation

It is non propagating that is, it remains confined locally and declines with time.
It is initiated spontaneously or by neurotransmitter or environmental stimulus.
It has no threshold or refractory period.
It can be either a depolarizing or hyperpolarizing response.
Self propagating potentials are action potentials.
They show all or none phenomenon.
It has a threshold and refractory period.
Ref: Textbook of physiology by A.K. Jain, 2nd edition, Vol 1,2 unit I, XI, Ch. 4,2, pg 36, 832 respectively

Q. 172. The cell junctions allowing exchange of cytoplasmic molecules between the two cells are called (ALL INDIA/03)
(a) Gap junctions
(b) Tight junctions
(c) Anchoring junctions
(d) Focal junctions

Ans. (a)

Note
Gap junctions:
There is a 2mm space between the opposing membranes. This gap is filled with densely packed particles through each of which there appears to be a channel that connects the two cells. Other advantages are:
a. It permits rapid propagation of electrical potential changes from one cell to another, e.g. cardiac and smooth muscle cells.
b. It permits direct transfer of ions and other smaller molecules between cells without traversing the extracellular space.

Tight junction:
The membrane of two cells become opposed and outer layer of the membranes fuse, thus obliterating the space between the two cells.
It forms a barrier to the movement of ions and other solutes from one side to other.
Ref: Textbook of physiology by A.K. Jain, 2nd edition, Vol 1, unit 1, Ch. 1, pg 7,8

Q. 173. SI unit for measuring blood pressure is (ALL INDIA/02)
(a) Torr
(b) BmrnHg
(c) kPa
(d) Bar

Ans. (c)
Note
The SI unit for measuring blood pressure is Pascal (Pa) and measured in kPa.
Ref: Principles and practice of medicine, Davidson, 19th edition, Ch. 23, Page 1215

Q. 174. Glucose mediated insulin release is mediated through (ALL INDIA/02)
(a) ATP dependent K+ channels
(b) cAMP
(c) Carrier modulators
(d) Receptor phosphorylation

Ans. (a)
Note
The process by which insulin secretion occurs normally requires glucose metabolism, possibly for formation of ATP. It also depends upon cAMP and requires presence of Ca^{2+} and K^+
Ref: Textbook of physiology by A.K. Jain, 2nd edition, Vol 2, unit IX, Ch. 7, pg 723

Q. 175. Sudden decrease in serum calcium is associated with (ALL INDIA/02)
(a) Increased thyroxine and PTH secretion
(b) Increased phosphate
(c) Increased excitability of muscle and nerve
(d) Cardiac conduction abnormalities

Ans. (c)
Note
Sudden decrease in calcium concentration is usually associated with hypoparathyroidism due to damage to the parathyroid gland during thyroidectomy. There is a decrease in ionized plasma Ca^{2+} level. As calcium exerts a stabilizing effect on the cell membrane of excitable tissues, therefore in hypocalcemia there is increased excitability of muscle and Nerve membrane, leading to tetany characterized by:
- Neuromuscular hyperexcitibility
- Facial irritability
- Carpopedal spasm

Ref: Textbook of physiology by A. K. Jain, 2nd edition, Vol 2, unit IX, Ch. 4, pg 684

Q. 176. Ablation of the 'somatosensory area I' of the cerebral cortex leads to (ALL INDIA/02)
(a) Total loss of pain sensation
(b) Total loss of touch sensation
(c) Loss of tactile localization but not of two point discrimination
(d) Loss of tactile localization and two point discrimination

Ans. (d)
Note
The cortical lesion
Primary sensory area or somatosensory area or S1 is situated in the post central gyrus containing Broadman's area 3, 2,1.
Area 3 neurons respond to light touch while area 1 and 2 neurons respond to pressure and joint movements and receive a few thalamic fibers. The arrangement of thalamic projection is such that the body is represented upside down.
It's removal produces defects in fine touch, position sense and discriminatory power and deficits in sensory processing.
Ref: Textbook of physiology by A.K. Jain, 2nd edition, Vol 2, unit XI, Ch. 5, pg 871
Other lesions of central nerves system with their peculiar nature are as under:

Thalamic lesion
Thalamus acts as great integrating and relay centre where information from all over is received and projected to cerebral cortex. Besides integrating the information it has some degree of ability to perceive exteroceptive sensations especially pain. Therefore lesion of thalamus causes impairment of all types of sensibilities. The control is contralateral.

Brainstem lesion (Lateral Medullary syndrome)
It results in loss of pain and temperature on ipsilateral face and opposite side of body.

Spinal cord lesion
Paraparesis or quadriparesis, with spasticity, hyperreflexia and Babinski sign
Bilateral sensory loss up to a level, bladder bowel and sexual dysfunction.

Q. 177. Non shivering thermogenesis in adults is due to (ALL INDIA/02)
(a) Thyroid hormone
(b) Brown fat between the shoulders
(c) Noradrenaline
(d) Muscle metabolism

Ans. (c)
Note
The non-shivering thermogenesis in adults is due to Noradrenaline as they do not have a certain type of fat tissue called 'Brown fat'. Neonates are endowed with considerable number of 'Brown fat'. When these cells are stimulated by sympathetic nerves; the mitochondria present in these cells produce large amount of heat. This is called non-shivering thermogenesis. In adults sympathetic stimulation releases norepinephrines and epinephrine which acts directly on muscle and liver cell resulting in glycogenolysis and heat production, it is also a non-shivering thermogenesis.

Q. 178. In metabolic acidosis, which of the following changes are seen (ALL INDIA/02)
(a) Increased K^+ excretion
(b) Decreased K^+ excretion
(c) Increased Na^+ excretion
(d) Increased Na^+ reabsorption

Ans. (b)
Note
In metabolic acidosis there is increased H^+ secretion. There is an inverse relation between K^+ and H^+ i.e. when H^+ secretion increases K^+ excretion decreases. Therefore answer should be b.
Ref: Textbook of physiology by A.K. Jain, 2nd edition, Vol 1, unit V, Ch. 9, pg 344

Q. 179. Tropomyosin (ALL INDIA/02)
(a) Helps in the fusion of actin and myosin
(b) Covers myosin and prevents attachments of actin and myosin
(c) Slides over myosin
(d) Causes Ca^{2+} release

Ans. (b)
Note
Tropomyosin- These are long filaments located in groove between 2 chains in the actin. It covers the binding site of actin where myosin head comes in contact with actin i.e. prevents the interaction between actin and myosin filaments.
Ref: Textbook of physiology by A.K. Jain, 2nd edition, Vol 1, unit III, Ch. 6, pg 152,153

Q. 180. TRH stimulation testing is useful in diagnosis of disorders of following hormones (ALL INDIA/02)
(a) Insulin
(b) ACTH
(c) Prolactin
(d) PTH

Ans. (c)

Note
The TRH stimulation results in release of; TSH, Prolactin, Growth Hormone therefore, in reference to above TRH stimulation testing is useful in supporting a diagnosis of disorders of 'Prolactin'.

Also see
High TRH levels stimulate prolactin releasing factor and increase prolactin. It is also considered as a galactogogue, hence we can do TRH stimulation test to diagnose disorders of prolactin hormone release.
Ref: Textbook of physiology by A.K. Jain, 2nd edition, Vol 2, unit IX, Ch. 2, pg 643

Q. 181. During muscular exercise all are seen except
(a) Increase in blood flow to muscles
(b) Stroke volume increases
(c) O_2 dissociation curve shifts to left
(d) O_2 consumption increases

Ans. (c)
Note
Oxygen dissociation curve is a curve relating percentage O_2 saturation of Hb to the pO_2. It has a characteristic sigmoid shape. If at any pO_2 the O_2 content that can be held by blood decreases there is unloading of O_2 from Hb and the curve shifts to right.
During muscular activity the oxygen requirement of muscles increases and it diffuses from Hb to combine with myoglobin. Thus saturation of Hb decreases and the curve shifts to the left.
Ref: Textbook of physiology by A.K. Jain, 2nd edition, Vol 1, unit VI, Ch. 3, pg 432,433

Q. 182. Tidal volume is calculated by (ALL INDIA/01)
(a) Inspiratory capacity minus the inspiratory reserve volume.
(b) Total lung capacity minus the residual volume.
(c) Functional residual capacity minus residual volume.
(d) Vital capacity minus expiratory reserve volume.

Ans. (a)
Note
Tidal volume is the volume of air inspired and expired during a quiet respiration.
Inspiratory reserve volume: It is the maximal volume of air which can be inspired after completing a normal tidal inspiration.
Inspiratory capacity is the maximal volume of air which can be inspired after completing a tidal expiration.
It can be computed as:
IC = TV + IRV
Therefore tidal vol can be calculated TV=IC-IRV
Ref: Textbook of physiology by A.K. Jain, 2nd edition, Vol 1, unit VI, Ch. 2, pg 411, 412

Q. 183. Surfactant production in lungs starts at (ALL INDIA/01)
(a) 28 weeks
(b) 32 weeks
(c) 34 weeks
(d) 36 weeks

Ans. (a)
Note
Surfactant is made by the cells in the airways and consists of phospholipids and protein. It begins to be produced in the fetus at about 24 to 28 weeks of pregnancy. Surfactant is found in amniotic fluid between 28 and 32 weeks. By about 35 week's gestation, most babies have developed adequate amounts of surfactant. Therefore neonates less than 35 weeks are prone to develop respiratory distress syndrome (RDS).

Q. 184. Initiation of nerve impulse occurs at the axon hillock because (ALL INDIA/01)
(a) It has a lower threshold than the rest of the axon
(b) It is unmyelinated
(c) Neurotransmitter release occurs here
(d) None of the above

Ans. (a)

Note
Hillock is the initial segment of axon. And it has a lower threshold than the rest of axon.

Q. 185. Albumin contributes the maximum to oncotic pressure because it has (ALL INDIA/01)
    (a)   High molecular weight, low concentration
    (b)   Low molecular weight, low concentration
    (c)   High molecular weight, high concentration
    (d)   Low molecular weight, high concentration

Ans. (d)

Note
The colloidal osmotic pressure due to plasma colloids is called as oncotic pressure.
Osmotic pressure across the capillary wall can be exerted both by:
a.   crystalloids- urea, Na^+, glucose
b.   colloids- plasma proteins
However capillary wall is permeable to crystalloids therefore they hardly contribute to the capillary osmotic pressure.
COP is inversely proportional to the molecular size and shape and is directly related to concentration of molecules.
Therefore 80% of COP is due to albumin which has the least molecular weight and maximum concentration.
Ref: Textbook of physiology by A.K. Jain, 2nd edition, Vol 1, unit I ,II, Ch. 2, pg 11, 47

Q. 186. After 5 days of fasting a man undergoes oral GTT, true is all except (ALL INDIA/01)
    (a)   GH levels are increased
    (b)   Increased glucose tolerance
    (c)   Decreased insulin levels
    (d)   Glucagon levels are increased

Ans. (b)

Note
After 5 days of fasting a man undergoes oral GTT, true is all except – (b) Increased glucose tolerance.

Q. 187. Metalloproteins help in jaundice by the following mechanism (ALL INDIA/01)
    (a)   Increased glucoronyl transferase activity
    (b)   Inhibit heme oxygenase
    (c)   Decrease RBC lysis
    (d)   Increase Y and Z receptors

Ans. (b)

Note
Metalloproteins help in jaundice by the mechanism; (b) Inhibit heme oxygenase.

Q. 188. Which protein prevents contraction by covering binding sites on actin and myosin (ALL INDIA/01)
    (a)   Troponin
    (b)   Calmodulin
    (c)   Thymosin
    (d)   Tropomyosin

Ans. (d)

Note
Tropomyosin are long filaments located in groove between 2 chains in the actin. It covers the binding site of actin where myosin head comes in contact with actin i.e. prevents the interaction between actin and myosin filaments.
Ref: Textbook of physiology by A.K. Jain, 2nd edition, Vol 1, unit III, Ch. 6, pg 152,153

Q. 189. Which of the following is not correct regarding capillaries (ALL INDIA/01)
(a) Greatest cross sectional area
(b) Contain 25% of blood
(c) Contains less blood than veins
(d) Have single layer of cells bounding the lumen

Ans. (b)

Note
All of above are correct about capillaries except; that it contains 25% of blood.
At a time only 5% of circulating blood is in the capillaries which allow continous exchange of oxygen, carbon dioxide, nutrients and waste products between the blood and interstitial fluid.
Ref: Textbook of physiology by A.K. Jain, 2nd edition, Vol 1, unit V, Ch. 10, pg 351

Q. 190. A 0.5 liter blood loss in 30 minutes will lead to (ALL INDIA/01)
(a) Increase in HR, decrease in BP
(b) Slight increase in HR, normal BP
(c) Decrease in HR and BP
(d) Prominent increase in HR

Ans. (b)

Note
When a normal subject with 5 liters of blood, losses 500 ml it amounts to be 20% of his blood volume. Normally loss of 20% of blood is well tolerated and there may be slight rise in heart rate but BP will be maintained to a normal limits. However, most of the people who donate blood, after donation of blood do not find any difficulty with blood pressure and pulse rate.

Q. 191. Single most important factor in control of automatic contractility of heart is (ALL INDIA/01)
(a) Myocardial wall thickness
(b) Right atrial volume
(c) SA node pacemaker potential
(d) Sympathetic stimulation

Ans. (d)

Note
The single most important factor in control of autonomic contractility of heart is sympathetic stimulation. Sympathetic supply to the heart is by sympathetic nerve cells located in the interomedial horn of the spinal horn of the spinal cord extending from T1 to T5 spinal segments. Fibers pass to the cardiac ganglia, from here post-ganglionic fibers pass to supply:
 -Nodal Tissues: SAN and AVN
 -Muscles of atria and ventricles
Sympathetic stimulation to the heart causes:
 -Increased H.R. – chronotropic action
 -Increased speed and force of contraction of myocardium- ionotropic action
 -Increased conductivity in conduction tissues- dromotropic action
 -Increased excitability of heart- bathmotropic action
Ref: Textbook of physiology by A.K. Jain, 2nd edition, Vol 1, unit V, Ch. 6, pg 319, 320

Q. 192. Which of the following is not mediated through negative feedback mechanism (ALL INDIA/01)
(a) TSH release
(b) GH formation
(c) Thrombin formation
(d) ACTH release

Ans. (c)

Note
The negative feedback mechanism includes following:
- Aldosterone K⁺ secretion
- Cortisol secretion
- Glucose regulation
- GH secretion
- BP regulation

Therefore, (c) thrombin formation is not a part of negative feedback mechanism.

Q. 193. Force generating proteins are (ALL INDIA/01)
(a) Myosin and myoglobin
(b) Dynein and kinesin
(c) Calmodulin and G protein
(d) Troponin

Ans. (b)

Note
Microtubles guide transport of proteins and vesicular material e.g., in nerves and Dyenin and Kinesin provide the force behind such movements.

Q. 194. Which is true about measurement of BP with sphygmomanometer versus intra-arterial pressure measurements (ALL INDIA/01)
(a) Less than intravascular pressure
(b) More than intravascular pressure
(c) Equal to intravascular pressure
(d) Depends upon blood flow

Ans. (b)

Note
The measurement of BP through sphygmomanometer is more than interavascular pressure.

Q. 195. Secondary hyperparathyroidism due to vitamin D deficiency shows (ALL INDIA/01)
(a) Hypocalcemia
(b) Hypercalcemia
(c) Hypophosphatemia
(d) Hyperphosphatemia

Ans. (c)

Note
The secondary hyperparathyroidism due to vitamin D deficiency results from decreased serum calcium because of decreased amount of active vitamin D. It prompts for release of hyperparathyroid hormone – which shows its activities to increase serum Ca^{++}, which takes place at the cost of loss of phosphate from the body – hypophosphatemia.

Also see
Increase in parathyroid hormone secretion leads to increase in calcium and phosphate absorption from GIT and decreased phosphate absorption from PCT and increased excretion in DT. This leads to decreased S. Phosphate.
Ref: Textbook of physiology by A.K. Jain, 2ⁿᵈ edition, Vol 2, unit IX, Ch. 4, pg 683

Q. 196. Maximum absorption of water takes place in (ALL INDIA/01)
(a) Proximal convoluted tubule
(b) Distal convoluted tubule
(c) Collecting duct
(d) Loop of Henle

Ans. (a)

Note
-In PCT passive reabsorption of 75-80% of water takes place along the osmotic gradient set by active transport of solutes.
-Loop of Henle: the descending limb of loop of Henle is permeable to water but ascending limb is impermeable. 5-10% of filtered water is removed so approximately 15% of filtered water enters DT.
-DCT- early part of DCT is relatively impermeable to water. Approximately 5-8% of the filtered water is removed passively.
-In terminal DCT and CT water is reabsorbed according to ADH secretion. Under the influence of ADH another 10-12% water is reabsorbed.
Ref: Textbook of physiology by A. K. Jain, 2nd edition, Vol 2, unit VII, Ch. 2, pg 517, 518

Q. 197. Consider the following (UPSC-06)
1. Reduced haemoglobin
2. Reduced serum ferritin
3. Elevated serum iron
4. Markedly reduced plasma LDH

Which of those given above is/are the diagnostic features of megaloblastic anaemia?
(a) 3 Only
(b) 1, 2 and 4 only
(c) 1 and 3 only
(d) 1, 2, 3 and 4

Ans. (c)
Note
IF with EF forms haematinic principle required for maturation of RBCs. Megaloblastic anaemia occurs due to absence of any of them. Blood changes in megaloblastic anemia are:
-Decreased RBC count to <1 million/mm^3
-Hb <12 mg%
-RBC diameter increases to 8.2 μm
-MCV increases to 95-160 μm^3 (n- 78-94 μm^3)
-MCH increases to 50pg
-MCHC is usually normal
♦ Peripheral smear shows nucleated RBCs with marked anisopoikilocytosis
♦ Reticulocyte count >5%
♦ Decreased life span of RBCs
♦ Increased S. Fe because of underutilization
♦ S. bilirubin increased to >1mg%
Ref: Textbook of physiology by A. K. Jain, 2nd edition, Vol 1, unit II, Ch. 4, pg 66,67

Q. 198. Match List I with List II and select the correct answer using the code given below the lists (UPSC-06)

List- I (Hemoglobin)	List-II (Amount of Blood)
A. Hb. in Male	1. 14 -18 gm%
B. Hb. in Female	2. 23 gm%
C. Hb. in newborn	3. 12.5 gm%
D. Hb. at the end of one year	4. 12 – 14 gm%

Code

	A	B	C	D
(a)	1	2	4	3
(b)	1	4	2	3
(c)	3	2	4	1
(d)	3	4	2	1

Ans. (b)

Note
Normal values of Hb
- At birth: 23g%
- At end of 3 months: 10.5mg%
- At 3 months to 1 year: 12.5mg%
- Adults: M: 14-18 g% & F: 12 – 15mg%

Ref: Textbook of physiology by A. K. Jain, 2nd edition, Vol 2, unit II, Ch. 3, pg 52

Q. 199. Posterior pituitary secrets which of the following hormones? (UPSC-06)
    (a)   ADH and Oxytocin
    (b)   ACTH and LH
    (c)   FSH and LH
    (d)   TSH

Ans. (a)

Note
Anterior pituitary secretes:
- TSH
- ACTH
- GH
- FSH
- LH
- LTH or prolactin
- ß- lipoproteins

Posterior pituitary secretes:
- Vasopressin (ADH) and Oxytocin

Intermediate lobe of pituitary secretes:
- Alpha and beta melanocyte stimulating hormone

Ref: Textbook of physiology by A. K. Jain, 2nd edition, Vol 2, unit IX, Ch. 2, pg 633

Bibliography

Books
Textbook of physiology by A. K. Jain, 2nd edition

Websites
www.similima.com
www.fleshandbones.com

Chapter 5
HOMEOPATHIC PHARMACY

Q. 1. Which one of the following drugs is prepared form "Indian Turnip"? (UPSC-02)
    (a) Aurum metallicum
    (b) Arum triphyllum
    (c) Artemisia vulgaris
    (d) Acalypha indica

Ans. (b)

Note
Arum triphyllum (Arum-t). Common name-Indian turnip.
Natural order- Araceae. Preparation - Tincture of fresh tuber or corn.
(Ref :Clarke)

Q. 2. Match the list –I (Drugs) with the list-II (part used for preparation of medicine) and select the correct answer using the codes given below the list (UPSC-02)

List I (DRUG)	List II (PARTS USED)
A. Arnica montana	1. Fresh flowering tops and leaves
B. Bryonia alba	2. The bark
C. Cinchona officinalis	3. Fresh root before flowering
D. Calendula officinalis	4. Entire fresh plant including root

Code

A	A	B	C	D
	1	3	2	4
B	A	B	C	D
	4	2	3	1
C	A	B	C	D
	1	2	3	4
D	A	B	C	D
	4	3	2	1

Ans. (d)

Note
The correct order:

List I (DRUG)	List II (PARTS USED)
A. Arnica montana	4. Entire fresh plant including root
B. Bryonia alba	3. Fresh root before flowering
C. Cinchona officinalis	2. The bark
D. Calendula officinalis	1. Fresh flowering tops and leaves

Ref: Text book of Homeopathic pharmacy 2nd Edition by DD Banerjee Pg- 606

Q. 3. The drugs prepared from healthy tissues or organs or their secretions are called (UPSC-02)
   (a)   Nosodes
   (b)   Imponderabilia
   (c)   Sarcodes
   (d)   Hormones

Ans. (c)

Note

In Greek the term 'sarcode' means fleshy. Sarcodes imply protoplasm of animals as distinguished from vegetable protoplasm. They are obtained from healthy endocrine or ductless gland.
Ref: Text book of Homeopathic pharmacy 2nd edition by DD Banerjee Pg 38, Ch-1.3

Q. 4. Which drug contains conine as an active alkaloid? (UPSC-02)
   (a)   Cinchona officinalis
   (b)   Conium maculatum
   (c)   Cannabis indica
   (d)   Cocculus indicus

Ans. (b)

Note

Conium maculatum contains conine as an active alkaloid.
Ref: Text Book of Homeopathic Pharmacy by Mandal & Mandal- Chapter 23Q.

Q. 5. Which one among the following contains strychnine as an active constituent? (UPSC-02)
   (a)   Stramonium
   (b)   Stannum metallicum
   (c)   Ignatia amara
   (d)   Nux vomica

Ans. (d)

Note

Nux vomica contains strychnine as an active constituent.

Ref: Text Book of Homeopathic Pharmacy by Mandal & Mandal-Chapter- 23Q.

Q. 6. In homeopathy, a process which brings about a quantitative reduction in the drug substance but a qualitative increase in its medicinal or therapeutic property is known as (UPSC-04)
   (a)   Potentisation
   (b)   Succession
   (c)   Ionization
   (d)   Dilution

Ans. (a)

Note

Potentisation is a process used exclusively in homeopathy which brings about a quantitative reduction in the drug substance but a qualitative increase in its medicinal or therapeutic property.
Ref: Text Book of Homeopathic Pharmacy by Mandal & Mandal, Chapter- 12

Q. 7. Consider the following statements (UPSC-04)
1. 10 minims of tincture and 90 minims of alcohol give 1st centesimal potency.
2. 6 minims of tincture and 99minims of dilute alcohol, the drug power of tincture being 1/6 give 1st centesimal potency.
3. Preparation of mother tincture consists in three steps viz; Estimation of plant moisture content, maceration and percolation.
4. Drugs like Bufo rana, Murex, Apis, Phytolacca, Helleborous and Naja, all belong to animal kingdom.

MCQ's in Homeopathic Pharmacy 315

Which of the statement /s given above is / are correct? (UPSC-02)
- (a) (1) and (3)
- (b) (3) only
- (c) (2) and (4)
- (d) (4) only

Ans. (a)

Note

The correct choice is (a) –(1) and (3):
1. **Correct** - 10 minims of tincture and 90 minims of alcohol give 1st centesimal potency – this is the preparation of medicine according to the -Class IV- this class includes dry plants, herbs, animal substances – dried or fresh.
2. **Incorrect** – As here the preparation is according to the –Class III - this class includes those plants which are less juicy. Preparation - Centesimal scale – 6 minims of mother tincture and 94 minims of dilute alcohol and ten downwards strokes of equal strength give 1st Centesimal potency having drug power of 1/6.
3. **Correct** - Preparation of mother tincture consists of three steps i.e. Estimation of plant moisture content, maceration and percolation.
4. **Incorrect**- Drugs like Bufo rana, Murex, Apis, and Naja, all belong to animal kingdom whereas Helleborous and Phytolacca belong to plant kingdom.

Ref: Text Book of Homeopathic Pharmacy by Mandal & Mandal, Chapter 10

Q. 8. Match List –I (Medicine) with List –II (Source of Medicine) and select the correct answer using the codes give below the lists (UPSC-04)

List –I (Medicine)	List –II (Source of Medicine)
A. Aranea diadema	1. Orange Spider
B. Mygale lasiodora	2. Spanish Spider
C. Tarentula hispanica	3. Papal Cross Spider
D. Theridion	4. Black Cuban Spider

Code

	A	B	C	D
A	3	2	4	1
B	1	4	2	3
C	3	4	2	1
D	1	2	4	3

Ans. (c)

Note

The correct answer is as under:

List –I (Medicine)	List –II (Source of Medicine)
A. Aranea diadema	3. Papal Cross Spider
B. Mygale lasiodora	4. Black Cuban Spider
C. Tarentula hispanica	2. Spanish Spider
D. Theridion	1. Orange Spider

Q. 9. Poison hemlock is the common name of (UPSC-04)
    (a) Cicuta virosa
    (b) Conium maculatum
    (c) Rhus toxicodendron
    (d) Cimicifuga

Ans. (b)
Note
Poison hemlock is the common name of Conium maculatum.
Ref: Allen's Key Notes

Q. 10. Ipecacuanha roots have (UPSC-04)
    (a) Transverse constriction or fissures externally
    (b) Smooth external surface
    (c) Longitudinal ridges
    (d) Spiral ridges on surface

Ans. (a)
Note
Ipecacuanha – Roots are torturous, seldom more than 15 cm long, 06 materia medica thick, from dark brick red to very dark brown closely annulated external ridges rounded and completely encircling the root.

Ref: Text Book of Homeopathic Pharmacy by Mandal & Mandal Chapter -27

Q. 11. Berberin is found in (KPSC/Lect/Pharm-04)
    (a) Berberis vulgaris
    (b) Argemone mexicana
    (c) Both the above
    (d) None of the above

Ans. (a)
Note
Berberis vulgaris contains the alkaloid– Berberine
Ref: Text Book of Homeopathic Pharmacy By Mandal & Mandal- Chapter -2

Q. 12. In LM potency preparation the size of globules used is (KPSC/Lect/Pharm-04)
    (a) 5 - Size
    (b) 20-Size
    (c) 30-Size
    (d) 40-Size

Ans. Use your discretion
Note
5- Size.
Ref: Text Book of Homeopathic Pharmacy by Mandal & Mandal- Chapter-10
Also see
But if only one such globule be taken, of which 100 weigh one grain, and dynamize it with 100 drops of alcohol, the proportion of 1 to 50,000 and even greater will be had, for 500 such globules can hardly absorb one drop, for their saturation.
Ref: Augmented Textbook of Homeopathic Pharmacy By D. D. Banerjee, 2nd Ed, Pg-565
Also see at § 270 Organon 6th Edition

Q. 13. Which species of Aloe is used in homeopathy? (KPSC/Lect/Pharm-04)
    (a) Aloe zizibar
    (b) Aloe coraco
    (c) Aloe socotrina
    (d) Aloe vera

Ans. (c)

Note
Species of Aloe used in homeopathy is 'Aloe socotrina', common name- aloes / ghritakumari, family-Liliaceae, part used- inspissated juice of the leaves.
Ref: Augmented Textbook of Homeopathic Pharmacy 2nd Edition by. Dr. D. D. Banerjee,–Page-598,605

Q. 14. The abbreviation for "Use if necessary" is (KPSC/Lect/Pharm-04)
    (a)   AC
    (b)   SOS
    (c)   CM
    (d)   HSS
Ans. (b)

Note
S.O.S. = Si opus sit = If necessary

Q. 15. The method used for separating volatile solid from non-volatile solid is called (KPSC/Lect/Pharm-04)
    (a)   Evaporation
    (b)   Sublimation
    (c)   Crystallization
    (d)   Decantation
Ans. (b)

Note
Sublimation
It is a process of converting a solid substance directly into vapor on heating without being converted to the liquid state and reconversion of the vapor to the solid state again through condensation.
Application
Sublimation is useful for purification of some solids like iodine, camphor etc. This process helps in separation of such solids from other common (non-volatile) solids like sand or charcoal.
Ref: Text Book of Homeopathic Pharmacy by Mandal & Mandal.Ch –6

Q. 16. Spermaceti physical nature is (KPSC/Lect/Pharm-04)
    (a)   Solid
    (b)   Liquid
    (c)   Semisolid
    (d)   Vapours
Ans. (c)

Note
Spermaceti (USP)
Synonyms - Cetaceum, Sp Esperma de Ballena
Source: It is a waxy substance obtained from the head of sperm whale Physeter macrocephalus Linn. (Family: Physeteridae)
Ref: Text Book of Homeopathic Pharmacy by Mandal & Mandal, Ch -8

Q. 17. Centesimal potency is discussed in (KPSC/Lect/Pharm-04)
    (a)   Vth Edition of Organon
    (b)   VIth Edition of Organon
    (c)   Materia medica pura
    (d)   Chronic diseases
Ans. (a)

Note
Centesimal scale
This scale was introduced by the founder of homeopathy Dr Hahnemann in Aphorism 270, 5th Edition of Organon of Medicine in1833
Ref: Text Book of Homeopathic Pharmacy By Mandal & Mandal, Ch -9

Q. 18. Metallic hard and stony hard drugs are triturated for 1x or 1c, for (KPSC/Lect/Pharm-04)
    (a)   One hour
    (b)   Two hours
    (c)   Three hours
    (d)   Four hours
Ans. (a)

Note
Master Hahnemann classified the substances taken for trituration into three categories as in Class –VII (includes dry insoluble medicinal substances like Calc.), Class- VIII (includes liquid insoluble substances like venoms) and Class IX (It includes fresh vegetables and animal substances like Agar.).
In Class VII; trituration process consists of three stages of 20 minutes each totaling 1 hour for preparing1x and 1c.
Ref: Text Book of Homeopathic Pharmacy by Mandal & Mandal, Ch –12

Q. 19. Class V of old class deals with (KPSC/Lect/Pharm-04)
    (a)   Mother tinctures
    (b)   Alcoholic solutions
    (c)   Aqueous solutions
    (d)   Mother solutions
Ans. (c)

Note
Old Method – Class V - Aqueous solution – Includes (Class –V (A) and Class V (B) Page No: 126
Ref: Text Book of Homeopathic Pharmacy by Mandal & Mandal, Ch-10.

Q. 20. Mullein oil is (KPSC/Lect/Pharm-04)
    (a)   An oil extract
    (b)   Alcoholic extract
    (c)   Aqueous extract
    (d)   Glycerin extract
Ans. Use your discretion

Note
Glycerine is used for preparation of mullein oil.
Ref: Text Book of Homeopathic Pharmacy by Mandal & Mandal, Pg-107 Ch-10
The alcoholic tincture is prepared from the fresh plant, chopped and pounded to a pulp.
Ref: Hering's Guiding Symptoms
Tincture of fresh plant at the commencement of flowering. ("Mullein Oil" is prepared by placing the crushed yellow blossoms in a bottle, which is corked and allowed to stand in the sun (Cushing), or by steeping the blossoms in oil and keeping in a warm place till the oil has absorbed them).
Cushing prepared from the flowers,"oil" (1) by putting the blossoms in a bottle and laying the bottle in the sun, and later (2) by expression.
Ref: Clarke's materia medica
External application – Oil Mullein; Source: The flower extract of Verbascum thapsus of family Scrophulariaceae.
Method of preparation: though the preparation is known as Mullein oil, it contains no oil excepting the essential oil present in the flower itself Solvents used are: Glycerine, alcohol and other inert substances 1 part of the flower yields to10 parts of Mullein essence.
Ref: Text Book of Homeopathic Pharmacy by Mandal & Mandal, Pg-117 Ch-13.

Note
It appears that both the options (b) and (d) are valid. Use your discretion

Q. 21. Inspissated Juice is used from (KPSC/Lect/Pharm-04)
    (a)   Arnica
    (b)   Grindelia
    (c)   Aloe
    (d)   Guaicum
Ans. (c)

Note
Extractions:
  -Aloe socotrina: It is extracted from inspissated juice of leaves.
  -Guaiacum officinale: It is extracted from the resins.
Ref: Text Book of Homeopathic Pharmacy by Mandal & Mandal, Ch-2

Q. 22. Binding material used for the tabloid preparation is (KPSC/Lect/Pharm-04)
  (a) Starch
  (b) Sugar
  (c) Glycerin
  (d) Calcium powder

Ans. (b)
Note
The tablets are unit forms of solid medicinal substances with or without suitable diluents prepared by compressing or moulding.
Source: These are prepared from pure refined sugar of milk.
Ref: Text Book of Homeopathic Pharmacy, Mandal and Mandal, Pg-109, Ch-8.

Q. 23. Globules are manufactured in a machine called (KPSC/Lect/Pharm-04)
  (a) Rotary
  (b) Evaporator
  (c) Coating pan
  (d) Granulator

Ans. (c)
Note
Globules or pilules are made by a mechanically rotating stainless steel globule making pan or pill-tube, containing granulated cane sugar, which has been properly moistened with purified water or Syrup simplex and then coated with a thin layer of super-finely crushed cane sugar (of not less than 300 mesh).
Ref: Augmented Textbook of Homeopathic Pharmacy, 2nd Edn by D. D. Banerjee, Pg-76, Ch 2.2

Also see
Globules preparations from cane sugar
Granulated cane sugar is placed in a rotating stainless steel globule making pan or pill tube and rolled until the granules are formed to spherical shape.
Ref: Textbook of Homeopathic Pharmacy, Mandal and Mandal Pg-76, Ch-8.

Q. 24. 1 grain powder is equal to (KPSC/Lect/Pharm-04)
  (a) 65 mg
  (b) 80 mg
  (c) 90 mg
  (d) 100 mg

Ans. (a)
Note
1 Grain = 0.0648gm. = 65 milligrams (approx.).
(Ref: Text Book of Homeopathic Pharmacy 2nd Edition by D.D. Banerjee, Chapter-4.2, Pg-237)
Weights and Measures- Table of Approximate equivalences adopted in stating doses: 1 Grain = 60 milligrams.
Text Book of Homeopathic Pharmacy by Mandal & Mandal- Chapter-17

Also See
There is difference in stating doses in both the above references. Use your discretion. However author's suggestion for answer is (a).

Q. 25. 1 ml of alcohol can give (KPSC/Lect/Pharm-04)
  (a) 46 drops
  (b) 17 drops
  (c) 20 drops
  (d) 35 drops

Ans. (b)

Note
Relations of metric and imperial system
1 millilitre (ml.) = 16.984 minims

Domestic/ household measure (approximate)	English Equivalents	Metric Equivalents
1 Drop	= 1 minim	=0.6 ml

Ref: Text Book of Homeopathic Pharmacy 2nd Edition by D.D. Banerjee - Chapter-4.2. Pg-237, 238.

Q. 26. Homeopathic drugs prepared by using other systems drug are called (KPSC/Lect/Pharm-04)
    (a)   Isopathic drugs
    (b)   Tautopathic drugs
    (c)   Homeopathic drugs
    (d)   Allopathic drugs
Ans. (b)

Note
Tautopathy
It is the system of medical therapeutics where a patient suffering from the adverse effects of a drug (usually allopathic) is given the same drugs in the potentized form to counteract / neutralize / antidote the adverse drug effects.

Though these drugs are prepared form drugs commonly used in the allopathic system of medicine yet after potentisation they are used according to the homeopathic principles.

Q. 27. Sepia is prepared by using the method of (KPSC/Lect/Pharm-04)
    (a)   Mother tincture
    (b)   Alcoholic solution
    (c)   Aqueous solution
    (d)   Trituration
Ans. (d)

Note
Sepia is prepared from the dried inky juice found in a bag like structure in the abdomen of the cuttle fish. This ink is insoluble in alcohol and water. According to old method of preparation of drug substances Class VII - which includes dry medicinal substances which in their crude state are neither soluble in purified water nor in alcohol; Sepia is prepared by triturating 1 part by weight of dried ink to 99 parts (in centesimal scale) or 9 parts (in decimal scale) by weight of sugar of milk to give 1st trituration. The following triturations are prepared by adding one part by weight of the preceding trituration to 99 or 9 parts of sugar of milk. The 4c liquid potency in centesimal scale is prepared from 3rd trituration and 8x liquid potency in decimal scale is prepared from 6x trituration.

Ref: Augmented Textbook of Homeopathic Pharmacy, 2nd Edn by D. D. Banerjee, Pg-485 Ch- 9.1, Pg-265 Ch- 5.2

Q. 28. The latest Bi-nominal system of nomenclature is introduced by (KPSC/Lect/Pharm-04)
    (a)   Linneus
    (b)   Bentham and Hooker
    (c)   TakhatJ'an
    (d)   Gibs
Ans. (b)

Note
The latest Bi-nominal system of nomenclature is introduced by Bentham and Hooker.

Q. 29. The earliest homeopathic pharmaceutical industry established in Philadelphia USA was: (KPSC/Lect/Pharm-04)
    (a)   Boericke & Tafel
    (b)   Boiron
    (c)   Madus
    (d)   Willmar Schwabe

Ans. (a)
Note
The earliest homeopathic pharmaceutical industry established in Philadelphia USA was Boericke & Tafel

Q. 30. Manufacture of Homeo drugs dealt in sub rule (KPSC/Lect/Pharm-04)
    (a)   85
    (b)   92
    (c)   67
    (d)   71

Ans. (a)
Note
Manufacture for sale of homeopathic medicines is dealt in sub rule 85:
85-A: Manufacture of more than one set of premises.
85-B: Application for license to manufacture homeopathic medicines.
85-C: Application to manufacture 'new homeopathic medicines'.
85-D: Form of license to manufacture homeopathic medicines.
85-E: Conditions for the grant or renewal of a license in Form –C.
85-F: Duration of license.
85-G: Certificate of renewal.
85-H: Conditions of license.
85-I: Cancellation and suspension of license.
Ref: Augmented Textbook of Homeopathic Pharmacy, 2nd Edn by D. D. Banerjee, Pg-542 Ch.10.1

Q. 31. Which type of solutions throw out crystals (KPSC/Lect/Pharm-04)
    (a)   Perfect solutions
    (b)   Unsaturated solutions
    (c)   Over saturated solutions
    (d)   Aqueous solutions

Ans. (c)
Note
Over saturated solutions throw out crystals.

Q. 32. Loganiaceae family members are (KPSC/Lect/Pharm-04)
    (a)   Nux vomica
    (b)   Ignatia amara
    (c)   Both of the above
    (d)   None of the above

Ans. (c)
Note
Nux vomica: Poison nut – Family: Loganiaceae
Ignatia amara: St Ignatius bean – Family: Loganiaceae
Ref: Augmented Textbook of Homeopathic Pharmacy, 2nd Edn by D. D. Banerjee, Pg-608,609 Ch-12.4**Q.**

Q. 33. Cephalandra and Bryonia belongs to (KPSC/Lect/Pharm-04)
    (a)   Compositae
    (b)   Solanaceae
    (c)   Cucurbitaceae
    (d)   Asteraceae

Ans. (c)

Note
Cephalandra belongs to the family Cucurbitaceae Ref: Boericke's materia medica
Bryonia belongs to the family Cucurbitaceae Ref: Allen's Key Notes

Q. 34. In Anacardium occidentale the part used is (KPSC/Lect/Pharm/2004)
    (a)   Seeds
    (b)   Kernel
    (c)   Fruit
    (d)   Juice of Epicarp

Ans. (d)

Note
Anacardium occidentale (Anac-oc).
Cashew nut. (West Indies.) Natural order: Anacardiaceae. Tincture of the black juice between outer and inner shell. (This nut is kidney shaped, that of Anacardium orientale is heart-shaped.)
Ref: Clarke's materia medica

Q. 35. In which year the first Homeopathic Pharmacopoeia was published? (KPSC/Lect/Pharm-04)
    (a)   1790
    (b)   1786
    (c)   1805
    (d)   1825

Ans. (d)

Note
In 1825 the first Homeopathic Pharmacopoeia "Dispensatorium Homeopathicum" was published by Dr. Carl W. Caspari of Leipzig Germany.
Ref: Text Book of Homeopathic Pharmacy 2nd Edition by D.D. Banerjee; Ch-1.1, Pg 6.

Q. 36. A substance which can cure a disease is called (KPSC/Lect/Pharm-04)
    (a)   Drug
    (b)   Medicine
    (c)   Remedy
    (d)   All the three

Ans. (b)

Note
Drug
A substance which alters the function or nutrition of a part or parts of the body. It has the capacity to effect a change in the humans or animals in health or disease.

Medicine
When a drug has been proved on healthy human beings of different ages and of both sexes and their subjective and objective symptoms have been thoroughly known it is called a medicine. It is prepared as per homeopathic pharmaceutical technique, as is administered to a patient as per law of 'similars'.

Remedy
If a medicine is administered to a patient according to the symptom similarity to perform a cure it is called remedy: According to aphorism 3 of Organon of Medicine by Hahnemann. "An indicated medicine is remedy".
Ref: Text Book of Homeopathic Pharmacy 2nd Edition by D.D. Banerjee

Q. 37. A mother tincture is (KPSC/Lect/Pharm-04)
    (a)   An alcoholic solution
    (b)   Alcoholic extract
    (c)   Dilution of the drug
    (d)   Aquo alcoholic extract

Ans. (d)

Note
Glossary
Mother tincture: The strongest liquid preparation used in homeopathy and is made by maceration of the drug or portion of it in alcohol or water.
In acids it means the 1st decimal dilution, i.e., one part of the acid to 9 parts of distilled water.
Ref: Text Book of Homeopathic Pharmacy 2nd Edition by D.D. Banerjee. Pg-664.

Q. 38. Glonoine is the drug prepared from (KPSC/Lect/Pharm-04)
(a) Glycerin trichloride
(b) Nitroglycerin
(c) Triglycerides
(d) Benzene

Ans. (b)
Note
Glonoine is Nitro-glycerine, $C_3H_5(NO_2)O_3$
Ref: Allen's Key Note.

Q. 39. Chemical formula of camphor is (KPSC/Lect/Pharm-04)
(a) $C_{10}H_{140}$
(b) $C_{10}H_{16}O$
(c) $C_{10}H_{10}N_{4}O$
(d) $C_3H_5N_3O_9$

Ans. (b)
Note
Camphor. $C_{10}H_{16}O$. Natural order: Lauracae. A gum obtained from Laurus camphora. Solution in rectified spirit.
Ref; Clarke's materia medica.

Q. 40. Graminaceae members are (KPSC/Lect/Pharm-04)
(a) Avena sativa
(b) Cynodon dactylon
(c) Both the two
(d) None of the above

Ans. (c)
Note
Avena sativa (Aven). Common name: Oat. N. O. Gramineae. Tincture of fresh plant in flower.
Ref: Clarke's materia medica
Cynodon dactylon. Common name: Durba. N.O. Gramineae.
Ref: Boericke's materia medica.

Q. 41. Ficus religiosa belongs to (KPSC/Lect/Pharm-04)
(a) Meliaceae
(b) Moraceae
(c) Urticaceae
(d) Myrtaceae

Ans. (b)
Note
Ficus religiosa (Fic-r.). Common Name: Pipal, Ashwath, Natural Order: Moraceae. Tincture made from tender leaves.
Ref: Text Book of Homeopathic Pharmacy 2nd Edition by D.D. Banerjee –Pg-608.

Q. 42. Cinnabaris is a (KPSC/Lect/Pharm-04)
(a) Zinc compound
(b) Lead compound
(c) Copper compound
(d) Mercuric compound

Ans. (d)

Note
Cinnabaris is a mercurial compound – Mercuric sulphide.
Ref: Boericke's materia medica

Also see
The common name of Cinnabaris is Mercurius sulphuratus ruber.
Ref: Clarke's materia medica

Q. 43. % of the dispensing alcohol is (KPSC/Lect/Pharm-04)
  (a) 95%
  (b) 88%
  (c) 75%
  (d) 91%

Ans. (b)

Note
Dispensing alcohol contains 88% by volume or 83.1% by weight of ethyl alcohol and 12% by volume of purified water.
Ref: Text Book of Homeopathic Pharmacy by Mandal & Mandal- Chapter – 8 –Vehicles –Pg-102

Q. 44. 60° O.P. alcohol % is (KPSC/Lect/Pharm-04)
  (a) 94.5 %
  (b) 91.4%
  (c) 60%
  (d) 57%t

Ans. (b)

Note
(60° OP) is rectified spirit it contains 91.29% by volume of ethyl alcohol.
Ref: Text Book of Homeopathic Pharmacy By Mandal & Mandal –Chapter – 8-Vehicles

Q. 45. Arbor vitae is the common name for (KPSC/Lect/Pharm-04)
  (a) Abrotanum
  (b) Arbus precatorius
  (c) Thalaspi bursa pastoris
  (d) Thuja

Ans. (d)

Note
Abrotanum = Southern wood
Arbrus prectorius = Jequirity = Crab's eye vine
Thalaspi bursa pastoris = Shepherd's purse
Thuja = Arbor vitae

Ref: Text Book of Homeopathic Pharmacy By Mandal & Mandal – Chapter -31 – List of drugs with their common name, family, distribution, and parts Used Pg-306

Q. 46. Lachesis male snake is (KPSC/Lect/Pharm-04)
  (a) Larger than the female
  (b) Equal is size
  (c) Smaller than the female
  (d) All possible

Ans. (c)

Note
Lacheis male snake is smaller than the female snake.

Q. 47. Morbid products with which drugs are prepared are called (KPSC/Lect/Pharm-04)
(a) Sarcodes
(b) Nosodes
(c) Medicines
(d) Remedies

Ans. (b)

Note
The homeopathic preparation from pure microbial culture obtained from diseased tissues and clinical material (Discharges, secretions)
Ref: HPI Volume IV. Text Book of Homeopathic Pharmacy By Mandal & Mandal – Chapter -2– Sources of Homoeoapthic drugs.

Nosodes:
The term '*nosode*' is derived from two Greek words, '*noses*' means disease, and '*cidos*' means appearance. The treatment of disease by means of its causal agent or a product of the same disease is called nosodes.
Ref: Text Book of Homeopathic Pharmacy 2nd Edition by D.D. Banerjee. Pg-40

Q. 48. Posology is the doctrine of (KPSC/Lect/Pharm-04)
(a) Medicine
(b) Potency
(c) Dosage
(d) None

Ans. (c)

Note
Posology means the doctrine of doses of medicine.
Ref: Text Book of Homeopathic Pharmacy By Mandal & Mandal – Chapter -16 – Posology and Homeopathic Posology

Also See
The term, posology originates from the Greek terms '*posos*' and '*logos*'. *Poso*, means how much. To us it is the science or doctrine of doses. Logos means discourses or study.
Ref: Text Book of Homeopathic Pharmacy 2nd Edition by D.D. Banerjee. Chapter – 6.4. Posology and Homeopathy Pg-347.

Q. 49. What are the sources of homeopathic pharmacy? (KPSC/Lect/Pharm-04)
(a) Materia Medica Pura
(b) Organon of Medicine
(c) Chronic diseases
(d) All of the above

Ans. (d)

Note
The sources of homeopathic pharmacy are:
    a. MM Pura parts – 1-6
    b. Organon of medicine – 1st to 6th Editions
    c. Chronic disease – Part I – IV
    d. Lesser writings of Hahnemann:
        i. Essay on New Principle for ascertaining the curative power of drug and some examination of previous principles
        ii. On value of speculative system of medicine, specially in connection with various systems of practice
        iii. On the preparation and dispensing of medicines of Homoeoapthic Physicians

Ref: Text Book of Homeopathic Pharmacy By Mandal & Mandal – Chapter -1 – Pharmacoepia and Pharmacy – Pg-3

Q. 50. When a medicine exhibits affinity for a particular system or organ in the body it is called (KPSC/Lect/Pharm-04)
    (a) Polychrest remedy
    (b) Indicated medicine
    (c) Organopathic drug
    (d) Proved drug

Ans. (c)

Note
Dr William Sharp suggests that the seat of lesion in disease or a seat of action of medicine should be the basis of remedy selection. He called it organopathy.

Q. 51. In which aphorism of Organon VI edition 50 millesimal potencies are discussed? (KPSC/Lect/Pharm-04)
    (a) § 207
    (b) § 250
    (c) § 270
    (d) §170

Ans. (c)

Note
The 50 millessimal scale was introduced by Dr. Hahnemann in the 6th edition *Organon of Medicine* in § 270
Details of the new and latest process of dynamisation of drugs according to Hahnemann; the method is described below in the foot note to this section.
Ref: Organon of Medicine 6th Edition
Potencies are prepared under this method are named by Dr. Pierre Schmidt of Geneva as, 'Fifty Millesimal Potencies' as the material part of the medicine is said to be decreased by 50,000 times for each degree of dynamisation, Hahnemann himself termed this new method as, '*renewed dynamisation*' (§161)
In footnote 1, § 132 he writes, '*New altered but perfected method*' – '*New dynamisation method*' etc. of Organon.
Ref: Text Book of Homeopathic Pharmacy 2nd Edition by D.D. Banerjee. Chapter – 6.1. Study of Different Scales of Preparation. Pg-327.

Q. 52. How many scales use triturations? (KPSC/Lect/Pharm-04)
    (a) One
    (b) Two
    (c) Three
    (d) All

Ans. (b)

Note
Scales of trituration are
    a. Decimal scale
    b. Centesimal scale
Ref: Text Book of Homeopathic Pharmacy By Mandal & Mandal – Chapter – 9 – Different scales of Preparation of Drugs

Also Note
Trituration
It is the mechanical process of potentisation of minerals, inorganic substances, which are insoluble in liquid vehicles.
Substances for Trituration

a. Class VII
The dry medicinal substances insoluble in purified water and alcohol like Arsenic, Alumina, Graphites, Corallium. Here the trituration ratio for centesimal scale is 1:99 (Drug substance; Sugar of milk). The 99 parts of milk sugar is divided into 3 equal parts of 33 parts each. Trituration takes place by the 3 usual stages of 20 minutes each.

b. **Class VIII**
These are liquid insoluble medicinal substances like Petroleum, Naja, Crotalus, and Lachesis. Trituration ratio for centesimal scale is 1:99. Here, 99 parts of milk sugar should not be divided into 3 equal parts as the quantity of milk sugar is very less. Hence, the entire sugar of milk should be taken at a time in the mortar and the drug substance is poured over it so that the oily dry substance doesn't stick to the surface of mortar.

c. **Class IX**
This includes fresh vegetable and animal substances like Psorinum, Medorrhinum, Blatta, and Agaricus. Here the ratio of drug substance to milk sugar is 2:99 as per centesimal scale as there is always some loss of drug substance by evaporation during trituration.

Two scales are used for trituration
a. Decimal
b. Centesimal

Ref: Text Book of Homeopathic Pharmacy 2nd Edition by D.D. Banerjee. Chapter – 6.2. Study of Potentisation Pg-338.

Q. 53. To get 1 X trituration the drug and sugar of milk are taken in a ratio of (KPSC/Lect/Pharm-04)
(a) 1:9
(b) 1:99
(c) 1:4
(d) 1:2

Ans. (a)
Note
Ref: Text Book of Homeopathic Pharmacy By Mandal & Mandal – Chapter – 9- Different scales of preparation of drugs

Also see
Decimal scale of trituration
Principle
For making the 1st Decimal drug strength, on part by weight of the crude drug with 9 parts weight of milk sugar taken.
Ref: Text Book of Homeopathic Pharmacy 2nd Edition by D.D. Banerjee. Chapter – 6.2. Study of Potentisation Pg-339.

Q. 54. Can the solid trituration be converted in to liquid dilution at (KPSC/Lect/Pharm-04)
(a) 6X
(b) 8X
(c) 10 X
(d) All the above

Ans. (a)
Note
Trituration is done upto 6x potency and then 8x liquid potency is prepared Ref: Text Book of Homeopathic Pharmacy By Mandal & Mandal – Chapter-9-Different scales of preparation of drugs Pg-117

Also see
Fluxion potency
It is a special and peculiar process where potency, obtained by trituration is converted to 8x potency by succussion without producing 7x potency. Hence, fluxion potency is also known as 'jumping potency'.
It is the potency of the homeopathic medicines, derived by displacement. Hahnemann directed that all metallic substances must be powdered and triturated into the corresponding solid potencies. As because up to 6x or 3 centesimal triturations, the medicinal content of the drugs are neither soluble in alcohol nor purified water.
Ref: Text Book of Homeopathic Pharmacy 2nd Edition by D.D. Banerjee. Chapter – 6.2 Study of Potentisation Pg-343.

Q. 55. Succussion is the process used for potentising (KPSC/Lect/Pharm-04)
(a) Solid drugs
(b) Insoluble drugs
(c) Soluble drugs
(d) All the above

Ans. (c)

Note
Succussion is a process of potentization of medicinal substances which are soluble in liquid vehicles particularly alcohol.
Ref: Text Book of Homeopathic Pharmacy By Mandal & Mandal – Chapter – 12 – Potentisation – Pg-166

Q. 56. What is the drug power of mother tinctures in Class III ? (KPSC/Lect/Pharm-04)
    (a)   1/2
    (b)   1/6
    (c)   1/10
    (d)   1/100

Ans. (b)
Note
Ref: Text Book of Homeopathic Pharmacy By Mandal & Mandal – Chapter – 10 –Method preparing Homoeoapthic drugs (Class – III) Pg-138
Also see
Class III

This class includes plants which are less juicy. They are mostly American plants. However, some European plants are also included in this class.

Preparation of Mother Tincture
Principle
Prepare the tincture by adding two parts by weight of alcohol to one part of the plant or plant part.
Calculation of Drug Power
Ratio of medicinal substance: Strong alcohol = 1:2
But loss of medicinal substance in 1c.c. = 2/3 c.c.
Net Medicinal Substance = (2-2/3) c.c. =1/3 c.c.
Vehicle loss in 1c.c. = 1.6 c.c.
Vehicle loss in 2 c.c. = 2x 1/6 c.c. =1/3 c.c.
    Net vehicle = (2-1/3) c.c. = 5/3 c.c.

Net Medicinal Substance	Solvent / Vehicle (Strong Alcohol)	Mother Tincture
1/3 c.c.	5/3 c.c.	(1/3+5/3) c.c. = 2 c.c.

In 2 c.c. Mother tincture, net medicinal substance = 1/3 c.c.
In 1 c.c. Mother tincture, net medicinal substance = 1/3 x ½ c.c. = 1/6 c.c.
Drug Power (D.P.) = 1/6 c.c.
Ref: Text Book of Homeopathic Pharmacy 2nd Edition by D.D. Banerjee. Chapter – 5.2 Method of Preparation of Homeopathic Drugs Pg-254, 255.

Q. 57. According to old method most juicy plants belong to? (KPSC/Lect/Pharm/2004)
    (a)   Class I
    (b)   Class II
    (c)   Class III
    (d)   Class IV

Ans. (a)
Note
Ref: Text Book of Homeopathic Pharmacy By Mandal & Mandal – Chapter – 10- Methods of preparing Homoeoapthic drugs – (Class –I –Pg-128)

Also see
Old Method of preparation of Mother tincture –Class I.
The plants in class-I, contain a large quantity of juice. It includes most of the European plants. The tincture is prepared by mixing equal parts by weight of the drug juice and alcohol (i.e., 1:1 ratio).
Ref: Text Book of Homeopathic Pharmacy 2nd Edition by D.D. Banerjee. Chapter – 5.2 Pg-250.

MCQ's in Homeopathic Pharmacy

Q. 58. The fundamental rule for the Class III Mother Tincture is discussed in Materia Medica Pura under (KPSC/Lect/Pharm-04)
(a) Bryonia
(b) Cactus
(c) Silicea
(d) Squilla

Ans. (d)

Note
CLASS III
The tinctures in this class are prepared with two parts by weight of alcohol to one part of plant, or part thereof. The fundamental rule for this class is contained in Hahnemann's Mat. Med. Pura, under Scilla. It is applicable to viscid (mucilaginous) material or scanty in juice.
The fresh plant, or part thereof, is pounded to a fine pulp and weighed. Then two parts by weight of alcohol are taken, and after thoroughly mixing the pulp with one-sixth part of it, the rest of the alcohol is then added. After having stirred the whole, and having filled it into a well-stoppered bottle, it is allowed to stand for eight days, in a dark, cool place. The tincture is then separated by decanting, straining and filtering. Drug power of the tincture is 1/6.
Ref: Homeopathic Pharmacy, Chapter 5.

Q. 59. What is the drug strength of Sulphur mother tincture? (KPSC/Lect/Pharm/2004)
(a) 1/2
(b) 1/10
(c) 1/1000
(d) 1/5000

Ans. (d)

Note
Mother tincture drug strength of Sulphur is 1/5000.
Ref: Hompath; Pharmacy Chapter 15.

Q. 60. What is the drug strength of Cactus grandiflorus mother tincture? (KPSC/Lect/Pharm/2004)
(a) 1/10
(b) 1/20
(c) 1/2
(d) 1/100

Ans. (b)
Cactus mother tincture; Drug Strength 1/20
Ref: Hompath; Pharmacy Chapter 15.

Also see
Ref: Text Book of Homeopathic Pharmacy 2nd Edition by D.D. Banerjee. Chapter – 12.8 Pg-646.

Q. 61. Calcarea carbonica is prepared from which layer of oyster shell? (KPSC/Lect/Pharm-04)
(a) Inner layer
(b) Middle layer
(c) Outer layer
(d) All of them

Ans. (b)

Note
The substance used by Hahnemann was an impure carbonate of lime as it exists in the oyster shell. Take well selected, tolerably *thick oyster shells, clean and break into small piece. The pure middle layer is selected, washed carefully with purified water, dried over a water bath and reduced to a fine powder using non-metallic instruments.* It is fine, white, microcrystalline powder, odorless, tasteless.
Ref: Hompath; Pharmacy Chapter 15.

Q. 62. Desiccator is used for removing the (KPSC/Lect/Pharm/2004)
    (a)   Dust
    (b)   Moisture
    (c)   Acidity
    (d)   None of them

Ans. (b)
Note
Desiccator is used for desiccation i.e., removing moisture from substances for keeping hygroscopic material i.e., which absorbs moisture from atmosphere.
Ref: Text Book of Homeopathic Pharmacy By Mandal & Mandal – Chapter- 4- Homeopathic pharmaceutical instruments and appliances – pg-40

Q. 63. Which part of the plant Bryonia is used for preparing mother tincture? (KPSC/Lect/Pharm/2004)
    (a)   Roots
    (b)   Bark
    (c)   Stem
    (d)   Leaves

Ans. (a)
Note
The roots of the plant Bryonia is used for preparing mother tincture.
Ref: Text Book of Homeopathic Pharmacy By Mandal & Mandal – Chapter – 31- List of drugs with their common names, family, distribution and parts used – Pg-303

Q. 64. Rhododendron is prepared from (KPSC/Lect/Pharm-04)
    (a)   Leaves
    (b)   Flowers
    (c)   Flower buds and leaves
    (d)   Fruit

Ans. (a)
Note
A native of Siberia grows in the mountains and flowers in July the tincture is prepared from the fresh leaves.
Ref: Hering's guiding Symptoms

Q. 65. Lac felinum is the milk obtained from a healthy (KPSC/Lect/Pharm/2004)
    (a)   Dog
    (b)   Cat
    (c)   Cow
    (d)   Horse

Ans. (b)
Note
Dog's Milk is   =   Lac caninum
Cat milk is   =   Lac felinum
Cow's Milk is   =   Lac vaccinum
Ref: Text Book of Homeopathic Pharmacy By Mandal & Mandal – Chapter – 2- Sources of Homeopathic drugs – Pg-16

Q. 66. For preservation of Fluoric acid the glass bottles which are used are (KPSC/Lect/Pharm-04)
    (a)   Amber colour
    (b)   White colour
    (c)   Blue colour
    (d)   Gutta purcha

Ans. (d)

Note
For preservation of Fluoric acid 'Gutta purcha' glass bottles are used.
Ref: Text Book of Homeopathic Pharmacy By Mandal & Mandal – Chapter – 14- Preservation of drugs and potentised medicines – Pg-183

Also see
For storing fluoric acid; Gutta purcha bottles are used, otherwise it may dissolve the glass.
Ref: Text Book of Homeopathic Pharmacy 2nd Edition by D.D. Banerjee. Chapter – 1.5 Pg-51.

Q. 67. What is the molecular weight of water? (KPSC/Lect/Pharm/2004)
    (a)   16
    (b)   18
    (c)   20
    (d)   22

Ans. (b)
Note
The molecular weight of water is 18.
Ref; Ref; Text Book of Homeopathic Pharmacy By Mandal & Mandal – Chapter – 8- vehicles (Liquid vehicles) –Pg-91

Q. 68. When a boiled solution of sugar of milk containing starch is treated with solution of iodine will turn it (KPSC/Lect/Pharm/2004)
    (a)   Red
    (b)   Brown
    (c)   White curdy
    (d)   Blue

Ans. (d)
Note
Ref: Text Book of Homeopathic Pharmacy By Mandal & Mandal – Chapter-7- Brief study of standardization of drugs and medicines – Pg-82

Also see
The most common impurity in sugar of milk is starch, which is easily detected by adding to its aqueous solution a 'solution of iodine'. If starch is present, the solution will turn blue.
Ref: Text Book of Homeopathic Pharmacy 2nd Edition by D.D. Banerjee. Chapter – 2.2, Pg-73.

Q. 69. If chloride to be tested the silver nitrate is added to give a (KPSC/Lect/Pharm/2004)
    (a)   Green PPT
    (b)   Red PPT
    (c)   Whitecurdy PPT
    (d)   Brown PPT

Ans. (c)
Note
If presence of sodium chloride is to be tested in sugar of milk, add silver nitrate solution, a precipitate will form which is insoluble in nitric acid.
Ref: Text Book of Homeopathic Pharmacy 2nd Edition by D.D. Banerjee. Chapter – 2.2, Pg-74.

Q. 70. What is the formula of Ethanol? (KPSC/Lect/Pharm/2004)
    (a) CH_3CHO
    (b) C_2H_5OH
    (c) C_3H_7OH
    (d) CH_2CH_3COOH

Ans. (b)
Note
Ref; Text Book of Homeopathic Pharmacy By Mandal & Mandal – Chapter-8- Vehicles (Ethyl alcohol) –Pg-95

Also see
The formula of Ethanol is C_2H_5OH.
Ref: Text Book of Homeopathic Pharmacy 2nd Edition by D.D. Banerjee. Chapter – 2.3, Pg-87.

Q. 71. Boiling point of ethyl alcohol is (KPSC/Lect/Pharm/2004)
    (a)   78.5 °C
    (b)   90.5 °C
    (c)   85.2 °C
    (d)   100 °C

Ans. (a)

Note
Ref: Text Book of Homeopathic Pharmacy By Mandal & Mandal – Chapter- 8- vehicles –Pg-98
Also see
The boiling point of ethyl alcohol is 78.5 °C.
Ref: Text Book of Homeopathic Pharmacy 2nd Edition by D.D. Banerjee. Chapter – 2.3, Pg-87.

Q. 72. Glycerin vehicle is obtained from (KPSC/Lect/Pharm/2004)
    (a)   Mineral source
    (b)   Plant source
    (c)   Animal source
    (d)   All the three

Ans. (d)

Note
Ref: Text Book of Homeopathic Pharmacy by Mandal & Mandal – Chapter-8 Vehicles (Glycerine) –Pg-105

Q. 73. Venoms are preserved in (KPSC/Lect/Pharm/2004)
    (a)   Alcohol
    (b)   Water
    (c)   Glycerin
    (d)   Acetone

Ans. (c)

Note
Venoms are preserved in 'Glycerin'.
Ref: Text Book of Homeopathic Pharmacy By Mandal & Mandal – Chapter-14- Preservation of drugs and potentised medicines – Pg-186
Glycerin is used in preparations of mother tincture and dilutions of certain poisonous products i.e., Apis, Naja, Tarentula, etc.
Ref: Text Book of Homeopathic Pharmacy 2nd Edition by D.D. Banerjee. Chapter – 2.3 Pg-103.

Q. 74. The fundamental principle for the dose should be (KPSC/Lect/Pharm-04)
    (a)   Singleness
    (b)   Simpleness
    (c)   Similarity
    (d)   All the three

Ans. (d)

Note
§246
The curative effect of the remedy may continue for ten, twenty, thirty, forty, or even one hundred days. Good results may be obtained by following these three conditions, viz:
1st. Select the appropriate homeopathic remedy simillimum.
2nd. Use smallest dose capable of getting action minimum.
3rd. Repeat single remedy at proper intervals simplex.
This practice gets the best results.

§247
Dose may be repeated in 14, 12, 10, 7 days in chronic cases but in acute cases repetition will be at much shorter intervals, 24, 12, 3, 4 hours and in very acute cases 1 or 2 hours or every five minutes varying with the nature of the case and the remedy. In the sixth and last edition of the Organon Hahnemann revised his earlier teachings with regard to the repetition of the dose. Prompted by the information acquired by prolonged observation he advises the repetition of the well selected remedy in gradually increasing potencies. This revised paragraph and the appended foot notes in the sixth edition deserve careful study. The advice to increase the potency of the succeeding doses is also again emphasized in the succeeding paragraph No. 248.
Ref: Organon Of Art Of Healing By Baldwin
§272
In the treatment of disease only one simple medicinal substance should be used at a time in any single prescription.
§273
A mixture of medicines is irrational.
Ref: Organon Of Art Of Healing By Baldwin
§ 274
As the true physician finds in simple medicines, administered singly and uncombined, all that he can possibly desire (artificial disease-forces which are able by homeopathic power completely to overpower, extinguish, and permanently cure natural diseases).
Ref: Organon 6th edition.

Q. 75. Volume II of HPI contain the drug monographs ranging (KPSC/Lect/Pharm-04)
    (a)   108
    (b)   115
    (c)   100
    (d)   170
Ans. (c)
Note
HPI – Vol-II Year of publication of – 1974. Ref; Text Book of Homeopathic Pharmacy By Mandal & Mandal– Chapter-2-Pharmacopeia and Pharmacy-Pg-2

Q. 76. Liniments are prepared from (KPSC/Lect/Pharm-04)
    (a)   Alcohol
    (b)   Distilled water
    (c)   Olive oil
    (d)   Rosmary oil
Ans. (c)
Note
Liniments are prepared from 'Olive oil'.
Ref: Text Book of Homeopathic Pharmacy By Mandal & Mandal – Chapter-13-External Applications- Pg-173
Also see
Olive oil is used in preparations of liniments for external applications.
Ref: Text Book of Homeopathic Pharmacy 2nd Edition by D.D. Banerjee. Chapter – 2.3 Pg-104.

Q. 77. Which part is called the body of the prescription? (KPSC/Lect/Pharm/2004)
    (a)   Superscription
    (b)   Subscription
    (c)   Inscription
    (d)   Signature
Ans. (c)
Note
a.   Superscription include – Name of patient / Age / Sex / Address / Rx
b.   Inscription includes – Name of Remedy / Potency / Quantity and name and quantity of vehicle (It is the body of the prescription)
c.   Subscription includes – Direction to the compounder

d.   Signature – It is put in the end of subscription
Ref: Text Book of Homeopathic Pharmacy By Mandal & Mandal – Chapter- 18- Rx writing

Also see
Signature contains:
- Direction for taking the medicine
- When to come for a follow up
- Any advise regarding diet, any precaution, lab examination etc.
- Signature of the physician with date and seal

Ref: Text Book of Homeopathic Pharmacy 2nd Edition by D.D. Banerjee. Chapter – 7.1 Pg-357.

Q. 78. Legally important part of the Signature is (KPSC/Lect/Pharm-04)
    (a)   Signature of the physician
    (b)   Registration No.
    (c)   Date
    (d)   All the three

Ans. (d)
Note
Signature of the physician with date and registration number obtained from the Central Council of Homeopathy (Legally speaking – the Signature, date, and registration number is important part of prescription) Ref; Text Book of Homeopathic Pharmacy By Mandal & Mandal – Chapter-18 – Rx writing –Pg-208

Q. 79. In old classification triturations are discussed in (KPSC/Lect/Pharm-04)
    (a)   Class VII
    (b)   Class VIII
    (c)   Class IX
    (d)   All the three

Ans. (d)
Note
Ref: Text Book of Homeopathic Pharmacy By Mandal & Mandal – Chapter- 10-Methods of preparing Homeopathic drugs – Pg-126

Also see
Preparation of mother substance – Mother substance is defined as a drug pharmaceutically prepared from a drug substance which is insoluble in liquid vehicles and is prepared by the process of trituration with sugar of milk. Mother substances are represented as 0 (Zero). Class VII, Class VIII, and Class IX are included in this category.
Class VII includes; dry insoluble substances.
Cass VIII includes; liquid insoluble substances
Class IX includes; fresh vegetables and animal substances.
Ref: Text Book of Homeopathic Pharmacy 2nd Edition by D.D. Banerjee. Chapter – 5.2- Pg-264.

Q. 80. Drugs can be standardized by (KPSC/Lect/Pharm-04)
    (a)   Physical assaying
    (b)   Chemical assaying
    (c)   Biological assaying
    (d)   All the three

Ans. (d)
Note
Ref; Text Book of Homeopathic Pharmacy By Mandal & Mandal – Chapter-7- Brief study of Standardization of Drugs and Medicines.

Q. 81. First Homeopathic Pharmacopeia was compiled by (KPSC/Lect/Pharm/2004)
    (a)   Close
    (b)   Caspari
    (c)   Herring
    (d)   Staff

Ans. (b)

Note
The First Homeopathic Pharmacopeia was published by Dr Carl W Caspari of Leipzig Germany in 1825 Ref; Ref; Text Book of Homeopathic Pharmacy By Mandal & Mandal – Chapter-1 Pharmacopeia and Pharmacy.

Q. 82. Placebo is discussed in the Organon in article (KPSC/Lect/Pharm/2004)
    (a)   § 270
    (b)   § 267
    (c)   § 281
    (d)   § 247

Ans. (c)
Note
§ 281
To ascertain whether the reappearing symptoms belong to the original natural disease or artificial medicinal disease, the best way is to discontinue the medicine or to *give only unmedicated globules for few more days* and then watch the effects. If the symptoms are due to medicinal aggravation they will automatically pass off in a few days or hours. If no symptoms of the original disease persist in the patient who is still observing proper hygienic rules, it is most probable that he is cured. But if the traces of the original disease symptoms continue during the later period of treatment it may be inferred that the original disease has not been extinguished in its totality and treatment should be continued with higher potencies (in gradually ascending series) of the previously indicated remedy. In case of a hyper-susceptibility in patients, the doses of medicine should be gradually raised to higher potencies; whereas a patient with less susceptibility will require rapid repetetion of the remedy in ascending scales of potency in accordance with Hahnemann's latest instructions.
Ref: Organon by Sarkar 6th Edition Pg-280 – 81

Also see
§ 91
The symptoms and feelings of the patient during a previous course of medicine do not furnish the pure picture of the disease; but, on the other hand , those symptoms and ailments which he suffered from before the use of the medicines, or after they had been discontinued for several days, give the true fundamental idea of the original form of the disease, and these especially the physician must take note of. When the disease is of a chronic character, and the patient has been taking medicine up to the time he is seen, the physician may with advantage leave him some days quite without medicine, or in the meantime *administer something of an unmedicinal nature* and defer to a subsequent period the more precise scrutiny of the morbid symptoms, in order to be able to grasp in their purity the permanent uncontaminated symptoms of the old affection and to form a faithful picture of the disease.
Ref: Organon of Medicine – 6th Edition (this aphorism is same in the 5th and 6th edition of Organon)

Q. 83. Ethanol is chemically (KPSC/Lect/Pharm/2004)
    (a)   Monohydric
    (b)   Dihydric
    (c)   Trihydric
    (d)   Tetrahydric

Ans. (a)
Note
Ref: Text Book of Homeopathic Pharmacy By Mandal & Mandal – Chapter-8- Vehicles – Alcohol – Pg 95

Q. 84. Lachesis is introduced by (KPSC/Lect/Pharm/2004)
    (a)   Kent
    (b)   Boenninghausen
    (c)   Hering
    (d)   Lippe

Ans. (c)
Note
The first trituration, and dilution in alcohol, of the snake poison, Trigonecephalus Lachesis, was made by Hering, on July 28th, 1828 The first cases were published in the Archives, in 1835 In 1837 this remedy was introduced into our Materia Medica.

Q. 85. Petroselinum belongs to (KPSC/Lect/Pharm/2004)
 (a) Mineral source
 (b) Plant source
 (c) Chemical source
 (d) Animal source

Ans. (b)
Note
Common Name: Garden parsley prepared from whole plant.
Ref: Text Book of Homeopathic Pharmacy By Mandal & Mandal – Chapter-31- List of Drugs with their common names, family, distribution and parts used

Q. 86. All mother tinctures are standardized at 1/10 DS by (KPSC/Lect/Pharm/2004)
 (a) Hahnemann
 (b) New method
 (c) Pharmacopeia
 (d) Organon of medicine

Ans. (b)
Note
Ref: Text Book of Homeopathic Pharmacy By Mandal & Mandal – Chapter-10- Method preparing Homeopathic drugs (Modern method) –Pg142

Also see
In Hahnemann's method (Old method) of preparation, the drug strength of various classes of drug substances are different owing to the difference in the solubility of the drugs in various solvents. To overcome this lack of uniformity of drug strength, Homeopathic Pharmacopeia of United States (H.P.U.S.) in 1941, barring a few exceptions *prescribed a uniform standard of 10% drug strength* for most medicinal preparations. This is the 'modern or new method' of preparation of tinctures and potencies, in which the tincture contains 1 gm. of the dry drug substance in 10 c.c. of tincture. The tincture hence contains $1/10^{th}$ part of medicinal substance i.e. a drug strength of 1/10, which corresponds to 1x trituration.
Ref: Text Book of Homeopathic Pharmacy 2nd Edition by D.D. Banerjee. Chapter – 5.3- Pg-269.

Q. 87. Club moss is the common name for:(KPSC/Lect/Pharm/2004)
 (a) Thuja occidentalis
 (b) Fucus
 (c) Lycopodium clavatum
 (d) Arnica montana

Ans. (c)
Note
Ref: Text Book of Homeopathic Pharmacy By Mandal & Mandal – Chapter-31- List of Drugs with their common name, family, distribution and parts used – Pg 305

Q. 88. M. Bhattacharya & Co.'s Pharmacopoeia was published in (KPSC/Lect/Pharm/2004)
 (a) 1900
 (b) 1893
 (c) 1920
 (d) 1972

Ans. (b)
Note
In India the first book was published by M Bhattacharya and Co, Calcutta in 1893 named 'Pharmaceutics Manual' Ref; Text Book of Homeopathic Pharmacy By Mandal & Mandal – Chapter-1- Pharmacopeia and Pharmacy – Pg 3

Also see
In India, the first unofficial pharmacopoeia, named 'Pharmaceutics Manual' was published by M. Bhattacharya and Co. Calcutta, in 1893. Since then it has run into several editions. The tenth edition published in 1944 incorporated about 70 of the important Indian drugs.

A thoroughly revised and enlarged 12th edition was published in July 1962, under the name and style of "M. Bhattacharya & Co.'s Homeopathic Pharmacopeia'.
Ref: Text Book of Homeopathic Pharmacy 2nd Edition by D.D. Banerjee. Chapter – 1.1- Pg-8.

Q. 89. Purification of commercial lactose was developed by (KPSC/Lect/Pharm/2004)
    (a)   Stapf
    (b)   Coolen
    (c)   Lavoishe
    (d)   Dunham

Ans. (a)
Note
It was given by Johann Ernest Stapf; Text Book of Homeopathic Pharmacy By Mandal & Mandal – Chapter-8- Vehicles – (Solid vehicles) – Pg 85

Q. 90. To separate the solute from solvent the method used is (KPSC/Lect/Pharm/2004)
    (a)   Filtration
    (b)   Distillation
    (c)   Sublimation
    (d)   Decantation

Ans. (b)
Note
Ref: Text Book of Homeopathic Pharmacy By Mandal & Mandal – Chapter-6- General Laboratory and Laboratory Methods – Pg 56

Also see
Filtration
It is a technique where suspended solid particles in a fluid are removed by passing the mixture through a porous barrier, usually paper or cloth. The particles are retained by the paper or cloths in the form of residue and the fluid passes through to make up the filtrate. (Pg-140)
Distillation
It is the process of purification of liquid substances by first converting it into its vapor state through the application of heat or by reduction of pressure. This is known as vaporization and then converting the vapor into the liquid state by cooling.
This is a rapid process where liquid (solvent) can be separated from solute. However, the main disadvantage is that some substances, which may be dissolved may get decomposed, if they are unstable at the boiling point of the liquid, and hence, the dissolved substance may not be obtained in its pure original form. (Pg-143)
Sublimation
It is the conversion of a solid to its vapor state without passing through the liquid phase on heating and vice versa, on cooling. It helps separate these solid from other common non-volatile solid like charcoal, sand etc. (Pg-145)
Decantation
It is the process in which the heavier particles in a suspension settle down when it is allowed to stand for sometime. The supernatant liquid can be easily decanted without disturbing the sediment. (Pg-140)
Ref: Text Book of Homeopathic Pharmacy 2nd Edition by D.D. Banerjee. Chapter – 3.3.

Q. 91. In class IX of old method the drug and vehicle ratio is (KPSC/Lect/Pharm/2004)
    (a)   1:9
    (b)   1:99
    (c)   2:9
    (d)   1:4

Ans. (c)
Note
Ref: Text Book of Homeopathic Pharmacy By Mandal & Mandal – Chapter-10- Methods of Preparing Homeopathic drugs– Pg 140

Also see
Class IX; this class deals with preparation of medicine from vegetables and animal substances by trituration, in solid form.

Principle

2 parts by weight of the medicinal substance is triturated with 99 parts (centesimal scale) or 9 parts (decimal scale) by weight of sugar of milk to produce the 1st trituration.

Note

Here the ratio or the medicinal substance and sugar of milk is 2:99 (centesimal scale) or 2:9 (decimal scale). The reason for taking 2 parts by weight of the medicinal substance is to compensate the loss of medicinal substance by evaporation during trituration.

Ref: Text Book of Homeopathic Pharmacy 2nd Edition by D.D. Banerjee. Chapter – 5.2- Pg-268.

Ref: Text Book of Homeopathic Pharmacy 2nd Edition by D.D. Banerjee. Chapter – 5.2- Pg-264.

Q. 92. Digitalis belongs to the family (KPSC/Lect/Pharm/2004)
- (a) Compositae
- (b) Scrophluraceae
- (c) Solanaceae
- (d) Rananculaceae

Ans. (b)

Note

Digitalis purpurea belongs to the family is Scrophluraceae some more information in respect of Digitalis purpurea is as under:

Common name: Fox glove Leaves of the 2nd year growth are used for preparation.

Ref: Text Book of Homeopathic Pharmacy By Mandal & Mandal – Chapter-31- List of Drugs with their common name, family, distribution and parts used– Pg 304

Q. 93. Bufo Rana is the drug prepared from (KPSC/Lect/Pharm/2004)
- (a) Toad
- (b) Snail
- (c) Snake
- (d) Lizard

Ans. (a)

Note

It is prepared from poison of toad.

Ref: Text Book of Homeopathic Pharmacy By Mandal & Mandal – Chapter-2- Sources of Homoeoapthic drugs – Pg 16

Also see

Bufo rana is the drug prepared from toad poison which is obtained from the dorsal glands of toad.

Ref: Text Book of Homeopathic Pharmacy 2nd Edition by D.D. Banerjee. Chapter – 1.3 - Pg-32.

Q. 94. Santonin is the active principle of (KPSC/Lect/Pharm-04)
- (a) Belladonna
- (b) Santalum album
- (c) Cina maritima
- (d) Pulsatilla nigricans

Ans. (c)

Note

Santoninum [Santoin]: General; Santonin is the active principle of Santonica, the unexpanded flower heads of Artemisia maritime; cina (Ref; Boericke materia medica)

Q. 95. Rule 67 of Sale of Homeo drugs the duration of licence is discussed in (KPSC/Lect/Pharm-04)
- (a) 67—C
- (b) 67—D
- (c) 67—E
- (d) 67—B

Ans. (c)

Note
Rule 67-E
Duration of license is one year for sale of homeopathic drugs.
Ref; Text Book of Homeopathic Pharmacy By Mandal & Mandal – Chapter-32- General Knowledge of Legislation in relation to Homoeoapthic Pharmacy – Pg 309

Also see
Rule 67-C
A license to sell, stock or exhibit for sale or distribute homeopathic medicines by retail or by wholesale shall be issued in Forms 20-C or 20-D, as the case may be.
Rule 67-D
Sale at more than one place – If drugs are sold or stocked for sale at more than one place, separate applications shall be made and a separate licence shall be obtained in respect to each place.
Rule 67-E
Duration of licences- an original licence or a renewed licence unless it is sooner suspended or cancelled, shall be valid up-to the 31st December of the year following the year in which it is granted or renewed:
Provided that if the application for renewal of the licence in force is made before its expiry or it the application is made and the additional fee paid within one month of its expiry, the licence shall continue to be in force until order are passed on the application. The licence shall be deemed to have expired, if application for its renewal is not made within one month after its expiry.
Rule 67-B
    -NA- (No such rule is given)
Ref: Text Book of Homeopathic Pharmacy 2nd Edition by D.D. Banerjee. Chapter – 10.1- Pg-540.

Q. 96. Route of administration of drugs is dealt in (KPSC/Lect/Pharm-04)
    (a)   Pharmacognosy
    (b)   Pharmacology
    (c)   Pharmaconomy
    (d)   Pharmacoproxy

Ans. (c)
Note
The route of administration of drug is dealt in 'Pharmaconomy'.
Also see
a.   Pharmacognosy
    It is a science which deals with history, source, cultivation, collection, preparation, distribution, identification, composition, purity, preservation and commerce of crude drugs of vegetable and animal origin.
b.   Pharmacology
    It is a branch which deals with drugs their sources, appearance, chemistry, preparation, actions and therapeutics.
c.   Pharmaconomy
    Deals with route or channel of administration of drugs and   medicines.
d.   Pharmacoproxy
    It is the art or science by which cruds drug substances are   converted into real medicines.
Ref: Text Book of Homeopathic Pharmacy By Mandal & Mandal – Chapter-20- Drug administraion

Q. 97. One who conducts proving experiment is called (KPSC/Lect/Pharm-04)
    (a)   Prover
    (b)   Ideal prover
    (c)   Master prover
    (d)   None of the above

Ans. (c)
Note
Prover
The One on which medicines are proved, by giving medicines. He takes the medicine but has no knowledge about whether he is taking which drug or been supplied only placebo.
Ideal prover

Ideal prover is free from all diseases, he is intelligent and of delicate, irritable temperament. Sensitive in nature and trustworthy.
Ref: Text book of Homeopathic Pharmacy, By D. D. Banerjee, 2nd Edition. Pg-399-400.

Also see
Best Prover
Aphorism 141.Comments about the ideal / best prover as under:
The healthy unprejudiced physician of fine perception makes the best prover. Every homeopathic physician should take an active part in proving some drugs as a part of the preparation for the practice of his art.
Master prover
-He is the one who designs and conducts the drug proving experiment, and has complete knowledge about the coded medicines, which code contains the medicine or placebo.

Q. 98. Temporary hardness of water is because of the presence of (KPSC/Lect/Pharm-04)
(a) Sulphates
(b) Phosphates
(c) Carbonates
(d) Chlorides

Ans. (c)
Note
Temporary hardness of water is because of presence of carbonates.

Q. 99. Decimal potencies are explained in (KPSC/Lect/Pharm-04)
(a) V edition of Organon
(b) VI edition of Organon
(c) Both the two
(d) None of the above

Ans. (d)
Note
The decimal potency was introduced by Dr. Constantine Hering to potentise snake venom. The centesimal scale was introduced by Dr Hahnemann in Vth edition of Organon of Medicine in aphorism 270.

Ref: Text Book of Homeopathic Pharmacy By Mandal & Mandal – Chapter-9- Different scales of preparation of drugs – Pg 116-7

Q. 100. Night blooming cereus is the name for (KPSC/Lect/Pharm/2004)
(a) Helianthus anus
(b) Cactus grandiflorus
(c) Calendula
(d) Chamomilla

Ans. (b)
Note
Night blooming cereus is the name for Cactus grandiflorus.

Ref: Text Book of Homeopathic Pharmacy By Mandal & Mandal – Chapter-31- List of Drugs, common name, family, distribution and parts used– Pg 303

Q. 101. Passiflora incarnata the part used is (KPSC/Lect/Pharm-04)
(a) Leaves
(b) Roots
(c) Flowers
(d) Fruits

Ans. (a)
Note
Passion Flower. N. O. Passifloraceae (of the Violal alliance) Tincture of fresh or dried leaves gathered in May Fluid Hydro-alcoholic extract powdered inspissated juice.
Ref: Clarke's materia medica

MCQ's in Homeopathic Pharmacy

Q. 102. Skunk is the material obtained from (KPSC/Lect/Pharm-04)
    (a) Musk deer
    (b) Toad skin
    (c) Anal gland of wild cat
    (d) Snake venum

Ans. (c)

Note
Skunk or Mephitis is prepared from the fluid secretions of the anal gland of wild cat.
Ref: Text Book of Homeopathic Pharmacy By Mandal & Mandal – Chapter-2- Sources of Homeopathic drugs– Pg 14

Q. 103. Propanetriol is the chemical name of (KPSC/Lect/Pharm-04)
    (a) Methyl alcohol
    (b) Ethyl alcohol
    (c) Glycerine
    (d) Benzene

Ans. (c)

Note
Propanetriol is the chemical name of glycerine.

Q. 104. Mercurialis perennis belongs to (KPSC/Lect/Pharm-04)
    (a) Animal kingdom
    (b) Mineral kingdom
    (c) Plant kingdom
    (d) Chemicals

Ans. (c)

Note
Mercurialis perennis – Synonym - Dog's Mercury Natural Order Euphorbiaceae. Tincture of whole fresh plant in flower.
Ref: Clarke materia medica

Q. 105. Vol – 1 of IHP contain Monographs of (KPSC/Lect/Pharm-04)
    (a) 170 Drugs
    (b) 210 Drugs
    (c) 118 Drugs
    (d) 180 Drugs

Ans. (d)

Note
Vol –I of IHP contain monographs of 180 drugs.

Q. 106. Extraction of mother tinctures from dry drug materials is carried out by the process of (KPSC/Lect/Pharm-04)
    (a) Filteration
    (b) Sublimation
    (c) Maceration
    (d) Percolation

Ans. (d)

Note
Extraction of mother tincture from dry drug material is carried out by the process of percolation.
Ref: Text Book of Homeopathic Pharmacy By Mandal & Mandal – Chapter-10- Methods of Preparing Homeopathic Drugs– Pg 146

Q. 107. Karl Fischer method of moisture estimation is otherwise known as (KPSC/Lect/Pharm-04)
  (a) Gravimetric method
  (b) Tolune method
  (c) Volumetric method
  (d) Titrimetric method

Ans. (d)

Note
Determination of moisture content for vegetable products:
  a. Gravimetric method.
  b. Volumetric method or Touene distillation method.
  c. Titrimetric Method or Karl Fischer Method
Ref: Text book of Homeopathic Pharmacy, By D. D. Banerjee, 2nd Edition. Chapter: 8.1.Pg-421.

Also see
Ref: Text Book of Homeopathic Pharmacy By Mandal & Mandal – Chapter-6- General Laboratory and Laboratory Methods - Pg 63

Q. 108. Imponderable drugs are introduced by Hahnemann in Organon of medicine in the article (KPSC/Lect/Pharm-04)
  (a) § 274
  (b) § 267
  (c) § 282
  (d) § 286

Ans. (d)

Note
§ 286

The dynamic force of mineral magnets, electricity and galvanism act no less powerfully upon our life principle and they are not less homeopathic than the properly so-called medicines which neutralize disease by taking them through the mouth, or by rubbing them on the skin or by olfaction. There may be diseases, especially diseases of sensibility, and irritability, abnormal sensations and involuntary muscular movements which may be cured by those means. But the more certain way of applying the last two as well as that of the so-called electro-magnetic machine lies still very much in the dark to make homeopathic use of them. So far both electricity and galvanism have been used only for palliation to the great damage of the sick. The positive, pure action of both upon the healthy human body have until the present time been but little tested.
Ref: Organon of Medicine 6th Edition

Q. 109. Homeopathic doses are synonymous for (KPSC/Lect/Pharm-04)
  (a) Infinitesimal doses
  (b) Microdoses
  (c) Minimal doses
  (d) Optimal doses

Ans. (a)

Note
Homeopathic doses are synonymous for 'infinistesimal doses'.

Also see
§16
The spirit-like dynamis, when disordered, is affected only by spirit-like morbid agencies. Hence dynamic action of remedial agencies must be used for purpose of cure. Life is the chemistry of the infinitesimal; the **infinitesimal** only can alter its processes or correct its disorder.
§269

The medicinal power of a crude substance is developed to an unparalleled degree by potentization. This process especially develops the medicinal powers of crude drugs, which in their crude state have no medicinal effect

on the human body. Recent discoveries of modern science have revealed many facts regarding the infinitesimal. The discovery of radium and its discernible radiant emanations and ......Cell chemistry is the chemistry of the infinitesimal, the potentized crude element. Thus Hahnemann, by his carefully devised process of potentization has stolen from nature her secret means of initiating life and correcting its defects.
Ref; Art of Healing by Baldwin.

Also see
By minutest subdivision, energy is liberated from inert mass - bulk-weight: from things palpable and manifest to our grosser senses. We are last beginning to realize the potentialities of the intangible and the imponderable. But the most sensitive thing in the world is the diseased cell or tissue for the remedy of like symptoms, in infinitesimal subdivision. And it is with this that we have to deal.
Ref: Homeopathy an Explanation of its Principles [Explanation]

Q. 110. Common name of Andrographis paniculata is (KPSC/Lect/Pharm-04)
(a) Babchi
(b) Somraj
(c) Kalmegh
(d) Kurchi

Ans. (c)
Note
Common name of Andrographis paniculata are: B. Klmegh; G. Kariyatu; H. Kiryat; M. kiryat, Nelavepu; Mar. Olikirayat; S. Bhunimba; T. Nilavembu; Te Nelavemu.
Ref: Text book of Homeopathic Pharmacy, By D. D. Banerjee, 2nd Edition. Chapter: 12.3 Pg-598.

Q. 111. Which drug belongs to Solanaceae? (KPSC- Re Exam/Lect/Organon-05)
(a) Dulcamara
(b) Drosera rotundifolia
(c) Equisetum hyemale
(d) Digitalis purpurea

Ans. (a)
Note
The above drugs belong to the family of:
    Dulcamara - Solanaceae
    Drosera - Droseraceae
    Equisetum - Equisetaceae
    Digitalis – Scrophulariaceae
Ref: Allen's key Notes

Q. 112. Of the below which is the correct one? (KPSC- Re Exam/Lect/Organon-05)
(a) When triturations attain the 3X potency then only it will be fit to be converted into liquid potency.
(b) When triturations attain the 5X potency then only it will be fit to be converted into liquid potency.
(c) When triturations attains the 6X potency, then only it will be fit to be converted into liquid potency.
(d) When triturations attains the 12X potency then only it will be fit to be converted into liquid potency.

Ans. (c)
Note
When trituration attains the 6X potency, then only it will be fit to be converted into liquid potency. This process is called 'Fluxion Potency'. It is a special and peculiar process where 6x potency, obtained by trituration is converted to 8x potency by succussion without producing 7x potency. It is basically used for the metallic substances or other drugs which in their crude form are neither soluble in alcohol nor purified water.
Ref: Text book of Homeopathic Pharmacy, By D. D. Banerjee, 2nd Edition. Chapter: 6.2 Pg-343.

Q. 113. Of the below statement which is correct? (KPSC- Re Exam/Lect/Organon-05)
(a) Potencies above 30th are high potencies
(b) Potencies above 1000th are high potencies
(c) Potencies above 200th are high potencies
(d) Potencies above 500th are high potencies

Ans. (a)

Note

Low potency	Medium Potency	High Potency
1c - 12c	12c - 30c	Above 30c

Ref: Organon by B.K. Sarkar Pg-426.

Q. 114. One fluid ounce is (KPSC/Lect/ Physiology-05)
(a) 6 fluid drachm
(b) 5 fluid drachm
(c) 8 fluid drachm
(d) 7 fluid drachm

Ans. (c)
Note
Imperial system (British)
Measures of Mass or Weights:
One fluid ounce is = 8 fluid drachms
Ref: Text book of Homoeopahic Pharmacy 2nd edition by D.D. Banerjee Chpater-4.2 Pg-236.

Q. 115. Croton tigrinum belongs to (KPSC/Lect/ Physiology-05)
(a) Euphorbiacea
(b) Umbiliferacea
(c) Solanacea
(d) Papaveracea

Ans. (a)
Note

Name	Synonyms	Family	Distribution	Part used
Croton tigrinum	Purging nut	Euphorbiaceae	Bengal, Assam, Burma	Oil from seeds

Ref: Text book of Homoeopahic Pharmacy 2nd edition by D.D. Banerjee Chpater-12.4 Pg-607.

Q. 116. Meaning of the abbreviation BID is (KPSC/Lect/ Physiology-05)
(a) Twice a day
(b) Twice daily
(c) Drink
(d) A large pill

Ans. (a)
Note
BID = Bis in die (In Latin or Greek) = Twice a day
Ref: Text Book of Homeopathic Pharmacy by Mandal & Mandal – Chapter-18- Prescription Writing Pg-204.
Ref: Text book of Homeopathic Pharmacy 2nd edition by D.D. Banerjee Chpater-7.1 Pg-359

Q. 117. Cantharis is prepared from (MD (Hom) Entr/ Paper-1-2001)
(a) Spanish fly
(b) Cockroach
(c) Home fly
(d) Honeybee

Ans. (a)

Note

Name	Common name	Class	Phylum	Part used
Cantharis vesicatoria	Spanish fly	Insecta	Arthropoda	Whole dried fly

Ref: Text book of Homeopathic Pharmacy 2nd edition by D.D. Banerjee Chpater-1.3, Pg-29. Also see at Pg- 484.

Q. 118. Stapf process is used in the purification of (MD (Hom) Entr/ Paper-1-01)
    (a)   Alcohol
    (b)   Water
    (c)   Sugar of milk
    (d)   Glycerine

Ans. (c)
Note
Stapf process is used in the purification of 'sugar of milk'.
Ref: Text Book of Homeopathic Pharmacy By Mandal & Mandal – Chapter-8- Vehicles– Purification of sugar of milk; Johann Ernst Staff Pg-85

Q. 119. 2nd volume of HPI published in the year (MD (Hom) Entr/ Paper-1-01)
    (a)   1892
    (b)   1971
    (c)   1974
    (d)   1992

Ans. (c)
Note
2nd volume of HPI published in the year 1974.
Ref: Text Book of Homeopathic Pharmacy by Mandal & Mandal – Chapter-1- Pharmacopeia and Pharmacy– Pg 2

Also see
HPI is the official pharmacopeia of India. Eight volumes have been published by the government of India (Ministry of Health and Family Welfare) by the Homeopathic Pharmacopeia Committee.

Volumes	No. of Monographs	Year of Publication
Vol. I of HPI	180	1971
Vol. II of HPI	100	1974
Vol. III of HPI	105	1978
Vol. IV of HPI	107	1984
Vol. V of HPI	114	1987
Vol. VI of HPI	104	1991
Vol. VII of HPI	105	1998
Vol. VIII of HPI	101	2000

Ref: Text book of Homoeopahic Pharmacy 2nd edition by D.D. Banerjee Chpater-1.1, Pg-7.

Q. 120. The branch of pharmacy which deals with the action of drugs (MD (Hom) Entr/ Paper-1-01)
    (a)   Pharmacology
    (b)   Pharmacopedia
    (c)   Pharmacopeia
    (d)   Pharmacography

Ans. (a)
Note
The branch of pharmacy which deals with the action of drugs is 'Pharmacology'.
Ref: Text Book of Homeopathic Pharmacy By Mandal & Mandal – Chapter-15- Pharmacology – Pg 187

Also see
Pharmacology
It is the science that deals with different aspects of the drugs. (Pg-666)
Pharmacopedia
The teaching of pharmacy and pharmacodynamics. (Pg-666)
Pharmacopeia
It is the standard authoritative book, containing a list of drugs and medicines, habitats, descriptions, collections and identification of drugs. It also provides directions for their preparations, combining, compounding and standardization. (Pg-6)
Pharmacography
A treatise on or description of drugs. (Pg-666)
Ref: Text book of Homoeopahic Pharmacy 2nd edition by D.D. Banerjee.

Q. 121. Symbol for if necessary (MD (Hom) Entr/ Paper-1-2001)
  (a) QID
  (b) PC
  (c) SOS
  (d) HS
Ans. (c)
Note

Abbreviation	Latin or Greek word	English Translation
SOS	Si opus sit	If necessary

Ref: Text book of Homoeopahic Pharmacy 2nd edition by D.D. Banerjee. Chapter 7.1, Pg-362.

Q. 122. Juice of the fresh plant is mixed with alcohol in (MtD (Hom) Entr/ Paper-1-2001)
  (a) Class IX
  (b) Class I
  (c) New Method
  (d) Potentisation
Ans. (b)
Note
Juice of the fresh plant is mixed with alcohol in Class I.
Also see
Class I: The plant in class I - contain large quantity of juice; it includes most of the European plants. The tincture is prepared by mixing equal parts by weight of the drug juice and alcohol i.e., 1:1 ratio.
Old method of preparation of drug substances
A. **Mother tincture**
  Class I: (Most juicy plants)
  Class II: (Medium juicy plants)
  Class III: (Least juicy plants)
  Class IV: (Dried vegetable and animal substances and also from fresh animals).
B. **Mother solution**
  Class V: Aqueous solutions
  Class V – A: These are easily soluble in water
  Class V – B: These are easily soluble, but require a large quantity of water.
  Class VI: Alcoholic solutions.
  Class VI – A : These are easily soluble in alcohol.
  Class VI – B: These are easily soluble but require a large quantity of alcohol.
C. **Triturations**
  Class VII : Trituration of insoluble medicinal substances.
  Class VIII: Trituration of liquids insoluble medicinal substance.
  Class IX : Trituration of fresh animal and vegetable substance.

Ref: Text book of Homeopathic Pharmacy 2nd edition by D.D. Banerjee. Chapter 5.2, Pg-248.

Q. 123. Vehicle for a liniment is (MD (Hom) Entr/ Paper-1-01)
(a) Paraffin
(b) Spermeceti
(c) Glycerine
(d) Vegetable oil

Ans. (d)
Note
Vehicle for a liniment is 'vegetable oil'.

Also see
Liniments they are spoken of as lubrication and are generally of oily, soapy, or spirituous consistency. They are mixture of solutions of different medicines (generally mother tincture) in oil, or are alcoholic solutions of soap or emulsions, and are suitable for external applications. The one part by weight or volume of mother tincture with 9 parts by weight or volume of olive oil.

Ref: Text book of Homeopathic Pharmacy 2nd edition by D.D. Banerjee. Chapter 7.5, Pg-385.

Q. 124. Polarimeter is used for determining (MD (Hom) Entr/ Paper-1-2001)
(a) Specific gravity
(b) PH
(c) Optical rotation
(d) Boiling point

Ans. (c)
Note
Polarimeter is used for determining 'optical rotation'.

Also see
The polarimetric method of analysis is based on the ability of substances to rotate the plane of polarization when polarized light passes through them.
Ref: Text book of Homeopathic Pharmacy 2nd edition by D.D. Banerjee. Chapter 3.4, Pg-209.

Q. 125. One tea-spoon is equal to (MD (Hom) Entr/ Paper-1-2001)
(a) 15 ml
(b) 10 ml
(c) 5 ml
(d) 2 ml

Ans. (c)
Note
One tea-spoon is equal to '5 ml'.
Ref: Text Book of Homeopathic Pharmacy By Mandal & Mandal – Chapter-17- Weights and measures– Pg 203

Also see
An average 1 teaspoon is equal to 5 ml.
Ref: Text book of Homeopathic Pharmacy 2nd edition by D.D. Banerjee. Chapter 4.2, Pg-238.

Q. 126. The name "50 Millesimal Scale" was given by (UPSC-06)
(a) Hahnemann
(b) Pierre Schmidt
(c) Kent
(d) Hering

Ans. (b)
Note
The name "50 Millesimal Scale" was given by 'Dr. Pierre Schmidt'.

Also see
The 50·millesimal scale has been mentioned in the sixth edition of Hahnemann's Organon of Medicine (Aphorism 270). This edition was published (1921) well after death of Hahnemann. Hahnemann himself termed this new method as, 'renewed dynamisation' in aphorism 161. However, the name '50 Millesimal

Scale' was later on given by Dr Pierre Schmidt, as the material part of the medicine is said to be decreased by 50,000 times for each degree of dynamisation.
Ref: Text book of Homeopathic Pharmacy 2nd edition by D.D. Banerjee. Chapter 6.1, Pg-327.

Q. 127. Refractive index of glycerine at 20 C is (UPSC-06)
    (a)   1.345 – 1.420
    (b)   1.459 - 1.470
    (c)   1.472 - 1.476
    (d)   1.481 - 1.495

Ans. (c)
Note
The refractive index of glycerine is: 1.471 to 1.473 at 20° C.(HPI)
Ref: Textbook of Homeopathic Pharmacy by DR. D.D. Banerjee 2nd edition. Chapter 2-3, Pg-102.

Q. 128. Match List I with List II and select the correct answer using the code given below the lists (UPSC-06)

List- I (Remedies)		List-II (Other names / Synonyms)
A	Actea racemosa	1 Cimicifuga
B	Anacardium orientale	2 Wild indigo
C	Apis mellifica	3 Honey bee
D	Baptisia tinctoria	4 Marking nut
E	Spongia tosta	5 Roasted sponge

Code

	A	B	C	D	E
(a)	1	2	3	4	5
(b)	5	4	1	2	3
(c)	1	4	3	2	5
(d)	5	2	1	4	3

Ans. (c)
Note
The correct sequence as under:

List- I (Remedies)		List-II (Other names / Synonyms)
A	Actea racemosa	1 Cimicifuga
B	Anacardium orientale	4 Marking nut
C	Apis mellifica	3 Honey bee
D	Baptisia tinctoria	2 Wild indigo
E	Spongia tosta	5 Roasted sponge

Ref: Textbook of Homeopathic Pharmacy by DR. D.D. Banerjee 2nd edition. Chapter 12.4, Pg-605.

Q. 129. Match List I with List II and select the correct answer using the code given below the lists: (UPSC-06)

Code

	A	B	C	D
(a)	2	3	1	4
(b)	2	1	3	4
(c)	4	3	1	2
(d)	4	1	3	2

Ans. (a)

Note

List-I (Common Name)	List-II (Remedy)
A Poke root	2 Phytolacca Decaudra
B Blood root	3 Sanguinaria
C Pink root	1 Spigelia
D Orange root	4 Hydrastis anadeusis

Ref: for A, B, & C from Pocket Manual of Homeopathic Materia Medica by William Boericke.
Ref: for D. Clarke's materia medica

Q. 130. Which part of plant is used for the preparation of "Sabina"? (UPSC-06)
    (a)   Stem
    (b)   Whole plant
    (c)   Fruit
    (d)   Bark

Ans. (a)

Note
Stem is used for the preparation of 'Sabina'.
Ref: Textbook of Homeopathic Pharmacy by DR. D.D. Banerjee 2nd edition. Chapter 1.3, Pg-19.

Q. 131. Fluxion potency is peculiar process when medicines prepared by trituration are converted into potency by succussion. What are the levels at which it is carried out? (UPSC-06)
    (a)   30 to 200
    (b)   2X to 4C
    (c)   6X to 8X
    (d)   12X to 14 X

Ans. (c)

Note
Fluxion potency is peculiar process when medicines prepared by trituration are converted into potency by succussion is at the level of 6x to 8x.
Ref: Text Book of Pharmacy 2nd Edition by D.D. Banerjee. Chapter 6.2 –Study of Potentisation. Pg-343.

Q. 132. Under which class (Old Method) is Aloe mother tincture prepared? (UPSC-06)
    (a)   Class II
    (b)   Class VI B
    (c)   Class VII
    (d)   Class V A

Ans. (c)

Note
Name of drug: Aloe socotrina
Part Used: Inspissated juice of leaves.
Class of Old method: IV and VII.
Ref: Text Book of Pharmacy 2nd Edition by D.D. Banerjee. Pg-648, 258, 265.

Q. 133. The source of "Tarentula hispanica" is (KPSC/Lect/Mat-Med-04)
    (a)   Spanish spider
    (b)   Cuban spider
    (c)   Black cuban spider
    (d)   Black hispania spider

Ans. (a)

Note
The source of "Tarentula hispanica" is 'Spanish spider'.

Also see
Spanish spider – Tarentula hispanica
Cuban spider – Tarentula cubensis
Black cuban Spider – Mygale lasiodora
Ref: Textbook of Homeopathic Pharmacy by DR. D.D. Banerjee 2nd edition. Chapter 1.3, Pg-28, 29.

Q. 134. The source of "Theridion" is (KPSC/Lect/Mat-Med-04)
  (a) White cuban spider
  (b) Cuban spider
  (c) Spanish spider
  (d) Orange spider

Ans. (d)

Note
The source of 'Theridion curassavicum' is Orange spider of 'Araneidease' family.
Ref: Allen's Key Note.

Also see
Cuban spider - Tarentula cubensis
Spanish spider – Tarentula hispanica
Orange spider - Theridion curassavicum
Ref: Textbook of Homeopathic Pharmacy by DR. D.D. Banerjee 2nd edition. Chapter 1.3, Pg- 29.

Q. 135. "Thyroidinum" is a (KPSC/Lect/Mat-Med-04)
  (a) Nosode
  (b) Sarcode
  (c) Imponderabilia
  (d) Plant product

Ans. (b)

Note
"Thyroidinum" is a 'Sarcode'.

Also see
Sarcodes are prepared from the secretion of healthy organism: Insulin - (B cells of the islets of Langerhans of the pancreas); Thyroidinum - (Thyroid gland).
Ref: Textbook of Homeopathic Pharmacy by Dr. D.D. Banerjee 2nd edition. Chapter 1.3, Pg-38.

Q. 136. The source of "Lobelia inflata" is (KPSC/Lect/Mat-Med-04)
  (a) Plant
  (b) Animal
  (c) Mineral
  (d) None of the above

Ans. (a)

Note
Lobelia inflata - Common name - Indian tobacco. Part used; whole fresh plant without roots.
Ref: Textbook of Homeopathic Pharmacy by DR. D.D. Banerjee 2nd edition. Chapter-1.3, Pg-18, 651.

Q.137. Mention the drug which is prepared from the normal secretion of a living animal ____ (PSC/WB/91)
  (a) Adrenalinum
  (b) Adonis vernalis
  (c) Actaea spicata
  (d) Agraphis nutans

Ans. (a)

Note
Adrenalinum is the drug which is prepared from the normal secretion of living animals.

Also see
Adrenalinum; extract of suprarenal bodies.
A Sarcode.
Tincture or trituration.
Ref: Clarke's Materia Medica.
Drug which is prepared from the normal secretion of living animal are known as sarcoids. Examples are: Cholesterin; Insulin - (B cells of the islets of Langerhans of the pancreas); Thyroidinum - (Thyroid gland). They have a great value in homoeopathic preparations. They are deep-acting remedies and have a property to set right the disturbed metabolism.
Ref: Pharmacy (Hompath).

Adonis vernalis
N. O. Ranunculaceae. Infusion or tincture of fresh plant, an extract, Adonidin. Clinical: abuminuria. Dropsy. Heart, affections of.
Ref: Clarke's Materia Medica.

Actaea spicata
Common name: Bane berry. Herb Christopher. (Europe and Asia.) N. O. Ranunculaceae. Tincture of root obtained in autumn. Clinical: Cancer of stomach. Fright, effects of. Hepatitis. Pleurisy. Rheumatism. Toothache.

Agraphis nutans
Common name: Bluebell. Wild Hyacinth. Scilla nutans. N. O. Liliaceae.
Tincture of fresh plant and growing shoots. Clinical: Adenoids. Catarrh. Deafness. Diarrhoea.

Q. 138. Medicine prepared from spider poisons _____ (PSC/WB/91)
    (a)   Cantharis vesicatoria
    (b)   Tarentula hispanica
    (c)   Bufo rana
    (d)   Murex purpurea

Ans. (b)

Note
Tarentula hispanica is prepared from spider poison.

Also see

Cantharis vesicatoria
Zoological name: Lytta vesicatoria Febricus.
Family: Cantharidae.
Distribution: It is commonly known as the Spanish fly and is found in the middle and south of Europe, and south-western Asia. It feeds on ash and other trees.
Part used: The whole dried fly.

Tarentula hispanica
Zoological Name: Tarentula hispanaica.
Family: Lycosidae
Description: A hairy spider, with six eyes and several pairs of legs, the third pair particularly being the shortest. The poison of the male and female spider are identical. According to Dr Mariano de la Paz Graells Pardo, Spain, the spider is most poisonous in the month of July.
Part used: The entire spider.
Ref: Pharmacy, Chapter– 15, Archives Hompath.

Bufo rana
Description: Homeopathic Bufo is made from the poison of the toad. The toad releases his poison when he is teased or irritated; it can paralyze a dog. The Chinese were the first to apply dried toad poison for a variety of complaints. American homeopath – J.T. Kent performed the first homeopathic provings with this substance.
Ref: http://www.realmagick.com/articles/90/1890.html

Murex purpurea

Zoological name: Murex purpurea.
Common name: Purple fish.
Natural order: Gastropoda.
Part used: Trituration of desiccated juice. Trituration or tincture of fresh juice (the fresh preparation is preferred, though the dried is the usual one).
Clinical: Abortion. Breasts, pains in. Cervix uteri, affections of. Climacteric sufferings. *(AQ) Diabetes. Dysmenorrhoea. Leucorrhoea. Menorrhagia. Metrorrhagia. Nymphomania. Pregnancy, affections of. Uterus, prolapse of.

Petroz first proved the Purple fish (Murex purpurea), which, like the Ink fish (Sepia officinalis), produces the chief intensity of its action on the female generative sphere.

Characteristics

They are chiefly distinguished in that Murex purpurea produces frantic sexual desire and tends to have excessive haemorrhage with large clots, Sepia officinalis having, in general, scanty flow. Another leading feature of Murex is – consciousness of the womb, sore pain in the uterus.
Ref: Clarke's Materia Medica.

Q. 139. Mention the vehicle by which we can prepare mother tincture _____ (PSC/WB/93)
    (a) Dilute alcohol
    (b) Rectified spirit
    (c) Strong alcohol
    (d) Absolute alcohol

Ans. (c)

Note

The vehicle by which we can prepare a mother tincture is strong alcohol.

Also see

Homeopathic dilute alcohol

It is prepared by adding three parts of distilled water to seven parts of alcohol of specific gravity 0.8075 that is strong alcohol. Wherever alcohol is mixed with water, there is a rise in temperature with shrinkage in volume to an extent of approximately 3 per cent. A little more water may have to be added to make the specific gravity stand at 0.90. It is used in the preparation of attenuations of drugs in the decimal scale. Official dilute alcohol is prepared by adding equal volumes of water and strong alcohol of specific gravity 0.8075 to 0.8104. The specific gravity of dilute alcohol is between 0.9139 and 0.9169 at 20°C.
Ref: Pharmacy, Chapter 3, Hompath.

Rectified spirit

In India, a pharmacist usually gets rectified spirit of 60° O.P. This needs to be redistilled to the strength of absolute (99 per cent by volume) or strong (94.4 per cent by volume) alcohol.

Strong alcohol

Whenever alcohol is mentioned, it is this alcohol, with 95 per cent volume, also called Alcohol fortier, fortis or strong alcohol, in homeopathy. Its main features are:
    (a) It is a transparent, colourless, mobile, volatile liquid having a pleasing aroma and a burning taste.
    (b) It is neutral to all indicators when pure.
    (c) Specific gravity of this alcohol at 25° is 0.8075 to 0.8104.
    (d) It is miscible with water, acetone, chloroform, ether and many other organic solvents.
    (e) It is identified by adding 10 ml of 0.5 per cent v/v solution to 2 ml of 4 per cent w/v solution of NaOH, and then slowly allowing it to run along a solution of Iodine. A yellow precipitate will collect, giving the identification of alcohol.
    (f) Refractive index is $nD20$ 1.3637 to 1.3639.

In homeopathic pharmacy, this alcohol, which is known as strong alcohol, is used for the preparation of mother tinctures.
Ref: Pharmacy, Chapter 3, Hompath.

Absolute alcohol
In India, a pharmacist usually gets rectified spirit of 60° O.P. This needs to be redistilled to the strength of absolute (99 per cent by volume) or strong (94.4 per cent by volume) alcohol.
Ref: Pharmacy, Chapter 3, Hompath.

Q. 140. The meaning of abbreviation HS is ____ (RSC/08) (RPSC/08)
    (a)   At bed time
    (b)   In the morning
    (c)   Tomorrow evening
    (d)   Every hour

Ans. (a)
Note
The meaning of abbreviation HS is at bed time.

Also see
Abbreviation HS means 'Hora somni' in Latin. The English translation is 'at bedtime.'
Ref: Augmented Textbook of Homoeopathic Pharmacy, by D.D. Banerjee, page 360, second edition.

Q. 141. Mention which one is published by the Authority of Government of India (PSC/WB/93)
    (a)   Pharmacy
    (b)   Pharmacology
    (c)   Pharmacodynamics
    (d)   Pharmacopoeia

Ans. (d)
Note
Pharmacopoeia is published by the Government of India.

Also see
Homoeopathic Pharmacopoeia of India (HPI) is the official pharmacopoeia of India. Eight volumes have been published by the Government of India (Ministry of Health and Family Welfare) by the Homoeopathic Pharmacopoeia Committee. The Homoeopathic Pharmacopoeia Committee was appointed by the Central Government in September 1962 under the chairmanship of Dr B. K. Sarkar.

Volumes	No. of Monographs	Year of Publication
Vol. I of HPI	180	1971
Vol. II of HPI	100	1974
Vol. III of HPI	105	1978
Vol. IV of HPI	107	1984
Vol. V of HPI	114	1987
Vol. VI of HPI	104	1991
Vol. VII of HPI	105	1998
Vol. VIII of HPI	101	2000

Ref: Homoeopathic Pharmacy, by D.D. Banerjee, page 7 and 8, second edition.

Homoeopathic Pharmaceutical Codex.
By India. Homoeopathic Pharmacopoeia Committee; India. Homoeopathic Pharmacopoeia Laboratory India;
Book : National government publication
Language: English

Publisher: New Delhi: Homoeopathic Pharmacopoeia Committee, Government of India, Department of ISM and Homoeopathy, 2002

Homoeopathic pharmacopoeia of India (HPI)

By India. Homoeopathic Pharmacopoeia Committee; India. Ministry of Health; India. Ministry of Health and Family Welfare; India.

Book
Language: English
Publisher: Delhi : Controller of Publications, 1971 that is, 1974-<2006>

Q. 142. Mention the name of the drug which is to be triturated from a liquid substance (PSC/WB/93)
    (a)   Acidum benzoicum
    (b)   Guaiacum officinale
    (c)   Petroleum
    (d)   Iodium

Ans. (c)

Note

From the choice given above, the drug which is to be triturated from liquid substance is Pertroleum.

Also see

The drugs are prepated mainly by three processes:
    (1)   By preparying mother tinctures.
    (2)   By preparying mother solutions.
    (3)   By triturating medicinal substances with sugar of milk.

Methods of prepaing homeopathic drugs under Class VIII includes those medicinal substances which are neither soluble in purified water, nor in alcohol. They are subjected to trituration with sugar of milk.

Drugs in (Class VIII):
    (1)   *Animal sources*:
    (a)   *Venoms*: Crotalus horridus, Elaps corallinus, Lachesis mutus, Naja tripudians, Vipera berus, Bufo rana, Bungarus krait, etc.
    (b)   *Other animals*: Aranenunum
    (2)   *Vegetable sources*: Myristica sebifera, Croton tiglium, etc.
    (3)   *Nosodes*: Lysainum, Malandrinum; Vaccininum; Variolinum.
    (4)   *Minerals*: Petroleum.

Ref: Textbook of Homoeopathic Pharamcy, by Mandal and Mandal, page139 and 140, repring edition.

Q. 143. Mention the vehicle by which you can prepare a liniment____ (PSC/WB/91) (RPSC/08
    (a)   Distilled H_2O
    (b)   Alcohol
    (c)   Glycerine
    (d)   Olive oil

Ans. NA

Use your discretion – you can prepare a liniment by using the vehicle glycerine as well as olive oil.

Note

Glycerine

It is a trihydric alcohol, containing not less than 98 per cent of $C_3H_8O_3$ (HPI). It is a common constituent of all animal and vegetable oils and fats, for example, coconut oil, olive oil, tallow, cod-liver oil, etc. in small quantities. It is formed during alcoholic fermentation of sugars and is present in minute amounts in normal blood.

Uses:

External application – Glycerine is an excellent solvent for various things like fixed alkalies, several salts, vegetables, acids, pepsin, tannin, some active principles of plants, gums, etc. Hence it is a good

vehicle for applying these substances on the skin and over sores. It is used in various skin diseases like eczema, herpes, etc.
Ref: Augmented Textbook of Homoeopathic Pharmacy, by D.D. Banerjee, page 103, second edition.

Olive oil:
From the ripe fruits of Olea Europea, family Oleaceae, found in southern Europe and around the Mediterranean sea.

It is an organic compound, a fixed oil, consisting of glycerides of fatty acids, chiefly oleic acid and smaller amounts of linolic, myristic, palmetic and stearic acid.

Uses:
It is used as an excellent external application for burns and skin diseases. It is applied externally for getting a smoothening effect on superficial ulcers. On rubbing upon the skin, it renders the skin smoother, softer and more flexible. It is used in the preparation of liniments for extrenal application.
Ref: Augmented Textbook of Homoeopathic Pharmacy, by D.D. Banerjee, page 104 and 105, second edition.

Q. 144. Drug power of Class III is (MD/NIH/98) –
    (a)   1/6
    (b)   1/2
    (c)   1/10
    (d)   1/100

Ans. (a)
Note
    Drug power of Class III is 1/6.

Also see
    Drugs under Class III
    This class includes plants which are less juicy.
    Drug power: It comes to 1/6 c.c.
    Ref: Augumented Textbook of Homoeopathic Pharmacy, by D. D. Baneerjee, page 255, second edition.
    Ref: Text Book of Homoeopathic Pharmacy, by Mandal and Mandal, Chapter–Method of Preparing Homoeopathic Drugs, page 131.

Q.145 'Spanish fly' is the common name of _____ (MD/NIH/98)
    (a)   Causticum
    (b)   Cantheris vesicatoria
    (c)   Terebinthiniae oleum
    (d)   Tarentula cubensis

Ans. (b)
Note
Spanish fly is the common name of Cantharis vesicatoria.
Ref: Allen's Keynotes.

Also see

Common name	Medicine	Reference
Hahnemann's tinctura acris sine Kali	Causticum	Ref: Allen's Keynotes.
Oil of turpentine, a volatile oil	Terebinthiniae oleum	Ref: Allen's Keynotes.

| Cuban spider | Tarentula cubensis | Ref: Boericke's Materia Medica |
| Spanish fly | Cantharis vesicatoria | Ref: Allen's Keynotes. |

Q. 146 HPI has ____ (MD/NIH/98)
    (a) 4 volumes
    (b) 5 volumes
    (c) 6 volumes
    (d) 8 volumes

Ans. (d)

Note

HPI has 8 volumes.

Also see

HPI is the official pharmacopoeia of India. Eight volumes have been published by the Government of India (Ministry of Health and Family Welfare) by the Homoeopathic Pharmacopoeia Committee.
Ref: Augmented Textbook of Homoeopathic Pharmacy, by D.D. Banerjee, page 7 and 8, second edition.

Q. 147. Source of Sepia officinalis is ____ (PSC/WB/93)
    (a) Vegetable kingdom
    (b) Mineral kingdom
    (c) Animal kingdom
    (d) Nosodes

Ans. (c)

Note

Sepia officinalis belongs to the animal kingdom.

Also see

Sepia officinalis; Cuttle fish. (Mollusca)
Ref: Allen's Keynotes.

Q. 148. The best time to administer an antipsoric medicine to a female is ____ (PSC/WB/91)
    (a) Immediately before menses are expected
    (b) During menstrual flow
    (c) After third day, from the day menses have set in
    (d) At midcycle

Ans. (c)

Note

The best time to administer an antipsoric medicine to females is after the third day, from the day menses have set in.

Also see

The dose of antipsoric medicine must not be taken by females shortly before their menses are expected, nor during their flow; but the dose can be given, if necessary, four days that is, about ninety six hours after the menses have set in. But in case the menses previously have been premature or too profuse, or dragged on too long, it is often necessary to give on this fourth day a small dose of Nux vomica (one very small pellet, moistened with a high dynamization) to be smelled, and then, on the fourth or sixth day following, the antipsoric. However, if the female is very sensitive and has weak nerves, she ought, until she comes near her full restoration, to smell such a pellet once almost every seventy-two hours after the beginning of her menses, notwithstanding her continued antipsoric treatment.

Ref: An Affair to Remember.
http://www.hpathy.com/papersnew/verspoor-affair.asp

Q.149. Hahnemann recommended the potency___ as the best to investigate the medicinal power of a drug (PSC/WB/91)
    (a)   Mother tincture
    (b)   30 C
    (c)   Decimal
    (d)   LM

Ans. (b)

Note
Hahnemann recommended 30 centesimal potency as the best potency to investigate the medicinal power of a drug.

Also see
In aphorism 128 (fifth edition) Hahnemann actually recommends carrying out provings in 30C.

Aphorism 128
The most recent observations have shown that medicinal substances, when taken in their crude state by the experimenter for the purpose of testing their peculiar effects, do not exhibit nearly the full amount of the powers that lie hidden in them which they do when they are taken for the same object in high dilutions potentized by proper trituration and succussion, by which simple operations the powers which in their crude state lay hidden, and, as it were, dormant, are developed and roused into activity to an incredible extent. In this manner we now find it best to investigate the medicinal powers even of such substances as are deemed weak, and the plan we adopt is to give to the experimenter, on an empty stomach, daily from four to six very small globules of the thirtieth potentized dilution of such a substance, moistened with a little water, and let him continue this for several days.
Ref: http://www.sciencebasedmedicine.org/?p=21

In aphorism 129 he suggests, if sufficient symptoms are not exhibited, increase the number of 30C 'globules' taken rather than using a lower potency.

Aphorism 129
If the effects that result from such a dose are but slight, a few more globules may be taken daily, until they become more distinct and stronger and the alterations of the health more conspicuous; for all persons are not effected by a medicine in an equally great degree; on the contrary, there is a vast variety in this respect, so that sometimes an apparently weak individual may be scarcely at all affected by moderate doses of a medicine known to be of a powerful character, whilst he is strongly enough acted on by others of a much weaker kind. And, on the other hand, there are very robust persons who experience very considerable morbid symptoms from an apparently mild medicine and only slighter symptoms from stronger drugs. Now, as this cannot be known beforehand, it is advisable to commence in every instance with a small dose of the drug and, where suitable and requisite, to increase the dose more and more from day to day.
Ref: http://www.vithoulkas.com/content/view/1170/lang,en/

Q. 150. The limitation of drug proving _____ (PSC/91)
    (a)   Highly poisonous substances
    (b)   Proving cannot be extended with the gross pathological changes
    (c)   Non-availability of idiosyncratic provers
    (d)   None of the above

Ans. (b)
From the choices given above, the most suitable answer is (b).

Note
The limitation of drug proveing is that proving cannot be extended with the gross pathological changes.

Also see
Aphorism 137
The more moderate, within certain limits, the doses of the medicine used for such experiments are – provided we endeavour to facilitate the observation by the selection of a person who is a lover of truth, temperate in

all respects, of delicate feelings, and who can direct the most minute attention to his sensations – so much the more distinctly are the primary effects developed, and only these, which are most worth knowing, occur without any admixture of secondary effects or reactions of the vital force. When, however, excessively large doses are used there occur at the same time not only a number of secondary effects among the symptoms, but the primary effects also come on in such hurried confusion and with such impetuosity that nothing can be accurately observed; let alone the danger attending them, which no one who has any regard for his fellow-creatures, and who looks on the meanest of mankind as his brother, will deem an indifferent manner.
Ref: Organon of Medicine.

Q. 151. Largest source of drug substances in homeopathy is from____ (PSC/WB/93)
  (a) Animal kingdom
  (b) Plant kingdom
  (c) Mineral kingdom
  (d) Synthetic kingdom

Ans. (b)

Note
Largest source of drug substances in homeopathy is from the Plant kingdom.

Q. 152. Which of the following mother tinctures can be identified by smell only___ (PSC/WB/93)
  (a) Kreosotum
  (b) Nux vomica
  (c) Aconitum napellus
  (d) Camphora officinalis

Ans. (a)

Note
Camphora officinalis tincture can be identified by smell only.

Also see
Kreosotum
Has a penetrating, smoky odour.
Ref: Pharmacopoeia, by Dr P.N. Verma and Dr Indu Vaid, page 1470, second edition.

Camphora officinalis
It has a strong, characteristic and pungent odour.
Ref: Pharmacopoeia, by Dr P.N. Verma and Dr Indu Vaid, page 621, second edition.

Extended information
Camphora officinalis contains more of polycyclic aromatic compounds and therefore, it is more odourous pungent compound.
Ref: (AQ)

Q. 153. The process of dynamisation of the liquid drug is known as _____(PSC/WC/91)
  (a) Trituration
  (b) Hydrolysis
  (c) Succussion
  (d) Exsiccation

Ans. (c)

Note
The process of dynamization of liquid drugs is known as succussion.

Also see
Succussion
This is a process of potentization for all soluble substances, it may be in water or alcohol. Excepting a few cases, alcohol is used as a vehicle in most of the drug preparations. Water soluble drugs, when they attain 3C attenuation, are converted into alcoholic preparations. This transfer is necessary for the preservation of drug substances.
Ref: Pharmacy, Chapter 8, Hompath.

Extended information
Aphorism 270
Thus, two drops of the fresh vegetable juice mingled with equal parts of alcohol are diluted with ninety eight drops of alcohol and potentized by means of two succussions, whereby the first development of power is formed and this process is repeated through twenty nine more phials, each of which is filled three-quarters full with ninety nine drops of alcohol, and each succeeding phial is to be provided with one drop from the preceding phial (which has already been shaken twice) and is in its turn twice shaken[1], and in the same manner at last the thirtieth development of power (potentized decillionth dilution X) which is the one most generally used.
Ref: Organon of Medicine.

Q. 154. Common name of Abrotanum is _____.
    (a)   Monk's hood
    (b)   Southern wood
    (c)   Red onion
    (d)   Surukuku

Ans. (b)
Note
Common name of Abrotanum is Southern wood.
Also see

Common Name	Latin Names
Monk's hood	Aconitum napellus
Southern wood	Abrotanum
Red onion	Allium cepa
Surukuku	Lachesis mutus

Ref: Allen's Keynotes.

Bibliography

Books
- Augmented Textbook of Homeopathic Pharmacy by DR. D.D. Banerjee 2nd Ed. – B. Jain Publishers (P) Ltd., New Delhi
- Homeopathic Software: Hompath; Pharmacy
- Text Book of Homeopathic Pharmacy by Mandal & Mandal
- Organon 5th and 6th Edition – B. Jain Publishers (P) Ltd., New Delhi
- Chronic Diseases their Peculiar Nature & their Hom. Cure – B. Jain Publishers (P) Ltd., New Delhi.
- Pocket Manual of Hom. Materia Medica & Repertory – Boericke – B. Jain Publishers (P) Ltd., New Delhi.
- Allen's Key Notes – B. Jain Publishers (P) Ltd., New Delhi.
- Condensed Hom. Materia Medica and Repertory – J. H. Clarke – B. Jain Publishers (P) Ltd., New Delhi.

Websites
www.similima.com

Softwares
RADAR
HOMPATH

Chapter 6
PATHOLOGY

Q. 1. In which one of the following conditions is serum alkaline phosphatase not raised? (UPSC-02)
    (a) Hypothyroidism
    (b) Paget's disease
    (c) Hepatic disease resulting from certain drugs
    (d) Osteoblastic bone disease

Ans. (a)
Note
Normal Range: 44 to 147 IU/L
Raised in: Anemia, biliary obstruction, bone disease, healing fracture, hepatitis, hyperparathyroidism, leukemia, liver diseases, osteoblastic bone cancers, osteomalacia, paget's disease, rickets.
Lower than normal: Malnutrition, protein deficiency.

More information:
Elevation of serum alkaline phosphatase is found in diseases of bone, liver and in pregnancy.
Reference; Textbook of pathology by Harsh Mohan 4th Edition, chapter 17 – GIT, pg 572

Q. 2. Casoni's intradermal test is done for the diagnosis of (UPSC-02)
    (a) Schistosomiasis
    (b) Hydatid cyst
    (c) Fish tapeworm infestation
    (d) Fascioliasis

Ans. (b)
Note
The diagnosis of hydatid cyst is made by peripheral blood eosinophilia, radiologic examination and serological test such as indirect haemagglutination test and casoni's skin test.
Ref; Textbook of pathology by Harsh Mohan, 4th Edition, chapter 17 – GIT, pg 598

Q. 3. Leiomyosarcoma is a malignant tumour originating from (UPSC-02)
    (a) Bone marrow
    (b) Striated muscle
    (c) Fibrous tissue
    (d) Smooth muscle

Ans. (d)
Note
Leiomyosarcoma is a malignant smooth muscle neoplasm and may present as soft tissue tumours but about 95% leiomyomas and substantial fraction of the malignant counterparts as well occur within female genital tract.
Ref: Robbin's pathologic basis of disease, 4th Edition, Ch 28- The Musculoskeletal System, pg 1377

Q. 4. Consider the following features (UPSC-02)
    (a) Pleomorphism
    (b) Loss of polarity
    (c) Atypical mitosis
    (d) Atypical nuclear cytoplasmic ratio

Which of these features is / are helpful for confirmation of a malignant tumor?
    (a) a and b
    (b) c only
    (c) b, c, and d
    (d) a and d

Ans. (d)

Note
As a result of neoplasia, noticeable alteration in neoplastic cells are observed.
1. Pleomorphism- means variation in size and shape of tumour cells.
2. Nucleocytoplasmic changes- nuclei of malignant tumour cells are enlarged, disproportionate to cell size so that nucleocytoplasmic ratio is increased.
Reference; Textbook of pathology by Harsh Mohan, 4th Edition, Chapter 7- Neoplasia, Pg 180

Q. 5. During his study on filariasis, Manson observed that laboratory workers in the night shifts were better because they identified lots of microfilaria, while the day workers did not identify even a single microfilaria. Thus he excluded all the day workers from the blood test. This action was not justified because: (UPSC-02)
   (a) Microfilaria are formed during night
   (b) Mosquitoes introduce microfilaria during night
   (c) Microfilaria appears in peripheral blood at night
   (d) Microfilaria is destroyed by daylight

Ans. (c)
Note
Wuchereria bancrofti
Ref: Parasitology by K.D. Chatterjee, Ch- Nematohelminthes.

Q. 6. For the diagnosis of Hodgkin's disease during histological examination one should confirm the presence of (UPSC-02)
   (a) Lymphocytes
   (b) Reed sternberg cells
   (c) Macropolycytes
   (d) Shikata cells

Ans. (b)
Note
Hodgkin's disease is a disorder involving primarily lymphoid tissues. It is characterized morphologically by the presence of distinctive neoplastic giant cells called Reed sternberg cells, admixed with a variable inflammatory infiltrate.
Ref: Robbin's pathologic basis of disease, 4th Edition, chapter 15- Diseases of white cells, LN& spleen, pg 717
For the diagnosis of Hodgkin's disease the detection of Reed-Sternberg cells on histological examination of biopsy is diagnostic.

Q. 7. Cloudy swelling occurs in all except (UPSC-02)
   (a) Heart
   (b) Kidney
   (c) Liver
   (d) Lung

Ans. (d)
Note
In reversible cell injury, cellular swelling or cloudy swelling occurs. Cloudy swelling results from impaired regulation of cellular volume, especially for sodium. Injurious agent may interfere with regulatory mechanism and result in accumulation of sodium in cell which in turn leads to inflow of water and hence cellular swelling occurs. The affected organ such as kidney, liver or heart muscle is enlarged due to swelling.
Ref: Textbook of pathology by Harsh Mohan, 4th Edition, Chapter 2- Cell injury & Cellular adaptation, Pg 25

Q. 8. Cholesterol level in blood does not increase in case of (UPSC-02)
   (a) Nephrotic syndrome
   (b) Obstructive jaundice
   (c) Hypoparathyroidism
   (d) Hyperthyroidism

Ans. (d)

Note
Normal Value: 140 -220 mg/dl
Increased levels occur in: Familial hyperlipidemias, hypothyroidism
Nephrotic syndrome, uncontrolled diabetes.
Decreased levels may indicate: hyperthyroidism, liver disease, malabsorption, malnutrition, pernicious anemia, sepsis.
Ref: Essentials of Biochemistry by U. Satyanarayana, Pg-167

Also see

INCREASED LIPOPROTEIN CLASS	INCREASED LIPID CLASS	DISORDER
LDL	Cholesterol	Nephrotic syndrome, hyperthyroidism
LDL and VLDL	Cholesterol and triglycerides	Nephrotic syndrome, stress, diet

Ref: Robbin's pathologic basis of disease, 4th Edition, chapter 12-Blood Vessels, pg 561

Q. 9. The light brown perinuclear pigment seen on H & E staining of the cardiac muscle fibres in the grossly normal appearing heart of an 83 year old man at autopsy is due to deposition of (AIIMS/May-03)
 (a) Hemosiderin
 (b) Lipochrome
 (c) Cholesterol metabolite
 (d) Anthracotic pigment

Ans. (b)
Note
Lipofuscin is an insoluble pigment known as lipochrome and wear & tear or aging pigment. In tissue sections it appears as a yellow brown, finely granular intracytoplasmic pigment. It is seen in cells undergoing slow, regressive changes and is particularly prominent in liver and heart of ageing patients or patients with severe malnutrition and cancer cachexia.
Ref: Robbin's pathologic basis of disease, 4th Edition, chapter 1- Cellular injury & adaptation, pg 25

Q. 10. Dystrophic gene mutation leads to (AIIMS/May-03)
 (a) Myaesthenia gravis
 (b) Motor neuron disease
 (c) Poliomyelitis
 (d) Duchenne muscular dystrophy

Ans. (d)
Note
Duchenne muscular dystrophy is caused by a mutation of the gene that encodes dystrophin, a 427-kDa protein localized to the inner surface of the sarcolemma of the muscle fiber. The dystrophin gene is more than 2000 kb in size and thus is one of the largest identified human genes. It is localized to the short arm of the X chromosome at Xp21.
Ref; Harrison 15th Edition.
Duchenne muscular dystrophy is most common dystrophy. It occurs due to defective gene on short arm of X chromosome. The product of normal gene found within muscle fiber prove to be a 400- kilodalton protein called dystrophin, which is present in only very small quantities in normal muscle but is deficient in patients with Duchene dystrophy
Ref: Robbins pathologic basis of disease, 4th Edition, chapter 28- The Musculoskeletal System, pg 1369

Q. 11. A 60 year old man presented with fatigue, weight loss and heaviness in left hypochondrium for 6 months The haemogram showed Hb- 10 gm/dL, TLC 5 lakhs/mm³, platelet count 4 lakhs/mm³, DLC: neutrophil 55%, lymphocytes 4%, monocytes 2%, basophils 6%, metamyelocytes 10%, myelocytes 18%, promyelocytes 2% and blast cells 3%. The most likely cytogenetic abnormality in this case is (AIIMS/May-03)
 (a) t (1;21)
 (b) t (9;22)

(c) t (15;17)
(d) Trisomy 21

Ans. (b)

Note
Chronic myeloid leukemia presents with marked leucocytosis. It consists of excessive proliferation of myeloid cells of intermediate grade (myelocytes and metamyelocytes) and mature segmented neutrophils. Myeloblasts usually do not exceed 10% of cells in peripheral blood and bone marrow. Increase in basophils is characteristic. Cytogenetic studies show characteristic chromosomal abnormality called Philadelphia chromosomal abnormality formed by reciprocal translocation between long arm of chromosome 22 and part of long arm of chromosome 9 t(9,22)

Reference
Textbook of pathology by Harsh Mohan, 4th Edition, chapter 12- The Hematopoietic System, page 388.

Q. 12. A renal biopsy from a 56 year old woman with progressive renal failure for the past 3 years shows glomerular and vascular deposition of pink amorphous material. It shows apple-green birefringence under polarized light after Congo red staining. These deposits are positive for lambda light chains. The person is most likely to suffer from (AIIMS/May-03)
  (a) Rheumatoid arthritis
  (b) Tuberculosis
  (c) Systemic lupus erythematosus
  (d) Multiple myeloma

Ans. (d)

Note
In multiple myeloma which is plasma cell dyscrasia, generalized amyloidosis occurs and there is deposition of amyloid which has affinity for congo red stain. If stain section is viewed in polarized light, the amyloid characteristically shows apple-green birefringence.
Ref: Textbook of Pathology by Harsh Mohan, 4th Edition, Chapter 3- Immunopathology & amyloidosis, Pg-70

Q. 13. A 40 year old male has chronic cough with fever for several months. The chest radiograph reveals a diffuse reticulonodular pattern. Microscopically on transbronchial biopsy there are focal areas of inflammation containing epitheloid cell granuloma, Langerhans giant cells, and lymphocytes. These findings are typical for which of the following type of hypersensitivity immunologic responses (AIIMS/May-03)
  (a) Type I
  (b) Type II
  (c) Type III
  (d) Type IV

Ans. (d)

Note
Ref: Textbook of Pathology by Harsh Mohan, 4th Edition, Chapter 3- Immunopathology, Pg-57

Q. 14. An adult old man gets burn injury to his hands. Over few weeks, the burned skin heals without the need for skin grafting. The most critical factor responsible for the rapid healing in this case is (AIIMS/May-03)
  (a) Remnant skin appendages
  (b) Underlying connective tissues
  (c) Minimal edema and erythema
  (d) Granulation tissue

Ans. (a)

Note
Full thickness burn implies total destruction of the entire skin and dermal appendages, obliterating the possibility of epithelial regeneration save from the margins (implying the need for skin grafting).
Ref: Robbin's pathologic basis of disease, 4th Edition, chapter 9-Environmental pathology, pg 502

Q. 15. On sectioning of an organ at the time of autopsy, a focal, wedge-shaped firm area is seen accompanied by extensive hemorrhage, with a red appearance. The lesion has a base on the surface of the organ. This finding is typically of (AIIMS/May-03)
- (a) Lung with pulmonary thromboembolism
- (b) Heart with coronary thrombosis
- (c) Liver with hypovolemic shock
- (d) Kidney with septic embolus

Ans. (a)

Note
Pulmonary emboli cause infarction when circulation is already inadequate. The pulmonary infarct is classically haemorrhagic and appears as raised, red blue area in early stages. The red cells begin to lyse within 48 hours and infarct becomes paler and eventually red brown, eventually infarct converts into a scar. Histologically the diagnostic feature of pulmonary infarction is ischaemic necrosis of lung substance.
Ref: Robbins pathologic basis of disease, 4th Edition, Ch 16- The Respiratory System, Pg 762

Q. 16. "Tophus" is the pathognomic lesion of which of the following condition (AIIMS/May-03)
- (a) Multiple myeloma
- (b) Cystinosis
- (c) Gout
- (d) Eale's disease

Ans. (c)

Note
The tophus is the pathognomic lesion of gout- a mass of urates, crystalline or amorphous, surrounded by an intense inflammatory reaction, composed of macrophages, lymphocytes, fibroblasts and extraordinary foreign body giant cells.
Ref: Robbin's pathologic basis of disease, 4th Edition, chapter 28- The Musculoskeletal System, pg 1358

Q. 17. Infertility is a common feature in "Sertoli cell only" syndrome because (AIIMS/May-03)
- (a) Too many sertoli cells inhibit spermatogenesis via inhibin
- (b) Proper blood-testis barrier is not established
- (c) There is no germ cells in this condition
- (d) Sufficient number of spermatozoa are not produced

Ans. (c)

Note
The 'Sertoli cell only' is another name for 'Germ cell aplasia'. In this condition there are no germ cells so there cannot be any spermatogenesis.

Q. 18. The most common infectious agent associated with chronic pyelonephritis is (AIIMS/May-03)
- (a) Proteus vulgaris
- (b) Klebsiella pneumoniae
- (c) Staphylococcus aureus
- (d) Escherichia coli

Ans. (d)

Note
Chronic pyelonephritis is chronic tubulointerstitial disease resulting from repeated attacks of inflammation and scarring. The most common pathogenic organism is E.Coli followed in decreasing frequency by enterobacter, klebsiella, pseudomonas, and proteus.
Ref: Textbook of pathology by Harsh Mohan, 4th Edition, Chapter 19- The Kidney & Lower Urinary Tract, Pg-666

Q. 19. The presence of small sized platelets on the peripheral smear is characteristic of (AIIMS/Nov-03)
- (a) Idiopathic thrombocytopenic purpura
- (b) Bernard Soulier syndrome
- (c) Disseminated intravascular coagulation
- (d) Wiskott-aldrich syndrome

Ans. (d)

Note
Wiskott-Aldrich syndrome; This X-linked disease characterized by eczema, thrombocytopenia, and repeated infections, is caused by mutations in the WASP gene. The platelets are small and have a shortened half-life. Affected male infants often present with bleeding, and most do not survive childhood, dying of complications of bleeding, infection, or lymphoreticular malignancy.
Ref: Harrison's 15th Edition, Chapter- Disorders of the immune system.

Q. 20. In malignant hyperthermia the increased heat production is due to (AIIMS/Nov-03)
- (a) Increased muscle metabolism by excess of calcium ions
- (b) Thermic effect of food
- (c) Increased sympathetic discharge
- (d) Mitochondrial thermogenesis

Ans. (a)
Note
Malignant hyperthermia occurs in individuals with an inherited abnormality of skeletal-muscle sarcoplasmic reticulum that causes a rapid increase in intracellular calcium levels in response to halothane and other inhalational anesthetics or to succinylcholine. Elevated temperature, increased muscle metabolism, rigidity, rhabdomyolysis, acidosis, and cardiovascular instability develop rapidly. This condition is often fatal.
Ref: Harrison's 15th Edition, Chapter- Cardinal Manifestations and Presentation of disease.

Q. 21. A 7 year old boy presented with generalized edema. Urine examination revealed marked albuminuria. Serum biochemical examination showed hypoalbuminemia with hyperlipidaemia. Kidney biopsy was undertaken. On light microscopic examination, the kidney appeared normal. Electron microscopic examination is most likely to reveal (AIIMS/Nov-03)
- (a) Fusion of foot processes of the glomerular epithelial cells.
- (b) Rarefaction of glomerular basement membrane.
- (c) Deposition of electron dense material in the basement membrane.
- (d) Thin basement membrane.

Ans. (a)
Note
Minimal change disease accounts for 80% cases of nephrotic syndrome in children less than 16 years of age with preponderance in boys. By electron microscopy, the most characteristic feature of disease is identified which is diffuse flattening of foot processes of visceral epithelial cells (podocytes)?
Ref: Textbook of Pathology by Harsh Mohan, 4th Edition, chapter 19- The Kidney & Lower Urinary Tract, pg 654

Q. 22. The following cereals should be avoided in patients with celiac disease, except (AIIMS/Nov-03)
- (a) Wheat
- (b) Barely
- (c) Maize
- (d) Rye

Ans. (c)
Note
Celiac sprue is important cause of malabsorption and is characterized by significant loss of villi in small intestine and hence diminished absorptive surface. In this there is genetic abnormality resulting in sensitivity to gluten and its derivative gliadin, present in diets such as wheat, barley and rye. The symptoms are usually relieved on elimination of gluten from diet.
Reference; Textbook of pathology by Harsh Mohan, 4th Edition, chapter 17 – GIT, pg 551

Q. 23. Obstruction to the flow of CSF at the aqueduct of Sylvius will most likely lead to enlargement of (AIIMS/Nov-03)
- (a) All of the ventricles
- (b) Only lateral ventricle
- (c) Only fourth ventricle
- (d) Both lateral and third ventricles

Ans. (d)

Note
CSF is mainly produced by choroids plexus in the lateral, third and fourth ventricle. CSF formed in the lateral ventricles flows through the foramina of Munro to the third ventricle and from there by aqueduct of sylvius to fourth ventricle. The fluid then passes through foramina of Magendie and Luschka of the fourth ventricle to subarachnoid space of brain.
Reference: Textbook of pathology by Harsh Mohan, 4th Edition, chapter -27- The Nervous System, pg 854

Q. 24. CD-95 has a major role in (AIIMS/Nov-03)
    (a) Apoptosis
    (b) Cell necrosis
    (c) Interferon activation
    (d) Proteolysis

Ans. (a)
Note
Apoptosis is a form of coordinated and internally programmed cell death. The final outcome of apoptotic regulators in the programmed cell death involves Fas receptor activation. Cell surface receptor Fas (CD95) is present on cytotoxic T-cells. On coming in contact with target cell, the Fas receptor is activated which leads to activation of caspases and subsequent proteolysis.
Ref: Textbook of pathology by Harsh Mohan, 4th Edition, chapter 2- Cell injury & Cellular adaptation, pg 37

Q. 25. Tectal breaking is seen in (AIIMS/Nov-03)
    (a) Dandy-Walker malformation
    (b) Arnold-Chiari malformation
    (c) Aqueductal stenosis
    (d) Third ventricular tumor

Ans. (b)
Note
Arnold Chiari Malformation
It is the Herniation of tonsils of cerebellum and medulla oblongata through foramen magnum into vertebral canal. It causes blockage of foramen megendie and Lushaka leading to hydrocephalus.
There is dorsal kink in the cervicomedullary junction and breaking of the quadrigeminal plate. (Quadrigeminal plate is the dorsal part of the midbrain and it is also called as Tectum).

Q. 26. Which of the following is not a complication of infective endocarditis? (AIIMS/Nov-03)
    (a) Myocardial ring abscess
    (b) Suppurative pericarditis
    (c) Myocardial infarction
    (d) Focal and diffuse glomerulonephritis

Ans. (c)
Note
Cardiac complications of infective endocarditis are:
    -Valvular stenosis
    -Perforation, rupture and aneurysm of valve leaflet
    -Abscess in valve ring
    -Myocardial abscess
    -Suppurative pericarditis
    -Cardiac failure
Extracardiac complications are:
    -Petechiae, emboli, Focal necrotizing glomerulonephritis.
Ref: Textbook of pathology by Harsh Mohan, 4th Edition, chapter 11-The Heart, pg310

Q. 27. All of the following are the classical presentation of craniovertebral junction anomalies except (AIIMS/Nov-03)
    (a) Pyramidal signs
    (b) Low hairline

(c) Short neck
(d) Pupillary asymmetry

Ans. (d)
Note
The craniovertebral anomalies include anomalies at the base of skull and atlanto-occipital region. The S/S of craniovertebral junctional anomaly is related to the abnormalities and symptomatology referable to following structures:
   a. Pons
   b. Medulla
   c. Cervicomedullary junction and upper cervical spinal cord
   d. Lower cranial nerves
   e. Cervical nerve roots

Pupillary asymmetry usually results due to defects in 2nd (Optic) and 3rd (Occulomotor) cranial nerves.
The 2nd CN directly comes from the cerebrum and 3rd comes from midbrain therefore their symptoms or sings are not referable to they cannot be affected by craniovertebral junctional anomaly.

Q. 28. An Rh –ve woman became pregnant with Rh +ve fetus. Within few days after birth, the infant developed jaundice, ascites, hepatomegaly and edema. The likely substance(s) deposited in skin and sclera in jaundice is/are given below Which is the best possible Ans.? (AIIMS/Nov-03)
   (a) Biliverdin
   (b) Conjugated and unconjugated bilirubin
   (c) Unconjugated bilirubin
   (d) Conjugated bilirubin

Ans. (b)
Note
The above clinical presentation points to be a case of 'Erythroblastosis fetalis'. There is an excessive RBC breakdown and increase in unconjugated bilirubin in comparison to conjugated bilirubin. The both types of bilirubin gets deposited into the skin and sclera to produce yellow discoloration.

Q. 29. Which of the following is the most likely inheritance pattern in the pedigree given below? (AIIMS/May-04)

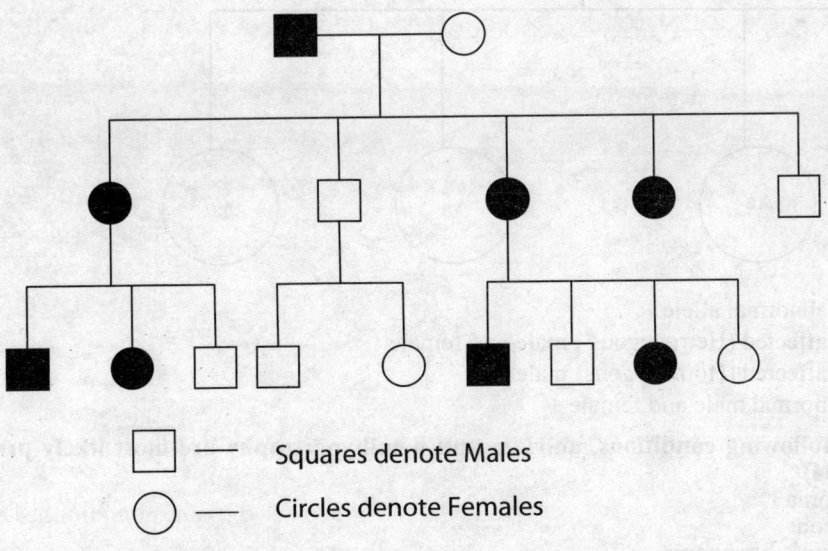

(a) Autosomal dominant
(b) Mitochondrial
(c) Autosomal recessive
(d) X-linked dominant

Ans. (d)
Note
The features suggestive of X linked dominant pattern are:
-A single abnormal X chromosome is capable to express the disease
-All the female offsprings of disease male will receive the abnormal X chromosome and express the disease, whereas the male offspring will be spared as they do not receive the X chromosome from their father.

-On the other hand mother having the disease can transmit the abnormal chromosome to both daughter and son equally.

Q. 30. If both husband and wife are suffering with achondroplasia, what are their chances of having a normal child (AIIMS/May-04)
(a) 0%
(b) 25%
(c) 50%
(d) 100%

Ans. (b)
Note
The achondroplasia is an autosomal dominant disease. Here both the parents have achondroplasia and out of four offsprings only one is the normal child. That suggests 25% is the change of having a normal child.

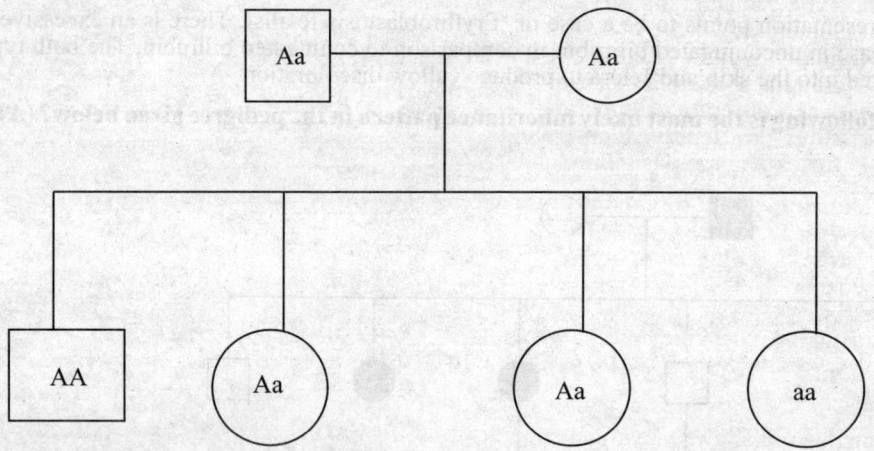

'A' - Denotes abnormal allele
aa - Denotes affected (Hetrozygous) male and female
AA - Denotes affected (Homozygous) male
Aa - Denotes normal male and female

Q. 31. In which of the following conditions, aniridia and hemihypertrophy are most likely present? (AIIMS/May/2004)
(a) Neuroblastoma
(b) Wilms' tumour
(c) Non-Hodgkin's lymphoma
(d) Germ cell tumour

Ans. (b)

Note
The wilm's tumour is associated with three groups of congenital malformations:
a. WAGR Syndrome; it consists of :
    -*Aniridia*
    -*Genital anomalies*
    -*Mental retardation*
b. Demus –Drash Syndrome; it consists of :
    -*Gonadal dysgenesis*
    -*Nephropathy leading to renal failure*
c. Bekwith-Wiedeman syndrome; it consists of:
    -*Enlargement of body organs*
    -*Hemihypertrophy*
    -*Renal medullary cysts*
    -*Abnormal large cells in adrenal cortex.*

Q. 32. Wire loop lesions are often characteristic for the following class of lupus nephritis (AIIMS/May-04)
    (a)   Mesangial proliferative glomerulonephritis(WHO class II)
    (b)   Focal proliferative glomerulonephritis (WHO class III)
    (c)   Diffuse proliferative glomerulonephritis (WHO class IV)
    (d)   Membranous glomerulonephritis (WHO class V)

Ans. (c)
Note
Wire loop lesions are characteristic of type IV or diffuse proliferative glomeruonephritis. Wire loop lesion denotes active disease and generally indicate a poor prognosis. However, wire loop lesions can also be seen in Type II focal type and Type V membranous type of glomerulonephritis.
WHO categorization of glomerular disease in systemic lupus erythematosus is:
    a. Class I: Normally by light electron and immunoflorescene.
    b. Class II: Mesangial glomerulonephritis
    c. Class III: Focal proliferative glomerulonephritis
    d. Class IV: Diffuse proliferative glomerulonephritis
    e. Class V: Diffuse membranous glomerulonephritis

Q. 33. Which of the following would be the best morphological feature to distinguish ulcerative colitis from Crohn's disease? (AIIMS/May-04)
    (a)   Diffuse distribution of pseudopolyps
    (b)   Mucosal edema
    (c)   Crypt abscesses
    (d)   Lymphoid aggregates in the mucosa

Ans. (a)
Note
In ulcerative colitis, the mucosa shows linear and superficial ulcers, usually not penetrating muscular layer. The intervening intact mucosa may form inflammatory pseudopolyps. Whereas in Crohn's disease the mucosa shows serpiginous ulcers while intervining surviving mucosa is swollen giving cobblestone appearance.
Ref: Textbook of pathology by Harsh Mohan, 4th Edition, chapter 17 – GIT, Pg- 545

Q. 34. In chronic viral hepatitis (AIIMS/May-04)
    (a)   Hepatitis A virus infection is a common cause in children.
    (b)   Morphological classification into chronic active hepatitis and chronic persistent hepatitis are important.
    (c)   Fatty change is pathognomic of hepatitis C virus infection.
    (d)   Grading refers to the extent of necrosis and inflammation.

Ans. (d)
Note
    (a)   HAV does not cause chronic hepatitis.
    (b)   Morphological classification into chronic persistent and chronic active hepatitis is no more valid.

(c) Fatty changes in hepatitis 'C' are moderated.
(d) Chronic hepatitis is defined as continuing or relapsing hepatic disease for more than six months with symptoms along with biochemical, serologic and histopathologic evidence of inflammation and necrosis. As such no grading in reference to extent of necrosis and inflammation is mentioned in TB of Pathology by Harsh Mohan.

Ref: Textbook of pathology by Harsh Mohan, 4th Edition, Chapter 18- The Liver, Biliary tract & Exocrine Pancreas, Pg 593

Q. 35. Mesangial deposits of monoclonal kappa/lambda light chains is indicative of (AIIMS/May-04)
    (a) Mesangioproliferative glomerulonephritis
    (b) Focal and segmental glomerulosclerosis
    (c) Kimmelsteil-Wilson lesions
    (d) Amyloidosis

Ans. (d)
Note
Amyloidosis is the term used for a group of diseases characterized by extracellular deposition of fibrillar proteinaceous substance called amyloid. Fibril proteins comprise about 90% of amyloid. AL protein of fibrils consists of polypeptides which are made of whole immunoglobulin light chains. In any case either lambda or kappa light chains form AL fibril protein.
Ref: Textbook of Pathology by Harsh Mohan, 4th Edition, Chapter 3- Immunopathology & amyloidosis, Pg-67

Q. 36. The liver biopsy in acute hepatitis due to hepatitis B virus is likely to show all of the following, except (AIIMS/May-04)
    (a) Ballooning change of hepatocytes
    (b) Ground glass hepatocytes
    (c) Focal or spotty necrosis
    (d) Acidophil bodies

Ans. (b)
Note
In acute hepatitis, liver biopsy shows:
    -Ballooning degeneration
    -Focal or spotty necrosis (dropout necrosis/ bridging necrosis)
    -Counciloman body or acidophil body
Whereas:
    -Ground glass appearance is not a part of acute hepatitis.
Ref: Textbook of pathology by Harsh Mohan, 4th Edition, chapter 18- The Liver, Biliary tract & Exocrine Pancreas, pg 593

Q. 37. Troponin-T is a marker of (AIIMS/May-04)
    (a) Renal diseases
    (b) Muscular dystrophy
    (c) Cirrhosis of liver
    (d) Myocardial infarction

Ans. (d)
Note
The enzyme most widely used in the detection of myocardial infarction is creatine kinase. More sensitive and cardio-specific enzymes are; CKMB, and Troponin –T&I.
Ref: Davidson's principle & practice of medicine, 19th Edition, Ch- Cardiovascular disease, pg 436

Q. 38. The following statements are true about tumor suppressor gene p 53 except (AIIMS/Nov-04)
    (a) It regulates certain genes involved in cell cycle regulation.
    (b) It's increased levels can induce apoptosis.
    (c) Its activity in the cells decreases following UV irradiation and stimulates cell cycle.
    (d) Mutations of the p 53 gene are the most common genetic alteration seen in the human cancer.

Ans. (c)

Note
The p53 is the tumour suppressor gene and is located on small arm of chromosome 17. p 53 is most common target for mutation or deletion in human tumours. Normally p 53 is a negative regulator of cell division. Mutation of p53 permits cells with damaged DNA to progress through cell cycle. Deletion of both alleles of p 53 is seen in 80% cases of colorectal cancer
Ref: Textbook of pathology by Harsh Mohan, 4th Edition, Ch 2- Cell injury & Cellular adaptation, pg 37, Chapter-7, Neoplasia, pg206

Q. 39. Increased susceptibility to breast cancer is likely to be associated with a mutation in the following gene (AIIMS/Nov/2004)
    (a)   p 53
    (b)   BRCA-1
    (c)   Retinoblastoma (Rb)
    (d)   H-Ras
Ans. (b)
Note
10% of human breast cancers can be linked directly to germline mutations. Several genes have been implicated in familial cases. The Li-Fraumeni syndrome is characterized by inherited mutations in the p 53 tumor suppressor gene, which lead to an increased incidence of breast cancer, osteogenic sarcomas, and other malignancies. Another tumor suppressor gene, *BRCA-1*, has been identified. Women who inherit a mutated allele of this gene from either parent have an approximately 60 to 80% lifetime chance of developing breast cancer and about a 33% chance of developing ovarian cancer. Men who carry a mutant allele of the gene have an increased incidence of prostate cancer but usually not of breast cancer.
Ref: Harrison's 15th Edition, Part six – Oncology and hematology – Section 1 – Neoplastic disorders – 89 Breast cancers.

Q. 40. Calcification of soft tissues without any disturbance of calcium metabolism is called (AIIMS/Nov-04)
    (a)   Ionotrophic calcification
    (b)   Monotrophic calcification
    (c)   Dystrophic calcification
    (d)   Calcium induced calcification
Ans. (c)
Note
Pathologic calcification implies the abnormal deposition of calcium salts, together with small amounts of iron, magnesium and other mineral salts. When deposition occurs in nonviable or dying tissues, it is known as dystrophic calcification; it may occur despite normal serum levels of calcium and in absence of derangements in calcium metabolism.
Ref: Robbins pathologic basis of disease, 4th Edition, Ch 1- Cellular injury & adaptation, pg 35

Q. 41. All of the following are examples of tumor markers, except (AIIMS/Nov-04)
    (a)   Alpha-HCG (α-HCG)
    (b)   Alpha-fetoprotein
    (c)   Thyroglobulin
    (d)   β2-microglobulin
Ans. (a)
Note
Alpha HCG is Human Chorionic Gonadotropin, a placental hormone.
Ref: Textbook of Pathology by Harsh Mohan, 4th Edition, Chapter-7, Neoplasia, Pg-214

Q. 42. Which of the following combinations of cytogenetic abnormality and associated leukemia/lymphoma is incorrect? (AIIMS/Nov-04)
    (a)   t(8;14) Burkitt's lymphoma
    (b)   t(15;17) AML-M3
    (c)   t(9;22) CML
    (d)   t(9;20) ALL
Ans. (d)

Note
ALL- acute lymphoblastic leukaemia. About 20 to 25% of pre B-cell ALL have t(1;19) translocation.
Ref: Robbins pathologic basis of disease, 4th Edition,Ch 15- Diseases of white cells, LN & spleen, Pg 724

Q. 43. Endoscopic biopsy from a case of H pylori related duodenal ulcer is most likely to reveal (AIIMS/Nov-04)
    (a)   Antral predominant gastritis
    (b)   Multifocal atrophic gastritis
    (c)   Acute erosive gastritis
    (d)   Gastric atrophy

Ans. (a)
Note
Helicobacter pylori gastritis- there is great evidence to suggest that increased density of H. pylori in the antrum is associated with greater likelihood of development of duodenal ulcer.
Reference; Textbook of pathology by Harsh Mohan, 4th Edition, chapter 17 – GIT, pg 527

Q. 44. Early gastric cancer generally indicates (AIIMS/Nov-04)
    (a)   Gastric adenocarcinoma detected early
    (b)   Gastric adenocarcinoma confined to the mucosa
    (c)   Gastric adenocarcinoma confined to the mucosa and submucosa
    (d)   Gastric adenocarcinoma less than 1 cm in size

Ans. (c)
Note
Early gastric carcinoma is term used to describe cancer limited to mucosa and submucosa.
Reference; Textbook of pathology by Harsh Mohan, 4th Edition, chapter 17 – GIT, pg 533

Q. 45. All of the following arteries are common sites of occlusion by a thrombus except (AIIMS/May-05)
    (a)   Anterior interventricular
    (b)   Posterior interventricular
    (c)   Circumflex
    (d)   Marginal

Ans. (d)
Note
Anterior ventricular artery (Left anterior descending coronary artery) is prone to occlusion leading to infarct involving ant wall of left ventricle near apex, anterior part of interventricular septum.
Posterior interventricular artery is a branch of right coronary artery and when occluded cause infarct of inferior wall of left ventricle posterior part inter-ventricular septum, inferior posterior right ventricle.
Circumflex artery infarct involves lateral wall of left ventricle at apex.
Marginal artery which supplies anterior wall of right ventricle is not a common area known to suffer any infarct.

Q. 46. The tissue of origin of the Kaposi's sarcoma is (AIIMS/May-05)
    (a)   Lymphoid
    (b)   Vascular
    (c)   Neural
    (d)   Muscular

Ans. (b)
Note
Kaposi's sarcoma is a malignant angiomatous tumour. Grossly the lesions in skin, gut, and other organs form prominent, irregular, purple, dome-shaped plaques or nodules. Histologically, in early patch stage, there are irregular vascular spaces separated by interstitial inflammatory cells and extravasated blood and haemosiderin.
Reference; Textbook of pathology by Harsh Mohan, 4th Edition, chapter 10, Blood vessels & lymphatics, pg 276

Q. 47. For which one of the following tumors gastrin is a biochemical marker? (AIIMS/May-05)
    (a) Medullary carcinoma of thyroid
    (b) Pancreatic neuroendocrine tumor
    (c) Pheochromocytoma
    (d) Gastrointestinal stromal tumor

Ans. (b)
Note
Zollinger Ellison syndrome is classically composed of triad of recalcitrant peptic ulcer disease, gastric hyper-secretion, and pancreatic islet cell tumour. Gastrin has been demonstrated in these tumours by radioimmunoassay.
Ref; Robbins pathologic basis of disease, 4th Edition, chapter 20- The Pancreas, pg1007

Q. 48. Which of the following is known as the "guardian of the genome"? (AIIMS/May-05):
    (a) p 53
    (b) Mdm2
    (c) p14
    (d) ATM

Ans. (a)
Note
The p 53 is a tumor suppressor gene. When DNA damage takes place, the p 53 level is increased and it also becomes activated, and assists in DNA damage control.

Q. 49. Chemotherapeutic drugs can cause (AIIMS/May-05):
    (a) Only necrosis
    (b) Only apoptosis
    (c) Both necrosis and apoptosis
    (d) Anoikis

Ans. (c)
Note
The chemotherapeutic drugs cause both necrosis and apoptosis. Apoptosis is a process by which single cells are removed from the living tissue.

Q. 50. An example of a tumour suppressor gene is (ALL INDIA-05)
    (a) Myc
    (b) Fos
    (c) Ras
    (d) Rb

Ans. (d)
Note
Cancer suppressor gene (anti-oncogene) – the mutation required to produce retinoblastoma involve the Rb gene
Ref; Robbin's pathologic basis of disease, 4th Edition, chapter 6- Neoplasia, pg 291

Q. 51. A simple bacterial test for mutagenic carcinogens is (ALL INDIA-05)
    (a) Ames test
    (b) Redox test
    (c) Bacteriophage
    (d) Gene slicing

Ans. (a)
Note
Test of a chemical compound for its carcinogenicity is usually done by mes test (test for mutagenicity). Ames test evaluates the ability of a chemical to induce mutation in the mutant strain of Salmonella typhimurium that cannot synthesise histidine.
Reference: Textbook of Pathology by Harsh Mohan, 4th Edition, Chapter 7- Neoplasia, Pg 194

Q. 52. The classification proposed by the International Lymphoma Study Group for non-Hodgkin's lymphoma is known as (ALL INDIA-05)
    (a)   Kiel classification
    (b)   REAL classification
    (c)   WHO classification
    (d)   Rappaport classification

Ans. (b)
Note
International Lymphoma Study Group in 1994 had proposed another classification called Revised European-American classification of Lymphoid neoplasms abbreviated as R.E.A.L. classification.
Reference: Textbook of pathology by Harsh Mohan, 4th Edition, Chapter 13- The Lymphoid System, pg 416

Q. 53. All of the following features are seen in the viral pneumonia except (ALL INDIA-05)
    (a)   Presence of interstitial inflammation
    (b)   Predominance of alveolar exudates
    (c)   Bronchiolitis
    (d)   Multinucleate giant cells in the bronchiolar wall

Ans. (b)
Note
Histologically, the hallmark of viral pneumonia is interstitial nature of the inflammatory reaction. The microscopic features are interstitial inflammation, necrotizing bronchiolitis, reactive changes (the lining epithelial cells of bronchioles and alveoli proliferate in the presence of virus and may form multinucleate giant cells) and in severe cases alveolar edema, scanty exudates.
Reference; Textbook of pathology by Harsh Mohan, 4th Edition, chapter 14- The Respiratory System, pg-443

Q. 54. Aschoff's nodules are seen in (ALL INDIA-05)
    (a)   Subacute bacterial endocarditis
    (b)   Libman-Sacks endocarditis
    (c)   Rheumatic carditis
    (d)   Non-bacterial thrombotic endocarditis

Ans. (c)
Note
The Aschoff's nodules are spheroidal or fusiform distinct microscopic structures occurring in interstitium of heart in rheumatic fever. They are specially found in vicinity of small vessels in myocardium and endocardium.
Ref: Textbook of Pathology by Harsh Mohan, 4th Edition, Chapter 11- The Heart, Pg 302

Q. 55. Pulmonary surfactant is secreted by (ALL INDIA-05)
    (a)   Type I pneumoncytes
    (b)   Type II pneumocytes
    (c)   Clara cells
    (d)   Bronchila epithelial cells

Ans. (b)
Note
The alveolar epithelium consists of two types of cells- Type 1 pneumocytes and Type 2 pneumocytes. Type 2 pneumocytes are essentially reserve cells which undergo hyperplasia when Type 1 pneumocytes are injured and are source of pulmonary surfactant rich in lecithin
Ref: Textbook of Pathology by Harsh Mohan, 4th Edition, Ch. 14- The Respiratory System, Pg-432

Q. 56. Which one of the following conditions commonly predisposes to colonic carcinoma? (ALL INDIA-05)
    (a)   Ulcerative colitis
    (b)   Crohn's disease
    (c)   Diverticular disease
    (d)   Ischemic colitis

Ans. (a)

Note
Colorectal cancer comprises 98% of all malignant tumours of large intestine. Presence of certain pre-existing diseases such as inflammatory bowel disease especially ulcerative colitis and diverticular disease for long duration increase the risk of developing colorectal cancer.
Reference: Textbook of pathology by Harsh Mohan, 4th Edition, Chapter 17 – GIT, pg 563

Q. 57. Fibrinoid necrosis may be observed in all of the following except (ALL INDIA-05)
(a) Malignant hypertension
(b) Polyarteritis nodosa
(c) Diabetic glomerulosclerosis
(d) Aschoff's nodule

Ans. (c)
Note
a. In malignant hypertension, microscopically necrotizing arteriolitis develops on hyaline arteriosclerosis and vessel wall shows fibrinoid necrosis
b. In polyarteritis nodosa, microscopically in acute stage there is fibrinoid necrosis in centre of nodule located in media
c. In diabetic glomerulosclerosis, hyaline arteriosclerosis is there but not fibrinoid necrosis
d. In Aschoff's nodule, the early stage of fibrinoid change is followed by proliferation of cells
Reference: Textbook of Pathology by Harsh Mohan, 4th Edition, Ch- 24-The Endocrine System Pg 807, Chapter 10, Blood vessels & lymphatics, Pg-265, Chapter 11- The Heart, Pg-305, Chapter19- The Kidney & Lower Urinary Tract, Pg- 674

Q. 58. In which of the following conditions bilateral contracted kidneys are characteristically seen? (ALL INDIA-05)
(a) Amyloidosis
(b) Diabetes mellitus
(c) Rapidly progressive (crescentic) glomerulonephritis
(d) Benign nephrosclerosis

Ans. (d)
Note
In benign nephrosclerosis, grossly both kidneys are affected equally and are reduced in size and weight
Ref: Textbook of Pathology by Harsh Mohan, 4th Edition, Chapter 19- The Kidney & Lower Urinary Tract, Pg- 673

Q. 59. All of the following vascular changes are observed in acute inflammation, except (ALL INDIA-05)
(a) Vasodilatation
(b) Stasis of blood
(c) Increased vascular permeability
(d) Decreased hydrostatic pressure

Ans. (d)
Note

In acute inflammation in early stages vasodilatation and increased hydrostatic pressure may result in some degree of transudation. This is soon overshadowed by increased vascular permeability and exudation of plasma proteins, the mark of acute inflammatory oedema.
Ref: Robbins Pathologic basis of disease, 4th Edition, Ch -2 - Inflammation & Repair, Pg-41

Q. 60. Which type of amyloidosis is caused by mutation of the transthyretin protein? (ALL INDIA-05)
(a) Familial mediterranean fever
(b) Familial amyloidotic polyneuropathy
(c) Dialysis associated amyloidosis
(d) Prion protein associated amyloidosis

Ans. (b)

Note
Transthyretin is a serum protein that transports thyroxine and retinol normally, while a variant of transthyretin is deposited in familial amyloid polyneuropathies and in senile amyloidosis.
Ref: Textbook of Pathology by Harsh Mohan, 4th Edition, Chapter -3-Immunopathology & amyloidosis, Pg-67

Q. 61. Which one of the following stains is specific for amyloid? (ALL INDIA-05)
    (a) Periodic acid schiff (PAS)
    (b) Alzerian red
    (c) Congo red
    (d) Von-Kossa
Ans. (c)

Note
All types of amyloid have affinity for congo red stain. The stain may be used on both gross specimens and microscopic sections; amyloid stains an orange colour. If the stained section is viewed in polarized light, amyloid characteristically shows apple green birefringence.
Ref: Textbook of Pathology by Harsh Mohan, 4th Edition, Chapter- 3-Immunopathology & amyloidosis, Pg-73

Q. 62. Which one of the following diseases characteristically causes fatty changes in liver? (ALL INDIA-05)
    (a) Hepatitis B virus infection
    (b) Wilson's disease
    (c) Hepatitis C virus infection
    (d) Chronic alcoholism
Ans. (d)

Note
Alcoholic liver disease is used to describe the spectrum of liver injury associated with acute and chronic alcoholism. There are three stages in alcoholic liver disease – alcoholic steatosis (fatty liver), alcoholic hepatitis and alcoholic cirrhosis.
Ref: Textbook of Pathology by Harsh Mohan, 4th Edition, Chapter 18 - The Liver, Biliary tract & Exocrine Pancreas, Pg- 603

Q. 63. The following is not a feature of Alzheimer's disease (ALL INDIA-04)
    (a) Neurofibrillary tangles
    (b) Senile (neuritic) plaques
    (c) Amyloid angiopathy
    (d) Lewy bodies
Ans. (d)

Note
Alzheimer's disease – the major microscopic features are neurofibrillary tangles, senile (neuritic) plaques, amyloid angiopathy, granulovacuolar degeneration and hirano bodies.
Lewy bodies is not a feature of Alzheimer's disease.
Ref: Robbins pathologic basis of disease, 4th Edition, Ch -The Nervous System, Pg- 1427

Q. 64. All of the following are good prognostic features for Hodgkin's disease, except (ALL INDIA-04)
    (a) Hemoglobin > 10 g/dl
    (b) WBC count < 15,000/mm3
    (c) Absolute lymphocyte count < 600/µl
    (d) Age < 45 years
Ans. (c)

Note
Following are poor prognostic factors for advanced Hodgkin's disease:
- a. Male gender
- b. Age > 45 years
- c. Stage IV disease
- d. Hemoglobin < 10.5 g/dl
- e. Leucocytosis with WBC > 15,000
- f. Lymphocytopenia either or both of
- i. Absolute Lymphocyte count < 600 /μl
- ii. Lymphocytes < 8% of WBC
- g. A serum albumin level < 4g/dl

Q. 65. A 60 year old male presented with acute chest pain of 4 hours duration. Electrocardiographic examination revealed new Q wave with ST segment depression. He succumbed to his illness within 24 hours of admission. The heart revealed presence of a transmural haemorrhagic area over the septum and anterior wall of the left ventricle. Light microscopic examination is most likely to reveal (ALL INDIA-04)
- (a) Edema in between normal myofibres
- (b) Necrotic myofibres with presence of neutrophils
- (c) Coagulative necrosis of the myocytes with presence of granulation tissue
- (d) Infiltration by histiocytes with haemosiderin laden macrophages

Ans. (c)

Note
In myocardial infarction- light microscopic changes observed are:
- By 12 hours; coagulative necrosis of myocardial fibers sets in and neutrophils begin to appear at margin of infarct.
- During first 24 hours; coagulative necrosis progresses further and the neutrophilic infiltrate at margin of infarct is slight.
- During first 48 to 72 hours, coagulative necrosis is complete and neutrophilic infiltrate is well developed.

Reference- Textbook of pathology by Harsh Mohan, 4th Edition, Chapter- 11- The Heart, Pg- 293

Q. 66. All of the following statements about Hairy cell leukaeumia are true, except (ALL INDIA-04)
- (a) Splenomegaly is conspicuous.
- (b) Results from an expansion of neoplastic T lymphocytes.
- (c) Cells are positive for Tartarate Resistant Acid Phosphatase (TRAP).
- (d) The cells express CD 25 consistently.

Ans. (b)

Note
Hairy cell leukemia is an uncommon form of chronic leukaemia in which there is presence of abnormal mononuclear cells with hairy cytoplasmic projections in the bone marrow, peripheral blood and spleen.These leukemic cells have characteristically positive staining for tartrate resistant acid phosphatase (TRAP).The controversy on origin of hairy cells whether these cells represent neoplastic T cells, B cells or monocytes, is settled with molecular analysis of these cells which assigns them B cell origin expressing CD19 and CD20 antigen. The disease often runs a chronic course and splenectomy is considered beneficial in many cases.
Ref: Textbook of Pathology by Harsh Mohan, 4th Edition, Chapter 12- The Hematopoietic System, Pg- 390

Q. 67. The blood in the vessels normally does not clot because (ALL INDIA-04)
- (a) Vitamin K antagonists are present in plasma
- (b) Thrombin has a positive feedback on plasminogen
- (c) Sodium citrate in plasma chelates calcium ions
- (d) Vascular endothelium is smooth and coated with glycocalyx

Ans. (d)

Note
The vascular endothelium is smooth and coated with glycocalyx.
Ref: Gray's Anatomy, Edition 38 Pg-1456.

Q. 68. A 37 year old multipara construction labourer has a blood picture showing hypochromic anisocytosis. This is most likely indicative of (ALL INDIA/04)
    (a)   Iron deficiency
    (b)   Folic acid deficiency
    (c)   Malnutrition
    (d)   Combined iron and folic acid deficiency

Ans. (a)
Note
In iron deficiency anemia, blood picture shows red cells in blood film are hypochromic and microcytic and there is anisocytosis and poikilocytosis.
Ref: Robbin's pathologic basis of disease, 4th Edition, Chapter- 8- Nutritional Disease, Pg- 460

Q. 69. Disseminated intravascular coagulation (DIC) differs from thrombotic thrombocytopenic purpura. In this reference the DIC is most likely characterized by (ALL INDIA-04)
    (a)   Significant numbers of schistocytes
    (b)   A brisk reticulocytosis
    (c)   Decreased coagulation factor levels
    (d)   Significant thrombocytopenia

Ans. (c)
Note
Disseminated intravascular coagulation is an acute, subacute or chronic thrombohemorrhagic disorder. It is characterized by activation of coagulation sequence that leads to formation of microthrombi throughout microcirculation of body. As a consequence of thrombotic diathesis, there is consumption of platelets, fibrin and coagulative factors and secondarily activation of fibrinolytic mechanisms.
Ref: Robbin's pathologic basis of disease, 4th Edition, Chapter- 14- Diseases of red cells & bleeding disorders, Pg- 698

Q. 70. The epitheloid cells and multinucleated gaint cells of granulomatous inflammation are derived from (ALL INDIA-02)
    (a)   Basophils
    (b)   Eosinophils
    (c)   CD4 T lymphocytes
    (d)   Monocytes-macrophages

Ans. (d)
Note
In chronic granulomatous inflammation, granulomas are small, 0.5 to 2 mm collections of modified macrophages called epitheloid cells usually surrounded by a rim of lymphocytes. Like all macrophages, epitheloid cells are derived from blood monocytes. Another feature of granuloma is presence of foreign body type giant cells and these are formed by coalescence of epitheloid cells.
Ref: Robbin's pathologic basis of disease, 4th Edition, Chapter- 2- Inflammation & Repair, Pg- 65

Q. 71. The following host tissue responses can be seen in acute infection, except (ALL INDIA-02)
    (a)   **Exudation**
    (b)   Vasodilatation
    (c)   Margination
    (d)   Granuloma formation

Ans. (d)
Note
Acute inflammation is of relatively short duration, lasting for a few minutes, several hours, or one or two days and its main characteristics are exudation of fluids and plasma proteins and the emigration of leucocytes,

predominantly neutrophils. In early stages, vasodilatation and increased hydrostatic pressure may result in some degree of transudation. However this is soon overshadowed by increased vascular permeability and exudation of plasma proteins, the mark of acute inflammatory oedema.
Ref: Robbin's pathologic basis of disease, 4th Edition, Chapter- 2- Inflammation & Repair, Pg- 40

Q. 72. The following feature is common to both cytotoxic T cells and NK cells (ALL INDIA-02)
    (a)   Synthesize antibody
    (b)   Require antibodies to be present for action
    (c)   Effective against virus infected cells
    (d)   Recognize antigen in association with HLA class II markers

Ans. (c)
Note
T Cell mediated cytotoxicity- in response to certain antigens including virus infected cells, tumor cells and incompatible tissue cells, the immune system responds by generation of cytotoxic T cells.
NK cells (natural killer cells): These cells are capable of lysing a variety of tumor cells, virus infected cells and some normal cells without proper sensitization.
Ref: Robbin's pathologic basis of disease, 4th Edition, Chapter- 5 – Diseases of immunity, Pg-183

Q. 73. In the intra-epithelial region of the mucosa of intestine, the predominant cell population is that of (ALL INDIA-02)
    (a)   B cell
    (b)   T cells
    (c)   Plasma cells
    (d)   Basophils

Ans. (b)
Note
The intra-epithelial region of mucosa of intestine has predominant population of T cells (Lymphocytes).

Q. 74. In primary tuberculosis, all of the following may be seen except (ALL INDIA-02)
    (a)   Cavitation
    (b)   Caseation
    (c)   Calcification
    (d)   Langerhan giant cell

Ans. (a)
Note
In primary tuberculosis, Ghon's focus is formed. Ghon's focus is an area of inflammatory consolidation circumscribed from surrounding lung parenchyma. The consolidated focus becomes granulomatous and then develops a soft casseous necrotic centre by second week. In most cases, primary tuberculosis does not progress and undergoes shrinkage with fibrosis, calcification and sometimes ossification with fibrous scarring and puckering of pleural surface.
Ref: Robbin's pathologic basis of disease, 4th Edition, Chapter- Infectious Diseases, Pg- 376

Q. 75. A myocardial infarct showing early granulation tissue has most likely occurred (ALL INDIA-02)
    (a)   Less than 1 hours
    (b)   Within 24 hours
    (c)   Within 1 week
    (d)   Within 1 month

Ans. (c)
Note
In myocardial infarction granulation tissue appears at the end of seven days. By the end of first week, the process of resorption of necrosed muscle by macrophages begins. Simultaneously, there is onset proliferation of capillaries and fibroblast from margin of infarct.
Ref: Textbook of Patholgoy, Harsh Mohan 4th Edition, Chapter 11, The Heart, Pg-293

Q. 76. A 10 year old boy, died of acute rheumatic fever. All the following can be expected at autopsy except (ALL INDIA-02)
    (a)   Aschoff's nodules
    (b)   Rupture of chordae tendinae
    (c)   Mc Callum patch
    (d)   Fibrinous pericarditis

Ans. (b)
Note
In rheumatic fever, rheumatic endocarditis, myocarditis and pericarditis occurs. In rheumatic mural endocarditis, Mac Callum patch is seen which is region of endocardial surface in the posterior wall of left atrium just above posterior leaflet of mitral valve. In rheumatic myocarditis, microscopically characteristic feature is presence of Aschoff bodies. In rheumatic pericarditis, grossly usual finding is fibrinous pericarditis.
Ref: Textbook of Pathology by Harsh Mohan, 4th Edition, Chapter- 11- The Heart, Pg- 302

Q. 77. All of the following are seen in asbestosis except (ALL INDIA-02)
    (a)   Diffuse alveolar damage
    (b)   Calcified pleural plaques
    (c)   Diffuse pulmonary interstitial fibrosis
    (d)   Mesotheliomas

Ans. (a)
Note
In asbestosis disease, histologically following changes are observed:
    -There is non specific interstitial fibrosis
    -Presence of asbestos bodies
    -Visceral pleural fibrosis
    -Fibrocalcific pleural plaques are most common lesions
Malignant mesothelioma is an uncommon tumour but association with asbestos exposure is present in 30% to 80% of cases with mesothelioma.
Ref: Textbook of Pathology by Harsh Mohan, 4th Edition, Chapter- 14- The Respiratory System, Pg-463

Q. 78. Macrophages containing large quantities of undigested and partial digested bacteria in intestine are seen in (ALL INDIA-02)
    (a)   Whipple's disease
    (b)   Amyloidosis
    (c)   Immunoproliferative small instetinal disease
    (d)   Vibrio cholerae infection

Ans. (a)
Note
Whipple's disease is an uncommon bacterial disease involving not only the intestines but also various other systems. Histologically the affected tissues show presence of characteristic macrophages containing PAS positive granules and rod shaped micro-organisms (Whipple's bacilli). These macrophages are predominantly present in the lamina propria of small intestine and mesenteric lymph nodes.
Ref: Textbook of Pathology by Harsh Mohan, 4th Edition, Chapter- 17 – GIT, Pg- 552

Q. 79. The histological features of coeliac disease include all of the following, except: (ALL INDIA-02)
    (a)   Crypt hyperplasia
    (b)   Increase in thickness of the mucosa
    (c)   Increase in intraepithelial lymphocytes
    (d)   Increase in inflammatory cells in lamina propria

Ans. (b)
Note
Celiac sprue is most important cause of primary malabsorption. The condition is characterised by significant loss of villi in the small intestine and hence diminished absorptive surface area. Histologically there is variable degree of flattening of mucosa. The surface epithelial cells are cuboidal or low columnar type. There may be

partial villous atrophy or subtotal villous atrophy characterized by flat mucosal surface. Lamina propria shows increased number of plasma cells and lymphocytes.
Ref: Textbook of pathology by Harsh Mohan, 4th Edition, Chapter- 17 – GIT, Pg- 551

Q. 80. In a chronic alcoholic all the following may be seen in the liver except (ALL INDIA-02)
- (a) Fatty degeneration
- (b) Chronic hepatitis
- (c) Granuloma formation
- (d) Cholestatic hepatitis

Ans. (c)
Note
In alcoholic liver disease, following morphological lesions are seen:
- Alcoholic steatosis (fatty liver)
- Alcoholic hepatitis
- Alcoholic cirrhosis

Ref: Textbook of pathology by Harsh Mohan, 4th Edition, Chapter- 18- The Liver, Biliary tract & Exocrine Pancreas, Pg- 601

Q. 81. Crescent formation is characteristic of the following glomerular disease (ALL INDIA-02)
- (a) Minimal change disease
- (b) Rapidly progressive glomerulonephritis
- (c) Focal and segmental glomerulosclerosis
- (d) Rapidly non prgressive glomerulonephritis

Ans. (b)
Note
Rapidly progressive glomerulonephritis (Crescentric glomerulonephrits) presents with an acute reduction in renal function resulting in acute renal failure in few weeks or months. It is characterized by formation of crescents outside the glomerular capillaries. Crescents are formed from proliferation of parietal epithelial cells lining Bowman's capsule with contribution from visceral epithelial cells and the invading mononuclear cells.
Ref: Textbook of pathology by Harsh Mohan, 4th Edition, Chapter- 19- The Kidney & Lower Urinary Tract, Pg-652

Q. 82. Necrotizing papillitis may be seen in all of the following conditions except (ALL INDIA-02)
- (a) **Sickle cell disease**
- (b) **Tuberculous pyelonephritis**
- (c) **Diabetes mellitus**
- (d) **Analgesic nephropathy**

Ans. (b)
Note
In tuberculous pyelonephritis, TB of kidney occurs due to haematogenous spread of infection from another site, most often from lungs. Grossly, lesions are often bilateral, usually involving medulla with replacement of papillae by caseous tissue.
Ref: Textbook of pathology by Harsh Mohan, 4th Edition, Chapter- 19- The Kidney & Lower Urinary Tract, Pg-668

Q. 83. Disease or infarction of neurological tissue causes it to be replaced by (ALL INDIA-02)
- (a) Fluid
- (b) Neuroglia
- (c) Proliferation of adjacent nerve cells
- (d) Blood vessel

Ans. (b)
Note
Infarction is the process of tissue necrosis resulting from some form of circulatory insufficiency. In case of infarct brain, there is liquefactive necrosis which heals by gliosis.
Ref: Textbook of pathology by Harsh Mohan, 4th Edition, Chapter- 4- Haemodynamic disorders, Pg- 111

Q. 84. Flat small vegetations in the cusps of both tricuspid and mitral valves are seen in (ALL INDIA-02)
    (a)   Viral myocarditis
    (b)   Libman Sacks endocarditis
    (c)   Rheumatic carditis
    (d)   Infective endocarditis

Ans. (b)
Note
Atypical Verrucous (Libman – Sacks) Endocarditis is characterized by sterile endocardial vegetations. Grossly, characteristic vegetations occur most frequently on mitral and tricuspid valves. The vegetations are small, granular, multiple and tend to occur on both surfaces of affected valves.
Ref: Textbook of pathology by Harsh Mohan, 4th Edition, Chapter- 11- The Heart, Pg- 307

Q. 85. Enzyme that protects the brain from free radical injury is (ALL INDIA-01)
    (a)   Myeloperoxidase
    (b)   Superoxide dismutase
    (c)   MAO
    (d)   Hydroxylase

Ans. (b)
Note
Free radicals are formed in physiological as well as pathological processes. However oxygen radicals are basically unstable and are destroyed spontaneously. The rate of spontaneous destruction is determined by catalytic action of certain enzymes such as superoxide dismutase, catalase and glutathione peroxidase.
Ref: Textbook of pathology by Harsh Mohan, 4th Edition, Chapter- 2- Cell injury & Cellular adaptation, Pg- 24

Q. 86. Autoimmune haemolytic anemia is seen in (ALL INDIA-01)
    (a)   ALL
    (b)   AML
    (c)   CLL
    (d)   CML

Ans. (c)
Note
In chronic lymphocytic leukemia, anemia is usually mild to moderate and normocytic normochromic in type. About 20% cases develop a Coomb's positive autoimmune haemolytic anemia.
Ref: Textbook of pathology by Harsh Mohan, 4th Edition, Chapter- 12- The Hematopoietic System, Pg- 389

Q. 87. All of the following are correct about thromboxane A2 except (ALL INDIA-01)
    (a)   Low dose aspirin inhibits its synthesis
    (b)   Causes vasoconstriction in blood vessels
    (c)   Causes bronchoconstriction
    (d)   Secreted by WBC

Ans. (d)
Note
Thromboxane A2 is a vasoconstrictor and bronchoconstrictor and enhances inflammatory cell function by causing platelet aggregation.
Ref: Textbook of pathology by Harsh Mohan, 4th Edition, Chapter- 5- Inflammation & Healing, Pg- 122

Q. 88. Which of the following complications is likely to result after several units of blood have been transfused (ALL INDIA-01)
    (a)   Metabolic alkalosis
    (b)   Metabolic acidosis
    (c)   Respiratory alkalosis
    (d)   Respiratory acidosis

Ans. (a)

Note
As sodium citrate is present in anticoagulant solution of blood which is metabolised to bicarbonate in liver causing metabolic alkalosis after several units of blood transfusion.

Q. 89. The mother has sickle cell disease and father is normal, chances of children having sickle cell disease and sickle cell trait respectively are (ALL INDIA-01)
(a) 0 and 100%
(b) 25 and 25%
(c) 50 and 50%
(d) 10 and 50%

Ans. (a)
Note
However the explanation is:
a. Sickle cell disease is the homozygous state of HbS(SS) where S stands for gene coding HbS
b. Sickle cell trait is the heterozygous state of HbS (SA) where A stands for absent gene.
c. Normal individuals have no gene for HbS (AA)
If the mother has sickle cell disease 'SS' and father is normal 'AA' all the offsprings will be 'SA' – thus % of sickle cell disease (SS) will be zero and that of sickle cell trait (SA) will be 100%.

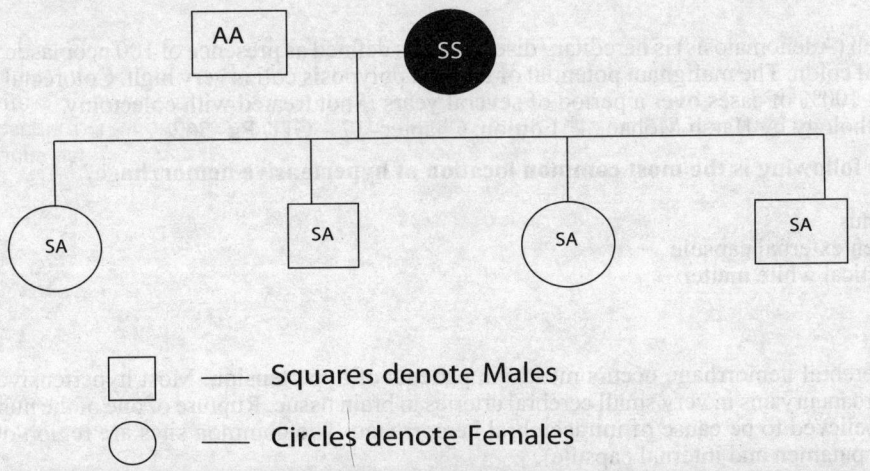

Q. 90. Father has a blood group B, mother has AB; children are not likely to have the following blood group (ALL INDIA/01)
(a) O
(b) A
(c) B
(d) AB

Ans. (a)
Note

BLOOD GROUP	ANTIGENS ON RED CELLS	NATURALLY OCCURING SERUM ANTIBODIES
AB	AB	None
A	A	Anti-B
B	B	Anti-A
O	O	Anti-A, Anti-B

Ref: Textbook of pathology by Harsh Mohan, 4th Edition, Chapter- 12- The Hematopoietic System, Pg- 404

Q. 91. An increased incidence of cholangiocarcinoma is seen in all of the following, except
    (a)   Hydatid cyst of liver
    (b)   Polycystic disease of liver
    (c)   Sclerosing cholangitis
    (d)   Liver flukes

Ans. (a)
Note
Complications of hydatid cyst include its rupture (e.g., into peritoneal cavity, bile ducts and lungs), secondary infection and hydatid allergy.
Ref: Textbook of Pathology by Harsh Mohan, 4th Edition, Chapter- 8- The Liver, Biliary tract & Exocrine Pancreas, Pg- 598

Q. 92. Strong correlation with colorectal cancer is seen in
    (a)   Peutz-Jeghers polyp
    (b)   Familial polyposis coli
    (c)   Juvenile polyposis
    (d)   Hyperplastic polyp

Ans. (b)
Note
Familial polyposis coli (Adenomatosis) is hereditary disease and is defined as presence of 100 neoplastic polyps on mucosal surface of colon. The malignant potential of familial polyposis coli is very high. Colorectal cancer develops virtually in 100% of cases over a period of several years if not treated with colectomy.
Ref: Textbook of pathology by Harsh Mohan, 4th Edition, Chapter- 17 – GIT, Pg- 562

Q. 93. Which of the following is the most common location of hypertensive hemorrhage?
    (a)   Pons
    (b)   Thalamus
    (c)   Putamen/external capsule
    (d)   Subcortical white matter

Ans. (c)
Note
Spontaneous intra-cerebral hemorrhage occurs mostly in patients of hypertension. Most hypertensives over middle age have microaneurysms in very small cerebral arteries in brain tissue. Rupture of one of the numerous microaneurysms is believed to be cause of intracerebral hemorrhage. The common sites are region of basal ganglia (particularly putamen and internal capsule).
Ref: Textbook of pathology by Harsh Mohan, 4th Edition, Chapter- 27- The Nervous System, Pg- 862

MICROBIOLOGY

Q. 94. Streptococcal toxic shock syndrome is due to the following virulence factor (AIIMS May 03):
    (a)   M protein
    (b)   Pyrogenic exotoxin
    (c)   Streptolysin O
    (d)   Carbohydrate cell wall

Ans. (b)
Note
The streptococcal toxic shock syndrome is caused due to the release of pyrogenic exotoxins or erythrogenic exotoxins. These exotoxins are produced only by few stains of beta hemolytic group A streptococci. Usually these toxins cause scarlet fever but sometimes these stains produce exotoxins that are super antigens. These super antigens (exotoxins) directly superstimulate T cells to pour out inflammatory cytokines. This causes streptococcal toxic shock syndrome.

MCQ's in Pathology

Q. 95. The virulence factor of Neisseria gonorrheae includes all of the following except (AIIMS May 03)
(a) Outer membrane proteins
(b) IgA protease
(c) M-proteins
(d) Pilli

Ans. (c)
Note
Neisseria gonorrhea contains several proteins called outer membrane proteins responsible for its pathogenecity.

Q. 96. A 'malignant pustule' is a term used for (AIIMS May 03)
(a) An infected malignant melanoma
(b) A carbuncle
(c) A rapidly spreading rodent ulcer
(d) Anthrax of the skin

Ans. (d)
It is the lesion in cutaneous anthrax. The lesion starts as papule, and then turns into vesicle and finally a painless round black lesion with a rim of edema. This lesion is called malignant pustule.

Q. 97. The following statements are true regarding botulism except (AIIMS May03)
(a) Infant botulism is caused by ingestion of preformed toxin.
(b) Clostridium botulinum A, B, C and F cause human disease.
(c) The gene for botulinum toxin is encoded by a bacteriophage.
(d) Clostridium baratti may cause botulism.

Ans. (a)
The botulinum toxin is heat resistant.

Q. 98. A 20 year old male had pain in abdomen and mild fever followed by gastroenteritis The stool examination showed presence of pus cells and RBC's on microscopy. The etiological agent responsible is most likely to be (AIIMS May03)
(a) Enteroinvasive E coli
(b) Enterotoxigenic E coli
(c) Enteropathogenic E coli
(d) Entroaggregative E coli

Ans. (a)
Note
The enteroinvasive strain E. Coli causes dysentery; blood in stool.

Q. 99. There has been an outbreak of food borne salmonella gastroenteritis in the community and the stool samples have been received in the laboratory. Which is the enrichment medium of choice? (AIIMS May03)
(a) Cary Blair medium
(b) VR medium
(c) Selenite "F" medium
(d) Thioglycholate medium

Ans. (c)
Note
The enrichment culture of choice for salmonella is Selenite 'F' medium.

Q. 100. Which of the following hepatitis viruses is a DNA virus? (AIIMS May 03)
(a) Hepatitis C virus
(b) Hepatitis B virus
(c) Delta agent
(d) Hepatitis E virus

Ans. (b)

Note
Hepatitis B is a DNA Virus.

Q. 101. All of the following are true regarding Hemophilus influenzae virus except (AIIMS Nov 03)
(a) It can be a part of the normal flora in some persons.
(b) The serotyping is based on the bacterial outer membrane proteins.
(c) It requires haemin and NAD for growth in culture medium.
(d) Type b is responsible for invasive disease.

Ans. (b)
Note
The serotyping is based on the bacterial outer membrane proteins.

Q. 102. A patient made a self-diagnosis of athlete's foot (tinea pedis) and began using a product advertised on television. The condition improved but did not clear and then the patient showed himself to a dermatologist. A skin scraping was sent to the laboratory for culture, including culture for fungi. The fungal culture yielded a slow growing colony, which produced a few small mitochondira. This is consistent with isolation of a dermatophyte of the genera (AIIMS Nov 03)
(a) Trichophyton
(b) Microsporum
(c) Epidermophyton
(d) Trichosporon

Ans. (a)
Note
Trichophyton have an abundant mitochondria which are arranged in clusters, whereas they have relatively scanty mitochondria.

Q. 103. All of the following are the most common nosocomial (infections acquired in hospitals) infections, except (AIIMS Nov 03)
(a) Staph aureus
(b) P. aeruginosa
(c) Enterobacteriaceae
(d) Mycobacterium

Ans. (d)
Note
Most common hospital infections are:
a. Staph aureus: It is mostly associated with pneumonia and infection of surgical wounds.
b. P. aeruginosa: Associated with nosocomial pneumonia.
c. Enterobacteriaceae: Associated with nosocomial pneumonia.

Q. 104. A 40 year old man underwent kidney transplantation for end stage renal disease. Two months after transplantation, he developed fever and features suggestive of bilateral diffuse interstitial pneumonia. Which one of the following is the most likely aetiological agent? (AIIMS Nov 03)
(a) Herpes simplex virus
(b) Cytomegalovirus
(c) Epstein-Barr virus
(d) Varicella-zoster virus

Ans. (b)
Note
Cytomegalovirus is mainly responsible for the infection occurring within one to four months, in patients undergoing renal transplant.

Q. 105. An elderly diabetic has left sided orbital cellulites CT scan of paranasal sinuses shows evidence of maxillary sinusitis. Gram stained smear of the orbital exudates shows irregularly branching septate hyphae. The following is the most likely aetiological agent (AIIMS Nov 03)
(a) Aspergillus
(b) Rhizopus

(c) Mucor
(d) Candida

Ans. (a)
Note
The septate hyphae is a classical feature of aspergillus and it can also cause sinusitis.

Q. 106. A patient, resident of Himachal Pradesh presented with a series of ulcers in a row, on his right leg. The biopsy from the affected area was taken and cultured on Sabauraud's dextrose agar. What would be the most likely causative organism ? (AIIMS Nov 03)
(a) Sporothrix schenckii
(b) Cladosporium spp
(c) Pseudoallescheria boydii
(d) Nocardia brasielensis

Ans. (a)
Note
The most common causative organism for causing erythmatous papules or nodules / ulcers in a linear arrangement along the lymphatic channel is a characteristic feature of Sprothrix schenckii. The organism are introduced as a result of trauma.
Ref: Harrison; 15th Edition. Section 9- Alterations in the Skin.

Q. 107. A 50 year old chronic alcoholic male agricultural worker presented with high grade fever of one week duration with spells of chills and rigor. Examination of the respiratory system revealed bilateral crepitations with scattered ronchi. Multiple subcutaneous nodules were found on the extensor surface of the left forearm, arm and left leg. Direct microscopy of the pus aspirated from the skin nodule revealed plenty of Gram negative bacilli with bipolar staining. Culture revealed distinct rough corrugated grey-white colonies on blood agar. The organisms were motile and oxidase positive The most likely diagnosis is (AIIMS Nov 03)
(a) Plague
(b) Melioidosis
(c) Bartonellosis
(d) Actinomycosis

Ans. (b)
Note
Melioidosis is a infection caused by *B. pseudomallei*. It causes a broad spectrum of acute or chronic, local or systemic, clinical or subclinical disease processes collectively called *melioidosis*.

B. pseudomallei is a free-living, small, motile, aerobic, gram-negative bacillary saprophyte normally found in soil, ponds, and rice paddies. Humans contract the disease through soil contamination of abrasions, ingestion, or inhalation leading to 'Pulmonary infection', which may give rise to hematogenous dissemination. This progression is more likely in chronically debilitated patients i.e., diabetes mellitus or alcoholism. Septicemic patients may present with severe tachypnea, confusion, headache, pharyngitis, diarrhea, and pustular lesions of the head, trunk, and extremities.
Ref: Harrison 15th Edition; Section 6 – Diseases caused by Gram- Negative Bactria.

Q. 108. Which one of the following statements is false? (AIIMS Nov 03)
(a) The presence of ingested erythrocytes is seen only in Entamoeba histolytica.
(b) Young adult male of low socioeconomic status are most commonly affected by invasive amoebiasis.
(c) A low iron content in the diet predisposes to invasive ameobiasis.
(d) The pathogenic and non-pathogenic strains of E histolytica can be differentiated by the electrophoretic study of zymodemes.

Ans. (c)
Note
The iron content of diet has no relationship with invasive ameobiasis.

Q. 109. The following phenomenon is responsible for antibiotic resistance in bacteria due to slime production (AIIMS Nov 03)
    (a)   Coaggregation
    (b)   Biofilm formation
    (c)   Mutation evolving an altered target site for antibiotics
    (d)   Mutation evolving a target bypass mechanism

Ans. (b)
Note
The phenomenon responsible for antibiotic resistance in bacteria due to slime production –that is by biofilm formation.
Slime is an extra-cellular secretion of some bacteria which remains around the bacteria providing a matrix in which formation of bio-film takes place. The bio-film formation helps in thin layer spreading of the bacterial colony and thus provides resistance to antibiotics by restricting access of drugs to the bacterium.

Q. 110. The protection against small pox by previous infection with cowpox represents (AIIMS May 04)
    (a)   Antigenic cross-reactivity
    (b)   Antigenic specificity
    (c)   Passive immunity
    (d)   Innate immunity

Ans. (a)
Note
The protection against small pox by previous infection with cowpox represents antigenic cross-reactivity.

Q. 111. Which of the following infestations lead to malabsorption? (AIIMS May 04)
    (a)   Giardia lamblia
    (b)   Ascaris lumbricoides
    (c)   Necator americana
    (d)   Ancylostoma duodenale

Ans. (a)
Note
Giardiasis range from asymptomatic carriage to fulminant diarrhea and malabsorption.
Ref: Harrison 15th Editon Section 17- protozoal infections.

Q. 112. Hepatitis C virus is a (AIIMS May 04)
    (a)   Togavirus
    (b)   Flavivirus
    (c)   Filovirus
    (d)   Retrovirus

Ans. (b)
Note
Hepatitis C virus is a Flavivirus.

Q. 113. A 23-year old male had unprotected sexual intercourse with a commercial sex worker. Two weeks later, he developed a painless, indurated ulcer on the glans that exuded clear serum on pressure Inguinal lymph nodes in both groins were enlarged and not tender. The most appropriate diagnostic test is (AIIMS May 04)
    (a)   Gram's stain of ulcer discharge
    (b)   Dark field microscopy of ulcer discharge
    (c)   Giemsa stain of lymph node aspirate
    (d)   ELISA for HIV infection

Ans. (b)
Note
The dark field microscopy of ulcer discharge for syphilis is the investigation of choice in the case sited above.

Q. 114. Which of the following is the most predominant constituent of sulphur granules of Actinomycosis (AIIMS May 04/01)
    (a)   Organisms
    (b)   Neutrophils and monocytes
    (c)   Monocytes and lymphocytes
    (d)   Eosinophils

Ans. (a)
Note
The organisms forming the colonies are recognized by sulphur granules of Actinomycosis.

Q. 115. An outbreak of streptococcal pharyngitis has occurred in a remote village. In order to carry out the epidemiological investigations of the outbreak it is necessary to perform the culture of the throat swab of the patients suffering from the disease. The transport media of choice would be (AIIMS Nov 04)
    (a)   Salt mannitol media
    (b)   Pike's media
    (c)   Stuart's media
    (d)   Cary Blair media

Ans. (b)
Note
The transport media of choice would be Pike's media (blood agar with crystal violet and sodium azide).

Q. 116. A fourteen year old boy is admitted with history of fever, icterus, conjunctival suffusion and hematuria for twenty days. Which of the following serological test can be of diagnostic utility? (AIIMS Nov 04)
    (a)   Widal test
    (b)   Microscopic agglutination test
    (c)   Paul Bunnel test
    (d)   Weil Felix reaction

Ans. (b)
Note
Severe leptospirosis, characterized by jaundice, renal dysfunction, and hemorrhagic diathesis, is referred to as *Weil's syndrome*.
A definite diagnosis of leptospirosis is based on seroconversion or a rise in antibody titer in the microscopic agglutination test (MAT). For a presumptive diagnosis of leptospirosis, an antibody titer of e"1:100 in the MAT or a positive macroscopic slide agglutination test in the presence of a compatible clinical illness is required. Antibodies generally do not reach detectable levels until the second week of illness.
Ref: Harrison, 15th Editon, Part seven – Infectious diseases.

Q. 117. The following methods of diagnosis utilize labelled antibodies except (AIIMS/May-05)
    (a)   ELISA (Enzyme linked immunosorbent assay)
    (b)   Hemagglutination inhibition test
    (c)   Radio immunoassay
    (d)   Immunofluorescence

Ans. (b)
The known facts that an antigen reacts only with antibody elicited by its own kind or by a closely related antigen is used in immunological technique now termed as labeled antibodies in order to locate and identify antigens in a given sample. Following methods use these labeled antibodies.
    a.   ELISA
    b.   Radio immunoassay
    c.   Immunofluorescence
Ref: Anantnaryan

Q. 118. Reduviid bug is a vector for the transmission of (AIIMS May 2005)
(a) Relapsing fever
(b) Lyme's disease
(c) Scrub typhus
(d) Chagas disease

Ans. (d)

Note
Reduviid bug is a vector for the transmission of Chagas' disease (American trypanosomiasis). Causative organism is a protozoan parasite *Trypanosoma cruzi*. In its acute form Chagas' disease is usually a mild febrile illness which resolves spontaneously, however, in the indeterminate phase of chronic Chagas' disease, the person remains infected for rest of the life. Few chronically infected patients develop cardiac and gastrointestinal lesions which may result in serious morbidity and even death.
Ref: Harrison 15th edition, section 17 – Protozoal infections.

Q. 119. All of the following are a part of the innate immunity except (AIIMS May 2005)
(a) Complement
(b) NK cells
(c) Macrophages
(d) T cells

Ans. (d)

Note
Innate immunity; it is the first line of defense against infectious agents. It is *nonspecific*, present since birth and is independent of prior exposure to a particular microorganism. It is devoid of immunological memory and is effective against a wide range of infectious agents. It has following components:
a. Compliment components
b. Cellular components – NK cells; Neutrophils, Eosinophils, Macrophages etc.
c. Antimicrobial peptides
d. Cytokines
e. Pattern recognition receptors (PRR)

If the innate immunity is breached then adaptive immunity or acquired immunity is called into action which is *specific* and mediated by antibody or lymphocytes. It provides immunological memory and is also acquired after exposure to an agent. Components of adaptive immune system are:
a. Cellular - thymus lymphocytes (T Cells).
b. Humoral - bone marrow derived B lymphocytes (B Cells)
c. Cytokines.

Q. 120. The following is the etiological agent of Rocky mountain spotted fever (AIIMS May 2005)
(a) Rickettsia rickettsii
(b) Rochalimaea quintana
(c) Rickettsia tsutsugamushi
(d) Coxiella burnetii

Ans. (a)

Note
The etiological agent of Rocky mountain spotted fever is 'Rickettsia rickettsii'. Discovered in the American West in the late nineteenth century, the Rocky Mountain Spotted Fever (RMSF) is at present documented in 48 states, Canada, Mexico, Costa Rica, Panama, Colombia, and Brazil. It is transmitted by *Dermacentor variabilis*, the American dog tick,
Ref: Harrison 15th Edition, Section 10- Rickettsia, Mycoplasma, and Chlamydia.

Q. 121. Intraspecies competition is the competition among (AIIMS May 2005)
(a) Species
(b) Individuals of a population
(c) Individuals of a community
(d) Populations and their regulatory factors

Ans. (b)

Note
Intraspecies competition is the competition among individuals of a population.

Q. 122. A woman with infertility receives an ovary transplant from her sister who is an identical twin what type of graft it is?
    (a)   Xenograft
    (b)   Autograft
    (c)   Allograft
    (d)   Isograft

Ans. (d)
Note
Isograft
A graft of tissue that is obtained from a donor genetically identical to the recipient.
Ref; http://www.thefreedictionary.com/isograft

Q. 123. The following statements are true regarding melioidosis except
    (a)   It is caused by Burkholderia mallei.
    (b)   The agent is a grain negative aerobic bacteria.
    (c)   Bipolar staining of the aetiological agent is seen with methylene blue stain.
    (d)   The most common form of melioidosis is pulmonary infection.

Ans. (a)
Note
Melioidosis is a infection caused by *B. pseudomallei*. It causes a broad spectrum of acute or chronic, local or systemic, clinical or subclinical disease processes collectively called *melioidosis*.

Q. 124. Which of the following viral infections is transmitted by tick?
    (a)   Japanese encephalitis
    (b)   Dengue fever
    (c)   Kyasanur forest disease (KFD)
    (d)   Yellow fever

Ans. (c)
Note
Kyasanur forest disease is a tick-born disease.
Ref: Harrison Table 198 -1.

Q. 125. Chlamydia trachomatis is associated with the following except
    (a)   Endemic trachoma
    (b)   Inclusion conjunctivitis
    (c)   Lymphogranuloma venereum
    (d)   Community acquired pneumonia

Ans. (d)
Note
Trachoma is associated with chronic conjunctivitis with infection by Chlamydia trachomatis.

Inclusion conjunctivitis is an acute ocular infection caused by sexually transmitted C. trachomatis.

Lymphogranuloma venereum is a sexually transmitted infection caused by C. trachomatis.
Ref: Harrison, 15t Editon.

Q. 126. The following statements are true regarding Clostridium perfringens except
    (a)   It is commonest cause of gas gangrene.
    (b)   It is normally present in human faeces.
    (c)   The principal toxin of C. perfringens is the alpha toxin.
    (d)   Gas gangrene producing strains of C. perfringens produce heat resistant spores.

Ans. (d)

Note
Cl. perfringens spores can usually be destroyed by boiling.
Ref: Harrison 15th Edition Section 5 Diseases caused by Gram Positive bactria 145. Gas gangrene.

Q. 127. The most common organism amongst the following that causes acute meningitis in an AIDS patients is
    (a)   Streptococcus pneumoniae
    (b)   Streptococcus agalactiae
    (c)   Cryptococcus neoformans
    (d)   Listeria monocytogenes

Ans. (c)
Note

Crytococcus neoformans; is a common cause of meningitis in AIDS.

L. monocytogenes is an intracellular pathogen. Predilection for causing illness in persons with deficient cell-mediated immunity. The organism can be found as part of the gastrointestinal flora in healthy individuals. The increased risk of *L. monocytogenes* infection in pregnant women may be due to both systemic and local immunologic changes associated with pregnancy. For example, local immunosuppression at the maternal-fetal interface of the placenta may facilitate intrauterine infection following transient maternal bacteremia.
Harrison 15th Edition, Infection caused by L. monocytogenes.
Streptococcus pneumoniae; is a common cause of community acquired bacterial meningitis.
Ref: Harrison, 15th Edition 372- Bactrial meningitis.
S. agalactiae in past was responsible for meningitis predominantly in neonates.
Ref: Harrison, 15th Edition 372- Bactrial meningitis.

Q. 128. A bacterial disease that has been associated with the 3 "Rs" i.e., rats, ricefields, and rainfall is
    (a)   Leptospirosis
    (b)   Plague
    (c)   Melioidosis
    (d)   Rodent-bite fever

Ans. (a)
Note
It suits most in case of leptospirosis as rat is a common rodent which is acts as carrier, its urine can contaminate the water for long period of time therefore ricefield worker can get the infection through the abrassed skin.

Q. 129. A child was diagnosed to be suffering from diarrhoea due to Campylobacter jejuni Which of the following will be the correct environmental conditions of incubation of the culture plates of the stool sample?
    (a)   Temperature of 42°C and microaerophilic
    (b)   Temperature of 42°C and 10% carbon dioxide
    (c)   Temperature of 37°C and microaerophilic
    (d)   Temperature of 37°C and 10% carbon dioxide

Ans. (a)
C. jejuni requires inoculation of fresh stool onto selective growth medium and incubation at 42°C in a microaerophilic atmosphere.
Ref: Harrison 15th Edition, 131. Acute infectious diarrheal diseases and Bacterial food poisoning.

Q. 130. Type I hypersensitivity is mediated by which of the following immunoglobulins?
    (a)   IgA
    (b)   IgG
    (c)   IgM
    (d)   IgE

Ans. (d)
Note
Coombs and Gell classified hypersensitivity reaction into 4 types:

Type 1 (Anaphylaxis, IgE or reagin dependant): Antibodies are fixed on the surface of tissue cells (Mast cells and basophils) in a sensitized individual. The antigen combines with the cell fixed antibody, leading to release of vasoactive amines which produce the clinical reaction.

Type 2 (Cytotoxic or cell stimulating): Initiated by IgG (rarely IgM) antibodies that react with cell surface or tissue antigen.

Type 3 (Immune complex or toxic complex disease): Here the damage is caused by antigen antibody complexes. These may precipitate in and around small blood vessels causing damage to the cells secondarily or on the membranes causing interference with their function.

Type 4 – (Delayed or cell mediated hypersensitivity): This is a cell mediated response. The antigen activates superficially sensitized CD4 and CD8 cells leading to lymphokine secretion.

Ref: Textbook of Microbiology, by: R. Ananthanarayan, 6th Edition, Chapter 18, Pg-150

Q. 131. Which of the following statements is true about hapten?
(a) It induces brisk immune response.
(b) It needs carrier to induce immune response.
(c) It is a T-independent antigen.
(d) It has no association with MHC.

Ans. (b)

Note
Haptens are substances that are incapable of producing antibodies by themselves but can react superficially with them. Haptens become immunogenic on combining with a larger molecule *carrier*. Haptens may be simple or complex.
Complex: These can precipitate with specific antibodies.
Simple: They are non precipitating.
Ref: Textbook of Microbiology, by: R. Ananthanarayan, 6th Edition, Chapter 11, Pg- 75

Q. 132. Regarding gas gangrene, one of the following is correct
(a) It is due to Clostridium botulinum infection.
(b) Clostridial species are gram-negative spore forming anaerobes.
(c) The clinical features are due to the release of protein endotoxin.
(d) Gas is invariably present in the muscle compartments.

Ans. (d)

Note
Clostridium consists of gram positive, anaerobic sporulating bacillus. The clostridia which usually cause gas gangrene are Clostridium perfringes and Cl. Welchii.
Gas gangrene is a rapidly developing oedematous myonecrosis occurring in connection with severe wounds of extensive muscle masses. It is associated with clostridial invasion and abundant exotoxin formation. The crushing of tissues and arteries produces anoxia of muscles. The clostridia elaborate toxins which further damage tissues. Lecithinases damage cell membrane and increases permeability leading to extravasation and increased tension in muscles. Collagenases also destroy collagen barriers in the tissues further damaging the tissues and muscles.
Ref: Textbook of Microbiology, by: R. Ananthanarayan, 6th Edition, Chapter 28, Pg- 230-236

Q. 133. The following statements are true about DPT vaccine except
(a) Aluminium salt has an adjuvant effect.
(b) Whole killed bacteria of bordetella pertussis has an adjuvant effect.
(c) Presence of acellular pertussis component increases its immunogenicity.
(d) Presence of H influenza type B component increases its immunogenicity.

Ans. (c)

Note
-Two preparations of DPT are in use: Formol toxoid and adsorbed toxoid. Formol toxoid is prepared by incubating the toxins with formaline at pH of 7.4 to 7.6.
Adsorbed toxoid is purified toxoid adsorbed onto insoluble aluminium compounds usually aluminium phosphate. It is much more immunogenic than formol toxoid.
-In the triple vaccine the Bordetella pertussis component acts as an adjuvant.

- Acellular vaccines containing the protective components of pertussis bacillus are now used in certain parts especially in case of older children.
- No reference could be found for effect of H influenza type B on DPT.

Ref: Textbook of Microbiology, by: R. Ananthanarayan, 6th Edition, Chapter 26, 38, page 220, 316

Q. 134. A 20 year-old man presented with hemorrhagic colitis The stool sample grew Escherichia coli in pure culture. The following serotype of E. coli is likely to be the causative agent
- (a) O157 : H7
- (b) O159 : H7
- (c) O107 : H7
- (d) O55 : H7

Ans. (a)

Note
Diarrheagenic E. coli is of 5 types:
i. Enteropathogenic E. coli: Causes diarrhea in infants and children. EPEC are identified by serotyping by their O and B Ag. (For eg. O26: B6, O55:B5, O111:B4)
ii. Enterotoxigenic E. coli: It is endemic in developing countries and tropics among all age groups in the local population. Serotypes responsible are: -O6, O8, O15, O25, O27, O167.
iii. Enetroinvasive E. coli: It resembles shigellosis ranging from mild diarrhea to frank dysentery.
iv. Enterohaemorrhagic E. coli: They produce toxins like verocytotoxin leading to diarrhea ranging from mild to fatal hemorrhagic colitis and hemolytic uraemic syndrome particularly in young children and elderly. The serotype responsible is O157:H7, O26:H1
v. Enteroinvasive E. coli: -Associated with persistent diarrhea especially in developing countries.

Ref: Textbook of Microbiology, by: R. Ananthanarayan, 6th edition, Chapter 30, page 256-257

Q. 135. A 30 year-old woman with a bad obstetric history presents with fever. The blood culture from the patient grows Gram-positive small to medium coccobacilli that are pleomorphic, occurring in short chains. Direct wet mount from the culture shows tumbling motility. The most likely organism is
- (a) Listeria monocytogenes
- (b) Corynebacterium sp
- (c) Enterococcus sp
- (d) Erysipelothrix rhusiopathiae

Ans. (a)

Note

Listeria monocytogenes
It is a small coccoid gram positive bacillus with a tendency to occur in chains. It exhibits a characteristic slow tumbling motility when grown at 25 degree Celsius but when grown at 37 degree Celsius it is immotile. Colonies are haemolytic on blood agar. It ferments glucose, maltose and L. rhamnose. It occurs as a saphrophyte in soil, water and sewage. Listerosis in humans presents as:
- Meningitis and meningoencephalitis in neonates and elderly
- Infection of pregnant women may lead to abortion or stillbirth
- Asymptomatic infection of the genital tract may lead to infertility
- It may also present as abscess, conjunctivitis, urethritis, pneumonia, infectious mononucleosis-like syndrome, endocarditis or septicemia.

Erysipelothrix rhusiopathiae
It is a slender non motile non-sporing non-capsulated gram positive rod. Human infection occurs by hands or fingers of persons handling fishes and animal products. The lesions are painful, oedematous and erythematous, usually involving the local lymphnodes and joints.

Ref: Textbook of Microbiology, by: R. Ananthanarayan, 6th Edition, Chapter 45, Pg- 372, 373

Q. 136. The most common agent associated with neonatal bacterial meningitis is
- (a) Haemophilus influenzae type b
- (b) Neisseria meningitidis
- (c) Streptococcus pneumoniae
- (d) Streptococcus agalactiae

Ans. (d)

MCQ's in Pathology

Note
Streptococcus agalactiae is a group B streptococcus and has assumed great clinical significance as the single most common cause of neonatal meningitis in the west. Infection usually occurs within a week of birth. Infection is usually acquired during birth from the maternal vagina. The most common early presentations are: -Septicemia, meningitis or pneumonia and is often fatal.
Other group B infections in neonates are: arthritis, osteomyelitis, conjunctivitis, respiratory infections, omphalitis and peritonitis.
Ref: Textbook of Microbiology, by: R. Ananthanarayan, 6th Edition, Chapter 23, Pg-195

Q. 137. In all of the following bacterial diarrheas toxins are implicated as a major pathogenetic mechanism, except
    (a)   Vibrio cholerae
    (b)   Shigella sp
    (c)   Vibrio parahaemolyticus
    (d)   Staphylococcus aureus

Ans. (c)
Note
V. parahaemolyticus is an enteropathogenic halophilic vibrio originally isolated as a causative agent of an outbreak of food poisoning due to sea food. It inhabits the coastal areas where it is found in fishes, crabs, shrimps and oysters. It resembles cholera vibrio and has a tendency to pleomorphism. No enterotoxin has been identified. The vibrio is believed to cause enteritis by invasion of the intestinal epithelium. It also causes acute diarrhea unassociated with food poisoning. Abdominal pain, diarrhea, vomiting and fever are the usual signs. Feces contain cellular exudates and blood. Cases are more common in summer and in adults than in children.
Ref: Textbook of Microbiology, by: R. Ananthanarayan, 6th Edition, Chapter 33, Pg- 292

Q. 138. A young pregnant woman presents with fulminant hepatic failure. The most likely aetiological agent is
    (a)   Hepatitis B virus
    (b)   Hepatitis C virus
    (c)   Hepatitis E virus
    (d)   Hepatitis A virus

Ans. (c)
Note

The Hepatitis E virus accounts for a large number of cases of enterically transmitted acute hepatitis in developing countries. It often appears as epidemics especially in the Indian subcontinent, Central America and North Africa. The source of infection is fecally contaminated drinking water and the environment. It has a fatality rate of 20-40% in pregnant women, especially in the last trimester of pregnancy.
The clinical presentation is similar to Hepatitis A.
Ref: Textbook of Microbiology, by: R. Ananthanarayan, 6th Edition, Chapter 59, Pg- 519

Q. 139. All of the following clinical features are associated with enteroviruses, except
    (a)   Myocarditis
    (b)   Pleurodynia
    (c)   Herpangina
    (d)   Hemorrhagic fever

Ans. (d)
Note
Enteroviruses belong to the family picornavirus and parasitize the enteric tract. They include the Poliovirus, Cox Sackie virus and Echovirus.

Cox Sackie virus produce a variety of clinical syndromes in humans.
    -Herpangina- Vesicular pharyngitis is a common clinical manifestation. It is a severe febrile pharyngitis with headache, vomiting and pain in abdomen. Characteristic lesions are small vesicles on fauces and posterior pharyngeal wall.
    -Aseptic meningitis

- Minor upper respiratory tract infection
- Orchitis
- Juvenile diabetes
- Epidemic pleurodynia or Bornholm's disease: febrile illness with a stitching pain in chest and abdomen
- Myocarditis and pericarditis
- Post viral fatigue syndrome

Ref: Textbook of Microbiology, by: R. Ananthanarayan, 6th Edition, Chapter 54, Pg- 453, 459, 460

Q. 140. Which of the following statements is true regarding ARBO viruses?
    (a)   Yellow fever is endemic in India.
    (b)   Dengue virus has only one serotype.
    (c)   Kyasanur Forest disease (KFD) is transmitted by ticks.
    (d)   Mosquito of Culex vishnui-complex is the vector of dengue fever.

Ans. (c)

Note
a. Yellow fever is a native of Africa and is spread by Aedes aegypti and from there it was transported to Europe and America. It presents with acute fever, chills, headache, nausea and vomiting. Signs are: slow pulse with high temperature, jaundice, hemorrhagic manifestations and albuminuria.
Ref: Textbook of Microbiology, by: R. Ananthanarayan, 6th edition, Chapter 57, page 490
b. Dengue virus has 4 serotypes: DEN 1, DEN 2, DEN 3, and DEN 4. It is transmitted by Aedes aegypti.
Ref: Textbook of Microbiology, by: R. Ananthanarayan, 6th edition, Chapter 57, page 491
c. Kyanusur Forest Disease is a tick borne hemorrhagic disease occurring in Karnataka state. It is characterized by fever, headache, conjunctivitis, myalgia and severe prostration. Some cases develop hemorrhages into skin, mucosa and viscera.
Ref: Textbook of Microbilogy, by: R. Ananthanarayan, 6th edition, Chapter 57, page 492
d. The mosquito Culex vishnoi complex transmits Japanese Enkephalitis.
Ref: Textbook of Microbiology, by: R. Ananthanarayan, 6th edition, Chapter 57, Pg 488

Q. 141. Laboratory diagnosis of viral respiratory tract infections can be established by all of the following tests, except
    (a)   Detection of virus specific IgM antibodies in single serum specimen.
    (b)   Demonstration of viral antigens by indirect immuno-fluorescence assay in nasopharyngeal washings.
    (c)   Isolation of viruses using centrifugation enhanced culture.
    (d)   Detection of viral hemagglutination inhibiting (HAI) antibodies in a single serum specimen.

Ans. (d)

Note
Laboratory diagnosis of viral diseases can be made by the following techniques:
a. Microscopy- It involves the use of direct and indirect fluorescent antibody techniques for examination of material from the lesions as well as for early demonstration of viral antigen in tissue cultures inoculated with specimens.
b. Demonstration of viral antigen: In cases where viral antigen is abundant in the lesions, its demonstration by serological methods such as precipitation in gel or immunoflorescence offers a rapid method of diagnosis. Also techniques like radioimmunoassay, ELISA, PCR have found a wide application.
c. Isolation of virus.
d. Serological diagnosis: Demonstration of a rise in titre of antibodies to a virus during the course of a disease is a strong evidence that it is the etiological agent.Examination of a single sample of a serum for antibodies may not be very useful except in cases where IgM specific tests are done. The serological tests done are: -neutralisation, complement fixation, ELISA, haemagglutination inhibition tests.
Ref: Textbook of Microbiology, by: R. Ananthanarayan, 6th Edition, Chapter 49, Page 421, 422

Q. 142. All of the following statements are true regarding poliovirus, except
(a) It is transmitted by feco-oral route.
(b) Asymptomatic infections are common in children.
(c) There is a single serotype causing infection.
(d) Live attenuated vaccine produces herd immunity.

Ans. (c)

Note

Polio virus is an enterovirus that parasitizes the GIT. It has three strains.
- Type 1 strain is the most common and causes epidemics.
- Type 2 strain causes endemic infections.
- Type 3 strains have also caused epidemics.

Immunity
- It is conferred by a infection and is type specific.

Transmission
- The virus is transmitted through faeco-oral route through ingestion.

Clinical features
- Following exposure 90-95% develop only inapparent infection.
- Clinical illness develops only in 5-10% of the individuals.
- Minor illness or abortive polio characterized by fever, headache, sore throat, malaise, etc.
- Sometimes the disease may progress to aseptic meningitis or *non paralytic poliomyelitis*.
- In very few cases assymetrical flaccid paralysis develops.

Two types of vaccines are available:
- Live attenuated vaccine developed by Sabin which not only confers systemic immunity but also gut immunity and hence along with protecting the individual also protects the community.

Ref: Textbook of Microbilogy, by: R. Ananthanarayan, 6th Edition, Chapter 54, Pg- 454-458

Q. 143. A 25 year old woman had premature rupture of membranes and delivered a male child who became lethargic and apneic on the 1st day of birth and went into shock. The mother had a previous history of abortion one year back. On culture, her vaginal swab growth of β-hemolytic colonies on blood agar was found. On staining these were found to be gram positive cocci. Which of the following is the most likely etiological agent?
(a) Streptococcus pyogenes
(b) Streptococcus agalactiae
(c) Peptostreptococci
(d) Enterococcus faecium

Ans. (b)

Note

Refer note for Q no 8

Q. 144. A farmer presenting with fever off-and-on for the past 4 years was diagnosed to be suffering from chronic brucellosis. All of the following serological tests would be helpful in the diagnosis at this stage, except
(a) Standard agglutination test
(b) 2 Mercapto-ethanol test
(c) Complement fixation test
(d) Coombs' test

Ans. (a)

Note

Blood cultures are the most definitive method of diagnosis of brucellosis.
a. The standard agglutination test is performed usually for acute infection. Most patients with brucellosis develop titers of 640 or more by 3-4 weeks of illness. Titres tend to decline after acute phase of the illness. The agglutination tests are positive in acute infection but are only weakly positive or even negative in chronic cases.

b. Cholera also causes agglutination, which may be differentiated from brucellosis by the agglutinin absorption test and also as they are removed by treatment with 2-mercapto-ethanol
c. The complement fixation test is more useful in chronic cases as it detects IgG antibody also.
d. As the serum often contains blocking antibodies, the most reliable method for obviating this is the antiglobulin or Coomb's test.

Ref: Textbook of Microbiology, by: R. Ananthanarayan, 6th Edition, Chapter 38, Pg- 321, 322

Q. 145. A man, after skinning a dead animal, developed a pustule on his hand. A smear prepared from the lesion showed the presence of gram positive bacilli in long chains which were positive for McFadyean's reaction. The most likely aetiological agent is
    (a)   Clostridium tetani
    (b)   Listeria monocytogenes
    (c)   Bacillus anthracis
    (d)   Actinomyces sp

Ans. (c)

Note
Cutaneous anthrax is most often found on exposed areas of skin. It result from contact with animals that have anthrax e.g., during skinning, butchering, or dissecting.
Harrison 15th Edition, Section 5- Diseases caused by Gram positive Bacteria.

Q. 146. Heat labile instruments for use in surgical procedures can be best sterilized by
    (a)   Absolute alcohol
    (b)   Ultra violet rays
    (c)   Chlorine releasing compounds
    (d)   Ethylene oxide gas

Ans. (d)

Note
Ethylene oxide is a colourless liquid which is gas at room temperature. It is due to alkylating action on amino, carboxyl, hydroxyl and sulphydryl groups in protein molecules. In addition, it also reacts with RNA and DNA.
It is used for sterelising heart-lung machines, respirators, sutures, dental equipment, books and clothings. It is unsuitable for fumigation because of its explosive nature. Materials which can be sterelised using it are: glass, metal, paper surfaces, clothing, plastics, soil some foods and tobacco.
Ref: Textbook of Microbiology, by: R. Ananthanarayan, 6th Edition, Chapter 3, Pg- 30

Q. 147. Thirty-eight children consumed eatables procured from a picnic party. Twenty children developed abdominal cramps followed by vomiting and watery diarrhea 6-10 hours after the party. The most likely etiology for the outbreak is
    (a)   Rotavirus infection
    (b)   Entero-toxigenic E. coli infection
    (c)   Staphylococcal toxin
    (d)   Clostridium perfringens infection

Ans. (c)

Note
The enterotoxin produced by staphylococcus is responsible for the manifestations of staphylococcal food poisoning: nausea, vomiting and diarrhea 2-6 hrs after consuming contaminated food containing the preformed toxin. The toxin is relatively heat stable, resisting 100 degrees for 10-40 minutes. Meat, milk and milk products cooked and left at room temperature after contamination with staphylococci are common items responsible.
Ref: Textbook of Microbiology, by: R. Ananthanarayan, 6th Edition, Chapter 22, Pg- 182

Q. 148. The following are true for Bordetella pertussis except
    (a)   It is a strict human pathogen.
    (b)   It can be cultured from the patient during catarrhal stage.
    (c)   It leads to invasion of the respiratory mucosa.
    (d)   Infection can be prevented by a acellular vaccine.

Ans. (c)

Note

Bordetella pertussis is a small, ovoid cocco bacillus. It is an obligate human parasite but infection can be produced experimentally in animals.

The pertussis toxin produced by the bacillus is believed to have an important role to play in the pathogenesis of whooping cough. The infection is limited to the respiratory tract and the bacteria do not invade the blood stream.

C/F

Catarrhal: Low grade fever, catarrhal symptoms and a dry irritating cough.

Paroxysmal stage: Intensity of cough increases and comes on in bouts followed by a characterized whoop.

Convalescence: Intensity and frequency of cough decreases.

Diagnosis: The bacilli are seen most abundantly during the early stage of the disease. Their number gradually decreases during the paroxysmal stage and during the convalescence they are not demonstrable.

Ref: Textbook of Microbiology, by: R. Ananthanarayan, 6th Edition, Chapter 37, Pg- 313-316

Q. 149. A chest physician performs bronchoscopy in the procedure room of the out patient department. To make the instrument safe for use in the next patient waiting outside, the most appropriate method to disinfect the endoscope is by
- (a) 70% alcohol for 5 min
- (b) 2% gluteraldelyde for 20 min
- (c) 2% formaldehyde for 10 min
- (d) 1% sodium hypochlorite for 15 min

Ans. (b)

Note

Gluteraldehyde is specifically effective against tubercle bacilli, fungi and viruses. It is less toxic and irritant than formaldehyde. It has no deleterious effect on the lens and cement of bronchoscope or cytoscope. It can be safely used to treat corrugated rubber anesthetic tubes and face masks, plastic endotracheal tubes, metal instruments and polythene tubing.

Ref: Textbook of Microbiology, by: R. Ananthanarayan, 6th Edition, Chapter 3, Pg- 29

Q. 150. Which of the following statements is true about endemic typhus
- (a) Is caused by R rickettsii.
- (b) Is transmitted by the bite of fleas.
- (c) Has no mammalian reservoir.
- (d) Can be cultured in chemical defined culture medium.

Ans. (b)

Note

Endemic typhus is caused by R. typhii which is transmitted by the rat flea, Xenopsylla cheopis. Humans acquire the disease through bite of the infected rat flea. Rickettsiae are unable to grow in cell free media. Growth generally occurs in cytoplasm of infected cells. They are readily cultivated in the yolk sac of developing chick embryo.

Ref: Textbook of Microbiology, by: R. Ananthanarayan, 6th Edition, Chapter 46, Pg- 380,381,385

Q. 151. The organism most commonly causing genital filariasis in most parts of Bihar and eastern UP is
- (a) Wuchereria bancrofti
- (b) Brugia malayi
- (c) Onchocerca volvulus
- (d) Dirofilaria

Ans. (a)

The most commonly causing genital filariasis in most parts of Bihar and eastern UP is Wuchereia bancrofti. In chronic bancroftian filariasis, the main clinical features are hydrocele, elephantiasis and chyluria. Elephantiasis may affect the legs, scrotum, arms, penis, vulva and breasts, usually in that order of decreasing frequency. The prevalence of chyluria is usually very low.

In chronic brugian filariasis is generally similar to bancroftian filariasis, but strangely the genitalia are rarely involved, except in areas where brugian filariasis occurs with bancroftian filalriasis.

Park and Park 16th Edition, Pg-201

Onchocerca volvulus may range from 1 to 10 cm in diameter and occur largely in persons bitten by *Simulium* flies in Africa. The nodules contain the adult worm encased in fibrous tissue. Migration of microfilariae into the eyes may result in blindness.

Ref: Harrison, 15th Edition- 128- Infection of skin muscle and soft tissue

Dirofilariae that affect primarily dogs, cats, and raccoons and *Brugia* parasites that affect small mammals occasionally infect humans incidentally. Because humans are an abnormal host, the parasites never develop fully. Pulmonary dirofilarial infection caused by the canine heartworm. ***Dirofilaria*** *immitis* generally presents in humans as a solitary pulmonary nodule. Chest pain, hemoptysis, and cough are uncommon

Ref: Harrison, 15th Edition- 221- Filariasis and related infections

Q. 152. Bacteria may acquire characteristics by all of the following except
(a) Taking up soluble DNA fragments across their cell wall from other species
(b) Incorporating part of host DNA
(c) Through bacteriophages
(d) Through conjugation

Ans. (b)
Note
Transmission of genetic material in the bacillus can occur by the following methods:
a. Transformation: It is the transfer of genetic material through the agency of Free DNA.
b. Transduction: Transfer of a portion of DNA from one bacterium to another by a bacteriophage. Transduction is limited not only to DNA but also episomes and plasmids may also be transduced.
c. Lysogenic conversion: The bacteriophage DNA becomes integrated with the bacterial chromosome as the prophage, which multiplies synchronously with the host DNA and is transferred to the daughter cells. This process is called as *lysogeny*.
d. Conjugation: It is a process whereby a donor bacterium makes physical contact with a recipient bacterium and transfers genetic elements into it.
e. Tranfer can also take place by F factor, colicinogenic factor.

Ref: Textbook of Microbiology, by: R. Ananthanarayan, 6th Edition, Chapter 8, Pg- 53-54

Q. 153. Neonatal thymectomy leads to (ALL INDIA/02)
(a) Decreased size of germinal center
(b) Decreased size of paracortical areas
(c) Increased antibody production by B cells
(d) Dcreased bone marrow production of lymphocytes

Ans. (b)
Note
Thymus gland is the major site for lymphocyte proliferation. T lymphocytes are selectively seeded into certain sites in the peripheral lymphatic tissues being found in the white pulp of the spleen, around the central arterioles and paracortical areas of the L.N. these regions have been termed as thymus dependant as they are grossly depleted in neonatal thymomectomy.

Ref: Textbook of Microbiology, by: R. Ananthanarayan, 6th edition, Chapter 15, page 110,111

Q. 154. Staphylococcus aureus differs from staphylococcus epidermidis by (ALL INDIA/02)
(a) Is coagulase positive
(b) Forms white colonies
(c) A common cause of UTI
(d) Causes endocarditis in drug addicts

Ans. (a)
Note
Staphylococcus aureus is coagulase positive, whereas staphylococcus epidermidis is coagulase negative.
Ref: Textbook of Microbiology, by: R. Ananthanarayan, 6th Edition, Chapter 22, Pg- 181, 185,186.

MCQ's in Pathology

Q. 155. Positive Shick's test indicates that person is (ALL INDIA/02)
  (a) Immune to diphtheria
  (b) Hypersensitive to diphtheria
  (c) Susceptible to diphtheria
  (d) Carrier of diphtheria

Ans. (c)

Note
Shick's test is the susceptibility test for diphtheria. It is done by injecting 0.2 ml of diphtheria toxin in left forearm (test arm) intra-dermally. Simultaneously 0.2 ml of heat inactivated toxin is injected in the right form arm (Control arm) first reading is taken after 24 – 48 hours and second reading after 5 – 7 days.

Type of Reaction	Observation	Interpretation
Positive reaction	No reaction on right arm. Circumscribed erythmatous reaction on let arm.	No hypersensitivity. Patient is susceptible.
Negative reaction	No reaction on either arm.	No hypersensitivity. No susceptibility.
Pseudo-Reaction	Diffuse erythmatous reaction on both arms. (which appears in 24 hours and fades by 4th day).	Patient is hypersensitive but not susceptible.
Combined Reaction	Pseudo reaction, followed by positive reaction on left arm.	Patient is susceptible as well as hypersensitive.

Ref: Textbook of Microbiology, by: R. Ananthanarayan 6th Edition. Pg-214

Q. 156. In a patient with typhoid, diagnosis after 15 days of onset of fever is best done by (ALL INDIA/02)
  (a) Blood culture
  (b) Widal
  (c) Stool culture
  (d) Urine culture

Ans. (b)
Investigations in case of suspected case of typhoid are
First week:
  -TLC: leucopenia
  -DLC: relative lymphocytosis
  -Blood culture: positive at end of week
Second week:
  -Widal test: positive
  -Blood culture: positive
Third week:
  -Widal test: positive
  -Stool culture: positive
  -Urine culture: positive
Diagnostic validity of widal test:
  -A widal test done in the 1st week of fever, may serve as baseline, and by itself is not diagnostic of enteric fever.
  -Only a four fold rise in the antibody titers of both the O type and the specific H type should be considered as definitely suggestive of enteric fever.
  -However widal in the 3rd week is quite suggestive investigation.

Q. 157. Which of the following is transmitted by rat urine? (ALL INDIA/02)
    (a)   Leptospira
    (b)   Listeria
    (c)   Legionella
    (d)   Mycoplasma

Ans. (a)
Note

Leptospirosis is a zoonosis having a worldwide distribution. It affects about 160 mammalian species. Rats are the most important reservoir. However, other wild mammals, dogs, fish, and birds may also harbor these microorganisms. Leptospires can persist in the renal tubules for years. Transmission of leptospira occurs from direct contact with urine, of an infected animal, or exposure to a contaminated environment. Human-to-human transmission is rare. Leptospira passed in the urine and can survive in water for many months, therefore the water is an important vehicle in their transmission.
Ref: Harrison, 15ht Edition, Part sever – Infectious diseases, Section 9- Spirocheatal diseases. 174. Leptospirosis.

Q. 158. All of the following are true about listeria except (ALL INDIA/02)
    (a)   Transmitted by contaminated milk
    (b)   Gram negative bacteria
    (c)   Causes abortion in pregnancy
    (d)   Causes meningitis in neonates

Ans. (b)
Note

It is a gram positive rod. Human disease due to *L. monocytogenes* mostly occurs in pregnancy or immunosuppression caused by illness or medication. Human listeriosis are attributable to the food-borne transmission. It causes invasive syndromes, such as meningitis, sepsis, chorioamnionitis, and stillbirth.
Ref: Harrison 15th Edition – Part Seve –Infectious diseases. Section 5 – Diseases caused by gram positive bacteria 142. Infections caused by Listeria

Q. 159. Which of the following statement is true about bacteroides (ALL INDIA/02)
    (a)   It is gram positive bacilli.
    (b)   It is strictly aerobic.
    (c)   It may cause peritonitis.
    (d)   Presence in stool culture indicates need for treatment.

Ans. (c)
Note
Most anaerobic gram –negative bacilli found in human infections are the members of 'Bacteroid family'. Members of this group are part of normal bowel flora.
Harrison, 15th Edition, Section 7 – Miscellaneous Bacterial Infections 167. Infections due to mixed anaerobic organisms.

Q. 160. Heat stable enterotoxin causing food poisoning is caused by all the following except (ALL INDIA/02)
    (a)   Bacillus cereus
    (b)   Yersinia enterocolitica
    (c)   Staphylococcus
    (d)   Clostridium perfringens

Ans. (d)
Note
Bacillus cereus, Staphylococcus and Yersinia enterocolitica produce enterotoxins which are heat stable, whereas Clostridium perfringens has been shown to produce a heat labile enterotoxin.
Ref: Ananthnarayan 6th Edition Pg-182, 233

MCQ's in Pathology

Q. 161. HIV virus contains (ALL INDIA/02)
    (a)   Single stranded DNA
    (b)   Single stranded RNA
    (c)   Double stranded DNA
    (d)   Double stranded RNA

Ans. (b)
Note
HIV virus contains single stranded RNA.
Ref: Ananthnarayan 6th Pg-540

Q. 162. Regarding HIV which of the following is not true (ALL INDIA/02)
    (a)   It is a DNA retrovirus.
    (b)   Contains reverse transcriptase.
    (c)   May infect host CD_4 cells other than T-lymphocytes.
    (d)   Causes a reduction in host CD_4 cells at late stage of disease.

Ans. (a)
Note
The HIV is a RNA virus.
Ref: Ananthnarayan 6th Pg-540

Q. 163. CMV retinitis in HIV occurs when the CD_4 counts fall below (ALL INDIA/02)
    (a)   50
    (b)   100
    (c)   200
    (d)   150

Ans. (a)
Note
AIDS patients are predisposed to CMV retinitis. HIV Patients at high risk of CMV retinitis when CD_4+ T cell count <100/uL, therefore they must undergo an ophthalmologic examination every 3 to 6 months. Most of the cases of CMV retinitis occur when a CD_4+ T cell count <50/uL. CMV retinitis is a painless, progressive loss of vision. Patients C/O blurred vision, and floaters. Both eyes are affected. The characteristic retinal appearance is that of perivascular hemorrhage and exudates.
Harrison 15th Edition, - 309- Human Immunodefiiency virus.

Q. 164. Epstein barr virus causes all the following except (ALL INDIA/02)
    (a)   Infectious mononucleosis
    (b)   Measles
    (c)   Nasopharyngeal carcinoma
    (d)   Non Hodgkin's lymphoma

Ans. (b)
Note
Measles virus is a member of the genus *Morbillivirus* and the family Paramyxoviridae. Apart from measles Epstein barr virus casues (a), (b) and (c).

Q. 165. In a patient, corneal scraping reveals narrow angled septate hyphae Which of the following is the likely aetiological agent? (ALL INDIA/02)
    (a)   Mucor
    (b)   Aspergillus
    (c)   Histoplasma
    (d)   Candida

Ans. (b)
Note
Aspergillus is a mold with septate hyphae about 2 to 4 um in diameter.
Ref: Harrison, 15th Edition, Section -15- Fungal and fungal infections.

Q. 166. Which of the following is true regarding globi in a patient with lepromatous leprosy? (ALL INDIA/02)
 (a) Consists of lipid laden macrophages
 (b) Consists of macrophages filled with AFB
 (c) Consists of neutrophils filled with bacteria
 (d) Consists of activated lymphocytes

Ans. (b)
Note
In lepromatous laprosy the dermis contains macrophages filled with acid-fast bacilli (AFB) forming clumps known as Globi.

Also see
In LL leprosy, bacilli are numerous in the skin (as many as 10^9/g), where they are often found in large clumps (globi), and in peripheral nerves, where they initially invade Schwann cells, resulting in foamy degenerative myelination and axonal degeneration
Ref: Harrison, 15t edition, Section 8- Mycobacterial diseases. 170 Leprosy

Q. 167. The following diagnostic tests are useful for corresponding purposes except (ALL INDIA/02)
 (a) Zeil-Neelson staining – Detection of mycobacteria
 (b) Immunoflorescence – Detection of influenza virus
 (c) Specific IgM antibodies – Immunity against rubella
 (d) Specific IgM antibodies – Detection of acute infection

Ans. (c)
Note
a. Zeil Neelson technique is used for microscopic study of the smear prepared from sputum, wherein the AFB are seen as bright red rods against a blue yellow or green background. For demonstration at least 10,000 AFB should be present per ml. of sputum. A positive report can be given only if 2 or more typical bacilli are seen.
Chapter 39, page 330
b. Immunoflorescence is used for serotyping the parainfluenza virus
Chapter56, page 478
c. IgM Ab tests help to identify current or recent infection in rubella (however it is not diagnostic). Presence of IgM in fetus or newborn indicates intrauterine infection and its detection is useful in diagnosis of congenital infections like syphilis and rubella.
Chapter 60, page 524

Also Note
Specific IgM antibody test are important in identifying current or recent infection in a patient. They are useful in assessing immune response but are in no way markers of immunity.
d. Demonstration of IgM antibodies in the serum indicates a recent infection.
Ref: Textbook of Microbiology, by: R. Ananthanarayan, 6th Edition, Chapter 12, Pg- 84

Q. 168. Confirmation of diagnosis of rota virus infection is by
 (a) Antigen detection in stool by ELISA
 (b) Antibody titres in serum
 (c) Antigen detection by immunoflurescence
 (d) Antigen detection in serum by ELISA

Ans. (a)
Note
Rota virus belongs to the family of Reoviridae. It is responsible for acute infantile gastroenteritis. The methods originally used for diagnosis were electron microscopy and immunoelectron microscopy. However these are complicated and expensive procedures. Serological tests for demonstration of the virus in stools are simpler and as sensitive. CF, CIE, ELISA and passive agglutination have been used for this purpose. IgM and IgG antibodies can be demonstrated in the blood of infected children.
Ref: Textbook of Microbiology, by: R. Ananthanarayan, 6th edition, Chapter 60, Pg- 529

Q. 169. Adenosine deaminase deficiency is seen in the following
(a) Common variable immunodeficiency
(b) Severe combined immunodeficiency
(c) Chronic granulomatous disease
(d) Nezelof syndrome

Ans. (b)

Note
Adenosine deaminase deficiency is a severe combined immunodeficiency disease associated with an enzyme deficiency. ADA catalyses the conversion of adenosine to inosine, an important step in the purine metabolism pathway. The range of immunodeficiency varies from complete absence to mild abnormalities of B and T cell functions. The condition is associated with chondrocyte abnormalities.
Ref: Textbook of Microbiology, by: R. Ananthanarayan, 6th Edition, Chapter 17, Pg- 146

Q. 170. False statement about the streptococcus is
(a) M protein is responsible for production of mucoid colonies.
(b) M protein is the major surface protein of group A streptococci.
(c) Mucoid colonies are virulent.
(d) Endotoxin causes rash of scarlet fever.

Ans. (a)

Note
a. Several protein Ags have been identified in the outer part of the cell wall. Str. pyogenes can be typed on the basis of surface proteins M, T, R. The M protein is the most important of these. It acts as a virulence factor by inhibiting phagocytosis. It is antigenic. The Ab to M protein promotes phagocytosis of the coccus and is therefore protective. It is heat stable but susceptible to tropic digestion.
b. Cultural characteristics of Str. pyogenes: Virulent strains on fresh isolation from lesions produce a matt colony, while avirulent strains produce glossy colonies. Strains with well marked capsules produce mucoid colonies corresponding in virulence to matt type.
c. The toxin is an exotoxin and not an endotoxin.
Pyrogenic toxin produced by Str. pyogenes produces an erythematous reaction. This was used to identify children susceptible to scarlet fever which is a type of an acute pharyngitis with extensive erythematous rash caused by Str. pyogenes strains that produce this toxin.
Ref: Textbook of Microbiology, by: R. Ananthanarayan, 6th edition, Chapter 23, page 189-191

Q. 171. Toxin involved in the streptococcal toxic shock syndrome is
(a) Pyrogenic toxin
(b) Erythrogenic toxin
(c) Hemolysin
(d) Neurotoxin

Ans. Use your discretion

Note
Ans. (a) and (b) both pyrogenic and erythrogenic toxin are one and the same thing.

Also see
This toxin is an exotoxin; it is called as erythrogenic toxin because its intradermal injection into susceptible individual produces a characteristic erythematous reaction. This was used to identify children susceptible to scarlet fever which is a type of an acute pharyngitis with extensive erythematous rash caused by Str. pyogenes. Strains that produce this toxin. The primary effect of this toxin is induction of fever and thus it was renamed as streptococcal pyrogenic exotoxin. SPEs are superantigens which induce massive release of inflammatory cytokines causing fever, shock and tissue damage.
Ref: Textbook of Microbiology, by: R. Ananthanarayan, 6th edition, Chapter 23, Pg-191.

Q. 172. A child presents with a white patch over the tonsils; diagnosis is best made by culture in (ALL INDIA /01)
(a) Loeffler medium
(b) LJ medium

(c) Blood agar
(d) Tellurite medium

Ans. (a)
Note
Child seems to be suffering from diphtheria. For growing the organism best culture mediums are: Loeffler's Serum Slope, Tellurite Blood Agar or a plate of ordinary blood agar. However, diphtheria bacilli grow on Loeffler's Serum Slope very rapidly and colonies can be seen in 6-8 hours. Colonies are at first small circular white opaque discs but enlarge on continued incubation and acquire a yellow tint.
Ref: -Textbook of Microbiology, by: R. Ananthanarayan, 6th edition, Chapter 26, page 214, 215

Q. 173. A patient with 14 days of fever is suspected of having typhoid. What investigation should be done? (ALL INDIA /01)
(a) Blood culture
(b) Widal test
(c) Stool culture
(d) Urine culture

Ans. (b)
Note
Widal test has highest positivity in the 3rd week.

Q. 174. In which stage of filariasis are microfilaria seen in peripheral blood?
(a) Tropical eosinophilia
(b) Early adenolymphangitis stage
(c) Late adenolymphangitis stage
(d) Elephantiasis

Ans. (b)
Note

Few of the infected individual have overt clinical manifestations of filarial infection despite large number of circulating microfilaria are present in the peripheral blood. It presents as acute denolymphagnitis and is characterised by fever, lymphatic inflammation and transient local edema, during this period.
Ref; Harrison, Filariasis and related infections.

Q. 175. All of the following are true except
(a) E coli is an aerobe and facultative anaerobe.
(b) Proteus forms uric acid stones.
(c) E coli is motile by peritrichate flagella.
(d) Proteus causes deamination of phenylalanine to phenylpyruvic acid.

Ans. (b)
Note
Proteus is responsible for 10 to 15% of cases of complicated UTI, due to the ability of *Proteus* to produce high levels of urease, which hydrolyzes urea to ammonia and results in alkalization of the urine. This in turn, leads to precipitation of organic and inorganic compounds, with the formation of struvite and carbonate-apatite crystals, and the development of calculi. Therefore, an unexplained alkaline urine should be cultured for *Proteus*, and identification of a *Proteus* species should prompt an evaluation for calculi.
Ref: Harrison 15th Edition, Section 6- Diseases caused by gram negative bactria.
Uric Acid Stones: These stones form because the urine becomes supersaturated with undissociated uric acid. In gout, idiopathic uric acid lithiasis, and dehydration, the average pH is usually below 5.4 and often below 5.0. Hyperuricosuria, when present, increases supersaturation, but urine of low pH can be supersaturated with undissociated uric acid even though the daily excretion rate is normal. Myeloproliferative syndromes, chemotherapy of malignant tumors, and the Lesch-Nyhan syndrome cause such massive production of uric acid and consequent hyperuricosuria that **stones** and **uric acid** sludge form even at a normal urine pH. Plugging of the renal collecting tubules by uric acid crystals can cause acute renal failure.
Ref; Harrison 15th Editon, Nephtolithiasis.

MCQ's in Pathology

Q. 176. Consumption of uncooked pork is likely to cause which of the following helminthic disease?
  (a) Tinea saginata
  (b) Tinea solium
  (c) Hydatid cyst
  (d) Trichuris trichura

Ans. (b)
Note
For the **pork** tapeworm *T. solium* humans are the only definitive hosts for pigs are the usual intermediate hosts. Humans acquire infections that lead to intestinal tapeworms by ingesting undercooked **pork** containing cysticerci.
Harrison 15th Edition, Section 18 – Helminthic Infections.

Q. 177. Vegetations on undersurface of AV valves are found in
  (a) Acute rheumatic carditis
  (b) Libman Sack's endocarditis
  (c) Non thrombotic bacterial endocarditis
  (d) Chronic rheumatic carditis

Ans. (b)
Note
Libman-Sacks endocarditis can be a cause of embolic stroke. These conditions overlap with the antiphospholipid syndrome, which probably requires long-term anticoagulation to prevent further stroke.
Ref: Harrison, 15th Edition, 361 – Cerebrovascular diseases.

Endothelial injury (e.g., at the site of impact of high-velocity jets or on the low-pressure side of a cardiac structural lesion) causes aberrant flow and allows either direct infection by virulent organisms or the development of an uninfected platelet-fibrin thrombus a condition called *nonbacterial thrombotic endocarditis* (NBTE). The thrombus subsequently serves as a site of bacterial attachment during transient bacteremia. The cardiac lesions most commonly resulting in NBTE are mitral regurgitation, aortic stenosis, aortic regurgitation, ventricular septal defects, and complex congenital heart disease. These lesions result from rheumatic heart disease (particularly in the developing world, where rheumatic fever remains prevalent), mitral valve prolapse, degenerative heart disease, and congenital malformations.
Ref: Harrison, 15th Edition, 126-Infectie endocarditis.

Q. 178. Triage means
  (a) Sorting out of cases on availability of medical resources and severity of patient's condition
  (b) Patients are divided into 3 groups
  (c) Severely injured patients are attended first in military camps
  (d) None of the above

Ans. (a)
Note
Triage is sorting out of cases on availability of medical resources and severity of patient's condition.
Currently many laboratory tools are available to evaluate the very common problem of chronic diarrhea. But these are costly, invasive and are extensive. Therefore one opts for lab investigation it is very much desirable to have a diagnostic evaluation based on careful history and physical examination. The simple triage tests are utilized before complex investigations are undertaken; the history, physical examination, and routine blood studies in an attempt to characterize the mechanism of diarrhea, identify diagnostically helpful associations, and assess the patient's fluid/electrolyte and nutritional status.
Ref: Harrison 15th Edition; 42- Diarrhoea and constipation.

Q. 179. Bronchiectasis is a condition of permanent abnormal dilatation of (UPSC-06)
  (a) Alveolar sac
  (b) Large bronchii
  (c) Bronchioles
  (d) lungs

Ans. (b)

Note
Bronchiectasis is a destructive lung disease characterized by chronic dilatation of the bronchi associated with persistent though variable inflammatory process in the lungs.
Ref: Medicine for Students By Golawalla, 20th Edition, Pg-238.
Bronchiactasis is defined as abnormal and irreversible dilatation of the bronchi and bronchioles developing secondarily to inflammatory weakening of the bronchial walls. The most characteristic clinical manifestation is persistent cough with expectoration of copious amounts of foul smelling purulent sputum.
Ref: Textbook of pathology, Harsh Mohan, 4th Edition, Chapter 14, Pg- 455

Q. 180. Consider the following features (UPSC-06)
  I. Axonal degeneration of both myelinated and unmyelinated fibers.
  II. Thinning of Schwann cell basal lamina.
  III. Thinning of basement membrane.
  IV. Patchy segmental myelination.

Which of the above features is/ are helpful for the confirmation of histopathology of diabetic neuropathy?
  (a) I only
  (b) II,III and IV
  (c) II and III only
  (d) I,II and III

Ans. (a)

Note
Diabetic neuropathy may affect all parts of the nervous system but symmetric peripheral neuropathy is most characteristic. The basic pathological lesion is segmental demyelination, Schwann cell injury and axonal damage.
Ref: Textbook of pathology, Harsh Mohan, 4th Edition, Chapter 24, Pg- 807

Bibliography

Books
- Textbook of pathology, Harsh Mohan, 4th Edition
- Textbook of Microbiology, by: R. Ananthanarayan, 6th Edition
- Harrison 15th Edition

Websites
www.similima.com
www.fleshandbones.com

Chapter 7
FORENSIC MEDICINE

Q. 1. The xiphoid process unites with the body of the sternum at the age of (UPSC-02)
    (a) 60 years
    (b) 40 years
    (c) 25 years
    (d) 16 years

Ans. (b)
Note
In cartilaginous sternum 5 bony centers appear from above downwards during the 5th, 6th, 7th, 8th and 9th fetal months. Fusion is complete by 25 years of age. In only about 10% of subjects fusion may occur in old age. The center for xiphoid process appears during the 3rd year or later. It fuses with the body at about 40 years.
Ref: B. D. Chaurasia's human anatomy, 3rd Edition, Vol 1, Chapter 13, Pg-172.

Q. 2. Where does rigor mortis start from? (UPSC-02)
    (a) Heart
    (b) Kidneys
    (c) Stomach
    (d) Eye

Ans. (a)
Note
Rigor mortis- after death the muscles of the body pass through three stages:
    (1) Primary relaxation or flaccidity
    (2) Rigor mortis or cadaveric rigidity
    (3) Secondary flaccidity
Rigor mortis is the state of stiffening of the muscles sometimes with slight shortening of the fibers. All the muscles of body are affected - voluntary or involuntary. It appears first in the involuntary muscles; the myocardium becomes rigid in an hour. Then in the lower jaws, eyelids and neck, and passes upward to the muscles of face and downwards to the muscles of chest, upper limbs, abdomen, lower limbs and lastly fingers.
Ref: The Essentials of Forensic Medicine and Toxicology, by Dr K. S. Narayan Reddy, 21st Edition, Chapter 7, Pg- 131,132

Q. 3. Which of the following are used for the detection of seminal stains (UPSC-04)
    I. Takayama's test
    II. Barberio's test
    III. Florence test
    IV. Acid phosphatase test

Select the correct answer using the codes given below:
    (a) I, II and III
    (b) II, III and IV
    (c) I, III and IV
    (d) I, II and IV

Ans. (b)
Note
I) Takayama's test: Is done to identify blood stains.
II) Barberio's test: A saturated aqueous or alcoholic solution of picric acid when added to spermatic fluid, produces- yellow needle shaped rhombic crystals of spermine picrate.

III) **Florence test:** The stain is extracted by 10% hydrochloric acid and a drop is placed on a glass slide and allowed to dry. It is stained with Florence solution (potassium iodide, iodine and water). If semen is present dark brown crystals of choline iodide appear immediately.

IV) **Acid phosphatase test:** In this test the level of acid phosphatase in the seminal fluid is determined. Undiluted semen has an acid phosphatase level of 340-360 bodansky units/ml, which gradually falls with vaginal secretion, and positive reactions are found for a period of 36 hours.

Other tests done to identify seminal fluid are
- Creatinine phosphokinase
- Semen specific glycoprotein
- Ammonium molybdate test
- Choline and spermine

Ref: The Essentials of Forensic Medicine and Toxicology, by Dr K. S. Narayan Reddy, 21st Edition, Chapter17,20 Pg- 355,356,386

Q. 4. Of the below which is the minimum age of a girl who can give valid consent in writing in the presence of one witness for medical examination in case of rape or kidnapping? (KPSC/Lect/Organon-05)
    (a)   A girl of 14 years of age
    (b)   A girl of 13 years of age
    (c)   A girl of 12 years of age
    (d)   A girl of 15 years of age

Ans. (c)
Note
In case of rape the victim should not be examined without proper requisition from the investigating police officer or the magistrate. The written witnessed consent of the woman is required. If she is under 12 years of age or of unsound mind the consent of her parents or guardian must be taken in writing.
Ref: The Essentials of Forensic Medicine and Toxicology, by Dr K. S. Narayan Reddy, 21st Edition, Chapter16, Pg- 340

Thus the minimum age for giving a written consent for examination is 12 years, thus the answer should be (c)

Q. 5. The most reliable diagnostic sign of drowning is (KPSC/Lect/Physio-05)
    (a)   Foreign bodies in air passages
    (b)   Water in stomach
    (c)   Cutis anserine
    (d)   Froth at nostrils

Ans. (d)
Note
The post mortem signs of drowning are variable and none of them are pathognomic.
A fine white, leathery froth or foam is seen at the mouth and nostrils, which is one of the most characteristic signs of drowning. The inhalation of water into the air passages causes irritation of the mucosa due to which the tracheal and bronchial glands secrete large quantities of tenacious mucous. Vigorous agitation of these secretions produces froth.
Other signs are:
- Cutis anserine or goose skin is produced by spasm of erector pilae muscles.
- Cadaveric spasm
- Washer woman's hands
- Water is present in the stomach in 70% cases, however it is possible that the victim may have drunk the same water shortly before death.
- There may be presence of substances such as sand, grit, diatoms and algae but their presence in trachea may be due to passive entry after death.

Ref: The Essentials of Forensic Medicine and Toxicology, by Dr K. S. Narayan Reddy, 21st Edition, Chapter14, Pg- 314-317

Q. 6. Ossification center appearing just before birth is (KPSC/Lect/Physio-05)
    (a)   Upper end of humerus
    (b)   Lower end of tibia
    (c)   Lower end of femur
    (d)   Scaphoid

Ans. (c)
Note
The femur ossifies from one primary and four secondary centres.
The center for shaft appears in the 7th week of intrauterine life. The secondary centers appear, one for the lower end at end of 9th month of intrauterine life.
One for head at First 6 months of life.
One for greater trochanter at 4th year.
One for lesser trochanter during the 12th year.
Ref: B.D. Chaurasia's human anatomy, 3rd Edition, Vol 2, chapter 1, Pg- 17

Q. 7. Most reliable method of identification of a person is by: (KPSC/Lect/Physio-05)
    (a)   DNA analysis
    (b)   Finger printing
    (c)   Scars
    (d)   Anthrapometry

Ans. (a)
Note
DNA typing or identification is a technique involving chemically dividing the DNA into fragments which form a unique pattern and then matching that identity profile with the pattern obtained. If the patterns match then, the possibility of error is less than one in 30 billion.
Ref: The Essentials of Forensic Medicine and Toxicology, by Dr K. S. Narayan Reddy, 21st Edition, Chapter20, Pg- 391
In case of finger printing there is a one in 64 thousand million chance of 2 persons having identical fingerprints.
Ref: The Essentials of Forensic Medicine and Toxicology, by Dr K. S. Narayan Reddy, 21st Edition, Chapter4, Pg- 71
By noting the information given in book DNA printing seems to be a better choice for identification.

Q. 8. The time required for the fixation of postmortem staining falls within one of the following ranges (KPSC/Lect/FMT-05)
    (a)   1 to 4 hours
    (b)   4 to 6 hours
    (c)   6 to 12 hours
    (d)   12 to 18 hours

Ans. (c)
Note
After death when coagulation in capillaries takes place, the stains become permanent- this is known as *fixation of post mortem staining*. This usually occurs in about 6 hours, but the condition of blood at the time of death exerts a considerable influence.
Ref: The Essentials of Forensic Medicine and Toxicology, by Dr K. S. Narayan Reddy, 21st Edition, Chapter7, Pg- 130

Q. 9. The most common type of inquest in India is (KPSC/Lect/FMT-05)
    (a)   Coroner
    (b)   Magistrate
    (c)   Procurator Fiscal
    (d)   Police

Ans. (d)
Note
Inquest is the investigation into the cause of death. It is conducted in cases of unusual death. Two types of inquests are carried out in India.

a. Police inquest: The officer-in charge of a police station conducts the inquest in any case of unnatural death in presence of 2 or more respectable inhabitants of the neighbourhood.
b. Magistrate's inquest: It is conducted by a district magistrate in case of
   -Death in custody
   -Dowry death
   -Death in prison, exhumation, death due to police firing.

Ref: The Essentials of Forensic Medicine and Toxicology, by Dr K. S. Narayan Reddy, 21st Edition, Chapter2, Pg- 5

Q. 10. One of the following statements is NOT true (KPSC/Lect/FMT-05)
(a) An Additional Sessions Judge can award any 'punishment authorized by law'.
(b) An Assistant Sessions Judge can award imprisonment for a term exceeding 10 years.
(c) Death sentence passed by an Additional Sessions Judge has to be confirmed by the High Court.
(d) An Assistant Sessions Judge cannot pass a death sentence.

Ans. (b)
Note
An Assistant Sessions Court can pass any sentence authorized by law except a death sentence or imprisonment for a term exceeding 10 years.
A sessions court can pass any sentence authorized by law but a death sentence passed by it must be confirmed by the high court.
Ref: The Essentials of Forensic Medicine and Toxicology, by Dr K. S. Narayan Reddy, 21st Edition, Chapter2, Pg- 6

Q. 11. Which of the following produces both physical and psychological dependence? (KPSC/Lect/FMT-05)
(a) Cocaine
(b) LSD
(c) Opium
(d) Marijuana

Ans. (c)
Note
Opium is derived from the dried juice of poppy. It's various derivatives are: heroin, morphine, codeine, pethidine etc.
Addiction to heroin is perhaps the worst because it produces a peculiar craving. With narcotics the psychic dependence is strong and tends to develop early. Tolerance occurs rapidly thus making it necessary to increase the amount of intake.
Ref: The Essentials of Forensic Medicine and Toxicology, by Dr K. S. Narayan Reddy, 21st Edition, Chapter30, Pg- 505-506
Park's Textbook of Preventive and Social Medicine, 17th Edition, Chapter17, Pg- 601

Q. 12. Foramen ovale in an infant gets closed in one of the following period after birth (KPSC/Lect/FMT-05)
(a) 1—2 weeks
(b) 2—4 weeks
(c) 1—2 months
(d) 2—3 months

Ans. (d)
Note
Normally this opening closes in the first year of life. When the lungs become functional at birth, the pulmonary pressure decreases and the left atrial pressure exceeds that of the right. This forces the septum primum against the septum secundum, functionally closing the foramen ovale. In time the septa eventually fuses, leaving a remnant of the foramen ovale, the fossa ovalis.
Ref: -http://en.wikipedia.org/wiki/Foramen_ovale_(heart)

Q. 13. In a court proceedings the judge can ask questions during (KPSC/Lect/FMT-05)
    (a) Examination-in-chief
    (b) Cross examination
    (c) Any stage of the examination
    (d) Re-examination

Ans. (c)
Note
Recording of evidence is done in the following sequence
    a. Oath
    b. Examination-in-chief
    c. Cross examination
    d. Re-examination
The judge can ask questions at any stage of the examination to clear up any doubts. The court is also empowered to recall and re-examine any witness already examined.
Ref: The Essentials of Forensic Medicine and Toxicology, by Dr K. S. Narayan Reddy, 21st Edition, Chapter2, Pg- 11-14

Q. 14. The Central Council of Homeopathy Act was passed in the year (KPSC/Lect/FMT-05)
    (a) 1971
    (b) 1972
    (c) 1973
    (d) 1974

Ans. (c)
Note
The Homeopathic Central Council Act was passed in both houses of parliament and was given ascent by the President of India on Dec 19th, 1973.
The central council was constituted in 1974 by the act of parliament called "The Homeopathy Central Council Act, 1973"
Ref: A treatise on Organon of medicine, A.K. Das, Part 3, chapter 31, Pg- 283, 284

Q. 15. Which of the following beverages contains the maximum percentage of alcohol? (KPSC/Lect/FMT-05)
    (a) Whisky
    (b) Brandy
    (c) Wine
    (d) Rum

Ans. (d)
Note
The approximate percentage of alcohol by volume in some of the common beverages is:
    -Rum, liquor: 50-60%
    -Whisky, gin, brandy-40-45%
    -Port, sherry- 20%
    -Wine-10-15%
    -Beer- 4-8%
Ref: The Essentials of Forensic Medicine and Toxicology, by Dr K. S. Narayan Reddy, 21st Edition, Chapter30, Pg- 490

Q. 16. The venom of krait is (KPSC/Lect/FMT-05)
    (a) Myotoxic
    (b) Cardiotoxic
    (c) Haemotoxic
    (d) Neurotoxic

Ans. (d)
Note
Krait belongs to the Elapid group of snakes. Elapid venoms are rich in cholinesterase, which catalyses the hydrolysis of A-Ch to choline and acetic acid. The symptoms of krait are similar to that of cobra, producing paralysis of the victim.

Ref: The Essentials of Forensic Medicine and Toxicology, by Dr K. S. Narayan Reddy, 21st Edition, Chapter29, Pg- 486

Q. 17. Touting means (KPSC/Lect/FMT-05)
(a) Using agents for procuring patients
(b) Splitting of fees received for professional service
(c) Assisting unqualified persons in treating patients
(d) Association of a doctor with a body of unqualified persons

Ans. (a)
Note
All of the following offences may lead to issual of a warning notice from the medical council of India.
a. Touting- Using agents for procuring patients.
b. Fee splitting or dichotomy- receiving or giving commission or some other benefits to a professional colleague or manufacturer or trader.
c. Assisting an un-qualified person to attend treat or perform an operation is called covering.
Other offences are; adultery, misconduct, issuing a false certificate, with-holding information from health authorities, disclosing secrets of a patient, advertising, unlawful abortion, association with manufacturing firms.
Ref: The Essentials of Forensic Medicine and Toxicology, by Dr K. S. Narayan Reddy, 21st Edition, Chapter3, Pg- 22-23

Q. 18. One of the following is NOT a delayed cause of death from injury (KPSC/Lect/FMT-05)
(a) Tetanus
(b) Fat embolism
(c) Thromboembolism
(d) Air embolism

Ans. NA
Note
All of the above choices are included as remote causes of death:
Remote causes of death:
- Infection (Cl. tetani, Cl. welchii, c. diphtheriae, streptococci)
- Gangrene
- Necrosis
- Crush syndrome
- Neglect of an injured person
- Surgical operation
- Supervention of disease from traumatic lesion
- Thrombosis and embolism
- Fat embolism
- Supra renal hemorrhage
- Air embolism
- ARSD
- DIC

Ref: The Essentials of Forensic Medicine and Toxicology, by Dr K. S. Narayan Reddy, 21st Edition, Chapter10, Pg- 255-260

Q. 19. Avulsion is a type of (KPSC/Lect/FMT-05)
(a) Chop wound
(b) Incised wound
(c) Laceration
(d) None of the above

Ans. (c)
Note
An avulsion is a laceration produced by sufficient force (shearing force) delivered at an acute angle to detach a portion of traumatized surface from its attachment. In laceration produced by shearing forces the skin may not a show sign of injury, but the underlying soft tissue is avulsed from the underlying fascia or connective tissue.

Ref: The Essentials of Forensic Medicine and Toxicology, by Dr K. S. Narayan Reddy, 21st Edition, Chapter8, Pg- 157

Q. 20. In judicial hanging, fracture of vertebral column is usually seen between (KPSC/Lect/FMT-05)
  (a) C1 and C2
  (b) C2 and C3
  (c) C4 and C5
  (d) C5 and C6

Ans. (b)
Note
In India legal death is carried out by hanging the criminal. The knot of the rope is place under the angle of jaw. The person is then dropped to the length of the rope. The sudden stoppage of moving body associated with the position of knot causes the head to be jerked violently. This causes fracture-dislocation at the level of C2-C3 or C3-C4. This results in rupture of the brain stem between the pons and the medulla and instantaneous and irreversible loss of consciousness and apnoea.
Ref: -The Essentials of Forensic Medicine and Toxicology, by Dr K. S. Narayan Reddy, 21st Edition, Chapter14, Pg- 295

Q. 21. Medullary index of hair is used to determine (KPSC/Lect/FMT-05)
  (a) Age
  (b) Race
  (c) Sex
  (d) Species

Ans. (d)
Note
The medulla of a hair is made of cells that run through the center of the cortex like a canal. In humans, this is a very small layer. The medulla may not be a continuous canal: it can be interrupted, fragmented, or absent.

Forensic scientists determine the medullary index of a hair: the diameter of the medulla relative to the diameter of the hair, expressed as a fraction. Humans have a medullary index of less than 1/3. The medullary index of animals is 1/2 or greater.

http://www.geocities.com/jordanscience2001/Hair_Identification.html
  -Medulla of human hair varies considerably; it is usually narrow; continuous, fragmented or entirely absent.
  -In animals it is continuous and wider.
Ref: The Essentials of Forensic Medicine and Toxicology, by Dr K. S. Narayan Reddy, 21st Edition, Chapter4, Pg- 78

Q. 22. Which one of the following biological fluids is NOT studied for estimating postmortem interval? (KPSC/Lect/FMT-05)
  (a) Vitreous humor
  (b) Urine
  (c) CSF
  (d) Blood

Ans. (b)
Note
The time interval between death and time of examination of body is known as post-mortem interval, the longer the post-mortem interval wider is the range of estimate. The chemical methods for estimating the time of death are:
  -Vitreous humor: Gradual linear increase in the potassium concentration and decrease in sodium concentration during the first 85 hours after death. But there is a wide variation.
  -CSF: Lactic acid concentration rises from the normal 15 mg% to over 200 mg% in 15 hours following death. Upto +/- 3 hours
  -Blood: Potassium, phosphorus and magnesium levels rise after death and sodium and chloride levels fall.
Ref: The Essentials of Forensic Medicine and Toxicology, by Dr K. S. Narayan Reddy, 21st Edition, Chapter7, Pg- 145-147

Q. 23. Finger prints can be permanently altered by (KPSC/Lect/FMT-05)
   (a) Eczema
   (b) Leprosy
   (c) Psoriasis
   (d) Scleroderma

Ans. (b)
Note
Incomplete atrophy of the ridges is seen in dermatitis. Ridge alteration is seen in eczema, acanthosis nigricans, Scleroderma, and dry or atrophic skin.
Permanent impairment of the pattern is seen in leprosy, electric injury and after exposure to radiation.
Ref: The Essentials of Forensic Medicine and Toxicology, by Dr K. S. Narayan Reddy, 21st Edition, Chapter 4, Pg- 72

Q. 24. Brush burn results from (KPSC/Lect/FMT-05)
   (a) Impact
   (b) Graze
   (c) Pressure
   (d) Dry heat

Ans. (b)
Note
Abrasion involves destruction of skin, which involves the superficial layers of the epidermis only. These are caused by a lateral rubbing action by a blow, a fall on a rough surface. Types:
   -Scratches
   -Grazes; sliding, scraping or a grinding abrasion, these are the commonest type of abrasions. An abrasion caused by violent lateral rubbing against a surface as in dragging over the ground is called as a brush burn.
   -Pressure abrasion
   -Impact abrasion
Ref: The Essentials of Forensic Medicine and Toxicology, by Dr K. S. Narayan Reddy, 21st Edition, Chapter 8, Pg- 148-149

Q. 25. Haptic hallucinations are seen in chronic poisoning with (KPSC/Lect/FMT-05)
   (a) Cocaine
   (b) Cannabis
   (c) LSD
   (d) Heroin

Ans. (a)
Note
Haptic hallucinations
These may be sensations of being touched or strangled, feeling that insects are crawling beneath the skin or feelings of sexual stimulation. The sensation of insects beneath the skin may occur in cocaine abusers, but it may also occur in schizophrenia.
Ref: http://www.gpnotebook.co.uk/simplepage.cfm?ID=-113967071
Ref: The Essentials of Forensic Medicine and Toxicology, by Dr K. S. Narayan Reddy, 21st Edition, Chapter 21, Pg- 399

Q. 26. Poisoning with one of the following produces clinical features similar to viper bite (KPSC/Lect/FMT-05)
   (a) Abrus precatorius
   (b) Ricinus communis
   (c) Semecarpus anacardium
   (d) Cerbera thevetia

Ans. (a)

Note
Abrus precatorius or jequirity or ganja.
The seeds contain an active principle abrin, a toxalbumen, which is similar to venom of viperine snakes. All parts of the plant are poisonous. The seeds are used for poisoning cattle and rarely for homicide.
Signs and symptoms include:
- Abdominal pain, nausea, vomiting
- Diarrhea
- Weakness
- Cold perspiration
- Trembling of hands
- Weak rapid pulse
- Rectal bleeding

Ref: The Essentials of Forensic Medicine and Toxicology, by Dr K. S. Narayan Reddy, 21st Edition, Chapter 29, Pg- 478

Q. 27. A First Class Judicial Magistrate can award imprisonment for a maximum period of (KPSC/Lect/FMT-05)
    (a)   3 years
    (b)   5 years
    (c)   7 years
    (d)   10 years

Ans. (a)
Note
Chief judicial magistrate: Can award a sentence of 7 years imprisonment and unlimited fine.
I class judicial magistrate: Can award imprisonment upto 3 years + fine upto Rs 5000
II class judicial magistrate: Can award imprisonment upto 1 year + fine upto Rs 3000
Ref: The Essentials of Forensic Medicine and Toxicology, by Dr K. S. Narayan Reddy, 21st Edition, Chapter 2, Pg- 6

Q. 28. A fetus is considered viable during the following month of intrauterine life (KPSC/Lect/FMT-05)
    (a)   5th
    (b)   6th
    (c)   7th
    (d)   8th

Ans. (c)
Note
Children born at or after 210 days of intrauterine life are viable, i.e. are born alive and able to survive. Children born after 180 days of uterine life may be viable and capable of continuing independent existence apart from their mothers.
Ref: The Essentials of Forensic Medicine and Toxicology, by Dr K. S. Narayan Reddy, 21st Edition, Chapter 16, Pg- 334

Q. 29. The section of IPC that define an injury (KPSC/Lect/FMT-05)
    (a)   44
    (b)   319
    (c)   320
    (d)   324

Ans. (a)
Note
An injury is any harm whatever illegally caused to any person in the body, mind, reputation or property. (sec. 44, IPC)
Ref: -The Essentials of Forensic Medicine and Toxicology, by Dr K. S. Narayan Reddy, 21st Edition, Chapter 8, Pg- 148

Q. 30. The usual postmortem interval required for the appearance of marbling (KPSC/Lect/FMT-05)
    (a)   18 hours
    (b)   24 hours
    (c)   36 hours
    (d)   48 hours

Ans. (c)
Note
Putrefaction is the final stage following death, produced mainly by the action of bacterial enzymes, mostly anaerobic organisms derived from the bowel. The characteristic features are: -
- Evolution of gases
- Liquefaction of tissues
- Colour changes: bacteria spread from the bowel into the tissue of abdominal wall. At early stage of putrefaction the haemoglobin diffuses into the surrounding tissue from the vessels giving a red colour.

This colour gradually changes to green (due to conversion of haemoglobin to sulphmethaemoglobin). This then spreads over the entire body. The colour changes to dark green then purple and finally dark blue. The superficial vessels are stained greenish-brown due to hemolysis of RBC's and infiltrates into the surrounding tissue giving it a marbled appearance.
Ref: The Essentials of Forensic Medicine and Toxicology, by Dr K. S. Narayan Reddy, 21st Edition, Chapter 7, Pg- 135,136

Q. 31. Homicidal hanging is also known as (KPSC/Lect/FMT-05)
    (a)   Mugging
    (b)   Lynching
    (c)   Garroting
    (d)   Burking

Ans. (b)
Note
a. Mugging: Strangulation caused by holding the neck of the victim in the bend of the elbow joint. Pressure is exerted either on the front of the larynx or at one or both sides of the neck by the forearm and upper arm.
b. Lynching: It is a homicidal hanging. Sometimes a suspect, accused or enemy is hanged by a rope from a tree, etc., by the mob.
c. Garroting: The victim is attacked from behind without warning. The throat may be grasped, or ligature is thrown over the neck and quickly tightened, by twisting it with a lever.
d. Burking: It is a method of homicidal smothering and traumatic asphyxia. Named after William Burk who killed 16 persons by throwing the victim to the ground and sitting on the chest and closing the nose and mouth with his hands, while his accomplice. Hare used to pull the victim around the room.
Ref: The Essentials of Forensic Medicine and Toxicology, by Dr K. S. Narayan Reddy, 21st edition, chapter 14, Pg- 294,300,309

Q. 32. Minimata disease is seen in poisoning with (KPSC/Lect/FMT-05)
    (a)   Copper
    (b)   Lead
    (c)   Mercury
    (d)   Antimony

Ans. (c)
Note
This disease was found in people living in Minimata bay, Japan as a result of dumping of large quantities of organic mercury in the sea, which resulted in poisoning. Individuals, began to have numbness in their limbs and lips. Some had difficulty hearing or seeing. Others developed shaking (tremors) in their arms and legs, difficulty walking, even brain damage. Others seemed to be going crazy, shouting uncontrollably.
Ref: http://rarediseases.about.com/od/rarediseases1/a/102304.htm

MCQ's in Forensic Medicine

Q. 33. McEwan's pupil is seen in poisoning with (KPSC/Lect/FMT-05)
    (a)   Ethyl alcohol
    (b)   Opium
    (c)   Barbiturates
    (d)   Chloral Hydrate

Ans. (a)
Note
There are three stages of alcohol intoxication:
-Stage of excitement
-Stage of in-coordination
-Stage of coma: In the stage of coma the motor and sensory cells are deeply affected, speech becomes thick and slurred, giddiness and fall occurs. The pulse is rapid, pupils are contracted but stimulation of the person e.g., pinching causes them to dilate with slow return.
Ref: The Essentials of Forensic Medicine and Toxicology, by Dr K. S. Narayan Reddy, 21st Edition, Chapter 30, Pg- 492, 493

Q. 34. Excusable homicide includes (KPSC/Lect/FMT-05)
    (a)   Judicial Execution
    (b)   Homicide committed by an insane person
    (c)   Infanticide by mother
    (d)   Death following police firing

Ans. (b)
Note
Excusable homicide is homicide caused unintentionally by an act done in good faith. This includes:

-Killing in self-defence when attacked, provided there is no other means of defense
-Causing death by accident or misadventure
-Death following a lawful operation
-Homicide by an insane person
Ref: The Essentials of Forensic Medicine and Toxicology, by Dr K. S. Narayan Reddy, 21st Edition, Chapter 10, Pg- 244

Q. 35. The clinical features of lucid interval is commonly seen in one of the following types of intracranial hemorrhage (KPSC/Lect/FMT-05)
    (a)   Subdural
    (b)   Extradural
    (c)   Intracerebral
    (d)   Subarachnoid

Ans. (b)
Note
In a typical case of extra-dural hemorrhage there is history of head injury which starts the bleeding and which will usually cause temporary loss of consciousness. This is followed by a period of normal consciousness the "lucid interval" of a few hours to a week.
As the pressure of the brain increases the patient becomes confused and then sleepy. Coma may finally ensue.
Ref: The Essentials of Forensic Medicine and Toxicology, by Dr K. S. Narayan Reddy, 21st Edition, Chapter 9, Pg- 215

Q. 36. The commonest type of finger print pattern (KPSC/Lect/FMT-05)
    (a)   Loops
    (b)   Whorls
    (c)   Arches
    (d)   Composite

Ans. (a)

Note
Classification of finger print pattern:
- Loops (67%) can be radial or ulnar
- Whorls (25%) can be concentric, spiral, double spiral, almond shaped
- Arches (6-7%) can be plain, tented or exception
- Composite (1-2%) can be central pocket loops, lateral pocket loops, twinned loops, and accidentals

Ref: The Essentials of Forensic Medicine and Toxicology, by Dr K. S. Narayan Reddy, 21st Edition, Chapter 4, Pg- 71

Q. 37. The blood is cherry red colour in poisoning with (KPSC/Lect/FMT-05)
   (a) Nitrites
   (b) Cyanides
   (c) Carbon monoxide
   (d) Phosphorous

Ans. (c)
Note
The hypostatic areas have distinct colour in certain cases of poisoning e.g.:
- CO poisoning- cherry red
- Hydrocyanic acid poisoning, burns- bright red
- Poisoning by nitrites, potassium chlorate, potassium bicarbonate, aniline – red brown
- Phosphorous- dark brown

Ref: The Essentials of Forensic Medicine and Toxicology, by Dr K. S. Narayan Reddy, 21st Edition, Chapter 7, Pg- 128, 130, 131

Q. 38. The most reliable criteria in Gustafson's technique for age estimation is (KPSC/Lect/FMT-05) (All India-03 & 05)
   (a) Attrition
   (b) Cementum apposition
   (c) Root resorption
   (d) Root transparency

Ans. (d)
Note
Gustafson's method: It is used for age estimation of adults over 21 years of age depending upon the physiological age changes in each of the dental tissues.
The various criteria are:
a. Attrition: Due to wear and tear from mastication, occlusional surface of the teeth is destroyed gradually, 1st involving the enamel, then dentin and at last the pulp.
b. Paraodontosis: Regression of gums and periodontal tissues surrounding the teeth takes place in advancing age.
c. Secondary dentine: May develop from the walls within the pulp cavity and decrease the size of the cavity.
d. Cementum apposition: The cementum increases in thickness particularly due to changes in the tooth position especially near the end of the root.
e. Root resorption: Absorption of the root starts at the apex and extends upwards, it usually occurs in the late age.
f. Transparency of roots: Canals in the dentin are at first wide, with age they are filled with minerals so that they become invisible. It is the most reliable method.

Ref: The Essentials of Forensic Medicine and Toxicology, by Dr K. S. Narayan Reddy, 21st Edition, Chapter 4, Pg- 58

Q. 39. Delirium tremens is seen in chronic abuse of (KPSC/Lect/FMT-05)
   (a) Alcohol
   (b) Cocaine
   (c) Datura
   (d) Heroin

Ans. (a)

Note
It usually results from long continued action of the poison on the brain. It occurs in chronic alcoholics due to:
- Temporary excess
- Sudden withdrawal of alcohol
- Shock after receiving an injury
- From acute infection

It begins 72-96 hours after last drink. There is an acute attack of insanity with coarse muscular tremors of the face, tongue and hands, insomnia, loss of memory, fear, and tendency to commit suicide or homicide.
Ref: The Essentials of Forensic Medicine and Toxicology, by Dr K. S. Narayan Reddy, 21st Edition, Chapter30, Pg- 501

Q. 40. Compressing the neck by the bend of the elbow-is (KPSC/Lect/FMT-05)
- (a) Mugging
- (b) Bansdola
- (c) Burking
- (d) Choking

Ans. (a)
Note
Mugging
Strangulation caused by holding the neck of the victim in the bend of the elbow joint. Pressure is exerted either on the front of the larynx or at one or both sides of the neck by the forearm and upper arm is called mugging.

Bansdola
One strong bamboo or stick is placed across the back of the neck and another across the front. Both the ends are tied with a rope due to which the victim is squeezed to death.

Burking
It is a method of homicidal smothering and traumatic asphyxia. Named after William Burk who killed 16 persons by throwing the victim to the ground and sitting on the chest and closing the nose and mouth with his hands, while his accomplice Hare used to pull the victim around the room.
Ref: The Essentials of Forensic Medicine and Toxicology, by Dr K. S. Narayan Reddy, 21st Edition, Chapter14, Pg- 300,309

Q. 41. The commonest site of traumatic rupture of intestines is (KPSC/Lect/FMT-05)
- (a) Jejunum
- (b) Ileum
- (c) Duodenum
- (d) Caecum

Ans. (a)
Note
The injuries to the stomach and intestine may be caused by any of the following:
- Forces of compression or crushing forces
- Forces of traction or tearing forces
- Forces of disruption

These can cause contusions or ruptures. The ruptures are often multiple and occur along the length of the anti mesenteric border of the bowel. The jejunum is the commonest site of rupture followed by duodenum, caecum and large intestine.
Ref: The Essentials of Forensic Medicine and Toxicology, by Dr K. S. Narayan Reddy, 21st Edition, Chapter9, Pg- 226

Q. 42. One of the following skeletal indices is used to determine the race of an individual (KPSC/Lect/FMT-05)
- (a) Ischiopubic
- (b) Sciatic notch
- (c) Cephalic
- (d) Medullary

Ans. (c)

Note
Race can be determined by
- Complexion
- Eyes
- Hair
- Skeleton- by calculating the cephalic index

It is calculated as follows:
Maximum breadth of skull X 100
Maximum length of the skull

Ref: The Essentials of Forensic Medicine and Toxicology, by Dr K. S. Narayan Reddy, 21st Edition, Chapter4, Pg- 50

Q. 43. All the following injuries amount to Grievous hurt except (KPSC/Lect/FMT-05)
    (a) Permanent privation of sight of either eye
    (b) Privation of any member or joint
    (c) Disfiguration of head or face
    (d) Fracture or dislocation of any bone or tooth

Ans. NA

Note
Grievous hurt: According to sec 320, IPC; any of the following constitute grievous hurt:
- Emasculation
- Permanent privation of sight of one eye
- Permanent privation of hearing of either ear
- Permanent privation of any member or joint
- Destruction or permanent impairing of power of any member or joint
- Permanent disfigurement of head or face
- Fracture or dislocation of a bone or tooth
- Any hurt that endangers life

Thus none of the given options can qualify as the right answer
Ref: The Essentials of Forensic Medicine and Toxicology, by Dr K. S. Narayan Reddy, 21st Edition, Chapter10, Pg- 244

Q. 44. Bluish discolouration of vaginal mucosa in pregnancy is known as (KPSC/Lect/FMT-05)
    (a) Goodell's sign
    (b) Bame's sign
    (c) Hegar's sign
    (d) Jacquemier's sign

Ans. (d)

Note
Goodell's sign
From second month onwards there is softening of cervix known as goodell's sign.
Hegar's sign
It is elicited 6th week onwards. One hand placed on the abdomen and 2 fingers in the vagina. The firm hard cervix is felt and above it the elastic body of the uterus is felt. Between the two the isthmus is felt as a soft compressible area.
Jacquemier's sign
The mucous membrane of the vagina changes from pink to violet as a result of increased vascularity. It is also called as Chadwick's sign.
Ref: The Essentials of Forensic Medicine and Toxicology, by Dr K. S. Narayan Reddy, 21st Edition, Chapter16, Pg- 331,332

Q. 45. Which one of the following is NOT an aggravated form of rape? (KPSC/Lect/FMT-05)
    (a) Gang rape
    (b) Rape on a pregnant woman
    (c) Rape on a woman in police custody
    (d) Rape on a girl below 15 years of age

Ans. (d)

Q. 46. Of the following causes of impotence in males, which is the commonest one? (KPSC/Lect/FMT-05)
    (a)   Diabetes mellitus
    (b)   Large hernias
    (c)   Emotional disturbances
    (d)   Orchitis following mumps

Ans. (c)
Note
The causes of impotency in males:
    -Age
    -Defects of development and acquired abnormalities: Intersexuality, hypospadias and other structural abnormalities.
    -Local diseases: Hernias, Phimosis, Elephantiasis, Hydrocele, Cancer, Syphilis, TB, Trauma.
    -General diseases: Diabetes, Chronic nephritis, Pulmonary TB.
    -Diseases of CNS: Disseminated sclerosis, Locomotor ataxia etc.
    -Psychical causes: They greatly outnumber all other causes.
Ref: The Essentials of Forensic Medicine and Toxicology, by Dr K. S. Narayan Reddy, 21st Edition, Chapter15, Pg- 323, 324

Q. 47. One of the following types of injury is characteristic of run-over accidents (KPSC/Lect/FMT-05)
    (a)   Avulsion
    (b)   Stretch laceration
    (c)   Patterned abrasion
    (d)   Split laceration

Ans. (a)
Note
If a person is run over by a vehicle and dragged, impact injuries may not be found, but the clothes are torn and avulsion of skin and compression injuries of internal organs are present. The body or clothing of the victim may show oil and rust from the under surface of the vehicle.
Ref: The Essentials of Forensic Medicine and Toxicology, by Dr K. S. Narayan Reddy, 21st Edition, Chapter9, Pg- 240

Q. 48. The most definite method of identification of an individual is (KPSC/Lect/FMT-05)
    (a)   DNA finger printing
    (b)   Neutron activation analysis
    (c)   Cheiloscopy
    (d)   Dactylography

Ans. (d)
Note
DNA typing or identification is a technique involving chemically dividing the DNA into fragments which form a unique pattern and then matching that identity profile with the pattern obtained. If the patterns match then the possibility of error is less than one in 30 billion.
Ref: The Essentials of Forensic Medicine and Toxicology, by Dr K. S. Narayan Reddy, 21st Edition, Chapter20, Pg- 391
In case of finger printing there is a one in 64 thousand million chance of 2 persons having identical fingerprints.
Ref: The Essentials of Forensic Medicine and Toxicology, by Dr K. S. Narayan Reddy, 21st Edition, Chapter4, Pg- 71
By noting the information given in book DNA printing seems to be a better choice for identification.
Dactylography
However, the information gathered from internet about dactylography us as under:
    -It remains the most commonly used forensic evidence worldwide - in most jurisdictions fingerprint examination cases match or outnumber all other forensic examination casework combined.
    -Dactylograpy outperforms DNA and all other human identification systems to identify more murderers

rapists and other serious offenders (fingerprints solve ten times more unknown suspect cases than DNA in most jurisdictions).
-Dactylography (Fingerprint) identification effects far more positive identifications of persons worldwide daily than any other human identification procedure.

Thus by this information we can say that the correct answer is (d).
Ref: http://experts.about.com/e/f/fi/fingerprint.htm

Q. 49. Hydrocution is due to (KPSC/Lect/FMT-05)
    (a)   Electrolyte imbalance
    (b)   Vagal inhibition
    (c)   Reflex laryngeal spasm
    (d)   Ventricular fibrillation

Ans. (b)
Note
Immersion syndrome or hydrocution: in this, death results from cardiac arrest due to vagal inhibition as a result of:
- Cold water stimulating the nerve endings
- Water striking against the epigastrium
- Cold water entering the eardrum, nasal passages and the pharynx and larynx, which causes stimulation of, nerve endings of the mucosa.

Falling or diving into water, feet first or diving involving horizontal entry into the water with a consequent blow on the abdomen cause such an accident. Alcohol increases such effects, due to generalized vasodilation of the skin vessels, and possibly by some effects on the vasomotor center.
Ref: The Essentials of Forensic Medicine and Toxicology, by Dr K. S. Narayan Reddy, 21st Edition, Chapter14, Pg- 313

Q. 50. All the following are clinical signs of brain stem death except (KPSC/Lect/FMT-05)
    (a)   Dilated and fixed pupils
    (b)   Absence of pulse
    (c)   Absence of vestibulo occular reflexes
    (d)   Absence of spontaneous breathing

Ans. (b)
Note
Diagnosis of brain stem death is done by: -
a.   The cause of death must be irremediable structural damage.
b.   Brain stem reflexes should be absent such as
    -Pupillary reflex should be absent
    -Vestibulo-occular reflex
    -Corneal reflex
    -No grimacing in response to painful stimuli
c.   Patient should be deeply commatose.
d.   The tests should be determined by 2 doctors
e.   Since brain stem is responsible for respiration therefore in brain stem death there will be absence of spontaneous respiration.
Ref: The Essentials of Forensic Medicine and Toxicology, by Dr K. S. Narayan Reddy, 21st Edition, Chapter6, Pg- 112,113

Q. 51. Quickening is felt by the mother during the following period of pregnancy (KPSC/Lect/FMT-05)
    (a)   10—12 weeks
    (b)   12—16 weeks
    (c)   16—20 weeks
    (d)   20—24 weeks

Ans. (c)

Note
From about the 16th- 20th week, the pregnant woman feels slight fluttering movements in the abdomen, which gradually increases in intensity. These are due to movements of the foetus and their first appearance is known as quickening.
Ref: The Essentials of Forensic Medicine and Toxicology, by Dr K. S. Narayan Reddy, 21st Edition, Chapter16, Pg- 331

Q. 52. A doctor disclosing the syphilitic condition of his patient to any one concerned is an example of (KPSC/Lect/FMT-05)
    (a)   Therapeutic privilege
    (b)   Ethical negligence
    (c)   Privileged communication
    (d)   Therapeutic misadventure

Ans. (c)
Note
It is the statement made bonafide upon any subject matter by a doctor to the concerned authority due to his duty to protect the interest of the community or the state.
To be privileged the communication must be made to a person having interest in it or in reference to which he has a duty. e.g.:
    a.   In case of infectious diseases.
    b.   Servants, employees or employers of a person suffering from epilepsy, hypertension, alcoholism, drug addiction etc.
    c.   In patients suffering from venereal diseases, the spouse may be informed about the state of the patient.
Ref: The Essentials of Forensic Medicine and Toxicology, by Dr K. S. Narayan Reddy, 21st Edition, Chapter3, Pg- 27,28

Q. 53. One of the following statements regarding MTP Act, 1971 is NOT true (KPSC/Lect/FMT-05)
    (a)   Consent of the husband is necessary
    (b)   Termination may be carried out in any maternity hospital
    (c)   Pregnancy may be terminated on grounds of contraceptive failure
    (d)   Above 12 weeks of pregnancy, two doctors have to opine jointly regarding applicability of an indication

Ans. (a)
Note
Under the Medical Termination Of Pregnancy Act of 1971 pregnancy can be terminated under the following conditions:
    a.   Therapeutic: when the continuation of pregnancy endangers the life of the mother
    b.   Eugenic: when there is a risk of the child being born with serious physical or mental abnormality
    c.   Humanitarian: when the pregnancy has been caused by rape
    d.   Social: when the pregnancy has been caused by contraceptive failure
Non-governmental organizations can take up abortions if a license has been obtained from the chief medical officer of the district.
Consent of the woman is required; if she is a minor then consent of the guardian is required. Consent of husband is not required.
If below 12 weeks it can be terminated on the opinion of a single doctor, if between 12-22 weeks- two doctors must concur (jointly give opinion) that there is an indication.
Ref: The Essentials of Forensic Medicine and Toxicology, by Dr K. S. Narayan Reddy, 21st Edition, Chapter18, Pg- 358,359

Q. 54. Florence test detects the following constituent of semen (KPSC/Lect/FMT-05)
    (a)   Spermine
    (b)   Choline
    (c)   Fructose
    (d)   Acid phosphatase

Ans. (b)

Note
Florence test
- The stain is extracted by 10% hydrochloric acid and a drop is placed on a glass slide and allowed to dry. It is stained with Florence solution (potassium iodide, iodine and water). If semen is present dark brown crystals of choline iodide appear immediately.

Additional information:
Acid phosphatase test
- In this test the level of acid phosphatase in the seminal fluid is determined. Undiluted semen has an acid phosphatase level of 340-360 bodansky units/ml, which gradually falls with vaginal secretion, and positive reactions are found for a period of 36 hours.

Barberio's test
- A saturated aqueous or alcoholic solution of picric acid when added to spermatic fluid, produces- yellow needle shaped rhombic crystals of spermine picrate.

Ref: The Essentials of Forensic Medicine and Toxicology, by Dr K. S. Narayan Reddy, 21st Edition, Chapter17, Pg- 355,356

Q. 55. Marsh's test is diagnostic of poisoning with (KPSC/Lect/FMT-05)
- (a) Arsenic
- (b) Copper
- (c) Lead
- (d) Mercury

Ans. (a)

Note
The Marsh's test is diagnostic of poisoning with arsenic

Marsh's Test: When the compounds of arsenic, except the metal and its sulphides are introduced into a hydrogen generator, arseniuretted hydrogen is liberated and may be burned in a jet together with the escaping hydrogen. The flame is bluish or greenish, violet or purple and emits garlic like odour. If the flame is suddenly cooled as by placing a piece of cold porcelain in the flame, arsenic is deposited as a blackish-brown stain of metallic luster. This stain is soluble in a solution of hypochlorite, while addition of ammonium sulphide does not dissolve, but detaches it from the porcelain. This is a very delicate test and detects arsenic upto one thousandth of a milligram.

However, another chemical tests used for identification of arsenic is - Reinsch's Test.

Ref: The Essentials of Forensic Medicine and Toxicology, by Dr K. S. Narayan Reddy, 21st Edition, Chapter27, Pg- 465

Q. 56. The punishment awarded to a doctor found guilty of professional criminal negligence is (KPSC/Lect/FMT-05)
- (a) Imprisonment for 2 years
- (b) Fine
- (c) Imprisonment for 7 years
- (d) 2 years imprisonment and fine

Ans. (d)

Note
Sec 304 A., IPC deals with it. "Whoever causes death of any person by doing any rash or negligent act not amounting to culpable homicide shall be punished with imprisonment up to 2 years, or with fine, or with both"

Criminal negligence is when a doctor:
- Shows gross absence of skill, inattention, negligence or care during treatment resulting in serious injury to or death of the patient by acts of omission or commission.
- Performs an illegal act
- When an assaulted person dies and the defense attributes his death to the negligence of the doctor or undue interference in the treatment of the deceased by the doctor.

Most of such cases are associated with drunkenness or with impaired efficiency due to use of drugs by doctors.

Ref: The Essentials of Forensic Medicine and Toxicology, by Dr K. S. Narayan Reddy, 21st Edition, **Chapter**3 Pg- 33

Q. 57. Cheiloscopy is the study of the prints of (KPSC/Lect/FMT-05)
(a) Foot
(b) Lip
(c) Fingers
(d) Palate

Ans. (b)
Note
Lip prints or cheiloscopy are useful in personal identification. Lip prints are divided into eight patterns, which are specific to the individual;
Vertical, branched, intersected, reticular patterns, etc. minor differences can be noted between the left and right and upper and lower lips.
Ref: The Essentials of Forensic Medicine and Toxicology, by Dr K. S. Narayan Reddy, 21st Edition, Chapter4 Pg- 73

Q. 58. The term "whiplash injury" refers to that involving the (KPSC/Lect/FMT-05)
(a) Spine
(b) Long bones
(c) Skull
(d) Rib cage

Ans. (a)
Note
Whiplash injury sustained commonly by the occupant of the front seat of car. When the vehicle comes to a stop; the forward thrust produces a state of acute hyperflexion, but this is converted to acute hyperextension as the forehead strikes the window, which causes injury to the cervical column. In such cases, and also due to a sharp blow against the spinous process of an upper cervical vertebra, fatal contusion or laceration of the spinal cord may occur without fracture of spine.
Ref: The Essentials of Forensic Medicine and Toxicology, by Dr K. S. Narayan Reddy, 21st Edition, Chapter9 Pg- 222

Q. 59. The central council of Homeopathy Amendment Act was passed in the year (KPSC/Lect/FMT-05)
(a) 2000
(b) 2001
(c) 2002
(d) 2004

Ans. (c)
Note
The Homeopathy Central Council (Amendment) Act, 2002 Act No. 51 OF 2002
[8th December 2002.]
It is an Act further to amend the Homeopathy Central Council Act, 1973.
Ref: http://www.austlii.edu.au/~andrew/CommonLII/IN-num_act/hcca2002367/

Q. 60. The preservative routinely used for preserving viscera for chemical examination is (KPSC/Lect/FMT-05)
(a) Normal saline
(b) 10 % Formalin
(c) Saturated saline
(d) Formol saline

Ans. (c)
Note
The preservatives used for preserving viscera are:
a. Saturated solution of sodium chloride.
b. Rectified spirit, except in cases of suspected poisoning by alcohol, acetic acid, phenol, phosphorus, paraldehyde

c. 10 mg/ml of sodium or potassium fluoride and 3 mg potassium oxalate should be used for preserving blood. Fluoride 10 mg for every 1 ml should also be added to urine and vitreous humour if alcohol estimation is required, and also to samples for analysis for cocaine, cyanide and CO.

The viscera should not be preserved in formaldehyde because extraction of poison, especially non-volatile organic compounds becomes difficult.

Ref: The Essentials of Forensic Medicine and Toxicology, by Dr K. S. Narayan Reddy, 21st Edition, Chapter5 Pg- 104

Q. 61. Ochronosis is seen in poisoning with (KPSC/Lect/FMT-05)
- (a) Nitric acid
- (b) Oxalic acid
- (c) Carbolic acid
- (d) Acetic acid

Ans. (c)

Note

Ochronosis is seen in poisoning with carbolic acid. In body the phenol is partly oxidized to hydroquinone and pyrocatechol, which with unchanged phenol is excreted in urine. The hydroquinone and pyrocatechol may cause pigmentation in the cornea and various cartilages, a condition called as ochronosis. It is associated with alkaptonuria, in which homogentisic acid gets deposited in cartilages, ligaments and fibrous tissue.

Ref: The Essentials of Forensic Medicine and Toxicology, by Dr K. S. Narayan Reddy, 21st Edition, Chapter26 Pg- 459

Q. 62. The following documents are exceptions to oral evidence in court except (KPSC/Lect/FMT-05)
- (a) Postmortem reports
- (b) Dying declaration
- (c) Reports of Mint Officers
- (d) Chemical Examiner's reports

Ans. (a)

Note

Exceptions to oral evidence:
- a. Dying declaration.
- b. Expert opinion expressed in a treatise may be proved in a court by producing such book if the author is dead or cannot be found without unreasonable delay or expense.
- c. Evidence of a doctor recorded in lower court is accepted in a higher court provided it is recorded and attested by Magistrate in presence of the accused.
- d. Evidence given by a witness in a previous judicial proceeding is admissible in subsequent judicial proceeding when the witness is dead or cannot be found.
- e. Evidence of mint officers or an officer of the India Security Press.
- f. Reports of certain government officers-chemical examiner, chief inspector of explosives, director of finger print bureau, etc.
- g. Public records.
- h. Hospital records.

Ref: The Essentials of Forensic Medicine and Toxicology, by Dr K. S. Narayan Reddy, 21st Edition, Chapter2 Pg- 10

Q. 63. One of the following tests is used for the detection of old blood stains (KPSC/Lect/FMT-05)
- (a) Takayama's test
- (b) Spectroscopy
- (c) Microscopy
- (d) Kastle Mayer test

Ans. (b)

Note
a. *Takayama's test*
It is a good test for detection of both old and new stains. Place a small drop of suspected material on the slide and 2-3 drops of Takayama reagent is added and covered with a coverslip. Pink feathery crystals of hemochromogen or reduced alkaline hematin crystals appear in 1-6 min.
b. *Spectroscopy*
It is the most delicate and reliable test for the determination of presence of bloodstains whether new or old. Less than 0.1ml of blood is sufficient.
c. *Kastle Mayer Test*
It is a chemical method used for examination of bloodstains. Also called as phenolphthalein test: To a solution extracted from the stain with distilled water. Add 10-20 drops of phenolphthalein reagent (phenolphthalein 2g+ sodium hydroxide 20g + distilled water 100 ml) and then a drop or 2 of 10 volumes hydrogen peroxide. If blood is present pink to purple color develops.
Ref: The Essentials of Forensic Medicine and Toxicology, by Dr K. S. Narayan Reddy, 21st Edition, Chapter20, Pg- 381,382

Q. 64. Which one of the following statements are NOT true regarding firearm exit wound? (KPSC/Lect/FMT-05)
(a) Everted margins
(b) Larger than the diameter of the bullet
(c) Presence of abrasion collar
(d) Presence of grease collar

Ans. (c) & (d)
Note

S. No.	Trait	Entrance wound	Exit wound
1	Size	Smaller than the diameter of bullet	Bigger than the bullet
2	Edges	Inverted	Everted, puckered or torn
3	Bruising, abrasion & grease collar	Present	Absent
4	Burning, blackening tattooing	May be seen around the wound	Absent
5	Bleeding	Less	More
6	Fat	No protrusion	May protrude
7	Tissues within and around the wound	May be cherry red due to CO of explosive gases	No colour change
8	Fibres of clothing	Turned in and may be carried into the wound	Turned out
9	Lead ring or metal ring	May be seen around the wound by microscopic examination	Absent

Ans both c and d are not seen in exit wounds
Differences between entrance and exit bullet wounds are:

Ref: The Essentials of Forensic Medicine and Toxicology, by Dr K. S. Narayan Reddy, 21st Edition, Chapter8 Pg- 187

Q. 65. The colour of postmortem staining is bright red in poisoning with (KPSC/Lect/FMT-05)
(a) Carbon monoxide
(b) Phosphorous
(c) Cyanides
(d) Carbon dioxide

Ans. (c)

Note
The hypostatic areas have distinct colour in certain cases of poisoning e.g.:
CO poisoning- Cherry red.
Hydrocyanic acid poisoning, burns- Bright red.
Poisoning by nitrites, potassium chlorate, potassium bicarbonate, aniline – Red brown
Phosphorous- dark brown.
Ref: The Essentials of Forensic Medicine and Toxicology, by Dr K. S. Narayan Reddy, 21st Edition, Chapter7, Pg- 128,130,131

Q. 66. False sense of perception without an external object is (KPSC/Lect/FMT-05)
    (a)   Illusion
    (b)   Hallucination
    (c)   Phobia
    (d)   Delusion
Ans. (b)
Note
    a.   Illusion: False interpretation by the senses of an external object or stimulus which has a real existence
    b.   Hallucination: It is a false sense of perception without any external object or stimulus to produce it. They may be visual, auditory, olfactory, gustatory, or tactile.
    c.   Phobia: Is an excessive irrational fear of a particular object or situation.
    d.   Delusion: False belief in something which is not a fact and which persists even after its falsity has been demonstrated.
Ref: The Essentials of Forensic Medicine and Toxicology, by Dr K. S. Narayan Reddy, 21st Edition, vChapter21, Pg- 398,399,400

Q. 67. The bite of one of the following snakes can produce clinical features similar to Crush syndrome (KPSC/Lect/FMT-05)
    (a)   Krait
    (b)   King Cobra
    (c)   Russel's Viper
    (d)   Sea Snake
Ans. (d)
Note
Crush syndrome
It results from severe crushing injury to the muscles especially those of the lower limbs. Severe ischaemia leads to necrosis of muscles (Rhabdomyolysis). The cause is obscure but may involve disturbance of the renal blood flow (leading to renal tubular necrosis) and ischaemia. Death usually occurs in 1-2 weeks after injury.
Ref: The Essentials of Forensic Medicine and Toxicology, by Dr K. S. Narayan Reddy, 21st Edition, Chapter10, Pg- 256
Sea snake bites: Pathophysiology:
The primary neurotoxin causes peripheral paralysis by competitively binding to postsynaptic nicotinic acetylcholine receptors at the neuromuscular junction. Potent myotoxins account for the significant muscle necrosis, with consequent myoglobinemia and hyperkalemia that may occur following envenomation. Sea snake venom does not affect blood coagulation to a significant degree.
D/D is
    -Guillain-Barré Syndrome
    -Rhabdomyolysis
    Ref: http://www.emedicine.com/emerg/topic543.htm

Q. 68. Anteroposterior compression fracture of hyoid bone is seen in (KPSC/Lect/FMT-05)
    (a)   Gagging
    (b)   Throttling
    (c)   Traumatic asphyxia
    (d)   Hanging
Ans. (d)

MCQ's in Forensic Medicine

Note
Hyoid bone fracture can be classified into 3 groups:
- Inward compression fractures
- Antero-posterior compression fracture
- Avulsion fracture

In case of hanging the hyoid bone is forced directly backwards, due to which the divergence of greater horns is increased which may fracture with outward displacement of the posterior small fragment. A-P compression fracture may occur either in the greater horn or at its junction with the body, and it may be bilateral.
Ref: The Essentials of Forensic Medicine and Toxicology, by Dr K. S. Narayan Reddy, 21st Edition, Chapter14, Pg- 306

Q. 69. Adipocere formation requires one of the following environmental conditions (KPSC/Lect/FMT-05)
  (a) Cold and Moist
  (b) Warm and Dry
  (c) Cold and Dry
  (d) Warm and Moist

Ans. (d)
Note
Adipocere formation is a modification of putrefaction. In this, fatty tissues of the body change into substance similar to soaps, known as adipocere. It is seen most commonly in bodies immersed in water or in damp environment. The change is due to gradual hydrolysis and hydrogenation of pre-existing fats, such as olein into higher fatty acids, which combine with calcium and ammonium ions to form insoluble soaps, which being acidic, inhibit putrefactive bacteria. The process starts under the influence of intrinsic lipases, and is continued by the bacterial enzymes of the clostridia group, mainly Cl. Perfringens, as the bacteria produce lecithinase, which facilitates hydrolysis and hydrogenation.
Ref: The Essentials of Forensic Medicine and Toxicology, by Dr K. S. Narayan Reddy, 21st Edition, Chapter7, Pg- 141

Q. 70. In India, the time limit for exhumation is (KPSC/Lect/FMT-05)
  (a) 5 years
  (b) 10 years
  (c) 20 years
  (d) No time limit

Ans. (d)
Note
Exhumation is the digging out of an already buried body from the grave. There is no time limit for exhumation in India. Autopsies are performed on exhumed bodies:
a. In criminal cases, such as homicide, suspected homicide disguised as suicide or other types of death, suspicious poisoning, death as a result of criminal abortion and criminal negligence.
b. In civil cases, such as accidental death claim, insurance, workmen's compensation claim, inheritance claims etc.
Ref: The Essentials of Forensic Medicine and Toxicology, by Dr K. S. Narayan Reddy, 21st Edition, Chapter5, Pg- 110

Q. 71. All the following conditions of the husband are indications for artificial insemination by donor except (KPSC/Lect/FMT-05)
  (a) Impotence
  (b) Sickle cell disease
  (c) Sterility
  (d) Rh incompatibility

Ans. (a)
Note
Indications of artificial insemination from husband are:
When the husband is impotent; and is unable to deposit semen into the vagina due to hypospadiasis, epispadiasis.

Artificial insemination by donor is indicated:
- When the husband is sterile
- When the husband is Rh incompatible to the wife
- When the husband is suffering from a hereditary disease.

Ref: The Essentials of Forensic Medicine and Toxicology, by Dr K. S. Narayan Reddy, 21st Edition, Chapter15, Pg- 326

Q. 72. The minimum age for giving valid consent for medical examination (KPSC/Lect/FMT-05)
- (a) 10 years
- (b) 12 years
- (c) 14 years
- (d) 18 years

Ans. (b)

Note
A child under 12 years cannot give a valid consent to suffer any harm, which may result from an act done in good faith and for its benefit. The consent of the parent or the guardian should be taken (Sec 89, IPC). If they refuse the doctor cannot treat the patient even to save his life.

Ref: The Essentials of Forensic Medicine and Toxicology, by Dr K. S. Narayan Reddy, 21st Edition, Chapter3, Pg- 42

Q. 73. Mee's lines are seen in chronic poisoning with (KPSC/Lect/FMT-05)
- (a) Lead
- (b) Arsenic
- (c) Copper
- (d) Mercury

Ans. (b)

Note
In chronic arsenic poisoning certain skin changes take place which include:
Pigmentation: Finely mottled brown changes mostly on the skin flexures, temples, eyelids and neck. (Rain drop type pigmentation), which persists for many months. There may be a rash resembling fading measles rash.
In prolonged contact hyperkeratosis of the palms and soles with irregular thickening of the nails and developments of bands of opacity in the fingernails called Aldrich-Mees lines are seen.

Ref: -The Essentials of Forensic Medicine and Toxicology, by Dr K. S. Narayan Reddy, 21st Edition, Chapter27, Pg- 464

Q. 74. The most commonly accepted hypothesis of SIDS is (KPSC/Lect/FMT-05)
- (a) Respiratory infection
- (b) Sleep Apnoea
- (c) Hypoganunaglobulinaemia
- (d) Cow's milk allergy

Ans. (b)

Note
Various theories have been put forward to explain SIDS (Sudden Infant Death Syndrome):
The commonly accepted hypothesis suggests that some infants have prolonged sleep apnoea (a periodic failure to breathe during sleep), which may make the patient susceptible to hypoxia which leads to bradycardia and finally cardiac arrest.
Nasal edema, mucous secretion may further narrow down the passage.
An element of laryngeal spasm has also been suggested.
Other possible causes are:
Conduction defects, mechanical upper airway obstruction, adrenal insufficiency, GERD leading to bradycardia.

Ref: The Essentials of Forensic Medicine and Toxicology, by Dr K. S. Narayan Reddy, 21st Edition, Chapter19, **Pg- 378**

Q. 75. In the Mental Health Act, the term "lunatic" is replaced by (KPSC/Lect/FMT-05)
(a) Mental patient
(b) Mentally ill patient
(c) Mentally disordered patient
(d) Mentally unsound patient

Ans. (b)

Note
The Mental Health Act, 1987 was enacted to consolidate and amend the law relating to the treatment and care of mentally ill persons to make better provision with respect to their property and affairs, and for that matters connected therewith. This act repeals the Indian Lunacy Act, 1912.
Ref: The Essentials of Forensic Medicine and Toxicology, by Dr K. S. Narayan Reddy, 21st Edition, Chapter21, Pg- 406

Q. 76. A toxalbumen is produced by one of the following plants (KPSC/Lect/FMT-05)
(a) Semecarpus anacardium
(b) Croton tiglium
(c) Plumbago rosea
(d) Calotropis gigantea

Ans. (b)

Note
Croton tiglium (jamalgota or naepala) seeds contain *crotin*, a toxalbumen that is not expressed with the oil. The oil is brown viscid, has unpleasant odour and acrid, burning taste. Crotonoside, a glycoside is also present, it is less poisonous.
Circumstances of poisoning are:
Accidental poisoning.
Suicide and homicide are rare.
The root and oil are sometimes taken internally as an abortifacient.
The oil is used as an arrow poison.
Ref: The Essentials of Forensic Medicine and Toxicology, by Dr K. S. Narayan Reddy, 21st Edition, Chapter29, Pg- 477,478

Q. 77. In case of death in prison, inquest will be conducted by (KPSC/Lect/FMT-05)
(a) Police
(b) Executive magistrate
(c) Jail superintendent
(d) Doctor

Ans. (b)

Note
A case in which a Magistrate conducts an inquest is:
a. Death in prison
b. Death in police custody and while under police interrogation
c. Death due to police firing
d. Exhumation
e. Dowry deaths
Ref: The Essentials of Forensic Medicine and Toxicology, by Dr K. S. Narayan Reddy, 21st Edition, Chapter2, Pg- 5

Q. 78. Fat embolism can be caused by (KPSC/Lect/FMT-05)
(a) Subclavian vein catheterisation
(b) Caesarean section
(c) Fracture of long bones
(d) Incised wounds of lower cervical region

Ans. (c)

Note
Fat embolism is caused by:
   a. Fracture of long bones
   b. An injury to the adipose tissue which forces the liquid fat into the damaged blood vessels
   c. Injecting oil into the circulation as in criminal abortion
   d. Occasionally in certain diseases due to trauma without any trauma
   e. In cases of burns

In every injury involving bone or subcutaneous tissue, fat embolism occurs to some extent, especially in crushing injuries of the buttocks and breasts.
Ref: The Essentials of Forensic Medicine and Toxicology, by Dr K. S. Narayan Reddy, 21st Edition, Chapter10, Pg- 256

Q. 79. Epidemic dropsy is caused by consuming (KPSC/Lect/FMT-05)
   (a) Mushrooms
   (b) Lathyrus sativus
   (c) Mustard oil
   (d) Argemone oil

Ans. (d)
Note
Mushrooms
It is characterized by irritant symptoms such as constriction of throat, burning pain in the throat, vomiting and diarrhea, cyanosis, collapse, slow pulse, and finally death.
Lathyrus sativus
It is a neurotoxin and characterized by progressive spastic paraplegia. It progresses irreversibly in four stages to physical disability.
Argemone Mexicana
It is a wild growing plant found all over India. The seeds are dark-brown in color, globular and slightly smaller than mustard seeds. The oil contains two alkaloids- sanguinarine and dihydro sanguinarine. All parts of the plant are poisonous. The oil causes epidemic dropsy characterized by:
Pedal edema, myocardial damage and dilatation of heart. Liver may be palpable and tender. Patient becomes breathless. Jerks are feeble. Dimness of vision, bluish mottling of the skin. Death occurs from severe damage to the heart.
It is used to adulterate mustard oil.
Ref: The Essentials of Forensic Medicine and Toxicology, by Dr K. S. Narayan Reddy, 21st Edition, Chapter38, Pg- 552,553

Q. 80. Which one of the following is NOT a constituent of Universal Antidote? (KPSC/Lect/FMT-05)
   (a) Animal charcoal
   (b) Tannic acid
   (c) Magnesium oxide
   (d) Potassium permanganate

Ans. (d)
Note
Ref: The Essentials of Forensic Medicine and Toxicology, by Dr K. S. Narayan Reddy, 21st Edition, Chapter24, Pg- 444

Q. 81. Fracture-a-la-signature is a (KPSC/Lect/FMT-05)
   (a) Ring fracture
   (b) Depressed fracture
   (c) Sutural diastasis
   (d) Comminuted fractures

Ans. (b)
Note
Depressed fractures are caused by local deformation of skull. In this fracture the bone is driven inwards into the skull cavity. The fractured bone is driven inwards into the skull cavity. The outer table is driven into the

diploe, the inner table is fractured irregularly and to a greater extent and may be comminuted. They are also called as *fractures- a -la- signature* as their pattern often resembles the weapon or agent which caused it.
Ref: The Essentials of Forensic Medicine and Toxicology, by Dr K. S. Narayan Reddy, 21st Edition, Chapter9, Pg- 204

Q. 82. The structure which has got minimum molecular life (KPSC/Lect/FMT-05)
- (a) Nervous tissue
- (b) Connective tissue
- (c) Skeletal tissue
- (d) Cardiac muscle

Ans. (a)
Note
Molecular death means death of cells and tissues individually, which takes place usually one or two hours after stoppage of the vital functions. Molecular death occurs piecemeal. Individual cells will live for a variable time after the circulation has stopped till their residual oxygen is exhausted. Nervous tissues die rapidly, the vital centers of the brain in about 5 min, but the muscles live upto 1 to 2 hours.
Ref: The Essentials of Forensic Medicine and Toxicology, by Dr K. S. Narayan Reddy, 21st Edition, Chapter6, Pg- 113

Q. 83. Criminal responsibility of an insane is defined in the following section of IPC (KPSC/Lect/FMT-05)
- (a) 82
- (b) 84
- (c) 85
- (d) 87

Ans. (b)
Note
The Mc Naughten Rule which states that "An accused person is not legally responsible if it is clearly proved that at the time of committing such a crime, he was suffering from such a defect of reason from abnormality of mind, that he did not know the nature and quality of the act he was doing, or that what he was doing was wrong."
This legal text has also been accepted in India and is included in Sec. 84, IPC.
Ref: The Essentials of Forensic Medicine and Toxicology, by Dr K. S. Narayan Reddy, 21st Edition, Chapter21, Pg- 411

Q. 84. Burtonian line is seen in chronic poisoning with (KPSC/Lect/FMT-05)
- (a) Lead
- (b) Arsenic
- (c) Barium
- (d) Manganese

Ans. (a)
Note
Signs and symptoms of lead poisoning are:
- a. Lead line: A stippled blue line known as the Burtonian line is seen on the gums in 50-70% of cases. It appears due to subepithelial deposit of granules at the junction with teeth only near dirty or carious teeth, within a week of exposure, especially on upper jaw.
- b. Anaemia
- c. Facial pallor
- d. Colic and constipation
- e. Lead palsy
- f. Encephalopathy
- g. Hypertension, chronic arteriosclerotic nephritis
Ref: The Essentials of Forensic Medicine and Toxicology, by Dr K. S. Narayan Reddy, 21st Edition, Chapter27, Pg- 467,468

Q. 85. All the following are features of a still born foetus except (KPSC/Lect/FMT-05)
(a) Born after 28 weeks of pregnancy
(b) Was alive in utero
(c) Will show signs of maceration
(d) Severe moulding of head

Ans. (c)
Note
A still born child is one which is born after the 28th week of pregnancy, and which did not breathe or show any other signs of life, at any time after being completely born. The child was alive in utero, but dies during the process of birth. The incidence is about 5%. It is born in sterile condition, and as such, putrefaction occurs from without inwards. Signs of prolonged labour, i.e., edema and bleeding into scalp, a caput succedaneum, and severe moulding of the head indicate stillbirth or death from natural causes shortly after birth.
Ref: The Essentials of Forensic Medicine and Toxicology, by Dr K. S. Narayan Reddy, 21st Edition, Chapter19, Pg- 368

Q. 86. Chapter III of the Central Council of Homoeopathy Act deals with (KPSC/Lect/FMT-05)
(a) Recognition of medical qualifications
(b) Central register
(c) Miscellaneous
(d) Number of seats allocated in Central Council in each state

Ans. (a)
Note
The IIIrd Chapter of Central Council of Homeopathy Act includes:
a. Recognition of medical qualification granted by certain medical institutions in India.
b. Recognition of medical qualifications granted by medical institutions in States or countries outside India.
c. Rights of persons possessing qualifications included in Second or the Third Schedule to be enrolled.
d. Power to require information as to courses of study and examinations.
e. Inspectors at examinations.
f. Visitors at examinations.
g. Withdrawal of recognition.
h. Minimum standards of education in Homeopathy.
Ref: http://www.indialawinfo.com/bareacts/hoca.html

Q. 87. The Indian Lunacy Act of 1912 has been replaced by the Mental Health Act of
(a) 1986
(b) 1987
(c) 1988
(d) 1989

Ans. (b)
Note
The Mental Health Act, 1987 was enacted to consolidate and amend the law relating to the treatment and care of mentally ill persons to make better provision with respect to their property and affairs, and for that matters connected therewith. This act replaces the Indian Lunacy Act, 1912.
Ref: The Essentials of Forensic Medicine and Toxicology, by Dr K. S. Narayan Reddy, 21st Edition, Chapter21, Pg- 406

Q. 88. Constricted pupils are seen in poisoning with
(a) Datura
(b) Cocaine
(c) Cannabis
(d) Opium

Ans. (d)
Note
There are 3 stages of opium poisoning:
a. Stage of excitement:
There is increased sense of well being, anxiety, restlessness, flushing of face, hallucinations.

b. Stage of stupor:
    The patient goes into stupor with giddiness and drowsiness. The pupils are constricted and face and lips are cyanosed.
c. Stage of coma:
    Muscles become flaccid and relaxed, all reflexes are abolished, the face is pale and conjunctiva is congested. Pupils are contracted to pinpoint size and do not react to light.
    Ref: The Essentials of Forensic Medicine and Toxicology, by Dr K. S. Narayan Reddy, 21st Edition, Chapter30, Pg- 506

Q. 89. The "thing or fact that speaks for itself" is legally termed
  (a) Res judicata
  (b) Vis Major
  (c) Respondent superior
  (d) Res ipsa loquitur

Ans. (d)
Note
The doctrine of Res Ipsa Loquitur states that ordinarily the professional negligence of a physician must be proved in Court by the expert evidence of another physician. The patient need not prove negligence where the rule of Res Ipsa Loquitur applies, which means "the thing or the fact speaks for itself". The rule is applied when the following conditions are satisfied:
    -In the absence of negligence the injury would have not occurred ordinarily.
    -The doctor had exclusive control over the injury producing instrument.
    -The patient was not guilty of contributory negligence.
Ref: The Essentials of Forensic Medicine and Toxicology, by Dr K. S. Narayan Reddy, 21st Edition, Chapter3, Pg- 32

Q. 90. All of the following are differential diagnosis of Battered Baby Syndrome except
  (a) Scurvy
  (b) Osteomyelitis
  (c) Congenital syphilis
  (d) Osteogenesis Imperfecta

Ans. NA
Note
It is also known as child abuse syndrome or Caffey's syndrome. A battered baby is one who has received repetitive physical injuries as a result of non-accidental violence, produced by a parent or guardian. In addition to physical injury, there may be non-accidental deprivation of nutrition, care and affection.
Differential Diagnosis:
Scurvy, congenital syphilis, osteomyelitis, leukaemia, rickets, juvenile osteoporosis with stress fractures, paralytic disease with fracture, infantile cortical hyperosteoses and osteogenesis imperfecta.
Ref: The Essentials of Forensic Medicine and Toxicology, by Dr K. S. Narayan Reddy, 21st Edition, Chapter19, Pg- 375,377
Comment: All above appear to be correct.

Q. 91. Punishment for murder is prescribed in one of the following sections of the IPC
  (a) 302
  (b) 304
  (c) 306
  (d) 309V

Ans. (a)
Note
Death or imprisonment for life, and also fine is the sentence awarded for murder under sec 302, IPC.
Ref: The Essentials of Forensic Medicine and Toxicology, by Dr K. S. Narayan Reddy, 21st Edition, Chapter10, Pg- 245

Q. 92. One of the following statements is NOT true regarding dying declaration (KPSC/Lect/FMT-05)
  (a) Oath is not required
  (b) Cross examination is allowed
  (c) A doctor should preferably be present during the recording
  (d) The statement can be recorded by any person

Ans. (b)
Note
It is a written or verbal statement of a person, who is dying as a result of some unlawful act, relating to the material facts of the cause of his death or bearing on the circumstances. If there is time, a magistrate is called to record the declaration. A doctor should certify that the person is conscious and his mental faculties are normal. If time does not permit to call a doctor then the statement may be recorded by the village headman, police or any other person but its value will be less.
When recording it, oath is not administered because of the belief that a dying person doesn't lie.

If a point is not clear questions may be asked to make it clear, but the actual question asked and the answer given should be recorded.
Ref: The Essentials of Forensic Medicine and Toxicology, by Dr K. S. Narayan Reddy, 21st Edition, Chapter2, Pg- 9

Q. 93. Incised looking lacerated wounds are (KPSC/Lect/FMT-05)
  (a) Split lacerations
  (b) Stretch lacerations
  (c) Cut lacerations
  (d) Tears

Ans. (a)
Note
Incised looking lacerated wounds are produced without excessive skin crushing and may have relatively sharp margins. Blunt force where the skin is close to bone and the subcutaneous fat is scanty may produce a wound, which by linear splitting of the tissues, may look like an incised wound. The commonest sites are: scalp, eyebrows, cheekbones, lower jaw, iliac crest, perineum, and shin.
Ref: The Essentials of Forensic Medicine and Toxicology, by Dr K. S. Narayan Reddy, 21st Edition, Chapter8, Pg- 156

Q. 94. The most conclusive evidence of antemortem drowning is the presence of (KPSC/Lect/FMT-05)
  (a) Water in the stomach
  (b) Emphysema aquosum
  (c) Foreign bodies in air passages
  (d) Persistent froth at mouth

Ans. (c)
Note
On cross section of the lungs there is an edematous condition of the lungs due to presence of a large amount of watery, frothy, blood stained fluid. This has been described as emphysema aquosum. It is seen in about 80% cases and is presumptive evidence of death from drowning.
Ref: The Essentials of Forensic Medicine and Toxicology, by Dr K. S. Narayan Reddy, 21st Edition, Chapter14, Pg- 315

Q. 95. Sex of a developing fetus can be determined in the following month of intrauterine life (KPSC/Lect/FMT-05)
  (a) 3rd
  (b) 4th
  (c) 5th
  (d) 6th

Ans. (c)
Note
The most accurate medical way to tell if one is pregnant with a boy or girl is to have a sonogram done at about 20 weeks gestation.
Ref: http://pediatrics.about.com/od/weeklyquestion/a/04_baby_gender.htm

Q. 96. Railway spine refers to one of the following types of injury to the spinal cord (KPSC/Lect/FMT-05)
    (a)   Confusion
    (b)   Laceration
    (c)   Concussion
    (d)   Transection

Ans. (c)
Note
Concussion of the spinal cord
This commonly occurs in railway and motor car collision and is known as RAILWAY SPINE. It also occurs from severe blows to the back, compression from dislocation or fracture of the vertebrae, damage by effusion of blood, fall from height or a bullet injury. It produces temporary paralysis, affecting the arms and hands or bladder, rectum or lower extremities. There are headaches, giddiness, restlessness, sleeplessness, neurasthenia, weakness in the limbs, amnesia, loss of sexual power and derangement of special senses. The paralysis is temporary and recovery occurs in about 48 hours.
Ref: The Essentials of Forensic Medicine and Toxicology, by Dr K. S. Narayan Reddy, 21st Edition, Chapter9, Pg- 223

Q. 97. In typical hanging, the position of the knot on the neck is (KPSC/Lect/FMT-05)
    (a)   At the nape of the neck
    (b)   Under the chin
    (c)   Anywhere other than the back of neck
    (d)   Just beneath the angle of jaw

Ans. (a)
Note
In a typical hanging the ligature runs from the midline above the thyroid cartilage symmetrically upwards on both sides of the neck to the occipital region. Thus the knot is at the back of the neck.
Ref: The Essentials of Forensic Medicine and Toxicology, by Dr K. S. Narayan Reddy, 21st Edition, Chapter14, Pg- 288

Q. 98. The first permanent tooth to erupt is the (KPSC/Lect/FMT-05)
    (a)   Canine
    (b)   Lateral incisor
    (c)   First molar
    (d)   Central Incisor

Ans. (c)
Note
Eruption of permanent teeth

Tooth	Eruption
First molar	6-7 years
Central incisor	6-8 years
Lateral incisor	7-9 years
First premolar	9-11 years
Second premolar	10-12 years
Canine	11-12 years
Second molar	12-14 years
Third molar	17-25 years

Ref: The Essentials of Forensic Medicine and Toxicology, by Dr K. S. Narayan Reddy, 21st Edition, Chapter4, Pg- 57

Q. 99. Statutory rape, is rape on a girl below (KPSC/Lect/FMT-05)
  (a) 10 years
  (b) 12 years
  (c) 15 years
  (d) 16 years

Ans. (d)
Note
Statutory rape: It is the normal physiologic intercourse with a girl below 16 years of age even with her consent.
Ref: The Essentials of Forensic Medicine and Toxicology, by Dr K. S. Narayan Reddy, 21st Edition, Chapter17, Pg- 338

Q. 100. The irresistible desire to steal articles is known as (KPSC/Lect/FMT-05)
  (a) Kleptomania
  (b) Dipsomania
  (c) Pyromania
  (d) Mutilomania

Ans. (a)
Note
An impulse is a sudden and irresistible force compelling a person, to the conscious performance of some action without motive or forethought.
Types
Kleptomania: An irresistible desire to steal articles of little value.
Pyromania: An irresistible desire to set fire to things.
Mutilomania: An irresistible desire to mutilate animals.
Dipsomania: An irresistible desire for alcoholic drinks at frequent intervals.
Sexual impulses
Suicidal and homicidal impulses.
Ref: The Essentials of Forensic Medicine and Toxicology, by Dr K. S. Narayan Reddy, 21st Edition, Chapter21, Pg- 399

Q. 101. All the following are true regarding a lacerated wound except (KPSC/Lect/FMT-05)
  (a) Irregular margins
  (b) Hemorrhage is more
  (c) Bruising of margins
  (d) Bridging of tissues

Ans. (b)
Note
Lacerated wounds are produced by application of blunt force to broad area of the body, which crush or stretch tissues beyond the limits of their elasticity. They are characterized by:
 -Irregular, ragged and uneven margins.
 -Pointed or blunted ends with minute tears at the margins.
 -Bruising is seen either in the skin or the subcutaneous tissue around the wound.
 -Deeper tissues are unevenly divided with tags of tissues at the bottom of the wound bridging across the margin.
 -Hemorrhage is less because the arteries are crushed and torn across irregularly, and thus the wound retracts and the blood clots readily.
Ref: The Essentials of Forensic Medicine and Toxicology, by Dr K. S. Narayan Reddy, 21st Edition, Chapter8, Pg- 156-158

Q. 102. A bullet which strikes an intervening object before hitting a target is called (KPSC/Lect/FMT-05)
  (a) Dumdum
  (b) Yawing
  (c) Tandem
  (d) Ricochet

Ans. (d)

Note
Dumdum bullet
It is open at the base and has the point covered with the jacket. When it strikes an object, the lead at the point expands or mushrooms, and produces a large hole.
Yawning bullet
A bullet traveling in an irregular fashion instead of traveling nose on is called Yawning bullet.
Tandem bullet
In some defective firearms the bullet may fail to come out from the muzzle. When it is fired again then the second bullet goes off carrying the first bullet with it, and both bullets enter the body through the same entry wound.
Ricochet bullet
It is one, which before striking the object aimed at strikes some intervening object first, and then after ricocheting and rebounding from these, hits the object. The path of ricochet is completely unexpected. It is usually seen with inferior firearms and low velocity bullets.
Tumbling bullet
A bullet that rotates end-on-end during its motion is called a tumbling bullet
Ref: The Essentials of Forensic Medicine and Toxicology, by Dr K. S. Narayan Reddy, 21st Edition, Chapter 8, Pg-177, 189, 190

Q. 103. Barberio's test is used to detect
   (a)   Animal blood
   (b)   Human blood
   (c)   Vaginal fluid
   (d)   Semen

Ans. (d)
Note
Barberio's test
A saturated aqueous or alcoholic solution of picric acid when added to spermatic fluid, produces- yellow needle shaped rhombic crystals of spermine picrate.
Other tests done to identify seminal fluid are:
   -Florence test
   -Acid phosphatase test
   -Creatinine phosphokinese
   -Semen specific glycoprotein
   -Ammonium molybdate test
   -Choline and spermine
Ref: The Essentials of Forensic Medicine and Toxicology, by Dr K. S. Narayan Reddy, 21st Edition, Chapter17, Pg- 355,356

Q. 104. Generalised convulsions are seen in poisoning with
   (a)   Nux-vomica
   (b)   Mercury
   (c)   Lead
   (d)   Arsenic

Ans. (c)
Note
Lead poisoning: The convulsions are preceded by prodromal symptoms such as increased acuity of perception, rigidity of muscles and muscular twitching. Convulsions are produced due to direct action on the reflex centers of the spinal cord, and affect all the muscles at a time. These are first clonic but eventually become tonic. During the convulsions, the face becomes cyanosed and has anxious look, eyes are staring and pupils are dilated. The convulsions are most marked in the anti-gravity muscles so that the body arches in hyperextension. Consciousness is not lost and mind remains clear till death.
Ref: The Essentials of Forensic Medicine and Toxicology, by Dr K. S. Narayan Reddy, 21st Edition, Chapter35, Pg- 534,535

Q. 105. Abrasion collar is seen with
   (a) Rifle bullet
   (b) Dum-Dum bullet
   (c) Richochetto wound
   (d) None of the above

Ans. (a)

Note
Rifle weapons include:
- Air and gas operated rifles
- Revolvers
- Automatic pistols
- Machine guns, etc.

An abrasion collar is seen when the bullet first strikes the skin. It first indents and then stretches the skin surface, so that perforation takes place through a tense area. After the bullet has perforated the skin, the elasticity of the skin causes the skin to contract. The skin is abraded around the hole due to rubbing of the gyrating body of the bullet against the inverted epidermis and heat of the bullet.
Ref: The Essentials of Forensic Medicine and Toxicology, by Dr K. S. Narayan Reddy, 21st Edition, Chapter 8, Pg- 171,184

Q. 106. Inquest which is not carried out in India is
   (a) Coroner's inquest
   (b) Police inquest
   (c) Magistrate inquest
   (d) Medical examiner's inquest

Ans. (d)

Note
Inquest is the investigation into the cause of death. It is conducted in cases of unusual death. Two types of inquests are currently carried out in India.
- Police inquest: The officer-in charge of a police station conducts the inquest in any case of unnatural death in presence of 2 or more respectable inhabitants of the neighbourhood.
- Magistrate's inquest: It is conducted by a district magistrate in case of
    - death in custody
    - dowry death
    - death in prison, exhumation, death due to police firing.

Ref: The Essentials of Forensic Medicine and Toxicology, by Dr K. S. Narayan Reddy, 21st Edition, Chapter 2, Pg- 5

In India, the Coroner's inquest is no more done now. It was actually a legacy of the English *Raj* that we had for over 200 years. Coroner used to be a special officer appointed by the government to inquire into causes of unnatural deaths. The Coroner was required to have a legal qualification and was usually an advocate, attorney, pleader, or first class magistrate, or a transferred metropolitan magistrate (all of whom must have a minimum of five years experience in the legal field). He held the rank of a First Class Judicial Magistrate. He presided over the Coroner's court and was governed by the provisions of the Coroner's Act 1871.
Ref: http://www.geradts.com/anil/ij/vol_002_no_001/ug002_001_1.html

Q. 107. Rigor mortis simulate
   (a) Cadaveric spasm
   (b) Livor mortis
   (c) Algur mortis
   (d) Mummification

Ans. (a)

Note
Conditions simulating cadaveric spasm are:
   a. Heat stiffening
   b. Cold stiffening

c. Cadaveric spasm: It is also called as cataleptic rigidity. In this, the muscles that were contracted during life become stiff and rigid immediately after death without passing into a stage of primary relaxation. As such, the change preserves the exact attitude of the person at the time of death for several hours afterwards. It occurs especially in cases of sudden death, excitement, fear, severe pain, exhaustion, cerebral haemorrhage, injury to the nervous system, firearm wound of the head, convulsant poisons, such as strychinine. This is usually limited to a single group of muscles and frequently involves the hands.

Ref: The Essentials of Forensic Medicine and Toxicology, by Dr K. S. Narayan Reddy, 21st Edition, Chapter7, Pg- 134

Q. 108. Test for detection of old blood stain is
    (a) Precipitin test
    (b) Benzidine test
    (c) Gel diffusion
    (d) Absorption elution

Ans. (b)
Note
    (a) Precipitin and
    (b) Gel diffusion tests:
These are used to identify if the blood is human or from a lower animal.
Ref: The Essentials of Forensic Medicine and Toxicology, by Dr K. S. Narayan Reddy, 21st Edition, Chapter20, Pg- 383
    (c) Benzidine test:
A test for blood; the suspected fluid is treated with glacial acetic acid and ether, and the latter is then decanted and treated with hydrogen peroxide and a solution of benzidine in acetic acid; the presence of blood is indicated by a bluish colour turning to purple.
Synonym: Adler's test.
Ref: http://cancerweb.ncl.ac.uk/cgi-bin/omd?benzidine+test
    (d) Absorption elution test:
A method based on the absorption elution technique shown to be applicable for the detection of M and N blood groups of dried bloodstains on cotton cloth.
Ref: http://www.astm.org/cgibin/SoftCart.exe/JOURNALS/FORENSIC/PAGES/1281.htm?E+mystore

Thus by exclusion we can say that the correct answer is benzidine test.

Q. 109. Medical negligence falls under following except
    (a) Sec 304 A
    (b) Indian Contract Act
    (c) IPC 312
    (d) IPC 351

Ans. (d)
Note
a. Sec 304 A
Causing death by negligence: Whoever causes the death of any person by doing any rash or negligent act not amounting to culpable homicide, shall be punished with imprisonment of either description for a term which may extend to two years, or with fine, or with both.
Ref: -http://www.indialawinfo.com/bareacts/ipc.html
b. Contract Act
Consists of limiting factors subject to which contract may be entered into, executed and breach enforced. It only provides a framework of rules and regulations which govern the formation and performance of contract.
Ref: -http://dateyvs.com/gener03.htm
c. IPC 312. Causing miscarriage
Whoever voluntarily causes a woman with child to miscarry, shall, if such miscarriage be not caused in good faith for the purpose of saving the life of the woman, be punished with imprisonment of either

description for a term which may extend to three years, or with fine, or with both; and, if the woman be quick with child, shall be punished with imprisonment of either description for a term which may extend to seven years, and shall also be liable to fine.

d. *IPC 351. Assault*
Whoever makes any gesture, or any preparation intending or knowing it to be likely that such gesture or preparation will cause any person present to apprehend that he who makes that gesture or preparation is about to use criminal force to that person, is said to commit an assault.
Ref: http://www.indialawinfo.com/bareacts/ipc.html

Q. 110. Aseptic autolysis is seen in
    (a)   Maceration
    (b)   Mummification
    (c)   Putrefaction
    (d)   Saponification

Ans. (a)
Note
a. *Maceration*
It is the process of aseptic autolysis seen in dead born children. This occurs when a dead born child remains in utero for about 3-4 days surrounded by liquor amnii but with the exclusion of air. The earliest sign of maceration is slippage, which can be seen in 12 hours after the death of the child in utero. The macerated fetus is soft, flaccid and flattens out when placed on a level surface. The skin is red or purple with large blebs containing serous fluid. The epidermis detaches easily and leaves moist gray areas. The abdomen is distended. Bones are flexible and the joints are abnormally mobile.
(Chapter 19, Pg- 368.)

b. *Mummification*
It is a modification of putrefaction. There is dehydration and shriveling of the cadaver, but the natural appearances are preserved. The factors necessary for its production are-
-Absence of moisture and air
-Continuous action of dry or warmed air.
(Chapter 7, Pg- 142)

c. *Putrefaction*
It is the final stage following death, produced mainly by the bacterial enzymes.

d. *Saponification*
It is a modification of putrefaction; in this the fatty tissues of the body change into a substance similar to soaps, known as adipocere. It is seen in bodies immersed in water or in a damp, warm environment.
(Chapter 7, Pg- 141)
Ref: The Essentials of Forensic Medicine and Toxicology, by Dr K. S. Narayan Reddy, 21st Edition

Q. 111. Widmark formula is used in
    (a)   Alcohol
    (b)   Barbiturates
    (c)   Cannabis
    (d)   Opium

Ans. (a)
Note
Widmark evolved a formula, which takes into account the size, and sex of the person and the type of person and the type of alcoholic liquor consumed. The formula is $A = PCR$, where:
A: is the weight of alcohol in grams of the body.
P: is the body weight in kg.
C: is the concentration of alcohol in the blood in mg/ kg.
R: is the constant (0.6 for men and 0.5 for women)
Ref: The Essentials of Forensic Medicine and Toxicology, by Dr K. S. Narayan Reddy, 21st Edition, Chapter30, Pg- 498,499

Q. 112. Section 191 IPC deals with
(a) Rape
(b) Giving false evidence
(c) Grievous hurt
(d) Assault

Ans. (b)

Note
Sec 191 defines a hostile witness as one who is supposed to have some interest or motive for concealing part of the truth, or for giving completely false evidence.
Ref: The Essentials of Forensic Medicine and Toxicology, by Dr K. S. Narayan Reddy, 21st Edition, Chapter2, Pg- 11

Q. 113. In typical hanging, the position of knot on the neck is
(a) At the nape
(b) Under the chin
(c) Anywhere other than the back of neck
(d) Just beneath the angle of jaw

Ans. (a)

Note
In a typical hanging the ligature runs from the midline above the thyroid cartilage symmetrically upwards on both sides of the neck to the occipital region.
Thus the knot is at the back of the neck.
Ref: The Essentials of Forensic Medicine and Toxicology, by Dr K. S. Narayan Reddy, 21st Edition, Chapter14, Pg- 288

Q. 114. Species identification is done by (AIIMS/May-03)
(a) Neutron activation analysis (NAA)
(b) Precipitin test
(c) Benzidine test
(d) Spectroscopy

Ans. (b)

Note
Serological examinations are done to determine whether the blood is of animal or human origin.
Precipitin test is an immunological test. Blood serum contains proteins in colloidal suspension, and when human serum is injected into an animal, the animal becomes immunized against these proteins and antibodies develop in his blood. If human serum is then brought into contact with this animal serum the antibodies will react with the proteins in the human serum and a visible precipitate forms.
Ref: The Essentials of Forensic Medicine and Toxicology, by Dr K. S. Narayan Reddy, 21st Edition, Chapter20, Pg- 383

Q. 115. A dead born fetus does not have (AIIMS/May-03)
(a) Rigor mortis at birth
(b) Adipocere formation
(c) Maceration
(d) Mummification

Ans. (b)

Note
The dead born fetus shows the following sign after it is born:
    -Rigor mortis at delivery
    -Maceration
    -Mummification
Ref: The Essentials of Forensic Medicine and Toxicology, by Dr K. S. Narayan Reddy, 21st Edition, Chapter19, Pg- 368,369
Adipocere formation is a modification of putrefaction; in this the fatty tissues of the body change into a substance similar to soaps, known as adipocere. It is seen in bodies immersed in water or in a damp, warm environment

Ref: -The Essentials of Forensic Medicine and Toxicology, by Dr K. S. Narayan Reddy, 21st edition. Chapter 7, Pg- 141

Q. 116. In a suspected case of death due to poisoning where cadaveric rigidity is lasting longer than usual, it may be a case of poisoning due to (AIIMS/May-03)
(a) Lead
(b) Arsenic
(c) Mercury
(d) Copper

Ans. (b)
Note
Arsenic delays putrefaction, thus we can say that it'll cause prolonged cadaveric spasm.
Ref: The Essentials of Forensic Medicine and Toxicology, by Dr K. S. Narayan Reddy, 21st edition chapter 27, Pg- 463

Q. 117. Which one of the following tissues putrefies late? (AIIMS/Nov-03)
(a) Brain
(b) Prostate
(c) Liver
(d) Stomach

Ans. (b)
Note
Prostate
It resists putrefaction for a long time.
Liver
It becomes soft and flabby within 12 to 24 hours of death. Multiple blisters appear around 24-36 hours. clostridium welchii forms characteristic small clumps in a tissue space and produce gas, which soon increase in size. When bubbles develop, the organ has a honeycombed, vesicular or "foamy" appearance. The greenish discoloration spreads to the whole organ, which finally becomes coal black.
Stomach
The stomach and intestines putrefy in 24-36 hours in summer and 3-5 days in winters. Dark red irregular patches involving the whole thickness of the wall are first seen on the posterior wall and then on the anterior wall. Gas blebs are formed in the submucous layer. They become softened, dark brown and change into dark, soft, pulpy mass. Other breakdown products reacting with sulphur may stain the mucosa green or black.
Ref: The Essentials of Forensic Medicine and Toxicology, by Dr K. S. Narayan Reddy, 21st edition chapter 7, Pg- 139, 140

Q. 118. Rule of Hasse is used to determine (AIIMS/Nov-03)
(a) The age of fetus
(b) Height of an adult
(c) Race of a person
(d) Identification

Ans. (a)
Note
Rule of Hasse (1895): This is a rough method of calculating the age of the fetus. The length of the fetus is measured from the crown to heel in centimeters.
-During the first five months the square root of the length gives the approximate age of the fetus in months.
-During the last five months, the length in cm divided by 5 gives the age of the fetus in months.
After birth, the length of an infant is fifty cm; sixty cm at the end of 6 months: 68 cm at the end of first year, and 100 cm at the end of 4th year.
Birth weight doubles at the end of 5 months of age and triples by about 1 year.
Ref: The Essentials of Forensic Medicine and Toxicology, by Dr K. S. Narayan Reddy, 21st edition chapter 4, Pg- 70

Q. 119. In which of the following weapons empty cartridge case is ejected after firing? (AIIMS/Nov-03)
(a) Shot gun
(b) Revolver
(c) Pistol
(d) Rifle

Ans. (c)
Note
Shot gun
It may be single barreled or double barreled. It is intended to fire a single shot at a time. The weapon is made to break open on the hinge across the breech facing for the insertion and extraction of cartridge cases.
Revolver
The cartridges are kept in chambers in a metal cylinder, which revolves or rotates before each shot to bring the next cartridge opposite the barrel, ready to be fired.
Pistol
It is a hand arm in which the cartridge is loaded directly into the chamber of the barrel. When a cartridge if fired, the empty cartridge case falls on the ground several metres away, and a new cartridge slips into the breech automatically by a spring.
Rifle
It is a gun with a long barrel, the bore of which is rifled. It may be self-loading or automatic or both.
Ref: The Essentials of Forensic Medicine and Toxicology, by Dr K. S. Narayan Reddy, 21st edition chapter 8, Pg-, 172,174, 175

Q. 120. In freshwater drowning the death occurs within 4-5 minutes of submersion due to ventricular fibrillation, which of the following reasons is responsible for this? (AIIMS/May-04)
(a) Total asphyxia is produced due to fresh water.
(b) Laryngospasm causing vagal inhibition.
(c) Hemoconcentration of blood caused by the osmotic pressure effect.
(d) Hemodilution, overloading of heart and hemolysis resulting in release of potassium.

Ans. (d)
Note
In drowning in fresh water, water passes rapidly from the lungs to the blood, leading to hemolysis and dilution of the blood. The blood volume may increase by 50% within a minute causing a great strain on the heart due to hypervolaemia. The concentration of electrolytes decreases in the serum. Proteins and Hb are also reduced. The serum potassium increases. This increased load causes rapid overburdening of the heart and produces pulmonary edema. Cardiac arrhythmia leads to ventricular tachycardia and fibrillation leading to death.
Ref: The Essentials of Forensic Medicine and Toxicology, by Dr K. S. Narayan Reddy, 21st edition chapter 14, Pg- 313

Q. 121. A 25 years female was found in room with 100% burns on her body. The tongue was protruding out; body was in pugilistic attitude with heat ruptures, peeling of skin, and heat hematoma and heat fractures of skull. Carboxy hemoglobin was 25% and soot particles were present in trachea. Which of the combinations of two findings will establish that the burns were antemortem in nature? (AIIMS/May-04)
(a) Heat hematoma & heat ruptures
(b) Heat fracture of skull and peeling of skin
(c) Heat hematoma and pugilistic attitude
(d) Carboxy hemoglobin (25%) and soot particles in trachea

Ans. (d)
Note
In death due to burns, the CO levels in the blood will be more than ten percent and may reach upto 70-80%, though children and old persons die at levels of 30-40%.
Presence of raised blood CO and soot or carbon particles in the air passages are an absolute proof that the person was alive at the time when fire occurred.
Pugilistic attitude is a posture adopted by the body on exposure to great heat. The arms are flexed at the elbows

and the wrists, legs are flexed at the knees and hip, head is slightly extended and all fingers are hooked like claws. This occurs due to coagulation of proteins, it occurs irrespective of whether the person was alive or dead at the time of fire.

Heat ruptures occur when great heat is applied and skin contracts either before or after death.

Ref: The Essentials of Forensic Medicine and Toxicology, by Dr K. S. Narayan Reddy, 21st edition chapter 12, Pg- 273,275

Q. 122. The phenomenon of suspended animation may be seen in (AIIMS/May-04)
(a) Throttling
(b) Drowning
(c) Strangulation
(d) Brain hemorrhage

Ans. (b)
Note
Suspended animation or apparent death: In this condition signs of life are not found as the functions are interrupted for some time, or are reduced to a minimum. However life continues and resuscitation is successful in such cases. The metabolic rate is so reduced that the requirement of individual cell is satisfied through the use of oxygen dissolved in the body fluids. It can occur in
- Freezing - Electrocution
- Newborn infants - Cholera
- Drowning - After anesthesia
- Shock - Cerebral concussion
- Insanity - Severe drug poisoning

Ref: The Essentials of Forensic Medicine and Toxicology, by Dr K. S. Narayan Reddy, 21st edition chapter 7, Pg- 126

Q. 123. A lady died due to unnatural death within seven years after her marriage The inquest in this case will be done by (AIIMS/May-04)
(a) Forensic medicine expert
(b) Deputy superintendent of police
(c) Sub-divisional magistrate
(d) Coroner

Ans. (c)
Note
As per sec 304-B; IPC where the death of a woman is caused by any burn or bodily injury or occurs otherwise than under normal circumstances within 7 years of marriage and it is shown that soon before her death she was subjected to cruelty or harassment by her husband or any relative of her husband for, or in connection with any demand for dowry, such a death shall be called "dowry death", and such husband or relative shall be deemed to have caused her death.

Ref: The Essentials of Forensic Medicine and Toxicology, by Dr K. S. Narayan Reddy, 21st edition chapter 10, Pg- 246

In such case of dowry death a District magistrate, Subdivisional Magistrate or any other Executive Magistrate, carries out the inquest.

Ref: The Essentials of Forensic Medicine and Toxicology, by Dr K. S. Narayan Reddy, 21st edition chapter 2, Pg- 5

Q. 124. Cheiloscopy is the study of prints of (AIIMS/May-04)
(a) Foot
(b) Fingers
(c) Palate
(d) Lips

Ans. (d)
Note
Lip prints or Cheiloscopy
This is a technique used for personal identification. Lip prints are divided into eight patterns, which are specific to the individual; vertical, branched, intersected, reticular patterns, etc. Minor differences are noted between the upper and lower lips and the right and left halves.

Ref: The Essentials of Forensic Medicine and Toxicology, by Dr K. S. Narayan Reddy, 21st edition chapter 4, Pg- 73

Q. 125. When a person has suspended himself by applying ligature around neck so that the point of suspension (knot) is situated in the region of the occiput. Such a hanging is called as (AIIMS/Nov-04)
(a) Typical
(b) Atypical
(c) Partial
(d) Incomplete

Ans. (a)
Note
In a case of typical hanging the ligature runs from the midline above the thyroid cartilage symmetrically upwards on both sides of the neck to the occipital region. Thus the point of suspension is the occipital region.
The knot therefore should be placed in the occiput.
Ref: The Essentials of Forensic Medicine and Toxicology, by Dr K. S. Narayan Reddy, 21st edition chapter 14, Pg- 288

Q. 126. Which of the following statements about blood grouping is not correct? (AIIMS/Nov-04)
(a) It can be used to resolve confusion of identity in alleged exchange of babies in maternity unit.
(b) It is the method to conclusively fix the paternity.
(c) It can assist in matching fragmented human remains in mass disaster.
(d) It can help to show whether blood stain on the weapon belongs to the suspect or victim.

Ans. (b)
Note
The tests for blood grouping may exclude a person as the possible father of the child but cannot definitely establish paternity. They can only indicate its possibilities. The exclusion of putative father is based upon the principle that a specific agglutinogen cannot appear in a child unless it was present in one of its parents.
Ref: The Essentials of Forensic Medicine and Toxicology, by Dr K. S. Narayan Reddy, 21st edition chapter 20, Pg- 387

Q. 127. The dead body of a murdered person is brought for preservation in mortuary. Which of the following statements is not correct? (AIIMS/Nov-04)
(a) The body should be stored averagely at 4°C.
(b) The body can be embalmed before postmortem.
(c) The body should be never undressed before the forensic doctor has seen it.
(d) The body can be stored at –20°C to preserve it for long duration.

Ans. (b)
Note
Embalming alters the appearance of the body, tissues and organs, making it difficult to interpret any injury or disease. Embalming completely destroys cyanide, alcohol and many other substances. Determination of the presence of many of the alkaloids and organic poisons becomes very difficult. The fixation process makes it difficult to extract drugs. Blood grouping cannot be made out. Thrombi and emboli will be dislocated and washed away. Thus embalming should not be done before post mortem.
Ref: The Essentials of Forensic Medicine and Toxicology, by Dr K. S. Narayan Reddy, 21st edition chapter 7, Pg- 143

Q. 128. An eleven year old rape victim is brought to causalty for medical examination. The medical officer is required to do the following things, except (AIIMS/Nov-04)
(a) The consent is to be taken from the patient.
(b) The patient should be examined in presence of a female attendant.
(c) The patient should be given necessary emergency treatment.
(d) All the necessary forensic samples should be collected.

Ans. (a)

Note
The following is the outline of a planned procedure in case of a victim of rape:
a. The victim should not be examined without requisition from the investigating officer or magistrate.
b. The written witnessed consent of the woman should be taken, if she is of unsound mind or less than 12 years of age, the consent of her parents is necessary.
c. The victim should be identified and all preliminary data about her should be noted.
d. Examination should be done without delay.
e. The victim is examined in the presence of a third person preferably a female attendant or a nurse.
f. The general demeanor of the patient should be noted along with the gait, physical development, etc.
Ref: The Essentials of Forensic Medicine and Toxicology, by Dr K. S. Narayan Reddy, 21st edition chapter 17, Pg- 340

Q. 129. A body is brought for autopsy with history of poisoning. On postmortem examination, there is dark brown postmortem staining and garlic odour in stomach. In this case the poisoning is most likely due to (AIIMS/Nov-04)
(a) Hydrocyanic acid
(b) Carbon dioxide
(c) Aniline dye
(d) Phosphorus

Ans. (d)
Note
The gastric and the intestinal contents in case of phosphorus poisoning may smell like that of garlic.
Other post mortem features are- signs of irritation of gastric and intestinal mucosa. The mucous membrane of the stomach and intestine are yellowish or grayish-white in colour and softened, thickened, inflamed and corroded or destroyed in patches. Multiple smaller haemorrhages are seen in the skin, subcutaneous tissues. The liver becomes swollen, yellow, soft, fatty and easily ruptured. The kidneys are yellow, greasy, and show hemorrhages on the surface. Fat emboli may be found in the pulmonary arterioles and capillaries.
Ref: The Essentials of Forensic Medicine and Toxicology, by Dr K. S. Narayan Reddy, 21st Edition, Chapter7, Pg- 131, 474

Q. 130. The ideal place to record temperature in dead body is from (AIIMS/Nov-05)
(a) Axilla
(b) Groin
(c) Rectum
(d) Mouth

Ans. (c)
Note
For measuring the temperature a laboratory thermometer 25 cm long, with a range of 0 – 50 degree Celcius is used. The rectum is the ideal place to record temperature except in case of sodomy. The thermometer should be inserted 8 – 10 cm and left there for two minutes. The temperature can also be recorded by making a small midline incision into the peritoneal cavity and inserting the thermometer in contact with the inferior surface of the liver. The external auditory meatus or the nasal passages can also be used to record the temperature.
A rough idea of the approximate time in hours of death can be obtained by using the formula:
Normal body temperature - rectal temperature
Rate of temperature fall per hour.
Ref: The Essentials of Forensic Medicine and Toxicology, by Dr K. S. Narayan Reddy, 21st Edition, Chapter7, Pg- 127

Q. 131. Diffusion of oxygen at the tissue level is affected in all the following poisonings except (AIIMS/Nov-05)
(a) Carbon monoxide
(b) Curare
(c) Phosgene
(d) Cyanides

Ans. (b)

MCQ's in Forensic Medicine

Note
a. Carbon monoxide: It has two hundred times more affinity towards Hb than that of O_2. It displaces oxygen from its combination with hemoglobin and forms a relatively stable compound known as carboxyhemoglobin. It thus reduces the oxygen content of the blood, and hence that of the tissues. (Chapter 37, Pg- 545)
b. c) Phosphorus is a protoplasmic poison, which affects cellular oxidation. (Chapter 28, Pg- 473)
c. d) Cyanide inhibits the action of cytochrome oxidase, carbonic anhydrase and probably of other enzyme systems. It blocks the final step of oxidative phosphorylation and prevents formation of ATP. It acts by reducing the oxygen carrying capacity of the blood and preventing the uptake of oxygen for cellular respiration. (Chapter 36, Pg 542)
Ref: The Essentials of Forensic Medicine and Toxicology, by Dr K. S. Narayan Reddy, 21st edition

Q. 132. Postmortem caloricity may be seen in all the following causes of death except (AIIMS/Nov-05)
    (a) Septicemia
    (b) Barbiturate poisoning
    (c) Strychnine poisoning
    (d) Tetanus

Ans. (b)
Note
In postmortem caloricity the temperature of the body remains raised for the first two hours or so after death. This occurs:
a. When the regulation of heat production has been severely disturbed before death, as in sunstroke and in some nervous disorders.
b. When there has been a great increase in heat production in the muscles due to convulsions, as in tetanus and strychnine poisoning, etc.
c. When there has been excessive bacterial activity, as in septicaemic condition, cholera and other fevers.
Ref: The Essentials of Forensic Medicine and Toxicology, by Dr K. S. Narayan Reddy, 21st Edition, Chapter7, Pg- 128

Q. 133. When a group of muscles of a dead body were in state of strong contraction immediately prior to death and remain so even after death, the condition is termed as (AIIMS/Nov-05)
    (a) Gas stiffening
    (b) Rigor mortis
    (c) Cadaveric spasm
    (d) Cold stiffening

Ans. (c)
Note
Cadaveric spasm is also called as cataleptic rigidity. In this, the muscles that were contracted during life become stiff and rigid immediately after death without passing into a stage of primary relaxation. As such, the change preserves the exact attitude of the person at the time of death for several hours afterwards. It occurs especially in cases of sudden death, excitement, fear, severe pain, exhaustion, cerebral hemorrhage, injury to the nervous system, firearm wound of the head, convulsant poisons, such as strychinine. This is usually limited to a single group of muscles and frequently involves the hands.
Ref: The Essentials of Forensic Medicine and Toxicology, by Dr K. S. Narayan Reddy, 21st Edition, Chapter7, Pg- 134

Q. 134. 'Patterned' abrasion is a variety of (AIIMS/Nov-05)
    (a) Linear abrasion
    (b) Pressure abrasion
    (c) Sliding abrasion
    (d) Superficial bruise

Ans. (b)

Note
Impact abrasions and pressure abrasions reproduce the pattern of the object causing it and are called as patterned abrasions. They are produced by force applied at right angles to the surface of the skin. If the skin is srtuck with a weapon having a patterned surface, the ridges of the object damage the epidermis, and the skin may be compressed into the cavities of the pattern causing intradermal bruise. Examples of patterned abrasions are- imprint of bicycle chain, ropes & serrated knife.
Ref: The Essentials of Forensic Medicine and Toxicology, by Dr K. S. Narayan Reddy, 21st Edition, Chapter8, Pg- 150

Q. 135. In a firearm injury, there is burning, blackening, toattooing around the wound, along with cherry red colour of the surrounding tissues and is cruciate in shape, the injury is (All INDIA-05)
  (a) Close shot entry
  (b) Close contact exit
  (c) Contact shot entry
  (d) Distant shot entry

Ans. (c)
Note
Contact wounds
They are usually round or oval, large, often ragged because of individual shot & tearing due to gases. CO in the gases combines with hemoglobin due to which wound of entry and the wound track becomes pink. Cruciate, stellate or ragged lacerations are seen especially if there is a thick bone immediately under the skin / muscle. The margins of the skin perforation are charred by flame, and the abraded border is usually soiled with minimum powder residue.
Ref: The Essentials of Forensic Medicine and Toxicology, by Dr K. S. Narayan Reddy, 21st Edition, Chapter8, Pg- 178

Q. 136. In methyl alcohol poisoning there is CNS depression, cardiac depression and optic nerve atrophy. These effects are produced due to (All INDIA-05)
  (a) Formaldehyde and formic acid
  (b) Acetaldehyde
  (c) Pyridine
  (d) Acetic acid

Ans. (a)
Note
Methanol is oxidized to formaldehyde (which is 33 times more toxic than methanol), which is further metabolized to formic acid (6 times more toxic than methanol) in the liver. This is responsible for metabolic acidosis and renal toxicity. Death is mainly due to acidosis from the production of organic acids, CNS depression is a minor factor.
Ref: The Essentials of Forensic Medicine and Toxicology, by Dr K. S. Narayan Reddy, 21st Edition, Chapter30, Pg- 504

Q. 137. In chronic arsenic poisoning the following samples can be sent for laboratory examination except (All INDIA-05)
  (a) Nail clippings
  (b) Hair samples
  (c) Bone biopsy
  (d) Blood sample

Ans. (d)
Note
For the purpose of exposure evaluation, arsenic can be measured in blood, hair, fingernails, and urine. Measurement of arsenic in blood is not considered to be a reliable indicator of chronic exposure to low levels of arsenic because arsenic is cleared from the blood within a few hours. Because of large inter-individual variability and potential contamination from other sources, nail and hair samples are not considered to be reliable indicators. Urine arsenic is considered to be the most reliable method for measuring exposure to

arsenic–particularly exposures occurring within a few days of the specimen collection. Fluctuations in urine excretion rates make a 24-hour collection the optimal sample.
Ref: -http://www.lycos.com/info/arsenic—arsenic-exposure.html

Q. 138. Which of the following statements is not correct regarding diatom? (All INDIA-05)
  (a) Diatoms are aquatic unicellular plant.
  (b) Diatoms has an extracellular coat composed of magnesium.
  (c) Acid digestion technique is used to extract diatoms.
  (d) Presence of diatoms in the femoral bone marrow is an indication of antemortem inhalation of water.

Ans. (b)

Note
Diatoms are microscopic unicellular or colonial algae. They have a complex structure of their cell walls, which are usually strongly impregnated with silica and contains chlorophyll and diatomin, a brown pigment. They secrete a hard siliceous outer box-like skeleton called a frustule. They resist heat and acid. Diatoms measuring up to sixty microns in diameter are said to enter the pulmonary circulation during drowning. A live body with active transportation can transport the diatoms to the brain, bone marrow, liver and other viscera and skeletal muscle. The bone marrow is highly suitable and reliable.
This is tested by taking a 5 gm sample of bone marrow and covering it with 5 times the volume of concentrated nitric acid and left at room temperature for 1-2 days to allow digestion. The tube is then centrifuged and supernatent acid is poured off and replaced by distilled water. The deposit is then examined under a microscope.
Ref: The Essentials of Forensic Medicine and Toxicology, by Dr K. S. Narayan Reddy, 21st Edition, Chapter14, Pg- 317,318

Q. 139. In India, magistrate inquest is done in the following cases except (All INDIA-05)
  (a) Exhumation cases
  (b) Dowry deaths within 5 years of marriage
  (c) Murder cases
  (d) Death of a person in police custody

Ans. (c)

Note
Magistrate's inquest: It is conducted by a district magistrate in case of:
  -Death in custody
  -Dowry death
  -Death in prison, exhumation, death due to police firing.
Ref: The Essentials of Forensic Medicine and Toxicology, by Dr K. S. Narayan Reddy, 21st Edition, Chapter2, Pg- 5

Q. 140. At autopsy, the cyanide poisoning case will show the following features, except (All INDIA-05)
  (a) Characteristic bitter lemon smell
  (b) Congested organs
  (c) The skin may be pinkish or cherry red in colour
  (d) Erosion and hemorrhages in oesophagus and stomach

Ans. (a)

Note
The post mortem appearances of cyanide poisoning are:
The eyes are bright, glistening and prominent with dilated pupils. The colour of cheeks and post mortem staining may be cherry red in about half the cases, because oxygen remains in the cells as oxyhemoglobin, and due to the formation of cyanmethaemoglobin. The odour of hydrocyanic acid may be noticed on opening the body. There is congestion of visceras and edema of lungs. The serous cavities are ecchymosed. The mucosa of the stomach and intestine is red and congested. The mucosa of the stomach may be eroded and blackened due to the formation of alkaline haematin. The stomach may contain frank or altered blood from the erosions and hemorrhages in the walls.

Ref: The Essentials of Forensic Medicine and Toxicology, by Dr K. S. Narayan Reddy, 21st Edition, Chapter36, Pg- 544

Q. 141. The most reliable criteria in Gustafson's method of identification is (All INDIA-05)
- (a) Cementum apposition
- (b) Transparency of root
- (c) Attrition
- (d) Root resorption

Ans. (b)

Note

Gustafson's method: It is used for age estimation of adults over 21 years of age depending upon the physiological age changes in each of the dental tissues.

The various criteria are:
a. Attrition: Due to wear and tear from mastication, occlusional surface of the teeth is destroyed gradually, 1st involving the enamel, then dentin and at last the pulp.
b. Paraodontosis: Regression of gums and periodontal tissues surrounding the teeth takes place in advancing age.
c. Secondary dentine: May develop from the walls within the pulp cavity and decrease the size of the cavity
d. Cementum apposition: The cementum increases in thickness particularly due to changes in the tooth position especially near the end of the root.
e. Root resorption: Absorption of the root starts at the apex and extends upwards, it usually occurs in the late age
f. Transparency of roots: Canals in the dentin are at first wide, with age they are filled with minerals so that they become invisible. It is the most reliable method.
Ref: The Essentials of Forensic Medicine and Toxicology, by Dr K. S. Narayan Reddy, 21st Edition, Chapter4, Pg- 58

Q. 142. The minimum age at which an individual is responsible for his criminal act is (All INDIA-05)
- (a) 7 years
- (b) 12 years
- (c) 16 years
- (d) 21 years

Ans. (a)

Note

Any act, which is done by a child under 7 years of age, is not an offence (Sec 82, IPC). A child between the age of 7 and 12 years is presumed to be capable of committing a crime, if he has attained sufficient maturity of understanding to judge the nature and consequences of his conduct on that occasion. (Sec 83, IPC)
Ref: The Essentials of Forensic Medicine and Toxicology, by Dr K. S. Narayan Reddy, 21st Edition, Chapter4, Pg- 68

Q. 143. BAL is useful in treating poisoning due to all, except (All INDIA-04)
- (a) Lead
- (b) Organic mercury
- (c) Cadmium
- (d) Arsenic

Ans. (c)

Note

B.A.L. (British Anti-Lewsite) or dimercaprol:
It is used as a physiological antidote to arsenic, lead, bismuth, copper, mercury, gold and other heavy metals. Many heavy metals have a great affinity for sulphydryl (SH) radicals, which combine with them in tissues and deprive the body of the use of respiratory enzymes of tissue cells. The compound formed by this heavy metal and dimercaprol is relatively stable, which is carried into the tissue fluids particularly plasma, and excreted in the urine. In severe poisoning a dose of 3-4 mg/kg is given. It should not be used when the liver is damaged.

Ref: The Essentials of Forensic Medicine and Toxicology, by Dr K. S. Narayan Reddy, 21st Edition, Chapter 24, Pg- 444,445

Q. 144. Counter-coup injuries are seen in (All INDIA-04)
(a) Brain
(b) Heart
(c) Liver
(d) Pancreas

Ans. (a)
Note

Coup means that the injury is located beneath the area of impact, and results directly by the impacting force. Counter-coup means that the lesion is present in an area opposite the side of impact. A certain amount of shear strain may occur below the point of impact, particularly if the skull is fractured, which accounts for the coup. Counter-coup injuries are not seen if the head is well fixed and cannot rotate. It is caused when a moving head is suddenly decelerated by hitting a firm surface. The sudden arrest of the head results in the brain striking against the arrested skull. Another factor responsible for the formation of counter-coup injuries is formation of cavity or vacuum in the cranial cavity on the opposite side of impact, as the brain lags behind the moving skull. This exerts a suction effect, which damages the brain.

Ref: The Essentials of Forensic Medicine and Toxicology, by Dr K. S. Narayan Reddy, 21st Edition, Chapter 9, Pg- 210,211

Q. 145. Disputed maternity can be solved by using the following tests except (All INDIA-04)
(a) Blood grouping
(b) HLA typing
(c) Preciptin test
(d) DNA fingerprinting

Ans. (c)
Note

When the same child is claimed by two women, or when two children are interchanged either by accident or by design in maternity home or hospital the case of disputed maternity arises. In such cases the blood grouping tests are useful. These include:
- Red cell antigens (ABO, P system, Rh system, etc.)
- White cell antigens (HL-A, B, C, D and DR)
- Serum protein polymorphism
- Red cell Enzyme polymorphisms

Ref: The Essentials of Forensic Medicine and Toxicology, by Dr K. S. Narayan Reddy, 21st Edition, Chapter 20, Pg- 389

Q. 146. Deep blue colour of hypostasis is seen in death due to poisoning by (All INDIA-04)
(a) Potassium cyanide
(b) Phophorus
(c) Aniline dyes
(d) Carbon monoxide

Ans. (c)
Note

Aniline can be toxic if ingested, inhaled, or by skin contact. Aniline damages hemoglobin, a protein that normally transports oxygen in the blood. The damaged hemoglobin cannot carry oxygen. This condition is known as methemoglobinemia and its severity depends on how much you are exposed to and for how long. Methemoglobinemia is the most prominent symptom of aniline poisoning in humans, resulting in cyanosis (a purplish blue skin color) following acute high exposure to aniline. Dizziness, headaches, irregular heartbeat, convulsions, coma, and death may also occur. Direct contact with aniline can also produce skin and eye irritation.

Ref: -http://www.atsdr.cdc.gov/tfacts171.html
However as per the information given in Reddy's:
The post mortem hypostasis in aniline poisoning is dark brown or red-brown.
Ref: -The Essentials of Forensic Medicine and Toxicology, by Dr K. S. Narayan Reddy, 21st Edition, Chapter7, Pg- 131

Q. 147. A 25 year old person sustained injury in right eye. He developed right corneal opacity following the injury. Left eye was already having poor vision. Corneoplasty of right eye was done and vision was restored. Medicolegally such injury is labelled as (All INDIA-04)
- (a) Grievous
- (b) Simple
- (c) Dangerous
- (d) Serious

Ans. (b)
Note
a. *Grievous hurt*
According to sec 320, IPC- any of the following constitute grievous hurt:
-Emasculation
-*Permanent privation* of sight of one eye
-Permanent privation of hearing of either ear
-Permanent privation of any member or joint
-Destruction or permanent impairing of power of any member or joint
-Permanent disfigurement of head or face
-Fracture or dislocation of a bone or tooth
-Any hurt that endangers life

Thus none of the given options can qualify as the right answer
b. Simple injury: -All injuries, which are not grievous, are simple.
c. Dangerous injuries are those, which cause imminent danger to life, either by involvement of important organs or structures, or extensive area of the body. If no surgical aid is available, such injuries may prove fatal. Some examples are:
-Stab on the abdomen or head or any vital part, hurt causing splenic rupture, squeezing testicles, incised wound of the neck, compound fractures of the skull, rupture of an internal organ, injury of a large blood vessel.
Ref: -The Essentials of Forensic Medicine and Toxicology, by Dr K. S. Narayan Reddy, 21st Edition, Chapter10, Pg- 244,245,246

Q. 148. A person was brought by police from the railway platform. He is talking irrelevant. He is having dry mouth with hot skin, dilated pupils, staggering gait and slurred speech. The most possible diagnosis is (All INDIA-04)
- (a) Alcohol intoxication
- (b) Carbamates poisoning
- (c) Organophosphorous poisoning
- (d) Datura poisoning

Ans. (d)
Note
Crushed or powdered seeds of datura are used for stupefying victims prior to a robbery or kidnapping. It is usually given in food, drinks, e.g. chapattis, curry, sweets, tea, liquor, etc. to travellers in railway stations, choultries.
Signs and symptoms are:
a. A bitter taste in mouth, dryness of mouth and throat, difficulty in talking, dysphagia, hoarseness of voice.
b. Congested face and conjunctiva, widely dilated pupils with loss of accommodation, photophobia, diplopia.
c. Mental changes are restlessness & agitation.
d. The patient becomes confused, giddy, staggering as if drunk.

e. Dry and hot skin, pulse rate- 120-140 per min., full and bounding.
f. Muscle tone and deep reflexes are increased and there may be muscle spasm.
g. Scarlatinal rash or exfoliation of skin.
h. Delirium, hallucination and delusions.

Ref: The Essentials of Forensic Medicine and Toxicology, by Dr K. S. Narayan Reddy, 21st Edition, Chapter33, Pg- 520,521

Q. 149. A convict whose family or relations were not known and no biological sample was available with jail authorities, escaped from the jail. A dead body resembling the convict was found in nearby forest, but due to mutilation of face, identity could not be established. The positive identity that he is the same convict who escaped from jail can be established by (All INDIA-04)
   (a) Blood grouping
   (b) DNA Profile
   (c) Anthropometry
   (d) HLA typing

Ans. (c)
Note
Since no biological sample of the patient is available, the only way out left is- Anthropometry.
It is also called as the Bertillon system.
It is based on the principle that after the age of 21 years, the dimensions of the skeleton remain unchanged and also that the ratio in size of different parts to one another varies considerably in different individuals. As such this is applicable to only to adults. This system includes:
   - Descriptive data such as colour of eyes, hair, complexion, shape of nose, ears, chin, etc.
   - Body marks: moles, scars, tattoo marks
   - Body measurements: height, antero-posterior diameter of head and trunk, span of outstretched arms, the length of left middle finger, left little finger, left forearm, left foot.
   - The photographs of the front view of the head and a profile view of the right side of head are also taken.

This has now been replaced by dactylography.
Ref: The Essentials of Forensic Medicine and Toxicology, by Dr K. S. Narayan Reddy, 21st Edition, Chapter4, Pg- 70

Q. 150. The cephalic index of Indian population is between (All INDIA-04)
   (a) 70-75
   (b) 75-80
   (c) 80-85
   (d) 85-90

Ans. (a)
Note
Cephalic index is calculated as follows:
X 100
Maximum breadth of skull x 100
Maximum length of the skull
The length and breadth are measured by calipers. The Indian skull is Caucasian with a few Negroid features.

Type of skull	Cephalic index	Race
Dolico-cephalic (long-headed)	70-75	Pure aryans, aborigines and Negroes
Mesaticephalic (medium headed)	75-80	Europeans and chinese
Brachycephalic (short headed)	80-85	mongolian

Ref: The Essentials of Forensic Medicine and Toxicology, by Dr K. S. Narayan Reddy, 21st Edition, Chapter4, Pg- 50

Q. 151. Mummification refers to (All INDIA-03)
    (a)   Hardening of muscles after death
    (b)   Colliquative putrification
    (c)   Saponification of subcutaneous fat
    (d)   Dessication of a dead body

Ans. (d)
Note
Mummification is a modification of putrefaction. There is dehydration and shriveling of the cadaver, but the natural appearances are preserved. The factors necessary for its production are-
    - Absence of moisture and air
    - Continuous action of dry or warmed air.

It begins in the exposed parts of the body like face, hands and feet and then extends to the entire body including the internal organs. The skin may be contracted, dry, brittle, leathery and shrunken. The skin becomes rusty-brown in colour, stretched tightly across the bony prominences, such as cheekbones, chin, costal margins. The entire body becomes thin; stiff, looses weight and becomes brittle. It occurs when the body is buried in shallow graves in dry sandy soils, where evaporation of body fluids is very rapid due to dry hot winds in summer.
Ref: The Essentials of Forensic Medicine and Toxicology, by Dr K. S. Narayan Reddy, 21st edition Chapter 7, Pg- 142,143

Q. 152. A patient has been allegedly bitten by cobra snake. The venom in such a bite would be (All INDIA-03)
    (a)   Musculotoxic
    (b)   Vasculotoxic
    (c)   Cardiotoxic
    (d)   Neurotoxic

Ans. (d)
Note
Cobra is included in the family - Elapidae. The venom of this snake is rich in cholinesterase. It catalyses the hydrolysis of acetylcholine to choline and acetic acid.
The signs and symptoms are:
    - Tenderness and pain in the bitten area.
    - The patient may feel sleepy, intoxicated, and weak and is reluctant to stand or move.
    - Weakness of muscles increases and develops into paralysis of the lower limbs. The paralysis spreads to the trunk, and affects the head, which falls forward. The eyelids also hang down.
    - After ½ hour there is excessive salivation and even vomiting.
    - This is followed by paralysis and swelling of the tongue and the larynx, due to which there is difficulty in speech and swallowing.
    - After about 2 hours there is complete paralysis, respiration slows down, coma sets in and finally the respiration stops with or without convulsions.
Ref: The Essentials of Forensic Medicine and Toxicology, by Dr K. S. Narayan Reddy, 21st edition Chapter 29, Pg- 483,486

Q. 153. All the following are related to legal responsibility of an insane person except (All INDIA-03)
    (a)   Mc Naughten's rule
    (b)   Durham's rule
    (c)   Curren's rule
    (d)   Rule of nine

Ans. (d)
Note
a.   *Mc Naughten's Rule*: An accused person is not legally responsible if it is clearly proved that at the time of committing the crime, he was suffering from such a defect of reason from abnormality of mind that he did not know the nature and quality of the act he was doing, or that what he was doing was wrong.
b.   *Durham's Rule*: According to this-"An accused person is not criminally responsible, if his unlawful act is a product of mental disease or mental defect". Here mental disease is referred to mental disorder, while the term mental defect refers to mental retardation.

c. *Curren's rule*: An accused person is not criminally responsible, if at the time of committing the act, he did not have the capacity to regulate his conduct to the requirements of the law, as a result of mental disease or defect.
d. *Rule of Nine*: It is used for estimation of the surface area of the body involved in case of burns.
-9%- head and each upper limb
-9%- for the front of each lower limb
-9%- for the back of each lower limb
-9%- for the front of chest
-9%- for the back of chest
-9%- for the back of abdomen
-9%- for the front of abdomen
-1% for the external genitalia

Ref: The Essentials of Forensic Medicine and Toxicology, by Dr K. S. Narayan Reddy, 21st edition Chapter 12,21, Pg- 272,411,412.413

Q. 154. Blackening and tattooing of skin and clothing can be best demonstrated by (All INDIA-03)
(a) Luminol spray
(b) Infrared photography
(c) Ultraviolet light
(d) Magnifying lens

Ans. (b)
Note
Blackening and tattooing can readily be demonstrated by infrared photography on both skin and clothing.
Ref: The Essentials of Forensic Medicine and Toxicology, by Dr K. S. Narayan Reddy, 21st edition Chapter 8, Pg- 179

Q. 155. In prenatal diagnostic technique Act 1994 which one of the following is not a ground for carrying out prenatal test? (All INDIA-03)
(a) Pregnant women above 35 years of age.
(b) History of two or more spontaneous abortion or fetal loss.
(c) When fetal heart rate is 160 per min at fifth and 120 per min at ninth month.
(d) History of exposure to potentially teratogenic drugs.

Ans. (c)
Note
According to the Prenatal Diagnostic Techniques Act, 1994, the tests should be carried out in the following cases:
a. Pregnant woman is above 35 years of age.
b. History of two or more spontaneous abortions or fetal loss.
c. History of exposure to teratogenic drugs, radiation, infections, or hazardous chemicals.
d. Family history of any mental disease, retardation or any other genetic abnormalities such as hemoglobinopathies, sex-linked disorders, congenital anomalies.

Ref: The Essentials of Forensic Medicine and Toxicology, by Dr K. S. Narayan Reddy, 21st edition Chapter 16, Pg- 534,535

Q. 156. Perjury means giving willful false evidence by a witness while under oath, the witness is liable to be prosecuted for perjury and the imprisonment may extend to seven years This falls under which section of IPC? (All INDIA-03)
(a) 190 of Indian Penal Code
(b) 191 of Indian Penal Code
(c) 192 of Indian Penal Code
(d) 193 of Indian Penal code

Ans. (d)
Note
Perjury means giving willful false evidence by a witness while under oath, or failure to tell what he knows or believes to be true.(s. 193, IPC and 344, Cr.P.C). The witness is liable to be prosecuted for perjury, and the imprisonment may extend for 7 years. (S. 193)

Ref: The Essentials of Forensic Medicine and Toxicology, by Dr K. S. Narayan Reddy, 21st edition Chapter 2, Pg- 12

Q. 157. What would be the race of individual if skull bone having following feature – rounded nasal opening, horseshoe shaped palate, round orbit & cephalic index above 80? (All INDIA-02)
(a) Negro
(b) Mongol
(c) European
(d) Aryans

Ans. (b)
Ref: The Essentials of Forensic Medicine and Toxicology, by Dr K. S. Narayan Reddy, 21st edition Chapter 4, fig (4-5), Pg- 50

Q. 158. Not a feature of brain death (All INDIA-02)
(a) Complete apnea
(b) Absent pupillary reflex
(c) Absence of deep tendon reflex
(d) Heart rate unresponsive to atropine

Ans. (c)
Note
Diagnosis of brain stem death is done by:
a. The cause of death must be irremediable structural damage.
b. Brain stem reflexes should be absent such as
 -Pupillary reflex should be absent
 -Vestibulo-occular reflex
 -Corneal reflex
 -No grimacing in response to painful stimuli
c. Patient should be deeply comatose.
d. The tests should be determined by 2 doctors.
e. Since brain stem is responsible for respiration therefore in brain stem death there will be absence of spontaneous respiration.

It is also characterized by cessation of spontaneous cardiac rhythm without assistance, absence of all reflexes except the spinal reflexes and bilateral dilation and fixation of pupils
Ref: The Essentials of Forensic Medicine and Toxicology, by Dr K. S. Narayan Reddy, 21st Edition, Chapter6, Pg- 112,113

Q. 159. At autopsy, a body is found to have copious fine leathery froth in mouth & nostrils which increased on pressure over chest. Death was likely due to (All INDIA-02)
(a) Epilepsy
(b) Hanging
(c) Drowning
(d) Opium poisoning

Ans. (c)
Note
The characteristic feature of drowning is appearance of a fine, white, lathery froth or foam at the mouth or nostrils. The inhalation of water irritates the mucous membrane of the air passages due to which the tracheal and bronchial glands secrete large amounts of mucous. The froth consists of protein and water. It is usually white but may be blood stained because of slight admixture with blood. If wiped away it gradually reappears, especially if pressure is applied on the chest.
Ref: The Essentials of Forensic Medicine and Toxicology, by Dr K. S. Narayan Reddy, 21st Edition, Chapter14, Pg- 314

Q. 160. In fire arm injury, entery-wound blackening is due to (All INDIA-02)
  (a) Flame
  (b) Hot gases
  (c) Smoke
  (d) Deposition from bullet

Ans. (d)
Note
In case of an entry wound caused by a gun fired from a distance of 30 cm, the tissues surrounding the wound are singed by flame and blackened by smoke, and tattooed by unburnt or partially burnt powder granules. The deposit of smoke is known as smudging or blackening.
Ref: The Essentials of Forensic Medicine and Toxicology, by Dr K. S. Narayan Reddy, 21st Edition, Chapter8, Pg- 179

Q. 161. Tentative cut is a feature of
  (a) Fall from the height
  (b) Homicidal assault
  (c) Accidental injury
  (d) Suicidal attempt

Ans. (d)
Note
Tentative cut are also known as hesitation marks or trial wounds. They are multiple cuts, which are small and superficial often involving only the skin, and are seen at the beginning of the incised wound. The sites of election of suicidal incised wounds are: throat, wrist and front of chest.
Ref: The Essentials of Forensic Medicine and Toxicology, by Dr K. S. Narayan Reddy, 21st Edition, Chapter8, Pg- 161

Q. 162. Gastric lavage is indicated in all cases of acute poisoning ideally because of (All INDIA-02)
  (a) Fear of aspiration
  (b) Danger of cardiac arrest
  (c) Danger of respiratory arrest
  (d) Inadequate ventilation

Ans. (d)
Note
In all cases of acute poisoning endotracheal intubation is highly recommended, for securing of the airway and to prevent aspiration. Even with intubation, there have been documented cases of patients aspirating gastric contents post extubation (14). However, the act of intubation itself may cause gagging leading to aspiration. Another common recommendation is to have the patient in the left lateral decubitus position for the lavage process. Realistically, however, if a patient is at any level of consciousness he/she will resist the "hose", and not remain in this position. Currently, the most common clinical practice is to have the patient sitting in an upright position when performing lavage.
Ref: http://enw.org/Research-GastricLavage.htm

Q. 163. All of the following are the methods used for detecting heavy metals, except (All INDIA-02)
  (a) Harrison & Gilroy test
  (b) Paraffin test
  (c) Neutron activation analysis
  (d) Atomic adsorption spectroscopy

Ans. (b)
Note
All these tests (a, c, d) are used for detecting fire arm discharges residues.
Harrison and Gilroy Test:
This detects the presence of antimony, barium and lead. A cotton swab moistened with molar hydrochloric acid is used.
Neutron activation analysis:
It is a chemical method used for the identification of minute traces of elements present in the hair, nails soil,

glass pieces etc. The residue from the suspects, hand is collected and moistened with 5% nitric acid. Antimony and copper are detected by this method.
Atomic absorption spectrometry:
This analytical system utilizes high temperatures to vaporize the metallic elements and to detect and quantitate them.
Ref: The Essentials of Forensic Medicine and Toxicology, by Dr K. S. Narayan Reddy, 21st Edition, Chapter8, Pg- 196

Q. 164. The sensation of creeping, bugs over the body is a feature of poisoning due to (All INDIA-02)
  (a) Cocaine
  (b) Diazepam
  (c) Barbiturates
  (d) Brown sugar

Ans. (a)
Note
This symptom is known as cocaine bugs. In this there is the characteristic feeling of presence of grains of sand under the skin or some insects creeping on the skin, giving rise to an itching sensation (Tactile hallucination). It is also called as Magnan's symptom.
Ref: -The Essentials of Forensic Medicine and Toxicology, by Dr K. S. Narayan Reddy, 21st Edition, Chapter33, Pg- 525

Q. 165. Which type of cattle poisoning occurs due to ingestion of linseed plant (All INDIA-02)
  (a) Aconite
  (b) Pilocarpine
  (c) Atropine
  (d) Hydro cyanic acid

Ans. (d)
Note
The seeds of some strains of linseed plant contain cyanogenic glycosides. Though the toxicity is low, especially if the seed is eaten slowly, it becomes more toxic if water is drunk at the same time. The cyanogenic glycosides are also present in other parts of the plant and have caused poisoning to livestock.
Ref:-http://www.ibiblio.org/pfaf/cgi-bin/arr_html?Linum+usitatissimum&CAN=COMIND

Q. 166. A 10 years old child presents in casualty with snake bite since six hours. On examination no systemic signs are found & laboratory investigation are normal except localized swelling over the leg < 5 cm. Next step in management would be (All INDIA-02)
  (a) Incision & suction of local swelling
  (b) IV antivenom
  (c) Subcutaneous antivenom at local swelling
  (d) Observe the patient for progression of symptoms; wait for antivenom therapy

Ans. (d)
Note
First aid management in snake bite includes:
  -Apply firm pressure over the bite area.
  -Wrap a firm bandage above the site of bite, which should be loosened every 10 min. for 10 sec.
  -Immobilize the limb.
  -Clean the wound with sterile saline or water.
  -Make parallel incisions through fang marks, about 1 cm. long, and 3mm deep.
Ref: The Essentials of Forensic Medicine and Toxicology, by Dr K.S. Narayan Reddy, 21st Edition, Chapter29, Pg- 487
Suspected pit viper bite management:
  - Observe asymptomatic patients for 12 hours after bite.
  - Mark leading edge of bite site swelling every 30 minutes.

Indications for discharge:
- No proximal spread of extremity findings.
- Normal laboratory studies.
- Patient able to return immediately in case of worsening.

Suspected coral snake bite management:
- Observe asymptomatic patient for at least 24 hours
- Requires immediate treatment and antivenom.

Ref: -http://www.fpnotebook.com/ER8.htm

Q. 167. 'Gold chloride' test is done in poisoning with (All INDIA-02)
   (a) Heroin
   (b) Barbiturates
   (c) Cocaine
   (d) Heavy metals

Ans. (c)
Note
The crystal test suggested by Allen and others [40] involves addition of a known cocaine enantiomer to a sample and then an acidic gold chloride reagent is used to form characteristic crystals. If the cocaine enantiomer added is different from the one originally present, crystals characteristic of the racemate will form rather than those characteristic of the pure enantiomer. It is important when performing this test that the amount of cocaine added is at least roughly the same as the amount present in the sample. It may be difficult to achieve this when dealing with a highly adulterated sample. Should any difficulty arise in discriminating between crystal types, an infrared spectrophotometry spectrum can be obtained that may facilitate the identification.
Ref:-http://www.unodc.org/unodc/bulletin/bulletin_1985-01-01_1_page006.html#s18

Q. 168. Gettler's test is done for death by (All INDIA-01)
   (a) Drowning
   (b) Hanging
   (c) Bums
   (d) Phophorus poisoning

Ans. (a)
Note
Gettler's test is done to study alterations in the blood after drowning. Normally, the chloride content is almost equal in the right and left chambers of the heart, and is about 600mg per 100 ml. When drowning occurs in fresh water, water tends to pass from the lungs to the blood and the blood gets diluted by as much as 72% in 3 minutes, and the blood in the left side of heart will show chloride content up to 50% lower than usual. In drowning in seawater, water is absorbed from the pulmonary circulation into the alveolar spaces, which may be upto 42%, and due to the hemoconcentration, the chloride content in the left side of the heart shows an increase up to 30-40%. A 25% difference in chloride is significant. The test is of doubtful value.
Hemodilution is far more dangerous than hemoconcentration. The red cells are crenated in seawater drowning and lysed in fresh water drowning and potassium sodium ratio is greatly increased.
Ref: The Essentials of Forensic Medicine and Toxicology, by Dr K. S. Narayan Reddy, 21st Edition, Chapter14, Pg- 317

Q. 169. Feature indicative of antimortem drowning is (All INDIA-01)
   (a) Cutis anserina
   (b) Rigor mortis
   (c) Washer woman's feet
   (d) Grass and weeds grasped in the hand

Ans. (d)
Note
The post mortem signs in case of drowning are variable and none of them are pathognomic.
A fine white, leathery froth or foam is seen at the mouth and nostrils, which is one of the most characteristic signs of drowning. The inhalation of water into the air passages causes irritation of the mucosa due to which

the tracheal and bronchial glands secrete large quantities of tenacious mucuous. Vigorous agitation of these secretions produces froth.

a. Other signs are: Cutis anserine or goose skin is produced by spasm of erector pilae muscles.
b. Cadaveric spasm
c. Washer woman's hands
d. Water is present in the stomach in 70% cases, however it is possible that the victim may have drunk the same water shortly before death.
e. There may be presence of substances such as sand, grit, diatoms and algae but their presence in trachea may be due to passive entry after death.
f. Weeds, gravel, grass, twigs, leaves etc may be grasped in the hands due to cadaveric spasm indicating that the person was alive at the time of drowning.

Ref: The Essentials of Forensic Medicine and Toxicology, by Dr K. S. Narayan Reddy, 21st Edition, Chapter14, Pg- 314-317

Q. 170. A boy has 20 permanent teeth and 8 temporary teeth His age is likely to be (All INDIA-01)
(a) 9 years
(b) 10 years
(c) 11 years
(d) 12 years

Ans. (c)
Note
By the time the child is 11 years old, the temporary teeth left are:
- Canines- 4(age of exfoliation- 9-12 years)
- 2nd molar- 4 (age of exfoliation- 10-12 years)
Making a total of 8
The permanent teeth, which have erupted, are:
First molar- 4 (age of eruption- 6-7 years)
Central incisor- 4 (age of eruption- 6-8 years)
Lateral incisor- 4 (age of eruption- 7-9 years)
1st PM- 4 (age of eruption- 9-11 years)
2nd PM- 4 (age of eruption- 10-12 years)
Thus making a total of 16
Ref: The Essentials of Forensic Medicine and Toxicology, by Dr K. S. Narayan Reddy, 21st Edition, Chapter4, Pg- 57

Q. 171. A person comes in contact with other. This is called (All INDIA-01)
(a) Locard's principle
(b) Quetlet's rule
(c) Petty's principle
(d) None of the above

Ans. (a)
Note
Locard's principle states that when any two objects come in contact, there is always a transfer of material from each object on the other. Thus traces from the scene of crime may be carried away on the person or tools of criminal, and at the same time traces from all or any of these may be left at the scene.
Ref: The Essentials of Forensic Medicine and Toxicology, by Dr K. S. Narayan Reddy, 21st Edition, Chapter23, Pg- 421

Q. 172. A boy attempts suicide. He is brought to a private doctor and he is successfully cured. Doctor should (All INDIA-01)
(a) Inform police
(b) Not required to inform police
(c) Report to magistrate
(d) Refer to a psychiatrist

Ans. (b)

Note
If a doctor treats a person who has attempted suicide, he is not legally bound to report, but if the person dies he is bound to inform the police.
Ref: The Essentials of Forensic Medicine and Toxicology, by Dr K. S. Narayan Reddy, 21st Edition, Chapter3, Pg- 29

Q 173. Which one of the following poisons results in bright cherry red coloured post-mortem lividity? (UPSC-02)
   (a) Opium
   (b) Potassium chloride
   (c) Carbon monoxide
   (d) Phosphorus

Ans. (c)
Note
Post mortem lividity or hypostasis is the bluish-purple or purplish-red discoloration, which appears under the skin in the most superficial layers of the dermis of the dependent parts of the body after death; due to capillo-venous distention. The hypostatic areas have distinct colour in certain cases of poisoning e.g.:
CO poisoning- cherry red
Hydrocyanic acid poisoning, burns- bright red
Poisoning by nitrites, potassium chlorate, potassium bicarbonate, aniline – red brown
Phosphorous- dark brown
Ref: The Essentials of Forensic Medicine and Toxicology, by Dr K. S. Narayan Reddy, 21st Edition, Chapter7, Pg- 128,130,131

Q. 174. Tactile hallucination is seen in chronic cases of poisoning with (KPSC-Lect/Physio-Bio/05)
   (a) Cocaine
   (b) Opium
   (c) LSD
   (d) Cannabis

Ans. (a)
Note
The tactile hallucinations are seen in cocaine poisoning. Magnan's symptom or cocaine bugs is characteristic in which there is a feeling as if grains of sand are lying under the skin or some small insects are creeping on the skin giving rise to itching sensation.
Ref: The Essentials of Forensic Medicine and Toxicology – By Dr. K.S. Narayan Reddy –19th Edition, Pg-503

Bibliography

Books
The Essentials of Forensic Medicine and Toxicology – By Dr. K.S. Narayan Reddy –19th Edition

Websites
www.similima.com
www.fleshandbones.com

Chapter 8
COMMUNITY MEDICINE

Q. 1. The percentage of available chlorine in bleaching powder
(a) 30%
(b) 33%
(c) 43%
(d) 45%

Ans. (b)

Note
Ref: Preventive and Social Medicine 17th Ed by Park and Park Pg 499.

Q. 2. In drinking water admissible amount of E. Coli is
(a) Nil
(b) 10
(c) 100
(d) 20

Ans. (a)

Note
Ref: Preventive and Social Medicine 17th Ed by Park and Park Pg 403.

Q 3. Minimum airspace for each worker as per Indian factories act is
(a) 200 cft
(b) 300 cft
(c) 500 cft
(d) 700 cft

Ans. (b)

Note
Most of the standards of ventilation have been based on the efficiency of ventilation in removing body odour. Different workers have advocated standards for the minimal fresh air supply of 300 c.ft. to 3000 c.ft. per hour per person.
Ref: Preventive and Social Medicine 16th Ed By Park and Park –Ventilation - Pg 516.

Q. 4. Small pox was eradicated in the year
(a) 1978
(b) 1977
(c) 1980
(d) 1989

Ans. (c)

Note
The last indigenous case in India occurred on 17th May 1975 in Bihar. On 24th May 1975 India's Last known case of small pox, an importation from Bangladesh occurred. On 5th July 1975, India was proclaimed to be no longer a small pox – endemic country. Finally in April 1977, India was declared smallpox free by an International commission for assessment of smallpox eradication. The world's last case of small pox was reported in 1978 and after 2 years WHO in 1980 declared that smallpox has been eradicated.
Ref: Preventive and Social Medicine 17th Ed By Park and Park Pg115 .

Q. 5. Commonest cause of neonatal mortality in India is (AIIMS/May-03)
   (a) Diarrheal diseases
   (b) Birth injuries
   (c) Low birth weight
   (d) Congenital anomalies

Ans. (c)
Note
The principal causes of infant mortality in India are low birth weight, respiratory infections, diarrheal diseases, congenital malformation and cord infection.
Birth weight is a major determinant of infant and perinatal mortality and morbidity. Virtually all infants weighting less than 1000 g at birth succumb.
Ref: Preventive and Social Medicine 16th Ed by Park and Park Pg387.
Ref; Park and Park -17th Ed .Pg 393 See Tables 18.

Q. 6. In calculating dependency ratio, the numerator is expressed as (AIIMS/May-03)
   (a) Population under 10 years and 60 and above
   (b) Population under 15 years and 60 and above
   (c) Population under 10 years and 65 and above
   (d) Population under 15 years and 65 and above

Ans. (d)
Note
The proportions of persons above 65 Years of age and children below 15 years of age are considered to be dependant on the economically productive age groups (15-64 years).
Ref: Preventive and Social Medicine 16th Ed By Park and Park Pg-323
Ref; Park and Park 17th Ed. Pg 329.

Q. 7. Which of the following is the 'Least common' complication of measles? (AIIMS- May-06)
   (a) Diarrhoea
   (b) Pneumonia
   (c) Otitis media
   (d) SSPE - Sub-acute Sclerosing Pan-Encephalitis

Ans. (d)
Note
The least common complication of measles is sub acute sclerosing pan-encephalitis.
Ref; Park and Park. 16th Ed -Pg-119

Q. 8. Residents of three villages with three different types of water supply were asked to participate in a study to identify cholera carrier. Because several cholera deaths had occurred in the recent past, virtually everyone present at the time submitted to examination. The proportion of residents in each village who were carriers was computed and compared. This study is a (AIIMS/May-03)
   (a) Cross-sectional study
   (b) Case-control study
   (c) Concurrent cohort study
   (d) Non-concurrent

Ans. (a)
Note
(a) *Cross Sectional Study*
   It is simplest form of an observational study. It is based on a single examination of a cross section of a population at point in time – the results of which can be projected on the whole population provided the sampling has been done correctly. It is also known as 'Prevalence Study".
Ref: Park and Park 16th Ed –Pg- 59. The 17th Ed-Pg-60.
(b) *Case Control Study*
   It is often called as 'retrospective study'; a common first approach to test causal hypothesis. By definition, a case control study involves two populations – cases and control.
Ref: Park and Park 16th Ed Pg- 60. The 17th Ed Pg-61.

(c) *Concurrent Cohort study*
A prospective cohort study (current cohort study) is one in which the outcome (disease) has not yet occurred at the time the investigations begin.
Ref: Park and Park 16th Ed Pg-65. 17th Ed Pg-66.
(d) *Non-concurrent study*
A retrospective cohort study (historical cohort study) is one in which the outcomes have occurred before the start of the investigation.
Ref: Park and Park 16th Ed Pg-65. The 17th Ed Pg-66.

Q 9. The following is true about the term 'new families' (AIIMS/May-03)
(a) It is a variant of the 3-generation family.
(b) It is applied to all nuclear families of less then 10 years duration.
(c) It is a variant of the joint family.
(d) It is applied to all nuclear families of less then 2 years duration.

Ans. (b)
Note
Ref. Park and Park 16th Ed Pg-466. The 17th Ed Pg-473.

Q. 10. A drug company is developing a new pregnancy- test kit for use on an outpatient basis. The company used the pregnancy test on 100 women who are known to be pregnant. Out of 100 women, 99 showed positive test. Upon using the same test on 100 non-pregnant women, 90 showed negative result. What is the sensitivity of the test? (AIIMS/May-03)
(a) 90%
(b) 99%
(c) Average of 90 & 99
(d) Cannot be calculated from the given data

Ans. (b)
Note
Sensitivity
Sensitivity is defined as the ability of the test to identify all those who have the disease i.e.,' True positive'. As per the data presented for developing a new pregnancy test results:

Screening test result	Pregnant / Diseased	Not Diseased/ Non-Pregnant	Total
Positive	99 (True Positive)	10 (False Positive)	
Negative	1 (False Negative)	90 (True Negative)	
Total	100 Cases	100 Cases	

Evaluation of screening test:
Sensitivity = True positive / Total number of cases = 99/100 = 99%
Therefore the sensitivity of the test is 99%.
Ref: Park and Park 17th Ed Pg-111, Table – 3A.

Q. 11. A man presents with fever and chills 2 weeks after a louse bite. There was a maculo-papular rash on the trunk which spread peripherally. The cause of this infection can be (AIIMS/May-03)
(a) Scrub typhus
(b) Endemic typhus
(c) Rickettsial pox
(d) Epidemic typhus

Ans. (d)
Note
Epidemic typhus is caused by R. Prowazekii and is spread by louse bite. Humans are known reservoir. Infection is characterised by fever, headache, malaise, prostration, skin rash and enlargement of spleen and liver.
Ref: Park and Park 17th Ed, Pg -229.

Q. 12. All of the following statements are true regarding Q fever except (AIIMS/May-03)
(a) It is a zoonotic infection.
(b) Human disease is characterized by an interstitial pneumonia.
(c) No rash is seen.
(d) Weil Felix reaction is very useful for diagnosis.

Ans. (d)
Note
Q fever is a highly infectious zoonotic disease. There is no skin lesion. Clinical picture is one of influenza or non-baterial pneumonia rather than a typhus fever.
Ref: Park and Park 17th Ed Pg-231.

Q. 13. Reservoir of Indian kala-azar is (AIIMS/May-03)
(a) Man
(b) Rodent
(c) Canine
(d) Equine

Ans. (a)
Note
Indian Kala-azar is considered to be a non-zoonotic infection with man as the sole reservoir.
Ref: Park and Park 17th Ed, Pg-234.

Q. 14. All of the following features are suggestive of asbestosis except (AIIMS/May-03)
(a) Occurs within five years of exposure.
(b) The disease progresses even after removal of contact.
(c) Can lead to pleural mesothelioma.
(d) Sputum contains asbestos bodies.

Ans. (a)
Note
Asbestosis does not usually appear until after 5 to 10 years of exposure. Ref; Park and Park 17th Ed Pg 578.

Q. 15. Brucellosis can be transmitted by all of the following except (AIIMS-May-06)
(a) Contact with infected placenta
(b) Ingestion of raw vegetables from infected farms
(c) Person to person transmission
(d) Inhalation of infected dust or aerosol

Ans. (c)
Note
There is no evidence for person to person transmission of Brucellosis.
The routes of spread are:
a. Contact infection; direct contact with infected tissues, blood, urine, vaginal discharge, aborted fetuses, and especially placenta. Infection takes place through abraded skin, mucosa or conjunctiva. This type of spread is largely occupational and involves workers handling livestock and slaughter house worker.
b. Food borne infection; Infection may take place by the ingestion of raw milk or dairy products from infected animals.
c. Air borne infection; the environment of a cowshed which is heavily infected and persons living there may get the infection.
Ref: Park and Park 16th Ed Pg-218.

Q. 16. Which of the following statements about lepromin is not true? (AIIMS-May-06)
(a) It is negative in most children in first 6 months of life.
(b) It is a diagnostic test.
(c) It is an important aid to classify type of leprosy disease.
(d) BCG Vaccination may convert lepra reaction from negative to positive.

Ans. (c)

Note
Value of the lepromin test
It is not a diagnostic test. As it may give positive result in normal subjects and negative results in lepromatous case. It's usefulness is as under:
    a.   To evaluate the immune status of leprosy patient.
    b.   To classify the leprosy
    c.   To estimate the prognosis in case of leprosy patient.
Ref: Park and Park 16th Ed Pg-245

Q. 17. The usefulness of a screening test depends upon its (AIIMS/May-03)
    (a)   Sensitivity
    (b)   Specificity
    (c)   Reliability
    (d)   Predictive value

Ans. (a)

Note
The most important criteria for a screening test is 'sensitivity' of the test.
Most important criteria for a confirmatory test is 'specificity' of the test.
Ref: Park and Park 16th Ed, Disease.Pg-107-113

Q. 18. Lice are not the vector of (AIIMS-May-06)
    (a)   Relapsing fever
    (b)   Q fever
    (c)   Trench fever
    (d)   Epidemic typhus

Ans. (b)

Note
Q fever is highly infectious zoonotic disease. It occurs mainly in persons associated with sheep, goats, cattle or other domestic animals. It is present in human and animal population in Haryana, Punjab, Delhi, Rajasthan. The causative agent is *Coxiella burnetii*. Q fever differs from rickettsial infections as there is no arthropod involved in its transmission to man.
Transmission results from (a) inhalation of infected dust from soil previously contaminated by urine or faeces of diseased animals.
Ref: Park and Park 16th Ed. Pg- 228

Q. 19. For the field diagnosis of trachoma, the WHO recommends that follicular and intense trachoma inflammation should be assessed in (AIIMS/May-03)
    (a)   Women aged 15-45 years
    (b)   Population of 10 to 28 years range
    (c)   Children aged 0-10 years
    (d)   Population above 25 years of age irrespective of sex

Ans. (c)

Note
Host factor for trachoma: in endemic areas children may show signs of disease at the age of only a few months but typically, children from age of 2-5 years are the most infected and this contributes to the high rate of blindness but also to the rate of occurrence among children.
Ref: Park and Park 17th Ed- Pg-237.

Q. 20. The following statements are true regarding leptospirosis, except (AIIMS-May 06)
    (a)   It is a zoonosis.
    (b)   Man is the dead end of host.
    (c)   Man is an accidental host.
    (d)   Lice act as reservoirs of infection.

Ans. (d)

Note
Leptospirosis is essentially animal infection and transmitted to man under certain environmental conditions. Source of infection: Leptospira are excreted in the urine of animals infected for a long time. Human infections are usually due to occupational exposure to the urine of infected animals e.g., agricultural and livestock farmers, workers in rice fields, sugarcane fields, and underground sewers, abattoir workers, meat and animal handlers, veterinarians. Leptospira can enter the body through skin abrasions or through intact mucous membrane by direct contact. Infection can also occur through inhalation as when milking infected cows or goats by breathing air polluted with droplets of urine.
Ref: Park and Park 16th Ed, Pg-219

Q. 21. Under the National Programme for Control of Blindness in India, medical colleges are classified as eye care centers of (AIIMS /Nov-03)
 (a) Primary level
 (b) Secondary level
 (c) Tertiary level
 (d) Intermediate level

Ans. (c)

Note
Refer to National Programme for control of blindness (see infra-structural development)
Ref: Park and Park 16th Ed Pg-312 and 17th Ed Pg-317.

Q. 22. Taking the definition of blindness as visual acuity less than 3/60 in the better eye, the number of blind persons per 100,000 population in India is estimated to be (AIIMS /Nov-03)
 (a) 500
 (b) 700
 (c) 1000
 (d) 1500

Ans. (b)

Note
Prevalence of blindness in India is (%) of total population i.e.,-7%.
Ref: Park and Park 17th Ed Pg-301.

Q. 23. If the prevalence is very low as compared to the incidence for a disease, it implies (AIIMS /Nov-03/ May-03)
 (a) Disease is very fatal and/or easily curable
 (b) Disease is non fatal
 (c) Calculation of prevalence and incidence is wrong
 (d) Nothing can be said, as they are independent.

Ans. (a)

Note
If the disease is acute and of short duration either because of rapid recovery or death the prevalence rate will be relatively low compared with the incidence rate.
Ref: Park and Park 17th Ed Pg-53.

Q. 24. The following is true about prevalence and incidence (AIIMS /Nov-03/May-03)
 (a) Both are rates
 (b) Prevalence is a rate but incidence is not
 (c) Incidence is a rate but prevalence is not
 (d) Both are not rates

Ans. (c)

Note
Although referred to as a rate, prevalence rate is really a ratio.
Ref: Park and Park 17th Ed Pg-52.

Q. 25. The rate adjusted to allow for the age distribution of the population is (AIIMS /Nov-03/May-05)
- (a) Perinatal mortality rate
- (b) Crude mortality rate
- (c) Fertility rate
- (d) Age-standardized mortality rate

Ans. (d)

Note

Perinatal mortality rate: It includes both late fetal deaths (still births) and early neonatal deaths.

Crude mortality rate: It is defined as "the number of deaths (from all causes) per 1000 estimated mid – year population in one year, in a given place.

Fertility rate: It is number of live births per 1000 women in the reproductive age group (15 -44 or 49 years) in a given year.

Age- standardized morality rate: It is used for comparing the death rates of two populations with different age composition, the crude death rate is not the right yardstick.

Ref: Park and Park 17th Ed Pg- 390, 48, 333, 50

Q. 26. The mechanisms by which cholera might be maintained during the intervals between peak cholera seasons is (AIIMS-May 2006)
- (a) Carrier status in animals
- (b) Carrier status in man
- (c) An environmental reservoir
- (d) Continuous transmission in man

Ans. (d)

Note

Cholera occurs at intervals even in endemic areas. For the fate of V. Cholera in the inter-epidemic periods. Following are three explanations:
   a. The existence of long term carriers.
   b. The existence of continuous transmission involving asymptomatic cases.
   c. The persistence of organism in a free living, in the environment.

To further explain:

Reservoir of infection: The human being is the only known reservoir of cholera infection. He may be a case of carrier. It is the mild and asymptomatic cases that play a significant role in maintaining endemic reservoir. Carriers; the carriers are usually temporary, rarely chronic.

From above it becomes clear that the 'Continuous transmission in man' is the only mechanism by which cholera might be maintained during the interval between peak cholera seasons.

Ref: Park and Park 16th Ed, Pg-165.

Q 27. The age and sex structure of a population may be best described by a (AIIMS /Nov-03/May-05)
- (a) Life table
- (b) Correlation coefficient
- (c) Population pyramid
- (d) Bar chart

Ans. (c)

Note

The age and sex distribution of a population is best represented by population pyramid.
Ref; Park and Park 17th Ed Pg-328.

Q. 28. In a double blind clinical drug trial (AIIMS /Nov-03)
- (a) Each patient receives a placebo.
- (b) Each patient receives both (double) treatments.
- (c) The patients do not know which treatment they are receiving.
- (d) The patients do not know that they are in a drug trial.

Ans. (c)

In a double blind trial doctor as well as the patient both do not know the group allocated and the treatment received.
Ref: Park and Park 17th Ed Pg-73

Q. 29. The most sensitive index of recent transmission of malaria in a community is (AIIMS /Nov-03)
    (a)   Spleen rate
    (b)   Infant parasite rate
    (c)   Annual parasite incidence
    (d)   Slide positivity rate

Ans. (b)
Note
Infant parasite rate: It is defined as the percentage of infants below the age of one year showing malaria parasites in their blood films. It is regarded as the most sensitive index of recent transmission of malaria in a locality.
Ref; Park and Park 17th Ed Pg-198.

Q. 30. Additional daily energy requirement during the first six months for a lactating woman is (AIIMS /Nov/ 2003)
    (a)   350 K calories
    (b)   450 K calories
    (c)   550 K calories
    (d)   650 K calories

Ans. (c)
Note
Refer the table 24 recommended daily intake for energy.
Ref: Park and Park 17th Ed Pg-432.

Q. 31. Bagassosis is most likely caused due to the inhalation of the dust of (AIIMS /Nov/ 2003)
    (a)   Free silica
    (b)   Coal
    (c)   Sugar cane
    (d)   Cotton fibre

Ans. (c)
Bagassosis is the name given to an occupational disease of the lungs caused by inhalation of bagasse or sugarcane dust.
Ref: Park and Park 17th Ed Pg-577.

Q. 32. In defining 'general fertility rate', the denominator is (AIIMS /Nov-03)
    (a)   Population between 15 and 49 years of age
    (b)   Women between 15 and 49 years of age
    (c)   Mid year population
    (d)   Live births

Ans. (b)
Note
General fertility rate is 'number of live births per 1,000 women in the reproductive age group (15-45 or 49 years) in a given year.
Ref: Park and Park 17th Ed Pg-333.

Q. 33. Mites are the vectors of the following diseases except (AIIMS /Nov-03)
    (a)   Scabies
    (b)   Scrub typhus
    (c)   Rickettsial pox
    (d)   Kyasanur forest disease

Ans. (d)
Note
Kyasanur forest disease is a febrile disease associated with hemorrhages caused by an arbovirus, flavivirus and transmitted to man by the bite of infected ticks.
Ref: Park and Park 17th Ed Pg-219.

Q. 34. Which one of the following methods is used for the estimation of chlorine demand of water? (AIIMS/ May-06)
  (a) Chlorometer
  (b) Horrock's apparatus
  (c) Berkfeld filter
  (d) Double pot method

Ans. (b)

Note
Chlorine demand of water is the amount of chlorine that is needed to destroy bacteria and to oxidize all the organic matter and ammoniacal substances present in the water. The chlorine demand of water can be estimated by Horrock's apparatus.
Ref: Park and Park 18th Ed.Pg-530

Q. 35. The national level system that provides annual national as well as state level reliable estimates of fertility and mortality is called (AIIMS /Nov-03/May-05)
  (a) Civil registration system
  (b) Census
  (c) Adhoc survey
  (d) Sample registration system

Ans. (d)

Note
Sample registration system was initiated in the mid 1960's to provide reliable estimates of birth and death rates at the national and state levels.
Ref: Park and Park 17th Ed Pg-605.

Q. 36. Which of the following is an example of Disability limitation? (AIIMS-May-2006)
  (a) Reducing occurrence of polio by immunization.
  (b) Arranging for schooling of child suffering from PRPP.
  (c) Resting affected limbs in neutral position.
  (d) Providing calipers for walking.

Ans. (c)

Note
When a patient reports late in the pathogenesis phase of the disease, the mode of intervention is disability limitation. The object of this intervention is to prevent or halt the transition of the disease process from impairment to handicap.

Impairment
Impairment is defined as 'Loss or abnormality of psychological, physiological, or anatomical structure or function'.

Disability
Because of impairment, the affected person may be unable to carry out certain activities considered normal for his age, sex etc. this inability to carry out certain activities is called as 'disability'.

Handicap
Handicap can be explained as:
Accident (Disease / disorder) → e.g.,Loss of foot (Impairment –extrinsic) → cannot walk (Disability – Objectified) -→ Unemployed (Handicap)

Disability prevention
It relates to all the levels of prevention:
  a. Reducing the occurrence of impairment i.e., immunization against polio (Primary prevention)
  b. Disability limitation by appropriate treatment (Secondary prevention)
  c. Preventing the transition of disability into handicap (Tertiary prevention)

Rehabilitation
It is defined as 'the combined and coordinated use of medical, social, educational and vocational measures for training and retraining the individual to the highest possible level of functional ability'. Following are the area's of concern in rehabilitation:

a. Medical rehabilitation; restoration of function
b. Vocational rehabilitation; restoration of the capacity to earn a livelihood.
c. Social rehabilitation; restoration of family and social relationships.
d. Psychological rehabilitation; restoration of personal dignity and confidence.
Ref: Park and Park 16th Ed, Pg-36

Q. 37. Mean hemoglobin of a sample of 100 pregnant women was found to be 10 mg% with a standard error of 1.0 mg%. The standard error of the estimate would be (AIIMS /May-04)
    (a) 0.01
    (b) 0.1
    (c) 1.0
    (d) 10.0

Ans. (b)
Note

$$\text{Standard error of mean} = \frac{\text{Standard deviation}}{\sqrt{\text{Sample size}}}$$

$$\frac{1}{\sqrt{100}}$$

$$\frac{1}{10} = 0.1$$

Ref: Park and Park 16th Ed Pg-597

Q. 38. For every 1,00,000 population, the highest prevalence of blindness in the world is seen in (AIIMS /May-04)
    (a) Sub-Saharan Africa
    (b) South Asia
    (c) Eastern Europe
    (d) Latin America

Ans. (a)
Note
Prevalence of blindness varies between countries from .2% or less in developed countries to more than 1% in some Sub-Saharan countries.
Ref: Park and Park 17th Ed Pg-301.

Q. 39. All of the following statements about plague is wrong, except (AIIMS /May -04)
    (a) Domestic rat is the main reservoir.
    (b) Bubonic is the most common variety.
    (c) The causative bacillus can survive up to 10 years in the soil of rodent burrows.
    (d) The incubation period for pneumonic plague is one to two weeks.

Ans. (b)
Note
Correct statements about plague are:
(a) Wild rodents are the main reservoir.
(b) Bubonic is most common type of plague.
(c) The infected fleas may live upto a year and certain species survive in the burrow microclimate for as long as four years.
(d) The incubation period of Bubonic plague is 2- 7 days, Septicaemic plague- 2- 7 days and pneumonic plague – 1-3 days.

Ref: Park and Park 16th Ed Pg-223

Q. 40. National Health Policy of India-2002 includes all of the following as goals, except (AIIMS /May-04)
(a) Eradicated polio and yaws by the year 2005
(b) Achieve zero level transmission of HIV/AIDS by year 2010
(c) Eliminate kala-azar by year 2005
(d) Eliminate lymphatic filariasis by year 2015

Ans. (c)
Note
To eliminate kala-azar by 2010.
Ref: Park and Park 17th Ed Pg-635.

Q. 41. The incubation period of yellow fever is (AIIMS /May-04)
(a) 3 to 6 days
(b) 3-4 weeks
(c) 1 to 2 weeks
(d) 8-10 weeks

Ans. (a)
Note
The incubation period of yellow fever is 3-6 days.
Ref: Park and Park 17th Ed Pg-216.

Q. 42. Mode of transmission of Q fever is (AIIMS /May-04)
(a) Bite of infected louse
(b) Bite of infected tick
(c) Inhalation of aerosol
(d) Bite of infected mite

Ans. (c)
Note
Transmission of Q fever results from
(i) Inhalation of infected dust from the soil previously contaminated by urine or faeces of diseased animals. The organism can also be transmitted by aerosols.
(ii) The organism can also gain entry into the body through abrasions, conjunctivae or ingestion of contaminated foods such as meat, milk and milk products.
Ref: Park and Park 17th Ed Pg-231.

Q. 43. The following are characteristic features of staphylococcal food poisoning, except (AIIMS /May-04)
(a) Optimum temperature for toxin formation is 37°C
(b) Intradietetic toxins are responsible for intestinal symptoms
(c) Toxins can be destroyed by boiling for 30 minutes
(d) Incubation period is 1-6 hours

Ans. (c)
Note
The toxins are relatively heat stable and resist boiling for 30 minutes or more.
Ref: Park and Park 17th Ed Pg-182.

Q. 44. Which of the following is the best indicator of severity of a short duration acute disease (AIIMS /May-04, All INDIA-05)
(a) Cause specific death rate
(b) 5-year survival
(c) Case fatality rate
(d) Standardized mortality ratio

Ans. (c)
Note
Case fatality rate is typically used in acute infectious diseases (food poisoning, cholera, and measles). It's usefulness for chronic diseases is limited.
Ref: Park and Park 17th Ed Pg-49.

MCQ's in Community Medicine

Q. 45. Which of the following is the most common cause of maternal mortality in India? (AIIMS /May-04/May-05)
(a) Hemorrhage
(b) Anemia
(c) Abortion
(d) Sepsis

Ans. (a)
Note
The single most common cause accounting for a quarter of all maternal deaths is obstetric hemorrhage generally occurring post-partum which can lead to death vary rapidly in the absence of prompt life saving care.
Ref: Park and Park 17th Ed Pg-388.

Q. 46. Which of the following is the nodal ministry for Integrated Child Development Services (ICDS) Programme Centre? (AIIMS /May-04)
(a) Ministry for Human Resource Development
(b) Ministry for Rural Development
(c) Ministry for Health and Family Welfare
(d) Ministry for Social Justice

Ans. (a)
Note
ICDS programme was started in 1975 under the ministry of social and women's welfare.
Ref: Park and Park 16th Ed Pg-407. However, now the nodal agency for this programme is Department of Women and Child Development, under Ministry of Human Resource Development.

Q. 47. The systematic distortion of retrospective studies that can be eliminated by a prospective design is (AIIMS /May-04)
(a) Confounding
(b) Effect modification
(c) Recall bias
(d) Measurement bias

Ans. (c)
Note
Refer to bias in case control studies.
Ref: Park and Park 17th Ed Pg-64.

Q. 48. Vitamin A deficiency is considered a public health problem if prevalence rate of night blindness in children between 6 months to 6 years is more than
(a) 0.01%
(b) 0.05%
(c) 0.1%
(d) 1.0%

Ans. (d)
Note
The formulation of effective intervention programme for prevention of vitamin A deficiency begins with the characterization of the problem. This is done by population survey involving the preschool children (6 month to 6 years) who are at special risk.
The criteria recommended by WHO is as under:

Criteria	Prevalence in population at risk (6 months to 6 years)
Night blindness	More than 1 per cent
Bitot's spots	More than 0.5 per cent
Corneal xerosis / Corneal ulceration / Keratomalacia	More than 0.01 per cent
Corneal ulcer	More than 0.05 per cent
Serum retinol (less than 10 mcg/dl)	More than 5 per cent

Ref: Park and Park 16th Ed, Pg- 410.

Q. 49. If a new effective treatment is initiated and all other factors remain the same; which of the following is most likely to happen? (AIIMS /May-04)
(a) Incidence will not change
(b) Prevalence will not change
(c) Neither incidence nor prevalence will change
(d) Incidence and prevalence will change

Ans. (a)

Note
The improvement in treatment may decrease the duration of illness and thereby decrease prevalence of a disease.
Ref: Park and Park 17th Ed Pg-53.

Q. 50. Which one of the following relationships shown between different parameters of a performance of a test, is correct (AIIMS /May-04)
(a) Sensitivity = 1 – specificity
(b) Positive predictive value = 1 – negative predictive value
(c) Sensitivity is inversely proportional to specificity
(d) Sensitivity = 1 – positive predictive value

Ans. (c)

Note
Sensitivity is inversely proportional to specificity.
Ref: Park and Park 17th Ed Pg-112.

Q. 51. The highest percentage of polysaturated fatty acids are present in
(a) Groundnut oil
(b) Soyabean oil
(c) Margarine
(d) Palm oil

Ans. (b)

Note
The fatty acid content % of different fats is as under:

Fats	Saturated fatty acids	Monosaturated fatty acids	Polysaturated fatty acids
Groundnut oil	19	50	31
Soyabean oil	14	24	62
Margarine	25	25	50
Palm oil	46	44	10

Ref: Park and Park 16th Ed Pg-407

Q. 52. Indicators of Physical Quality of Life Index, includes all of the following except (AIPGME -99-& 06-May-06)
a) Infant mortality
b) Life expectancy at age one
c) Literacy
d) Per-capita gross national product

Ans. (d)

Note
The PQLI is consolidated by (a), (b) and (c).
Ref: Park & Park, 16th Ed, Pg- 15

MCQ's in Community Medicine

Q. 53. All of the following are true about break point chlorination, except (AIIMS /May-04)
    (a)   Free chlorine is released in water after break point chlorination.
    (b)   Chlorine demand is the amount needed to kill bacteria, oxidize organic matter and neutralize ammonia.
    (c)   1 ppm free chlorine should be present in water after break point has reached.
    (d)   Contact period of 1 hour is necessary.

Ans. (c)

Note
The minimum recommended concentration of free chlorine is .5 gm per liter for one hour.
The breakpoint chlorination; it is the point at which the residual chlorine appears and when all the combine chlorines have been completely destroyed. Ref: Park and Park 17th Ed Pg-498

Q. 54. Tablets supplied by Govt. of India contain the following amount of iron and folic acid (AIIMS /May-04)
    (a)   60 mg elemental iron + 500 μg FA
    (b)   100 mg elemental iron + 500 μg FA
    (c)   200 mg elemental iron + 1 mg FA
    (d)   100 mg elemental iron + 5 mg FA

Ans. (a)

Note
The Government of India has initiated a programme in which 60 mg of elemental iron and 500 mcg of folic acid are being distributed daily to pregnant women through antenatal clinics, primary health centers and their sub-centers.
Ref: Park and Park 17th Ed Pg-363.

Q. 55. Weight of an Indian reference woman is (AIIMS/Nov-04)
    (a)   45 Kg
    (b)   50 Kg
    (c)   55 Kg
    (d)   60 Kg

Ans. (b)

Note
An Indian Reference Women is between 20 and 39 years of age, healthy and weights 50 kg.
Ref: Park and Park 17th Ed Pg-431

Q. 56. Orthotolidine test is used to determine (AIIMS/Nov-04)
    (a)   Nitrates in water
    (b)   Nitrites in water
    (c)   Free and combined chlorine in water
    (d)   Ammonia content in water

Ans. (c)

Note
Orthotolidine test enables both free and combined chlorine in water to be determined with speed and accuracy.
Ref: Park and Park 17th Ed Pg-498.

Q. 57. The analytical study where population is the unit of study is (AIIMS/Nov-04)
    (a)   Cross sectional
    (b)   Ecological
    (c)   Case-control
    (d)   Cohort

Ans. (b)

Note
Epidemiological studies can be classified as observational studies and experimental studies with further subdivisions:
1. Observational studies
    a. Descriptive studies
    b. Analytical studies
        i. Ecological or Correlational, with populations as unit of study.
        ii. Cross sectional or Prevalence, with Individual as unit of study.
        iii. Case Control or Case reference, with individual as unit of study.
        iv. Cohort or Follow up, with individuals as unit of study.
2. Experimental studies intervention studies
    a. Randomized controlled trials or Clinical trials – With patients as unit of study.
    b. Field trials or Community intervention studies – With healthy people as unit of study.
    c. Community trials: With communities as unit of study.
Ref: Park and Park 16th Ed, Page 52-53.

Q. 58. Which one of the following arbovirus diseases has not been reported in India? (AIIMS/Nov-04)
(a) Japanese encephalitis
(b) Yellow fever
(c) Chikungunya fever
(d) Kyasanur forest disease

Ans. (b)

Note
Paradoxically there is no evidence that yellow fever has ever been present in Asia.
Ref: Park and Park 17th Ed Pg-216.

Q. 59. In all of the following diseases chronic carriers are found except (AIIMS/May -06)
(a) Measles
(b) Typhoid
(c) Hepatitis B
(d) Gonorrhoea

Ans. (a)

Note
Source of infection; the only source of infection is a case of measles, carriers are not known to occur.
Ref: Park and Park 16th Ed- Pg-118

Q. 60. Study of time, place and person is called as
(a) Experimental epidemiology
(b) Analytical epidemiology
(c) Descriptive epidemiology
(d) Randomized controlled trial

Ans. (c)

Note
(a) *Experimental epidemiology*
 -This is similar to control studies except that these studies involve some active intervention or manipulation in the experimental group while making no change in the control group:
    a. Randomized Control Trial is also a type of Experimental study.
(b) *Analytical epidemiology*
 -This the second major type of epidemiological studies.
 -The objective here is not to 'describe' the disease but to 'analyze' or test the hypothesis formulated in descriptive studies. These comprise:
    a. Case control studies
    b. Cohort studies

(c) *Descriptive epidemiology*
    -This is the first phase of an epidemiological investigation
    -It involves the 'Description' of disease in reference to time of occurrence, place and person.
Ref: Park & Park, 16th Ed, Pg- 55

Q. 61. All of the following statements regarding dracunculiasis are true except (AIIMS/Nov-04)
(a) India has eradicated this disease.
(b) Niridazole prevents transmission of the disease.
(c) The disease is limited to tropical and subtropical regions.
(d) No animal reservoir has been proved.

Ans. (b)
Note
The India was declared free of guineaworm disease in 1999.
The drugs available for the treatment are Niridazole, Mebendazole and Metronidazole. None of these drugs have any effect in preventing transmission of the disease.
Ref: Park and Park 17th Ed Pg-189.

Q. 62. In which of the Indian states the maximum number of AIDS cases has been reported till now? (AIIMS/Nov-04)
(a) Delhi
(b) Kerala
(c) Tamil Nadu
(d) Bihar

Ans. (c)
Note
Ref: Park and Park 16th Ed Fig. 1. Shows the diversity of epidemic in different states of India. P-259

Q. 63. All of the following statements about mosquito are true except (AIIMS/Nov-04)
(a) It is a definitive host in malaria.
(b) It is a definitive host in filaria.
(c) Its life cycle is completed in 3 weeks.
(d) The female can travel up to 3 kilometers.

Ans. (b)
Note
Man is a definite host and mosquito is intermediate host in filariasis.
Ref: Park and Park 17th Ed Pg-202.

Q. 64. All of the statements about quarantine are true except (AIIMS/Nov-04)
(a) It is synonymous with isolation.
(b) Absolute quarantine is restriction during the incubation period.
(c) Exclusion of children from schools is an example of modified quarantine.
(d) Quarantine should not be longer than the longest incubation period.

Ans. (a)
Note
In contrast to isolation, quarantine, applied to restrictions on the healthy contacts of an infectious disease.
Ref: Park and Park 17th Ed Pg-98.

Q. 65. A total of 5000 patients of glaucoma are identified and surveyed by patient interviews regarding family history of glaucoma. Such a study design is called (AIIMS/Nov-04)
(a) Case series report
(b) Case-control study
(c) Clinical trial
(d) Cohort study

Ans. (a)

Note
Case series; it is a description of cases. There are no comparison groups, only patient's characteristics are studied. It doses not provide any useful information.

Q. 66. In a 3 × 4 contingency table, the number of degrees of freedom equals to (AIIMS/Nov-04)
    (a)   1
    (b)   5
    (c)   6
    (d)   12

Ans. (c)
Note
The (degree of freedom) df = (c-1) (r-1)'
c = Number of columns
r = Number of rows
Therefore: df = (3-1) (4-1) = 2x3=6.
Ref: Park and Park 17th Ed Pg-616.

Q. 67. The literacy rate of Indian population as per Census 2001 is (AIIMS/Nov-04)
    (a)   54.5%
    (b)   65.4%
    (c)   85.8%
    (d)   75.5%

Ans. (b)
Note
The literacy rate of Indian Population as per census 2001 is 65.38%.
Ref: Figure-6, Park and Park 17th Ed Pg-330.

Q. 68. Niacin deficiency in a maize eating population is due to (AIPG/95/97)
    (a)   High Trytophan
    (b)   High Isoleucine
    (c)   High Leucine
    (d)   High Phenylalamine

Ans. (c)
Note
Corn based diet predispose to niacin deficiency due to low tryptophan and niacin content, and high leucine content which interferes in conversion of tryptophan into niacin.

Q. 69. Which of the following vitamins is supposed to prevent congenital neural tube defects? (AIPG/1995/147)
    (a)   Thiamine
    (b)   Riboflavin
    (c)   Folic acid
    (d)   Pyridoxine

Ans. (c)
Note
Folate supplementation reduces the incidence of fetal **neural tube** defects.
Ref: Harrison, 15th Ed. Medical disorders during pregnancy.

Q. 70. The earliest change in iron deficiency anemia is (AIPGME/95/97, All INDIA-01)
    (a)   Decreased serum iron
    (b)   Decreased serum ferritin
    (c)   Decreased TIBC
    (d)   Decreased hemoglobin

Ans. (b)

Note
As long as iron stores are present and can be mobilized, the serum iron, total iron-binding capacity (TIBC) remains within normal limits. At this stage, red cell morphology and indices are normal. When iron stores become depleted, the serum iron begins to fall. Gradually, the TIBC increases. The serum ferritin level correlates with total body iron stores; thus, the serum ferritin level is the most convenient laboratory test to estimate iron stores. As iron stores are depleted, the serum ferritin falls to 15 µg/L. Such levels are virtually always diagnostic of absent body iron stores. As long as the serum iron remains within the normal range, hemoglobin synthesis is unaffected despite the dwindling iron stores. Once the transferrin saturation falls to 15 to 20%, hemoglobin synthesis becomes impaired. Therefore the earliest change in iron deficiency anaemia is decreased serum ferritin level.
Ref: Harrison 15th Ed – Iron deficiency.

Q. 71. The National health policy is based on (AIPG/1995/149)
    (a)   Comprehensive health care
    (b)   Subsidized health care
    (c)   Socialized medicine
    (d)   Equitable distribution of health resources

Ans. (a)
Note
The National health policy lays stress on:
a. Need of establishing 'comprehensive primary health care' services to reach the population in the remotest areas of the country.
b. The policy emphasizes the Preventive promotive and rehabilative aspects of public health care.
c. It views health and human development as a vital component of overall, integrated socio-economic development, decentralized system of health care delivery with maximum community and individual self reliance and participation.
Ref: Park and Park 16th Ed Pg-617

Q. 72. The most common cancer, affecting both males and females of the world, is (AIIMS/May-05)
    (a)   Cancer of the pancreas
    (b)   Buccal mucosa cancer
    (c)   Lung cancer
    (d)   Colo-rectal cencer

Ans. (c)
Note
Table-4. Ranking order by site of 8 selected cancers.
Ref: Park and Park 17th Ed Pg-288.

Q. 73. Which one of the following statements regarding pre and post clinical trial is most appropriate? (AIIMS/May-05)
    (a)   They cannot be randomized.
    (b)   They are useful studies involving mortality.
    (c)   They use the patient as his or her own control.
    (d)   They are usually easier to interpret than the comparable parallel clinical trial.

Ans. (c)
Note
The statement 'They use the patient as his or her own control' regarding pre-and post clinical trial is most appropriate to 'the use the patient as his or her own control'- as one can compare the incidence of disease before and after introduction of a interventive measure. The experiment serves it's own control and therefore eliminates all possibilities of group difference.

Q. 74. All are true about classical dengue fever except (AIPGME-1994/131)
    (a)   Case fatality is low
    (b)   Breakbone fever
    (c)   Positive tourniquet test
    (d)   It is a self limiting disease

Ans. (c)

Note
A positive 'tourniquet test' is indicative of dengue hemorrhagic fever and it is not a part of classical dengue fever.
Ref: Park and Park 16th Ed Pg-187

Q. 75. The safe limit of Fluorine in drinking water is (AIPGME -94)
    (a)   0.2 -0.5 mg/L
    (b)   0.5 -0.8 mg/L
    (c)   0.8 -1.2 mg/L
    (d)   1.2 -2.0 mg/L

Ans. (b)

Note
The recommended level of fluorides in drinking water in this country is accepted as 0.5 to 0.8 mg per liter.
Ref: Park and Park 16th Ed Pg-418.

Q. 76. Rabies can be transmitted by all the following routes except: (AIPG/94)
    (a)   Aerosol
    (b)   Bites
    (c)   Ingestion
    (d)   Licks

Ans. (c)

Note
The ingestion is not implicated in transmission of rabies. Mode of transmission of rabies is as under:
a.   Animal bites- the saliva must contain virus.
b.   Licks- licks on abraded skin or mucous membrane.
c.   Aerosol- especially observed in nature only in certain caves harboring rabies infected bats.
d.   Person to person- by corneal and organ transplant.
Ref: Park and Park 16th Ed, Pg-205-206

Q. 77. National Family Health Survey has successfully completed (AIIMS/May-05)
    (a)   One round
    (b)   Two round
    (c)   Three round
    (d)   Four round

Ans. (b)
Two surveys have been completed till now. First round in 92-93, and second round in 98-99.

Q. 78. In an epidemic of Poliomyelitis, the best way to stop spread is by
    (a)   Injection of killed vaccine
    (b)   OPV Drops to all children
    (c)   Isolation of cases
    (d)   Chlorination of all wells

Ans. (b)

Note
The advantages of OPV are:
a.   Easy to administer, do not require a highly trained person.
b.   Induces both humoral and intestinal immunity
c.   Antibody is quickly produced in a large proportion of vaccines, even a single dose elicits substantial immunity.
d.   The vaccine excretes the virus and so infects others who are also immunized thereby.
e.   Useful in controlling epidemics.
Ref: Park and Park 16th Ed Pg-154

MCQ's in Community Medicine

Q. 79. The following disease requires isolation to break transmission except (AIPGME/99)
    (a)   Measles
    (b)   Mumps
    (c)   Chicken pox
    (d)   Tetanus

Ans. (d)

Note
Tetanus is not a communicable disease; hence it will not require any isolation to break the transmission.
Ref: Park and Park 16th Ed Pg-236

Q. 80. In India, the vector of Japanese encephalitis is (AIPGME/1994/132)
    (a)   Aedes aegypti
    (b)   Aedes culcifaciens
    (c)   Cluex vishnui
    (d)   Mansonoides

Ans. (c)

Note
The Culex vishnui, Culex gelidus and Culex tritaeniorhynchus (especially in south India) has been implicated as the most important vector for transmission of JE to men.
Ref: Park and Park 16th Ed Pg-216.

Q. 81. A one day census of inpatients in a mental hospital could (AIIMS/May/05)
    (a)   Give good information about the patients in that hospital at that time.
    (b)   Give reliable estimates of seasonal factors in admissions.
    (c)   Enable us to draw conclusions about the mental hospitals of India.
    (d)   Enable us to estimate the distribution of different diagnosis in mental illness in the local area.

Ans. (a)
It gives information about the patient in that hospital at that period of time.

Q. 82. Highest biological value of protein is seen in (AIPGME/94)
    (a)   Eggs
    (b)   Fish
    (c)   Soyabean
    (d)   Gram

Ans. (a)

Note
Egg protein has all the nine essential amino acids needed by the body in right proportions. Nutritionists consider egg protein as the best among food proteins.
Ref: Park and Park 16th Ed Pg-422

Q. 83. Sputum examination for AFB is a type of (AIPG/95)
    (a)   Primary prevention
    (b)   Secondary prevention
    (c)   Tertiary prevention
    (d)   Primordial prevention

Ans. (b)

Note
The sputum examination for AFB is a test to diagnose the case in early stages. And secondary prevention is defined as 'action which halts the progress of a disease at its incipient stage and prevents complications'. The specific interventions are early diagnosis and adequate treatment.
Ref: Park and Park 16th Ed Pg-34

Q. 84. A bacterium can divide every 20 minutes. Beginning with a single individual, how many bacteria will be there in the population if there is exponential growth for 3 hours? (AIIMS/May-05)
    (a)   18
    (b)   440
    (c)   512
    (d)   1024

Ans. (c)
Note
According to law of exponential growth:
-Number of bacteria after 180 minutes (3 Hours) = $2^{180/20}$
= 2^9
= 512

Q. 85. The carrying capacity of any given population is determined by its (AIIMS/May-05)
    (a)   Population growth rate
    (b)   Birth rate
    (c)   Death rate
    (d)   Limiting resource

Ans. (d)
Note
The carrying capacity is 'number of individuals who can be supported in a given area within natural resource limits, and without degrading natural, social, cultural and economic environment for present and future generations.
Internet.
Ref: Internet

Q. 86. Which of the following is characteristic of a single exposure common vehicle outbreak? (AIIMS/May-05)
    (a)   Frequent secondary cases
    (b)   Severity increases with increasing age
    (c)   Explosive
    (d)   Cases occur continuously beyond the longest incubation period

Ans. (c)
Note
Characteristic of a single exposure common vehicle outbreak is (c) Explosive.
It is characterised by:
    -Epidemic tends to be explosive
    -All cases develop within same incubation period
    -Curve rises and falls rapidly
    -No secondary waves
The Bhopal gas tragedy fulfills the 'Point Source Epidemic' criteria:
    -It was single exposure to agent / Bhopal gas
    -All cases developed simultaneously within one incubation period.
Other examples are:
    -Food poisoning
    -Minamala disease in Japan
Ref: Park & Park, 16th Ed, Pg- 56

Q. 87. Which of the following is a zoonotic disease (AIPG/95)
    (a)   Hydatid cyst
    (b)   Malaria
    (c)   Filariasis
    (d)   Dengue fever

Ans. (a)

MCQ's in Community Medicine

Note
The zoonotic diseases are those where animals are involved in it's transmission or in maintaining the infection within the environment.

Q. 88. Which of the following statements is true about BCG vaccination (AIIMS/May-05)
(a) Distilled water is used as diluent for BCG vaccine.
(b) The site for injection should be cleaned thoroughly with spirit.
(c) Mantoux test becomes positive after 48 hours of vaccination.
(d) WHO recommends Danish 1331 strain for vaccine production.

Ans. (d)
Note
The (a), (b) and (c) are incorrect.
Ref; Park and Park 17th Ed Pg-149.

Q. 89. Which of the following is false about whooping cough? (AIPG/95)
(a) Affects children 1 year of age.
(b) Contagious in the catarrhal stage.
(c) Carriers are the most important source of infection.
(d) Secondary attack rate is high.

Ans. (c)
Note
A chronic carrier stage of whooping cough does not exist.
Ref: Park and Park 16th Ed Pg-129

Q. 90. Which one of the following pulses has the highest content of iron? (AIIMS/May-05)
(a) Bengal gram
(b) Black gram
(c) Red gram
(d) Soya bean

Ans. (d)
Note
Soya bean has 10.4 mg per 100 gm iron which is the highest.
Ref; Park and Park 17th Ed Pg-428.

Q. 91. Human development index is measured by all except (AIIMS/May-05)
(a) Under five mortality
(b) Life expectancy at birth
(c) Literacy
(d) Per capita income

Ans. (a)
Note
Human development index is defined as a composite index combining indicators representing three dimensions
- Longevity (Life expectancy at birth),
- Knowledge (Adult literacy rate and mean years of schooling), and
- Income (Real GDP per capita in purchasing power – parity dollars).
Ref: Park and Park 17th Ed Pg-15.

Q. 92. 'Endemic disease' means that a disease (AII INDIA-05)
(a) Occurs clearly in excess of normal expectancy.
(b) Is constantly present in a given population group.
(c) Exhibits seasonal pattern.
(d) Is prevalent among animals.

Ans. (b)

Note
Endemic disease refers to the constant presence of a disease or infectious agent within a given geographic area or population group without importation from outside.
Ref; Park and Park 17th Ed Pg-82.

Q. 93. Which of the following is not true about the 'Tuberculin Test'? (AIPG/95)
(a) It is only tool available for estimating the prevalence of TB in a community.
(b) Induration of 10 mm indicates a positive test.
(c) It is a specific test.
(d) New cases occur more commonly in patients who are tuberculin reactors.

Ans. (c)

Note
'Tuberculin Test' is not a specific test as positive test can be interpreted in following manner:
a. On the basis of positive test one cannot diagnose the case as of tuberculosis.
b. It cannot specify about the susceptibility or immune status of a person for tuberculosis.
c. It measures the prevalence of TB in a community.

Q. 94. Which one of the following statements about influence of smoking on risk of coronary heart disease (CHD) is not true? (AII INDIA-05)
(a) Influence of smoking is independent of other risk factors for CHD.
(b) Influence of smoking is only additive to other risk factors for CHD.
(c) Influence of smoking is synergistic to other risk factors for CHD.
(d) Influence of smoking is directly related to number of cigarettes smoked per day.

Ans. (b)

Note
The degree of risk of developing CHD is directly related to the number of cigarettes smoked per day. There is evidence that the influence of smoking is not only independent of but also synergistic with other risk factors such as hypertension and elevated serum cholesterol. This means that the effects are more than addictive.
Ref; Park and Park 17th Ed Pg-275.

Q. 95. Diseases in which herd immunity does not protect an individual is (AIPG/95)
(a) Measles
(b) Tetanus
(c) Polio
(d) Diphtheria

Ans. (b)

Note
In case of Tetanus herd immunity does not protect the individual.
Ref: Park and Park 16th Ed Pg-90.

Q. 96. All of the following statements are true about congenital rubella except (AII INDIA-05)
(a) It is diagnosed when the infant has IgM antibodies at birth.
(b) It is diagnosed when IgG antibodies persist for more than 6 months.
(c) Most common congenital defects are deafness, cardiac malformations and cataract.
(d) Infection after 16 weeks of gestation results in major congenital defects.

Ans. (d)

Note
Infection in the second trimester may cause deafness but those infected after 16 week suffer no major abnormalities.
Ref; Park and Park 17th Ed Pg-122.

MCQ's in Community Medicine

Q. 97. The recommended daily energy intake of an adult woman with heavy work is (AII INDIA-05)
    (a)   1800
    (b)   2100
    (c)   2300
    (d)   2900

Ans. (d)
Note
Recommended daily energy of adult women is 2925 K cal per day.
Ref; Park and Park 17th Ed Pg-432.

Q. 98. All of the following methods are antilarval measures except (AII INDIA 05)
    (a)   Intermittent irrigation
    (b)   Paris green
    (c)   Gamusia affinis
    (d)   Malathion

Ans. (d)
Note
As a low volume spray malathiom has been widely used for killing adult mosquitoes to prevent or interrupt dengue hemorrhagic fever and mosquito borne encephalitis epidemics.
Ref; Park and Park 17th Ed Pg-558.

Q. 99. All of the following are true about the herd immunity for infectious diseases except (AII INDIA-05)
    (a)   It refers to group protection beyond what is afforded by the protection of immunized individuals.
    (b)   It is likely to be more for infections that do not have a sub-clinical phase.
    (c)   It is affected by the presence and distribution of alternative animal hosts.
    (d)   In the case of tetanus it does not protect the individual.

Ans. (b)
Note
Herd immunity implies group protection beyond that afforded by the protection of immunized individuals. Herd immunity provides an immunological barrier to the spread of disease in human herd.
Elements which contribute to herd immunity are:
a.   Occurrence of clinical and subclinical infection in the herd.
b.   Immunization of herd.
c.   Herd structure: It is subject to variation because of births, deaths ad population mobility. An ongoing immunization programme will keep up the herd immunity at a very high level.
The herd structure includes not only the hosts belonging to herd species but also the presence and distribution of alternative animal hosts and possible insect vectors as well as those environmental and social factors that favor or inhibit the spread of infection from host to host.
In the case of tetanus, however, herd immunity does not protect the individual.
Ref: Park and Park 16th Ed, Pg-89, 99.

Q. 100. The best indicator for monitoring the impact of Iodine Deficiency Disorder Control Programme is (AII INDIA-05)
    (a)   Prevalence of goitre among school children
    (b)   Urinary iodine levels among pregnant women
    (c)   Neonatal hypothyroidism
    (d)   Iodine level in soil

Ans. (c)
Note
Neonatal hypothyroidism is a sensitive pointer to environmental Iodine Deficiency and can thus be an effective indicator for monitoring the impact of Iodine Deficiency Disorder Control Programme.
Ref: Park and Park 16th Ed, Pg-433

Q. 101. What is the color-coding of bag in hospitals to dispose off human anatomical wastes such as body parts (AII INDIA-05)
 (a) Yellow
 (b) Black
 (c) Red
 (d) Blue

Ans. (a)

Note
Human anatomical wastes are disposed in yellow plastic bag and disposed by incineration or deep burial. The types of waste and their disposal procedures are as under:

Category	Type of Waste	Disposal
Cat-1:	Human anatomical waste; tissue, organs, body parts	Incineration / Deep burial
Cat-2:	Animal waste; tissue, organs, carcasses, bleeding parts, fluids, experimental animals used in research, waste generated by veterinary hospitals colleges, discharges from hospitals, animal house.	Incineration / Deep burial
Cat-3:	Microbiology and biotechnology waste.	Local autoclaving / microwaving / incineration
Cat-4:	Waste sharps; needles, syringes, blades, glass.	Disinfection / Autoclaving / Microwaving / Mutilation / shredding
Cat-5:	Discarded medicines and cytotoxic drugs.	Incineration destruction and rugs disposal in secured landfills
Cat-6:	Solid waste; items contaminated with blood, cotton, dressings, soiled plaster casts, linen, beddings.	Incineration, autoclaving / microwaving
Cat-7:	Solid waste; other than sharp, i.e., tubing, catheters, intravenous sets etc.	Disinfection by chemical treatment/ Autoclaving / Microwaving and mutilation / shredding
Cat-8:	Liquid waste; from laboratory, washing cleaning, housekeeping and disinfecting activity	Disinfection by chemical treatment and discharge into drains
Cat-9:	Incineration ash from any bio-medical waste.	Disposal in municipal landfill
Cat-10:	Chemicals used in production of biological, chemicals, used in disinfection, as insecticides.	Chemical treatment and discharge into drains for liquids and secured landfill for solids

Color coding for waste disposal:

Color Code	Type of Container	Category of waste	Disposal
Yellow	Plastic bag	Cat: 1, 2, 3 and 6	Incineration / Deep burial
Red	Plastic bag / Disinfected container	Cat: 3, 6, 7	Autoclaving / Microwaving / Chemical treatment
Blue / White translucent	Plastic bag / Puncture proof container	Cat: 4, 7	Autoclaving / Microwaving / Chemical treatment and Destruction / Shredding
Black	Plastic bag	Cat: 5, 9, 10	Disposal in secured landfills

Q. 102. WHO defines adolescent age between (AII INDIA-05)
 (a) 10-19 years of age
 (b) 10-14 years of age
 (c) 10-25 years of age
 (d) 9-14 years of age

Ans. (a)

Note
Adolescent: 10 - 19 Years
Youth: 15 – 24 years

Young People: 10 – 24 Years
Ref: Ghai

Q. 103. India belong to which stage of demographic cycle (AIPG/95)
    (a)   Slow stationary
    (b)   High stationary
    (c)   Early expanding
    (d)   Late Expanding

Ans. (d)
Note
India has entered 'Late Expanding' phase of Demographic cycle.
There is a demographic cycle of five stages through which a nation passes and they are as under:
a.   *First stage (High Stationary)*
    High birth rate and high death rate.
b.   *Second stage (Early Expanding)*
    Death rate declines, birth rate remains unchanged.
c.   *Third stage (Late Expanding)*
    Death rate further declines, birth rate begins to fall, Birth exceeds death.
    (India has entered this phase)
d.   *Fourth Stage (Low Stationary)*
    Low birth rate and low death rate. Very low growth rates / almost zero.
e.   *Fifth Stage (Declining)*
    Birth rate lower than death rate.
Ref: Park and Park 16th Ed Pg-319

Q. 104. The following tests are used to check the efficiency of pasteurization of milk except (AII INDIA - 05)
    (a)   Phosphatase test
    (b)   Standard plate count
    (c)   Coliform count
    (d)   Methylene blue reduction test

Ans. (d)
Note
Following three are the tests of pasteurized milk:
a.   Phosphatase Test: It detects inadequate pasteurization.
b.   Standard Plate Count: It determines the bacteriological quality of pasteurized milk.
c.   Coliform Count: The coliform organisms are usually completely destroyed by pasteurization, therefore their presence in pasteurized milk indicates improper pasteurization or post pasteurization contamination.
Park and Park 16th Ed Pg- 443

Q. 105. What will be the BMI of a male whose weight is 89 kg and height is 172 cm? (AII INDIA-05)
    (a)   27
    (b)   30
    (c)   33
    (d)   36

Ans. (b)
Note
The BMI = Weight (Kg) / Height (m)^2
Ref: Park and park 16th Ed P-297

Q. 106. The most common side effect of IUD insertion is (AII INDIA-05)
    (a)   Bleeding
    (b)   Pain
    (c)   Pelvic infection
    (d)   Ectopic pregnancy

Ans. (a)

Note
The commonest complaint of women fitted with an IUD (inert or medicated) is increased vaginal bleeding. It accounts for 10 – 20 % of all IUD removals.
Ref: Park and park 16th Ed P-335

Q. 107. For the treatment of case of class III dog bite, all of the following are correct except (AII INDIA-05)
    (a)   Give immunoglobulins for passive immunity
    (b)   Give ARV
    (c)   Immediately stitch wound under antibiotic coverage
    (d)   Immediately wash wound with soap and water

Ans. (c)
Note
Bite wound should not be immediately sutured to prevent additional trauma which may help spread the virus into deeper tissues. If suturing is necessary, it should be done 24 to 48 hours later, applying minimum possible stitches, under the cover of antirabies serum locally.
Ref: Park and Park 16th Ed Pg-207-208.

Q. 108. A 2-year-old female child was brought to a Primary Health Clinic with a history of cough and fever for 4 days with inability to drink for last 12 hours. On examination, the child was having weight of 5 kg and respiratory rate of 45/minute with fever. The child will be classified as suffering from (AII INDIA -05)
    (a)   Very severe disease
    (b)   Severe pneumonia
    (c)   Pneumonia
    (d)   No pneumonia

Ans. (a)
Note
This 2 year old female baby has history of cough and fever 4 days with inability to drink for last 12 hours. It falls in category of 'very severe disease' and the danger sign is 'not able to drink'.
Ref: Park and Park 16th Ed Pg-134, 135.

Q. 109. The information technology has revolutionized the world of medical sciences. In which of the following year the Information Technology Act was passed by the Government of India? (A I I INDIA-05)
    (a)   1998
    (b)   2000
    (c)   2001
    (d)   2003

Ans. (b)
Note
Information Technology Act, 2000- it came into force from Oct 17th 2000.

Q. 110. Transplantation of Human Organs Act was passed by Government of India in (AII INDIA-05)
    (a)   1996
    (b)   1993
    (c)   1998
    (d)   1994

Ans. (d)
Note
The Transplantation of Human Organs Act was passed in 1994.

Q. 111. The growth pattern of a population with an annual growth rate of 1.5% to 2.0% is (AIPG/95)
    (a)   Slow growth
    (b)   Moderate growth
    (c)   Rapid growth
    (d)   Very rapid growth

Ans. (d)

Note

Rating	Annual Rate of Growth %
a. Slow Growth	Less than 0.5
b. Moderate Growth	0.5 – 1.0
c. Rapid Growth	1.0 – 1.5
d. Very Rapid Growth	1.5 – 2.0

Ref: Park and Park 16th Ed, Pg-320

Q. 112. An IQ between 50 – 70 would be classified as what kind of mental retardation (AIPG/95)
    (a)   Mild
    (b)   Moderate
    (c)   Severe
    (d)   Borderline

Ans. (a)

Note
Intelligence quotient (IQ)- It is obtained by dividing the mental age by chronological age and multiplying with 100.

$$IQ = \frac{Mental\ Age}{Chronological\ Age} \times 100$$

When the mental age is the same as chronological age, the IQ is 100. Higher the IQ more brilliant the child. Similarly if a child is 10 years of age and his mental age level is 5 years, the IQ is 50.

Level of Intelligence	IQ Range
Idiot	0 - 24
Imbecile	25 - 49
Moron	50 - 69
Border line	70 - 79
Low Normal	80 - 89
Normal	90 - 109
Superior	110 - 119
Very Superior	120 - 139
Near Genius	140 and above

Ref: Park and Park 16th Ed Pg-462
WHO classification of IQ:

Level of Intelligence	IQ Range
Mild	50 - 70
Moderate	35 - 49
Severe	20 - 34
Profound	< 20

Ref: Park and Park 17th Ed Pg-327

Q. 113. The screening method of choice in an area where the prevalence of leprosy is 1/1000 is (AIPG/95)
    (a)   Contact survey
    (b)   Group survey
    (c)   Mass survey
    (d)   Any of the above

Ans. (b)
The Choice of case finding method is related to the prevalence rate of leprosy in the region and is as under:
a.   Contact surveys: Most suitable for low prevalence rate which is less than 1/1000.
b.   Group surveys: Most suitable for moderate prevalence which is 1/1000 or higher.
c.   Mass survey: It is most suitable for Hyper-endemic area where the prevalence rate is 10/1000 or high.
Ref: Park and Park 16th Ed Pg-246

Q. 114. In Niacin deficiency, all of the following are seen except (AIPG/96)
    (a)   Deafness
    (b)   Diarrhea
    (c)   Dementia
    (d)   Dermatitis

Ans. (a)

Note
Pellagra is due to deficiency of Niacin and is characterised by diarrhea, dementia and dermatitis.
Ref: Park and Park 16th Ed Pg-413

Q. 115. Measures of Primary prevention of Hypertension includes all of the following except (AIPG/97)
    (a)   Weight reduction
    (b)   Exercise promotion
    (c)   Reduction of salt intake
    (d)   Early diagnosis of hypertension

Ans. (d)

Note
The early diagnosis is part of secondary prevention.

Q. 116. Vitamin B12 is not found in (AIPG/97)
    (a)   Soyabean
    (b)   Milk
    (c)   Meat
    (d)   Fish

Ans. (a)

Note
Vitamin B12 is not found in vegetable origin foods.

Q. 117. First indices to change in iron deficiency anemia is (AIPG/97)
    (a)   S. iron
    (b)   Total Iron Binding Capacity
    (c)   S. Ferritin
    (d)   S. hemoglobin concentration

Ans. (c)

Note
See Q No 70 and 218.

MCQ's in Community Medicine   495

Q. 118. Maize is deficient in (AIPG/97)
(a) Tryptophan
(b) Threonine
(c) Methionine
(d) Leucine

Ans. (a)
Note
See Q. No 68

Q. 119. Sanguinarine is derived from (AIPG/97)
(a) Fusorium incamatum
(b) Argemone oil
(c) Jhunjujia seeds
(d) Khesari dhal

Ans. (b)
Note
Epidemic dropsy cases are reported in India from time to time. The cause of this was not known before 1926. Sarkar attributed it to the contamination of mustard oil with 'Argemone oil'. Lal and Roy (1937) and Chopra et.al., (1939) gave experimental proof of the epidemic dropsy. Mukherji et. Al., (1941) isolated the toxic alkaloid, 'Sanguinarine' from argemone oil. This substance interferes with the oxidation of pyruvic acid which accumulates in the blood.
Ref: Park and Park 16th Ed Pg- 445

Q. 120. The most common cancer affecting Indian urban women in Delhi, Mumbai and Chennai is (AII INDIA-05)
(a) Cervical cancer
(b) Ovarian cancer
(c) Breast cancer
(d) Uterine cancer

Ans. (c)
Note
Cancer incidences in females at Delhi, Mumbai and Chennai:

City	Ca Breast	Ca Cervix	Ca Ovary
Delhi	29.8	24.1	10.0
Mumbai	28.0	17.0	8.2
Chennai	26.0	29.8	5.8

The overall incidence of cancer breast is more common in Delhi, Mumbai and Chennai.
Ref: Park and Park 17th Ed, Pg-299.

Q. 121. The most common malignant tumor of adult males in India is (AII INDIA-04)
(a) Oropharyngeal carcinoma
(b) Gastric carcinoma
(c) Colo-rectal carcinoma
(d) Lung cancer

Ans. (a)

Q. 122. The National Population Policy of India has set the following goals except (AII INDIA-04)
(a) To bring down total fertility rate (TFR) to replacement levels by 2015.
(b) To reduce the infant mortality rate to 30 per 1000 live births.
(c) To reduce the maternal mortality rate to 100 per 100,000 live births.
(d) 100 percent registration of births, deaths, marriages and pregnancies.

Ans. (a)

The objective of National Population Policy 2000 is to bring TFR to replacement level by 2010.
Ref: Park and Park 17th Ed Pg- 337

Q. 123. The following statements are true about intrauterine devices (IUD), except (AII INDIA-04)
    (a)   Multiload Cu-375 is a third generation IUD.
    (b)   The pregnancy rate of Lippe's loop and Cu-T 200 are similar.
    (c)   IUD can be used for emergency contraception within 5 days.
    (d)   Levonorgestrol releasing IUD has an effective life of 5 years.

Ans. (a)
Note
Multiload cu –375 is a second generation IUCD.
Ref: Park and Park 17th Ed Pg- 340

Q. 124. All of the following are used as proxy measures for incubation period except (AII INDIA-04)
    (a)   Latent period
    (b)   Period of communicability
    (c)   Serial interval
    (d)   Generation time

Ans. (a)
Note
1. Latent period: The term is used in non infectious as the equivalent of incubation period in infectious.
2. Period of communicability: The time during which an infectious agent may be transferred directly or indirectly from an infected person to another person, from an infected animal to man or from an infected person to an animal, including arthropods.
3. Serial interval: The gap in time between the onset of primary case and the secondary case.
4. Generation time: The interval between receipt of infection by a host and maximal infectivity of that host. In general it is roughly equal to the incubation period.
Ref: Park and Park 17th Ed Pg- 88

Q. 125. "Five clean practices" under strategies for elimination of neonatal tetanus include all except (AII INDIA-04)
    (a)   Clean surface for delivery
    (b)   Clean hand of the attendant
    (c)   New blade for cutting the cord
    (d)   Clean airway

Ans. (d)
Note
Over the last decade, most programmes in developing countries have concentrated on training the traditional birth attendants, providing home delivery kits and educating pregnant women about the "three cleans"- clean hands, clean delivery surface and clean cord care i.e. clean blade for cutting the cord, clean tie for the cord and no application on the cord stump.
Ref: Park and Park 17th Ed Pg- 241

Q. 126. The current recommendation for breast-feeding is that (AII INDIA-04)
    (a)   Exclusive breast-feeding should be continued till 6 months of age followed by supplementation with additional foods.
    (b)   Exclusive breast-feeding should be continued till 4 months of age followed by supplementation with additional foods.
    (c)   Colostrum is the most suitable food for a new born baby but it is best avoided in first 2 days.
    (d)   The baby should be allowed to breast-feed till one year of age.

Ans. (b)
Note
No other food is required to be given until 4 to 5 months after birth. At the age of 4 to 5 months, breast milk should be supplemented by additional foods rich in protein and the other nutrients.
Ref: Park and Park 17th Ed Pg- 366

MCQ's in Community Medicine

Q. 127. According to International Health Regulations, there is no risk of spread of yellow fever if the Aedes aegypti index remains below (AII INDIA-04)
- (a) 1%
- (b) 5%
- (c) 8%
- (d) 10%

Ans. (a)
Ref: Park and Park 17th Ed Pg- 217

Q. 128. The following statements about breast milk are true except (AII INDIA-04)
- (a) The maximum milk output is seen at 12 months
- (b) The coefficient of uptake of iron in breast milk is 70%
- (c) Calcium absorption of human milk is better than that of cow's milk
- (d) It provides about 65 Kcals per 100 ml

Ans. (a)

Note
Under normal conditions Indian mothers secrete 400 – 600 ml of milk daily. The maximum milk output is at 5 – 6 months (730 ml/ day) after which the output declines. At 12 months the output is 525 ml/day
Ref: Park and Park, 16th Ed, Pg-359

Q. 129. All of the following statements about leprosy are true except (AII INDIA-04)
- (a) Multibacillary leprosy is diagnosed when there are more than 5 skin patches.
- (b) New case detection rate is an indicator for incidence of leprosy.
- (c) A defaulter is defined as a patient who has not taken treatment for 6 months or more.
- (d) The target for elimination of leprosy is to reduce the prevalence to less than 1 per 10,000 population.

Ans. (b)

Note
Since a, c, d are true therefore b is false.
Ref: Park and Park 17th Ed Pg- 245, 242, 311

Q. 130. Multipurpose worker scheme in India was introduced following the recommendation of (AII INDIA-04)
- (a) Srivastava Committee
- (b) Bhore Committee
- (c) Kartar Singh Committee
- (d) Mudaliar Committee

Ans. (c)

Note
1. Shrivastav Committee, 1975: The Govt of India in the Ministry of Health and Family Planning had in Nov 1974 set up a group on medical education and support manpower popularly known as Shrivastav committee. Ref: Park and Park 16th Ed, Pg- 637
2. Bhore Committee, 1946: The Govt of India in 1943 appointed the Health Survey and Development Committee with Sir Joseph Bhore as Chairman to survey the then existing position regarding the health conditions and health organizations in the country, and to make recommendations for the future development. The committee met regularly for 2 years and submitted in 1946 its famous report, which runs into 4 volumes. Ref: Park and Park 16th Ed, Pg- 636
3. Kartar Singh Committee, 1973: The Govt of India constituted a Committee in 1972 known as "The Committee on Multipurpose Workers under Health and Family Planning "under the Chairmanship of Kartar Singh, Additional Secretary, Ministry of Health and Family Planning, Government of India. Ref: Park and Park 16th Ed, Pg- 637
4. Mudaliar committee: In 1959, the Govt of India appointed another committee known as "Health Survey and Planning Committee "popularly known as the Mudaliar Committee to survey the progress made

in the field of health since submission of the Bhore Committee's report and to make recommendations for the future development and expansion of health services.
Ref: Park and Park 17th Ed Pg- 636

Q. 131. The usefulness of a 'screening test' in a community depends on its (AII INDIA-04)
(a) Sensitivity
(b) Specificity
(c) Reliability
(d) Predictive value

Ans. (d)

Note
In addition to sensitivity and specificity, the performance of a 'screening test' is measured by its 'predictive value', which reflects the diagnostic power of the test.
Park and Park 16th Ed P-111.

Q. 132. If the grading of diabetes is classified as 'mild' 'moderate' and 'severe' the scale of measurement used is (AII INDIA-04)
(a) Interval
(b) Nominal
(c) Ordinal
(d) Ratio

Ans. (c)

Note
The grading of diabetes is classified as 'mild', 'moderate' and 'severe' the scale of measurement used is "Ordinal Scale". Here the data is placed in a meaningful order.

Q. 133. A study began in 1970 with a group of 5000 adults in Delhi who were asked about their alcohol consumption. The occurrence of cancer was studied in this group between 1990-1995. This is an example of (AII INDIA -04)
(a) Cross-sectional study
(b) Retrospective cohort study
(c) Concurrent cohort study
(d) Case-control study

Ans. (c)

Note
A prospective or concurrent cohort study is one in which the outcome (e.g. disease) has not occurred at the time the investigation begins.
Ref: Park and Park 17th Ed Pg- 66
The present study is 'alcohol consumption' to 'occurrence of cancer' and therefore falls in category of 'prospective / Concurrent cohort study.

Q. 134. The most appropriate test to assess the prevalence of tuberculosis infection in a community is (AII INDIA-04)
(a) Mass Miniature Radiography
(b) Sputum examination
(c) Tuberculin test
(d) Clinical examination

Ans. (c)

Note
Prevalence of tuberculosis is the percentage of individuals who show a positive reaction to the standard tuberculin test.
Ref: Park and Park 17th Ed Pg 140

MCQ's in Community Medicine

Q. 135. A 37 weeks pregnant woman attends an antenatal clinic at a primary health centre. She has not had any antenatal care till now. The best approach regarding tetanus immunization in this case would be to (AII INDIA-04)
  (a) Give a dose of tetanus toxoid (TT) and explain her that it will not protect the new born and she should take the second dose after four weeks even if she delivers in the meantime.
  (b) Do not waste the TT vaccine as it would anyhow be of no use in this pregnancy.
  (c) Given one dose of TT and explain that it will not be useful for this pregnancy.
  (d) Give her anti-tetanus immunoglobulin along with the TT vaccine.

Ans. (a)
Note
In unimmunized pregnant women, two doses of tetanus toxoid should be given, the first as early as possible during pregnancy and second at least a month later and at least 3 weeks before delivery. The golden rule is that no pregnant mother should be denied even one dose of tetanus toxoid if she is seen late in pregnancy.
Ref: Park and Park 17th Ed Pg 241

Q. 136. Dietary changes advocated by WHO for prevention of heart diseases include all of the following except (AII INDIA-04)
  (a) A decrease in complex carbohydrate consumption.
  (b) Reduction in fat intake to 20 to 30 percent of caloric intake.
  (c) Consumption of saturated fats be limited to less than 10 percent of total energy intake.
  (d) Reduction of cholesterol to below 100 mg per 1000 kcal per day.

Ans. (a)
Note
The WHO Expert Committee considered the following dietary changes to be appropriate for high incidence population:
  -Reduction of fat intake to 20-30 % of total energy intake.
  -Consumption of saturated fats must be limited to less than 10% of total energy intake.
  -A reduction of dietary cholesterol to below 100 mg per 1000 kcal per day.
  -Increase in complex, carbohydrate consumption (i.e. vegetables, fruits, whole grain and legumes).
  -Avoidance of alcohol consumption; reduction of salt intake to 5 g daily or less.
Ref: Park and Park 17th Ed Pg 276

Q. 137. Essential components of RCH Programme in India include all of the following except (AII INDIA-04)
  (a) Prevention and management of unwanted pregnancies.
  (b) Maternal care including antenatal, delivery & post-natal services.
  (c) Reduce the under five mortality to half.
  (d) Management of reproductive tract infections & sexually transmitted infections.

Ans. (c)
Ref: Park and Park 17th Ed Pg 320, 321

Q. 138. A child aged 4 months was brought to a health worker in the sub center with complaints of cough and fever. On examination, there was chest indrawing and respiratory rate was 45 per minute. Which of the following is best way to manage the child? (AII INDIA-04)
  (a) The child should be classified as a case of pneumonia.
  (b) Give an antibiotic and advise mother to give home care.
  (c) Reassess the child within 2 days or earlier if the condition worsens.
  (d) Refer urgently to hospital after giving the first dose of an antibiotic.

Ans. (d)
Note
The above clinical situation prompts that - the child should be referred urgently to hospital and given first dose of antibiotic.
Ref: Park and Park 17th Ed Pg 135,136
Severe pneumonia: The most important signs to consider when deciding if the child has pneumonia are the child's respiratory rate and whether or not there is chest indrawing.

Protocol for Classification and Management of Pneumonia in a child 2 months to 5 years of age is as:

Age	Criteria for fast breathing
Less than 2 Months	RR > 60/min
2 Months to 12 Months	RR > 50/min
12 Months to 5 years	RR 40/min

Evaluating Features			
No chest Indrawing No fast breathing	No chest Indrawing Fast Breathing Present	Chest indrawing present Nasal flare preset Grunting Present Cyanosis Present Wheezing Present	Chest Indrawing present -Not able to drink -Convulsions -Sleepy / Difficult to awake -Stridor -Severe malnutrition
Inference drawn			
No Pneumonia	Pneumonia	Severe Pneumonia	Very severe Pneumonia
Action suggested			
Home care	Home care Antibiotics Treat fever Treat wheezing	Give first dose of Antibiotic Refer to Hospital	Give first dose of antibiotic Refer urgently to hospital

Q. 139. All of the following are modes of transmission of leprosy, except (AII INDIA-04)
    (a) Breast milk
    (b) Insect bite
    (c) Transplacental spread
    (d) Droplet infection

Ans. (c)

Note
Mode of transmission of leprosy:
    -Droplet infection
    -Contact transmission
    -Other routes-breast milk, insect vectors, by tattooing needles
Ref: Park and Park 17th Ed Pg 244

Q. 140. Which of the following is the most reliable method of estimating blood alcohol level? (AII INDIA-04)
    (a) Cavett's test
    (b) Breath alcohol analyzer
    (c) Gas liquid chromatography
    (d) Thin layer chromatography

Ans. (c)

Note
Gas liquid chromatography provides qualitative and quantitative analysis of the alcohol present in bood.

Q. 141. The parameters of sensitivity and specificity are used for assessing (AII INDIA-03)
    (a) Criterion validity
    (b) Construct validity
    (c) Discriminant validity
    (d) Content validity

Ans. (a)

Ref: Park and Park 17th Ed Pg 111

MCQ's in Community Medicine

Q. 142. Chi-square test is used to measure the degree of (AII INDIA-03)
    (a) Causal relationship between exposure and effect
    (b) Association between two variables
    (c) Correlation between two variables
    (d) Agreement between two observations

Ans. (b)
Note
The test of association between two events is the most important application of Chi-square test.

Q. 143. Elements of primary health care include all of the following except (AII INDIA-03)
    (a) Adequate supply of safe water and basic sanitation
    (b) Providing essential drugs
    (c) Sound referral system
    (d) Health education

Ans. (c)
Note
Elements of primary health care:
- Education concerning prevailing health problems and methods of preventing and controlling them.
- Promotion of food supply and proper nutrition.
- An adequate supply of safe drinking water and basic sanitation.
- Maternal and child health care, including family planning.
- Immunization against major infectious diseases.
- Prevention and control of locally endemic diseases.
- Appropriate treatment of common diseases and injuries.
- Provision of essential drugs.

Ref: Park and Park 17th Ed Pg 650

Q. 144. Elemental iron and folic acid contents of pediatric iron-folic acid tablets supplied under Rural Child Health (RCH) program are (AII INDIA-03)
    (a) 20 mg iron & 100 micrograms folic acid.
    (b) 40 mg iron & 100 micrograms folic acid.
    (c) 40 mg iron & 50 micrograms folic acid.
    (d) 60 mg iron & 100 micrograms folic acid.

Ans. (a)
Note
Dosage of iron-folic acid supplementation in children: one tablet of iron and folic acid contain 20 mg of elemental iron (60 mg of ferrous sulphate) and 0.1 mg of folic acid.
Ref: Park and Park 17th Ed Pg 437

Q. 145. In the management of leprosy, lepromin test is most useful for (AII INDIA 2003)
    (a) Herd immunity
    (b) Prognosis
    (c) Treatment
    (d) Epidemiological investigations

Ans. (b)
Note
The lepromin test is of great value in estimating the prognosis in case of leprosy of all types.
Ref: Park and Park 17th Ed Pg 247

Q. 146. The following statements about meningococcal meningitis are true, except (AII INDIA-03)
    (a) The source of infection is mainly clinical cases
    (b) The disease is more common in dry and cold months of the year
    (c) Chemoprophylaxis of close contacts of cases is recommended
    (d) The vaccine is not effective in children below 2 years of age

Ans. (a)

Note
Meningococcal meningitis source of infection: the organism is found in the nasopharynx of cases and carriers. Clinical cases present only a negligible source of infection.
Ref: Park and Park 17th Ed Pg 132

Q. 147. The Protein Efficiency Ratio (PER) is defined as (AII INDIA-03)
(a) The gain in weight of young animals per unit weight of protein-consumed.
(b) The product of digestibility coefficent and biological value.
(c) The percentage of protein absorbed into the blood.
(d) The percentage of nitrogen absorbed from the protein absorbed from the diet.

Ans. (a)
Note
The protein efficiency ratio is gain in weight of young animal per unit weight of protein consumed.

Q. 148. The Vitamin A supplement administered in "Prevention of nutritional blindness in children programme" contains (AII INDIA-03)
(a) 25,000 I.U../ml
(b) 1 lakh I.U./ml
(c) 3 lakh I.U../ml
(d) 5 lakh I.U../ml

Ans. (b)
Note
The strategy is to administer a single massive dose of 200,000 IU of vitamin A in oil (retinol palmitate) orally every 6 months to pre school children (1 year to 6 years), and half that dose (100,000 IU) to children between 6 months and one year of age.
Ref: Park and Park 17th Ed Pg 417

Q. 149. A 5 year old boy passed 18 loose stools in last 24 hours and vomited twice in last 4 hours. He is irritable but drinking fluids. The optimal therapy for this child is
(a) Intravenous fluids
(b) Oral rehydration therapy
(c) Intravenous fluid initially for 4 hours followed by oral fluids
(d) Plain water add libitum

Ans. (b)
Ref: Park and Park 17th Ed Pg 172

Q. 150. The commonest cause of low vision in India is (AII INDIA-03)
(a) Uncorrected refractive error
(b) Cataract
(c) Glaucoma
(d) Squint

Ans. (b)
Note
Causes of blindness in India

Cause	Number %
Cataract	81 %
Trachoma and associated infections	0.2 %
Corneal opacity	3.0 %
Vitamin deficiency	0.04 %
Refractive error	7.0 %
Glaucoma	2.0 %
Other causes	6.76 %

Ref: Park and Park 16th Ed Pg-299

Q. 151. Most important epidemiological tool used for assessing disability in children is (AII INDIA-03)
    (a)   Activities of Daily Living (ADL) scale
    (b)   Wing's Handicaps, Behaviour and Skills (HBS) Schedule
    (c)   Binet and Simon IQ tests
    (d)   Physical Quality of Life Index (PQLI)

Ans. (b)
Note
Wing's Handicaps, behaviour and Skills (HBS) Schedule; has been used in epidemiological studies to assess the total child population in terms of detailed scales of specific ability and disabilities.

Q. 152. Scope of family planning services include all of the following except (AII INDIA-03)
    (a)   Screening for cervical cancer
    (b)   Providing services for unmarried mothers
    (c)   Screening for HIV infection
    (d)   Providing adoption services

Ans. (c)
Note
Screening for HIV infection is not included in the Family planning services. However, the scope of family planning services includes following:
    a.   Proper spacing and limitation of births
    b.   Advice for parenthood
    c.   Sex education
    d.   Screening for pathological conditions related to reproductive system i.e., Ca cervix
    e.   Genetic counseling
    f.   Premarital consultation and examination
    g.   Pregnancy test
    h.   Marriage counseling
    i.   Preparation of couple for arrival of their 1st child
    j.   Teaching home economics and nutrition
    k.   Provides adoption services
Ref: Park and Park 17th Ed Pg 335

Q. 153. Class II exposure in animal bites includes the following (AII INDIA-03)
    (a)   Scratches without oozing of blood
    (b)   Licks on a fresh wound
    (c)   Scratch with oozing of blood on palm
    (d)   Bites from wild animals

Ans. (b)
Note
Bites from animals are classed as under:

Class	Features
Class I	Licks on healthy unbroken skin Scratches without oozing of blood
Class II	Licks on fresh cuts Scratches with oozing of blood All bites except those on Head, Neck, Face, Palm and Fingers Minor wounds less than 5 in number
Class III	All bites and scratches with oozing of blood on neck, head, face, palm and fingers Lacerated wound on any part of the body Multiple wounds 5 or more in member Bites from wild animals

Ref: Park and Park 17th Ed Pg 212

Q. 154. Elemental iron and folic acid contents of iron and folic acid adult tablets supplied under the "National Programme for Anaemia Prophylaxis" are (AII INDIA-03)
    (a)   60 mg of elemental iron and 250 microgram of folic acid
    (b)   100 mg of elemental iron and 500 micrograms of folic acid
    (c)   20 mg of elemental iron and 750 micrograms of folic acid
    (d)   200 mg of elemental iron and 1000 micro-grams of folic acid

Ans. (b)
Note
In Iron and folic acid adults tablets the amount of elemental iron is 60 mg (180 mg ferrous sulphate) and folic acid is 500 micro grams
Ref: Park and Park 17th Ed Pg 439

Q. 155. Denominator while calculating the secondary attack rate includes (AII INDIA-03)
    (a)   All the people living in next fifty houses
    (b)   All the close contacts
    (c)   All susceptibles amongst close contact
    (d)   All susceptibles in the whole village

Ans. (c)
Note
Secondary attack rate is expressed as:
SAR= Number of exposed persons developing the disease within the range of the incubation period / total number of exposed or susceptible contacts x100
Ref; Park and Park 17th Ed Pg 88

Q. 156. The response which is graded by an observer on an agree or disagree continuum is based on (AII INDIA-03)
    (a)   Visual analog scale
    (b)   Guttman scale
    (c)   Likert scale
    (d)   Adjectival scale

Ans. (c)
Note
Likert scale; has a role in behavioural sciences and the subject's answers are recorded on a five point scale:
a.   Disagree strongly
b.   Disagree
c.   Neither agree or disagree
d.   Agree
e.   Agree strongly.

Q. 157. Leprosy is considered a public health problem if the prevalence of leprosy is more than (A I I INDIA-03)
    (a)   1 per 10,000
    (b)   2 per 10,000
    (c)   5 per 10,000
    (d)   10 per 10,000

Ans. (a)
Note
Prevalence of leprosy as one case per 10,000 populations is taken as a potential public health problem.
Ref: Park and Park 17th Ed Pg-311

Q. 158. For controlling an outbreak of cholera, all of the following measures are recommended except (AII INDIA-03)
    (a)   Mass chemoprophylaxis
    (b)   Proper disposal of excreta

(c) Chlorination of water
(d) Early detection and management of cases

Ans. (a)
Note
Mass chemoprophylaxis is not advised for the total community because in order to prevent one serious case of cholera, some 10,000 persons must be given medicines. Further the drug's effect is only short lived for a few days.
Ref: Park and Park 17th Ed Pg 173

Q. 159. Iron and folic acid supplementation forms (AII INDIA-02)
(a) Health promotion
(b) Specific protection
(c) Primordial prevention
(d) Primary prevention

Ans. (b)
Note
The following are some of the currently available interventions aimed at specific protection:
a. Immunization
b. Use of specific nutrients
c. Chemoprophylaxis
d. Protection against occupational hazards
e. Protection against accidents
f. Protection from carcinogens
g. Avoidance of allergens
Ref: Park and Park 17th Ed Pg 36

Q. 160. The most important function of sentinel surveillance is (AII INDIA-02)
(a) To find the total amount of disease in a population
(b) To plan effective control measures
(c) To determine the trend of disease in a population
(d) To notify disease

Ans. (a)
Note
Sentinel surveillance is a method for identifying the missing cases and thereby supplementing the notified cases. The sentinel data is extrapolated to the entire population to estimate the disease prevalence in the total population.
Ref: Park and Park 17th Ed Pg 34

Q. 161. Serial interval is (AII INDIA-02)
(a) Time gap between primary and secondary case
(b) Time gap between index and primary case
(c) Time taken for a person from infection to develop maximum infectivity
(d) The time taken from infection till a person infects another person

Ans. (a)
Note
Serial interval is the gap in the time between the onset of the primary case and the secondary case.
Ref: Park and Park 17th Ed Pg 88

Q. 162. About direct standardization all are true except (AII INDIA-02)
(a) Age specific death rates are not needed
(b) A standard population is needed
(c) Population should be comparable
(d) Two propulations are compared

Ans. (a)

Note
In direct standardization, a standard population is selected. A standard population is defined as one for which the numbers in each age and sex group are known. The standard population can also be created by combining 2 populations. The next step is to apply the standard population whose crude death rate is to be adjusted or standardized.
Ref: Park and Park 17th Ed Pg 50.

Q. 163. Which vaccine is contraindicated in pregnancy? (AII INDIA-02)
    (a)   Rubella
    (b)   Diphtheria
    (c)   Tetanus
    (d)   Hepatitis B

Ans. (a)

Note
Pregnancy is considered a contraindication to rubella immunization.
Ref: Park and Park 17th Ed Pg 123.

Q. 164. The infectivity of chicken pox lasts for (AII INDIA-02)
    (a)   Till the last scab falls off
    (b)   6 days after onset of rash
    (c)   3 days after onset of rash
    (d)   Till the fever subsides

Ans. (b)

Note
The period of communicability of patients with varicella is estimated to range from 1 to 2 days before the appearance of rash and 4 to 5 days thereafter.
Ref: Park and Park 17th Ed Pg 117.

Q. 165. Carriers are important in all the following except (AII INDIA 02)
    (a)   Polio
    (b)   Typhoid
    (c)   Measles
    (d)   Diphtheria

Ans. (c)

Note
Carriers are not important the only source of infection is a case of measles..
Ref: Park and Park 17th Ed Pg 119

Q. 166. Acute flaccid paralysis is reported in a child aged (AII INDIA 02)
    (a)   0-3 years
    (b)   0-5 years
    (c)   0-15 years
    (d)   0-25 years

Ans. (c)

Note
In AFP surveillance WHO recommends; reporting of every case of AFP in children aged less than 15 years.

Q. 167. A 2-year-old boy, presented with cough, fever & difficulty in breathing. His Respiratory Rate is 50/min. There was no chest indrawing. Auscultation of chest reveals bilateral crepitions. The most probable diagnosis is (AII INDIA-02)
    (a)   Very severe pneumonia
    (b)   Severe pneumonia

(c) Pneumonia
(d) No pneumonia

Ans. (c)

Note
The child is of 2 years of age and presenting with cough, fever and difficulty in breathing, respiratory rate is 50/min and there is no chest indrawing. He falls in the category of pneumonia.
Ref: Park and Park 16th Ed, Pg-134-35

Q. 168. Active and passive immunity should be given together in all except (AII INDIA-02)
    (a) Tetanus
    (b) Rabies
    (c) Measles
    (d) Hepatitis B

Ans. (c)

Note
Measles can be prevented by giving Ig early in incubation period.

Q. 169. Cereals and proteins are considered complementary because (AII INDIA-02)
    (a) Cereals are deficient in methionine.
    (b) Cereals are deficient in methionine and pulse are deficient in lysine.
    (c) Cereals are deficient in lysine and pulses are deficient in methionine.
    (d) Cereal proteins contain non-essential amino-acids, while pulse proteins contain essential amino acids.

Ans. (c)

Note
The cereals are deficient in lysine and pulses are deficient in methionine. Cereal proteins are poor in nutritive quality, being deficient in essential amino acid, lysine. The proteins of maize are still poorer, being deficient in lysine and tryptophan a precursur of niacin. However, if cereals are eaten with pulses, which is a traditional Indian diet, cereal and pulse protein complement each other and provide a more balanced and complete protein intake.
Ref: Park and Park, 16th Ed Pg-419.

Q. 170. For a 60 kg Indian male, the minimum daily protein requirement has been calculated to be 40 g (mean) & standard deviation is 10. The recommended daily allowance of protein would be (AII INDIA-02)
    (a) 60 g/day
    (b) 70 g/day
    (c) 40 g/day
    (d) 50 g/day

Ans. (a)

Q. 171. A population study showed a mean glucose of 86 mg/dl. In a sample of 100 showing normal curve distribution, what percentage of people have glocose above 86%? (AII INDIA-02)
    (a) 65
    (b) 50
    (c) 75
    (d) 60

Ans. (b)

Note
The above population has 86 mg% as the mean, in a normal distribution (Bell-shaped) Curve, 50% of subject fall on the right and 50% fall on the left side of the mean. Therefore, the most suitable answer is (b).

Q. 172. The best method to show the association between height and weight of children in a class is by (AII INDIA-02)
    (a)   Bar chart
    (b)   Line diagram
    (c)   Scatter diagram
    (d)   Histogram

Ans. (c)

Note
Scatter or Dot diagram is prepared after cross tabulation in which frequencies of at-least 2 variables have been cross classified. One variable being independent and other variable being dependent.

Q. 173. In a study, variation in cholesterol was seen before and after giving a drug. The test of significance would be (AII INDIA-02)
    (a)   Unpaired T test
    (b)   Paired T test
    (c)   Chi square test
    (d)   Fisher test

Ans. (b)

Note
Paired T – test it is applied to paired data when each individual gives a pair of observation. For example as above; the serum lipid levels were tested both before and after administering a hypolipidemic drug. Therefore a paired T – test is suitable in this case.

Q. 174. All of the following are common causes of post neonatal infant mortality in India, except (AII INDIA-02)
    (a)   Tetanus
    (b)   Malnutrition
    (c)   Diarrheal diseases
    (d)   Acute respiratory infection

Ans. (a)

Note
Tetanus is a cause of neonatal mortality but not a cause of post neonatal mortality.
Causes of infant mortality:

Neonatal Mortality (0 – 4 Weeks)	Post Neonatal Mortality (1 – 12 Months)
a. Low birth weight	a. Diarrheal diseases
b. Birth injury and difficult labour	b. Acute respiratory infections
c. Congenital abnormalities	c. Other communicable diseases
d. Hemolytic diseases of newborn	d. Malnutrition
e. Conditions of placenta and cord	e. Congenital abnormalities
f. Diarrheal diseases	f. Accidents
g. Acute respiratory infections	
h. Tetanus	

Ref: Park and Park 16th Ed Pg-387

Q. 175. True about 'total fertility rate' is (AII INDIA-02)
    (a)   Sensitive indicator of family planning achievement
    (b)   Completed family size
    (c)   Number of live births per 1000 married women in reproductive age group
    (d)   Average number of girls born to a woman

Ans. (b)

Note
'Total fertility rate represents' the average number of children a woman would have if she were to pass through her reproductive years bearing children at the same rates as the women now in each age group (28). It is computed by summing the age – specific fertility rate for all ages; if 5 – year age groups are used, the some of the rates is multiplied by 5. This measure gives the approximate magnitude of 'completed family size'.
Ref: Park and Park 16th Ed Pg-326

Q. 176. 'Silent epidemic' of the century is (AII INDIA-02)
    (a)   Coronary artery disease
    (b)   Chronic liver disease
    (c)   Chronic obstructive lung disease
    (d)   Alzheimer's disease

Ans. (d)

Note
In recent years there has been a steady increase in mental disorders. Alzheimer's disease described as the 'silent epidemic' of the century, is an important cause of morbidity and mortality.
Park and Park 16th Ed Pg-37

Q. 177. Basanti a 29 years aged female from Bihar presents with active tuberculosis. She delivers baby. All of the following are indicated except (AII INDIA-01)
    (a)   Administer INH to the baby
    (b)   Withhold breast feeding
    (c)   Give ATT to mother for 2 years
    (d)   Ask mother to ensure proper disposal of sputum

Ans. (a)

Note
Neonatal tuberculosis: Whenever the placenta shows tuberculous lesions or the new borne infant is only positively reactive to tuberculin test, the neonate should receive only INH (15 mgm /Kg/day) for nine months. If there is associated demonstrable tuberculous disease RIF (10 mgm/Kg/day) should be added. If the mother is tuberculous and the placenta is normal the new borne infant should be carefully observed, chest X-ray and tuberculin test (Mantoux) done. Isolation from the mother as long as the mother's disease is not adequately controlled.
Mother can breast feed the baby by covering her mouth. Such baby needs BCG vaccination.
Ref: Principles of Pediatrics by Dr. Tirthankar Datta. 1st Ed P-129.

Q. 178. Under the national TB programme, for a PHC to be called a PHC-R, requisite is (AII INDIA-01)
    (a)   Microscopy
    (b)   Microscopy plus radiology
    (c)   Radiology
    (d)   None of the above

Ans. (b)

Under the National T.B. Control Programme, all the PHC have microscopy facility whereas the PHC's with additional radiology facility were called PHC-R.

Q. 179. A person has received complete immunization against tetanus 10 years ago, now he presents with a clean wound without any lacerations from an injury sustained 3 hours ago. He should now be given (AII INDIA-01)
    (a)   Full course of tetanus toxoid
    (b)   Single dose of tetanus toxoid
    (c)   Human tetanus globulin
    (d)   Human tetanus globulin and single dose of toxoid

Ans. (b)

Note
For prevention of tetanus following are the recommendations:

Immunization status	Wounds less than 6 hours old, clean, non-penetrating and with negligible tissue damage	Other type of wounds
a. Complete course of tetanus toxoid (TT) or a booster dose within the past five years.	Nothing required	Nothing required.
b. Complete course of TT or a booster dose more than 5 years ago but less than 10 years.	TT one dose	TT one dose.
c. Complete course of TT or a booster dose more than 10 years ago.	TT one dose	TT one dose + Human tetanus globulin.
d. Had not completed course of TT or immunization status known.	TT complete course	TT complete course + Human tetanus globulin.

Ref: Park and Park 16th Ed, P- 238

Q. 180. The false statement regarding tetanus is (AII INDIA-01)
(a) Five doses of immunization provide life long immunity.
(b) TT affords no protection in the present injury.
(c) TIG is useful in lacerated wound.
(d) TT and Ig both may be given in suspected tetanus.

Ans. (a)

Q. 181. A certain community has 100 children out of whom 28 are immunised against measles. 2 of them acquired measles simultaneously. Subsequently 14 get measles. Assuming the efficacy of the vaccine to be 100%. What is the secondary attack rate? (AII INDIA-01)
(a) 5%
(b) 10%
(c) 20%
(d) 21.5%

Ans. (c)
Note
Secondary Attack Rate (SAR) is defined as 'number of exposed persons developing the disease within the range of the incubation period following exposure to the primary case.

$$SAR = \frac{\text{The number of exposed persons developing the disease within the range of incubation period}}{\text{Total number of exposed or susceptible contantacts}} \times 100$$

$$SAR = \frac{14}{100-28-2} \cdot 100$$

$$SAR = \frac{14}{70} \cdot 100$$

Ref: Park and Park 16th Ed P-87

Q. 182. A community has a population of 10,000 and a birth rate of 36 per 1000. 5 maternal deaths were reported in the current year. The MMR is (AII INDIA 01)
  (a)   14.5
  (b)   13.8
  (c)   20
  (d)   5

Ans. (b)

Maternal mortality rate measures the risk of women dying from puerperal causes and is defined as:

$$MMR = \frac{\text{Total number of female deaths due to complications of pregnancy, child birth or within 24 days of delivery from puerperal causes in an area during a given year}}{\text{Total number of live birth in the same area and year}} \times 1000$$

$$MMR = \frac{\text{Total number of female death}}{\text{Total number of live births}} \times 1000$$

$$MMR = \frac{5}{36} \times 1000 = 13.8$$

Ref: Park and Park 16th Ed Pg -380

Q. 183. 10 babies are born in a hospital on same day. All weigh 2.8 kg each. Calculate the standard deviation (AII INDIA-01)
  (a)   Zero
  (b)   One
  (c)   Minus one
  (d)   0.28

Ans. (a)

Note
The standard deviation is the most frequently used measure of deviation. In simple terms it is defined as Root – means – Square – Deviation.

$$S.D. = \frac{\sqrt{\Sigma(X - \bar{X})^2}}{n-1}$$

Since all the ten babies weight the same = 2.8 Kg, therefore, the arithmatic mean is also 2.8 therefore $x - \bar{x} = 2.8 - 2.8 = 0$ also $\Sigma = 0$ and $\sqrt{0/9} = 0$ thus standard deviation = 0.
Ref: Park and Park 16th Ed P-594

Q. 184. Out of 11 births in a hospital, 5 babies weighed over 2.5 kg and 5 weighed less than 2.5 kg. What value does 2.5 represent (AII INDIA-01)
(a) Geometric average
(b) Arithmatic average
(c) Median
(d) Mode

Ans. (c)
Note
Ref: Park and Park 16th Ed P-593

Q. 185. A man weighing 68 kg, consumes 325 gm carbohydrate, 65 gm protein and 35 gms fat in his diet. The most applicable statement here is (AII INDIA 01)
(a) His total calorie intake is 3000 kcal.
(b) The proportion of proteins, fats and carbohydrates is correct and in accordance with a balanced diet.
(c) He has a negative nitrogen balance.
(d) 30% of his total energy intake is derived from fat.

Ans. (b)
Note
For balanced diet see Park and Park 16th Ed Pg-424.

Q. 186. A country has a population of 1000 million; birth rate is 23 and death rate is 6. In which phase of the demographic cycle does this country lie (AII INDIA-01)
(a) Early expanding
(b) Late expanding
(c) Plateau
(d) Declining

Ans. (b)
Note
The figures for the said country point to 'late expanding phase of demographic cycle'.
However demographic cycles are reviewed as under:
(a) Early Expanding Phase: The death rate begins to decline while the birth rate remains unchanged.
(b) Late Expanding Phase: The death rate declines still further and the birth rate tends to fall. The population continues to grow because birth exceeds deaths.
(c) Plateau Phase: It can be high stationary or low stationary.
   a. The high stationary phase: Is characterised by high birth rate and a high death rate which cancel each other and the population remains stationary.
   b. Low stationary phase: It is characterised by the low birth rate and low death rate with the result the population remains stationary.
   c. Declining phase: The population begins to decline because birth rate is lower than death rate.
Ref: Park and Park 17th Ed Pg 325

Q. 187. In a population of 10,000 beta carotene was given to 6000; it was not given to the remainder. 3 out of the first group got lung cancer while 2 out of the other 4000 also got lung cancer. The best conclusion is (AII INDIA-01. 02)
(a) Beta carotene and lung cancer have no relation to one another
(b) The p value is not significant
(c) The study is not designed properly
(d) Beta carotene is associated with lung cancer

Ans. (a)
Note
-Beta carotene was given to 6000 and 3 developed Ca lung; therefore Ca developed = 1/ 2000 persons.
-Beta carotene was not taken by 4000 and 2 developed Ca lung, therefore Ca developed 1/2000.
It indicates that there was no benefit of taking beta carotene to prevent the Ca. It confirmed the statement 'beta carotene and lung cancer have no relation to one another'.

MCQ's in Community Medicine 513

Q. 188. A subcentre in a hilly area caters to a population of (AII INDIA-01)
    (a)   1000
    (b)   2000
    (c)   3000
    (d)   5000

Ans. (c)
Note
The sub-centre is the peripheral outpost of existing health delivery system in rural areas. They are being established on the basis of one sub-centre for every 5000 polulation in general and one for every 3000 population in hilly, tribal and backward areas. As on 30th June 1996, 132730 sub-centres were established in the country.
Ref: Park and Park 16th Ed Pg-639

Q. 189. In a community, an increase in new cases denotes (AII INDIA-01)
    (a)   Increase in incidence rate
    (b)   Increase in prevalence rate
    (c)   Decrease in incidence rate
    (d)   Decrease in prevalence rate

Ans. (a)
Note
Incidence rate is defined as the number of new cases occurring in a defined population during a specified period of time.
Ref: Park and Park 17th Ed Pg -52

Q. 190. Virulence of a disease is indicated by (AII INDIA-01)
    (a)   Proportional mortality rate
    (b)   Specific mortality rate
    (c)   Case fatality ratio
    (d)   Amount of GDP spent on control of disease

Ans. (c)
Note
Case fatality rate represents the killing power of diseases. It is simply the ratio of death to cases. The case fatality is closely related to virulence.
Ref: Park and Park 17th Ed Pg -49

Q. 191. Which of the following diseases needs not to be screened for in workers to be employed in a dye industry in Gujarat? (AII INDIA-01)
    (a)   Anemia
    (b)   Bronchial asthma
    (c)   Bladder cancer
    (d)   Precancerous lesion

Ans. (a)
Note
In case of dye industry it is risky to employ men suffering from; Asthma, skin, bladder and kidney diseases, precancerous lesions.
Ref: Park and Park 17th Ed Pg -582

Q. 192. Best test to detect iron deficiency in community is (AII INDIA-01)
    (a)   Serum transferrin
    (b)   Serum ferritin
    (c)   Serum iron
    (d)   Hemoglobin

Ans. (b)
Note
The best test to detect iron deficiency in community is Serum ferritin.
Ref: Park and Park 17th Ed Pg -424, also see Park 16th Ed Pg-417.

Q. 193. Which of the following is not a complete sterilization agent (AII INDIA-01)
(a) Glutaraldehyde
(b) Absolute alcohol
(c) Hydrogen peroxide
(d) Sodium hypochlorite

Ans. (b)

Note
The sterilization means removal of both bacteria and spores. However, alcohol is not a sporicidal, therefore it is not a complete sterilizing agent.

Q. 194. Seasonal trend is due to (AII INDIA-01)
(a) Vector variation
(b) Environmental factors
(c) Change in herd immunity
(d) All of the above

Ans. (b)

Note
Environmental factors / Physical environment: It includes non-living things and physical factors e.g., air, water, soil, housing, climate, geography, heat, light, noise, debris, radiation etc.
Ref: Park and Park 17th Ed Pg -31

Q. 195. Immunity develops after how many days of administering Japanese Encephalitis vaccination?
(a) 7 days
(b) 15 days
(c) 30 days
(d) 60 days

Ans. (c)

Note
A killed 'mouse brain' vaccine is available for primary immunization against Japanese Encephalitis. Two doses of 1 ml each (.5 ml for children under the age 3 years) should be administered subcutaneously at an interval of 7 to 14 days. A booster injection of 1 mm should be given after a few months (before one year) in order to develop full protection. The protective immunity develops in about a months time after the second dose.
Ref: Park and Park 17th Ed Pg 219

Q. 196. Which of the following vaccines are not to be given to a patient with AIDS?
(a) BCG
(b) DPT
(c) OPV
(d) Measles.

Ans. (a)

Note
Since the risks and known consequences of natural infection with tubercular bacilli are likely to be more serious than the risk associated with live attenuated vaccines, the WHO has recommended that all asymptomatic HIV infected children should receive the BCG vaccine and those with symptoms of AIDS related complex (ARC) / AIDS should not be given BCG.
Ref: Park and Park 16th Ed Pg-150

Q. 197. Bitot's spots are caused due to the deficiency of (UPSC-06)
(a) Vitamin A
(b) Vitamin D
(c) Vitamin E
(d) Biotin

Ans. (a)

Note
The signs of vitamin A deficiency are predominantly occular. They include night blindness, conjunctival xerosis, Bitot's spots, corneal xerosis and Keratomalacia.
Ref: Park and Park 16th Ed Pg-409

Q. 198. Consider the following statements (UPSC-06)
1. Human body has an excellent capacity to store vitamin B12
2. Milk is a good source of vitamin B12

Which of the statements given above is/are correct?
(a) 1 Only
(b) 2 Only
(c) Both 1 and 2
(d) Neither 1 nor 2

Ans. (c)
Note
The human body has good capacity to store vitamin B12, and it is available in dairy products- since only one choice is there and most of the Indians who are vegetarians they cannot have the access to this vitamin. Vegetarian do take milk – therefore it prevents deficiency and one can safely conclude that milk is a good source of vitamin B12.

Q. 199. Markedly retarded growth, edema of legs, lethargy, dry brittle hair, with flag sign, distended abdomen are clinical features of (UPSC-06)
(a) Marasmus
(b) Kwashiorkor
(c) Cretinism
(d) Rickets

Ans. (b)
Note
Edema of legs, lethargy, dry brittle hair, with flag sign, distended abdomen are the classical symptoms of PCM are there but the flag sign and edema are more in tune with Kwashiorkor.
Description:
The flag sign for protein malnutrition sometimes involves alternating light and dark bands of color along individual hair fibers. Other symptoms that may be present are hair loss, and thin, papery dark skin.

Q. 200. Physical quality of life Index (PQLI) includes all except (AIPGME-00)
(a) Gross Domestic Products
(b) Literacy rate
(c) Infant mortality rate
(d) Life expectancy at age 1 year

Ans. (a)
Note
The PQLI has not included the GNP into consideration to show that money is not everything.
Ref: Park and Park 16th Ed, Pg- 15.

Q. 201. Primary prevention does not include (AIPGME-00)
(a) Early diagnosis and treatment
(b) Health promotion
(c) Specific protection
(d) Health education

Ans. (a)
Note
Primordial prevention:
 -It is prevention of emergence of primary risk factors
 -Main intervention is individual and mass education
Primary Prevention:
a. Heath promotion:

- Health Education
- Environment modification
- Nutritional interventions
- Life style and behaviour changes

b. Specific Protection
- Immunization
- Chemoprophylaxis

Secondary Prevention:
- It is early diagnosis and treatment

Tertiary Prevention:
- It is disability limitation and rehabilitation.

Ref: Park and Park.

Q. 202. Primordial prevention is done in population (AIPGME-00)
(a) With risk factors
(b) Without risk factors
(c) Whole population with low prevalence of disease
(d) Population with disease

Ans. (b)

Note

Primordial prevention:
- It is prevention of emergence of primary risk factors.
- Main intervention is individual and mass education.

Aim of Primordial Prevention is:
- It is aimed at preventing the emergence of risk factors.

Intervention is:
- It is to be started when risk factors have not yet appeared in the – person, group, population, and country.
- Main effort is to cultivate a lifestyle in children which reduces the development of risk factors for health problem in future.

Mechanism:
- It is achieved through individual and mass education.

Ref: Park and Park.

Q. 203. The Gap between Primary and Secondary case is (AIPGME-00)
(a) Serial interval
(b) Generation time
(c) Incubation period
(d) Secondary attack rate

Ans. (a)

Note

a. *Serial interval*
- The gap between the onset of primary and secondary case is known as Serial interval.

b. *Generation Time*
- It is defined as 'the interval in time between receipt of infection by the host and maximum infectivity of that host.

c. *Incubation period*
- It is the time interval between invasion by an infectious agent and appearance of first sign or symptoms of disease in question.

d. *Latent Period*
- It is equivalent to incubation period, but while 'incubation period' is used for infectious diseases, the latent period is used for non-infectious diseases.

e. *Secondary attack role*
- It is the number of exposed persons developing the disease within the range of incubation period and has nothing to do with the 'gap' as in the question.

MCQ's in Community Medicine

Q. 204. In culex mosquito the type biological transmission for Filaria parasite is (AIPGME-00)
(a) Cyclo-developmental
(b) Cyclo-propagative
(c) Propagative
(d) Cyclical

Ans. (a)
Note
a. Cyclo-deveplomental: Agent undergoes only development and no multiplication i.e., Microfilaria in mosquito and Guinea worm in Cyclops.
b. Cyclo- progapative: The agent multiplies and changes in form, i.e., Malaria in mosquito.
c. Propagative: Agent merely multiply but no change in form i.e., Plague, bacilli in rat flea and yellow fever in mosquito.
Ref: Park and Park 16th Ed Pg- 87

Q. 205. All are true regarding point source Epidemic except (AIPGME-00)
(a) All cases occur abruptly and simultaneously
(b) Children are most commonly affected
(c) Occurs within a specific time period
(d) No secondary waves

Ans. (b)
Note
Point source epidemic results from infections:
 -An affected person and not necessarily a child
 -Contaminants of environment i.e., air, water, food, soil.
Features of point source epidemic:
 -Epidemic wave rises and falls sharply with no secondary waves.
 -Epidemic are explosive, with clustering of cases, within narrow interval of time.
 -All cases develop within one incubation period of disease.
Ref: Park and Park 16th Ed Pg- 54

Q. 206. False regarding propagated epidemic is (AIPGME-00)
(a) No secondary waves
(b) Spread depends on herd immunity
(c) Person to person transmission occurs
(d) Slow rise

Ans. (a)
Note
It is to be noted that 'absence of secondary wave is a feature of 'point source epidemic'.
The propagated epidemic; it has propagation which takes place from person to person. The features of propagated epidemic include:
 -Gradual rise and tails off over a long time period.
 -Speed of spread depends on; herd immunity and opportunities of contact & secondary contact.

Q. 207. Prevalence of clinical cases of polio can be estimated by multiplying the number of residual paralytic cases by (AIPGME-00)
(a) 1.33
(b) 1.25
(c) 3.00
(d) 1.99

Ans. (a)
Note
A rough estimate of all clinical cases of poliomyelitis could be made by multiplying the prevalence rate of residual paralysis due to poliomyelitis by 1.33.
Ref: Park and Park 16th Ed Pg-152

Q. 208. Reverse Cold Chain is used for (AIPGME-00)
(a) Carrying stool samples of polio patients from PHC.
(b) Transporting outdated vaccines from PHC to district hospital.
(c) Transporting vaccines to lab. To check its potency.
(d) Transporting vaccine from camps to sub-centre.

Ans. (a)

Note
Reverse Cold Chain is used for transportation of viable poliovirus in stool to an investigation centre.
Ref: WHO field Guide, for nodal officers, engaged in Polio Eradication / Surveillance.

Q. 209. Commonest complication of mumps is (AIPGME-00)
(a) Orchitis & oophritis
(b) Encephalitis
(c) Pneumonia
(d) Myocarditis

Ans. (a)

Note
Ref: Harrison 15th Ed. Pg-1147.

Q. 210. Vector control for yellow fever around an airport is done upto a distance of (AIPGME-00)
(a) 400 m
(b) 200 m
(c) 500 m
(d) 100 m

Ans. (a)

Note
The Airport and Seaports have to be kept free from the breeding of insect vectors (Ades mosquito) for a distance of 400 meters.
Ref: Park and Park 16th Ed – Pg-214

Q. 211. The best measure of incidence of T.B. in a community is (AIPGME-00)
(a) Tuberculin conversion index
(b) Mantoux positivity
(c) Sputum positivity
(d) Prevalence of tuberculosis

Ans. (a)

Note
In developing countries, every one percent of annual risk of infection is said to correspond to 50 new cases of smear – positive pulmonary tuberculosis, per year for 100,000 general population. Also known as "tuberculin conversion" index", this parameter is considered one of the best indicators for evaluating the tuberculosis problem and it's trend.
Ref: Park and Park 16th Ed Pg-139

Q. 212. Tuberculin test denotes (AIPGME-00)
(a) Previous or present sensitivity to tubercular proteins.
(b) Patient is resistant to tuberculosis.
(c) Person is susceptible to tuberculosis.
(d) Protective immune status of individual against tuberculosis.

Ans. (a)

Note
The tuberculin test was discovered by 'Von Pirquet' in 1907. A positive reaction to the test is generally accepted as evidence of past or present infection by M. *tuberculosis*.
Ref: Park and Park 16th Ed Pg-141

MCQ's in Community Medicine

Q. 213. Regarding rabies, true is (AIPGME-00)
    (a) Incubation period depends on the site of bite.
    (b) Diagnosis is by eosinophilic intra-nuclear infection.
    (c) It is a DNA virus.
    (d) Caused only by dogs.

Ans. (a)
Note
Rabies virus is a RNA virus.
Rabies can be caused by bite of dogs, cats, fox, bats etc.
Inclusion bodies in rabies are the 'Negri Bodies' these are intra-cytolpasmic round pink structures with characteristic basophilic inner bodies.
Ref: Park and Park 16th Ed, Pg-206

Q. 214. Definition of blindness by WHO includes (AIPGME-00)
    (a) Visual acuity < 3/60
    (b) Visual acuity <6/60
    (c) Visual acuity < 4/60
    (d) Visual acuity < 5/60

Ans. (a)
Note
WHO defines blindness as:
a. Visual acuity less than 3/60
    Or
b. Inability to count fingers in at a distance of 3 meters
Other criteria are:
a. Visual acuity less than 1/60 or inability to count fingers in daylight at 1 meter distance
b. No light perception
Ref: Park and Park 16th Ed, Pg-298

Q. 215. Bhopal gas tragedy is an example of (AIPGME-99)
    (a) Point source epidemic
    (b) Propagated epidemic
    (c) Continuous epidemic
    (d) Modern epidemics

Ans. (a)
Note
The main features of 'Point Source Epidemic' are:
    -Epidemic tends to be explosive
    -All cases develop within same incubation period
    -Curve rises and falls rapidly
    -No secondary waves
The Bhopal gas tragedy fulfills the 'Point Source Epidemic' criteria:
    -It was single exposure to agent / Bhopal gas
    -All cases developed simultaneously within one incubation period
Other examples are:
    -Food poisoning
    -Minamala disease in Japan
Ref: Park & Park, 16th Ed, Pg- 56

Q. 216. Following is true for CHD in India, except (AIPGME-99)
    (a) CHD presents a decade later than in western countries.
    (b) Diabetes mellitus is the commonest cause.
    (c) More common in males than females.
    (d) Heavy smoking is an etiological factor.

Ans. (a)

Note
The Pattern of 'Coronary Artery Disease' in India is as under:
a. CHD appears a decade earlier compared with age incidence in developed nations.
b. Males are affected more than females.
c. Hypertension and diabetes account for about 40% of all cases.
d. Etiologically heavy smoking is associated with CHD.
Ref: Park & Park, 16th Ed, Pg- 270

Q. 217. Commonest cause of infant mortality rate in India is (AIPGME-99)
    (a) Prematurity
    (b) Diarrhea
    (c) Respiratory infection
    (d) Congenital malformation

Ans. (a)
Note
Low birth weight is the most common cause of infant mortality in India. However, prematurity is associated with other factors therefore, 'Prematurity' is the most suitable choice in reference to the other variables.
Ref: Park & park 16th Ed, Pg-376.

Q. 218. Extra calorie requirements for a lactating mother are (AIPGME-99)
    (a) 300 Kcal/day
    (b) 400 Kcal/day
    (c) 550 Kcal/day
    (d) 600 Kcal/day

Ans. (c)
Note
The extra calorie requirement during pregnancy is 300 Kcal/day.
The extra calorie requirement during First 6 month is 550 Kcal/day.
The extra calorie requirement during Next 6 month is 400 Kcal/day.
Ref: Park & Park 16th Ed, Pg-415

Q. 219. Which of the following trace elements cannot be completely supplemented by diet in pregnancy? (AIPGME-99)
    (a) Fe
    (b) Ca++
    (c) Zn
    (d) Manganese

Ans. (a)
Note
Diet at it's best can provide 18 – 20 mg of Iron. The amount of iron absorbed from intestines and mobilized from body store is inadequate to meet the demand of pregnancy – especially the second half of pregnancy (last 12 weeks). Therefore, Iron supplementation is crucial and very important during the second half of pregnancy.
Ref: Text book of Obstetrics by D.C. Dutta 4th Ed, Pg-56

Q. 220. Colostrum is rich in the following constituents as compared to breast milk
    (a) Minerals
    (b) Proteins
    (c) Fats
    (d) Carbohydrates

Ans. (b)
Note
Colosturm is very rich in proteins Vit-A, sodium and chloride, though it also contains carbohydrate, fat, and potassium.
Ref: Text book of Obstetrics by D.C. Dutta 4th Ed – Pg-56

Q. 221. The child survival and safe mother hood (CSSM) Programme includes all except
    (a)   Essential newborn care
    (b)   Acute respiratory disease control
    (c)   Nutrition supplementation
    (d)   Universal immunization

Ans. (c)

Note
The CSSM programme has the following components:
    a.   Early registration of pregnancy
    b.   To provide minimum three antenatal check-ups
    c.   Universal converge of all pregnant women with TT immunization
    d.   Advise on food, nutrition and rest
    e.   Detection of high risk pregnancy and prompt referral
    f.   Clean deliveries by trained personnel
    g.   Birth spacing, and
    h.   Promotion of institutional deliveries
Ref: Park and Park 16th Ed Pg 315

Bibliography

Books
1. Principles of Pediatrics by Dr. Tirthankar Datta. 1st Ed
2. Preventive and Social Medicine Park and Park 16th Ed
3. Preventive and Social Medicine 17th Ed By Park and Park
4. Text book of Obstetrics by D.C. Dutta 5th Ed

Websites
www.similima.com
www.fleshandbones.com

Chapter 9
SURGERY

Q. 1. In a suspected case of Prostatic enlargement, which one of the following procedure is likely to confirm the diagnosis? (UPSC-04)
    (a)   Urine examination
    (b)   Rectal examination
    (c)   Ultrasonography
    (d)   Measuring water intake and output of urine

Ans. (c)
Note
In a suspected case of Prostatic enlargement 'ultrasonography' is the most suitable procedure to confirm the diagnosis out of above.

Also see
Urine examination has no value in suspected case of BHP. Rectal examination is an important procedure to confirm the enlarged prostatic gland, however if the median lobe is only enlarged then it may not give us a fair idea. The ultrasonography (U/S) examination is a non-invasive and better technique that gives the comprehensive idea about prostatic enlargement in its different lobes, total volume and post residual urine in the bladder which guides us for a better treatment planning and further evaluation. Similarly input and output chart have no scientific validity for judging the prostatic enlargement.

However, Trans Rectal Ultrasonography (TRUS) remains the most accurate method of staging the local disease. It can be used in early detection of tumors in screening program. Local disease can be diagnosed with increased sensitivity by TRUS as compared to rectal examination.
Ref: Bailey and Love's Short Practice of Surgery, 24th Ed, Chapter 66, Page 1252

Q. 2. Sub-dural haemorrhage is commonly because of rupture of (K/MD/Ent-II/01)
    (a)   Anterior cerebral artery
    (b)   Middle cerebral artery
    (c)   Posterior cerebral artery
    (d)   Dural sinuses

Ans. (d)
Note
It can occur due to head injury and caused by rupture of dural sinus or small veins between the dura mater and arachnoid mater.

Also see
Significant subdural hemorrhage is caused by rupture of superior cerebral veins. The cerebral hemisphere moves along with the lower part of superior cerebral veins, whereas upper parts of these veins are fixed to the superior sagittal sinus into which they drain.
Ref: Textbook of surgery, S. Das. 3rd Ed. Pg-545

Q. 3. Which one of the following structure in the neck is most likely to be mistaken for a carcinomatous lymph node? (UPSC-04)
    (a)   Sternomastid tendon
    (b)   Laryngeal cartilage
    (c)   Thyroid Gland
    (d)   Greater cornu of the hyoid bone

Ans. (d)
Note
Anatomical consideration

The hyoid bone lies in the anterior midline of the neck between the chin and the thyroid cartilage. At rest it lays at the level of C_3. It has three parts: body, greater cornu and lesser cornu.
Ref: -B.D.Chaurasia's human anatomy, Vol 3, 3rd Ed, chapter 1, page 30

Also see
A carcinomatous lymph node is fixed and has a bony consistency. Therefore, the most probable mistake which could take place while palpating the lymph nodes in submandibular area and mistaking a firm mass which is in reality is greater cornu of the hyoid bone.

Ref: A Manual Of Clinical Surgery, by S. Das, 5th Ed, Chapter 8, Page 82, Chapter – 27, Pg-288

Q. 4. A patient with a history of peptic ulcer presented with sudden onset of severe pain in upper abdomen. Routine blood examination and straight X-Ray of abdomen showed (UPSC-04)
1. Marked tenderness over upper abdomen
2. Absence of bowel sounds
3. Leucocytosis
4. Gas shadow under the diaphragm

Code:
    (a)   1 & 2
    (b)   1 & 3
    (c)   4 Only
    (d)   2 & 3

Ans. (c)
Note
Patient with history of (H/O) peptic ulcer with severe pain in abdomen whether developed perforation is confirmed on radiological findings; gas shadow under the diaphragm.

Ref: A Concise Textbook of Surgery, S. Das, 3rd Ed, Chapter 44, Pg 842

Q. 5. Which of the following is diagnosed by employing angiography? (UPSC-04)
    (a)   Angina
    (b)   Blockage of coronary arteries
    (c)   Myocarditis
    (d)   Pericarditis

Ans. (b)
Note
From the above 'blockage of coronary arteries' is diagnosed by employing angiography.

Also see

The angina, myocarditis, and pericarditis cannot be diagnosed by coronary angiography; however it is the blockage of coronary artery which will show its position and extent of obstruction. The answer suggested is (b).

Ref: Davidson's Principles and Practice of Medicine, 19th Ed, Chapter 12, Pg 426

Q. 6. Healing of a skin wound by first intention results in (UPSC-04)
    (a)   A small amount of granulation tissue and scar
    (b)   An intense inflammatory response
    (c)   Contracture
    (d)   Keloid

Ans. (a)
Note
Healing of a skin wound by first intention results in 'A small amount of granulation tissue and scar'.
Also see
Healing by first intention occurs in wounds having following characteristics:
    -Clean and uninfected wounds
    -Surgically incised
    -Without much loss of cells and tissue

Healing by first intention leads to rapid healing with a small neat scar.
Healing by second intention it is characterized by:
- Extensive loss of tissue
- A large tissue defect, or infection

The wound has to be left open.

Ref: Textbook of Pathology by Harsh Mohan, 4th Ed, Chapter 5, Pg 154,155

Q. 7. Which one of the following statement is not correct? (UPSC-04)
(a) Thyroglossal cyst moves upwards with the protrusion of tongue.
(b) In a case of head injury, bleeding from nose occurs in fracture of the anterior fossa.
(c) Dislocation of spine without fracture can occur only in the dorsal spine.
(d) In the passive SLR test if pain appear below 40, it suggests impingement of PID on a nerve root.

Ans. (c)
Note
The Choice of (c) - a, b, and d are correct.
Also see
a. The thyroglossal cyst is a cystic swelling developed in the remnant of thyroid gland. It moves down with deglutition as it is attached to hyoid bone by fibrous tissue, it also moves up with protrusion of tongue.
Ref: A Concise Textbook of Surgery, S. Das, 3rd Ed, Chapter 36, page 624-627
b. Fracture of anterior cranial fossa may cause bleeding and discharge of CSF through the nose. It may also cause a condition called black eye.
Ref: B.D. Chaurasia's Human Anatomy, Vol 3, chapter 1, page 17
c. Dislocation of spine without fracture cannot take place in dorsal spine as it is a fixed spine.
d. SLR is done with the patient lying supine on the examining table and raising the leg by flexing the hip and keeping the knees extended. If pain is evoked under an angle of 40 degrees it indicates impingement of the protruding disc on a nerve root.

Ref: A Concise Textbook of Surgery, S. Das, 3rd Ed, Chapter 30, Pg 512

Q. 8. Which is not a feature of cataract? (KPSC/Lect/Physio-05)
(a) Black spots
(b) Polyopia
(c) Coloured hallow
(d) Conjunctival congestion

Ans. (d)
Note
The all three a, b, c are the features of cataract.
Also see
Development of opacity in the lens is known as cataract.
C/F (Clinical Features):
- Glare
- Uniocular polyopia
- Colored halo
- Black spots
- Image blurred and distortion of images
- Doubling and trebling of objects
- Loss of vision

Ref: Ophthalmology by A.K. Khurana, 3rd Ed, Chapter 9, Pg 231

Q. 9. Commonest tumour of nasopharynx is (KPSC/Lect/Physio-05)
(a) Fibroma
(b) Chondroma
(c) Papilloma
(d) Adenoma

Ans. (a)

Note
The commonest tumor of nasopharynx is angiofibroma and antro-choanal polypus. Angio-fibroma is a misnomer. Both the tumors are benign in nature.
Ref: Bailey and Love's Short Practice of Surgery, 24th Ed, Chapter- 43. Pg-677

Also see
It is a rare tumor though it is the commonest benign tumor of the nasopharynx. Also called as benign nasopharyngeal angiofibroma. It is predominantly seen in adolescent males in the second decade of life.
C/F:
- Profuse and recurrent epistaxis
- Progressive nasal obstruction and the nasal speech
- Conductive hearing loss
- Mass in the nasopharynx
- Broadening of the bridge of the nose, proptosis and swelling of the cheek

Ref: Diseases of Ear Nose & Throat by P.L. Dhingra, Ch 50, Pg 299,300

Q. 10. Renal calculi is seen in (KPSC/Lect/Physio-05)
(a) Hyperthyroidism
(b) Hyperparathyroidism
(c) Cushing's disease
(d) Addison's disease

Ans. (b)
Note
Renal calculi is seen in 'hyperparathyroidism'.

Also see
The hyper-parathyroidism causes high serum calcium levels which is thrown out by kidneys. Therefore the non-specific symptoms of hyperparthyroidsm are; polyurea, polydipsia, and muscle weakness and weight loss – which is great clue to the diagnosis for a physician. Most of the time these patients do present with one sided complaint of renal calculi, as high concentrated urine will cause precipitation and renal calculi are formed.

Ref: Bailey and Love's Short Practice of Surgery, 24th Ed, Chapter- 45. Pg-736
Extended information:
Predisposing factors for renal calculi are:
1. Environmental and dietary: (low urine output):
   - High temperature
   - Low fluid intake
   - Diet- high in protein, Na and low in Ca
   - High citrate and oxalate excretion
2. Other medical conditions:
   - Hypercalcemia (hyperparathyroidism, malignancy, multiple myeloma, addison's disease)
   - Renal tubular acidosis
   - Ileal disease
3. Congenital and inherited conditions:
   - Familial hypercalciuria
   - Medullary sponge kidney

Ref: Davidson's Principles and Practice of Medicine, 19th Ed, Chapter 14, 16, page 632,716

Q. 11. A three years old boy presents with poor urinary stream. Most likely cause is (AIIMS/May-03)
(a) Stricture urethra
(b) Neurogenic bladder
(c) Urethral calculus
(d) Posterior urethral valve

Ans. (d)
Note
A three years old boy presents with poor urinary stream. Most likely cause is 'Posterior urethral valve'.

Also see

The three year old boy having stricture in urethra is very remote unless it is due to some congenital local or due to some iatrogenic cause. The poor urinary stream is most likely due to posterior urethral valve which causes obstruction to the flow of urine.

Congenital valves of posterior urethra are symmetrical folds of urothelium, which can cause obstruction to the urethra of boys. They behave as flap valves. Although urine does not flow normally a urethral catheter can be passed without difficulty. Treatment involves. Transurethral resection of valves using a pediatric rectoscope.

Ref: Bailey and Love's Short Practice of Surgery, 24th Ed, Chapter- 67 Pg-1257

Q. 12. There is a high risk of renal dysplasia in (AIIMS/May-03)
    (a)   Posterior urethral valve
    (b)   Bladder exostrophy
    (c)   Anorectal malformation
    (d)   Neonatal sepsis

Ans. (a)
Note
As posterior utrethral valve is one of the causes of obstruction to the flow of urine and the choice given in (a) appears to be right.

Also see
The term renal cystic dysplasia is used for conditions where there is defective renal differentiation with persistence of structures in the kidney not represented in normal nephrogenesis. Renal dysplasia is thus diagnosed on histological basis.

The pathogenesis of renal dysplasia is unknown. However renal dysplasia is commonly associated with obstructive abnormalities of the ureter and lower urinary tract. It is often discovered in new borns. It is hypothesized that the condition results from intrauterine obstruction and disorganized metanephrogenic differentiation.

Ref: Text Book of Pathology By Harshmohan. Chapter 19 – Pg-641

Q. 13. Hypochloremia, hypokalemia and alkalosis are seen in (AIIMS/May-03)
    (a)   Congenital hypertrophic pyloric stenosis
    (b)   Hirschsprung's disease
    (c)   Esophageal atresia
    (d)   Jejunal atresia

Ans. (a)
Note
Hypochloremia, hypokalemia and alkalosis are seen in 'Congenital pyloric stenosis'.
Characteristically the first-born male child is affected at 4 weeks after birth. Presenting symptom is projectile vomiting. The vomitus has milk but no bile. The metabolic effects are similar to GOO. Due to vomiting of gastric acid there is hypochloraemic alkalosis but with time the patient becomes progressively hyponatraemic and potassium excretion starts leading to hypokalemia.

Ref: Bailey and Love's Short Practice of Surgery, 24th Ed, Chapter 52, Pg 917

Also see
In infants the congenital hypertrophic pyloric stenosis occurs approximately 3 per 1000 infants. Symptoms appear several weeks after birth. The clinical presentation is: Vomiting- forcible and projectile, weight loss diarrhea (loose green stools), leading to hypochloremia, hypokalaemia and alkalosis. Constipation. Visible peristalsis usually from left to right side. On Palpation; lump in upper abdomen better felt after an episode of vomiting.

Q. 14. Post-dural puncture headache is typically (AIIMS/May-03)
    (a)   A result of leakage of blood into the epidural space
    (b)   Worse when lying down than in sitting position
    (c)   Bifrontal or occipital
    (d)   Seen within 4 hours of dural puncture

Ans. (c)

Note
Post-dural puncture headache is typically 'Bifrontal or occipital'.

Also see

The authors claim that epidural blood patches (EBPs) seal the puncture by initiating an inflammatory response, whereas in fact it has been shown that they do so by blood moving from the epidural toward the subarachnoid space through the orifice until a clot is formed that would act as a 'plug'. A gradient has to be established, increasing the epidural pressure to higher levels so the fluid passes into the intrathecal space and tampons the orifice. However, in most of these punctures, the superficial layer of the arachnoid is also perforated; this is precisely the meningeal layer that may initiate an inflammatory process that may progress to radiculitis (transient nerve root irritation) demonstrated by 'enhancement', and edema and swelling of the nerve roots
Ref: http://bja.oxfordjournals.org/cgi/content/full/92/5/767

Also see
A postdural puncture headache (PDPH) or "spinal headache" is usually described as a severe, dull, non-throbbing pain, usually fronto-occipital, which is aggravated in the upright position and diminished in the supine position.

Ref: http://www.soap.org/media/newsletters/fall2000/pathophysiology_management.htm

Q. 15. A young patient presents with history of dysphagia more to liquid than solids. The first investigation you will do is (AIIMS/May-03)
    (a)   Barium swallow
    (b)   Esophagoscopy
    (c)   Ultrasound of the chest
    (d)   CT scan of the chest

Ans. (a)
Note
The first investigation to be done is 'Barium swallow'.
In a patient presenting with dysphagia more to liquids than solids, the first investigation to be carried out is Barium swallow, it will provide a broad insight into the uncoordinated peristalsis as well as fairly good assessment of any growth in the oesophagus.
Ref: Davidon's Principles and Practice of Medicine, 18th Ed, Chapter – 9- Pg – 612, Fig- 9.12

Also see
When the patient first presents with dysphagia to liquids and then to solids it probably points to a diagnosis of cardio-spasm.
Barium meal is by far the most important investigation in dysphagia, what ever the cause.
Causes of dysphagia:
In the mouth:
    -Tonsillitis, quinsy, CA tongue, paralysis of soft palate
In the pharynx:
    -Lumen-foreign body
    -Wall- acute pharyngitis, malignancy, hysterical
    -Outside the wall- enlarged cervical LN (Lymph Node), enlarged thyroid
In the oesophagus:
    -Lumen-foreign body
    -Wall- stricture, atresia, achalasia, neoplasm
    -Outside the wall- mediastinal tumors, goiter, aortic aneurysm

Ref: A Concise Textbook of Surgery, S. Das, 3rd Ed, Chapter 31, Pg 323-325

Q. 16. Which of the following is not true of gas gangrene (AIIMS/May-03)
    (a)   It is caused by Clostridium perfringens.
    (b)   Clostridium perfringens is a gram-negative spore-bearing bacillus.
    (c)   Gas gangrene is characterized by severe local pain, crepitus and signs of toxemia.
    (d)   High dose penicillin and aggressive debridement of affected tissue is the treatment of established infection.

Ans. (b)

Note
From the above 'Clostridium perfringens is a gram-negative spore bearing bacillus' is not true of gas gangrene.

Also see
Gas gangrene is caused by clostridium perfringes, which is a gram positive sporulating bacillus found in nature, particularly in soil and faeces. The α toxin produced by the bacillus is important in its pathogenesis.
C/F:
-A brown foul smelling discharge escapes from the wound. Crepitus can be detected.
Ref: Bailey and Love's Short Practice of Surgery, 24th Ed, Chapter 8, Pg 91, 100, 101

Q. 17. In a blast injury, which of the following organ is least vulnerable to the blast wave? (AIIMS/May-03)
    (a)   GI tract
    (b)   Lungs
    (c)   Liver
    (d)   Ear drum

Ans. (c)
Note
In a blast injury, out of above 'liver' is least vulnerable to the blast wave.

Also see
When the body is impacted by a blast pressure wave, it sets up a series of stress events by entering the body, which is capable of injury particularly at the air fluid levels. Thus injury to the lungs, ear and to a lesser extent the GIT is notable.
The structures injured by the primary blast waves in order of prevalence, are the middle ear, the lungs and the bowels.
Ref: Bailey and Love's Short Practice of Surgery, 24th Ed, Chapter 18, Pg 288. 23rd Edition

Q. 18. Which of the following is not a contraindication for extra corporeal shockwave lithotripsy (ESWL) for renal calculi? (AIIMS/May-03)
    (a)   Uncorrected bleeding diathesis
    (b)   Pregnancy
    (c)   Ureteric stricture
    (d)   Stone in a calyceal diverticulum

Ans. (d)
Note
Out of the above 'Stone in a calyceal diverticulum' is not a contraindication for extra corporeal shockwave lithotripsy for renal calculi.

Also see
Stones in the renal pelvis and calyces are ideal for ESWL.
Patient selection-
Exceptions for ESWL:
-Pregnant women, abdominal aortic aneurysm, uncorrectable coagulation disorders.
Relative contraindications:
-Cystine and matrix stones, any distal obstruction in the urinary tract.
Ref: A Concise Textbook of Surgery, S. Das, 3rd Ed, Chapter 57 Pg 1175-1176

Q. 19. Which of the following is not an appropriate investigation for anterior urethral stricture? (AIIMS/May-03)
    (a)   Magnetic resonance imaging
    (b)   Retrograde urethrogram
    (c)   Micturating cysto-urethrogram
    (d)   High frequency ultrasound

Ans. (a)

Note
Out of the above 'Magnetic resonance imaging' is not an appropriate investigation for anterior urethral stricture'.
Urethrogram and voiding cystourethrogram will reveal the site, length of stricture or presence of diverticulum proximal to the stricture.
Excretory urograms may reveal urinary calculi.
Urethroscopy confirms diagnosis.
Ref: A Concise Textbook of Surgery, S. Das, 3rd Ed, Chapter 59, Pg 1263

Q. 20. The recommended treatment for preputial adhesions producing ballooning of prepuce during micturition in a 2-year-old boy is (AIIMS/May-03)
    (a)   Wait and watch policy
    (b)   Circumcision
    (c)   Dorsal slit
    (d)   Preputial adhesions release and dilatation

Ans. (b)
Note
The recommended treatment for preputial adhesions producing ballooning of prepuce during micturition in a 2-year-old boy is 'circumcision'.
Also see

The condition in which the orifice of the prepuce is too small to permit its normal retraction over the glans penis is called as phimosis. In children upto 3 yrs the prepuce may be normally adherent to the glans so that retraction is difficult.
C/F: (Clinical Features)
When the child micturates the prepuce balloons out and the urine comes out in a thin stream.
Indications of circumcision:
In infants and young boys: Circumcision is done apart from religious reasons for true phimosis with recurrent attacks of balanitis.
In adults: splitting of an abnormally tight frenulum, balanitis and penile carcinoma.
Ref: A Concise Textbook of Surgery, S. Das, 3rd Ed, Chapter 61 Pg 1300, 1301

Q. 21. Cells from the neural crest are involved in all except (AIIMS/May-03)
    (a)   Hirschsprung's disease
    (b)   Neuroblastoma
    (c)   Primitive neuroectodermal tumour
    (d)   Wilm's tumour

Ans. (d)
Note
Cells from the neural crest are involved in all of above except 'Wilm's tumor'.
Also see
a.   Hirschsprung's disease (Congenital megacolon): An obstruction of the large intestine caused by inadequate motility (Muscular movement of the bowel) that occurs as a congenital condition. This occurs due to absence of ganglionic cells in the neural plexus of intestinal wall. It results from failure of migration of neuroblasts into the gut from the vagal nerve trunks at the end of 1st trimester.
Ref: Bailey and Love's Short Practice of Surgery, 24th Ed, Chapter57, Page 1027
b.   Neuroblastoma:
A malignant tumor that develops from embryonic neural crest origin. The tumor appears in infancy or childhood.
Ref: Textbook of Pathology by Harsh Mohan, 4th Ed, Chapter 15 Pg 489
c.   Primitive neuroectodermal tumor:
May occur at any age many appear before 35 years of age.
    -Microscopically, the tumors resemble neuroblastomas.
    -They are composed of sheets of small round cells that resemble lymphocytes.
    -The cytoplasm is indistinct.
    -Mostly present as a mass attached to a nerve.

- As a result of attachment to nerve, neurological symptoms are often a presenting feature.
- The tumors are highly aggressive, and rapidly give rise to metastasis and death.
- Survival at 3 years has been reported at 50% or less.

Ref: http://pathweb.uchc.edu/eatlas/Bone/76.HTM

Wilm's tumor:
d. A cancerous tumor of the kidney that occurs in children. It is an embryonic tumor derived from primitive renal epithelial and mesenchymal components.

Ref: Textbook of Pathology by Harsh Mohan, 4th Ed, Chapter 19 Pg 683

Q. 22. A Warthin's tumour is (AIIMS/May-03, Nov-04)
- (a) An adenolymphoma of parotid gland
- (b) A pleomorphic adenoma of the parotid
- (c) A carcinoma of the parotid
- (d) A carcinoma of submandibular salivary gland

Ans. (a)

Note
A Warthin's tumour is 'An adenoma of parotid gland'.

Also see
A Warthin's tumour (Synonym; Adenolymphoma); is a benign tumor of the parotid gland seen more commonly in men from 4th to 7th decades of life.

Q. 23. Regarding testicular tumour, the following are false except (AIIMS/May-03/ Nov-04)
- (a) They are commonest malignancy in older man.
- (b) Seminomas are radiosensitive.
- (c) Only 25% of stage 1 teratomas are cured by surgery alone.
- (d) Chemotherapy rarely produces a cure in those with metastatic disease.

Ans. (b)

Note
Regarding testicular tumour, all of above are false except that 'saminomas are radiosensitive'.

Also see
Testicular tumors comprise 1-2% of malignant tumors in men. Depending on the cellular type they are classified into:
- Seminoma
- Teratoma
- Combination of 1 and 2
- Interstitial tumors
- Lymphoma and
- Other tumors

Seminomas are extremely radiosensitive and excellent results have been obtained by radiotherapy in stage 1 and 2.
Teratomas are less sensitive to radiotherapy.
Stage 1 teratomas are simply watched by monitoring the level of tumor markers and repeated tomography.
Teratomas of stage 2 to 4 are managed by chemotherapy.
Survival rate of stage 1 tumor for a period of 5 years is >85%

Ref: Bailey and Love's Short Practice of Surgery, 24th Ed, Chapter 68 Pg 1278-1280

Q. 24. Upper GI endoscopy and biopsy from lower esophagus in a 48 year old lady with chronic heart burn shows presence of columnar epithelium with goblet cells. The feature is most likely consistent with (AIIMS/May-03)
- (a) Dysplasia
- (b) Hyperplasia
- (c) Carcinoma in-situ
- (d) Metaplasia

Ans. (d)

Note
The above features are consistent with 'Metaplasia'.

Also see
Following reflux esophagitis the stratified squamous epithelium of the lower esophagus is replaced by columnar epithelium.
On microscopic examination we see that metaplastic columnar cells replace the squamous epithelium.
Ref: Textbook of Pathology by Harsh Mohan, 4th Ed, Chapter 17 Pg 515
Dysplasia; is disordered epithelial cells often associated with hyperplasia and metaplasia.
Ref: Textbook of Pathology by Harsh Mohan, 4th Ed, Chapter 2 Pg 43-45
Hyperplasia; It is the increase in the number of parenchymal cells resulting in enlargement of the organ.
Metaplasia; it is a reversible change of 1 type of epithelium or mesenchymal epithelial cells to another type of adult cells, usually in response to an abnormal stimulus.

Q. 25. Which of the following is not an oncological emergency (AIIMS/May-03)
- (a) Spinal cord compression
- (b) Superior vena caval syndrome
- (c) Tumor lysis syndrome
- (d) Carcinoma cervix stage III B with pyometra

Ans. (d)

Note
Out of the above 'Carcinoma cervix stage III B with Pyometra' is not an oncological emergency.

Also see
Following is the list of oncological emergencies:
a. Spinal Cord Compression (SCC): The prevalence of SCC is as high as 30% of patients with disseminated cancer that have spinal cord compression; however, only 5% experience cord dysfunction. The vast majority of lesions are metastatic. The most common causes are metastasis from various cancers, including lung, breast, prostate, multiple myeloma, and colon.
b. Superior Vena Cava Syndrome: The prevalence of Superior Vena Cava Syndrome (SVCS) is rare, occurring in approximately 5% of small cell lung cancer patients. Bronchiogenic carcinomas and lymphomas are the most common causes.
c. Tumor Lysis Syndrome: (TLS) has prevalence as high as 40% in high-grade non-Hodgkin's Lymphoma (6% of these are clinically significant). The TLS occurs in patients with myeloproliferative disorders such as leukemia and lymphoma, which require chemotherapy that causes lysis of a massive number of cells in a short period of time.
d. Syndrome Of Inappropriate Antidiuretic Hormone: Syndrome of (SIADH) is uncommon but occurs in 1% to 2% of cancer patients, most often with Small Cell Lung Cancer and occasionally caused by chemotherapy medications such as vincristine and cyclophosphamide.
e. Disseminate Intravascular Coagulation
f. Hypercalcemia
g. Thrombocytopenia
Ref: http://www.redorbit.com/news/display?id=145141&source=r_health

Q. 26. The intra-abdominal pressure during laparoscopy should be set between (AIIMS /Nov-03)
- (a) 5-8 mm of Hg
- (b) 10-15 mm of Hg
- (c) 20-25 mm of Hg
- (d) 30-35 mm of Hg

Ans. (b)

Note
The intra-abdominal pressure should be set between 10-15 mm of Hg.

Also see
To obtain exposure during laparoscopy the peritoneal cavity is insufflated with gas, usually carbon dioxide. Surgeons may either do this through a spring-loaded needle called a Veress needle, or by making a small

incision down to the peritoneum and directly placing the insufflating needle or catheter. Generally insufflation pressures greater than 20 mm Hg are not used because of the potential for cardiovascular compromise.
Ref:-http://www.rashaduniversity.com/lasu.html

Q. 27. On mammogram all of the following are the features of a malignant tumour except (AIIMS /Nov-03)
    (a)   Spiculation
    (b)   Microcalcification
    (c)   Macrocalcification
    (d)   Irregular mass

Ans. (c)
Note
On mammogram all of the above are the features of a malignant tumor except 'Macrocalfication'.
Also see
Mammography is an X-ray examination of the breast.
    a. It is especially useful as screening procedure.
    b. It is useful in obese women with large breasts where palpation is difficult.
    c. For examination of opposite breast in women who have been treated for CA in 1 breast.
    d. Swelling of breast where clinical diagnosis is not very certain.
Benign breast lesions:
These are well circumscribed and homogenous and often surrounded by a zone of fatty tissue. Calcium deposition if present is coarse and situated at the periphery of lesion.
In case of carcinoma:
The margins are poorly defined, edges are speculated or irregular. Finely stippled calcification in the soft tissues and peri-ductal region is very suggestive. Malignant lesions reveal themselves as localized fine or punctate calcification and small areas of increased stromal density and architectural distortion.
Ref: - A Concise Textbook of Surgery, S. Das, 3rd Ed, Chapter 39, Pg 719
Ref: -A Manual of Clinical Surgery, S. Das, Chapter 30, Pg 318

Q. 28. A 55 year old post menopausal woman, on hormone replacement therapy (HRT), presents with heaviness in both breasts. A screening mammogram reveals a high density spiculated mass with cluster of pleomorphic microcalcification and ipsilateral large axillary lymph nodes. The mass described here most likely represents (AIIMS /Nov-03)
    (a)   Cystosarcoma phylloides
    (b)   Lymphoma
    (c)   Fibroadenoma
    (d)   Carcinoma

Ans. (d)
Note
The mass described here most likely represents; Carcinoma.
Also see
Risk factors for breast cancer:
    -Age: Incidence increases with age.
    -Genetic factors: Family history of breast cancer has often showed an increased incidence in some families.
    -Child bearing and fertility: Single and nulliparous women have a higher risk Oral Contraceptive Pills and Hormone Replacement Therapy, if taken for long periods can increase the risk of Ca.
Diet: high fat diet.
Clinical Features: A painless lump is the presenting feature.
It is asymptomatic but if large it can cause discomfort.
Axillary lymph nodes may be palpable.
Ref: A Concise Textbook of Surgery, S. Das, 3rd Ed, Chapter 39, Pg 711-715

Q. 29. During repair of indirect inguinal hernia, while releasing the constriction at the deep inguinal ring, the surgeon takes care not to damage one of the following structures (AIIMS /Nov-03)
    (a)   Falx inguinalis (conjoint tendon)

(b) Interfoveolar ligament
(c) Inferior epigastric artery
(d) Spermatic cord

Ans. (c)

Note
Surgeon while repair of indirect inguinal hernia, takes care not to damage 'inferior epigastric artery'.

Also see
The inferior epigastric artery arises from the external iliac artery near its lower end and passes medial to the deep inguinal ring and enters the rectus sheath by passing in front of the arcuate line.
Thus during the process of herniography, while suturing, the inferior epigastric artery may get damaged.
Ref: A Concise Textbook of Surgery, S. Das, 3rd Ed, Chapter 56, Pg 1104
Ref: B.D.Chaurasia's Human Anatomy, 3rd Ed, Vol 2, Chapter 16, Pg 174

Q. 30. During bilateral adrenalectomy for Cushing's disease, intraoperative dose of hydrocortisone should be given after (AIIMS /Nov-03/Nov-04)
(a) On opening the abdomen
(b) Ligation of left adrenal vein
(c) Ligation of right adrenal vein
(d) Excision of both adrenal glands

Ans. (d)

Note
During bilateral adrenalectomy for Cushing's disease, intraoperative dose of hydrocortisone should be given after 'excision of both adrenal glands'.

Also see
-When bilateral adrenalectomy is considered corticosteroids should be administered pre- operatively 48 and 24 hours prior to the surgery. During surgery, at the time of removal of adrenal glands and an additional same dose at 8 and 16 hours post-operatively should be given.
Ref: A Concise Textbook of Surgery, S. Das, 3rd Ed, Chapter 38, Pg 688

Q. 31. Recurrent laryngeal nerve is in close association with (AIIMS /Nov-03)
(a) Superior thyroid artery
(b) Inferior thyroid artery
(c) Middle thyroid vein
(d) Superior thyroid vein

Ans. (b)

Note
Recurrent laryngeal nerve is in close association with 'inferior thyroid artery'.

Also see
The right recurrent laryngeal nerve arises from the vagus in front of right subclavian artery, winds backwards below the artery and then runs upwards and medially behind the subclavian and common carotid artery to reach the tracheo oesophageal groove. In upper part of the groove it is related to the inferior thyroid artery.
Ref: B.D.Chaurasia's Human Anatomy, Vol 3, Chapter 13, Pg 153

Q. 32. The treatment of choice for symptomatic, retained common bile duct stones, is (AIIMS /Nov-03)
(a) Immediate surgery
(b) Conservative treatment with antibiotics
(c) Endoscopic sphincterotomy
(d) Medical dissolution of the stones

Ans. (c)

Note
Choice for symptomatic, retained common bile duct stone is 'endoscopic sphincteroctomy'.

Also see
If after cholecystectomy a stone is present in the bile duct then it should be removed immediately by endoscopy.
Ref: A Concise Textbook of Surgery, S. Das, 3rd Ed, Chapter 46, Pg 912
Also see
Procedures used for Common Bile Duct stones are:
Choledochoscopy can be performed using either open or laparoscopic techniques. Small, flexible choledochoscopes are introduced through an open CBD or cystic duct. This enables direct visualization and extraction of CBD stones. Sensitivity for detection approaches 100% in expert hands. Choledochoscopy can be performed postoperatively through the tract of a T-tube 6 weeks after the T-tube was placed.
Endoscopic sphincterotomy: This procedure can be performed preoperatively or postoperatively for CBD stones. Usually, stones smaller than 1 cm pass spontaneously within a few days of the sphincterotomy. For extraction of larger stones, a basket or a balloon catheter is required. Endoscopic sphincterotomy is contraindicated in patients with coagulopathy and usually in patients with a long distal CBD.
Ref:- http://www.emedicine.com/med/topic350.htm

Q. 33. A 50 year old smoker male presents with pain along the left arm and ptosis. His chest radiograph shows soft tissue opacity at the left lung apex with destruction of adjacent ribs. The picture is suggestive of (AIIMS /Nov-03)
    (a)   Adenocarcinoma lung
    (b)   Bronchial carcinoid
    (c)   Pancoast tumour
    (d)   Bronchoalveolar carcinoma

Ans. (c)
Note
The above clinical features are in favour of 'Pancoast tumour'.
Also see
Bronchial carcinoma in the apex of the lungs may cause Horner's syndrome (ipsilateral partial ptosis, enophthalmos, a small pupil and ipsilateral anhydrosis) due to involvement of sympathetic chain.
Pancoast's syndrome: It is characterized by pain in shoulder and along the inner aspect of the arm caused by involvement of the lower part of the brachial plexus.
Ref: Davidson's Principles and Practice of Medicine, 19th Ed, Chapter 13, Pg 545

Q. 34. Breast conservation surgery for breast cancer is indicated in one of the following conditions (AIIMS /Nov-03)
    (a)   T1 breast tumor
    (b)   Multicentric tumor
    (c)   Extensive in situ cancer
    (d)   T4b breast tumor

Ans. (a)
Note
Breast conservation surgery for breast cancer is indicated in T1 breast tumor.
Also see
In conservative surgery of breast the tumor is removed and the breast is preserved.
Patients suitable for conservative surgery are:
    -A single clinical mammographic lesion measuring 4cm or less without signs of local involvement (T1, T2, <4cm) with no extensive nodal involvement (N1, N0) or metastasis (M0).
    -No age limit is there and elderly and fit patients are treated in the same way as younger patients
Contraindications:
    -Tumors >4cm in size
    -Distant metastasis, extensive nodal involvement
    -Fixity of the tumor to the underlying muscles
    -Multicentricity
    -Multifocality
    -Poor differentiation
Ref: A Concise Textbook of Surgery, S. Das, 3rd Ed, Chapter 39, Pg 723

MCQ's in Surgery

Q. 35. A 65 year old male was diagnosed with prostate cancer three years back and was treated by surgery and hormone therapy. Presently he has developed urinary symptoms and progressive backache. What is the tumor marker, which can be indicative of disease relapse? (AIIMS /Nov-03)
(a) CA 125
(b) Beta-HCG
(c) Carcinoembryonic antigen (CEA)
(d) PSA

Ans. (d)

Note
The tumor marker is PSA.

Also see
Prostate specific antigen or PSA is the most important tumor marker available for prostatic CA. If PSA titre is >10 nmol/ml, it is suggestive of prostatic CA. If >35nmol/ml it is a case of advanced prostatic cancer. A decrease in the level of PSA is a good prognostic sign.
Ref: A Concise Textbook of Surgery, S. Das, 3rd Ed, Chapter 59, Pg 1251
-CA 125 is elevated in ovarian tumors.
-CEA or carcino embryogenic Ag is elevated in CA bowel, pancreas and breast.
-HCG is elevated in trophoblastic tumors, non-seminomatous germ cell tumors.
Ref: Textbook of Pathology by Harsh Mohan, 4th Ed, chapter 7, Pg 214

Q. 36. Which of the following malignant disease of children has the best prognosis? (AIIMS /Nov-03)
(a) Wilm's tumor
(b) Neuroblastoma
(c) Rhabdomyosarcoma
(d) Primitive neuroectodermal tumor

Ans. (a)

Note
Childen have best prognosis in 'Wilm's Tumor'.

Also see
a. *Nephroblastoma or wilm's tumor*
It is an embryonic tumor derived from primitive renal epithelium and mesenchymal components. It is the most common abdominal malignancy of young children.
Prognosis: With a combination of nephrectomy and post-operative irradiation the prognosis has improved considerably, and the survival rate is more than 75%.
Ref: Textbook of Pathology by Harsh Mohan, 4th Ed, chapter 19, Pg 683

b. *Neuroblastoma*
It is confined to children and occurs during the first 2 years of life. It consists of masses of undifferentiated small round cells, which are known as neuroblasts.
Blood borne metastasis is quite common to bones, liver, skull or brain.
Abdominal mass is the most common presenting symptom.
Investigations are done for urinary excretion of catecholamines and elevated levels of VMA.
Treatment: -total excision of the gland.
Prognosis is hopeless however in a few cases benign changes may be seen.
Ref: A Concise Textbook of Surgery, S. Das, 3rd Ed, Chapter 38, Pg 681

c. *Rhabdomyosarcoma*
It is the commonest soft tissue sarcoma in children and is a highly malignant tumor arising out of rhabdomyoblasts.
Ref: Textbook of pathology by Harsh Mohan, 4th Ed, chapter 26, Pg 847

d. *Primitive neuro ectodermal tumor*
May occur at any age many appear before 35 years of age.
-They are composed of sheets of small round cells that resemble lymphocytes.
-The cytoplasm is indistinct.
-Mostly present as a mass attached to a nerve.
-As a result of attachment to nerve, neurological symptoms are often a presenting feature.

- The tumors are highly aggressive, and rapidly give rise to metastasis and death.
- Survival at 3 years has been reported at 50% or less.

Ref:-http://pathweb.uchc.edu/eatlas/Bone/76.HTM

Q. 37. A three year old male child presents with history of constipation and abdominal distension for the last two years. The plain radiograph of abdomen reveals fecal matter containing distended bowel loops. A barium enema study done subsequently shows a transition zone at the recto-sigmoid junction with reversal of recto-sigmoid ratio. The most probable diagnosis is (AIIMS /Nov-03)
- (a) Anal atresia
- (b) Malrotation of the gut
- (c) Hirschsprung's disease
- (d) Congenital megacolon

Ans. (c)

Note

The most probable diagnosis is 'Hirschsprung's disease'.

Also see

Hirschsprung's disease occurs due to absence of ganglionic cells in the neural plexus of intestinal wall. It results from failure of migration of neuroblasts into the gut from the vagal nerve trunks at the end of 1st trimester. In about 2/3rds of cases the bowel proximal to the aganglionic segment becomes gradually dilated and hypertrophied for a variable length as the peristaltic waves try to propel the stools through the obstructing aganglionic segment. There is a visible transition zone, 1-5 cm in length, between the dilated bowel and the normal sized aganglionic segment of bowel on the distal side.

The clinical picture varies from acute intestinal obstruction in children to chronic constipation in later life
X-ray shows distended loops of bowel

Ref: Bailey Bailey and Love's Short Practice of Surgery, 24th Ed, Chapter 57, Pg 1027
Ref: A Concise Textbook of Surgery, S. Das, 3rd Ed, Chapter 53, Pg 1013

Q. 38. Investigation of choice to diagnose Hirschsprung's disease is (AIIMS /Nov-03)
- (a) Rectal manometry
- (b) Barium enema
- (c) Rectal biopsy
- (d) Laparotomy

Ans. (c)

Note

Rectal biopsy for diagnosing Hirschsprung's disease will demonstrate absence of ganglionic cells in the intramural and submucous plexus. Biopsy should be taken at least 2cm above the dentate line.
Ref: A Concise Textbook of Surgery, S. Das, 3rd Ed, Chapter 53, Pg 1014

Q. 39. The tendency of colonic carcinoma to metastasize is best assessed by (AIIMS /Nov-03)
- (a) Size of tumor
- (b) Carcinoembryonic antigen (CEA) levels
- (c) Depth of penetration of bowel wall
- (d) Proportion of bowel circumference involved

Ans. (b)

Note

The tendency of colonic carcinoma to metastasize is best assessed by 'Carcinoembryonic antigen levels'.

Also see

Colorectal carcinoma comprises 98% of all malignant tumors of the large intestine. In the diagnosis of colorectal Ca apart from proctoscopy, Ba enema, CT scan, the role of tumor markers has been emphasized especially CEA, which is elevated in all cases of metastatic CA, while it is positive in 20-30 % of early lesions and 60-70% of advanced primary lesions. However these are only prognostic markers as they are also elevated in a number of other conditions such as of pancreas, ovaries, urinary bladder, lungs and breast.
Ref: Textbook of Pathology by Harsh Mohan, 4th Ed, Chapter 17, Pg 565

MCQ's in Surgery   537

Q. 40. A 40 year old patient has undergone an open cholecystectomy. The procedure was reported as uneventful by the operating surgeon. She has 100 ml of bile output from the drain kept in the gallbladder bed on the first post operative day. On examination she is afebrile and anicteric. The abdomen is soft and bowel sounds are normally heard. As an attending physician, what should be your best possible advice? (AIIMS /Nov-03)
  (a) Order an urgent endoscopic retrograde cholangiography and biliary stenting
  (b) Urgent laparotomy
  (c) Order an urgent hepatic iminodiacetic acid scintigraphy (HIDA)
  (d) Clinical observation

Ans. (d)
Note
The best advice in above situation is keeping the patient under 'Clincial observation'.

Also see
Drainage is must after cholecystectomy as there may be leakage of bile from some unknown duct, which may lead to Waltman-Walter's syndrome. This syndrome is manifested by chest pain or an upper abdominal pain, tachycardia and low B.P.
The drain is removed after 48 hrs. It may be kept for a longer period if the discharge continues.
Indications for exploration of CBD (Common Bile Dutt) are:
  -Intermittent jaundice or biliary colic.
  -When bile duct is dilated or thickened.
  -When on aspiration the bile appears white.
However since the patient has no such problems he should be kept under observation.
Ref: A Concise Textbook of Surgery, S. Das, 3rd Ed, Chapter 46, Pg 908

Q. 41. The following are true about hepatocellular carcinoma except (AIIMS /Nov-03)
  (a) It has a high incidence in East Africa and South-east Asia.
  (b) Its worldwide incidence parallels the prevalence of hepatitis B.
  (c) Over 80% of tumours are surgically resectable.
  (d) Liver transplantation offers the only chance of cure in those with irresectable disease.

Ans. (c)
Note
All of the above are true for hepatocellular carcinoma except that 'over 80% of tumors are surgically resectable'.

Also see
Hepatocellular carcinoma is the commonest primary malignancy of liver. It shows marked geographic variations in incidence, which is closely related to HBV infection. HCCA (Hepato Cellular Carcinoma) is the leading malignant tumor in SE Asia.
Peak incidence occurs in the 5th and 6th decade.
Treatment involves liver transplantation and surgical resection of the tumor.
Ref: Textbook of Pathology by Harsh Mohan, 4th Ed, Chapter 18, Pg 616-618
Ref: Bailey and Love's Short Practice of Surgery, 24th Ed, Chapter 52, Pg 950

Q. 42. A 50 year old woman presented with history of recurrent episodes of right upper abdominal pain for the last one year. She presented to casualty with history of jaundice and fever for 4 days. On examination, the patient appeared toxic and had a blood pressure of 90/60 mm Hg. She was started on intravenous antibiotics. Ultrasound of the abdomen showed presence of stones in the common bile duct. What would be the best treatment option for her? (AIIMS /Nov-03)
  (a) ERCP and bile duct stone extraction
  (b) Laparoscopic cholecystectomy
  (c) Open surgery and bile duct stone extraction
  (d) Lithotripsy

Ans. (a)
Note
The best treatment option for her in above given clinical situation is 'ERCP and bile duct stone extraction'.

Also see
In such cases the scheme of management is:
Conservative management: With antibiotics, analgesics, sphincter of Oddi relaxants, vitamin K, and IV fluids.
After the jaundice subsides operation should be done.
In case of jaundiced patients ERCP should be done.
Ref: A Concise Textbook of Surgery, S. Das, 3rd Ed, Chapter 46, Pg 915

Q. 43. Hypoparathyroidism following thyroid surgery commonly occurs within (AIIMS /Nov-03/Nov-04)
    (a)   24 hours
    (b)   2-5 days
    (c)   7-10 days
    (d)   2-3 weeks

Ans. (b)
Note
Hypoparathyroidism following thyroid surgery commonly occurs within '2-5 days'.
Also see
Damage to the parathyroid gland during thyroidectomy may lead to tetany. Majority of the patients present within 2-5 days after operation but a few may be delayed until 2-3 weeks.
Other complications:
Early - hemorrhage, infection, thyroid crises, recurrent laryngeal nerve palsy, respiratory obstruction
Late - thyroid insufficiency, recurrent thyrotoxicosis, keloid
Ref: A Concise Textbook of Surgery, S. Das, 3rd Ed, Chapter 37, Pg 657-658

Q. 44. A 69 year old male patient having coronary artery disease was found to have gall bladder stones while undergoing a routine ultrasound of the abdomen. There was no history of biliary colic or jaundice at any time. What is the best treatment advice for such a patient for his gallbladder stones? (AIIMS /Nov-03/ All India/03)
    (a)   Open cholecystectomy
    (b)   Laparoscopic cholecystectomy
    (c)   No surgery for gallbladder stones
    (d)   ERCP and removal of gallbladder stones

Ans. (c)
Note
The best advice in above situation is 'No surgery for gallbladder stones'.
Also see
Asymptomatic gallstones found accidentally do not usually cause any trouble and should not be operated upon.
Ref: Davidson's Principles and Practice of Medicine, 19th Ed, Chapter 18, Pg 884
In asymptomatic gallstone patients, the risk of developing symptoms or complications requiring surgery is quite small (in the range of 1 to 2% per year). The recommendation for cholecystectomy in a patient with gallstones is based on assessment of following factors:
    a.   The presence of symptoms those are frequent enough or severe enough to interfere with the patient's general routine.
    b.   The presence of a prior complication of gallstone disease, i.e., history of acute cholecystitis, pancreatitis, gallstone fistula, etc.
    c.   The presence of an underlying condition predisposing the patient to increased risk of gallstone complications (e.g., calcified or porcelain gallbladder and/or a previous attack of acute cholecystitis regardless of current symptomatic status).
    d.   Age under 50 years is a worrisome factor in asymptomatic gallstone patients. Few authorities would now recommend routine cholecystectomy in all young patients with silent stones.
    Since all above conditions do not apply to the above case therefore the most suitable choice is (c).
Ref: Harrison Section 2 Liver and Biliary disease, 302 diseases of the gall bladder and bile ducts

Q. 45. A 14 year old healthy girl of normal height and weight for age, complains that her right breast has developed twice the size of her left breast since the onset of puberty at the age of 12. Both breasts have a similar consistency on palpation with normal nipples areolae. The most likely cause for these findings is (AIIMS /Nov-03)
- (a) Cystosarcoma phylloides
- (b) Virginal hypertrophy
- (c) Fibrocystic disease
- (d) Early state of carcinoma

Ans. (b)
Note
The most likely cause for above findings is 'Virginal hypertrophy'.
Also see
This is a condition where the breasts enlarge excessively at the time of adolescence when breasts normally become sensitive to estrogen.
Enlargement is bilateral, and excessive although each breast is not necessarily equal in size.
Ref: http://www.wdxcyber.com/dxbrs001.htm
It is typical for a woman's breasts to be unequal in size particularly while the breasts are developing during puberty. Statistically it is slightly more common for the left breast to be the larger. In some rare cases, the breasts may be significantly different in size, or one breast may fail to develop entirely. A vast number of medical conditions are known to cause abnormal development of the breasts during puberty. Virginal breast hypertrophy is a condition which involves excessive growth of the breasts during puberty, and in some cases the continued growth beyond the usual pubescent
Ref: http://en.wikipedia.org/wiki/Breasts

Q. 46. Regarding varicose veins, which one of the following statements is true (AIIMS /Nov-03)
- (a) Over 20% are recurrent varicosities.
- (b) The sural nerve is in danger during stripping of the long saphenous vein.
- (c) The saphenous nerve is closely associated with the short saphenous vein.
- (d) 5% oily phenol is an appropriate sclerosant for venous sclerotherapy.

Ans. (d)
Note
Regarding varicose veins, amongst above '5% oily phenol is an appropriate sclerosant for venous sclerotherapy' is true statement.
Also see
Consider the above choices:
- (a) Not Clear
- (b) The sural nerve is in danger during striping of the long saphenous vein; Incorrect- The sural nerve is a branch of the tibial nerve. It descends between the two heads of gastrocnemius and pierces the deep fascia in the middle of the leg. It accompanies the small saphenous vein.
- (c) The sphenous nerve is closely associated with the short saphenous vein – Incorrect – sphenous nerve is a branch of posterior division of femoral nerve. It pierces the deep fascia on the medial side of the knee and descends close to the great saphenous vein either in front or it or behind it.
- (d) True; in sclerotherapy 5% Ethanolamine oleate is used to damage the intima of the vein and produce sclerosis.

References:
B.D.Chaurasia's Human Anatomy, 3rd Ed, Vol 2, Chapter 9, Pg 93
A Concise Textbook of Surgery, S. Das, 3rd Ed, Chapter 16, Pg 207,208

Q. 47. Dysphagia lusoria is due to (AIIMS /Nov-03)
- (a) Esophageal diverticulum
- (b) Aneurysm of aorta
- (c) Esophageal web
- (d) Compression by aberrant blood vessel

Ans. (d)

Note
Dysphagia lusoria is due to 'compression by aberrant blood vessel'.

Also see
Severe vascular anomalies may produce dysphagia by compression of the esophagus. Dysphagia lusoria is classically due to an aberrant right subclavian artery (Arteria lusoria). However, vascular rings such as a double aortic arch more commonly compress the esophagus. Dysphagia occurs in minority of cases and usually presents early in childhood, although it can occur in the late teens also. Treatment is by dividing of the non dominant component of the ring.
Ref: Bailey and Love's Short Practice of Surgery, 24th Ed, Chapter 50, Pg 858

Q. 48. Least malignant thyroid cancer is (AIIMS /Nov-03)
- (a) Papillary carcinoma
- (b) Follicular carcinoma
- (c) Medullary carcinoma
- (d) Anaplastic carcinoma

Ans. (a)

Note
The least malignant thyroid cancer is 'Papillary carcinoma'.

Also see
a. Papillary carcinoma: Overall mortality rate is 11%. Incidence of lymph node and vascular metastasis is 35% and 40% respectively
b. Follicular carcinoma: It appears to be macroscopically encapsulated but microscopically there appears to be invasion of the vascular spaces. Blood borne metastasis is almost twice as common and eventual mortality is twice as compared to papillary carcinoma.
c. Medullary carcinoma: Lymph node metastasis occurs in 50-60% cases and blood borne metastasis is common.
d. Undifferentiated carcinoma (Anaplastic carcinoma): Local infiltration is an early feature of these tumors which spread by lymphatics and blood stream. These are extremely lethal tumors and survival for more than 1-2 years after presentation is most unusual.

Ref: Bailey and Love's Short Practice of Surgery, 24th Ed, Chapter 40, Pg 728, 729,730 and 731

Q. 49. A blood stained discharge from the nipple indicates (AIIMS /Nov-03)
- (a) Breast abscess
- (b) Fibroadenoma
- (c) Duct papilloma
- (d) Fat necrosis of breast

Ans. (c)

Note
A blood stained discharge from the nipple indicates 'Duct papilloma'.

Also see
a. Breast abscess: The affected breast becomes painful, redness is limited to the area involved, edema & brawny induration.
b. Fibroadenoma: Presents as a slow growing painless solitary lump in the lower part of breast. Discharge is absent.
c. Duct Papilloma: This is a benign tumor arising from the lining epithelium of a principle lactiferous duct. It is of small size and said to be pre cancerous. Age group affected- 30-50. Bloody discharge from the nipple is the most frequent symptom. Small soft swelling palpable below the nipple.
d. Fat necrosis of breast: Occurs after some sort of injury and may be confused with a new growth.

Ref: A Concise Textbook of Surgery, S. Das, 3rd Ed, Chapter 39, Pg 693, 694, 707, 709, 710

Q. 50. The commonest site of carcinoma esophagus in India is (AIIMS /Nov-03)
- (a) Upper 1/3rd
- (b) Middle 1/3rd
- (c) Lower 1/3rd
- (d) GE junction

Ans. (b)

Note
The commonest site of carcinoma esophagus in India is 'Middle 1/3rd'.

Also see
- Squamous cell carcinoma usually affects the upper 2/3rds of the esophagus and adenocarcinoma affects the lower 1/3rd.
- SCCA (Squamoue Cell Carcinoma) is more common than Adenocarcinoma.

Answer could be (a) and (b) Both use your discretion.
Ref: Bailey and Love's Short Practice of Surgery, 24th Ed, Chapter 50, Pg 873

Q. 51. Which of the following substances is not used as an irrigant during transurethral resection of the prostate? (AIIMS /Nov-03)
    (a)   Normal saline
    (b)   15% glycine
    (c)   5% dextrose
    (d)   Distilled water

Ans. (a)

Note
'Normal saline' is not used as an irrigant during transurethral resection of the prostate.

Also see
During TURP, hyponatremia is avoided by using 1.5% isotonic glycine, which may be caused by continuous irrigation with sterile water. After the operation is over, the bladder is drained with a 3-way self-retaining catheter with isotonic saline.
Ref: A Concise Textbook of Surgery, S. Das, 3rd Ed, Chapter 59, Pg 1243

Q. 52. A 65-year-old smoker presents with hoarseness, hemoptysis and a hard painless lump in the left supraclavicular fossa. Which of the following is the most appropriate diagnostic step (AIIMS / May-04)
    (a)   Undertake an open biopsy of the neck lump
    (b)   Undertake a radical neck dissection
    (c)   Do fine needle aspiration cytology
    (d)   Give a trial of anti tuberculous therapy

Ans. (a)

Note
Most appropriate diagnostic step for above is 'Undertake an open biopsy of the neck lump'.

Also see
Supraclavicular lymph nodes are commonly enlarged in TB, Hodgkin's disease and in malignant growth of breast, arm and chest (here in this case carcinoma bronchus is most important cause it is causing hoarsness due to involvement of left recurrent laryngeal nerve most probably due to hilar lymph node enlargement causing compression).

The left supraclavicular nodes are involved in malignant growths of distant organs (area drained by thoracic duct). e.g., stomach, testes and other abdominal organs. Biopsy is very helpful in early diagnosis of such malignancy.
Ref: B.D. Chaurasia's Human Anatomy, 3rd Ed, Vol 3, Chapter 33, Pg 311

Q. 53. During surgery of hernia, the sac of a strangulated inguinal hernia should be opened at the (AIIMS /May-04)
    (a)   Neck
    (b)   Body
    (c)   Fundus
    (d)   Deep ring

Ans. (c)

Note
During surgery of hernia, the sac of a strangulated inguinal hernia should be opened at the 'fundus'.
Also see
In case of a strangulated hernia it is advisable to open it at the fundus before the constriction is relieved. This is done to avoid the risk of contaminating the peritoneal cavity with highly toxic fluid swarming with organisms in the sac containing devitalized tissue. Another advantage of opening the sac at fundus is that the contents of sac will not slip inside the abdomen before they are thoroughly examined.
Ref: A Concise Textbook of Surgery, S. Das, 3rd Ed, Chapter 56, Pg 1109

Q. 54. The most common site of a benign (peptic) gastric ulcer is (AIIMS /May-04)
    (a)   Upper third of lesser curvature
    (b)   Greater curvature
    (c)   Pyloric antrum
    (d)   Lesser curvature near incisura angularis

Ans. (d)
Note
The most common site of a benign (peptic) gastric ulcer is 'lesser curvature near incisura angularis'.

Also see
Chronic gastric ulcers are much more common in the lesser curvature, especially at the incisura angularis, than the greater curvature and even when high on the lesser curvature they tend to be at the boundary between the acid secreting and non-acid secreting epithelia.
Ref: Bailey and Love's Short Practice of Surgery, 24th Ed, Chapter 51, Pg 905

Q. 55. Which of the following is the most common endocrine tumour of pancreas (AIIMS /May-04)
    (a)   Insulinoma
    (b)   Gastrinoma
    (c)   Vipoma
    (d)   Glucagonoma

Ans. (a)
Note
'Insulinoma' is the most common endocrine tumour of pancreas.

Also see
Insulinoma
It is an insulin producing adenoma of the I^2-cells. It is the most common islet cell tumor. Majority of the patients are in the 4th & 7th decade of life. It is characterized by attacks of hypoglycemia.
The attacks principally consist of confusion, stupor and loss of consciousness and are promptly relieved by feeding glucose.
Ref: A Concise Textbook of Surgery, S. Das, 3rd Ed, Chapter 48, Pg 963

Q. 56. Cock's peculiar tumour is (AIIMS /May-04)
    (a)   An infected sebaceous cyst
    (b)   A malignant tumour of the scalp
    (c)   A metastatic lesion of the scalp
    (d)   An indicator of underlying osteomyelitis

Ans. (a)
Note
'An infected sebaceous cyst' is Cock's peculiar tumour.

Also see
This is a cyst of the sebaceous glands due to blockage of the duct of this gland, which opens mostly into the hair follicle, and thus the gland becomes distended by its own secretions.
Complications:
    -Infections
    -Ulceration

- Sebaceous horn
- Malignancy
- Calcification

After the cyst has ruptured and chronic infection spreads to the surrounding tissues from the sebaceous cyst, it may lead to a painful boggy fungating and discharging mass known as Cock's Peculiar Tumor.

Ref:
A Concise Textbook of Surgery, S. Das, 3rd Ed, Chapter 9, Pg 81
A Manual of Clinical Surgery, S. Das, Chapter 3, Pg 43

Q. 57. A 43-year-old lady presents with a 5 cm lump in right breast with a 3 cm node in the supraclavicular fossa. Which of the following TNM stage she belongs to as per the latest AJCC staging system (AIIMS /May-04)
    (a)   T2N0M1
    (b)   T1N0M1
    (c)   T2N3M0
    (d)   T2N2M0

Ans. (c)

Note
As per latest AJCC staging system she belongs to 'T2N3M0'.

Also see
The TNM system of staging is based on clinical observations relating to Tumor (T), Node (N) and Metastasis (M)

TUMOR
T_0 - No demonstrable tumor
Tis - CA in situ
T1 - Tumor 2cms or less
T_2 - Tumor 2cm- 5cm
T_3 - Tumor more than 5cms
T_4 - Tumor size is of any size with skin infiltration, ulceration, skin oedema, peau de-orange, pectoral muscle or chest wall involvement.

NODE
N_0 - No clinically palpable nodes
N_1 - Clinically palpable axillary nodes
N_2 - Clinically palpable and fixed nodes
N_3 - Homolateral supra or infra clavicular nodes

METASTASIS
M_0 - Metastasis absent
M_1 - Present

Ref: A Concise Textbook of Surgery, S. Das, 3rd Ed, Chapter 39, Pg 719

Q. 58. Which of the following statements about the Holmium:YAG laser is incorrect? (AIIMS / May-04)
    (a)   It has a wave length of 2100 nm.
    (b)   It's use for uric acid stones has caused deaths due to generation of cyanide.
    (c)   It is effective against the hardest urinary stones.
    (d)   It can even cut the wire of stone baskets.

Ans. (b)

Note
Incorrect statement about Holmium: YAG laser is 'It's use for uric acid stones has caused deaths due to generation of cyanide'.

Also see
The Holmium: YAG (Ho: YAG) and pulse-dye laser are used for fragmentation of urinary calculi through miniaturized rigid and flexible endoscopes. The Holmium: YAG laser is effective at fragmenting all stones types. However, it can also cut a stone basket or the wall of a ureter if contact occurs. Holmium: YAG laser utilizes a wavelength in the infrared zone (2100 microns). The laser works on the surface of the stone by

vaporizing water and organic matter in the stone resulting in destruction in the urinary calculus.

Advantages of Holmium: YAG Laser
1. This laser can make small stone fragments from large stones either by fragmentation or by vaporization.
2. This laser device is easy to use.
3. It is ready to use within one minute after it is turned on.
4. No special non-conduction solution is required.
5. The fiber can be placed with great precision and controlled action.
6. Protective eye ware does not compromise the ureteroscopic view of the stone or fiber.
7. The machine is readily moved from one operating room to another.
8. The laser fibers are versatile and can be used in rigid or flexible ureteroscopes.
9. This laser can be used with high efficacy regardless of stone composition.
10. This laser reduces the need for stone manipulation or basketing.

Disadvantages
1. Destruction of large stones can be tedious and time consuming.
2. The laser will melt the wires of a basket or guide wire if fired directly onto the wire making extraction of the basket or wire difficult.

Ref: http://www.urologystone.com/CH07TreatmentOptions/holmiumLaserLithotripsy.html

Q. 59. The treatment of choice for a mucocele of gall bladder is (AIIMS /May-04)
(a) Aspiration of mucous
(b) Cholecystectomy
(c) Cholecystostomy
(d) Antibiotics and observation

Ans. (b)

Note
'Cholecystectomy' is the choice for a mucocele of gall bladder.

Also see
Cholesterol type of stones impact in the cystic duct or neck of the gall bladder resulting in hydrops. The bile is absorbed and the gall bladder becomes filled and distended with mucous.
O/E:
    -The gall bladder is distended and tender
    -Slight jaundice may be seen
Treatment:
    -Cholecystectomy to avoid complications such as infection, perforation and gall stone ileus.
Ref: A Concise Textbook of Surgery, S. Das, 3rd Ed, Chapter 46, Pg 900

Q. 60. Virchow's triad includes all of the following, except (AIIMS /May-04)
(a) Venous stasis
(b) Injury to veins
(c) Blood hypercoagulability
(d) Venous thrombosis

Ans. (d)

Note
Virchow's triad includes all of the above, except 'Venous thrombosis'.

Also see
Humans possess an inbuilt system by which the blood remains in fluid state normally and guards against haemorrhage and thrombosis. However injury to the blood vessels initiates hemostasis. Virchow described three primary events, which predispose to thrombus formation called as Virchow's triad.
This includes:
    -Endothelial injury
    -Alteration in the flow of blood
    -Hypercoaguability of blood
Ref: Textbook of Pathology by Harsh Mohan, 4th Ed, Chapter 4, Pg 97

Q. 61. The most common cause of superficial thrombophlebitis is (AIIMS /May-04)
(a) Trauma
(b) Infection
(c) Varicosities
(d) Intravenous infusion

Ans. (d)
Note
'Intravenous infusion' is the most common cause of superficial thrombophlebitis.
Also see
It occurs more often in varicose veins or after I.V. infusion. It is also seen in association with polycythaemia, polyarteritis, Buerger's disease and visceral carcinoma.
Clinical features:
   -Firm cord can be palpated along the course of a non-superficial vein. There may be associated redness, tenderness and induration.
Ref: A Concise Textbook of Surgery, S. Das, 3rd Ed, Chapter 16, Pg 212

Q. 62. A man is rushed to casualty, nearly dying after a massive blood loss in an accident. There is not much time to match blood groups, so the physician decides to order for one of the following blood groups. Which one of the following blood groups should the physician decide? (AIIMS /May-04)
(a) O negative
(b) O positive
(c) AB positive
(d) AB negative

Ans. (a)
Note
Physician should decide for 'O Negative' blood group.
Also see
In case of emergency if time does not permit to do proper grouping and cross matching or to wait for the availability of the proper cross- matched blood then one can use blood group O.
Ref: A Concise Textbook of Surgery, S. Das, 3rd Ed, Chapter 4, Pg 40
However since the Rh status of patient is also not known therefore to prevent iso- immunization Rh negative blood should be used.

Q. 63. All of the following are risk factors for carcinoma gall bladder, except (AIIMS /May-04)
(a) Typhoid carriers
(b) Adenomatous gall bladder polyps
(c) Choledochal cysts
(d) Oral contraceptives

Ans. (d)
Note
All of the above are risk facators for carcinoma gall bladder, except 'Oral contraceptives'.
Also see
a. Typhoid gall bladder: Salmonella typhii can infect the gall bladder and cause acute cholecystitis. Occasionally gall stones may also be associated with typhoid gall bladder.
   Ref: Bailey and Love's Short Practice of Surgery, 24th Ed, 54, Page 978
   It is associated with an increased risk of bile duct carcinoma.
   Ref: A Concise Textbook of Surgery, S. Das, 3rd Ed, Chapter 46, Pg 921
b. Gall-bladder polyps: Gallbladder polyps are also thought to be risk factors for gallbladder cancer.
   Ref:http://www.surgery.usc.edu/divisions/tumor/pancreas_diseases/web%20pages/BILIARY%20SYSTEM/Gall bladder%20cancer.html
c. Choledochal cyst: It is due to specific weakness in a part of or whole wall of CBD. It appears that the anomaly is premalignant and CA of biliary tract is a well-recognized complication.
   Ref: Bailey and Loves Short Practice of Surgery, Chapter 54, Pg 973
   Therefore, the choice suggested is (d)

Q. 64. A posteriorly perforating ulcer in the pyloric antrum of the stomach is likely to produce initial localized peritonitis or abscess formation in the (AIIMS /Nov-04/ All INDIA-03)
    (a)   Greater sac
    (b)   Left subhepatic and hepatorenal spaces (Pouch of Morrison)
    (c)   Omental bursa
    (d)   Right subphrenic space

Ans. (c)
Note
A posteriorly perforating ulcer in the pyloric antrum of the stomach is likely to produce initial localized peritonitis or abscess formation in the 'Omental bursa'.

Also see
A posterior gastric ulcer may perforate into the lesser sac or omental bursa. The leaking fluid passes out through the epiploic foramen to reach the hepatorenal pouch. Sometimes in these areas the epiploic foramen is closed by adhesions. The lesser sac becomes distended and can be drained by a tube passed through the lesser omentum.
Ref: B.D. Chaurasia's Human Anatomy, 3rd Ed, Vol 2, Chapter 18, Pg 202

Q. 65. Which of the following is the investigation of choice for assessment of depth of penetration and perirectal nodes in rectal cancer? (AIIMS /Nov-04)
    (a)   Trans rectal ultrasound
    (b)   CT scan pelvis
    (c)   MRI scan
    (d)   Double contrast barium enema

Ans. (a)
Note
'Trans-rectal ultrasound' is the investigation of choice for assessment of dept of penetration and perirectal nodes in rectal cancer.

Also see
-Endorectal ultrasound is a powerful tool for the pre-operative staging of rectal CA. The accuracy of MRI and CT is less in assessing the depth of local invasion and involvement of meso-rectal lymph nodes. It is used to identify patients with locally advanced disease who may be considered for primary RT to down stage the disease.
Ref: A Concise Textbook of Surgery, S. Das, 3rd Ed, Chapter 61, Pg 1312

Q. 66. All of the following clinicopathologic features are seen more often in seminomas as compared to non-seminomatous germ cell tumours of the testis, except (AIIMS /Nov-04)
    (a)   Tumors remain localized to testis for a long time.
    (b)   They are radiosensitive.
    (c)   They metastasize predominantly by lymphatics.
    (d)   They are often associated with raised levels of serum alpha-feto protein and human chorionic gonadotrophin.

Ans. (d)
Note
It is the commonest malignant tumor of the testis and constitutes 45% of all germ cell tumors. Only 10% of these tumors are associated with increased AFP or hCG levels. They are extremely radiosensitive and tend to remain localized to the testes for a long time.
Ref: Textbook of Pathology by Harsh Mohan, 4th Ed, Chapter 20, Pg 697

Q. 67. The treatment of choice in renal cell carcinoma with the tumor of less than 4 cm in size is (AIIMS /Nov-04)
    (a)   Partial nephrectomy
    (b)   Radical nephrectomy
    (c)   Radial nephrectomy + post operative radiotherapy
    (d)   Radical nephrectomy + chemotherapy

Ans. (a)

Note
'Partial nephrectomy' is the treatment of choice in renal cell carcinoma with tumour of less than 4 cm in size.

Also see
-The definitive treatment for primary renal cell carcinoma (RCCA) is radical nephrectomy. The cases can be divided into 4 groups:
Group 1: Cases with no demonstrable metastases "radical nephrectomy with removal of perinephric fat and regional lymph nodes.
Group 2: Cases where there are no demonstrable metastases and tumor is too fixed. Treatment is X-ray therapy or chemotherapy.
Group 3: RCCA with solitary metastasis. Treatment is radical nephrectomy with excision of solitary metastasis
Group 4: Bilateral tumors "partial nephrectomy".
Ref: A Concise Textbook of Surgery, S. Das, 3rd Ed, Chapter 57, Pg 1191

Q. 68. A 40 year old woman has undergone a cholecystectomy. The histopathology reveals that she has a 3 cm adenocarcinoma in the body of the gallbladder infiltrating up to the serosa. Which of the following further management would you advise her? (AIIMS /Nov-04)
    (a) Chemotherapy
    (b) Radiotherapy
    (c) Radical cholecystectomy
    (d) Follow up with regular ultrasound examinations

Ans. (c)
Note
'Radical cholecystectomy' is the further course of management in above case.

Also see
Simple cholecystectomy is not the treatment of choice in gall bladder carcinoma even if the patient comes at an early stage. The choice lies between:
a. Extended cholecystectomy: This is a radical surgery and involves excision of the gall bladder with hepatic band and regional lymph nodes.
b. Extended right hepatic lobectomy.
Ref: A Concise Textbook of Surgery, S. Das, 3rd Ed, Chapter 46, Pg 921

Q. 69. Which one of the following is the treatment of choice for a 4 cm retroperitoneal lymph node mass in a patient with non seminomatous germ cell tumour of the testis? (AIIMS /Nov-04)
    (a) Radical radiotherapy alone
    (b) High orchidectomy + RPLND (Retroperitoneal Lymph Node Dissection)
    (c) RPLND alone
    (d) High orchidectomy alone

Ans. (b)
Note
High orchidectomy + RPLND (Retroperitoneal Lymph Node Dissection) is the treatment of choice in above clinical presentation.

Also see
As soon as the diagnosis is confirmed inguinal orchidectomy with high cord ligation at the deep inguinal ring is mandatory. As the histopathology shows the tumor to be non- seminomatous treatment depends upon the stage: Involvement of retro peritoneal lymph nodes indicates stage 2 therefore radical neck dissection or radiotherapy should be done.
Ref: A Concise Textbook of Surgery, S. Das, 3rd Ed, Chapter 60, Pg 1291, 1292

Q. 70. A 13 year old boy presents with acute onset right scrotal pain. The pain is not relieved on elevation of the scrotum and he has no fever or dysuria. The testis is enlarged and tender. His routine urinary examination is normal. There is no history of trauma. Which of the following is the most appropriate management? (AIIMS /Nov-04)
    (a) Immediate exploration
    (b) Antibiotics

(c) Psychiatric evaluation
(d) Antibiotics and scrotal elevation

Ans. (a)

Note

'Immediate exploration' is the most appropriate management.

Also see

The patient seems to be suffering from torsion of testis. This condition is commonly seen in pre-pubertal males.
Predisposing factors are:
 -Inversion of testes, undescended testes, long mesorchium, voluminous tunica vaginalis.
Initiating factors are:
 -Spasm of cremaster muscle, which may occur while lifting heavy weights, straining at stool, coitus, and during sleep.
Elevation of leg ameliorates the pain in epididymo-orchitis but not in torsion of testes.
Treatment:
 -Manual detorsion.
 -If this fails then surgical exploration should be done.
Ref: A Concise Textbook of Surgery, S. Das, 3rd Ed, Chapter 60, Pg 1273-1275

Q. 71. A 25 year old lady presents with spontaneous nipple discharge of 3-months duration. On examination the discharge is bloody and from a single duct. The following statements about management of this patient are true except (AIIMS /Nov-04)
(a) Ultrasound can be a useful investigation
(b) Radical duct excision is the operation of choice
(c) Galactogram, though useful, is not essential
(d) Majority of blood-stained nipple discharges are due to papillomas or other benign condition

Ans. (a)

Note

All of the above are true except 'Ultrasound can be a useful investigaiton'.

Also see

Causes of discharge of blood from nipples:
 -Pregnancy, duct papilloma, duct carcinoma.
 -Duct papilloma is a benign tumor arising from the lining epithelium of lactiferous duct.
 -Most patients are in the age group of 20-30 years.
 -Ductograms are useful in identifying ductal papilloma.
Treatment:
 -Complete excision of the duct involved along with the tumor, done by wedge resection.
Ref: A Concise Textbook of Surgery, S. Das, 3rd Ed, Chapter 39, Pg 710

Q. 72. All of the following statements are correct about renal transplantation except (AIIMS /Nov-04)
(a) Renal transplantation is heterotopic.
(b) Cyclosporine is the mainstay of immunosuppression.
(c) In India, organ harvesting from brain dead patients is not permitted by law.
(d) Kidney after removal is flushed with cold perfusion solution.

Ans. (c)

Note

All of the above statements are correct about renal transplantation except that 'In India, organ harvesting from brain dead patients is not permitted by law'.

Also see

 -To prevent rejection of the transplant immunosuppressive therapy is used. Most immunosuppressive protocols use a calcineurin blocker (cyclosporins or tacrolimus) as the main agent. This is often given with an anti proliferative agent and steroid.

-After dissection the organs to be preserved are perfused in situ. This produces rapid cooling of the organs, reduces their metabolic rate and preserves their viability. The abdominal organs are perfused with chilled organ preservation solution via an aortic or portal canula.

Ref: - Bailey and Love's Short Practice of Surgery, 24th Ed, Chapter 11, Page 136,132
-The Transplantation of Human Organs Act (Act no 42 of 1994) accepts the brain dead criterion
Ref: The Essentials of Forensic Medicine and Toxicology 21st Edition, by Dr. K. S. Narayan Reddy, Chapter 3, Pg 48

Q. 73. All of the following statements are true about repair of groin hernias except: (AIIMS /Nov-04)
- (a) Lichten-stein tension free repair has a low recurrence rate.
- (b) TEEP repair is an extraperitoneal approach to laproscopic repair of groin hernia.
- (c) In Shouldice repair, non-absorbable mesh is used.
- (d) The surgery can be done under local anaesthesia in selected cases.

Ans. (c)

Note
All of the above statements are true about repair of groin hernias except 'In shouldice repair, non-absorbable mesh is used'.

Also see
- (a) Lichten-Stein tension free repair is a technique of herniorraphy. It is often used as it is a relatively easy operation with less stay at the hospital, it may be performed under LA, with this technique the recurrence rate is less than 1% and patients recover rapidly with minimum post-operative pain.
- (b) Laparoscopic repair of hernia can be done by TEPA-totally extra-peritoneal approach or TAPP-Transabdominal peri peritoneal approach.
- (c) Shouldice repair is another method of hernoirraphy. The materials used are dexon and polypropylene. Dexon is an absorbable suture.
- (d) The operation for hernia can be done under general anesthesia, epidural or spinal anesthesia or local anesthesia.

Ref: A Concise Textbook of Surgery, S. Das, 3rd Ed, Chapter 56, Pg 1105, 1106
Ref: Bailey and Love's Short Practice of Surgery, 24th Ed, Chapter 42, 62, Pg 849, 850, 1147

Q. 74. A 25 year old male presents to emergency with history of road traffic accident two hours ago. The patient is hemodynamically stable, abdomen is soft. On catheterization of the bladder, hematuria is noticed. The next step in the management should be: (AIIMS /Nov-04)
- (a) Immediate laparotomy
- (b) Retrograde cystouretherography (RGU)
- (c) Diagnostic peritoneal lavage (DPL)
- (d) Contrast enhanced computed tomography (CECT) of abdomen

Ans. (d)

Note
The next step in the management should be Contrast enhanced computed tomography (CECT) of abdomen.

Also see
CT scanning is usually performed after simpler investigations such as plain films or USG. In many places however it is used as the primary investigation in evaluation of a patient with abdominal trauma and severe pancreatitis, it has a major role in cancer staging.
Ref: Bailey and Love's Short Practice of Surgery, Chapter 1, Pg 12,13

Q. 75. Which of the following statements best represents Ludwig's angina? (AIIMS /Nov-04)
- (a) A type of coronary artery spasm.
- (b) An infection of the cellular tissues around submandibular salivary gland.
- (c) Oesophageal spasm.
- (d) Retropharyngeal infection.

Ans. (b)

Note
Ludwig's angina is an infection of the cellular tissues around submandibular salivary gland.

Also see
Ludwig's angina is the infection of submandibular space, which lies between the mucous membrane of the floor of mouth and tongue on one side and superficial layer of the deep cervical fascia on the other.
Ref: Diseases of Ear Nose & Throat by P.L. Dhingra, Cp 45, Pg 277

Q. 76. Which of the following best represents 'ranula'? (AIIMS /Nov-04)
    (a)   A type of epulis
    (b)   A thyroglossal cyst
    (c)   **Cystic swelling in the floor of mouth**
    (d)   Forked uvula

Ans. (c)
Note
Cystic swelling in the floor of mouth represents the best out of above for 'ranula'.

Also see
It is a transparent cyst on the floor of the mouth on one side or other. The cyst is considered to be a mucous retention cyst arising from the glands of Blandin and Nuhn situated on the floor of mouth.
Ref: A Concise Textbook of Surgery, S. Das, 3rd Ed, Chapter 33, Pg 580

Q. 77. Complications of total thyroidectomy include all except (AIIMS /Nov-04)
    (a)   Hoarseness
    (b)   Airway obstruction
    (c)   Hemorrhage
    (d)   **Hypercalcemia**

Ans. (d)
Note
Complications of total thyroidectomy include all except 'Hypercalcemia'.

Also see
Damage to the parathyroid gland during thyroidectomy may lead to tetany.
Other complications: Early- hemorrhage, infection, thyroid crisis, recurrent laryngeal nerve palsy, respiratory obstruction
Late -thyroid insufficiency, recurrent thyrotoxicosis, and keloid
Ref: A Concise Textbook of Surgery, S. Das, 3rd Ed, Chapter 37, Pg 657-658

Q. 78. Treatment of choice for medullary carcinoma of thyroid is (AIIMS /Nov-04)
    (a)   **Total thyroidectomy**
    (b)   Partial thyroidectomy
    (c)   I131 ablation
    (d)   Hemithyroidectomy

Ans. (a)
Note
Treatment of choice for medullary carcinoma of thyroid is 'Total thyroidectomy'.

Also see
Medullary carcinoma shows a familial tendency and has an autosomal dominant inheritance. When associated with pheochromocytoma and parathyroid tumors it is known as MEN 2 syndrome.
Total thyroidectomy is the treatment of choice for medullary CA.
Ref: A Concise Textbook of Surgery, S. Das, 3rd Ed, Chapter 37, Pg 665-666

Q. 79. Thoracic extension of cervical goitre is usually approached through (AIIMS /Nov-04/All India-04)
    (a)   **Neck**
    (b)   Chest
    (c)   Combined cervico-thoracic route
    (d)   Thoracoscopic

Ans. (a)

Note
Thoracic extension of cervical goitre is usually approached through 'Neck'.

Also see
The treatment is by resection, which is done by first mobilizing the cervical part of goiter through the characteristic neck incision.
Ref: A Concise Textbook of Surgery, S. Das, 3rd Ed, Chapter 37, Pg 649, 650

Q. 80. Which of the following is not an indication for cholecystectomy? (AIIMS /Nov-04)
    (a)   70-year-old male with symptomatic gallstones
    (b)   20-year-old male with sickle cell anemia and symptomatic gallstones
    (c)   65-year-old female with a large gallbladder polyp
    (d)   55-year-old with an asymptomatic gallstone

Ans. (d)

Note
Out of above '55-year old with an asymptomtic gall stone' is not an indication for cholecystectomy.

Also see
Asymptomatic gall stones found accidentally are not normally treated because majority will never give symptoms. Symptomatic gall stones are best treated surgically.
Ref: Davidson's Principles and Practice of Medicine, chapter 18, page 884
-In case of gall bladder polyp if the patient is symptomatic then cholecystectomy should be done.
Ref: Bailey and Love's Short Practice of Surgery, 24th Ed, Chapter 54, Pg 978

Q. 81. The initial investigation of choice for a post cholecystectomy biliary stricture is (AIIMS / Nov-04)
    (a)   Ultrasound scan of the abdomen
    (b)   Endoscopic cholangiography
    (c)   Computed tomography
    (d)   Magnetic resonance cholangiography

Ans. (b)

Note
The initial investigation of choice for a post cholecystectomy biliary stricture is 'Endoscopic cholangiography'.

Also see
ERCP; Indications are:
    -Jaundice-persistent or recurrent.
    -Biliary tract problems: post-operative biliary problems.
    -Pancreatic diseases.
Ref: Bailey and Love's Short Practice of Surgery, 24th Ed, Chapter 46, Pg 912

Q. 82. The treatment of choice for an 8 mm retained common bile duct (CBD) stone is (AIIMS / Nov-04)
    (a)   Laparoscopic CBD exploration
    (b)   Percutaneous stone extraction
    (c)   Endoscopic stone extraction
    (d)   Extracorporeal shock wave lithotripsy

Ans. (c)

Note
The treatment of choice for an 8 mm retained common bile duct (CBD) stone is 'Endoscopic stone extraction'.

Also see
If after cholecystectomy a stone is present in the bile duct then it should be removed immediately by endoscopy.

Other post cholecystectomy problems are:
- Stricture of bile duct
- Cystic duct syndrome
- Biliary dyskinesia

Ref: A Concise Textbook of Surgery, S. Das, 3rd Ed, Chapter 46, Pg 912

Q. 83. The direction of flow of venous blood in conditions of valve incompetence affecting perforating veins of lower limb is (AIIMS /Nov-04)
- (a) Along gravity
- (b) Superficial to deep
- (c) Along osmotic gradient
- (d) Deep to superficial

Ans. (d)

Note
The direction of flow of venous blood in conditions of valve incompetence affecting perforating veins of lower limb is 'Deep to superficial'.

Also see
Under normal circumstances the blood flows from superficial venous system to the deep veins through the competent perforators and from deep veins to the heart by muscle pump. Only when the valves of perforators become incompetent the blood will flow in the opposite direction and thus leads to varicosity of the superficial veins.

Ref: Concise Textbook of Surgery by S. Das, 3rd Ed, Chapter – 16 Pg 201-2

Q. 84. According to the Glasgow coma scale (GCS) a verbal score of 1 indicates (ALL INDIA-05)
- (a) No response
- (b) Inappropriate words
- (c) Incomprehensible sounds
- (d) Disoriented response

Ans. (a)

Note
According to the Glasgow coma scale (GCS) a verbal score of 1 indicates 'No response'.

Also see
Systemic assessment of an unconscious patient is done using Glasgow coma scale; the criteria are:
1. Eye opening
2. Best motor response
3. Verbal response

Ref: Davidson's Principles and Practice of Medicine, 19th Ed, Chapter – 22 Pg-1143

Q. 85. In which one of the following perineural invasion in head and neck cancer is most commonly seen? (ALL INDIA-05)
- (a) Adenocarcinoma
- (b) Adenoid cystic carcinoma
- (c) Basal cell Adenoma
- (d) Squamous cell carcinoma

Ans. (b)

Note
Out of above in 'Adenoid cystic carcinoma' perineural invasion in head and neck cancer is most commonly seen.

Also see
Adenoid cystic carcinoma is a poorly encapsulated infiltrating tumor and is unique to being as common in submandibular gland as in parotid gland. These tumor show a tendency to reoccur and often involve the perineural spaces.

Ref: Concise Textbook of Surgery By S Das, 3rd Ed, Chapter 35 Pg 609

Q. 86. In which one of the following conditions the sialography is contraindicated? (ALL INDIA-05)
    (a)   Ductal calculus
    (b)   Chronic parotitis
    (c)   Acute parotitis
    (d)   Recurrent sialadenitis

Ans. (c)

Note
From above in case of 'acute parotitis' sialography is contraindicated.

Also see
In case of a recurrent sub acute or chronic parotitis a sialogram is always performed. It shows any radioluecent obstruction, narrowing or dilatation of ducts. Position or size of a salivary neoplasm can also be detected.
Ref: A Concise Textbook of Surgery by S. Das, 3rd Ed, Chapter 35 Pg 604

Q. 87. The most common site of leak in CSF rhinorrhea is (ALL INDIA-05)
    (a)   Sphenoid sinus
    (b)   Frontal sinus
    (c)   Cribriform plate
    (d)   Tegmen tympani

Ans. (c)

Note
The most common site of leak in CSF rhinorrhoea is 'Cribriform plate'.

Also see
CSF discharging from the nose is known as CSF rhinorrhoea. Cerebrospinal fluid is a clear colorless fluid that bathes the brain and spinal cord, cushioning them against trauma. In fact in literal terms the brain and spinal cord floats in the cerebrospinal fluid. The specific gravity of brain is only 4% of that of CSF, hence it could float easily in the CSF.
The high pressure leaks are commonly encountered in the cribriform area. This is due to the fragility and unique anatomy in this area i.e. (prolongation of the subarachnoid space along the olfactory filaments). The leak during these conditions functions as a safety valve alleviating the increased intracranial pressure. These high pressure leaks are associated with slow growing tumors and 1/4 of them have hydrocephalus.
Normal pressure leaks - These leaks are associated with congenital dehiscence or thin bone along the skull base. Commonly this type of leaks occur in the ethmoidal sinus adjacent to the cribriform plate.
Ref: http://www.drtbalu.co.in/csf_rhino.html
Other sites of leak are ethmoid air sinuses or frontal sinuses. CSF from the middle cranial fossa reaches the nose by sphenoid sinus.
Ref: Diseases of Ear Nose Throat by P.L. Dhingra. Chapter 30 Pg 202

Q. 88. Lumbar sympathectomy is of value in the management of (ALL INDIA-05)
    (a)   Intermittent claudication
    (b)   Distal ischaemia affecting the skin of the toes
    (c)   Arteriovenous fistula
    (d)   Back pain

Ans. (b)

Note
Lumbar sympathectomy is of value in the management of 'Distal ischaemia affecting the skin of the toes'.

Also see
The indications for sympathetectomy are:
    -Circulatory insufficiency- by doing it the smooth muscles of the arterial walls are released from their spasm.
    -Hyperhidrosis
Ref: A Concise Textbook of Surgery, S. Das, 3rd Ed, Chapter 18, Pg 256

Q. 89. The earliest manifestation of increased intracranial pressure following head injury is (ALL INDIA-05)
  (a) Ipsilateral papillary dilatation
  (b) Contralateral papillary dilatation
  (c) Altered mental status
  (d) Hemiparesis

Ans. (a)

Note
The earliest manifestation of increased intracranial pressure following head injury is 'ipsilateral papillary dilatation.

Also see
Pupil on the side of the injury will first constrict due to stretching of the occulomotor nerve, which is followed by dilatation due to paralysis of that nerve.
Ref: A Concise Textbook of Surgery, S. Das, 3rd Ed, Chapter 31, Pg 549

Q. 90. In which of the following conditions splenectomy is not useful? (ALL INDIA-05)
  (a) Hereditary spherocytosis
  (b) Porphyria
  (c) Thalassemia
  (d) Sickle cell disease with large spleen

Ans. NA

Note
In all of the above conditions splenectomy is useful.
Ref: A Concise Textbook of Surgery, S. Das, 3rd Ed, Chapter 47, Pg 934-935

Also see
Indications for splenectomy:
Trauma:
  -Commonest organ injured in blunt abdominal trauma
  -Associated with lower rib fractures
  -25% injuries are iatrogenic
Spontaneous rupture:
  -Usually seen in those with massive splenomegaly (e.g. infectious mononucleosis)
  -Often precipitated by minor trauma
Hypersplenism:
  -Hereditary spherocytosis or elliptocytosis
  -Idiopathic thrombocytopenic purpura
Neoplasia:
  -Lymphoma or leukaemic infiltration
  -Splenectomy not usually required for diagnosis
  -Only required if hypersplenism resistant to treatment
With other viscera:
  -Total gastrectomy
  -Distal pancreatectomy
Other indications:
  -Splenic cysts
  -Hydatid cysts
  -Splenic abscesses
Ref: http://www.surgical-tutor.org.uk/default home.htm?system/vascular/spleen.htm~right

Q. 91. The following is ideal for the treatment with injection of sclerosing agents (ALL INDIA-04/05)
  (a) External hemorrhoids
  (b) Internal hemorrhoids
  (c) Prolapsed hemorrhoids
  (d) Strangulated hemorrhoids

Ans. (b)

Note
'Internal hemorrhoids' are ideal for the treatment with injection of sclerosing agents.

Also see
Sclerosant injection has been the method of choice for treatment of small vascular hemorrhoids and is used to control all cases of primary hemorrhoids.
Ref: A Concise Textbook of Surgery, S. Das, 3rd Ed, Chapter 54, Pg 1058

Q. 92. In which of the following locations, carcinoid tumor is most common? (ALL INDIA-05)
    (a)   Esophagus
    (b)   Stomach
    (c)   Small bowel
    (d)   Appendix

Ans. (d)
Note
Carcinoid tumors are most common in 'appendix'.

Also see
Carcinoid tumors originate from argentaffin cells. They can occur anywhere in the GIT from the stomach to the anus. Appendix is the most frequently affected site (50%) followed by ileum (25%) and rectum (15%). Outside the GIT carcinoid tumor is found in bronchus and ovarian teratoma.
Ref: A Concise Textbook of Surgery, S. Das, 3rd Ed, Chapter 49, Pg 977

Q. 93. Pancreatitis, pituitary tumor and pheochromocytoma may be associated with (ALL INDIA-04/05)
    (a)   Medullary carcinoma of thyroid
    (b)   Papillary carcinoma of thyroid
    (c)   Anaplastic carcinoma of thyroid
    (d)   Follicular carcinoma of thyroid

Ans. (a)
Note
Pancreatitis, pituitary tumor and pheochromocytoma may be associated with 'Medullary Carcinoma of Thyroid'.

Also see
Medullary carcinoma of thyroid is associated with MEN-2 syndrome (multiple endocrine neoplasia), which includes primary hyperparathyroidism and pheochromocytoma.

Ref: Davidson's Principles and Practice of Medicine, 19th Ed, Chapter 16, Pg 688 and 704

Q. 94. Gardener's syndrome is a rare hereditary disorder involving the colon It is characterized by (ALL INDIA-05)
    (a)   Polyposis colon, cancer thyroid, skin tumours.
    (b)   Polyposis in jejunum, pituitary adenoma and skin tumours.
    (c)   Polyposis colon, osteomas, epidermal inclusion cysts and fibrous tumours in the skin.
    (d)   Polyposis of gastrointestinal tract, cholangiocarcinoma and skin tumours.

Ans. (c)
Note
Gardener's syndrome is characterized by polyposis colon, osteomas, epithermal inclusion cysts and fibrous tumours in the skin.

Also see
    -Gardener's syndrome is a variant of Familial Adenomatous Polyposis. In gardener's syndrome benign extra intestinal features like epidermoid cysts and osteomas are prominent.
Ref: Davidson's Principles and Practice of Medicine, 19th Ed, Chapter 17, Pg 822

Q. 95. All of the following are true for patients of ulcerative colitis associated with primary sclerosing cholangitis (PSC), except: (ALL INDIA-05)
    (a)   They may develop biliary cirrhosis.
    (b)   May have raised alkaline phosphatase.
    (c)   Increased risk of hilar cholangiocarcinoma.
    (d)   PSC reverts after a total colectomy.

Ans. (d)
Note
All of the above are true for patients of ulcerative colitis associated with primary sclerosing cholangitis (PSC), except 'PSC reverts after a total colectomy'.

Also see
Sclerosing cholangitis is a condition characterized by fibrotic obliteration of the intrahepatic and/or extra hepatic bile duct system and may be primary or secondary. Primary has no known cause but associated with ulcerative colitis, retroperitoneal fibrosis, HIV, infection and a variety of autoimmune disorders. Secondary biliary cirrhosis may result. There is a strong association with cholangiocarcinoma. S. Bilirubin, GGT, alkaline phosphatase is elevated.
Ref: Davidson's Principles and Practice of Medicine, 19th Ed, Chapter 18, Pg 874

Q. 96. The most common complication seen in hiatus hernia is (ALL INDIA-05)
    (a)   Esophagitis
    (b)   Aspiration pneumonitis
    (c)   Volvulus
    (d)   Esophageal stricture

Ans. (a)
Note
The most common complication seen in hiatus hernia is 'Esophagitis'.

Also see
Hiatus hernia causes reflux because the pressure gradient between the abdominal and thoracic cavities, which normally pinches the hiatus, is lost. In addition the oblique angle between the cardiac and esophagus disappears, almost all patients who develop esophagitis, Barrett's oesophagus or peptic strictures have hiatus hernia.
Ref: Davidson's Principles and Practice of Medicine, 19th Ed, Chapter 17, Pg 776

Q. 97. The most sensitive imaging modality for diagnosing ureteric stones in a patient with acute colic is (ALL INDIA-05)
    (a)   X-ray KUB region
    (b)   Ultrasonogram
    (c)   Non contrast CT scan of the abdomen
    (d)   Contrast enhanced CT scan of the abdomen

Ans. (c)
Note
The most sensitive imaging modality for diagnosing ureteric stones in a patient with acute colic is 'Non contrast CT scan of the abdomen'.

Also see
When the stone is in ureter IVU is most commonly used investigation but it shouldn't be given during acute colic.
Spiral C.T. gives the most accurate assessment.
Ref: Davidson's Principles and Practice of Medicine, 19th Ed, Chapter 14, Pg 633

Q. 98. Which one of the following is not used as a tumor marker in testicular tumors? (ALL INDIA-05)
    (a)   AFP
    (b)   LDH
    (c)   HCG
    (d)   CEA

Ans. (d)

Note
CEA is not used as a tumor marker in testicular tumors.

Also see
Tumor markers elevated in testicular tumors are:
HCG and AFP. In addition carcinoembryogenic Ag (CEA), HPL, Placental alkaline phosphatase, testosterone and leutinizing hormone may also be elevated.
Ref: Textbook of Pathology by Harsh Mohan, 4th Ed, Chapter 20, Pg 696

Q. 99. The commonest site of oral cancer among Indian population is (ALL INDIA-04)
- (a) Tongue
- (b) Floor of mouth
- (c) Alveobuccal complex
- (d) Lip

Ans. (d)

Note
The commonest site of oral cancer among Indian populaiton is Alveobuccal complex.

Q. 100. Which of the following is not an indication of RT in pleomorphic adenoma of parotid (ALL INDIA-04)
- (a) Involvement of deep lobe.
- (b) 2nd histologically benign recurrence.
- (c) Microscopically positive margins.
- (d) Malignant transformation.

Ans. (b)

Note
The 2nd histologically benign recurrence is not an indication for radiotherapy in reference to above.

Q. 101. Unilateral undescended testis is ideally operated around (ALL INDIA-04)
- (a) 2 months of age
- (b) 6 months of age
- (c) 12 months of age
- (d) 24 months of age

Ans. (d)

Note
Failure of descent of the testis into the scrotum at any point along the normal path of descent. Orchidopexy is the treatment of choice. It is unnecessary to perform this operation before the completion of the 2nd birthday of the child.
Ref: A Concise Textbook of Surgery, S. Das, 3rd Ed, Chapter 60, Pg 1270

Q. 102. The short bowel syndrome is characterized by all of the following, except (ALL INDIA-04)
- (a) Diarrhea
- (b) Hypogastrinemia
- (c) Weight loss
- (d) Steatorrhea

Ans. (b)

Note
The short bowel syndrome is characterized by all of the following, except 'Hypogastrinemia'.

Also see
Short bowel syndrome is defined as malabsorption resulting from extensive small intestinal resection. Clinical features; diarrhea, steatorrhea, dehydration and signs of hypovolaemia are common, as are weight loss, loss of muscle bulk and malnutrition.
Ref: Davidson's Principles and Practice of Medicine, 19th Ed, Chapter 17, Pg 796-797

Extended information
Fasting plasma gastrin levels measured by radioimmunoassay were found to be low in patients with hypothyroidism. The decreased gastrin level in patients with hypothyroidism was significantly improved after the thyroid function was normalized by treatment.
Ref: http://www.springerlink.com/content/x6q2804150340333

Q. 103. All of the following are significant risk factors for colonic carcinoma in an adenomatous polyp, except (ALL INDIA-04)
    (a)   Pedunculated polyp
    (b)   Villous histology
    (c)   Size >2 cm
    (d)   Atypia

Ans. (a)

Note
All of the above are significant risk factors for colonic carcinoma in an adenomatous polyp, except 'Pedunculated polyp'.

Also see
Risk factors for malignant change in colonic polyp are:
1. Large in size
2. Multiple polyps
3. Villous architecture
4. Dysplasia

Ref: Davidson's Principles and Practice of Medicine, 19th Ed, Chapter 17, Pg 820

Q. 104. Which one of the following preservatives is used while packing catgut suture? (ALL INDIA-04)
    (a)   Isopropyl alcohol
    (b)   Colloidal iodine
    (c)   Glutaraldehyde
    (d)   Hydrogen peroxide

Ans. (a)

Note
Isopropyl alcohol is used while packing catgut suture.

Also see
a. Isopropyl alcohol is used while packing catguts.
b. Colloidal iodine is used as a skin disinfectant.
c. 2 % glutaraldehyde is used for sterilizing Bronchoscope.
d. Use of hydrogen peroxide in surgical wards is a well known fact.
Ref: http://www.rxpgonline.com/article1516.htmla

Q. 105. Which of the following is not an important cause of hyponatraemia? (ALL INDIA-04)
    (a)   Gastric fistula
    (b)   Excessive vomiting
    (c)   Excessive sweating
    (d)   Prolonged Ryle's tube aspiration

Ans. (c)

Note
Excessive sweating is not an important cause of hyponatraemia.

Also see
The most frequent cause for sodium depletion in surgical practice is obstruction of small intestine with rapid loss of gastric, biliary, pancreatic and intestinal secretions by aperistalsis and ejection, vomiting or aspiration. Duodenal, total biliary, pancreatic and high intestinal external fistula is also causes of hyponatremia. Gastric aspiration is another cause.

Other causes are:
Hyperglycemia, tubulointerstitial diseases, psychogenic polydypsia, inappropriate ADH secretion, liver failure, renal failure, nephrotic syndrome.

Therefore the answer is (c).
Ref: Bailey and Love's Short Practice of Surgery, 24th Ed, Chapter 4, Page 42

Q. 106. Which of the following types of pancreatitis has the best prognosis? (ALL INDIA-04)
- (a) Alcoholic pancreatitis
- (b) Gall stone pancreatitis
- (c) Postoperative pancreatitis
- (d) Idiopathic pancreatitis

Ans. (b)
Note
Gall stone pancreatitis is having the best prognosis.

Also see
Biliary tract disease (gall stones) is the most common cause of acute pancreatitis. Other etiologies include penetrating peptic ulcer, trauma, post-ERCP, post-operative, metabolic (hypertriglyceridemia), and drug-induced. In approximately 85 to 90% of patients, this is self-limited and resolves completely in 3 to 7 days after treatment is instituted. Medical therapy is aimed at reducing pancreatic secretion, thereby "resting" the pancreas, and usually involves analgesia, intravenous fluids, eliminating oral intake, and occasionally nasogastric suction.
Ref: http://www.netmedicine.com/photo/pearls/ptod0016.htm

Q. 107. Chronically lymphoedematous limb is predisposed to all of the following, except (ALL INDIA-04)
- (a) Thickening of the skin
- (b) Recurrent soft tissue infections
- (c) Marjolin's ulcer
- (d) Sarcoma

Ans. (c)
Note
Chronically lymphoedematous limb is predisposed to all of the following, except 'Marjolin's ulcer'.

Also see
Marjolin's ulcer is the name given to a squamous cell carcinoma arising from a chronic benign ulcer or a scar.e.g. Venous ulcer.
Ref: A Concise Textbook of Surgery, S. Das, 3rd Ed, Chapter10, Pg 108

Q. 108. The most common site of intestinal obstruction in gall stone ileus is (ALL INDIA-04)
- (a) Jejunum
- (b) Ileum
- (c) Transverse colon
- (d) Sigmoid colon

Ans. (b)
Note
The most common site of intestinal obstruction in gall stone ileus is 'Ileum'.

Also see
If a gall stone larger than 2.5cm has migrated to the gut it may impact at the terminal ileum or occasionally in duodenum or sigmoid colon. The resultant intestinal obstruction is known as gall stone ileus.
Ref: Davidson's Principles and Practice of Medicine, 19th Ed, Chapter 18, Pg 884

Q. 109. For a rectal carcinoma at 5 cm from the anal verge the best acceptable operation is (ALL INDIA-04)
- (a) Anterior resection
- (b) Abdomino-perineal resection

(c) Posterior resection
(d) Local resection

Ans. (b)

Note
For a rectal carcinoma at 5 cm from the anal verge the best acceptable operation is 'Abdomino-peritoneal resection'.

Also see
The type of resection depends upon the site of carcinoma:
a. Proximal rectal carcinoma (junction with the sigmoid colon-15 to 16 cm above the anus to 11 cm above the anus) –Low anterior resection
b. Mid rectal carcinoma (from 11cm above the anus to 7cm above the anus)-abdominoperineal resection
c. Distal rectal carcinoma (in these cases abdominoperineal or perineo-abdominal resection is done)

Ref: A Concise Textbook of Surgery, S. Das, 3rd Ed, Chapter55, Pg 1067
Sabiston 15th Edition Chapter 32
Bailey 23rd Edition Pg 1108

In general, tumors within 7 to 8 cm. of the anal verge are treated by APR, whereas those more than 12 cm. from the anal verge are adequately managed by low abdominal resection. Lesions lying between 7 and 11 cm. from the anal verge may be managed by either procedure, depending on the size of the lesion, the size of the pelvis, and the differentiation of the tumor. In general, a lesion that is easily palpated with the examining finger is often removed by APR. However, if the neoplasm can be delivered to the level of the abdominal incision following mobilization of the rectum, an adequate resection may be performed. The use of circumferential stapling devices greatly facilitates the construction of the LAR.

Explanation
Bailey categorically says that tumours in lower 3rd of rectum are resected by abdominal perineal resection. You all know that the length of the rectum is about 12 to 15 cm and the anal canal is about 4 cm. Any tumour 5 cm from anal verge is at the lower 1/3rd of rectum and is treated by APR.

Q. 110. First treatment of rupture of varicose veins at the ankle should be (ALL INDIA-04)
(a) Rest in prone position of patient
(b) Application of a tourniquet proximally
(c) Application of a tourniquet distally
(d) Direct pressure and elevation

Ans. (d)

Note
First treatment of rupture of varicose veins at the ankle should be 'Direct pressure and elevation'.

Also see
Hemorrhage is a common complication of varicose veins; it may follow a minor trauma. Treatment is by elevation of the leg and application of pressure.

Q. 111. Bedsore is an example of (ALL INDIA-03)
(a) Tropical ulcer
(b) Trophic ulcer
(c) Venous ulcer
(d) Post thrombotic ulcer

Ans. (b)

Note
Bedsore is an example of 'Trophic ulcer'.

Also see
Trophic ulcers are caused by various factors such as impairment of nutrition of tissues, inadequate blood supply and neurological deficit. These ulcers have a punched out edge with slough in the floor thus resembling a gummatous ulcer.
Ref: A Concise Textbook of Surgery, S. Das, 3rd Ed, Chapter 11, Pg 128

MCQ's in Surgery

Q. 112. Marjolin's ulcer is (ALL INDIA-03)
    (a)   Malignant ulcer found on the scar of burn
    (b)   Malignant ulcer found on infected foot
    (c)   Trophic ulcer
    (d)   Meleney's gangrene

Ans. (a)
Note
Marjolin's ulcer is 'Malignant ulcer found on the scar of burn'.
Also see
Marjolin's ulcer is the name given to a squamous cell carcinoma arising from a chronic benign ulcer or a scar, e.g., venous ulcer. The scar, which may show malignant change, is the scar of a burn.
Ref: A Concise Textbook of Surgery, S. Das, 3rd Ed, Chapter10, Pg 108

Q. 113. If a patient with Raynaud's disease immersed his hand in cold water, the hand will (ALL INDIA-03)
    (a)   Become red
    (b)   Remain unchanged
    (c)   Turn white
    (d)   Become blue

Ans. (c)
Note
If a patient with Raynaud's disease immersed his hand in cold water, the hand will 'turn white'.
Also see
Following exposure to cold, in a patient suffering from raynaud's disease, the digital arteries go into spasm and the decreased blood flow is evidenced by blanching of the fingers.
Ref: A Concise Textbook of Surgery, S. Das, 3rd Ed, Chapter15, Pg 166

Q. 114. The best treatment for cystic hygroma is (ALL INDIA-03)
    (a)   Surgical excision
    (b)   Radiotherapy
    (c)   Sclerotherapy
    (d)   Chemotherapy

Ans. (a)
Note
The mainstay of treatment is surgical excision for cystic hygroma.
Also see
Cystic hygroma is the most common form of lymphangioma. Most are present in neck. In 20% cases it's present in the axilla. These are painless and soft swellings; showing fluctuation and fluid thrill. Excision is the only treatment available.
Ref: A Concise Textbook of Surgery, S. Das, 3rd Ed, Chapter17, Pg 222

Q. 115. Which of the following is most suggestive of neonatal small bowel obstruction? (ALL INDIA-03)
    (a)   Generalised abdominal distension
    (b)   Failure to pass meconeum in the first 24 hours
    (c)   Bilious vomiting
    (d)   Refusal of feeds

Ans. (c)
Note
Infant having bilious vomiting points to intestinal obstruciton.

Q. 116. What is most characteristic of congenital hypertrophic pyloric stenosis? (ALL INDIA-03)
    (a)   Affects the first born female child
    (b)   The pyloric tumour is best felt during feeding

(c) The patient is commonly marasmic
(d) Loss of appetite occurs early

Ans. (b)

Note
Most characteristic of congenital hypertrophic pyloric stenosis is that 'The pyloric tumour is best felt during feeding'.

Also see
It is classically the first-born male child that is most commonly affected. The condition is most commonly seen at the first 4 weeks after birth ranging from the 3rd to the 7th week. Forcible projectile vomiting of milk is present with weight loss. Diagnosis is made by test feed, which produces peristaltic waves.
Ref: Bailey and Love's Short Practice of Surgery, 24th Ed, Chapter 51, Pg 899
An enlarged pylorus, classically described as an "olive," can be palpated in the right upper quadrant or epigastrium of the abdomen. Palpation should reveal the pyloric olive just on or to the right of the midline. To be assured of the diagnosis, the physician should be able to roll the pylorus beneath the examining finger. The tumor (mass) is best felt after vomiting or during, or at the end of, feeding. The diagnosis is easily made if the presenting clinical features are typical, with projectile vomiting, visible peristalsis, and a palpable pyloric tumor.
Ref: http://www.emedicine.com/ped/topic1103.htm

Q. 117. Which of the following lasers is used for treatment of benign prostatic hyperplasia as well as urinary calculi? (ALL INDIA-03)
(a) CO2 laser
(b) Excimer laser
(c) Ho : YAG laser
(d) Nd : YAG laser

Ans. (c)

Note
Ho: YAG laser is used for treatment of benign prostatic hyperplasia as well as urinary calculi.

Also see
Long pulse Holmium: YAG (Ho: YAG) laser is an attractive alternative to other conventional laser lithotriptors Ho: YAG laser (2.12 µm) has been used extensively in urology for laser lithotripsy.
Ref: http://www.ece.utexas.edu/bell/xprojects/lithotripsy/aboutHoYAG.htm

Q. 118. What is the most appropriate operation for a solitary nodule in one lobe of thyroid? (ALL INDIA-03)
(a) Lobectomy
(b) Hemithyroidectomy
(c) Nodule removal
(d) Partial lobectomy with 1 cm margin around nodule

Ans. (d)

Note
Partial lobectomy with 1 cm margin around nodule is the most appropriate operation for a solitary nodule in one lobe of thyroid.

Also see
If there are no pressure symptoms or an acute increase in the size then it may be left alone. However, since there are chances of malignancy the treatment should be excision of the solitary nodule along with a margin of the normal thyroid tissue all around.
Ref: A Concise Textbook of Surgery, S. Das, 3rd Ed, Chapter37, Pg 651

Q. 119. A 65 year old male smoker presents with gross total hematuria. The most likely diagnosis is (ALL INDIA-03)
(a) Carcinoma urinary bladder
(b) Benign prostatic hyperplasia
(c) Carcinoma prostate
(d) Cystolithiasis

Ans. (a)

Note
The most likely diagnosis is carcinoma urinary bladder.

Also see
Increased risk of bladder cancer is seen with use of aniline dyes, cigarette smoking, S. hematobium, and Balkhan nephropathy.
C/F: Painless haematuria is by far the commonest symptom and should be regarded as indicating of bladder cancer unless proved otherwise.
Ref: Bailey and Love's Short Practice of Surgery, 24th Ed, Chapter 65, Pg-1229

Q. 120. A 10-mm calculus in the right lower ureter associated with proximal hydrouretero-nephrosis is best treated with (ALL INDIA-03)
(a) Extracorporeal shockwave lithotripsy
(b) Antegrade percutaneous access
(c) Open ureterolithotomy
(d) Ureteroscopic retrieval

Ans. (d)
Note
The best treatment for above clinical presentation is 'Ureteroscopic retrieval'.

Also see
The explanations for above options are as under:
a. Extracorporeal shockwave lithotripsy is used in cases of renal calculi (Pg 1187)
b. Antegrade percutaneous access is also used in case of renal calculi (Pg 1185)
c. Open ureterolithotomy indications are: repeated attacks of pain, enlarging stone, UTI, obstruction of kidney, and a very large stone. (Pg 1189)
d. Ureteroscopic retrieval is used to retrieve stones impacted in the ureter (Pg 1190)
Ref: Bailey and Love's Short Practice of Surgery, 24th Ed, Chapter 64

Q. 121. Semen analysis of a young man who presented with primary infertility revealed low volume, fructose negative ejaculate with azoospermia. Which of the following is the most useful imaging modality to evaluate the cause of his infertility? (ALL INDIA-03)
(a) Colour duplex ultrasonography of the scrotum
(b) Transrectal ultrasonography
(c) Retrograde urethrography
(d) Spermatic venography

Ans. (b)
Note
The most useful imaging modality to evaluate the cause of infertility is transrectal ultrasonography.

Also see
The fluid part of semen is contributed chiefly by the prostate and seminal vesicles. Fructose is contributed by seminal vesicles. Its main function is that it acts as a metabolic fuel for the sperms. So any pathology in seminal vesicle and prostate may contribute to infertility. Thus for preliminary investigation trans-rectal ultrasound is the best modality for investigation.
Ref: Textbook of Physiology Vol 2, unit 10, Ch 2, Pg-769

Q. 122. A 70 year old patient with benign prostatic hyperplasia underwent transurethral resection of prostate under spinal anaesthesia. One hour later, he developed vomiting and altered sensorium. The most probable cause is (ALL INDIA-03)
(a) Overdosage of spinal anaesthetic agent
(b) Rupture of bladder
(c) Hyperkalemia
(d) Water intoxication

Ans. (d)
Note
The most probable cause for above presentation is 'water intoxication'.

Also see
The absorption of water into circulation at the time of 'Transurethral resection' can give rise to congestive cardiac failure, hyponatremia, and hemolysis. The patient may therefore present with confusion and other cerebral events mimicking a stroke.
Ref: Bailey and Love's Short Practice of Surgery, 24th Ed, Chapter, Pg 66, 1247

Q. 123. The commonest cause of an obliterative stricture of the membranous urethra is (ALL INDIA-03)
    (a)   Fall-astride injury
    (b)   Road-traffic accident with fracture pelvis and rupture urethra
    (c)   Prolonged catheterization
    (d)   Gonococcal infection

Ans. (b)
Note
The commonest cause is traumatic particularly rupture of the membranous part of urethra following trauma to pelvis.

Also see
Various causes of stricture are:
    -Congenital
    -Traumatic
    -Inflammatory-post gonococcal, tuberculous, post urethral chancre
    -Instrumental- following endoscopy
    -Post-operative following amputation of penis, open prostatectomy
Ref: A Concise Textbook of Surgery, S. Das, 3rd Ed, Chapter 59, Pg 1262

Q. 124. Which of the following is an absolute indication for surgery in cases of benign prostatic hyperplasia (ALL INDIA-03)
    (a)   Bilateral hydroureteronephrosis
    (b)   Nocturnal frequency
    (c)   Recurrent urinary tract infection
    (d)   Voiding bladder pressures >50 cm of water

Ans. (a)
Note
Bilateral hydroureteronephrosis is an absolute indication for surgery in case of BHP.

Also see
Strong indications for treatment are:
    -Acute retention
    -Chronic retention with renal impairment-residual urine of 220 ml or more, hydroureter and hydronephrosis.
    -Hemorrhage
    -Low maximum flow rate (<10ml/sec) and an increase in residual volume of urine (100-200ml).
    -Bladder outflow obstruction-stone, infection
Ref: Bailey and Love's Short Practice of Surgery, 24th Ed, Chapter, Pg 66, and 1243

Q. 125. A 27 year old man presents with a left testicular tumor with a 10 cm retroperitoneal lymph node mass. The treatment of choice is (ALL INDIA-03)
    (a)   Radiotherapy
    (b)   Immunotherapy with interferon and inter-leukins
    (c)   Left high inguinal orchidectomy plus chemotherapy
    (d)   Chemotherapy alone

Ans. (c)
Note
Left high inguinal orchidectomy plus chemotherapy is the treatment of choice in above given case.

Also see
As soon as diagnosis is established inguinal orchidectomy with high cord ligation at the deep inguinal ring is mandatory. After that the treatment differs according to the histopathological type of tumor.
-In seminoma: If there's involvement of retro peritoneal lymph nodes then stage is 2nd and its treatment involves radiotherapy of 3500 rads.
-In Teratoma: Radical node dissection and radiotherapy are done.

Q. 126. The best time for surgery of hypospadias is (ALL INDIA-03)
    (a)   1-4 months of age
    (b)   6-10 months of age
    (c)   12-18 months of age
    (d)   2-4 years of age

Ans. (b)
Note
The best time for surgery of hypospadias is 6 – 10 months of age.

Also see
Hypospadias is a disorder in which the male urethral opening is not located at the tip of the penis. The urethral opening can be located anywhere along the urethra. Most commonly with hypospadias, the opening is located along the underside of the penis, near the tip. Hypospadias can be repaired with surgery. Usually, the surgical repair is done when the baby is between 6 and 12 months, when penile growth is minimal.
Ref: http://www.healthsystem.virginia.edu/uvahealth/peds_hrnewborn/hsp.cfm

Q. 127. The Hunterian Ligature operation is performed for (ALL INDIA-03)
    (a)   Varicose veins
    (b)   Arteriovenous fistulae
    (c)   Aneurysm
    (d)   Acute ischemia

Ans. (c)
Note
The Hunterian Ligature operation is performed for 'Aneurism'.

Also see
The process of arterial ligation is becoming absolute now-a-days since the collateral circulation maintains blood flow through aneurysm and if collateral circulation is inadequate, gangrene can occur. Different methods of ligation are:
    -Anel's method-ligation proximal to the sac
    -Brasdor's method-ligation just distal to the sac
    -Hunter's method-ligation applied immediately above the branch of the artery
    -Wardrop's method-immediately below a branch of the artery
Ref: A Concise Textbook of Surgery, S. Das, 3rd Ed, Chapter 15, Pg 191

Q. 128. Sympathectomy is indicated in all the following conditions except (ALL INDIA-03)
    (a)   Ischaemic ulcers
    (b)   Intermittent claudication
    (c)   Anhidrosis
    (d)   Acrocyanosis

Ans. (c)
Note
Sympathectomy is indicated in all of the above conditions except 'Anhidrosis'.

Also see
Indications of sympathetectomy are:
a.   Rest pain and minor ulceration
b.   Buerger's disease
c.   Raynaud's disease and other vasospastic conditions
d.   Senile gangrene
Ref: A Concise Textbook of Surgery, S. Das, 3rd Ed, Chapter 15, Pg 154, 169

Q. 129. A patient suddenly experienced pain radiating along the medial border of the dorsum of foot. Which of the following nerve is most likely to be accidently ligated? (ALL INDIA-02)
    (a)   Sural nerve
    (b)   Saphenous nerve
    (c)   Deep peroneal nerve
    (d)   Genicular nerve

Ans. (b)
Note
In above given presentation the most likely nerve involved is 'Saphenous nerve'.
Also see
The saphenous nerve is a branch of posterior division of the femoral nerve. It pierces the deep fascia on the medial side of the knee. It supplies the skin of the medial side of the leg and medial border of the foot up to the ball of the great toe.
Ref: B.D. Chaurasia's Human Anatomy, 3rd Ed, Vol 2, Chapter, Pg 8, 81

Q. 130. In an adult patient with pleural effusion, the most appropriate site for pleurocentesis done by inserting a needle is in (ALL INDIA-02)
    (a)   5th intercostal space in midclavicular line
    (b)   7th intercostal space in midaxillary line
    (c)   2nd intercostal space adjacent to the sternum
    (d)   10th intercostal space adjacent to the vertebral column

Ans. (b)
Note
In pleural effusion, the most appropriate site for pleurocentesis done by inserting a needle is in '7th intercostal space in midaxillary line'.
Also see
Pleurocentesis is performed under local anesthesia using aseptic precautions. The needle is introduced in 7th intercostal space in midaxillary line, just above the rib (to avoid damage to neurovascular bundle) at the point of maximum dullness. Fluid is withdrawn for diagnosis and symptomatic relief. Too much fluid should not be withdrawn as it causes pulmonary oedema.
Ref: Bailey and Love's Short Practice of Surgery, 24th Ed, Chapter 47, Pg 793, Fig 47.29

Q. 131. A 24 years old man falls on the ground when he is struck in the right temple by a baseball. While being driven to the hospital, he lapses into coma. He is unresponsive with the dilated right pupil when he reaches the emergency department. The most important step in initial management is (ALL INDIA-02)
    (a)   Craniotomy
    (b)   CT scan of the head
    (c)   X-ray of the skull and cervical spine
    (d)   Doppler ultrasound examination of the neck

Ans. (a)
Note
The most important step in intital management is 'craniotomy'.
Also see
The events in this case suggest right subdural haematoma.

Q. 132. Not a feature of de Quervain's disease (ALL INDIA-02)
    (a)   Autoimmune in etiology
    (b)   Raised ESR
    (c)   Tends to regress spontaneously
    (d)   Painful & associated with enlargement of thyroid

Ans. (a)
Note
'Autoimmune etiology' is not a feature of de Quervain's disease'.

Also see
Granulomatous thyroiditis or de Quervain's or sub acute thyroiditis is a self-limiting inflammation of the thyroid gland. Etiology of the condition is not known but clinical feature of prodromal phase and preceding respiratory infection suggests a viral etiology. Patient presents with painful thyroid gland, fever, and features of hyperthyroidism.
Ref: Textbook of Pathology by Harsh Mohan, 4th Ed, Chapter 24, Pg 790

Q. 133. A 35 years old woman has had recurrent episodes of headache and sweating. Her mother had renal calculi and died of thyroid cancer. Physical observations revealed a thyroid nodule and ipsilateral enlarged cervical lymph nodes. Before performing thyroid surgery the woman's physician should order (ALL INDIA-02)
    (a)   Thyroid scan
    (b)   Estimation of hydroxy indole acetic acid in urine
    (c)   Estimation of urinary metanephrines, VMA and catecholamines
    (d)   Estimation of TSH, and TRH levels in serum

Ans. (c)
Note
The investigations suggested in above situation are 'estimation of urinary metaphrines, VMA and catecholamines'.
Also see
Since the patient's mother had thyroid cancer; the patient may be suffering from multiple endocrine neoplasias. Patients are in the age group of 20-60 yrs. In this pheochromocytoma is associated with medullary carcinoma of thyroid, hyperparathyroidism, pituitary adenoma, and mucosal neuromas. The C/F is due to secretion of catecholamines. Most common feature is: -hypertension. Diagnosis is established by measuring 24 hr urinary catecholamines or their metabolites-metanephrine and VMA.
Ref: Textbook of Pathology by Harsh Mohan, 4th Ed, Chapter 24, Pg 785

Q. 134. All of the following are associated with thyroid storm, except (ALL INDIA-02)
    (a)   Surgery for thyroiditis
    (b)   Surgery for thyrotoxicosis
    (c)   Stressful illness in thyrotoxicosis
    (d)   I131 therapy for thyrotoxicosis

Ans. (a)
Note
All of above associated with thyroid storm, except 'Surgery for thyroiditis'.
Also see
Thyroid Storm
When the levels of thyroid hormones become very high in a patient who has hyperthyroidism, the symptoms get worse and can result in a serious condition called thyroid storm. One major sign of thyroid storm that differentiates it from plain hyperthyroidism is a marked elevation of body temperature, which may be as high as 105-106 °F
Causes of Thyroid Storm are:
    -Infections, especially of the lung
    -Thyroid surgery in patients with overactive thyroid gland
    -Stopping medications given for hyperthyroidism
    -Too high dose of thyroid
    -Treatment with radioactive iodine
    -Pregnancy
    -Heart attack or heart emergencies
Ref:-http://www.emedicinehealth.com/thyroid_storm/page2_em.htm

Q. 135. Needle biopsy of solitary thyroid nodule in a young woman with palpable cervical lymph nodes on the same sides demonstrates amyloid in stroma of lesion. Likely diagnosis is (ALL INDIA-02)
    (a)   Medullary carcinoma thyroid
    (b)   Follicular carcinoma thyroid

(c) Thyroid adenoma
(d) Multinodular goitre

Ans. (a)
Note
The likely diagnosis for above condition is 'Medullary carcinoma thyroid'.
Also see
Medullary tumor is tumor of the parafollicular cells derived from the neural crest. There is a high level of characteristic amyloid stroma. They produce high levels of calcitonin. Lymph node involvement occurs in 50-60% of the cases and blood borne metastasis is common.
Ref: Bailey and Love's Short Practice of Surgery, 24th Ed, Chapter, Pg 44, 731

Q. 136. A 26 years old woman presents with a palpable thyroid nodule, and needle biopsy demonstrates amyloid in the stroma of the lesion. A cervical lymph node is palpable on the same side as the lesion. The preferred treatment should be (ALL INDIA-02)
(a) Removal of the involved node, the isthmus, and the enlarged lymph node.
(b) Removal of the involved lobe, the isthmus, a portion of the opposite lobe, and the enlarged lymph node.
(c) Total thyroidectomy and modified neck dissection on the side of the enlarged lymph node.
(d) Total thyroidectomy and irradiation of the cervical lymph nodes.

Ans. (c)
Note
Treatment of medullary carcinoma is by total thyroidectomy and resection of the involved lymph nodes with either a radical or modified neck dissection.
Ref: Bailey and Love's Short Practice of Surgery, 24th Ed, Chapter, Pg 44, 732

Q. 137. The most common tumour of the salivary gland is (ALL INDIA-02)
(a) Mucoepidermoid tumor
(b) Warthin's tumor
(c) Acinic cell tumor
(d) Pleomorphic adenoma

Ans. (d)
Note
Pleomorphic adenoma is most common tumor of the salivary gland.
Also see
Pleomorphic adenoma accounts for >75% of parotid tumors, 50% of submandibular tumors. It is a benign tumor and very rarely after a number of years may undergo malignant transformation.
Ref: Bailey and Love's Short Practice of Surgery, Chapter 42, Pg 659

Q. 138. The premalignant condition with the highest probability of progression to malignancy is (ALL INDIA-02)
(a) Dysplasia
(b) Hyperplasia
(c) Leucoplakia
(d) Erythroplakia

Ans. (d)
Note
The premalignat condition with highest probability of progression to malignancy is 'Erythroplakia'.
Also see
(a) Dysplasia is an abnormality of development.
(b) Hyperplasia is increase in volume of a tissue or an organ caused by the formation and growth of new cells.
Ref: Dorland's Pocket Medcial Dictionary, 21st Ed.

(c) Leukoplakia: It is a small-circumscribed white plaque to an extensive lesion involving wide areas of oral mucosa. The incidence of ultimate malignant transformation increases with age.

(d) Erythroplakia: Any lesion of the oral mucosa that presents as a bright red velvety appearing plaque. In some cases it is associated with leukoplakia. The incidence of malignant transformation is 17-fold higher than leukoplakia.

Ref: Bailey and Love's Short Practice of Surgery, 24th Ed, Chapter 41, Pg 639

Q. 139. Corkscrew esophagus is seen in which of the following condition? (ALL INDIA-02)
    (a) Carcinoma esophagus
    (b) Scleroderma
    (c) Achalasia cardia
    (d) Diffuse esophagus spasm

Ans. (d)

Note
Corkscrew esophagus is seen in 'diffuse esophagus spasm'.

Also see
It is a condition in which there are incordinated contractions of the esophagus causing dysphagia and chest pain. The condition may be dramatic with spastic pressures on manometry of 400-500 mm of Hg, marked hypertrophy of circular muscle and a cork screw oesophagus on Barium swallow.

Ref: Bailey and Love's Short Practice of Surgery, 24th Ed, Chapter 50, Pg 885

Q. 140. Barrett's esophagus is (ALL INDIA-02)
    (a) Lower esophagus lined by columnar epithelium
    (b) Upper esophagus lined by columnar epithelium
    (c) Lower esophagus lined by ciliated epithelium
    (d) Lower esophagus lined by pseudostratified epithelium

Ans. (a)

Note
Barrett's esophagus is lower esophagus lined by columnar epithelium.

Also see
Barrett's esophagus is a metaplastic change in the lining of the esophagus in response to chronic GERD. In Barrett's esophagus the junction between the squamous esophageal mucosa and gastric mucosa moves proximally. There is a high risk of developing CA so the patients should be screened regularly.

Ref: Bailey and Love's Short Practice of Surgery, 24th Ed, Chapter 50, Pg 869

The most widely accepted theory for Barrett's esophagus is that damage to the squamous mucosa initiates a process of healing. There are cells lying deep in the wall of the esophagus that have the potential to transform themselves into a variety of shapes and take on special functions during this healing process. It is these cells that become the new columnar mucosa of the esophagus. Barrett's esophagus is caused by chronic reflux of acid from the stomach into the esophagus.

Ref: http://www.sts.org/doc/4490

Q. 141. The adenocarcinoma of esophagus develops in (ALL INDIA-02)
    (a) Barrett's esophagus
    (b) Long standing achalasia
    (c) Corrosive stricture
    (d) Alcohol abuse

Ans. (a)

Note
The adenocarcinoma of esophagus develops in 'Barrett's esophagus'.

Also see
In Barrett's esophagus several types of gastric mucosa may be found in lower esophagus. When intestinal metaplasia occurs there is an increased risk of adenocarcinoma of the esophagus about 25 times that of general population.

Ref: Bailey and Love's Short Practice of Surgery, 24th Ed, Chapter 50, Pg 869

Q. 142. The lowest recurrence of peptic ulcer is associated with (ALL INDIA-02)
  (a) Gastric resection
  (b) Vagotomy + drainage
  (c) Vagotomy + antrectomy
  (d) Highly selective vagotomy

Ans. (c)
Note
The lowest recurrence of peptic ulcer is associated with 'Vagotomy + antrectomy'.
Also see
In addition to a truncal vagotomy the antrum of the stomach is removed, thus removing the source of gastrin and the gastric remnant is joined to the duodenum. The recurrence rate is exceedingly low.
Ref: Bailey and Love's Short Practice of Surgery, 24th Ed, Chapter 51, Pg 910

Q. 143. Risk factor for development of gastric CA (ALL INDIA-02)
  (a) Blood group O
  (b) Duodenal ulcer
  (c) Intestinal hyperplasia
  (d) Intestinal metaplasia type III

Ans. (d)
Note
Risk factor for development of gastric CA is 'Intestinal metaplasia type III'.
Also see
a. Blood group O; Not a risk factor rather blood group A has predilection for gastric ulcer. Gastric ulcers develop into CA
b. Duodenal ulcer does not change into CA
c. Intestinal hyperplasia; NA
d. Intestinal metaplasia type III; Intestinal metaplasia occurs in chronic gastirtis and involves anteral mucosa, and it predisposes to CA
Ref; Textbook of Pathology by Harshmohan 4th Ed, Pg-524
Risk factors for gastric CA
  -H. pylori-associated with gastritis, intestinal metaplasia, and gastric atrophy
  -Pernicious anemia
  -Gastric atrophy and polyp
  -Peptic ulcer surgery
  -Intestinal metaplasia
  -Cigarette smoking and dust ingestion
  -Excessive salt intake, deficiency of anti-oxidants and exposure to N-nitroso compounds
Ref: Bailey and Love's Short Practice of Surgery, 24th Ed, Chapter 51, Pg 919

Q. 144. In a case of hypertrophic pyloric stenosis, the metabolic disturbance is (ALL INDIA-02)
  (a) Respiratory alkalosis
  (b) Metabolic acidosis
  (c) Metabolic alkalosis with paradoxical aciduria
  (d) Metabolic alkalosis with alkaline urine

Ans. (c)
Note
In a case of hypertrophic pyloric stenosis, the metabolic disturbance is 'Metabolic alkalosis with paradoxical aciduria'.
Also see
Vomiting of HCl leads to hypochloremic alkalosis. Initially the sodium and potassium may be relatively normal. However as dehydration progresses more profound metabolic abnormalities arise. Initially the urine has low chloride and high bicarbonate, but because of dehydration a phase of sodium retention follows and potassium and hydrogen are excreted in preference. This results in the urine becoming paradoxically acidic and hypokalemia ensues.
Ref: Bailey and Love's Short Practice of Surgery, 24th Ed, Chapter 51, Pg 917

MCQ's in Surgery 571

Q. 145. All of the following indicates early gastric cancer except (ALL INDIA-02)
    (a)   Involvement of mucosa
    (b)   Involvement of mucosa and submucosa
    (c)   Involvement of mucosa, submucosa and muscularis
    (d)   Involvement of mucosa, submucosa and adjacent lymph nodes

Ans. (c)
Note
All the following indicates early gastric cancer except 'involvement of mucosa, submucosa and muscularis'
Also see
Gastric CA can be divided into early and late. Early CA is limited to the mucosa and submucosa with or without involvement of the lymph nodes. This can be protruding, superficial or excavated.
Muscularis is involved in the late stages.
Ref: Bailey and Love's Short Practice of Surgery, 24th Ed, Chapter 51, Pg 922

Q. 146. In gastric outlet obstruction in a peptic ulcer patient, the site of obstruction is most likely to be (ALL INDIA-02)
    (a)   Antrum
    (b)   Duodenum
    (c)   Pylorus
    (d)   Pyloric canal

Ans. (b)
Note
In gastric outlet obstruction in a peptic ulcer patient, the site of obstruction is most likely to be 'duodenum'.
Also see
The two common causes of GOO (gastric outlet obstruction) are: - gastric cancer and pyloric stenosis secondary to peptic ulcer. Commonly when the condition is due to underlying peptic ulcer disease, the stenosis is found in the first part of duodenum.
Ref: Bailey and Love's Short Practice of Surgery, 24th Ed, Chapter 51, Pg 917

Q. 147. Ramesh met with an accident with a car and has been in 'deep coma' for the last 15 days. The most suitable route for the administration of protein and calories is by (ALL INDIA-02)
    (a)   Jejunostomy tube feeding
    (b)   Gastrostomy tube feeding
    (c)   Nasogastric tube feeding
    (d)   Central venous hyperalimentation

Ans. (a)
Note
The most suitable route for the administration of protein and calories is by 'Jejunostomy tube feeding'
Also see
It is of importance in controlling infusion rate of nutrients. Advantages are-more effective nutrient delivery decreased abdominal discomfort and decreased incidence of osmotic diarrhea.
Ref: Bailey and Love's Short Practice of Surgery, 24th Ed, Pg 69-70

Q. 148. A 10 months old infant present with acute intestinal obstruction. Contrast enema X-ray shows the intussusception. Likely cause is (ALL INDIA-02)
    (a)   Peyer's patch hypertrophy
    (b)   Mekel's diverticulum
    (c)   Mucosal polyp
    (d)   Duplication cyst

Ans. (a)
Note
The likely cause for above is 'Pyer's patch hypertrophy'.

Also see
Intussusception occurs when one portion of the gut becomes invaginated within an immediately adjacent segment. It is seen in children after weaning. It is believed to be due to hyperplasia of peyer's patches in the terminal ileum, which occurs secondary to weaning.
Ref: Bailey and Love's Short Practice of Surgery, 24th Ed, Chapter 58, Pg 1067

Q. 149. After undergoing surgery, for carcinoma of colon, a 44 year old patient developed single liver metastasis of 2 cm. What do you do next? (ALL INDIA-02)
(a) Resection
(b) Chemo-radiation
(c) Acetic acid injection
(d) Radiofrequency ablation

Ans. (a)
Note
The next option is liver resection.
Also see
Metastasis of colonic carcinoma is carried to the liver via the portal system. Patients with upto 2 or 3 liver metastasis confined to 1 lobe of the liver may be offered hepatic resection. In multiple painful hepatic metastasis cytotoxic drugs, cryotherapy or laser can achieve palliation.
Ref: Bailey and Love's Short Practice of Surgery, 24th Ed, Chapter 57, Pg 1050 & 1053

Q. 150. Ten days after a splenectomy for blunt abdominal trauma, a 23 years old man complains of upper abdominal and lower chest pain exacerbated by deep breathing. He is anorectic but ambulatory and otherwise making satisfactory progress. On physical examination, his temperature is 38.2°C (108°F) rectally, and he has decreased breath sounds at the left lung base. His abdominal wound appears to be healing well, bowel sounds are active and there are no peritoneal signs. Rectal examination is negative. The WBC count is 12,500 per mm^3 with a shift to left Chest X-ray shows plate like atelectasis of the left lung field. Abdominal X-rays show a nonspecific gas pattern in the bowel and an air-fluid level in the left upper quadrant serum amylase is 150 Somogyi units/dl (normal 60 to 80). The most likely diagnosis is (ALL INDIA-02)
(a) Subphrenic abscess
(b) Pancreatitis
(c) Pulmonary embolism
(d) Subfascial wound infection

Ans. (a)
Note
The most likely diagnosis for above is 'subphrenic abscess'.
Also see
As per the question patient has:
a. Pyrexia (108 F)
b. Decreased breath sounds of left lung base
c. Increased WBC counts
d. Collapse of base of left lung
e. Air fluid level in the left upper quadrant of abdomen
f. Level of S. amylase (Which is towards the upper limits of normal; however it should be much more in case of pancreatitis)
The all above features point to a diagnosis of subphrenic abscess
Ref: Bailey and Love's Short Practice of Surgery, 24th Ed, Chapter 56, Pg 1013

Q. 151. Sentinel lymph node biopsy is an important part of the management of which of the following conditions? (ALL INDIA-02)
(a) Carcinoma prostate
(b) Carcinoma breast
(c) Carcinoma lung
(d) Carcinoma nasopharynx

Ans. (b)

Note

Sentinel lymph node biopsy is an important part of the management of 'Carcinoma breast'.

Also see

Sentinel node biopsy is a technique currently under evaluation, which may well prove the way forward in the future in the management of the patients with clinically node negative disease. The sentinel node is localized perioperatively by the injection of patent blue dye and /or radioisotope labeled albumin near the tumor. In patients in whom there is no tumor involvement of sentinel node further axillary detection can be avoided.
Ref: Bailey and Love's Short Practice of Surgery, 24th Ed, Chapter 46, Pg 767

Q. 152. All of the following are the clinical features of thromboangitis obliterans except (ALL INDIA-02)
- (a) Raynaud's phenomenon
- (b) Claudication of extremeties
- (c) Absence of popliteal pulse
- (d) Migratory superficial thrombophlebitis

Ans. (c)

Note

All of the above are the clinical features of thromboangitis obliterans except 'Absence of popliteal pulse'.

Also see

Buerger's disease or thromboangitis obliterans is characterized by occlusive disease of small and medium sized arteries. Thrombophlebitis of superficial or deep veins and raynaud's phenomenon occurring in male patients of young age group.
In lower extremities the disease commonly affects arteries beyond the popliteal artery starting in tibial arteries extending to the vessels of foot.
Ref: Bailey and Love's Short Practice of Surgery, 24th Ed, Chapter 15, Pg 231
Ref: A Concise Textbook of Surgery, S. Das, 3rd Ed, Chapter Pg15, 173

Q. 153. Rani, a 16 years old girl who has non-pitting edema of recent onset affecting her right leg but no other symptoms is referred for evaluation.True statements about this patient include (ALL INDIA-02)
- (a) Prophylactic antibiotics are indicated.
- (b) A lymphagiongram will show hypoplasia of the lymphatics.
- (c) Elastic stocking and diuretics will lead to a normal appearance of the limb.
- (d) A variety of operations will ultimately lead to a normal appearance of the limb.

Ans. (b)

Note

True statements about this patient include 'A lymphagiongram will show hypoplasia of the lymphatics'.

Also see

Lymphoedema is the end result of insufficient lymphatic outflow due to aplasia, hypoplasia primary decreased lymphatic contractility or inflammatory obliteration. Contrast lymphangiography remains the standard by which all other lymphatic imaging is judged and provides precise information about the anatomy of the lymphatic system.
Ref: Bailey and Love's Short Practice of Surgery, 24th Ed, Chapter 17, Pg 258

Q. 154. All of the following statements about acute adrenal insufficiency are true except (ALL INDIA-02)
- (a) Hyperglycemia is usually present.
- (b) Acute adrenal insufficiency usually is secondary to exogenous glucocorticoid administration.
- (c) Acute adrenal insufficiency presents with weakness, vomiting, fever, and hypotension.
- (d) Hyponatremia occurs because of impaired renal tubule sodium resorption.

Ans. (a)

Note

All of the above statements about acute adrenal insufficiency are true except 'hyperglycemia is usually present'.

Also see
Acute adrenal crisis is a medical emergency caused by a lack of cortisol. Patients may experience lightheadedness or dizziness, weakness, sweating, abdominal pain, nausea and vomiting, or even loss of consciousness.
Adrenal crisis occurs if the adrenal gland is deteriorating (Addison's disease, primary adrenal insufficiency), if there is pituitary gland injury (secondary adrenal insufficiency), or if adrenal insufficiency is not adequately treated.
Risk factors for adrenal crisis include physical stress such as infection, dehydration, trauma, or surgery, adrenal gland or pituitary gland injury, and ending treatment with steroids such as prednisone or hydrocortisone too early.

Clinical features are:
- Headache
- Profound weakness
- Vomiting
- Low blood pressure
- Dehydration
- High fever
- Shaking chills
- Confusion or coma
- Joint pain
- Abdominal pain
- Unintentional weight loss
- Rapid respiratory rate (see tachypnea).
- Unusual and excessive sweating on face and/or palms.

Signs and test:
- An ACTH (cortisone) stimulation test shows low cortisol.
- The baseline cortisol level is low.
- Fasting blood sugar may be low.
- Serum potassium is elevated (usually primary adrenal insufficiency).
- Serum sodium is decreased (usually primary adrenal insufficiency).

Ref: http://www.nlm.nih.gov/medlineplus/ency/article/000357.htm

Q. 155. All of the following are correct statements about radiological evaluation of a pateint with Cushing's syndrome except (ALL INDIA-02)
  (a) MRI of the sella turcica will identify a pituitary cause for Cushing's syndrome.
  (b) Petrosal sinus sampling is the best way to distinguish a pituitary tumor from an ectopic ACTH producing tumor.
  (c) MRI of the adrenals may distinguish adrenal adenoma from carcinoma.
  (d) Adrenal CT scan distinguishes adrenal cortical hyperplasia from an adrenal tumor.

Ans. (a)
Note
All of the above are correct statements about radiological evaluation of a pateint with Cushing's syndrome except 'MRI of the sell a turcica will identify a pituitary cause for Cushing's syndrome'.

Also see
Pituitary CT has replaced other techniques for detection of pituitary macro adenomas in Cushing's disease.
B/L selective inferior petrosal venous sinus sampling for ACTH levels is a valuable method for confirmation of pituitary dependant Cushing's disease.
Ref: Bailey and Love's Short Practice of Surgery, 24th Ed, Chapter 45, Pg 743

Q. 156. A male aged 60 years has foul breath. He regurgitates food that is eaten 3 days ago. Likely diagnosis is (ALL INDIA-01)
  (a) Zenker's diverticulum
  (b) Meckel's diverticulum
  (c) Scleroderma
  (d) Achalasia cardia

Ans. (a)

Note
Likely diagnosis in above clinical presentation is 'Zenker's diverticulum'.

Also see
It is a pharyngo-esophageal diverticulum as it protrudes posteriorly above the cricopharyngeal sphincter through natural weak points between the oblique and horizontal fibres of inferior pharyngeal constrictor.
C/Fs are: -effortless regurgitation, cervical dysphagia, and gurgling sensation on swallowing.
Ref: A Concise Textbook of Surgery, S. Das, 3rd Ed, Chapter 43, Pg 804

Q. 157. Most common site for squamous cell carcinoma esophagus is (ALL INDIA-01)
- (a) Upper third
- (b) Middle third
- (c) Lower third
- (d) Gastro-esophageal junction

Ans. Use your discretion

Note
Most common site for squamous cell carcinoma esophagus is upper third and middle third. Ans both a and b could be equally correct.

Also see
Squamous cell carcinoma and adenocarcinoma are the commonest esophageal cancers. SCCA affects the upper 2/3rds of the esophagus and adenocarcinoma affects the lower 1/3rds of the esophagus.
Ref: Bailey and Love's Short Practice of Surgery, 24th Ed, Chapter 50, Pg 873

Q. 158. What is true regarding congenital hypertrophic pyloric stenosis? (ALL INDIA-01)
- (a) More common in girls
- (b) Hypochloremic alkalosis
- (c) Heller's myotomy is the procedure of choice
- (d) Most often manifests at birth

Ans. (b)

Note
What is true regarding congenital hypertrophic pyloric stenosis 'Hyperchloremic alkalosis'.

Also see
In pyloric stenosis vomiting of hydrochloric acid leads to hypochloremic alkalosis.
Ref: Bailey and Love's Short Practice of Surgery, 24th Ed, Chapter 51, Pg 917

Q. 159. A Patient presents with recurrent duodenal ulcer of 2.5 cm size. Procedure of choice is (ALL INDIA-01)
- (a) Truncal vagotomy and antrectomy
- (b) Truncal vagotomy and gastrojejunostomy
- (c) Highly selective vagotomy
- (d) Laparoscopic vagotomy and gastrojejunostomy

Ans. (a)

Note
The procedure of choice for above case is 'Truncal vagotomy and anterectomy'.

Also see
In this procedure truncal vagotomy in addition to removal of antrum of the stomach is done, thus removing the source of gastrin. The gastric remnant is joined to the duodenum. The recurrence rate is exceedingly low.
Ref: Bailey and Love's Short Practice of Surgery, 24th Ed, Chapter 51, Pg 910

Q. 160. All are features of hyperplastic tuberculosis of gastrointestinal tract except (ALL INDIA-01)
- (a) Presents with a mass in RIF (Right iliac fossa).
- (b) Barium meal shows pulled up caecum.
- (c) Most common site is ileocecal junction.
- (d) ATT is the treatment of choice.

Ans. (d)

Note
The entire above are features of hyperplastic tuberculosis of gastrointestinal tract except 'Most common site is ileocecal junciton'.

Also see
It affects the terminal 2 inches of the ileum and caecum. Infection first starts in the lymphoid follicles and spreads to the submucous and subserous planes. Patient presents with abdominal pain off and on due to sub-acute intestinal obstruction. A mass may be present in the right iliac fossa. Barium meal shows:
- Persistent narrowing of the affected segment.
- Caecum is pulled up.
- Ileocaecal angle is widened.

Treatment: If obstruction is present surgery is the method of choice.
Ref: A Concise Textbook of Surgery, S. Das, 3rd Ed, Chapter 49, Pg 967

Q. 161. A 56 year old woman has not passed stools for the last 14 days. X-ray shows no air/fluid levels. Probable diagnosis is (ALL INDIA-01)
    (a)   Paralytic ileus
    (b)   Aganglionosis of the colon
    (c)   Intestinal pseudo-obstruction
    (d)   Duodenal obstruction

Ans. (c)
Note
Probable diagnosis is 'intestinal pseudo-obstruction'.

Also see
Both duodenal obstruction and paralytic ileus show multiple air fluid levels therefore they have been excluded. **Abdominal** radiographs showing evidence of colonic obstruction with marked caecal distention characterize **pseudo-obstruction** of the colon. The presentation is in the form of acute or chronic intestinal obstruction.
Ref: Bailey and Love's Short Practice of Surgery, 24th Ed, Chapter 58, Pg 1074

Q. 162. A man aged 60 years has history of IHD and atherosclerosis. He presents with abdominal pain and maroon stools. Most likely diagnosis is (ALL INDIA-01)
    (a)   Acute intestinal obstruction
    (b)   Acute mesenteric ischemia
    (c)   Peritonitis
    (d)   Appendicitis

Ans. (b)
Note
Most likely diagnosis for above is 'Acute mesenteric ischaemia'.

Also see
Mesenteric vascular disease may be classified as acute intestinal ischaemia with or without occlusion. The superior mesenteric vessels are most likely to be affected.
Possible sources are:
a.   Left atrium associated with fibrillation
b.   A mural myocardial infarct
c.   An atheromatous plaque from aortic aneurysm & mitral valve vegetation.
Clinical features are:
- Abdominal pain-central
- Persistent vomiting and defecation
- Passage of altered blood in stool

Ref: Bailey and Love's Short Practice of Surgery, 24th Ed, Chapter 58, Pg 1074

Q. 163. True statement regarding 'fistula-in-ano' is (ALL INDIA-01)
    (a)   Posterior fistulae have straight tracks.
    (b)   High fistulae can be operated with no fear of incontinence.
    (c)   High and low divisions are made in relation to the pelvic floor.
    (d)   Intersphincteric is the most common type.

Ans. (d)

Note
'Intersphincteric is the most common type' is the true statement regarding 'fistula-in-ano'.

Also see
a. Fistulas with an external opening in relation to the anterior ½ of the anus tend to be of the direct type. Those with an external opening in relation to posterior ½ of the anus usually have curving tracks. (Pg 1137)
b. High fistula can only be treated by staged operations because there is a risk of incontinence.
c. Anal fistulas are of two types-High or Low depending on whether it is above or below the anorectal ring.

Ref: Bailey and Love's Short Practice of Surgery, 24th Ed, Chapter 61 Pg 1136, 1337

Q. 164. In a 27 year old male most common cause of a colovesical fistula would be (ALL INDIA-01)
    (a) Crohn's disease
    (b) Ulcerative colitis
    (c) TB
    (d) Cancer colon

Ans. (a)

Note
In a 27 year old male most common cause of a colovesical fistula would be 'crohn's disease'.

Also see
Fistulous connections between loops of affected bowel or between bowel & bladder, or vagina are specific complications of Crohn's disease.
Ref: Davidson's Principles and Practice of Medicine, 19th Ed, Chapter 17, Pg 812

Q. 165. Following trauma, a patient presents with a drop of blood at the tip of urinary meatus. He complaint's of inability to pass urine. Next step should be (ALL INDIA-01)
    (a) IVP should be done
    (b) MCU should be done
    (c) Catheterize, drain bladder and remove the catheter thereafter
    (d) Catheterize, drain bladder and retain the catheter thereafter

Ans. (d)

Note
Next step in above case should be 'catheterize, drain bladder and retain the catheter thereafter'.
Ref: Bailey and Love's Short Practice of Surgery, 24th Ed, Chapter 66, Pg 1258

Q. 166. Chandu, a 45 years male shows calcification on the right side of his abdomen in an AP view. In lateral view the calcification is seen to overlie the spine. Most likely diagnosis is (ALL INDIA-01)
    (a) Gallstones
    (b) Calcified mesenteric nodes
    (c) Renal stones
    (d) Calcified rib

Ans. (c)

Note
Most likely diagnosis for above is 'renal stone'.
Ref: Bailey and Love's Short Practice of Surgery, 24th Ed, Chapter 64, Pg 1184

Q. 167. CA prostate commonly metastasises to the vertebrae because (ALL INDIA-01)
    (a) Valveless communication exist with Batson's prevertebral plexus
    (b) Via drainage to sacral lymph node
    (c) Of direct spread
    (d) None of above

Ans. (a)

Note
Prostate is the most common site of origin for skeletal metastases.
Ref: Bailey and Love's Short Practice of Surgery, 24th Ed, Chapter 64, Pg 1184

Also see
The prostatic venous plexus communicates with vesicle plexus and internal pudendal vein. Valveless communications exist between the prostatic and vertebral venous plexus through which prostatic cancer can spread to the vertebral column and skull.
Ref: B.D. Chaurasia's Human Anatomy, 3rd Ed, Vol 2, Chapter 32, Pg 329

Q. 168. Following sexual intercourse, a person develops pain in the left testes that does not get relieved on elevation of scrotum. Diagnosis is (ALL INDIA-01)
    (a)   Epididymo-orchitis
    (b)   Torsion testis
    (c)   Fournier's gangrene
    (d)   Tumor testes

Ans. (b)
Note
The probable diagnosis for above clinical presentation is 'Torsion testis'.
Also see
The precipitating factors for torsion of testes are:
    -Straining at stool
    -Coitus
    -Lifting a heavy weight
Most commonly there is a sudden agonizing pain in the groin and lower abdomen. Elevation of testes reduces the pain of epididymo-orchitis but makes it worse in torsion of testes thus helping in their differentiation.
Ref: Bailey and Love's Short Practice of Surgery, 24th Ed, Chapter 68, Pg 1272-1273

Q. 169. A testicular tumor in a man aged 60 years is most likely to be (ALL INDIA-01)
    (a)   Germ cell tumor
    (b)   Sertoli cell tumor
    (c)   Teratocarcinoma
    (d)   Lymphoma

Ans. (d)
Note
A testicular tumor in a man aged 60 years is most likely to be 'lymphoma'.
Also see
a.   Germ Cell Tumor-Frequent before the age of 45.
b.   Sertoli Cell Tumor- They may occur at any age but are more frequently found in infants and children.
c.   Teratoma-They are common in infants and children.
d.   Lymphoma-It comprises 5% of testicular malignancy and is the commonest testicular tumor in elderly. Bilaterality is seen in ½ of the cases.
Ref: Textbook of Pathology by Harsh Mohan, 4th Ed, Chapter 20, Pg 699-701

Q. 170. A patient presents with bilateral proptosis, heat intolerance and palpitations. Most unlikely diagnosis here would be (ALL INDIA-01)
    (a)   Hashimoto's thyroiditis
    (b)   Thyroid adenoma
    (c)   Diffuse thyroid igoitre
    (d)   Reidel's thyroiditis

Ans. (d)
Note
Most unlikely diagnosis here would be 'Reidel's thyroiditis'.
Also see
a.   Main complaint is enlargement of neck with slight pain and tenderness in the region of neck. The patient may initially be hyperthyroid but hypothyroidism is inevitable. (Pg 667)
b.   Patient usually presents with slow growing swelling of neck. No other complaint is evident. (Pg 661)

MCQ's in Surgery   579

c. There is a tight sensation in the neck especially when swallowing. The goiter is soft and symmetrical and thyroid is enlarged 2-3 times its normal size. (Davidson's Principles and Practice of Medicine, 19th Ed, Chapter 17, Pg 702)
d. Occurs most frequently in women. Symptoms are due to compression of trachea, esophagus and recurrent laryngeal nerve. (Pg 668)

Ref: A Concise Textbook of Surgery, S. Das, 3rd Ed, Chapter 37

Q. 171. A patient with long standing multinodular goitre develops hoarseness of voice. Also, the swelling undergoes sudden increase in size likely diagnosis is (ALL INDIA-01)
(a) Follicular CA
(b) Papillary CA
(c) Medullary CA
(d) Anaplastic CA

Ans. (a)
Note
The diagnosis for above clinical presentation is 'Follicular CA'.
Also see
The follicular carcinoma tends to occur in older age group. Patient presents with a long-standing history of goiter. Sudden change in the form of increase in size or diffuse swelling into a firm swelling is characteristic. Pain and invasion to the adjacent structures is a late feature.
Ref: A Concise Textbook of Surgery, S. Das, 3rd Ed, Chapter 37, Pg 664

Q. 172. A patient presents with swelling in the neck following a thyroidectomy. What is the most likely resulting complication? (ALL INDIA-01)
(a) Respiratory obstruction
(b) Recurrent laryngeal nerve palsy
(c) Hypovolemia
(d) Hypocalcemia

Ans. (a)
Note
The most likely resulting complication for above is 'respiratory obstruction'.
Also see
Most cases of respiratory obstruction are due to laryngeal oedema; the commonest cause is tension hematoma. Other causes are:
  -Anesthetic intubation
  -Surgical manipulation
Ref: Bailey and Love's Short Practice of Surgery, 24th Ed, Chapter 44, Pg 725

Q. 173. A patient on the same evening following thyroidectomy presents with a swelling in the neck and difficulty in breathing. Next management would be (ALL INDIA-01)
(a) Open sutures immediately
(b) Intubate oro-tracheally
(c) Wait and watch
(d) Administer oxygen by mask

Ans. (a)
Note
Next management would be for the above case is 'open sutures immediately'.
Also see
Respiratory obstruction occurs due to tension hematoma, which leads to laryngeal oedema. So the tension hematoma should be released at once. If this doesn't help then intubation should be done.
Ref: Bailey and Love's Short Practice of Surgery, 24th Ed, Chapter 44, Pg 725

Q. 174. A patient undergoes thyroid surgery, following which he develops perioral tingling. Blood Ca^{2+} is 89 mEq. Next step is (ALL INDIA-01)
(a) Vitamin D orally
(b) Oral Ca^{2+} and vitamin D

(c) Intravenous calcium gluconate and serial monitoring
(d) Wait for Ca^{2+} to decrease to < 70 before taking further action

Ans. (c)

Note

The next step in above clinical presentation is 'Intravenous calcium gluconate and serial monitoring'.

Also see

The symptoms and signs given point to a diagnosis of hypoparathyroidism. It occurs due to infarction through damage to end-arteries.

It's mostly transient and treatment is by administration of 20ml 20% calcium gluconate.

Ref: Bailey and Love's Short Practice of Surgery, 24th Ed, Chapter 37, Pg 658

Q. 175. A case of blunt trauma is brought to the emergency in a state of shock. He is not responding to IV crystalloids. Next step in his management would be (ALL INDIA-01)
(a) Immediate laparotomy
(b) Blood transfusion
(c) Albumin transfusion
(d) Abdominal compression

Ans. (a)

Note

The next step in above case for his management would be 'Immediate laparotomy'.

Also see

The abdomen should neither be ignored nor the sole focus of the treating physician and surgeon. The most reliable signs and symptoms in alert patients are pain, tenderness, gastrointestinal hemorrhage, hypovolaemia, and evidence of peritoneal irritation. However, large amounts of blood can accumulate in the peritoneal and pelvic cavities without any significant or early changes in the physical examination findings. In an unstable patient, the question of abdominal involvement must be expediently addressed. This is accomplished by identifying free intra-abdominal fluid using diagnostic peritoneal lavage (DPL) or the Focused Assessment with Sonography for Trauma (FAST) examination. The objective is to rapidly identify patients who need a laparotomy. Indications for laparotomy in a patient with blunt abdominal injury include the following:
-Signs of peritonitis.
-Uncontrolled shock or hemorrhage.
-Clinical deterioration during observation.
-Hemoperitoneum findings after FAST or DPL examinations.

Ref: http://www.emedicine.com/MED/topic2804.htm

Q. 176. Babu is brought to the emergency as a case of road- traffic accident. He is hypotensive. Most likely ruptured organ is (ALL INDIA-01)
(a) Spleen
(b) Mesentery
(c) Kidney
(d) Rectum

Ans. (a)

Note

The most likely ruptured organ in above presentation is 'spleen'.

Also see

Splenic rupture should be considered after any trauma, but particularly if there has been a history of injury to the left upper quadrant of the abdomen. The patient may go into shock due to blood loss. Treatment involves laparotomy. Blood is evacuated and spleen inspected.

Ref: Bailey and Love's Short Practice of Surgery, 24th Ed, Chapter 53, PG 955, 956

Q. 177. A patient is brought to the emergency as a case of head injury, following a head on collision road traffic accident. His BP is 90/60 mmHg. Tachycardia is present. Most likely diagnosis is (ALL INDIA-01)
(a) EDH (Extradural Hemorrhage)
(b) SDH (Subdural Hemorrhage)

(c) Intracranial hemorrhage
(d) Intra-abdominal bleed

Ans. (d)

Note
Most likely diagnosis for above case is 'intra-abdominal bleed'.

Also see
No localizing sings for Extradural or Subdural hemorrhage or signs of intracranial hemorrhage are given in above case. However, the patient is presening with low BP and Tachycardia which points to blood loss and most probable concealed intra-abdominal blood loss can only be suspected in this given case.

Q. 178. Ulcer that may develop in burn tissue is (ALL INDIA-01)
(a) Marjolin's
(b) Rodent
(c) Melanoma
(d) Curling's

Ans. (a)
(Same as 131,141)

Note
Ulcer that may develop in burn tissue is 'Marjolin's ulcer'.

Also see
Marjolin's ulcer is the name given to a squamous cell carcinoma arising from a chronic benign ulcer or a scar.e.g. Venous ulcer or an old burn.
Ref: A Concise Textbook of Surgery, S. Das, 3rd Ed, Chapter10, Pg 108

Q. 179. An elderly man presents with history of abdominal pain. He is found to have a fusiform dilatation of the descending aorta. Likely cause is (ALL INDIA-01)
(a) Trauma
(b) Atherosclerosis
(c) Right ventricular failure
(d) Syphilitic aortitis

Ans. (b)

Note
Most likely cause for above presentation is 'Atherosclerosis'.

Also see
Dilatations of localized segment of arterial system are called as aneurysms. It can be grouped according to shape into –fusiform, saccular, dissecting
Or according to etiology into –atherosclerotic, traumatic, syphilitic, collagen disease.
The majority of aneurysms are atherosclerotic fusiform aneurysms.
Ref: A Concise Textbook of Surgery, S. Das, 3rd Ed, Chapter15, Pg 225

Q. 180. All of the following are correct regarding AV fistula except (ALL INDIA-01)
(a) Arterialization of the veins
(b) Proximal compression causes increase in heart rate
(c) Overgrowth of a limb
(d) Causes LV enlargement and LV failure

Ans. (b)

Note
All of the following are correct regarding AV fistula except 'Proximal compression causes increase in heart rate'.

Also see
Communication between arteries and veins is called as A-V fistula.
The structural effect is that the veins become dilated, tortuous and thick walled i.e. arterialised .Due to enhanced venous return and increased venous pressure LVH can occur.
A congenital fistula may cause overgrowth of the limb.

Pressure on the arteries proximal to the fistula causes swelling to decrease in size, the thrill and bruit to cease and pulse rate to fall.
Ref: Bailey and Love's Short Practice of Surgery, 24th Ed, Chapter 15, Pg 231

Q. 181. All of the following are correct about axillary vein thrombosis except (ALL INDIA-01)
    (a)   May be caused by a cervical rib.
    (b)   Treated with IV anticoagulant.
    (c)   Embolectomy is done in all cases.
    (d)   May occur following excessive exercise.

Ans. (c)
Note
All of the above are correct about axillary vein thrombosis except 'Embolectomy is done in all cases'.

Also see
Axillary venous thrombosis may occur following excessive exercise or as a complication of thoracic outlet syndrome. Its occurrence is associated with a cervical rib. The arm becomes swollen and veins are distended. Treatment is by anticoagulant.
Ref: Bailey and Love's Short Practice of Surgery, 24th Ed, Chapter 17, Pg 255

Q. 182. A 80 year old patient presents with a midline tumor of the lower jaw, involving the alveolar margin. He is edentulous. Treatment of choice is (ALL INDIA-01)
    (a)   Hemimandibulectomy
    (b)   Commando operation
    (c)   Segmental mandiblectbmy
    (d)   Marginal mandibulectomy

Ans. (c)
Note
Invasion in the edentulous mandible is almost always via deficiencies in cortical bone of alveolar crest. Marginal resection is the treatment of choice. Radiotherapy is used in adjuvant not clear manner.
Ref: Bailey and Love's Short Practice of Surgery, 24th Ed, Chapter 41, Pg 646

Q. 183. Most common cause of unilateral parotid swelling in a 27 year old male is (ALL INDIA-01)
    (a)   Warthin's tumor
    (b)   Pleomorphic adenoma
    (c)   Adenocarcinoma
    (d)   Hemangioma

Ans. (b)
Note
Most common cause of unilateral parotid swelling in a 27 year old male is 'Pleomorphic adenoma'.

Also see
Pleomorphic adenoma occurs at any age (mean being 42yrs). It accounts for at least 75% of parotid tumors and >50% of submandibular tumors.
Ref: Bailey and Love's Short Practice of Surgery, 24th Ed, Chapter 42, Pg 659

Q. 184. A 45 year old woman presents with a hard and mobile lump in the breast. Next investigation is (ALL INDIA-01)
    (a)   FNAC
    (b)   USG
    (c)   Mammography
    (d)   Excision biopsy

Ans. (a)
Note
The next investigation in above case is 'FNAC'.

Also see
The following algorithm is used for investigation of a breast lump:

CYSTIC	SOLID	
	Clinically benign	Clinically Malignant
FNA	FNA	FNA

Cytology	Cytology	Cytology	Cytology	Cytology
Benign, lump disappears	Malignant, lump disappears	Benign	Malignant	Benign
Follow-up	Urgent biopsy	Follow-up or excise	Treat cancer	Urgent biopsy

Ref: Bailey and Love's Short Practice of Surgery, 24th Ed, Chapter 46, Pg 760

Q. 185. A 45 years old man presents with progressive cervical lymph nodes enlargement since 3 months. Most diagnostic investigation is (ALL INDIA-01)
    (a)   X-ray soft tissue
    (b)   FNAC
    (c)   Lymph node biopsy
    (d)   None of the above
Ans. (c)
Note
Most diagnostic investigation for above is 'Lymph node biopsy'.
Also see
This is the most important special investigation. Biopsy should be called for in these cases.
Ref: A Concise Textbook of Surgery, S. Das, 3rd Ed, Chapter17, Pg 228, 229

Q. 186. All of the following are true about fibrolamellar carcinoma of the liver except (ALL INDIA-01)
    (a)   Equal incidence in males and females
    (b)   Better prognosis than HCC
    (c)   AFP levels always greater than > 1000
    (d)   Occur in younger individuals
Ans. (c)
Note
All of the above are true about fibrolamellar carcinoma of the liver except ' AFP levels always greater than > 1000.
Also see
Fibrolamellar carcinoma is a clinical variant of hepatocellular carcinoma (HCCA). It is found in young people of both sexes. The prognosis is better than in other forms of HCCA. It may remain undetected initially because it often occurs in patients with underlying cirrhosis. The patient has a tender palpable mass in the right upper abdomen. Ascites with RBCs and malignant cells is found in about ½ the patients. Lab findings include markedly elevated S. alkaline phosphatase and high S. AFP >500ng/ml.
Ref: Textbook of Pathology by Harsh Mohan, 4th Ed, Chapter 18, Pg 617

Q. 187. A child presents with an expansible swelling on medial side of the nose. Likely diagnosis is (ALL INDIA-01)
    (a)   Teratoma
    (b)   Meningocele
    (c)   Dermoid cyst
    (d)   Lipoma
Ans. (b)
Note
The most likely diagnosis of above condition is 'Meningocele'.

Also see
Encephalocele or meningoencephalocele- It is the herniation of brain tissue with meninges through a congenital bony defect.
An extra nasal meningoencephalocele presents as a subcutaneous pulsatile swelling in the midline at the root of nose, on the side of nose or on the antero-medial aspect of the orbit. Swelling shows cough impulse.
Ref: Diseases of Ear, Nose and Throat, by P.L. Dhingra, Chapter 26, Pg 177

Q. 188. Direct impact on the bone will produce a
    (a)   Transverse fracture
    (b)   Oblique fracture
    (c)   Spiral fracture
    (d)   Communited fracture

Ans. Use your discreation
Note
Direct impact on the bone will produce a (a) 'Transverse fracture' and (b) communited fractutre.
Also see
Fracture occurring due to direct trauma is called as a traumatic fracture. It can be of two types:

    -Tapping: This causes transverse fracture
    -Crush injury: It causes comminuted fracture
Ref: A Concise Textbook of Surgery, S. Das, 3rd Ed, Chapter 22, Pg 293, 294

Q. 189. A 12 year old girl complains of pain persisting in her leg for several weeks with a low grade fever. A radiograph reveals a mass in the diaphyseal region of the left femur with overlying cortical erosion and soft tissue extension. A biopsy of the lesion, shows numerous small round cells, rich in PAS positive diastase sensitive granules The most likely histological diagnosis is
    (a)   **Osteogenic sarcoma**
    (b)   **Osteoblastoma**
    (c)   **Ewing's sarcoma**
    (d)   **Chondroblastoma**

Ans. (c)
Note
The most likely histological diagnosis for above case is 'Ewing's sarcoma'.
Also see
a.   *Osteogenic sarcoma*
    It is the most common primary malignant tumor of the bone characterized by osteoid or bone formation.
    It is of two types: Medullary and Parosteal
    It presents with pain, tenderness and an obvious swelling of the affected extremity.
    X-ray shows a sunburst appearance due to osteogenesis.
b.   *Osteoblastoma*
    These are benign tumors occurring in children and young adults. It is >1cm, painless, located in the medulla and commonly seen in vertebra ribs and long bones.
c.   *Ewing's sarcoma*
    Occurs in patients between 5-20 yrs. It arises in medullary canal of diaphysis or metaphysis.
    Common sites are metaphysis of long bones particularly tibia, femur and humerus.
    C/F:
    -Pain, tenderness and swelling of affected area. TLC and ESR are elevated
    X-ray shows onion peel appearance
    Pathology:
    -It consists of small and uniform round cells having ill-defined cytoplasm which contains glycogen which stains with PAS reaction.
d.   *Chondroblastoma*
    Rare benign tumor arising from epiphysis of long bones. Occurs in patients <20 yrs of age and has a male preponderance.
Ref: Textbook of Pathology by Harsh Mohan, 4th Ed, Chapter 25, Pg 824, 829

Q. 190. 'Whip-lash' injury is caused due to
   (a)   A fall from a height
   (b)   Acute hyperextension of the spine
   (c)   A blow on top to head
   (d)   Acute hyperflexion of the spine

Ans. Use your discretion

Note
'Whip-lash' injury is caused due to 'Acute hyperflexion of the spine'.

Also see
The name or denomination 'Whiplash Injury' derives from the etiopathogenic description of the sudden sharp whipping movement of the head and neck, produced at the moment of a traffic accident, particularly subsequent to collisions from the rear, head-on or side collisions. In the case of a head-on collision, a forward displacement of the body is produced as a result of the inertia provoking tension upon the safety belt together with a neck hyper flexion followed by a hyperextension of it, thus producing "the whiplash". In the case of a collision from the rear, the mechanism is inverted, first hyperextension followed by hyper flexion of the neck. Thus answer should be both b and d.
Ref: http://www.vertigo-dizziness.com/english/whiplash_injury.html

Q. 191. The operative procedure known as "micro fracture" is done for the
   (a)   Delayed union of femur
   (b)   Non union of tibia
   (c)   Loose bodies of ankle joint
   (d)   Osteochondral defect of femur

Ans. (d)

Note
The operative procedure known as "micro fracture" is done for the 'osteochondral defect of femur'.

Also see
Micro fracture surgery is a procedure that involves an arthroscopic entry into the knee to repair defects in cartilage. Micro fracture surgery is designed to repair chondral defects in the knee, which are areas where cartilage has worn away leaving bone on bone. These defects in cartilage result in pain and swelling with minimal physical activity. The procedure involves fracturing the areas where cartilage is deficient. The result is a thick clot that forms in the fractured area. This clot eventually becomes the replacement cartilage
Ref: http://www.uwm.edu/People/taylortd/index.html

Q. 192. A thirty one year old male with nephrotic syndrome complains of pain in right hip joint of 2 months duration. The movements at the hip are free but painful terminally. The most likely diagnosis is
   (a)   Tuberculosis of hip
   (b)   Avascular necrosis of femoral head
   (c)   Chondrolysis of hip
   (d)   Pathological fracture of femoral neck

Ans. (d)

Note
The most likely diagnosis is 'Patholgical fracture of femoral neck'.

Also see
Nephrotic syndrome if progresses to CRF can lead to renal osteodystrophy due to diminished activity of 1-hydroxylase enzyme which leads to diminished intestinal absorption of calcium; hypocalcaemia & reduction of calcification of osteoid. This may lead to pathological fractures of the hip.
Ref: Davidson's Principles and Practice of Medicine, 19th Ed, Chapter 14, Pg 601

Q. 193. The most commonly affected component of the lateral collateral ligament complex in an "ankle sprain" is the
    (a)   Middle component
    (b)   Anterior component
    (c)   Posterior component
    (d)   Deeper component

Ans. (b)

Note
The most commonly affected component of the lateral collateral ligament complex in an "ankle sprain" is the 'Anterior component'.

Also see
The fibrous capsule of the ankle joint is supported on each side by strong collateral ligaments
    -Medial (deltoid)
    -Lateral (lateral ligament)
The lateral ligament is divided into –anterior, posterior and calcaneofibular component.
The true sprains of ankle joint are caused by forced plantar flexion, which leads to tearing of the anterior fibres of the capsule.
Ref: B.D.Chaurasia's Human Anatomy, 3rd Ed, Vol 2, Chapter 12, Pg 132-134

Q. 194. The stability of the ankle joint is maintained by all of the following, except
    (a)   Plantar calcaneonavicular (spring) ligament
    (b)   Deltoid ligament
    (c)   Lateral ligament
    (d)   Shape of the superior talar articular surface

Ans. (a)

Note
The stability of the ankle joint is maintained by all of the following, except, 'planter calcaneonavicular (spring) ligament'.

Also see
Structurally the ankle joint is very strong. The stability of the joint is ensured by:
    -Close interlocking of the articular surface.
    -Strong collateral ligament (medial and lateral)
    -Tendons that cross the joint
Ref: B.D.Chaurasia's Human Anatomy, 3rd Ed, Vol 2, Chapter 12, Pg 132-134

Q. 195. You have treated the simple and undisplaced fracture of shaft of right tibia in a nine year girl with above knee plaster cast. Parents want to know the prognosis of union of the fractured limb which was affected by poliomyelitis four years ago. What is the best possible advice will you offer to the parents?
    (a)   Fracture will unite slowly
    (b)   Fracture will not unite
    (c)   Fracture will unite normally
    (d)   Fracture will unite on attaining puberty

Ans. (c)

Note
The best possible advice offered to the parents is 'fractue will unite normally'.

Also see
a.   The causes of delayed union are:
    -Infection, type of injury, inadequate blood supply, inadequate immobilization, distraction of fractured segments, internal fixation, systemic diseases and pathological fractures.
b.   The causes of non-union are:

-Interposition of soft tissues, poor blood supply, distraction of the fragments. Therefore if the patient is managed properly the fracture should unite normally.
Ref: A Concise Textbook of Surgery, S. Das, 3rd Ed, Chapter 22, Pg 312, 313

Q. 196. A pole vaulter had a fall during pole vaulting and had paralysis of the arm. Which of the following investigations gives the best recovery prognosis?
    (a)   Electromyography
    (b)   Muscle biopsy
    (c)   Strength duration curve
    (d)   Creatine phosphokinase levels

Ans. (a)

Note
The investigation gives the best recovery prognosis in above case is 'Electromyography'.

Also see
As per the history the patient seems to have sustained a brachial plexus injury, which is caused by traction as a result of violent displacement of the shoulder girdle and the cervical spine. According to the degree of injury the damage ranges from complete paralysis of the arm to paralysis of a particular muscle group. Investigations include - Electromyography especially in supraclavicular injury.
Ref: Bailey and Love's Short Practice of Surgery, 24th Ed, Chapter 34, Pg 537

Q. 197. In a patient with a history of burning pain localized to the plantar aspect of the foot, the differential diagnosis must include
    (a)   Peripheral vascular disease
    (b)   Tarsal coalition
    (c)   Tarsal tunnel syndrome
    (d)   Planter fibromatosis

Ans. (c)

Note
In a patient with a history of burning pain localized to the plantar aspect of the foot, the differential diagnosis must include 'tarsal tunnel syndrome'.

Also see
Tarsal tunnel – entrapment of the posterior tibial nerve in the flexor retinaculum, which causes burning, numbness, and tingling in the distal sole and toes.
Ref: Davidson's Principles and Practice of Medicine, 19th Ed, Chapter 20, Pg 1005

Q. 198. An elderly woman was admitted with a fracture of the neck of right femur which failed to unite. On examination an avascular necrosis of the head of femur was noted. The condition would have resulted most probably from the damage to
    (a)   Superior gluteal artery
    (b)   Inferior gluteal artery
    (c)   Acetabular branch of obturator
    (d)   Retinacular branches of circumflex femoral arteries

Ans. (d)

Note
The avascular necrosis of head of femur is due to the damge of 'retinacular brances of circumflex femoral arteries'.

Also see
The obturator artery, medial and lateral circumflex arteries and superior and inferior gluteal arteries supply the hip joint. Retinacular arteries arise from this circle and supply the intracapsular part of the neck. Damage to retinacular arteries causes avascular necrosis of head of femur. Such damage is maximum in the sub capsular area.
Ref: B. D. Chaurasia's Human Anatomy, Vol 2, Chapter 12, Pg 122, 123

Q. 199. A 44-year-old man presented with acute onset of low backache radiating to the right lower limb. Examination revealed SLRT < 40° on the right side, weakness of extensor hallucis longus on the right side, sensory loss in the first web space of the right foot and brisk knee jerk. Which of the following is the most likely diagnosis?
(a) Prolapsed intervertebral disc L4-5
(b) Spondylolysis L5-S1
(c) Lumbar canal stenosis
(d) Spondylolisthesis L4-5

Ans. (a)

Note
For the above given clinical problem most likely diagnosis is 'prolapsed intervertebral disc L4-5'.

Also see
The roots affected are – L4, L5 & S1. In case of L5 involvement the sensory impairment is detected in the back of thigh, lateral aspect of leg and dorsum of the foot is +ve at >40 degrees, suggesting impingement of the protruding intervertebral disc.
Ref: A Concise Textbook of Surgery, S. Das, 3rd Ed, Chapter 30, Pg 511-512

Q. 200. A woman of 45, a known cause of pemphigus vulgaris on a regular treatment with controlled primary disease presented with pain in the right hip and knee. Examination revealed no limb length discrepancy but the patient has tenderness in the Scarpa's triangle and limitation of adduction and internal rotation of the right hip joint as compared to the other side. The most probable diagnosis is
(a) Stress fracture of neck of femur
(b) Avascular necrosis of femoral head
(c) Perthes' disease
(d) Transient synovitis of hip

Ans. (b)

Note
The most probable diagnosis is for the above clinical presentation is 'Avascular necrosis of femoral head'.

Also see
Causes of avascular necrosis of head of femur are:
a. Congenital- Sickle cell anaemia, thalassaemia
b. Drug induced – Steroids and alcohol
c. Trauma
d. Infections – Septic arthritis
e. Environmental- Caisson's disease
The patient complaints of sudden onset of pain in the hip joint. On examination nothing may be found except painful limitation of movement.
Ref: Bailey and Love's Short Practice of Surgery, 24th Ed, Chapter 23, Pg 376

Q. 201. A 24-year-old male, known epileptic, presented following a seizure with pain in the right shoulder region. Examination revealed that the right upper limb was adducted and internally rotated and the movements could not be performed. Which of the following is the most likely diagnosis?
(a) Posterior dislocation of shoulder
(b) Luxatio erecta
(c) Intrathoracic dislocation of shoulder
(d) Subglenoid dislocation of shoulder

Ans. (a)

Note
The most probable diagnosis is for the above clinical presentation is 'posterior dislocation of shoulder'.

Also see
The cause of dislocation is usually due to trauma.
a. Posterior dislocation is a rare phenomenon caused by forced internal rotation on the abducted arm. Persistant

internal rotation of humerus is pointing to posterior dislocation.
Ref: A Manual of Clinical Surgery, S. Das, Chapter 13, Pg 136

Q. 202. A 30-year-old male underwent excision of the right radial head. Following surgery, the patient developed inability to extend the fingers and thumb of the right hand. He did not have any sensory deficit. Which one of the following is the most likely cause?
    (a)   Injury to posterior interosseus nerve.
    (b)   Iatrogenic injury to common extensor origin.
    (c)   Injury to anterior interosseus nerve.
    (d)   High radial nerve palsy.

Ans. (a)
Note
The most probable diagnosis is for the above clinical presentation is 'injury to posterior interosseus nerve'.
Also see
Posterior interosseous nerve is the deep terminal branch of radial nerve given off at the cubital fossa, at the level of lateral epicondyle of the humerus. It may get damaged during an operation for exposure of the head of radius. Since the extensor carpi radialis longus and brevis are spared, wrist drop doesn't occur.
Ref: B.D.Chaurasia's Human Anatomy, 3rd Ed,Vol -1, Chapter 9, Pg 129,130

Q. 203. A 10-year-old boy presenting with a cubitus varus deformity and a history of trauma 3 months back. On clinical examination, has the preserved 3 bony point relationship of the elbow. The most probable diagnosis is
    (a)   Old unreduced dislocation of elbow
    (b)   Non-union lateral condylar fracture of humerus
    (c)   Malunited intercondylar fracture of humerus
    (d)   Malunited supracondylar fracture of humerus

Ans. (d)
Note
The most probable diagnosis is for the above clinical presentation is 'malunited supracondylar fracture of humerus'.
Also see
The supra-condylar fracture of humerus is of two types:
    Backward - Occurs by fall on the hand with elbow bent.
    Forward - Fall on the stretched hand with fully extended elbow so that the lower fragment is tilted forwards.
The victims are usually children and present with a gross swelling at the elbow on examination there may be bruising and posteriorly prominence of the elbow (backward)
Or a more extended elbow with forwardly tilted distal segment (forward).

Complications are cubitus valgus or varus, myositis ossificans traumatica, injury to the brachial vessels, volkmann's contracture, and nerve injury.
Ref: A Manual of Clinical Surgery, S. Das, Chapter 13, Pg 141

Q. 204. A 33-year-old man presented with a slowly progressive swelling in the middle 1/3rd of his right tibia. X-ray examination revealed multiple sharply demarcated radiolucent lesions separated by areas of dense and sclerotic bone. Microscopic examination of a biopsy specimen revealed island of epithelial cells in a fibrous stroma. Which of the following is the most probable diagnosis?
    (a)   Adamantioma
    (b)   Osteofibrous dysplasia
    (c)   Osteosarcoma
    (d)   Fibrous cortical defect

Ans. (a)
Note
The most probable diagnosis is for the above clinical presentation is 'adamantioma'.
Also see
Adamantioma is seen in tibia. It commences superficially or subperiosteally at either end of tibia. It is locally

destructive slow growing tumor presents with pain and tenderness though at times painless; swelling is the only presenting complaint. X-ray shows osteolytic lesion of the shaft with a well defined and an intact cortex. In the area of osteolytic lesion finely trabeculated lamellae may be found.
Treatment involves amputation through the proximal bone.
Ref: A Concise Textbook of Surgery, S. Das, 3rd Ed, Chapter 28, Pg 447

Q. 205. A 15-year-old boy presented with painful swelling over the left shoulder. Radiograph of the shoulder showed an osteolytic area with stippled calcification over the proximal humeral epiphysis. Biopsy of the lesion revealed an immature fibrous matrix with scattered giant cells Which of the following is the most likely diagnosis?
    (a)   Giant cell tumor
    (b)   Chondroblastoma
    (c)   Osteosarcoma
    (d)   Chondromyxoid fibroma

Ans. (b)

Note
The most probable diagnosis is for the above clinical presentation is 'chondroblastoma'.

Also see
Chondroblastoma: It is a benign tumor arising from epiphysis of long bones and upper tibia, upper humerus and femur. It occurs in patients under 20 yrs of age. X-ray shows sharply circumscribed lesions with multiple foci of calcification. It may be asymptomatic or produce local; pain, tenderness and discomfort.
Pathology: It is composed of small, round to polygonal mononuclear cells resembling chondroblasts and also contains multinucleate giant cells.

Q. 206. A 46-year-old known alcoholic, presented with pain in the dorsal spine. On examination there is tenderness at the dorso-lumbar junction. Radiograph shows destruction of the 12th dorsal vertebra with loss of the disc space between D12-L1 vertebrae. The most probable diagnosis is:
    (a)   Metastatic spine disease
    (b)   Pott's spine
    (c)   Missed trauma
    (d)   Multiple myeloma

Ans. (b)

Note
The most probable diagnosis is for the above clinical presentation is 'pott's disease'.

Also see
Spinal TB is more common in the lower thoracic region.
C/F: Pain; localized or referred, stiffness, swelling.
X-ray features are: Osteolytic lesion in the vertebral bodies adjacent to the vertebral discs.
Narrowing of the intervertebral disc.
Lytic lesions in bone of adjacent vertebra.

Q. 207. A 50-year-old man sustained posterior dislocation of left hip in an accident. Dislocation was reduced after 3 days. He started complaining of pain in left hip after 6 months X-rays of the pelvis were normal. The most relevant investigation at this stage will be
    (a)   CRP levels in blood
    (b)   Ultrasonography of hip
    (c)   Arthrography of hip
    (d)   MRI of hip

Ans. (d)

Note
The most relevant investigation at this stage will be 'MRI of hip'.

Also see
Common complications of posterior dislocation of hip are:
- Avascular necrosis of femoral head: Even if reduction is carried out within 8 hours of injury it happens in 15% cases X-ray appearance reveals itself about 2-3 years after injury.
- Sciatic nerve injury.
- Myositis ossificans.
- Other associated fractures- Posterior rim of acetabulum, neck of femur, head of femur, etc

Ref: A Concise Textbook of Surgery, S. Das, 3rd Ed, Chapter 24, Pg 360
Since X-Ray has not revealed anything the next best option would be MRI.
MRI scan should be done in 4-6 weeks to look for signs of osteonecrosis (Avascular necrosis). This is repeated at about 3 months.
Ref: http://www.emedicine.com/sports/topic47.htm

Q. 208. A 30-year old man involved in fisticuffs, injured his middle finger and noticed slight flexion of DIP joint. X-rays were normal. The most appropriate management at this stage is
 (a) Ignore
 (b) Splint the finger in hyperextension
 (c) Surgical repair of the flexor tendon
 (d) Buddy strapping

Ans. (b)

Note
The most appropriate management for the above clinical presentation is 'splint the finger in hyperextension'.

Also see
As per the history given the patient seems to be suffering from Mallet finger- that occurs if the fingertip is forcibly bent during active extension of the other joints of the finger when the extensor muscle is in full command.
C/F: The terminal joint is kept flexed.
Treatment: If radiologically no fracture is seen then the injury should be treated with a splint, which keeps the terminal phalanx in full extension for 6 weeks.
Ref: A Concise Textbook of Surgery, S. Das, 3rd Ed, Chapter 20, Pg 281

Q. 209. De Quervain's disease classically affects the
 (a) Flexor pollicis longus and brevis
 (b) Extensor carpi radialis and extensor pollicis longus
 (c) Abductor pollicis longus and brevis
 (d) Extensor pollicis brevis and abductor pollicis longus

Ans. (d)

Note
De Quervain's disease classically affects the 'extensor pollicis brevis and abductor pollicis longus'.

Also see
De Quervain's disease – It is the condition where fibrous sheath containing the extensor pollicis brevis and abductor pollicis longus tendons become fibrosed and thickened, so that the intrathecal lumen becomes narrowed. It is seen in middle aged people especially women. Main symptom is pain in the radial side of the wrist with weakness of the grip. Pain is aggravated by abduction and extension of thumb.
Ref: A Concise Textbook of Surgery, S. Das, 3rd Ed, Chapter 20, Pg 280

Q. 210. In trigger finger the level of tendon sheath constriction is found at the level of
 (a) Middle phalanx
 (b) Proximal interphalangeal joint
 (c) Proximal phalanx
 (d) Metacarpo-phalangeal joint

Ans. (d)

Note
In trigger finger the level of tendon sheath constriction is found at the level of 'Metacarpo-phalangeal joint'.

Also see
Trigger finger is a condition of stenosing tenovaginitis (tenosynovitis) of flexor tendons. In this condition there is obstacle to voluntary flexion or extension of finger. When the finger is extended it is difficult to do so initially, but when the portion of obstruction is crossed, the finger suddenly straightens with a snap hence called trigger finger.
Ref: A Concise Textbook of Surgery, S. Das, 3rd Ed, Chapter 20, Pg 280-281

Q. 211. What is pathognomic feature of rheumatoid arthritis?
    (a)   Rheumatoid factor
    (b)   Rheumatoid nodule
    (c)   Morning stiffness
    (d)   Ulnar drift of fingers

Ans. (b)

Note
The pathognomic feature of rheumatoid arthritis from above given options is 'rheumatoid nodule'.

Also see
Diagnostic criteria for RA are:
    -Morning stiffness (for more than an hour)
    -Rheumatoid nodule
    -Arthritis of three or more joint areas
    -Rheumatoid factor
    -Small joint arthritis
    -X-ray changes
    -Symmetrical arthritis
    -More than 6 weeks duration
Four of these have to be present to establish a diagnosis of RA
Ref: Davidson's Principles and Practice of Medicine, 19th Ed, Chapter 20, Pg 1003
However morning stiffness and RA factor are not specific to RA.
Other diseases in which RA factor may be present are: SLE, Scleroderma, etc.
Therefore we can say that rheumatoid nodule is diagnostic of RA.

Q. 212. Which one of the following bone tumors typically affects the epiphysis of a long bone?
    (a)   Osteosarcoma
    (b)   Ewing's sarcoma
    (c)   Chodroblastoma
    (d)   Chondromyxoid fibroma

Ans. (c)

Note
'Chondroblastoma' from above is the bone tumor which typically affects the epiphysis of a long bone.

Also see
The tumors, which arise from epiphysis of long bones, are: Chondroblastoma and Giant cell tumors.
Ref: Textbook of Pathology by Harsh Mohan, chapter 25, Pg 827-828

Q. 213. A young woman met with an accident and had mild quadriparesis. Her lateral X-ray cervical spine revealed C5-C6 fracture dislocation. Which of the following is the best line of management?
    (a)   Immediate anterior decompression
    (b)   Cervical traction followed by instrument fixation
    (c)   Hard cervical collar and bed rest
    (d)   Cervical laminectomy

Ans. (b)

Note
The best line of treatment from above for the management of 'cervical spine C5-C6 fracture dislocation' is 'cervical traction followed by instrument fixation'.

Also see
Injuries such as fracture dislocation of the cervical vertebrae are caused by flexion or flexion and rotation. These dislocations should be reduced as soon as possible. If the patient has a complete cord injury, the dislocation can be simply reduced by traction. Facet dislocations are unstable and once reduced internal fixation and bone grafting is recommended.
Ref: Bailey and Love's Sort Practice of Surgery, Chapter 33, Pg 511, 512

Q. 214. Which one of the following is the investigation of choice for evaluation of suspected Perthe's disease?
    (a) Plain X-ray
    (b) Ultrasonography (US)
    (c) Computed tomography (CT)
    (d) Magnetic resonance imaging (MRI)

Ans. (d)

Note
From above 'magnetic resonance imaging (MRI)' is the investigation of choice for evaluation of suspected Perthe's disease.

Also see
Perthe's disease is a type of crushing osteochondritis where the whole or a part of femoral head becomes avascular.
Ref: A concise textbook of surgery, S. Das, 3rd Ed, Chapter 29, page 466
In Perthe's disease early stage of disease is evident in X-Ray with increased joint space and head of femur stands away a little laterally. With onset of ischaemia the head shows an increased density – at first granular then uniform. As condition advances flattening of head with patchy fragmentation becomes obvious. The neck of femur becomes wide with a band of rarefaction and even a cystic appearance with surrounding sclerosis.
Ref: A manual of clinical surgery, S. Das, Chapter 16, Page 185

However for the evaluation of suspected Perthe's disease the MRI is most sensitive and specific means of detecting changes in avascular necrosis, sensitivity and specificity around 100%.

Q. 215. Neuronal degeneration is seen in all of the following except
    (a) Crush nerve injury
    (b) Fetal development
    (c) Senescence
    (d) Neuropraxia

Ans. (d)

Note
Neuronal degeneration is seen in all of the above except 'Neuropraxia'.

Also see
Nerve injury is of 3 types:
a. *Neuropraxia*
    - Local block to conduction of nerve impulse at a discrete area along the course of the nerve. The axons are in continuity therefore Wallerian degeneration doesn't occur. Nerve conduction distal to the site of injury remaining normal. It is caused by a mild injury.
b   *Axonotmesis*
    -There is anatomical disruption of the nerve, however the supporting conductive tissues are structurally intact.
c.   *Neurotmesis*
    -It is a state where the nerve has been completely affected so that recovery is not possible.
Ref: Bailey and Love's Short Practice of Surgery, 24th Ed, Chapter 34, Page 532

Q. 216. In Klippel-Feil syndrome, the patient has all of the following clinical features except
 (a) Low hair line
 (b) Bilateral neck webbing
 (c) Bilateral shortness of sternocleidomastoid muscles
 (d) Gross limitations of neck movements

Ans. (c)

Note
In Klippel-Feil syndrome, the patient has all of the above clinical features except 'Bilateral shortness of sternocleidomastoid muscles'.

Also see
Kippel-feil syndrome comprises of multiple congenital abnormalities in the cervical spine leading to a characteristic short, stiff neck with a low hairline. Torticollis, facial asymmetry and webbing of neck may be apparent.
Ref: Bailey and Love's Short Practice of Surgery, 24th Ed, Chapter 27, page 429

Q. 217. The most common sequelae of tuberculous spondylitis in an adolescent is
 (a) Fibrous ankylosis
 (b) Bony ankylosis
 (c) Pathological dislocation
 (d) Chronic osteomyelitis

Ans. (b)

Note
The most common sequelae of tuberculous spondylitis in an adolescent is 'bony ankylosis'.

Also see
Spinal tuberculosis / Pott's disease / Tuberular Spondylitis: involves two or more adjacent vertebral bodies. In children upper thoracic spine is most common to be affected, and lower thoracic and upper lumbar vertebrae are affected in adults. With advanced disease, collapse of vertebral bodies results in kyphosis (*gibbus*).
Ref: Harrison 15th Edition, Section 8-Myobacterial diseases.

Q. 218. In radionuclide imaging the most useful radio- pharmaceutical for skeletal imaging is
 (a) Gallium 67 (67Ga)
 (b) Technetium-sulphur-colloid (99mTc-Sc)
 (c) Technetium-99m (99mTc)
 (d) Technetium-99m linked to methylene disphosphonate (99mTc-MDP)

Ans. (d)

Note
In radionuclide imaging the most useful radio- pharmaceutical for skeletal imaging is 'Technetium-99m linked to methylene disphosphonate (99mTc-MDP)'.
The most common reasons for performing a bone scan is to detect areas of abnormal bone growth due to fractures, tumors, infection, or otherbone diseases. The radio pharmaceutical most commonly used is 99mTc-Medronate (MDP). MDP is injected into a vein, usually in the arm, where it is transported by the bloodstream to the bones.
Ref:-http://www.amershamhealth-us.com/patient/diaguide/bone.html

Q. 219. Heberden's arthropathy affects
 (a) Lumbar spine
 (b) Symmetrically large joints
 (c) Sacroiliac joints
 (d) Distal interphalangeal joints

Ans. (d)

Note
Heberden's arthropathy affects 'distal interphalangeal joints'.

MCQ's in Surgery   595

Also see
It is a manifestation of nodal Osteoarthritis; the affected joint develops postero-lateral swellings on each side of the extensor tendon. They enlarge and harden to become Heberdon's (Distal IPJs) and Bouchard's (Proximal IPJs) nodes.
Ref: Davidson's Principles and Practice of Medicine, 19th Ed, Chapter 20, page 998-999

Q. 220. Subtrochanteric fractures of femur can be treated by all of the following methods except
       (a)   Skeletal traction on Thomas' splint
       (b)   Smith Petersen nail
       (c)   Condylar blade plate
       (d)   Ender's nail

Ans. (b)
Note
Subtrochanteric fractures of femur can be treated by all of the following methods except 'Smith Petersen nail'.
Also see
Smith-Peterson nail is used for internal fixation in case of intracapsular fracture of femur.
    -In case of subtrochanteric fracture if the general condition of the patient is poor traction is offered by Thomas splint.
    -If general condition is good then internal fixation is done.
Ref: A Concise Textbook of Surgery, S. Das, 3rd Ed, Chapter 22, page 369 and 367

Q. 221. All of the following are true about fracture of the atlas vertebra, except
       (a)   Jefferson fracture is the most common type.
       (b)   Quadriplegia is seen in 80% cases.
       (c)   Atlanto-occipital fusion may sometimes be needed.
       (d)   CT scans should be done for diagnosis.

Ans. (d)
Note
All of the above are true about fracture of the atlas vertebra, except 'CT scan should be done for diagnosis.
Also see
Jefferson fracture is fracture of ring of C1 caused by axial loading. Although the fracture can usually be diagnosed on plain X-ray, CT is helpful in determining the fracture pattern and to be sure that there is no associated injury of the adjacent levels.
They are usually treated in a halo jacket for 3 months. Occassionally the fracture may fail to heal and persistent instability may be present. This requires posterior occipitocervical fusion.
Ref: -Bailey and love's short practice of surgery, chapter 33, page 510
Trauma to the cervical spine may lead to spinal cord compression which may in turn lead to UMN signs and sensory loss in all 4 limbs.
Ref: Davidson's Principles and Practice of Medicine, 19th Ed, Chapter 22, page 1187-1188

Q. 222. A 30-year-old man had road traffic accident and sustained fracture of femur. Two days later he developed sudden breathlessness. The most probable cause can be
       (a)   Pneumonia
       (b)   Congestive heart failure
       (c)   Bronchial asthma
       (d)   Fat embolism

Ans. (d)
Note
The most probable cause for his sudden breathlessness can be 'fat embolism'.
Also see
Due to bony injury the chylomicrons become aggregated and form large embolic fat globules in the circulation, lung capillaries are the first place where they lodge. Incidence of fat embolism is greatest following fracture of the femoral shafts. It affects the lungs, brain and skin.
It presents as

- Tachypnoea, dyspnoea and cyanosis.
- Confusion, agitation and stupor.
- Petechial hemorrhages on the chest, axilla and upper extremity.

Ref: A Concise Textbook of Surgery, S. Das, 3rd Ed, Chapter 22, page 310

Q. 223. A 45-year-old was given steroids after renal transplant. After 2 years he had difficulty in walking and pain in both hips. Which one of the following is most likely cause?
- (a) Primary osteoarthritis
- (b) Avascular necrosis
- (c) Tuberculosis
- (d) Aluminum toxicity

Ans. (b)

Note
Most likely cause for above given clinical presentation is 'avascular necrosis'.

Also see
Causes of avascular necrosis of head of femur are:
a. Congenital – Sickle cell anaemia, thalassaemia
b. Drug induced – Steroids and alcohol
c. Trauma
d. Infections – Septic arthritis
e. Environmental – Caisson's disease

The patient complains of sudden onset of pain in the hip joint. On examination nothing may be found except painful limitation of movement.

Ref: Bailey and Love's Short Practice of Surgery, 24th Ed, Chapter23, page 376

Q. 224. All of the following areas are commonly involved sites in pelvic fracture except
- (a) Pubic rami
- (b) Alae of ileum
- (c) Acetabula
- (d) Ischial tuberosities

Ans. (d)

Note
All of the above areas are commonly involved sites in pelvic fracture except 'ischial tuberosities'.

Also see
Pelvic fractures represent 3% of all skeletal fractures, with single pubic rami and avulsion fractures the most common.
Acetabular fractures most commonly involve disruption of the acetabular socket when the hip is driven backward in a motor vehicle accident.
http://www.emedicine.com/emerg/topic203.htm
Fracture of the ischial tuberosities is a kind of an avulsion fracture.
In general, they are uncommon injuries, seen almost exclusively in adolescent athletes with a 2:1 male to female preponderance.
 - They occur most often in track events like hurdling and sprinting, or games like soccer or tennis.
 - Most common to avulse is the ischial tuberosity followed by anterior inferior iliac spine (AIIS) and the anterior superior iliac spine (ASIS) about equally.

Ref:- http://www.learningradiology.com/archives06/COW%20205-Ischial%20Avulsion%20Fx/avulseischiumcorrect.html

Q.225. In some old fractures, cartilaginous tissue forms over the fractured bone ends with a cavity in between containing clear fluid. This condition is called as
- (a) Delayed union
- (b) Slow union
- (c) Non union
- (d) Pseudarthrosis

Ans. (d)

Note
The above condition is known as 'pseudarthrosis'.

Also see
Pseudoarthrosis is the formation of a false joint caused by the failure of the bones to fuse. This most commonly occurs when the bones do not heal properly after a fracture.

Pseudoarthrosis usually causes pain, because the two bones are moving against each other, instead of being fused together. This movement may cause problems with metal screws or other hardware used to fuse the bones together. Additional surgery may be required to align the bones and fuse them together.

Ref:- http://www.universityhealth.org/134506.cfm

Q. 226. All of the following can be the complications of a malunited Colle's fracture, except
    (a)   Rupture of flexor pollicis longus tendon
    (b)   Reflex sympathetic dystrophy (RSD)
    (c)   Carpal tunnel syndrome
    (d)   Carpal instability

Ans. (a)

Note
All of the above can be the complications of a malunited Colle's fracture, except 'Rupture of flexor pollicis longus tendon'.

Also see
In Colle's fracture nerve injury is not usually seen but median nerve compression may be seen on rare occasions.

Delayed rupture of extensor pollicis longus tendon sometimes occurs rarely after Colle's fracture. It is more common after undisplaced fracture rather than displaced fracture, and is due to ischaemic degeneration of the tendon following injury to the vascular supply of the tendons.

Ref: A Concise Textbook of Surgery, S. Das, 3rd Ed, Chapter 23, page 352

Q. 227. Tuberculosis of the spine commonly affects all of the following parts of the vertebra, except
    (a)   Body
    (b)   Lamina
    (c)   Spinous process
    (d)   Pedicle

Ans. (c)

Note
Tuberculosis of the spine commonly affects all of the above parts of the vertebra, except 'Spinous process'.

Also see
Tuberculosis can affect all the four
Clinically there are four types:
a. Para discal lesion begins in the metaphysis erodes the cartilage and destroys the disc, resulting in narrowing of the disc space.
b. Central type begins in the midsection of the body, which gets softened and yields under gravity and muscle action, leading to compression, collapse and bony deformation.
c. Anterior lesions lead to cortical bone destruction beneath the anterior longitudinal ligament. Spread of the infection is in the subperiosteal and sub ligamentous planes resulting in the loss of periosteal blood supply to the body with resultant collapse. Other factors such as periarteritis and endarteritis contribute to the collapses.
d. In appendicle type, the infection settles in the pedicles, the laminae, the articular processes or the spinous processes and causes initial ballooning of the structure followed by destruction

Ref: http://www.thamburaj.com/spinal_tuberculosis.html

Q. 228. An army recruit, smoker and 6 months into training started complaining of pain at posterior medial aspect of both legs. There was acute point tenderness and the pain was aggravated on physical activity. The most likely diagnosis is
    (a)   Buerger's disease
    (b)   Gout

(c) Lumbar canal stenosis
(d) Stress fracture

Ans. (d)

Note
The most likely diagnosis for the above clinical presentation is 'stress fracture'.

Also see
It is also known as fatigue fracture. Often repeated trauma or loads applied to the skeleton at the same site may cause such a fracture. This is commonest in the metatarsals but may also be found in the tibia, fibula, and neck of femur. In such a case the fracture site becomes painful and tender.
Ref: A Concise Textbook of Surgery, S. Das, 3rd Ed, Chapter 22, page 295

Q. 229. Management plan for osteogenic sarcoma of the lower end of femur must include
(a) Radiotherapy - amputation - chemotherapy
(b) Surgery alone
(c) Chemotherapy - limb salvage surgery - chemotherapy
(d) Chemotherapy + radiotherapy

Ans. (a)

Note
Management plan for osteogenic sarcoma of the lower end of femur must include 'Radiotherapy – amputation – chemotherapy'.

Also see
Majority of the patients with osteosarcoma should be treated with radiotherapy first followed by amputation provided they do not develop early lung metastasis.
Amputation- In case of lower femur growth disarticulation of hip should be considered.
Ref: A Concise Textbook of Surgery, S. Das, 3rd Ed, Chapter 28, page 441-442

Q. 230. The management of fat embolism includes all the following, except
(a) Oxygen
(b) Heparinization
(c) Low Molecular weight dextran
(d) Pulmonary embolectomy

Ans. (d)

Note
The management of fat embolism includes all the following, except 'Pulmonary embolectomy'.

Also see
Due to bony injury the chylomicrons become aggregated and form large embolic fat globules in the circulation.
Treatment consists of 2 components: -
a. Prophylaxis: Early stabilization of the fracture, IV infusion, electrolyte balance, O_2 therapy especially in low PaO_2. Heparin has also been suggested in the management of fat embolism.
b. Therapeutic: Corticosteroids therapy and ventilatory support along with positive pressure respiration with O_2.
Ref: A Concise Textbook of Surgery, S. Das, 3rd Ed, Chapter 22, page 310

Q. 231. A 25 year old male with roadside accident underwent debridement and reduction of fractured both bones right forearm under axillary block. On the second postoperative day the patient complained of persistent numbness and paraesthesia in the right forearm and the hand. The commonest cause of this neurological dysfunction could be all of the following except
(a) Crush injury to the hand and lacerated nerves.
(b) A tight cast or dressing.
(c) Systemic toxicity of local anaesthetics.
(d) Tourniquet pressure.

Ans. (c)

Note
The commonest cause of this neurological dysfunction could be all of the above except 'systemic toxicity of local anaesthetics'.

Also see
Nerve injury due to a tourniquet leads to local block to conduction of nerve impulses at a discrete area along the course of nerve. It is a mild type of injury. Recovery is complete. Similar is the case with a tight dressing or a cast.
A laceration or a stretch to the nerve leads to Axonotmesis.In, which degeneration of nerve occurs but supporting structure remains intact.
Ref: Bailey and Love's Short Practice of Surgery, 24th Ed, Chapter34, page 532

Q. 232. Commonest cause for neuralgic pain in foot is
    (a)   Compression of communication between medial and lateral plantar nerve
    (b)   Exaggeration of longitudinal arches
    (c)   Injury to deltoid ligament
    (d)   Shortening of plantar aponeurosis

Ans. (a)
Note
Commonest cause for neuralgic pain in foot is 'Compression of communication between medial lateral planter nerve'.

Also see
Compression of the communication between the lateral and medial plantar nerve causes neuralgic pain in the foot known as metatarsalgia. The cause of this is flat foot, which leads to: -
    -Loss of spring in the foot.
    -Loss of shock absorbing function.
    -Los of concavity of the sole leading to compression of nerves and vessels of the sole.
Medial and lateral plantar nerves are branches of the tibial nerve.
Medial nerve supplies the skin on the medial 3½ toes.
Lateral plantar nerve supplies lateral 1½ toes.
Ref: B.D.Chaurasia's human anatomy, 3rd Ed, Vol 2, chapter 13, page 142, and chapter 11, page 110

Q. 233. A ten-year old girl presents with swelling of one knee joint. All of the following conditions can be considered in the differential diagnosis, except
    (a)   Tuberculosis
    (b)   Juvenile rheumatoid arthritis
    (c)   Hemophilia
    (d)   Villonodular synovitis

Ans. (c)
Note
For the swelling of knee joint all of the above conditions can be considered in differential diagnosis except 'Hemophilia'.

Also see
Hemophilia is an X-linked recessive disorder. Thus on pedigree grounds girls are the carrier of the disease whereas boys suffer from the disease.
Ref: Davidson's Principles and Practice of Medicine, 19th Ed, Chapter 19, page 949

Q. 234. Avascular necrosis can be a possible sequelae of fracture of all of the following bones, except
    (a)   Femur neck
    (b)   Scaphoid
    (c)   Talus
    (d)   Calcaneum

Ans. (d)
Note
Avascular necrosis can be possible sequelae of fracture of all of the above bones, except 'Calcaneum'.

Also see
a) Complications of fracture neck of femur
The important complications are: a) Non-union b) Avascular necrosis of head of femur.
Ref: Bailey and Love's Short Practice of Surgery, Chapter 24, Pg- 377
b) Scaphoid: It is a fracture occurs after a fall on the out stretched hand. The bone fractures at right angle to the long axis. Its importance lies in the fact that it has a tendency to non-union and avascular necrosis of the body of the bone. Scaphoid normally has two nutrient arteries such a fracture may deprive the proximal ½ of its blood supply leading to avascular necrosis.
Ref: B.D.Chaurasia's human anatomy, 3rd Ed, Vol 2, chapter 2, page 23
c) Talus: Blood supply to the proximal half of the talus travels up the neck of this bone therefore a fracture across the neck leads to avascular necrosis.
Ref: Bailey and Love's Short Practice of Surgery, 24th Ed, Chapter24, page 399

The talus is predisposed to avascular necrosis (AVN), or bone death due to ischemia, owing to its unique structure, characteristic extraosseous arterial sources, and variable intraosseous blood supply. Both traumatic and atraumatic causes have been implicated in talar AVN. The risk of posttraumatic AVN can be predicted using the Hawkins classification system.
Ref: http://radiographics.rsnajnls.org/cgi/content/full/25/2/399

Q. 235. Sciatic nerve palsy may occur in the following injury
    (a) Posterior dislocation of hip joint
    (b) Fracture neck of femur
    (c) Trochanteric fracture
    (d) Anterior dislocation of hip

Ans. (a)

Note
Sciatic nerve palsy may occur in the injury 'Posterior dislocation of hip joint'.

Also see
Causes of sciatic nerve palsy:
Wounds – Fracture of pelvis, Posterior dislocation of the hip, Operation for hip replacement, and tumors, occasionally injure the sciatic nerve. The features present are:
Motor:
    -Paralysis of flexors of the knee.
    -Foot-drop may occur following complete paralysis below the knee.
Sensory:
    -Complete loss of sensations below the knee with the exception of skin supplied by saphenous nerve.
Ref: Bailey and Love's Short Practice of Surgery, 24th Ed, Chapter34, page 539

Q. 236. A 30-year old male was brought to the casualty following a road traffic accident. His physical examination revealed that his right lower limb was short, internally rotated and flexed and adducted at the hip. The most likely diagnosis is
    (a) Fracture neck of femur
    (b) Trochanteric fracture
    (c) Central fracture dislocation of hip
    (d) Posterior dislocation of hip

Ans. (d)

Note
The most likely diagnosis is for the above clinical presentation is 'Posterior dislocation of hip'.

Also see
Cause of dislocation is a force applied along the long axis of the shaft of femur when the hip is flexed and adducted.

On Inspection: -The leg is shorter, internally rotated and slightly flexed
Ref: A Concise Textbook of Surgery, S. Das, 3rd Ed, Chapter 24, page 358

MCQ's in Surgery   601

Q. 237. Which one of the following tests will you adopt while examining a knee joint where you suspect an old tear of anterior cruciate ligament?
    (a)   Posterior drawer test
    (b)   McMurray test
    (c)   Lachman test
    (d)   Pivot shift test

Ans. (c)
Note
Lachman test is suggested in suspected case of old tear of anterior cruciate ligament.

Also see
Three ways of assessing the anterior cruciate ligament are:
a.   Anterior drawer test.
b.   Lachman's test
c.   Pivot shift test (Macintosh test).
Lachman's test is more sensitive than is the anterior drawer sign.
The other situation where Lachman's test is used is during the examination of the acutely injured knee.
Ref: http://chpweb.weber.edu/hthsci/casestudies/ACL/examination_of_theanterior_cruci.html

Q. 238. An eight-year old boy presents with back pain and mild fever. His plain X-ray of the dorsolumbar spine reveals a solitary collapsed dorsal vertebra with preserved disc spaces. There was no associated soft tissue shadow. The most likely diagnosis is
    (a)   Ewing's sarcoma
    (b)   Tuberculosis
    (c)   Histiocytosis
    (d)   Metastasis

Ans. (c)
Note
The most likely diagnosis is for above clinical presentation is 'Histocytosis'.

Also see
It is a malignant proliferation of histiocytes and macrophages. There are three disorders included under it out of which the commonest is Eosinophilic granuloma. It is more common and most patients affected are children and young adults with a slight male preponderance. The condition presents as a solitary osteolytic lesion in the femur, skull, vertebra, ribs and pelvis. The lesions remain asymptomatic until erosion of the bone and pain occurs.
Ref: Textbook of Pathology by Harsh Mohan, 4th Ed, Chapter 13, Page 426

Q. 239. Kienbock's disease is due to avascular necrosis of
    (a)   Femoral neck
    (b)   Medial cuneiform bone
    (c)   Lunate bone
    (d)   Scaphoid bone

Ans. (c)
Note
Kienbock's disease is due to avascular necrosis of 'Lunate bone'.

Also see
The etiology is unclear but involves both ischaemia and microtrauma to the lunate causing sclerosis initially then collapse and finally arthritis. Many patients have a relatively short ulna.
Ref: Bailey and Love's Short Practice of Surgery, 4th Ed, Chapter30, Page 488

Q. 240. Pseudoclaudication is due to compression of
    (a)   Femoral artery
    (b)   Femoral nerve
    (c)   Cauda Equina
    (d)   Popliteal artery

Ans. (c)

Note
Pseudoclaudication is due to compression of 'Cauda Equina'.

Also see
In lumbar canal stenosis in elderly patients there is development of exercise induced weakness and paraesthesia in the legs. (Cauda equina claudication)
These symptoms progress with continous exertion and are relieved rapidly on taking a short rest. On examination peripheral pulses are normal.
Ref: Davidson's Principles and Practice of Medicine, 19th Ed, Chapter 22, page 1191

Q. 241. Carpel tunnel syndrome is due to compression of
    (a) Radial nerve
    (b) Ulnar nerve
    (c) Palmar branch of the ulnar nerve
    (d) Median nerve

Ans. (d)

Note
Carpel tunnel syndrome is due to compression of 'Median nerve'.

Also see
This is a condition in which the median nerve is compressed at the wrist when it passes through the carpal tunnel. It is characterized by formication of fingers – index and middle and sometimes thumbs. There may also be pain in the distribution of median nerve distal to the tunnel.
Ref: A Concise Textbook of Surgery, S. Das, 3rd Ed, Chapter 20, page 282

Q. 242. Most common nerve involved in the fracture of surgical neck of humerus is
    (a) Median
    (b) Radial
    (c) Ulnar
    (d) Axillary

Ans. (d)

Note
Most common nerve involved in the fracture of surgical neck of humerus is 'Axillary nerve'.

Also see
a. Median nerve is injured at the wrist or elbow due to fracture of the distal humerus or dislocation of the elbow joint.
b. Radial nerve: It is injured in the radial groove in association with the shaft of humerus or as a result of pressure as in Saturday night palsy due to falling into a heavy sleep with the arm over the sharp edge of the back of the chair.
c. Ulnar nerve is damaged by lacerations in the forearms or entrapment as it passes behind the medial epicondyle of the humerus.
d. Axillary or circumflex nerve is damaged in dislocations of shoulder joint.
Ref: Bailey and Love's Short Practice of Surgery, 24th Ed, Chapter 34, page 538-539

Q. 243. All of the following are associated with supracondylar fracture of humerus, except
    (a) It is uncommon after 15 years of age.
    (b) Extension type fracture is more common than the flexion type.
    (c) Cubitus varus deformity commonly results following malunion.
    (d) Ulnar nerve is most commonly involved.

Ans. (d)

Note
All of above are associated with supracondylar fracture of humerus, except 'ulnar nerve is most commonly involved'.

MCQ's in Surgery

Also see
Supracondylar fracture is the commonest fracture around the elbow in children and usually occurs in children under 10. The injury is usually due to a fall on the outstretched hand with an extended elbow and these results in a hyperextension injury with posterior angulation with or without posterior displacement of the distal fracture.

Complications are:
- Occlusion of the brachial artery.
- Radial and median nerve injury.
- Volkmann's ischaemic contracture.
- Malunion: A flexion or extension deformity will remodel. Varous deformity with gunstock deformity is unsightly but not a functional problem.

Ref: Bailey and Love's Short Practice of Surgery, 24th Ed, Chapter 22, page 357-359

Q. 244. A 40 years old man, was admitted with fracture shaft femur following a road traffic accident. On 2nd day he became disoriented. He was found to be tachypnoeic, and had conjunctival petechiae. Most likely diagnosis is
(a) Pulmonary embolism
(b) Sepsis syndrome
(c) Fat embolism
(d) Hemothorax

Ans. (c)

Note
Most likely diagnosis for above clinical presentation is 'fat embolism'.

Q. 245. Kumar, a 31 years old motorcyclist sustained injury over his right hip joint. X-ray revealed a posterior dislocation of the right hip joint. The clinical attitude of the affected lower limb will be
(a) External rotation, extension & abduction
(b) Internal rotation, flexion & adduction
(c) Internal rotation, extension & abduction
(d) External rotation, flexion & abduction

Ans. (b)

Note
In the above given presentation of posterior dislocation of right hip joint, clinical attitude of the affected lower limb will be 'internal rotation, flexion and adduction'.

Also see
Cause of dislocation is a force applied along the long axis of the shaft of femur when the hip is flexed and adducted.
On Inspection:
- The leg is shorter, internally rotated and slightly flexed.

Ref: A Concise Textbook of Surgery, S. Das, 3rd Ed, Chapter 24, page 358

Q. 246. Pappu, 7 years old young boy, had fracture of lateral condyle of femur. He developed malunion as the fracture was not reduced anatomically. Malunion will produce
(a) Genu valgum
(b) Genu varum
(c) Genu recurvatum
(d) Dislocation of knee

Ans. (a)

Note
In the above given presentation malunion of fracture of lateral condyle of femur will produce 'Genu valgum'.

Also see
Genu valgum or knock-knee means excessive adduction of the knee joint.

Causes:
- Bone softening as in rickets, osteomalacia.
- Laxity of ligaments – Particularly medial collateral ligament.
- Bone injury- Epiphyseal damage, fracture of the lateral tibial condyle.
- Thinned out cartilage – OA
- Muscle weakness
- Idiopathic

Ref: A Concise Textbook of Surgery, S. Das, 3rd Ed, Chapter 29, Pg- 484

Q. 247. Inversion injury at the ankle can cause all of the following except
(a) Fracture tip of lateral melleolus
(b) Fracture base of the 5th metatarsal
(c) Sprain of extensor digitorum brevis
(d) Fracture of sustentaculam tali

Ans. (c)

Note
Inversion injury at the ankle can cause all of the above except 'sprain of extensor digitorum brevis'.

Also see
Extensor digitorum brevis is a muscle situated on the lateral part of the dorsum of the foot arising out of calcaneum, inferior retinaculum and interosseous talocalcaneal ligament.
Its action is extension of the MTP joints of the 1st, 2nd, 3rd and 4th toe.
Ref: B.D.Chaurasia's human anatomy, 3rd Ed, Vol 2, chapter 8, page 87
Therefore it is unlikely to be injured in inversion injury of the foot

Q. 248. A previously healthy 45 years old laborer suddenly develops acute lower back pain with right-leg pain & weakness of dorsiflexion of the right great toe. Which of the following is true?
(a) Immediate treatment should include analgesics, muscle relaxants & back strengthening exercises.
(b) The appearance of the foot drop indicates early surgical intervention.
(c) If the neurological signs resolve within 2 to 3 weeks but low back pain persists, the proper treatment would include fusion of affected lumbar vertebra.
(d) If the neurological signs fail to resolve within 1 week, lumbar laminectomy and excision of any herniated nucleus pulposus should be done.

Ans. (b)

Note
In the above given clinical presentation 'the appearance of foot drop indicates early surgical intervention'.

Also see
The signs and symptoms given indicate that the prolapse is at the level of L4-L5. Immediate treatment involves absolute bed rest for at least 3 weeks. Surgery and fusion is indicated in cases if the neurological symptoms are progressing and there is no response to conservative treatment being given.
Ref: Davidson's Principles and Practice of Medicine, 19th Ed, Chapter 22, page 1191

Q. 249. Acute osteomyelitis is most commonly caused by
(a) Staphylococcus aureus
(b) Actinomyces bovis
(c) Nocardia asteroides
(d) Borrelia vincentii

Ans. (a)

Note
Acute osteomyelitis is most commonly caused by 'staphylococcus aureus'.

Also see
It is an acute infective and inflammatory process around the bone caused by pyogenic organisms. The commonest being staphylococcus aureus.

It is a disease of childhood and occurs frequently in the undernourished people with poor general resistance.
Ref: A Concise Textbook of Surgery, S. Das, 3rd Ed, Chapter 25, page 389

Q. 250. A 45 years male presented with an expansile lesion in the centre of femoral metaphysic. The lesion shows endosteal scalloping & punctuate calcifications. Most likely diagnosis is
- (a) Osteosarcoma
- (b) Chondrosarcoma
- (c) Simple bone cyst
- (d) Fibrous dysplasia

Ans. (b)

Note
Most likely diagnosis is for the above clinical presentation is 'chondrosarcoma'.

Also see
It is a malignant tumor of the chondroblasts arising within the diaphysis or metaphysis (central chondrosarcoma) and periosteum of metaphysis (peripheral chondrosarcoma). Both forms of chondrosarcoma occur in the 3rd – 6th decade with male preponderance.

They are found in central skeleton and around the knee joint. X-ray shows hugely expansile and osteolytic growth with foci of calcification. It is a slow growing tumor and comes to attention due to pain and gradual enlargement.
Ref: Textbook of Pathology by Harsh Mohan, 4th Ed, Chapter 25, Page 828

Q. 251. Raju, a 10 years old child, presents with predisposition to fractures, anemia, hepatosplenomegaly and a diffusely increased radiographic density of bones. The most likely diagnosis is
- (a) Osteogenesis imperfecta
- (b) Pyenodysotosis
- (c) Myelofibrosis
- (d) Osteopetrosis

Ans. (d)

Note
The most likely diagnosis for above clinical presentation is 'Osteopetrosis'.

Also see
Osteopetrosis is also known as the marble bone disease. It occurs due to defective osteoclast function. It is an autosomal dominant or recessive disorder.
There is overgrowth of calcified dense bone occupying the whole of marrow space available. There is hypocalcaemia. Despite this there is poor skeletal support and high susceptibility to fracture. The infantile malignant form is characterized by anaemia, thrombocytopenia, neutropenia and hepato-splenomegaly.
Osteogenesis imperfecta: Autosomal dominant or recessive disorder characterized by defective osteoblasts leading to thin cortices and irregular trabeculae. These fragile bones become liable to fracture.
Ref: Textbook of Pathology by Harsh Mohan, 4th Ed, Chapter 25, Page 817

Q. 252. In a patient with head injury, unexplained hypotension warrants evaluation of
- (a) Upper cervical spine
- (b) Lower cervical spine
- (c) Thoracic spine
- (d) Lumbar spine

Ans. (c)

Note
In a patient with head injury, unexplained hypotension warrants evaluation of 'thoracic spine'.

Also see
Hypotension in a patient with injury to the head could be possibly due to trauma to the thoracic spine. This leads to damage to the thoraco-lumbar sympathetic neurons from the medullary cardiovascular center producing a marked fall in the BP from a resting value of 100 to 40 mm of Hg.

Ref: Textbook of Physiology by A.K. Jain, vol-2, Unit- 9, Cp-8, Pg 906
This occurs due to loss of venous tone with pooling of the blood in the dilated peripheral venous system, therefore the heart doesn't fill properly and cardiac output falls.
Ref: A Concise Textbook of Surgery, S. Das, 3rd Ed, Chapter 2, page 8

Q. 253. Complete transection of the spinal cord at the C_1 level produces all of the following effects except
    (a)   Hypotension
    (b)   Limited respiratory effort
    (c)   Anaesthesia below the level of the lesion
    (d)   Areflexia below the level of the lesion

Ans. (b)
Note

Complete transection of the spinal cord at the C_1 level produces all of the following effects except 'limited respiratory effort'.

Also see
Complete transection of spinal cord at C_1 leads to loss of all functions below the level of transection, whereas the upper part remains normal.
Respiration is regulated by two mechanisms:
    a.   Autonomic regulation- by medulla and pons
    b.   Voluntary control- by cerebral cortex

Therefore a transection below or at the level of C_1 will not affect respiration.
Ref: Textbook of physiology by A.K. Das, vol-1, Unit- 6, Cp-4, Pg 442

Q. 254. Following anterior dislocation of the shoulder, a patient develops weakness of flexion at elbow and lack of sensation over the lateral aspect fore arm. Nerve injured is
    (a)   Radial nerve
    (b)   Musculocutaneous nerve
    (c)   Axillary nerve
    (d)   Ulnar nerve

Ans. (b)
Note
The nerve injury in above clinical presentation appears to be of 'musculocutaneous nerve'.

Also see
The musculocutaneous nerve is the main nerve of the front of the arm and continues below the elbow as lateral cutaneous nerve of the forearm. It is the branch of lateral cord of brachial plexus.
Actions: Muscular: supplies the coracobrachialis, biceps and brachialis.
Sensory- It supplies the skin on the lateral side of forearm from elbow to the wrist.
Ref: B.D.Chaurasia's human anatomy, 3rd Ed, Vol 1, chapter 8, page 81-82

Q. 255. Babloo a 10 years old boy presents with fracture of humerus. X-ray reveals a lytic lesion at the upper end. Likely condition is
    (a)   Unicameral bone cyst
    (b)   Osteosarcoma
    (c)   Osteoclastoma
    (d)   Aneurysmal bone cyst

Ans. (a)
Note
The likely condition for above given clinical presentation is 'unicameral bone cyst'.
Also see
Unicameral / simple /solitary bone cyst
It is a benign condition occurring in children and adolescents. It most frequently affects the metaphysis of upper end of humerus. The cyst expands the bone causing thinning of the overlying cortex.
C/F: It may remain asymptomatic or may cause pain due to fracture.

Osteosarcoma
Osteosarcoma is the most common type of malignant bone cancer, accounting for 35% of primary bone malignancies. There is a preference for the metaphyseal region of tubular long bones. 50% of cases occur around the knee.
Ref: http://en.wikipedia.org/wiki/Osteosarcoma
Osteoclastoma
Osteoclastoma: A type of bone tumor characterized by massive destruction of bone near the end (epiphysis) of a long bone. The site most commonly struck by this tumor is the knee - the far end of the femur and the near end of the tibia. The tumor is often coated by new bony growth. It causes pain and restricts movement. Treatment for osteoclastoma is surgery.
Osteoclastoma occurs more often than women than in men and has a peak incidence in the third decade of life. Osteoclastoma, also called giant cell tumor of bone. The tumor is full of large multinucleate cells (cells with more than one nucleus) that look gigantic when viewed magnified through a microscope.
Ref: http://www.medterms.com/script/main/art.asp?articlekey=11795
Aneurysmal bone cyst
It is an expanding osteolytic lesion filled with blood seen in patients less than 30 yrs of age. Bones frequently involved are shafts of metaphyses of long bones or vertebral column.

X-ray shows a characteristic ballooned out expansile lesion under the periosteum.
Ref: Textbook of pathology by Harsh Mohan, 4th Ed, chapter 25, page 822

Q. 256. A patient sustained injury to the upper limb 3 years back. He now presents with valgus deformity in the elbow and paraesthesia over the medial border of the hand. The injury is likely to have been
    (a)   Supracondylar fracture humerus
    (b)   Lateral condyle fracture humerus
    (c)   Medial condyle fracture humerus
    (d)   Posterior dislocation of the humerus

Ans. (b)

Note
The injury is likely to have been 'lateral condyle fracture humurus' as per the above given clical presentation.

Also see
Lateral condylar fracture is relatively common injury caused by a fall on the outstretched hand especially in children.
Complications:
Non-union occurring due to a missed fracture or inadequate fixation. This may lead to valgus deformity and tardy ulnar nerve palsy.
Ref: Bailey and Love's Short Practice of Surgery, 24th Ed, Chapter 22, page 359&360

Q. 257. A woman aged 60 years suffers a fall. Her lower limb is abducted and externally rotated. Likely diagnosis is
    (a)   Neck of femur fracture
    (b)   Intertrochanteric femur fracture
    (c)   Posterior dislocation of hip
    (d)   Anterior dislocation of hip

Ans. (d)

Note
A woman aged 60 years suffers a fall. Her lower limb is abducted and externally rotated Likely diagnosis is 'anterior dislocation of hip'.

Also see
It is caused when the hip is widely abducted and femur is externally rotated, e.g. when a weight falls on the back of a person who is working with abducted legs knees straight and bent forwards.
The attitude in ADH is characteristic- the hip is flexed, externally rotated and abducted.
Ref: A Concise Textbook of Surgery, S. Das, 3rd Ed, Chapter 24, page 360-361

Q. 258. Triple arthrodesis involves
(a) Calcaneocuboid, talonavicular and talocalcaneal
(b) Tibiotalar, calcaneocuboid and talonavicular
(c) Ankle joint, calcaneocuboid and talonavicular
(d) None of the above

Ans. (a)

Note
Triple arthrodesis involves 'Calcaneocubouid, talonavicular and talocalcaneal'.

Also see
A triple arthrodesis consists of the surgical fusion of the talocalcaneal (TC), talonavicular (TN), and calcaneocuboid (CC) joints in the foot. The primary goals of a triple arthrodesis are to relieve pain from arthritic, deformed, or unstable joints. Other important goals are the correction of deformity and creation of a stable, balanced plantigrade foot. A common feature of patients is the development of degenerative joint disease (DJD). Depending on the underlying pathology, the patient may present with a varus or valgus deformity or neither. Post-traumatic arthritis often presents with a rectus foot and complaints consistent with DJD of the STJ.
Ref: http://www.emedicine.com/orthoped/topic354.htm

Q. 259. Babu a 19 years old male has a small circumscribed sclerotic swelling over diaphysis of femur. Likely diagnosis is
(a) Osteoclastoma
(b) Osteosarcoma
(c) Ewing's sarcoma
(d) Osteoid osteoma

Ans. (d)

Note
Likely diagnosis for above is 'osteoid osteoma'.

Also see
The tumors affecting diaphysis are:
Benign- osteoid osteomas, enchondroma, adamantioma
Malignant- Ewing's sarcoma, chondrosarcoma, lymphoma

Osteoid osteoma
It is a commonly seen tumor in the young and is generally small and painful. It is located in the cortex of long bones. The tumor is clearly demarcated. On X-ray it appears as-a small radiolucent central focus or either surrounded by dense sclerotic bone.
Ref: Textbook of Pathology by Harsh Mohan, 4th Ed, Chapter 25, Page 823

Q. 260. Most common site of osteogenic sarcoma is
(a) Femur, upper end
(b) Femur, lower end
(c) Tibia, upper end
(d) Tibia, lower end

Ans. (b)

Note
Most common site of osteogenic sarcoma is 'femur lower end'.

Also see
It is the most common primary malignant tumor of the bone. It is seen in patients aged 10-20 yrs. Males are more frequently affected than females. They tumor arises in the epiphyses of long bones. Most commonly affected sites in descending order of frequency are:
a. Lower femur
b. Upper tibia
c. Upper humerus
d. Pelvis
e. Upper end of femur
f. Less frequently it also affects the jaw bones and vertebrae.
Ref: Textbook of Pathology by Harsh Mohan, 4th Ed, Chapter 25, page 824

Q. 261. Involvement of PIP joint, DIP joint and the carpometacarpal joint of base of thumb with sparing the wrist is seen in
 (a) Rheumatoid arthritis
 (b) Osteoarthritis
 (c) Psoriatic arthritis
 (d) Pseudogout

Ans. (b)
Note
Involvement of PIP joint, DIP joint and the carpometacarpal joint of base of thumb with sparing the wrist is seen in 'Osteoarthritis'.
Also see
Osteoarthrosis is a non-inflammatory degenerative disease of the joints characterized by focal loss of hyaline cartilage and simultaneous proliferation of new bone with remodeling of the joint contour. OA preferentially affects certain small and large joints. Large joints- knee, hip, intervertebral joints (cervical and lumbar). Small joints- MTP joints of the foot, 1st MCP, DIP and PIP joints.
Ref: Davidson's Principles and Practice of Medicine, 19th Ed, Chapter 20, page 996-999

Q. 262. The pivot test is for
 (a) Anterior cruciate ligament
 (b) Posterior cruciate ligament
 (c) Medial meniscus
 (d) Lateral meniscus

Ans. (a)
Note
The pivot test is for 'anterior cruciate ligament'.
Also see
Three ways of assessing the anterior cruciate ligament are:
a. Anterior drawer test
b. Lachman's test
c. Pivot shift test (Macintosh test)
Ref: http://chpweb.weber.edu/hthsci/casestudies/ACL/examination_of_theanterior_cruci.html

Q. 263. Iliotibial band contracture following polio is likely to result in
 (a) Extension at hip
 (b) Extension at knee
 (c) Flexion at hip and knee
 (d) Extension at hip and knee

Ans. (c)
Note
Iliotibial band contracture following polio is likely to result in 'Flexion at hip and knee'.
Also see
Poliomyelitis leads to certain patterns of deformities such as flexion contracture of the knee, hip and calcaneus of the hind foot. Patient with weak quadriceps and flexion conracture may develop knee-hand gait in which the hand supports the knee, which can't be locked into extension.
Ref: Bailey and Love's Short Practice of Surgery, 24th Ed, Chapter 27, page 453

ENT

Q. 264. Which of the following would be the most appropriate treatment for rehabilitation of a patient, who has bilateral profound deafness following surgery for bilateral acoustic schwannoma?
 (a) Bilateral high powered digital hearing aid
 (b) Bilateral cochlear implants
 (c) Unilateral cochlear implant
 (d) Brain stem implant

Ans. (d)

Note
Most appropriate rehabilitation for above given presentation would be 'brain stem implant'.
Also see
This procedure is used to treat deafness caused by damage to the vestibulocochlear nerve due to tumors or surgery.
In people with vestibulocochlear nerve damage, hearing is not improved by hearing aids or cochlear implants.
Auditory brain stem implants are electrodes placed in a part of the brain (the cochlear nucleus) responsible for processing sound signals carried to it from the ear through the vestibulocochlear nerve.
Ref: http://www.nice.org.uk/page.aspx?o=56897

Q. 265. Iatrogenic traumatic facial nerve palsy is most commonly caused during
    (a)   Myringoplasty
    (b)   Stapedectomy
    (c)   Mastoidectomy
    (d)   Ossiculoplasty

Ans. (c)
Note
Iatrogenic traumatic facial nerve palsy is most commonly caused during 'mastoidectomy'.
Also see
Facial nerve palsy is a common complication of cortical mastoidectomy. Other complications are:
    -Dislocation of incus
    -Injury to sigmoid sinus with profuse bleeding
    -Injury to the duramater of middle cranial fossa
    -Injury to horizontal semicircular canal
    -Post-operative wound infection
Ref: Diseases of Ear Nose & Throat by P.L. Dhingra, Cp 77, Pg 462

Q. 266. Which of the following is not the site for paraganglioma?
    (a)   Carotid bifurcation
    (b)   Jugular foramen
    (c)   Promontary in middle ear
    (d)   Geniculate ganglion

Ans. (d)
Note
Out of above 'geniculate ganglion' is not the site for paraganglioma.
Also see
Tumors originating from parasympathetic ganglion are called paraganglioma and are named according to location of tissue. The ones arising from the glomus jugulare bodies of middle ear are called as jugular paraganglioma and are the most common benign tumors of the middle ear.
Histologically similar tumors are found in carotid bodies at the bifurcation of CCA and vagus.
Ref: Textbook of Pathology by Harsh Mohan, 4th Ed, Chapter 15, Page 493

Q. 267. In complete bilateral palsy of recurrent laryngeal nerves, there is
    (a)   Complete loss of speech with stridor and dyspnea
    (b)   Complete loss of speech but no difficulty in breathing
    (c)   Preservation of speech with severe stridor and dyspnea
    (d)   Preservation of speech and no difficulty in breathing

Ans. (c)
Note
In complete bilateral palsy of recurrent laryngeal nerves, there is 'Preservation of speech with severe stridor and dyspnea'.
Also see
Commonest cause of bilateral recurrent laryngeal nerve palsy is neuritis or surgical trauma during thyroidectomy.

C/F: As both cords lie in median or paramedian position the airway is inadequate causing dyspnea and stridor but voice is good. Dyspnea and stridor are aggravated on exertion and crying.
Ref: Diseases of Ear Nose & Throat by P.L. Dhingra, Cp 60, Pg 361

Q. 268. "Gold standard" surgical procedure for prevention of aspiration is
    (a)   Thyroplasty
    (b)   Tracheostomy
    (c)   Tracheal division and permanent tracheostome
    (d)   Feeding gasgtrostomy/jejunostomy

Ans. (b)
Note
"Gold standard" surgical procedure for prevention of aspiration is 'tracheostomy'.
Also see
Tracheostomy
An opening is made into the anterior wall of trachea and convert it into a stoma on the skin surface.
Functions of tracheostomy:
a.   Protection of airways from pharyngeal secretions.
b.   Altered pathway for breathing.
c.   Permits removal of tracheo-bronchial secretions.
d.   Administration of anesthetics.
Ref: Diseases of ear nose & throat by P.L. Dhingra, Cp 64, Pg 381

Q. 269. Which of the following statement is not true for contact ulcer?
    (a)   The commonest site is the junction of anterior 1/3rd and middle 1/3rd of vocal cord and gastroesophageal reflux is the causative factor.
    (b)   Can be caused by intubation injury.
    (c)   The vocal process is the site and is caused/aggravated by acid reflux.
    (d)   Can be caused by adductor dysphonia.

Ans. (a)
Note
The statement 'the commonest site is the junction of anterior $1/3^{rd}$ and middle $1/3^{rd}$ of vocal cord and gastgroesophageal reflux is the causative factor' is not true for contact ulcer.
Also see
Contact ulcer is produced due to faulty voice production in which vocal processes of arytenoids hammer against each other resulting in ulceration and granuloma formation. Some cases are due to gastric reflux.
Chief complaints are:
      - Hoarseness of voice.
      - A constant desire to clear the throat.
      - Pain in throat worse on phonation.
On examination: Unilateral or bilateral ulcers with congestion of arytenoids cartilages. There may be granuloma formation.
Ref: Diseases of Ear Nose & Throat by P.L. Dhingra, Cp 61, Pg 318

Q. 270. All of the following cause a gray-white membrane on the tonsils, except
    (a)   Infectious mononucleosis
    (b)   Ludwig's angina
    (c)   Streptococcal tonsillitis
    (d)   Diphtheria

Ans. (b)
Note
All of the above cause a gray-white membrane on the tonsils, except 'Ludwig's angina'.
Also see
D/D of membrane formation over tonsils:
a.   Membranous tonsillitis
b.   Diphtheria
c.   Vincent's angina

d. Infectious mononucleosis
e. Agranulocytosis
f. Leukaemia
g. Aphthous ulcers
h. Malignancy of tonsils
i. Traumatic ulcer

Ref: Diseases of Ear Nose & Throat by P.L. Dhingra, Cp 52, Pg 313-315

Q. 271. A tracheostomised patient, with Portex tracheostomy tube, in the ward, developed sudden complete blockage of the tube. Which of the following is the best next step in the management?
 (a) Immediate removal of the tracheostomy tube
 (b) Suction of tube with sodium bicarbonate
 (c) Suction of tube with saline
 (d) Jet ventilation

Ans. (a)

Note
The best step in the management of above given case is 'immediate removal of the tracheostomy tube'.

Also see
This is usually due to viscid mucous blocking the tube.
Humidification will render the secretions less viscid. A sucker or a catheter is used to keep the tracheo-bronchial tree free of secretions. When mucous is very tenacious isotonic saline or a mucolytic agent may be advised through a nebuliser. If there is an inner tube it should be removed every 4 hrs and washed in sodium bicarbonate.
Ref: Bailey and Love's Short Practice of Surgery, 24th Ed, Chapter 43, page 692
Once the tube is out, administer oxygen through the stoma. Continue to assess respiratory rate, breathing effort, and the need for suctioning. If adequate spontaneous respirations can't be maintained or progress to respiratory arrest occurs, begin bagmask-valve ventilation with 100% oxygen. Place the bag-mask-valve device over his nose and mouth and occlude the stoma opening with a gloved finger or piece of gauze.
Prepare a second tracheostomy tube for insertion or clean the tube just removed. Assist in replacing the tracheostomy tube or inserting an endotracheal tube if the tracheostomy tube can't be reinserted..
Ref: http://www.findarticles.com/p/articles/mi_qa3689/is_200410/ai_n9431294

Q. 272. All of the following surgical procedures are used for allergic rhinitis, except
 (a) Radiofrequency ablation of the inferior turbinate
 (b) Laser ablation of the inferior turbinate
 (c) Submucosal placement of silastic in inferior turbinate
 (d) Inferior turbinectomy

Ans. (c)

Note
All of the above surgical procedures are used for allergic rhinitis, except 'Submucosal placement of silastic in inferior turbinate'.

Also see
Laser surgery, which is one type of surgical treatment for allergic and hypertrophic rhinitis.
Ref: - http://www.annals.com/abs/annals299.htm
Although allergic rhinitis is a medical condition, adjunctive surgery may be offered to alleviate obstructive symptoms in appropriate individuals. Examples are nasal polypectomy in the patients who have severe polyposis and various inferior turbinate reduction maneuvers in patients who have nasal obstruction caused by turbinate hypertrophy that persists despite maximal medical therapy.
Ref: http://www.emedicine.com/

Q. 273. Otoacoustic emissions arise from
 (a) Inner hair cells
 (b) Outer hair cells
 (c) Both inner and outer hair cells
 (d) Organ of Corti

Ans. (b)

Note
Otoacoustic emissions arise from 'outer hair cells'.

Also see
These are low intensity sounds produced by movement of outer hair cells of the cochlea and are produced either spontaneously or in response to the acoustic stimulation. Their absence indicates that the structure has been damaged or hair cells are non functional.
Ref: Diseases of ear nose & throat by P.L. Dhingra, Cp 5, Pg 36

Q. 274. A laryngocele arises from the
    (a)   True vocal cord
    (b)   Subglottis
    (c)   Saccule of the ventricle
    (d)   Anterior commissure

Ans. (c)
Note
A laryngocele arises from the 'Saccule of the ventricle'.

Also see
It is an air filled cystic swelling due to dilatation of the saccule. It may be
    -Internal- Confined to larynx and presents as distention of false cord
    -External- Distended saccule herniates through thyroid membrane
    -Combined/Mixed- Both internal and external components are present.
Ref: Diseases of ear nose & throat by P.L. Dhingra, Cp 61, Pg 367

Q. 275. Which one of the following statements truly represents Bell's paralysis?
    (a)   Hemiparesis and contralateral facial nerve paralysis.
    (b)   Combined paralysis of the facial, trigeminal and abducens nerves.
    (c)   Idiopathic ipsilateral paralysis of the facial nerve.
    (d)   Facial paralysis with a dry eye.

Ans. (c)
Note
Out of the above statement truly represents Bell's paralysis is 'Idiopathic ipsilateral paralysis of the facial nerve'.

Also see
Idiopathic facial nerve palsy or Bell's palsy is caused by damage to the portion of the facial nerve lying in facial canal, which leads to LMN symptoms on the affected side.
Ref: Davidson's Principles and Practice of Medicine, 19th Ed, Chapter 22, page 1183

Q. 276. All are true for Gradenigo's syndrome except
    (a)   It is associated with conductive hearing loss.
    (b)   It is caused by an abscess in the petrous apex.
    (c)   It leads to involvement of the cranial nerves V and VI.
    (d)   It is characterized by retro-orbital pain.

Ans. (a)
Note
All of the above are true for Gradenigo's syndrome except 'it is associated with conductive hearing loss'.

Also see
Gradenigo's syndrome is the classical presentation of petrositis, which is a complication of otitis media. It consists of a triad of:
    -External rectus palsy (6th cranial nerve)
    -Deep seated ear or retro-orbital pain (5th cranial nerve)
    -Persistent ear discharge
Fever, headache, malaise and neck rigidity may also be present.
Ref: Diseases of ear nose & throat by P.L. Dhingra, Cp 13, Pg 103

Q. 277. The most common and earliest manifestation of carcinoma of the glottis is
    (a)   Hoarseness
    (b)   Hemoptysis
    (c)   Cervical lymph nodes
    (d)   Stridor

Ans. (a)

Note
The most common and earliest manifestation of carcinoma of the glottis is 'hoarseness'.

Also see
In a vast majority of cases, laryngeal carcinoma originates in the glottic region. Free edge and upper surface of vocal cord in its anterior and middle third is the most frequent site.
Signs and symptoms are:
-Hoarseness of voice is an early sign because lesions of vocal cord affect its vibratory capacity. Increase in size of the growth with accompanying edema or cord fixation may cause stridor and laryngeal obstruction.
Ref: Diseases of ear nose & throat by P.L. Dhingra, Cp 62, Pg 371-372

Q. 278. Androphonia can be corrected by doing
    (a)   Type 1 Thyroplasty
    (b)   Type 2 Thyroplasty
    (c)   Type 3 Thyroplasty
    (d)   Type 4 Thyroplasty

Ans. (d)

Note
Androphonia can be corrected by doing 'type 4 Thyroplasty'.

Also see
The General information about the pitch of voice:
The frequency (or subjectively, the pitch) of a string is directly proportional to the tension in the string
So, when the vocal cord is shortened → Tension is decreased → Frequency decreases → Voice becomes more masculine.
When the vocal cord is lengthened → Tension increases → Frequency increase → Voice becomes more feminine.

The Question:
Here, the question says correction of "androphonia", which means that a person has a "male-ish" voice and the aim of the treatment would be to raise the frequency by lengthening the cord. That's why the answer is Type IV Isshiki Thyroplasty.

The distracters and the correct Ans.
Type 1 Thyroplasty is medialisation—In VC paralysis or VC atrophy.
Type 2 Thyroplasty is lateralisation- In severe adductor spasmodic dysphonia.
Type 3 Thyroplasty is relaxation of vocal fold to lower the vocal pitch— In lowering vocal pitch for excessive high pitch in males.
Type 4 Thyroplasty is tensing or stretching of vocal fold to raise the pitch by approximating cricothyriod.
Ref: http://www.rxpgonline.com/postt35407.html

Q. 279. Weber test is done by
    (a)   Placing the tuning fork on the mastoid process and comparing the bone conduction of the patient with that, of the examiner.
    (b)   Placing the tunning fork on the vertex of the skull and determining the effect of gently occluding the auditory canal on the threshold of low frequencies.
    (c)   Placing the tuning fork on the mastoid process and comparing the bone conduction in the patient.
    (d)   Placing the tuning fork on the forehead and asking him to report in which ear he hears it better

Ans. (d)

Note
Weber test is done by 'Placing the tuning fork on the forehead and asking him to report in which ear he hears it better'.
Also see
A vibrating tuning fork is placed on the middle of the forehead or vertex and the patient is asked in which ear the sound is heard normally it is heard equally in both ears.
It is lateralised to the worse ear in conductive deafness and the better ear in sensorineural deafness.
Ref: Diseases of ear nose & throat by P.L. Dhingra, Cp 5, Pg 30

Q. 280. On otological examination all of the following will have positive fistula test, except
    (a)   Dead ear
    (b)   Labyrinthine fistula
    (c)   Hypermobile stapes foot plate
    (d)   Following fenestration surgery
Ans. (a)
Note
On otological examination all of the following will have positive fistula test, except 'Dead ear'.
Also see
Fistula test
Basis of this test is to produce nystagmus by production of pressure changes in the external canal, which are transmitted to the labyrinth. Stimulation of labyrinth leads to nystagmus and vertigo.
Normally the test is negative because the pressure changes in the external auditory canal can't be transported to labyrinth. It is also absent when the labyrinth is dead.
It is positive in erosion of horizontal semicircular canal as in cholesteatoma or a surgically created window in it, abnormal opening in the oval window or the round window.
Ref: Diseases of ear nose & throat by P.L. Dhingra, Cp 7, Pg 53

Q. 281. Acute otitis media in children is most commonly due to
    (a)   Morexiella catarrhalis
    (b)   H influenzae
    (c)   Streptococcus pneumoniae
    (d)   Staphylococcus aureus
Ans. (c)
Note
Acute otitis media in children is most commonly due to 'Streptococcus pneumoniae'.
Also see
It is an acute inflammation of the middle ear caused by pyogenic organisms. It is common in children and adolescents of lower socio-economic class. Most common organism affected is streptococcus pneumoniae, hemophilus influenzae and morexiella catarrhalis.
Ref: Diseases of ear nose & throat by P.L. Dhingra, Cp 11, Pg 80

Q. 282. All of the following are true for Ramsay Hunt syndrome, except
    (a)   It has viral etiology
    (b)   Involves VII nerve
    (c)   May involve VIII nerve
    (d)   Results of spontaneous recovery are excellent
Ans. (d)
Note
All of the above are true for Ramsay Hunt syndrome, except 'Results of spontaneous recovery are excellent'.
Also see
Ramsay hunt syndrome or herpes zooster oticusis is a complication of varicella zooster infection in which there is facial palsy along with a vesicular rash in the external auditory meatus and pinna. There may also be anesthesia of face, giddiness and hearing impairment due to involvement of 5th and 8th cranial nerve.
Ref: Diseases of ear nose & throat by P.L. Dhingra, Cp 15, Pg 124

Q. 283. Rajesh, a 7 months old child, presents with failure to gain weight & noisy breathing which becomes worse when the child cries. Laryngoscopy shows a reddish mass in subglottis. Treatment modality may include all except
(a) Radiotherapy
(b) Steroids
(c) Tracheostomy
(d) Carbon dioxide laser treatment

Ans. (a)

Note
For the above clinical presentation treatment modality may include all above, except 'Radiotherapy'.

Also see
Infantile hemangioma involves the sub glottis and presents as stridor in the 1st 6 months of life. About 50% of such children have hemangiomas elsewhere in the body particularly in the head and neck. They tend to involute spontaneously but tracheostomy may be needed to release the obstruction. Most of them can be evaporated by CO_2 laser.
Ref: Diseases of Ear Nose & Throat by P.L. Dhingra, Cp 61, Pg 368

Q. 284. A 50 years old male chronic smoker complaints of hoarseness for the past 4 months. Microlaryngoscopic biopsy shows it to be keratosis of the larynx. All are suggested treatment modalities for this condition, except
(a) Laser vaporizer
(b) Stop smoking
(c) Stripping of vocal cord
(d) Partial laryngectomy

Ans. (d)

Note
For the above clinical presentation all are suggested treatment modalities for this condition, except 'partial laryngectomy'.

Also see
Keratosis / Leukoplakia
This is a localized form of epithelial hyperplasia involving the upper surface of one or both vocal cords. It appears as white plaque or warty growth on the vocal cord without affecting its mobility. It is a precancerous condition. Pressure symptoms are hoarseness. Treatment involves stripping of vocal cords and subjecting the tissue to biopsy. Chronic laryngeal irritants should be sought and eliminated.
Ref: Diseases of Ear Nose & Throat by P.L. Dhingra, Cp 61, Pg 367

Q. 285. The treatment of choice of a $T_1N_0M_0$ glottic carcinoma
(a) External beam radiography
(b) Brachytherapy
(c) Surgery
(d) Chemotherapy

Ans. (a)

Note
The treatment of choice of a $T_1N_0M_0$ glottic carcinoma is 'External beam radiography'.

Also see
T_1 *Stage*
The tumor is limited to vocal cords with normal motility. Biopsy should be done and if it shows invasive carcinoma radiotherapy should be done.
Ref: Diseases of Ear Nose & Throat by P.L. Dhingra, Cp 62, Pg 374

Q. 286. A 3 months old child presents with intermittent stridor. Most likely cause is
(a) Laryngotracheobronchitis
(b) Laryngomalacia
(c) Respiratory obstruction
(d) Foreign body aspiration

Ans. (b)

Note
The most likely cause for the above given case is 'Laryngomalacia'.

Also see
It is the most common congenital anomaly of the larynx. It is characterized by excessive flaccidity of the supra-glottic larynx which is sucked in during inspiration producing stridor and sometimes cyanosis. Stridor is increased on crying but subsides on placing the child in prone position cry is normal. It manifests itself soon after birth and disappears by the age of 2 years.
Ref: Diseases of Ear Nose & Throat by P.L. Dhingra, Cp 59, Pg 353

Q. 287. A patient presents with facial nerve palsy following head trauma with fracture of the mastoid. Best intervention here is
    (a)   Immediate decompression
    (b)   Wait and watch
    (c)   Facial sling
    (d)   Steroids

Ans. (a)
Note
Best intervention here is 'immediate decompression'.

Also see
Facial nerve can be paralysed following trauma due to fracture of the temporal bone, ear or mastoid surgery, parotid surgery and trauma to the face.
Other causes are:
Idiopathic/Bell's palsy
Herpes Zooster
Neoplasms (Intratemporal and parotid)
Systemic diseases
Ref: Diseases of Ear Nose & Throat by P.L. Dhingra, Cp 15, Pg 123-126

Q. 288. Chandu a 15 years aged boy presents with unilateral nasal blockade, mass in the cheek and epistaxis. Likely diagnosis is
    (a)   Nasopharyngeal CA
    (b)   Angiofibroma
    (c)   Inverted papilloma
    (d)   None of the above

Ans. (b)
Note
The most likely diagnosis in above given case is 'angiofibroma'.

Also see
Angiofibroma:
It is believed to arise from posterior part of nasal cavity close to the superior margin of sphenopalatine foramen from here the tumor grows into nasal cavity, nasopharynx and into the pterygopalatine fossa, running behind the posterior wall of maxillary sinus. It may extend into the nasal cavity, PNS, pterygo-maxillary fossa, orbits, and cranial cavity.
C/F: Epistaxis, nasal obstruction, Conductive hearing loss & Widening of nasal bridge
Ref: Diseases of Ear Nose & Throat by P.L. Dhingra, Cp 50, Pg 299-300

Q. 289. A 40 years old diabetic presents with blackish nasal discharge and a mass in the nose. Likely diagnosis is
    (a)   Mucormycosis
    (b)   Actinomycosis
    (c)   Rhinosporiodosis
    (d)   Histoplasmosis

Ans. (a)
Note
The most likely diagnosis for above is 'mucormycosis'.

Also see
Mucormycosis
It is a fungal infection of nose and PNS which may prove to be fatal. It is seen in uncontrolled diabetes mellitus or those on immuno-suppressive drugs. Typical finding is presence of black necrotic mass filling the nasal cavity and eroding the septum and hard palate.
Ref: Diseases of ear nose & throat by P.L. Dhingra, Cp 29, Pg 197

Rhinosporodiosis
It is a fungal granuloma affecting the nose and nasopharynx acquired through contaminated water of ponds also frequented by animals. In the nose the disease presents as leafy, polypoidal mass pink to purple in color and attached to nasal septum or lateral wall.

Q. 290. Most radiosensitive tumour of the following is
    (a)   Supraglottic CA
    (b)   CA glottis
    (c)   CA nasopharynx
    (d)   Subglottic CA

Ans. (c)
Note
Most radiosensitive tumour out of the above is 'Ca nasophrynx'.

Also see
In case of supra, sub and glottic carcinoma radiotherapy is the treatment of choice in early stages of carcinoma.
In naso-pharyngeal carcinoma irradiation is the treatment of choice. Recurrent or residual tumor requires a 2nd course of external radiotherapy.
Ref: Diseases of Ear Nose & Throat by P.L. Dhingra, Cp 50, Pg 305

Q. 291 In which of the following locations there is collection of pus in the quinsy?
    (a)   Peritonsillar space
    (b)   Parapharyngeal space
    (c)   Retropharyngeal space
    (d)   Within the tonsil

Ans. (a)
Note
Collection of pus in the quinsy takes place at 'Peritonsillar space'.

Also see
Quinsy is a collection of pus in the peritonsillar space which lies between the capsule of tonsil and superior constrictor muscle. It is usually seen in adults and rarely in children. It is usually unilateral.
C/F:
General: Fever, malaise, bodyache, nausea
Local: Odynophagia, throat pain, muffled and thick speech, foul breath, ipsilateral earache and trismus
Ref: Diseases of Ear Nose & Throat by P.L. Dhingra, Ch 53, Pg 318, 319

Q. 292. Meniere's disease is characterized by
    (a)   Conductive hearing loss and tinnitus
    (b)   Vertigo, ear discharge, tinnitus and headache
    (c)   Vertigo, tinnitus, hearing loss and headache
    (d)   Vertigo, tinnitus and hearing loss

Ans. (d)
Note
Meniere's disease is characterized by 'Vertigo, tinnitus and hearing loss'.

Also see
It is also called endolymphatic hydrops-The endolymphatic sac in the inner ear is distended. It is characterized by triad of vertigo, tinnitus and sensorineural deafness
Ref: Diseases of Ear Nose & Throat by P.L. Dhingra, Cp 16, Pg 129

MCQ's in Surgery 619

Q. 293. In right middle ear pathology Weber's test will be
    (a) Normal
    (b) Centralised
    (c) Lateralised to right side
    (d) Lateralised to left side

Ans. (c)
Note
Similar to 332
In right middle ear pathology Weber's test will be 'lateralised to right side'.
Also see
A vibrating tuning fork is placed on the middle of the forehead or vertex and the patient is asked in which ear the sound is heard normally it is heard equally in both ears.
It is lateralised to the worse ear in conductive deafness and the better ear in sensorineural deafness.
Ref: Diseases of Ear Nose & Throat by P.L. Dhingra, Cp 5, Pg 30

Q. 294. A 5 year old boy has been diagnosed to have posterior superior retraction pocket cholesteatoma. All would constitute part of the management, except
    (a) Audiometery
    (b) Mastoid exploration
    (c) Tympanoplasty
    (d) Myringoplasty

Ans. (a)
Note
All of above would constitute part of the management, except 'Audiometry'.
Also see
Surgical treatment is the mainstay of treatment:
    -Canal Wall Down Procedure-Operations performed are: Atticotomy, modified mastoidectomy and radical mastoidectomy
    -Canal Wall Up Procedure
    -Reconstructive surgery-Myringoplasty or tympanoplasty.
Ref: Diseases of ear nose & throat by P.L. Dhingra, Cp 12, Pg 94-95

Q. 295. A 31 year old female patient complains of bilateral impairment of hearing for the past 5 years. On examination, tympanic membrane is normal and audiogram shows a bilateral conductive deafness. Impedance audiometry shows As type of curve and acoustic reflexes are absent. All constitute part of treatment, except
    (a) Hearing aid
    (b) Stapedectomy
    (c) Sodium fluoride
    (d) Gentamicin

Ans. (d)
Note
All constitute part of treatment for above except, 'Gentamicin'.
Also see
Impedance audiometry consists of two parts:
Tympanometery
In this procedure a type As graph indicates that compliance is lower at or near ambient air pressure. It is seen in otosclerosis.
Acoustic reflex
A loud sound above the thresh-hold of hearing of a particular ear causes bilateral contraction of stapedial muscle. Thus stapedial otosclerosis leads to stapes fixation, which causes absence of acoustic reflex.
Treatment:
    -Medical treatment- sodium fluoride
    -Surgical: -Stapedectomy

-Hearing Aid
Ref: Diseases of Ear Nose & Throat by P.L. Dhingra, Cp 2 and 14, Pg 33, 34, 114, 116

Q. 296. A middle aged male comes to the out patient department (OPD) with the only complaint of hoarseness of voice for the past 2 years. He has been a chronic smoker for 30 years. On examination, a reddish area of mucosal irregularity overlying a portion of both cords was seen. Management would include all, except
    (a)   Cessation of smoking
    (b)   Bilateral cordectomy
    (c)   Microlaryngeal surgery for biopsy
    (d)   Regular follow-up

Ans. (b)
Note
For the above condition management would include all, except 'bilateral cordectomy'.

Q. 297. Type I thyroplasty is for
    (a)   Vocal cord medialization
    (b)   Vocal cord laterlization
    (c)   Vocal cord shortening
    (d)   Vocal cord lengthening

Ans. (a)
Note
Type I thyroplasty is for 'Vocal cord medialization'.
Also see
Type 1 Thyroplasty is for medialisation and undertaken in case of VC paralysis or VC atrophy.
Type 2 Thyroplasty is lateralization and undertaken in severe adductor spasmodic dysphonia.
Type 3 Thyroplasy is relaxation of vocal fold to lower the vocal pitch undertaken in lowering vocal pitch for excessive high pitch in males.
Type 4 thyroplasy is tensing or stretching of vocal fold in order to raise the pitch by approximating cricothyriod.
Ref:-http://www.rxpgonline.com/postt35407.html

OPHTHALMOLOGY

Q. 298. A patient has a miotic pupil, IOP= 25, normal anterior chamber, hazy cornea and a shallow anterior chamber. In fellow eye diagnosis is
    (a)   Acute anterior uveitis
    (b)   Acute angle closure glaucoma
    (c)   Acute open angle glaucoma
    (d)   Senile cataract

Ans. (a)
Note
The diagnosis for above given presentation is 'Acute anterior uveitis'.
Also see
Causes of miotic pupil:
    -Local mitotic drugs
    -Iridiocyclitis
    -Horner's syndrome
    -Head injury and
    -Strong light (Pg 22)
Causes of increased IOP:
    -An IOP >21 mmHg is indicative of glaucoma (Pg 25)
Causes of shallow anterior chamber:
    -Primary narrow angle glaucoma

-Hypermetropia
-Malignant glaucoma
-Postoperative shallow anterior chamber (Pg 21).

Hazy cornea: Transparency is lost in al of the following conditions:
-Oedema (uveitis, increased intra-occular pressure)
-Opacity
-Ulceration
-Dystrophies
-Degenerations, and
-Vascularization (Pg 20)

Ref: Ophthalmology by A.K. Khurana, 3rd Ed, Chapter 2

Q. 299. A woman complains of coloured haloes around lights in the evening, with nausea and vomiting, IOP is normal diagnosis is
    (a)   Incipient stage, glaucoma open angle
    (b)   Prodromal stage, closed angle glaucoma
    (c)   Migraine
    (d)   Raised ICT (Intra Cranial Tension)

Ans. (b)
Note
The diagnosis for above is 'Prodromal stage, closed angle glaucoma'.
Also see

During the prodromal phase of angle closure glaucoma there occurs an attack of transient rise of intra-occular pressure (40-60 mmHg) lasting for a few seconds precipitated by anxiety, overwork and fatigue.
Symptoms: During this phase patient experiences transient blurring of vision, colored halo around light due to corneal oedema and a mild headache.
Ref: Ophthalmology by A.K. Khurana, 3rd Ed, Chapter 9, Pg 231

Q. 300. Babloo, a 5 years old child, presents with large cornea, lacrimation and photophobia. Diagnosis is
    (a)   Megalocornea
    (b)   Congenital glaucoma
    (c)   Congenital cataract
    (d)   Anterior uveitis

Ans. (b)
Note
The diagnosis for above condition is 'Congenital glaucoma'.
Also see
It is due to high IOP which results from developmental anomaly of the angle of the anterior chamber, not associated with any other occular abnormalities.
C/Fs are:
-Photophobia, blepharospasm, lacrimation and eye rubbing
-Corneal signs- corneal edema and corneal enlargement
-Thin and blue sclera
-Deep anterior chamber
-Flat lens
-Increased IOP
Ref: Ophthalmology by A.K. Khurana, 3rd Ed, Chapter 9, Pg 220

Q. 301. Herpes zoster ophthalmicus causes all except:
    (a)   Nummular keratitis
    (b)   Vitreal hemorrhage
    (c)   Uveitis
    (d)   Cranial nerve palsies

Ans. (b)

Note
Herpes zoster ophthalmicus causes all of above except 'vitreal hemorrhage'.
Also see
It is an acute infection of the Gasserian ganglion of the 5th cranial nerve by Varicella-Zoster virus (VZV).
C/F:
General features:
 -Sudden onset with fever, malaise and severe neuralgia along the course of affected nerve.
Cutaneous lesions:
 -Skin, eyelids and other affected areas become red edematous followed by vesicle formation.
Occular lesions:
 -Conjunctivitis, zooster keratitis (it may be microdendritic, epithelial ulcers, nummular keratitis, disciform keratitis).
 -Iridiocyclitis, episcleritis and scleritis.
 -Secondary glaucoma.
Ref: Ophthalmology by A.K. Khurana, 3rd Ed, Chapter 5, Pg 126-127

Q. 302. Bilateral ptosis is not seen in
 (a) Marfan's syndrome
 (b) Myaesthenia gravis
 (c) Myotonic dystrophy
 (d) Kearns-Sayre syndrome

Ans. (a)
Note
Bilateral ptosis is not seen in 'Marfan's syndrome'.
Also see
Marfan's syndrome
It is inherited as an autosomal dominant trait. It causes skeletal defects i.e., tall, lanky frame with long arms and spider-fingers, chest abnormalities (Pectus excavatum). Common eye problem is nearsightedness (myopia) and dislocation of lens of eye. The white of the sclera may appear bluish. Cardiovascular abnormalities associated are aortic regurgitation and prolapse of mitral valve.
Myaesthenia gravis
Disorder is characterised by chronic weakness of voluntary muscles, which improves with rest and worsens with activity. Common eye complaints are double vision, and ptosis (may be unilateral if due to paralysis of the occulomotor nerve). It is bilateral in cases of occular myopathy.
Myotonic dystrophy
The affected patients have a typical "hatchet-faced' appearance due to temporalis, masseter, and facial muscle atrophy and weakness. Other features include; intellectual impairment, hypersomnia, posterior subcapsular cataracts, frontal baldness, donadal atrophy, insulin resistance.
Ref: Harrison- section 3- disorders of nerve and muscles
Kearns-Sayre syndrome (KSS)
It is a rare neuromuscular disorder with onset usually before the age of 20. It is the result of abnormalities in the DNA of mitochondria - small rod-like structures found in every cell of the body that produces the energy that drives cellular functions. KSS is characterized by progressive limitation of eye movements until there is complete immobility, accompanied by eyelid droop.
Ref: http://www.ninds.nih.gov/disorders/kearns_sayre/kearns_sayre.html
Ref: Hutchinson's clinical methods, chapter- 12, Pg 290
Options b, c and d are e.g. of myopathy.

Q. 303. Eye is deviated laterally and downwards and patient is unable to look up or medially. Likely nerve involved is
 (a) Trochlear
 (b) Trigeminal
 (c) Oculomotor
 (d) Abducent

Ans. (c)

Note
The nerve involved in above condition is 'occulomotor'.

Also see

If the eye deviates laterally and downwards then it means that the following muscles are paralyzed- superior, middle and inferior rectus and inferior oblique muscles because of which the inferior rectus and lateral rectus act uninhibitedly. This means that there is paralysis of the third cranial nerve, which, supplies these muscles.
Ref: Ophthalmology by A.K. Khurana, 3rd Ed, Chapter 13, Pg 294

Q. 304. An elderly male with heart disease presents with sudden loss of vision in one eye. Examination reveals cherry red spot. Diagnosis is
    (a)   Central retinal vein occlusion
    (b)   Central retinal artery occlusion
    (c)   Amaurosis fugax
    (d)   Acute ischemic optic neuritis

Ans. (b)
Note
The disgnosis for the above presentation is 'central retinal artery occlusion'.

Also see
Occlusive disorders of the retinal vessels are more common in patients suffering from hypertension and other cardiovascular diseases. Common causes of retinal artery occlusion are:
    -Thrombosis, embolism
    -Retinal arteritis with obliteration
    -Angiospasm is a rare cause of retinal artery occlusion
C/F:
Symptoms; sudden painless loss of vision
Signs; direct papillary reflex is lost. Retina becomes milky white due to edema. Central part of the macular area shows cherry-red spot due to vascular choroid shinning through the thin retina.
Ref: Ophthalmology by A.K. Khurana, 3rd Ed, Chapter 11, Pg 253

Q. 305. Which of the following, is not a feature in diabetic retinopathy on fundus examination
    (a)   Microaneurysms
    (b)   Retinal hemorrhages
    (c)   Arteriolar dilatation
    (d)   Neovascularisation

Ans. (c)
Note
'Arteriolar dilatation' is not a feature of diabetic retinopathy on fundus examination.

Also see
Over time, diabetes affects the circulatory system of the retina. The earliest phase of the disease is known as background diabetic retinopathy. In this phase, the arteries in the retina become weakened and leak, forming small, dot-like hemorrhages. These leaking vessels often lead to swelling or edema in the retina and decreased vision.
The next stage is known as proliferative diabetic retinopathy. In this stage, circulation problems cause areas of the retina to become oxygen-deprived or ischemic. New, fragile, vessels develop as the circulatory system attempts to maintain adequate oxygen levels within the retina. This is called neovascularization. Unfortunately, these delicate vessels hemorrhage easily. Blood may leak into the retina and vitreous, causing spots or floaters, along with decreased vision.
In the later phases of the disease, continued abnormal vessel growth and scar tissue may cause serious problems such as retinal detachment and glaucoma.
Ref: http://www.stlukeseye.com/Conditions/DiabeticRetinopathy.asp

Q. 306. All are true regarding optic neuritis except
    (a)   Decreased visual acuity
    (b)   Decreased pupillary reflex

(c) Abnormal electroretinogram
(d) Abnormal visual evoked response retinogram

Ans. (c)
Note
All of the above are true regarding optic neuritis except 'Abnormal electroretinogram'.
Also see
Optic neuritis involves inflammation and demyelination disorder of the optic nerve.
Clinical profile; it may present as papillitis, neuroretinitis and retro bulbar neuritis.
C/F:
- Decreased visual activity
- Impaired color vision
- Pupil shows ill-sustained constriction to light

On ophthalmoscopy:
- Hyperaemia of the disc, blurring of margins, splinter hemorrhages and fine exudates
- Visual field changes- development of centrocecal scotoma
- VER (visually evoked response) shows reduced amplitude and delay in transmission time.

Ref: Ophthalmology by A.K. Khurana, 3rd Ed, Chapter 12, Pg 281

Q. 307. Chalky white optic disc on fundus examination is seen in all except
(a) **Syphilis**
(b) Leber's hereditary optic neuropathy
(c) Post papilledema optic neuritis
(d) Traumatic injury to the optic nerve

Ans. (d)
Note
Chalky white optic disc on fundus examination is seen in all except 'traumatic injury to the optic nerve'.
Also see
Normal disc is pinkish in color with central pallor, whereas it becomes chalky white in optic atrophy
It results from lesions proximal to the optic disc without antecedent papilloedema retro-bulbar neuritis, leber's disease and other hereditary optic atrophy, toxic amblyopia and tabes dorsalis.
Ref: Ophthalmology by A.K. Khurana, 3rd Ed, Chapter 12, Pg 286-287

Q. 308. Polychromatic luster is seen in
(a) Complicated cataract
(b) Diabetes mellitus
(c) Post radiation cataract
(d) Congenital cataract

Ans. (a)
Note
Polychromatic luster is seen in 'complicated cataract'.
Also see
It refers to opacification of the lens secondary to some intra-occular disease. It presents in 2 forms:
a. Post cortical complicated cataract- secondary to affections of the posterior segment. In the beam of slit lamp the opacities have an appearance like breadcrumb. A very characteristic sign is appearance of iridescent colored particles- polychromatic halos.
b. Anterior cortical complicated cataract.
Ref: Ophthalmology by A.K. Khurana, 3rd Ed, Chapter 8, Pg 194-195

Q. 309. In which of the following conditions, severe itching of the eye with ropy discharge in a 10 year old boy with symptoms aggravating in summer season is most likely present?
(a) Trachoma
(b) Vernal keratoconjunctivitis
(c) Acute conjunctivitis
(d) Blepharitis

Ans. (b)

Note
The most likely cause of the above given clinical presentation is 'Vernal keratoconjunctivitis'.

Also see
Vernal keratoconjunctivitis
It is a recurrent bilateral interstitial self-limiting allergic inflammation of the conjunctiva having a periodic seasonal incidence.
Etiology
It is due to a hypersensitivity reaction to some exogenous allergen. It is seen in the age group of 4-20 years of age.
Season
Summers
C/F:
Burning itching aggravated in warm and humid weather.
Other associated symptoms are:
  -Photophobia, lacrimation, stringy discharge with heaviness of lids.
Ref: Ophthalmology by A.K. Khurana, 3rd Ed, Chapter 4, Pg 99

Q. 310. The most common condition of inherited blindness due to mitochondrial chromosomal anomaly is
    (a)   Retinopathy of prematurity
    (b)   Leber's Hereditary Optic neuropathy
    (c)   Retinitis pigmentosa
    (d)   Retinal detachment

Ans. (b)
Note
The most common condition of inherited blindness due to mitochondrial chromosomal anomaly is 'Leber's Hereditary Optic neuropathy'.

Also see
a)   Retrolental fibroplasias: It is a bilateral proliferative retinopathy occurring in premature infants exposed to high concentration of O_2 during the first 10 days of life.
    Ref: Ophthalmology by A.K. Khurana, 3rd Ed, Chapter 11, Page 258
b)   Leber's disease: It is a hereditary optic neuritis, which primarily affects males around 20 years of age.

    Female carriers transmit it. It is characterized by progressive visual failure. Eventually bilateral primary optic atrophy results.
    Ref: Ophthalmology by A.K. Khurana, 3rd Ed, Chapter 12, Page 282
c)   Retinitis pigmentosa: It is a hereditary disorder predominantly affecting the rods more than the cones. It is an autosomal dominant, recessive or X-linked disease.
    Ref: Ophthalmology by A.K. Khurana, 3rd Ed, Chapter 11, Page 260
d)   Retinal detachment: Risk factors are; a family history of retinal detachment, aucasian background, and male sex. This may be caused by trauma, the aging process, a tumor or an inflammatory disorder.
    Ref; Physician's Home assistant.

Q. 311. A two week old child presents with unilateral cataract. Which of the following statement represents the best management advice?
    (a)   The best age to operate him to get the best visual results is four weeks.
    (b)   The best age to operate him to get the best visual results is four months.
    (c)   The best age to operate him to get the best visual results is four years.
    (d)   The eye is already lost, only cosmetic correction is required.

Ans. (a)
Note
'The best age to operate him to get the best visual results is four weeks' is the best management advice for above case.

Also see
A congenital cataract occurs due to some disturbance in the normal growth of the lens. When the disturbance occurs before birth the child is born with a congenital cataract.

Treatment of a complete unilateral cataract involves removal preferably within a few weeks of birth.
Ref: Ophthalmology by A.K. Khurana, 3rd Ed, Chapter 8, Pg 189

Q. 312. Photodynamic therapy is used in the eye for the following disease
(a) Cataract
(b) Glaucoma
(c) Uveitis
(d) Wet AMD (Age related macular degeneration)

Ans. (d)
Note
Photodynamic therapy is used in the eye for the 'Wet AMD'.
Also see
It is also called senile macular degeneration. It is a bilateral disease.
It is of two types:
a. Non-exudative age related macular degeneration (ARMD)/ dry ARMD: It is characterized by occurrence of colloid bodies, pale areas of retinal pigment epithelium.
b. Wet/ exudative ARMD
Treatment involves - Laser photocoagulation is indicated in these patients to prevent further loss of vision.
Ref: Ophthalmology by A.K. Khurana, 3rd Ed, Chapter 11, Pg 264, 265

Q. 313. All are ocular emergencies, except
(a) Angle closure glaucoma
(b) Central serous retinopathy
(c) Retinal detachment
(d) Central retinal arterial occlusion

Ans. (b)
Note
All of above are ocular emergencies, except 'Central serous retinopathy'.
Also see
Central serous retinopathy (CSR) is characterized by spontaneous retinal detachment in the macular region with or without retinal pigment epithelial detachment.
C/F: sudden onset of painless loss of vision associated with micropsia, metamorphopsia and relative positive scotoma.
Ref: Ophthalmology by A.K. Khurana, 3rd Ed, Chapter 11, Pg 263

Q. 314. A two months old child presents with epiphora and regurgitation. The most probable diagnosis is
(a) Mucopurulent conjunctivitis
(b) Buphthalmos
(c) Congenital dacryocystitis
(d) Encysted mucocele

Ans. (c)
Note
The most probable diagnosis for the above presentation is 'congenital dacrocystitis'.
Also see
It is the inflammation of lacrimal sac occurring in a new born infant.
Etiology:
 -It follows stasis of secretions in the lacrimal sac due to congenital blockage of naso-lacrimal duct.
Other causes are:
 -Presence of epithelial debris
 -Membranous occlusion in upper end of lacrimal sac
 -Complete non-canalization
 -Bony occlusion
C/F:
 -Epiphora followed by copious muco-purulent discharge
Investigation:

-Regurgitation test-when pressure is applied on the lacrimal sac purulent discharge regurgitates from the lower punctum.
Ref: Ophthalmology by A.K. Khurana, 3rd Ed, Chapter 15, Pg 342

Q. 315. Which prominent ocular manifestation is associated with Marfan's syndrome?
    (a)   Microcornea
    (b)   Microspherophakia
    (c)   Megalocornea
    (d)   Ectopia lentis

Ans. (d)
Note
Ocular manifestation is associated with Marfan's syndrome is 'ectopia lentis'.
Also see
Marfan's syndrome is an autosomal dominant mesodermal dysplasia. In this condition lens is displaced upwards and temporarily. Systemic anomalies include- arachnodactyly, long extremities, hyper extensibility of joints, high arched palate and dissecting aortic aneurysm.
Ectopia lentis- displacement of lens from its normal position
Ref: Ophthalmology by A.K. Khurana, 3rd Ed, Chapter 8, Pg 210

Q. 316. An 18 year old boy comes to the eye casualty with history of injury with a tennis ball. On examination there is no perforation but there is hyphaema. The most likely source of the blood is
    (a)   Iris vessels
    (b)   Circulus iridis major
    (c)   Circulus iridis minor
    (d)   Short posterior ciliary vessels

Ans. (a)
Note
The most likely source of blood is 'iris vessels' in the above given case.
Also see
Hyphaemia is collection of blood in the anterior chamber from conjunctival or scleral vessels due to minor occular trauma or otherwise.
Ref: -Ophthalmology by A.K. Khurana, chapter 8, page 207
Traumatic hyphaemia occurs due to collection of blood in anterior chamber. It occurs due to injury to the iris or ciliary body blood vessels.
Ref: Ophthalmology by A.K. Khurana, 3rd Ed, Chapter 17, Pg 372

Q. 317. A 25 year old male gives history of sudden painless loss of vision in one eye for the past 2 weeks. There is no history of trauma. On examination the anterior segment is normal but there is no fundal glow. Which one of the following is the most likely cause?
    (a)   Vitreous hemorrhage
    (b)   Optic atrophy
    (c)   Developmental cataract
    (d)   Acute attack of angle closure glaucoma

Ans. (a)
Note
The most likely cause for above is 'vitreous hemorrhage'.
Also see
Vitreous hemorrhage occurs from retinal vessels and may present as pre-retinal or intra-gel hemorrhage
Causes:
    -Spontaneous
    -Traumatic
    -Inflammatory disease (chorioretinitis, periphlebitis retinae)
    -Vascular disorders
    -Metabolic diseases
    -Blood dyscrasias and bleeding disorders

-Neoplasms
C/F:
- Sudden development of floaters in small haemorrhage
- Sudden painless loss of vision in massive haemorrhages

Q. 318. The mother of a one and a half year old child gives history of a white reflex from one eye for the past 1 month. On computed tomography scan of the orbit there is calcification seen within the globe. The most likely diagnosis is
- (a) Congenital cataract
- (b) Retinoblastaoma
- (c) Endophthalmitis
- (d) Coats' disease

Ans. (b)
Note
The most likely diagnosis is 'retinoblastoma'.
Also see
Retinoblastoma
It is a common congenital malignant tumor arising from neurosecretory retina of one or both eyes.
C/F:
- Quiscent stage- leukocoria, squint, nystagmus and defective vision
- Glaucomatous stage
- Stage of extra-occular extension
- Stage of distant metastases

Histo-pathological features are:
- Flexner-Wintersteiner rosettes
- Homer-Wright rosettes

Other features are calcification and necrosis
Ref: Ophthalmology by A.K. Khurana, 3rd Ed, Chapter 11, Pg 268, 270

Q. 319. Under the WHO 'Vision 2020' programme, the 'SAFE' strategy is adopted for which of the following diseases?
- (a) Trachoma
- (b) Glaucoma
- (c) Diabetic retinopathy
- (d) Onchocerciasis

Ans. (a)
Note
The 'SAFE' strategy is adopted for 'trachoma'.
Also see
Effective interventions have been demonstrated for prevention of blindness in trachoma by SAFE strategy.
S- Surgical correction for deformity
A- antibiotics for acute infections and community control
F- Facial hygiene
E- Environmental change including improved access to water sanitation and health education.
Ref: Ophthalmology by A.K. Khurana, 3rd Ed, Chapter 20, Pg 432

Q. 320. Horner's syndrome is characterized by all of the following except
- (a) Miosis
- (b) Enophthalmos
- (c) Ptosis
- (d) Cycloplegia

Ans. (d)
Note
Horner's syndrome is characterized by all of the above except 'cycloplegia'.
Cycloplegia is paralysis of the ciliary muscle of the eye, resulting in a loss of accommodation.

Also see
Horner's syndrome occurs due to lesion of sympathetic supply and it leads to –
- Ptosis-partial
- Miosis
- Iris hetrochromia
- Ipsilateral anhidrosis

Ref: Davidson's Principles and Practice of Medicine, 19th Ed, Chapter 22, Pg 1156
Mnemonic:
PAM:
- Ptosis
- Anhidrosis
- Miosis

Q. 321. The superior oblique muscle is supplied by
   (a) 3rd cranial nerve
   (b) 4th cranial nerve
   (c) 5th cranial nerve
   (d) 6th cranial nerve

Ans. (b)
Note
The superior oblique muscle is supplied by 4th cranial nerve the 'trochlear'.
Also see
The superior oblique muscle arises from the bone above and medial to optic foramina. It runs forward and turns around a pulley and is inserted into the upper and outer part of sclera behind equator.
The superior oblique muscle is supplied by the 4th cranial nerve
It causes intorsion, depression and abduction of the eyeball
Ref: Ophthalmology by A.K. Khurana, 3rd Ed, Chapter 13, Pg 292, 294
Mnemonic:
SO4; Superior oblique is supplied by 4th cranial nerve (Trochlear)

Q. 322. Which of the following statement is true regarding Acanthamoeba keratitis?
   (a) For the isolation of the causative agent, corneal scraping should be cultured on a nutrient agar plate.
   (b) The causative agent, Acanthamoeba is a helminth whose normal habitat is soil.
   (c) Keratitis due to Acanthamoeba is not seen in the immunocompromised host.
   (d) Acanthamoeba does not depend upon a human host for the completion of its life-cycle.

Ans. (d)
Note
True regarding Acanthamoeba keratistis from the above statement is 'Acanthamoeba does not depend upon a human host for the completion of its life-cycle'.
Also see
It is a free lying amoeba found in the soil, fresh water, well water, sea water, sewage and air.
Infection results from direct contact with the contaminated material e.g, people using contact lenses and trauma.
C/F:
   -Severe pain, watering, photophobia and blurred vision.
Diagnosis is done by:
   -Corneal scrapings cultured in non-nutrient agar.
Ref: Ophthalmology by A.K. Khurana, 3rd Ed, Chapter 5, Pg 128

Q. 323. Contact lens wear is proven to have deleterious effects on the corneal physiology. Which of the following statements is incorrect in connection with contact lens wear?
   (a) The level of glucose availability in the corneal epithelium is reduced.
   (b) There is a reduction in hemidesmosome density.
   (c) There is increased production of CO_2 in the epithelium.
   (d) There is a reduction in glucose utilization by corneal epithelium.

Ans. Use your discretion

Note
It was discovered that lens wear induces a reduction in epithelial oxygen uptake and thickness, the induction of epithelial microcysts, stromal thinning, and increased endothelial polymegethism. Although the epithelial changes recovered within one month, the principle of ocular compromise during lens wear was firmly established.
Ref: http://www2.umist.ac.uk/optometry/dept/contact.htm
(The options given do not include the correct answer)

Q. 324. Painless sudden visual loss is seen in all except
  (a) CRAO
  (b) Retinal detachment
  (c) Vitreous hemorrhage
  (d) Angle closure glaucoma

Ans. (d)

Note
Painless sudden visual loss is seen in all except 'Angle closure glaucoma'.

Also see
Central retinal artery occlusion or CRAO occurs due to obstruction at the level of lamina cribrosa.
It causes sudden painless loss of vision.
Retina becomes white due to oedema and a cherry red spot is seen at the fovea.
Ref: Ophthalmology by A.K. Khurana, 3rd Ed, Chapter 11, Pg 253
Angle closure glaucoma
Angle closure glaucoma (also called closed-angle glaucoma) may present very differently from open-angle glaucoma. In contrast to open-angle glaucoma which is mostly asymptomatic, (acute) angle closure glaucoma may present suddenly with pain, nausea, and decreased vision.
Ref: http://www.medrounds.org/glaucoma-guide/2006/06/section-4-d-angle-closure-glaucoma.html

Q. 325. In which of the following conditions Berlin's edema is seen?
  (a) Open angle glaucoma
  (b) After cataract surgery
  (c) After concussional trauma
  (d) Diabetic retinopathy

Ans. (c)

Note
Berlin's edema is seen in 'after concussional trauma'.

Also see
Post traumatic maculopathies are usually produced by contusion, namely: rupture of the choroid, chorioretinitis sclopetaria, postraumatic macular hole, commotio retinae (Berlin's oedema) and Purtscher's retinopathy was reported.
Ref: http://www.medscape.com/medline/abstract/11178804?prt=true

Q. 326. Magnification obtained with direct ophthalmoscope for an emmetropic patient is
  (a) 5 times
  (b) 10 times
  (c) 15 times
  (d) 20 times

Ans. (c)
Note
Magnification obtained with direct ophthalmoscope for an emmetropic patient is 15 times.

Also see
Ophthalmoscopy is done to assess the state of fundus and detect the opacities of ocular media. In direct ophthalmoscopy the imgae formed is erect virtual and about 15 times magnified in emmetropes.
Ref: Ophthalmology by A.K. Khurana, 3rd Ed, Chapter 2, Pg 34

MCQ's in Surgery	631

Q. 327. Which laser is used in the management of after cataracts?
    (a)   Argon
    (b)   Krypton
    (c)   Nd-YAG
    (d)   Excimer

Ans. (c)

Note
Nd-YAG laser is used in the management of after cataracts.

Also see
After- cataract is a late post-operative complication of cataract surgery also known as secondary cataract.
Causes:
-Residual opaque lens matter may persist after cataract surgery when it is imprisoned between the remains of anterior and posterior capsule surrounded by fibrin or blood.
Treatment:
-YAG-laser capsulotomy or discission.
Ref: Ophthalmology by A.K. Khurana, 3rd Ed, Chapter 8, Pg 210

Q. 328. In human corneal transplantation, the donor tissue is
    (a)   Synthetic polymer
    (b)   Donated human cadaver eyes
    (c)   Donated eyes from live human beings
    (d)   Monkey eyes

Ans. (b)

Note
In human corneal transplantation, the donor tissue is 'Donated human cadaver eyes'.

Also see
Corneal transplantation or keratoplasty is an operation in which the patient's diseased cornea is replaced by the donor's healthy cornea.

Donor tissue should be removed within 6 hours of death for the transplant to be successful.
Ref: Ophthalmology by A.K. Khurana, 3rd Ed, Chapter 5, Pg 145

Q. 329. Which of the following best defines the "saccade"?
    (a)   Voluntary slow eye movements
    (b)   Involuntary slow eye movements
    (c)   Abrupt, involuntary slow eye movements
    (d)   Abrupt, involuntary rapid eye movements

Ans. (d)

Note
From the above '(d) - Abrupt, involuntary rapid eye movements' defines the "saccade".

Also see
Saccadic eye movements are jerky fast small movements that rapidly bring the eye from one fixation position to another to allow for a sweeping search of the visual fields.
Ref: Textbook of Physiology by A.K. Jain, 3nd Ed, Vol 2, Unit 9, Chapter 14 Pg 963

Q. 330. A 35 year old insulin dependent diabetes mellitus (IDDM) patient on insulin for the past 10 years complains of gradually progressive painless loss of vision. Most likely he has
    (a)   Cataract
    (b)   Vitreous hemorrhage
    (c)   Total hematogenous retinal detachment
    (d)   Traditional retinal detachment not involving the macula

Ans. (a)

Note
The above patient's presenting features go in favour of 'cataract'.

Also see
Diabetic cataract is of 2 types:
Senile cataract and true diabetic cataract.
Ref: Ophthalmology by A.K. Khurana, 3rd Ed, Chapter 8, Pg 194

Q. 331. A 56 year old man has painful weeping rashes over the upper eyelid and forehead for the last 2 days along with ipsilateral acute punctate keratopathy. About a year back, he had chemotherapy for Non-Hodgkin's lymphoma. There is no other abnormality. Which of the following is the most likely diagnosis?
    (a)   Impetigo
    (b)   Systemic lupus erythematosus
    (c)   Herpes zoster
    (d)   Pyoderma gangrenosum

Ans. (c)

Note
The most likely diagnosis for above clinical presentation is 'Herpes zoster'.

Also see
Anamnesis of above case includes:
    -A 56 yreas old man. (Aging weakens the immune system)
    -H/O Non-Hodgkin's lympha treated with chemotherapy a year back. (Chemotherapy also weakness the immunity)
    -P/C: Developed painful weeping rash over upper eyelid, forehead with acute ipsilateral punctate keratopathy (this rash appears to be an early feature of Herpes Zoster, which usually developed in immune compromised state and this is the background of above case – which is affecting the ophthalmic division of trigeminal nerve).

Extended information
Herpes Zoster
It is an acute infection of the Gasserian ganglion of the 5th cranial nerve by Varicella-Zoster virus (VZV). The infection is contracted in childhood and manifests as chicken pox. The virus then becomes latent in the sensory ganglion of trigeminal nerve. If the patient develops poor immunity the virus reactivates itself and replicates and travels down the branches of trigeminal nerve.
Ref: Ophthalmology by A.K. Khurana, 3rd Ed, Chapter 5, Pg 126, 127

Q. 332. An 18 years old girl was using spectacles for last 10 years, came with the history of photophobia and sudden loss of vision in right eye. Which one of the following clinical examinations should be performed to clinch the diagnosis?
    (a)   Cycloplegia refraction
    (b)   Indirect ophthalmoscopy
    (c)   Schiotz tonometry
    (d)   Gonioscopy

Ans. (b)

Note
Diagnosis can be clinched with 'indirect ophthalmoscopy'.

Also see
As per the history given the diagnosis seems to be primary retinal detachment. The predisposing factors are:
    -No age is a bar
    -M: F ratio is 3:2
    -Association with myopia is seen in 40% cases
    -Trauma
    -Aphakia
    -Retinal degeneration

Clinical features:
- Prodromal symptoms – Dark spots muscae volitantes and photophobia
- Symptoms of detached retina- sudden painless loss of vision.

O/E:
- Ophthalmoscopy both direct and indirect
- Electroretinography
- Plane mirror examination
- Visual field charting etc.

Ref: Ophthalmology by A.K. Khurana, 3rd Ed, Chapter 11, Pg 265, 266

Q. 333. A 25-year-old male gives a history of redness, pain and mild diminution of vision in one eye for past 3 days. There is also a history of low backache for the past one year. On examination there is circumcorneal congestion, cornea is clear apart from a few fine keratic precipitates on the corneal endothelium, there are 2+ cells in the anterior chamber and the intraocular pressure is within normal limits. The patient is most likely suffering from
- (a) Acute attack of angle closure glaucoma
- (b) HLA B-27 related anterior uveitis
- (c) JRA associated uveitis
- (d) Herpetic keratitis

Ans. (b)

Note
The above clinical presentation is in favour of 'HLA B-27 related anterior uveitis'.

Also see
Specifically in above presentation the patient is 25 years of age and having history of low backache for last one year. These featues are in favour of A.S.
In 40% of cases, ankylosing spondylitis is associated with iridocyclitis causing eye pain and photophobia (increased sensitivity to light).

Extended information
The symptoms point to a diagnosis of sero negative arthritis like reiter's disease or ankylosing spondilitis. They are HLA B 27 linked diseases seen in young males commonly and associated with articular and extra articular features such as uveitis.
Uveitis associated with AS:
- Acute recurrent, non-granulomatous type of iridocyclitis

Uveitis associated with Reiter's disease:
- Acute mucopurulent conjunctivitis with punctate keratitis or acute non-granulomatous iridocyclitis.

Ref: Ophthalmology by A.K. Khurana, 3rd Ed, Chapter 7, Pg 173, 174

Q. 334. A 3-year-old child presents with a right convergent squint of 6 months duration. What is the appropriate management?
- (a) Immediate surgical correction followed by amblyopia therapy.
- (b) Proper refractive correction, amblyopia therapy followed by surgical correction.
- (c) Prescribe spectacles and defer surgery until the child is 5 year old.
- (d) Botulinum toxin injection followed by occlusion therapy.

Ans. (b)

Note
The appropriate management for the above child is 'Proper refractive correction, amblyopia therapy followed by surgical correction'.

Also see
The child seems to be having an accommodation squint. It usually develops at the age of 2-3 years and is associated with a high hypermetropia (+4D to +7D). Mostly it is for near and distance.
Treatment modalities- In most cases correction of refractive error by spectacles completely cures the condition. Squint surgery is required in most cases to correct the deviation. However it should be instituted after the correction of refraction, treatment of amblyopia and orthoptic exercises.

Ref: Ophthalmology by A.K. Khurana, 3rd Ed, Chapter 13, Pg 303, 308

Q. 335. A young man aged 30 years, presents with difficulty in vision in the left eye for the last 10 days. He is immunocompetent, a farmer by occupation, comes from a rural community and gives history of trauma to his left eye with vegetative matter 10-15 days back. On examination, there is an ulcerative lesion in the cornea, whose base has raised soft creamy infiltrate. Ulcer margin is feathery and hyphate. There are a few satellite lesions also. The most probable etiological agent is
    (a) Acanthamoeba
    (b) Corynebacterium diphtheriae
    (c) Fusarium
    (d) Streptococcus pneumoniae

Ans. (c)
Note
The most probable etiological agent is for the above given clinical presentation is 'Fusarium'.
Also see
Fusarium is a filamentous fungus. The mode of infection is by means of crop leaf, branches of tree etc. The farm workers are more commonly affected.
C/F:
Signs
    -Dry, grey-white ulcer with rolled out edges.
    -Delicate feathery finger like extensions.
    -Sterile immune ring.
    -Multiple small, satellite lesions.
Ref: Ophthalmology by A.K. Khurana, 3rd Ed, Chapter 5, Pg 123

Q. 336. A patient presented with normal eyesight and absence of direct and consensual light reflexes. Which of the following cranial nerves is suspected to be lesioned?
    (a) Occulomotor
    (b) Trochlear
    (c) Optic
    (d) Abducent

Ans. (a)
Note
The clinical presentation from above is suggestive of involvement of 3rd Craial nerver the 'Occulomotor'.
Also see
Information about light travels in the optic nerve in optic tract to the superior colliculi, from here colliculo-nuclear fibres arise, which cross both in front and behind the aqueduct of sylvii and relay in both sides of 3rd cranial nerve. The fibres of the 3rd nerve relay in the ciliary ganglion and pass in short ciliary nerve to the sphincter pupillae.
Ref: Textbook of Physiology, AK Jain, vol-2, Unit 12, Chapter 4, Pg 1081
Because some fibres in the optic nerve decussate in the optic chiasma, light shone into one eye simultaneously stimulate the brain stem occulomotor nucleus bilaterally and causes constriction of both pupils simultaneously-Consensual light reflex.
(Thus both optic and occulomotor nerves are involved in reaction of the pupils to light. Since vision is normal therefore the lesion is probably at the level of occulomotor nerve)
Ref: Hutchinson's Clinical Methods, Chapter 11, Pg 247

Q. 337. A 20 year old man complains of difficulty in reading the newspaper with his right eye, three weeks after sustaining a gun shot injury to his left eye. The most likely diagnosis is
    (a) Macular edema
    (b) Sympathetic ophthalmia
    (c) Optic nerve avulsion
    (d) Delayed vitreous hemorrhage

Ans. (b)
Note
The most likely diagnosis for above presentation is 'Sympathetic ophthalmia'.

Also see
Sympathetic ophthalmia
It is a granulomatous uveitis (a kind of inflammation) of both eyes following trauma to one eye. It is the most dreaded complication of unilateral severe eye injury, as it can leave the patient completely blind. Symptoms may develop from days to several years after a penetrating eye injury.
Ref: http://en.wikipedia.org/wiki/Sympathetic_ophthalmia
A bullet injury is an e.g. of a penetrating injury of the eye. This may damage the eye by following mechanisms:
- Mechanical effects
- Infection
- Post-traumatic iridiocyclitis
- Sympathetic ophthalmitis

Ref: Ophthalmology by A.K. Khurana, 3rd Ed, Chapter 17, Pg 325

Q. 338. A recurrent bilateral conjunctivitis occurring with the onset of hot weather in young boys with symptoms of burning, itching, and lacrimation with polygonal raised areas in the palpebral conjunctiva is
    (a) Trachoma
    (b) Phlyctenular conjunctivitis
    (c) Mucopurulent conjunctivitis
    (d) Vernal keratoconjunctivitis

Ans. (d)
Note
The above features are in favour of 'Vernal keratoconjunctivitis'.
Also see
The child is suffering from vernal keratoconjunctivitis or spring catarrah.
It is a recurrent bilateral, interstitial, self-limiting, allergic inflammation of the conjunctiva having a periodic seasonal incidence.
Ref: Ophthalmology by A.K. Khurana, 3rd Ed, Chapter 4, Pg 99

Extended information
1. Trachoma has follicles.
2. Phlyctenular conjunctivitis is unilateral and itching is not marked.
3. Mucopurulent conjunctivitis may not be recurrent.
4. Vernal kerato conjunctivitis is the most appropriate choice.

Observation
The history and signs point classically to Vernal Conjunctivitis
Ref: www.targetpg.com/exams/aipg/2003/S11Ophthal.doc

Q. 339. A patient is on follow-up with you after enucleation of a painful blind eye. After enucleation of the eyeball, a proper sized artificial prosthetic eye is advised after a postoperative period of
    (a) About 10 days
    (b) About 20 days
    (c) 6 to 8 weeks
    (d) 12 to 24 weeks

Ans. (c)
Note
A proper sized artificial prosthetic eye is advised after a postoperative period of 6 – 8 weeks.
Also see
Patients are started on oral antibiotic medication for one week after surgery (enucleation). After the dressing is removed patients will be instructed to place an antibiotic ointment in their eye socket 2-3 times daily for several weeks. A conformer (plastic shell) will be placed under the eyelids after surgery to keep the eyelids from sticking to the underlying surface. Once the swelling in the conjunctiva has subsided in 6 to 8 weeks, patients are asked to see an occularist for final fitting of their occular prosthetic ("glass eye").
Ref: -http://www.texaseyeplastics.com/enucleation.htm

Q. 340. In a patient with AIDS chorioretinitis is typically caused by
    (a) Cytomegalovirus (CMV)
    (b) Toxoplasma gondii
    (c) Cryptococcus neoformans
    (d) Histoplasma capsulatum

Ans. (a)
Note
In a patient with AIDS chorioretinitis is typically caused by 'Cytomegalovirus'.
Also see
CMV infection is very common in patients suffering from AIDS. ¼th of the patients with CD4 counts < 100/cumm would proceed to develop active CMV Retinitis. Patients present with floaters, flashing lights, field defects or rarely diminished central visual acuity.
Ref: Davidson's Principles and Practice of Medicine, 19th Ed, Chapter 1, Pg 125

Extended information
    -CMV retinitis is an important cause of blindness in immunocompromised patients, particularly patients with advanced AIDS.
    -One of consequences of HIV infection is CMV retinitis.
    -Patients at high risk of CMV retinitis (CD4+ T cell count <100/uL).
    -Cases of CMV retinitis occur in patients with a CD4+ T cell count <50/uL.
    -CMV retinitis presents as a painless, progressive loss of vision, blurred vision.
    -The disease is usually bilateral, affecting one eye more than the other.
    -CMV infection of the retina results in visual loss that is irreversible.

Remarks
1. Cytomegalvirus causes chorioretinitis in 30 % of HIV Cases. (Harrison)
2. Chorioretinitis due to toxoplasmosis can be seen alone or, more commonly, in association with CNS toxoplasmosis, but is less common than CMV Chorioretinitis.
3. Cryptococcus neoformans causes meningitis.
4. Histoplasma capsulatum affects the lungs.

Q. 341. Vortex vein invasion is commonly seen in
    (a) Retinoblastoma
    (b) Malignant melanoma
    (c) Optic nerve gliomas
    (d) Medullo-epitheliomas

Ans. (b)
Note
Vortex vein invasion is more commonly seen in 'malignant melanoma'.
Ref: Ophthalmology by A.K. Khurana, 3rd Ed, Pg 181
Also see
1. Retinoblastoma also invades Vortex vaein, but less commonly than Malignant Melanoma.
2. Vortex vein invasion is commonly seen in Malignant melanoma.
3. Vortex vein invasion is not commonly seen in Optic nerve gliomas.
4. Vortex vein invasion is not commonly seen in Medullo-epitheliomas.
Ref: www.targetpg.com/exams/aipg/2003/S11Ophthal.doc

Q. 342. A child has got a congenital cataract involving the visual axis which was detected by the parents right at birth. This child should be operated
    (a) Immediately
    (b) At 2 months of age
    (c) At 1 year of age when the globe becomes normal sized
    (d) After 4 years when entire ocular and orbital growth become normal

Ans. (a)
Note
A complicated unilateral cataract should be removed within a few weeks of birth.

A complicated bilateral cataract should be removed as soon as possible.
Ref: Ophthalmology by A.K. Khurana, 3rd Ed, Chapter 8, Pg 189

Also see
LASIK or for that matter any surgery for correction of refractive error should be performed after the error has stabilized: preferably after the age of 20 years.
It is considered for correction of myopia upto −30 D.
Ref: Ophthalmology by A.K. Khurana, 3rd Ed, Chapter 3, Pg 76, 77

Q. 343. Fasanella Servat operation is specifically indicated in
    (a)   Congenital ptosis
    (b)   Steroid induced ptosis
    (c)   Myasthenia gravis
    (d)   Horner's syndrome

Ans. (d)
Note
Fasanella Servat operation is specifically indicated in 'Horner's syndrome'.

Also see
Horner's syndrome is an example of neurogenic ptosis. Conservative treatment is done for at least 6 months. Surgical treatment if required is:
    -Fasanella Sarvat operation
    -Levator resection
Ref: Ophthalmology by A.K. Khurana, 3rd Ed, Chapter 14, Pg 332, 333

Extended information
1. Congenital ptosis, if mild can be managed by Fasanella Serva operation.
2. Steroid induced ptosis.
3. Myasthenia gravis needs medical management or Thymectomy.
4. Fasanella Servan Operation is best suited for Horner's syndrome.
Ref: www.targetpg.com

Q. 344. In the normal human right eye, the peripheral field of vision is usually least
    (a)   On the left side (nasally)
    (b)   In the downward direction
    (c)   In the upward direction
    (d)   On the right side (temporally)

Ans. (a)
Note
In the normal human right eye, the peripheral field of vision is usually least on the left side (nasally).

Also see
The normal human visual field extends to approximately 35 degrees nasally (toward the nose, or inward) in each eye, to 90 degrees temporally (away from the nose, or outwards), and approximately 50 degrees above and below the horizontal meridian
Ref: http://en.wikipedia.org/wiki/Visual_field
By this we can say that peripheral visual field is least nasally

Q. 345. Tonography helps you to determine
    (a)   The rate of formation of aqueous.
    (b)   The facility of outflow of aqueous.
    (c)   The levels of intraocular presure at different times.
    (d)   The field changes.

Ans. (b)
Note
Tonography helps you to determine 'the facility of outflow of aqueous'.

Also see
Tonography is a non-invasive procedure for determination of facility of aqueous outflow. The C-value is expressed as aqueous outflow in microliter/ min/ml of Hg.
Ref: Ophthalmology by A.K. Khurana, 3rd Ed, Chapter 2, Pg 32, 33

Q. 346. Epiphora is
    (a)   Cerebrospinal fluid running from the nose after fracture of anterior cranial fossa.
    (b)   An epiphenomenors of a cerebral tumor.
    (c)   An abnormal overflow of tears due to obstruction of lacrimal duct.
    (d)   Eversion of lower eyelid following injury.

Ans. (c)
Note
Excessive watering of eyes due to obstruction to the outflow of normally secreted tears is called as Epiphora.
Ref: Ophthalmology by A.K. Khurana, 3rd Ed, Chapter 15, Pg 340

Q. 347. Occulomoter nerve palsy affects all of the following muscles, except
    (a)   Medial rectus
    (b)   Inferior oblique
    (c)   Lateral rectus
    (d)   Levetor palpabrae superioris

Ans. (c)
Note
Occulomoter nerve palsy affects all of the following muscles, except 'lateral rectus'.
Also see
Lateral rectus is supplied by the Abducens nerve (6th cranial nerve).
Occulomotor nerve supplies- medial rectus, inferior oblique, superior and inferior rectus and levator palpebrae superioris.
Ref: Textbook of Physiology by A.K. Jain, vol 2, Unit 12, and Chapter 4 Pg 1100

Q. 348. Kusum Lata presents with acute painful red eye and mildly dilated vertically oval pupil. Most likely diagnosis is
    (a)   Acute retrobulbar neuritis
    (b)   Acute angle closure glaucoma
    (c)   Acute anterior uveitis
    (d)   Severe keratoconjunctivitis

Ans. (b)
Note
Most likely diagnosis is 'Acute angle closure glaucoma'.
Also see
Acute angle closure glaucoma is characterized by severe pain in the eye, redness, photophobia, impaired vision and lacrimation.
Signs
    - Chemosed and congested conjunctiva.
    - On gonioscopy the angle is closed.
    - Cornea-oedematous and insensitive.
    - Pupil- semidilated, vertically oval and fixed.
Ref: Ophthalmology by A.K. Khurana, 3rd Ed, Chapter 9, Pg 232

Q. 349. An optic nerve injury may result in all of the following except
    (a)   Loss of vision in that eye
    (b)   Dilatation of pupil
    (c)   Ptosis
    (d)   Loss of light reflex

Ans. (c)

Note
An optic nerve injury may result in all of the following except 'ptosis'.

Also see
Optic nerve is a sensory nerve responsible for vision.
Ref: Textbook of physiology by A.K. Jain, Vol 2, Unit 11, Chapter 1 Pg 826

Q. 350. Enucleation of the eyeball is contraindicated in
    (a)   Endophthalmitis
    (b)   Panophthalmitis
    (c)   Intraocular tumours
    (d)   Painful blind eye

Ans. (b)
Note
Enucleation of the eyeball is contraindicated in 'Panophthalmitis'.

Also see
Enucleation is the excision of eyeball.
Absolute indication: Retinoblastoma and malignant melanoma.
Relative indications: painful blind eye following absolute glaucoma, endophthalmitis, mutilating orbital injuries, pthisis bulbi and anterior staphyloma.
Ref: Ophthalmology by A.K. Khurana, 3rd Ed, Chapter 18, Pg 410

Q. 351. Under the school eye screening programme in India, the initial vision screening of school children is done by
    (a)   School teachers
    (b)   Primary level health workers
    (c)   Eye specialists
    (d)   Medical officers

Ans. (a)
Note
Under the school eye screening programme in India, the initial vision screening of school children is done by 'school teachers'.

Also see
Under school health services health appraisal of children should be done by periodic medical examination and observation of children by the class teacher.
Ref: Park's Textbook of Preventive and Social Medicine, Chapter 9, Pg 400

Q. 352. All of the following are given global prominence in the VISION 2020 goals, except
    (a)   Refractive errors
    (b)   Cataract
    (c)   Trachoma
    (d)   Glaucoma

Ans. (d)
Note
All of the following are given global prominence in the VISION 2020 goals, except 'Glaucoma'.

Also see
VISION 2020:
The Right to Sight is a global initiative which aims to help to eliminate avoidable blindness by the year 2020, jointly launched by theWorld Health Organization and the International Agency for the Prevention of Blindness (IAPB) together with an international coalition of government agencies, institutions and non-governmental organisations concerned with eye care and the prevention and management of blindness.
The major causes include:
    -Cataract
    -Trachoma
    -Onchocerciasis

-Childhood blindness
-Refractive error
-Low vision
Ref: http://www.vision-2020.org/default.asp

Q. 353. All of the following types of lymphoma are commonly seen in the orbit except
    (a)   Non Hodgkin's lymphoma, mixed lymphocytic & histiocytic.
    (b)   Non Hodgkin's lymphoma, lymphocytic poorly differentiated.
    (c)   Burkitt's lymphoma.
    (d)   Hodgkin's lymphoma.

Ans. (d)
All of the following types of lymphoma are commonly seen in the orbit except 'Hodgkin's lymphoma'.

Also see
Orbits are more commonly involved by non-hodgkin's lymphoma. Other structures involved are: -lacrimal duct, lids and sub-conjunctival tissue.
Ref: Ophthalmology by A.K. Khurana, 3rd Ed, Chapter 16, Pg 366

Q. 354. All of the following muscles are innervated by facial nerve except
    (a)   Occipito-frontalis
    (b)   Anterior belly of digastric
    (c)   Risorius
    (d)   Procerus

Ans. (b)

Note
All of the above muscles are innervated by facial nerver except 'Ant. belly of Diagastric'.

Also see
The branches of facial nerve and the muscles supplied by them are:
i.   Nerve to Stapedius.
ii.   Chorda tympani – Carries the preganglionic secretomotor fibres to the submandibular glands.
iii.   Posterior auricular – Auricularis posterior, occipitalis, intrinsic muscles of the back of auricle.
iv.   Digastric muscle- Posterior belly of digastric muscle.
v.   Stylohyoid branch- Stylohyoid muscles.
vi.   Temporal branch- Auricularis anterior, auricularis superior, intrinsic muscles on the lateral side of the ear, frontalis, orbicularis occuli, corrugator supercilli.
vii.   Zygomatic branch- Orbicularis oculi.
viii.   Buccal branches- Muscles of buccal area.
ix.   Mandibular branches- Muscles of the lower lip and chin.
x.   Cervical branches- Platysma.
Ref: B.D.Chaurasia's Human Anatomy, 3rd Ed, Vol 3 Chapter 9, Pg 113, 114
The anterior belly of digastric is supplied by mylohyoid
Ref: B.D.Chaurasia's Human Anatomy, 3rd Ed, Vol 3, Chapter 11, Pg 128

Q. 355. Stapes foot plate covers
    (a)   Round window
    (b)   Oval window
    (c)   Inferior sinus tympani
    (d)   Pyramid

Ans. (b)

Note
Stapes foot plate covers 'Oval window'.

Also see
The middle ear has three ossicles- malleus, incus and stapes.

The stapes has a head, neck, anterior and posterior crura and a footplate held in oval window by anular ligament.
Ref: Diseases of Ear Nose & Throat by P.L. Dhingra, Cp 2 , Pg10

Q. 356. The treatment of choice for stage 1 cancer larynx is
    (a)   Radical surgery
    (b)   Chemotherapy
    (c)   Radiotherapy
    (d)   Surgery followed by radiotherapy

Ans. (c)
Note
The treatment of choice for stage 1 cancer larynx is 'radiotherepy'.
Also see
Radiotherapy is reserved for early lesions, which neither impair cord mobility nor invade cartilage or cervical nodes.
CA of vocal cords without impairment of mobility gives a 90% cure rate after irradiation and has advantage of preservation of voice.
Ref: Diseases of Ear Nose & Throat by P.L. Dhingra, Cp 62, Pg 373

Q. 357. The etiology of anterior ethmoidal neuralgia is
    (a)   Inferior turbinate pressing on the nasal septum
    (b)   Middle turbinate pressing on the nasal septum
    (c)   Superior turbinate pressing on the nasal septum
    (d)   Causing obstruction of sphenoid opening

Ans. (b)
Note
The etiology of anterior ethmoidal neuralgia is 'Middle turbinate pressing on the nasal septum'.
Also see
This uncommon condition occurs as a result of the middle turbinate pressing on the nasal septum so irritating the nerve as it enters the roof of the nose. Pain is felt at the roof of the nose and radiates to the forehead.
The ultimate treatment is anatomical correction. Temporary relief may be obtained by cocainisation of the nose.
Ref: http://www.gpnotebook.co.uk/cache/503709750.htm

Q. 358. All of the following signs could result from infection within the right cavernous sinus except
    (a)   Constricted pupil in response to light
    (b)   Engorgement of the retinal veins upon ophthalmoscopic examination
    (c)   Ptosis of the right eyelid
    (d)   Right ophthalmoplegia

Ans. (a)
Note
All the above signs could result from infection within the right cavernous sinus except 'Constricted pupil in response to light'.
Also see
Extension of infection into the cavernous sinus leads to cavernous sinus thrombosis, which has the following features-
a.   Severe pain of eye and forehead on the affected side.
b.   Conjunctiva swollen and congested.
c.   Fundus is normal however in advanced cases congestion occurs.
d.   Pupil fixed and dilated.
e.   Proptosis.
f. 3rd, 4th and 6th cranial nerve palsy.
g.   Edema of mastoid region.
Ref: Ophthalmology by A.K. Khurana, 3rd Ed, Chapter 16, Pg 357, 358
Ref: Diseases of Ear Nose & Throat by P.L. Dhingra, Cp 382, Pg 345

Q. 359. Marked tenderness with severe pain at Mcburney's point is a diagnostic feature of (UPSC-06)
    (a)   Salpingitis
    (b)   Appendicitis
    (c)   Ovaritis
    (d)   Cystitis

Ans. (b)

Note
Marked tenderness with severe pain at Mcburney's point is a diagnostic feature of 'Appendicitis'.

Also see
Classical presentation of appendicitis begins with colicky pain around the navel. As the inflammation increases the pain tends to move downward and to the right and localizes directly above the position of appendix at a point calle "McBurney's Point". It is denoted as – a line drawn from the navel to the Right anterior superior iliac spine – McBurney's Point is 2/3 away from the navel on this line.

Q. 360. Rectal bleeding in a child is likely to be (UPSC-06)
    (a)   Fissure
    (b)   Polyp
    (c)   Proctitis
    (d)   Hemorrhoids

Ans. (b)

Note
Rectal bleeding in a child is likely to be 'polyp'.

Also see
The child seems to be having juvenile polyp. These are bright red glistening pedunculated structures found in infants and children. It can cause bleeding or pain if it prolapses during defecation.
Ref: Bailey and Love's Short Practice of Surgery, 24th Ed, Chapter 60, page 1103

Q. 361. Which one of the following is the complication of "Meckel's Diverticulum"? (UPSC-06)
    (a)   Retinal detachment
    (b)   Hemorrhoids
    (c)   Peptic ulcer
    (d)   Corneal ulcer

Ans. (c)

Note
From the above 'Peptic ulcer' is the complication of "Meckel's Diverticulum".

Also see
Other complications are:
a.   Intestinal obstruction
b.   Bleeding from peptic ulcer
c.   Meckel's diverticulitis
d.   Chronic peptic ulcer
Ref: A Concise Textbook of Surgery, S. Das, 3rd Ed, Chapter 49, page 973

Q. 362. A ranula is found (UPSC-06)
    (a)   In the front of neck
    (b)   Laterally in the neck
    (c)   On the upper surface of tongue
    (d)   On the floor of the mouth

Ans. (d)

Note
A ranula is found 'on the floor of the mouth'.

MCQ's in Surgery   643

Also see
Ranula is a Latin word meaning "a small frog". This cyst is considered to be a mucus retention cyst on the floor of mouth. It is usually unilateral.
Ref: A Concise Textbook of Surgery, S. Das, 3rd Ed, Chapter 33, page 580

Q. 363. Acute pain in right hypochondrium with vomiting, tenderness and rigidity may occur in (UPSC-06)
    (a)   Acute Cholecystitis
    (b)   Cholelithiasis
    (c)   Acute hepatitis
    (d)   IInd week of typhoid

Ans. (a)

Note
Acute pain in right hypochondrium with vomiting, tenderness and rigidity may occur in 'Acute cholecystitis'.

Also see
Pain in acute cholecystitis is felt in the right upper quadrant of abdomen and may be referred to the inferior angle of scapula. Tenderness is usually present in right upper quadrant.
Ref: A Concise Textbook of Surgery, S. Das, 3rd Ed, Chapter 46, page 902

Q. 364. Which one of the following is the most common cause of 'Spontaneous Pneuothorax' in India? (UPSC-06)
    (a)   Rupture of subplerual emphysematous bulla.
    (b)   Rupture of a subpleural tubercular fous into the pleural space.
    (c)   Rupture of a staphylococcal lung abscess.
    (d)   Bronchial carcinoma.

Ans. Use your discretion

Note
Possible choice is in (a) and (b).
Most common causes are COPD and TB.
Classification of spontaneous pneumothorax.
Primary: Without any evidence of overt lung disease.
Secondary: Underlying lung disease most commonly COPD and TB are seen. Asthma, lung abscess, pulmonary infarct and bronchogenic CA are other causes.
Ref: Davidson's Principles and Practice of Medicine, 19th Ed, Chapter 13, Pg 570.

(Bibliography)

Books
1.   Bailey and Love's Short Practice of Surgery 24th Ed.
2.   B.D. Chaurasia's Human Anatomy 3rd Ed.
3.   A Concise Textbook of Surgery, S. Das, 3rd Ed.
4.   A Manual Of Clinical Surgery, by S. Das, 5th Ed.
5.   Ophthalmology by A.K. Khurana, 3rd Ed.
6.   Diseases of Ear Nose & Throat by P.L. Dhingra.

Websites
www.similima.com
www.fleshandbones.com

Chapter 10
OBSTETRICS AND GYNECOLOGY

Q. 1. Which one of the following should be choice of treatment for a lady who is mother of two children and suffering from profuse per vaginal bleeding at the time of climacteric, sonography revealing fibroid uterus? (UPSC-02)
    (a)   Regular blood transfusion
    (b)   Improving the general health
    (c)   Hysterectomy
    (d)   Treatment for fibroid

Ans. (d)
Note
The homeopathic concept of treatment is more conservative and consider the parts of the body whether un-useful (Uterus after menopause) or vestigial (Appendix) should not be taken out in the name of treatment unless it is life threatening and there is no other option left. As diseases express through these organs only and health is holistic, which is harmony in all the organ-systems, sensations and functions. As most of the time these fibroid do not cause any problem but are concomitant findings. These usually subside naturally in size, once the menopause occurs.

The homeopathic treatment plan is more of a conservative and in a way passive in intervention. Therefore, the logical step from the homeopathic point of view is to treat the patient homeopathically to achieve menopause in the most natural manner.

However, on the contrary, allopathic treatment plan is more aggressive and of active intervention. When the same case is taken up by allopathic physician he formulates the above case i.e., a mother of two children having profuse vaginal bleeding at the time of climacteric with fibroid uterus. The patient has complete family and menopause is the end of fertility period. There is no need of the uterus so; hysterectomy is the treatment of choice according to the current bio-medical practice. Also allopathic system of medicine has no concept of treating fibroid with internal medication.

Q. 2. Which one of the following is the commonest cause of abortion in the third trimester? (UPSC-02)
    (a)   Uterine malfunction
    (b)   Fibroid uterus
    (c)   Chronic maternal illness
    (d)   Cervical incompetence

Ans. (c)
Note
The question is ambiguous as:
a.   The term abortion is usually used in fetal loss in 1st and 2nd trimester.
b.   The term to be used in case of fetal loss in third trimester is IUD (intra-uterine death)
The causes of IUD may be different from the causes of abortion.
The most important cause of IUD are:
a.   Accidental / Trauma (External trauma, i.e. fall, injury in any form)
b.   Accidental placental separation / APH
c.   Diabetic mother
d.   Fetal anomalies
e.   Acute maternal infection causing hyperpyrexia (Malaria)
f.   Other obstetric causes (Intranatal)

Note
The definition of abortion is 'termination of product of conception before 20th weeks of pregnancy or weight of product of conceptus is less than 500 gms, as per WHO classification. Technically the word third trimester is wrong. The term abortion can be used upto 20th week of gestation. (The non-viability of foetus in 3rd trimester is labeled as 'intrauterine death' and not abortion).
Significance:
It has been observed that foetus of 20 weeks gestation is able to sustain life in extra-uterine environment (latest as per WHO report). Nearly all pregnancies are viable after the 27th week, and almost no pregnancies are viable before the 20th week.
Causes:
Apart from above, other causes for second and third trimester losses are more often the result of a maternal endocrine abnormality. Recognition and control of the metabolic disturbance are the goals of treatment.
Conclusion:
All above can be the causes of 2nd trimester abortion. However the chronic maternal debility is the most important cause of fetal death as well as abortion (which covers both 2nd and 3rd trimester fetal loss). Therefore, among the given choices most appropriate answer could be (c).

Q. 3. Apthous patches in vagina are found in (UPSC-02)
  (a) Caulophyllum and Alumina
  (b) Caulophyllum and Cocculus indicus
  (c) Sepia
  (d) Kreosotum

Ans. Use your Discretion

Note
Ref:
Rep: Kent, Chapter; Genitalia female: vagina, Rubric/Symptom; Aphthae; 1: Caul. (Only single drug is given in Kent's Repertory)
Also see
[boericke] [Female Sexual System]Vagina:Aphthous patches, ulcers, erosions:
Alumn, ARG-N, Carb-v, CAUL, GRAPH, HELON, HYDR, Ign, Kreos, Lyc, Lyss, Merc, Nat-m, NIT-AC, Rhus-t, SEP, Thuj.

Q. 4. During antenatal check-up the expected mother is identified as a high risk candidate as she is suffering from (UPSC-02)
  (a) Hypertension and nephritis
  (b) Hypertension and appendicitis
  (c) Nephritis and neuralgic pain
  (d) Neuralgic pain and headache

Ans. (a)

Note
The hypertension and nephritis both are important causes of pre-eclamptic toxaemia (PET) and eclampsia.

Q. 5. Which one among the following is most common type of ectopic pregnancy? (UPSC-02)
  (a) Ovarian
  (b) Primary abdominal
  (c) Interstitial
  (d) Tubal

Ans. (d)

Note
Common implantation sites of extrauterine ectopic pregnancy is as under:
Ovarian 0.5%
Abdominal 1%
Tubal:
  -Ampula 55%
  -Isthmus 25%

-Infundibular 16%
-Interstitial 20%
Ref: Textbook of Obstetric by D.C. Dutta 6th Edi, Pg-179

Q. 6. If the growth of fetus does not correlate with the period of amenorrhea, the medicine prescribed should be (UPSC-02)
   (a) Calcarea carbonica
   (b) Mercurius corrosivus
   (c) Secale cornutum
   (d) Baryta carbonica

Ans. (c)

Note
Repertory- Synthesis; Fetus -Arrested development of the: Sec.cor. is the only remedy given.

Q. 7. Match List –I (Character of vaginal discharge – leucorrhoea) with List – II (Pathology) and select the correct answer using the codes given below the lists (UPSC2002)

List I (Character of discharge - leucorrhea)	List II (Pathology)
A. Irritating discharge	1. Estrogen deficiency (senile vaginitis)
B. Yellow discharge	2. Candida albicans infection
C. Offensive discharge	3. Bacterial infection
D. Blood stained discharge	4. CA Cervix

Code

	A	B	C	D
(a)	2	3	4	1
(b)	4	3	2	1
(c)	2	1	4	3
(d)	4	1	2	3

Ans. (a)

Note
The sequential presentation is as under:

List I (Character of discharge - leucorrhea)	List II (Pathology)
A. Irritating discharge	2. Candida albicans infection
B. Yellow discharge	3. Bacterial infection
C. Offensive discharge	4. Ca. Cervix
D. Blood stained discharge	1. Estrogen deficiency (senile vaginitis)

Q. 8. The complication of the third stage of labour is caused by (UPSC-02)
(a) Retained placenta
(b) Obstructed labour
(c) Rigid os
(d) Elderly primigravida

Ans. (a)
Ref: Textbook of Obstetrics by D.C. Dutta 6th Edi-Pg-141

Q. 9. Hydatidiform mole is principally a disease of (UPSC-02)
(a) Amnion
(b) Chorion
(c) Ovum
(d) Decidua

Ans. (b)

Note
Hydatidiform mole is one of the gestational trophoblastic disease / tumor. Hydatidiform mole is a condition which develops when a pregnancy has many complications. The hydatidiform mole could be of following two varieties:
a. Complete mole; here the fetus doesn't grow at all and whole of the product of conception are replaced by grape like structure.
b. Incomplete (Partial) mole; in presence of foetus, part of placenta grows into grape like structure. Conception takes place; but the placental tissue itself grows very fast, rather than supporting the growth of a fetus. The result is a tumor, rather than a baby. This is known as a molar pregnancy.

Q. 10. Which one of the following is the commonest cause of PPH (Post Partum Hemorrhage)? (UPSC-02)
(a) Early primigravida
(b) Twin Pregnancy
(c) Obstructed Labour
(d) Retained placenta

Ans. (d)

Note
Once a baby is delivered, the uterus normally continues to contract (tightening of uterine muscles) and expels the placenta. After the placenta is delivered, these contractions help compress the bleeding vessels in the area where the placenta was attached. If the uterus does not contract strongly enough, called uterine atony, these blood vessels bleed freely and hemorrhage occurs. This is the most common cause of postpartum hemorrhage. If small pieces of the placenta remain attached, bleeding is also likely. It is estimated that as much as 600 ml (more than a quart) of blood flows through the placenta each minute in a full-term pregnancy.

Q. 11. Consider the following causes of hirsutism in females (UPSC-04)
1. Polycystic ovaries
2. Adrenal hyperplasia
3. Familial
4. Pregnancy

Which of the causes given above are correct?
(a) 1,3 and 4
(b) 1 and 2
(c) 2,3 and 4
(d) 1,2 and 3

Ans. (d)

Note
Hirsutism is defined as the excessive growth of thick dark hair in locations where hair growth in women usually is minimal or absent. Such male-pattern growth of terminal body hair usually occurs in androgen-stimulated locations, such as the face, chest, and areolae.
Causes:
Ovarian causes of hirsutism
    -PCOS is the most common cause of androgen excess and hirsutism.
Familial hirsutism
    -Familial hirsutism is not associated with androgen excess.
Drug-induced hirsutism
    -Drugs such as phenytoin, minoxidil, diazoxide, cyclosporine, streptomycin, psoralen, penicillamine, high-dose corticosteroids, metyrapone, phenothiazines, acetazolamide, and hexachlorobenzene presumably exert their effects independently of androgens.
Congenital adrenal hyperplasia (CAH)
    -Children with CAH, the classic form of adrenal hyperplasia, may exhibit hirsutism.

Q. 12. Consider following features (UPSC-04)
1. Rise of FSH level
2. Rise in LH level
3. Hot flushes and night sweats
4. Increased Vagina lubrication

Which of the above features point out to menopausal syndrome?
(a) 1,2 and 3
(b) 1,3 and 4
(c) 2, 3 and 4
(d) 1, 2 and 4

Ans. (a)
Note
The estrogen deficiency will lead to decrease vaginal secretion. Thus option 4 is incorrect.

Q. 13. Endometrial cancer most commonly presents as (UPSC-04)
(a) Abnormal vaginal bleeding
(b) Bowel obstruction
(c) Foul vaginal discharge
(d) Pelvic pain

Ans. (a)
Note
Endometrium is the inner lining of uterus. Endometrial cancer most often occurs among those above the age of 50. It can be detected at an early stage because it frequently produces post menopausal vaginal bleeding. If discovered early by removing the uterus surgically can eliminate the cancer.

Q. 14. Which one of the following is the most common type of ovarian malignancy? (UPSC-04)
(a) Serous cystadenocarcinoma
(b) Brenner's tumour
(c) Dysgerminoma
(d) Mucinous adenocarcinoma

Ans. (a)
Serous cystadenocarcinoma
These are amongst the most common cystic ovarian neoplasms, accounting about 50% of all ovarian tumours, of these 60% are benign, 15 % are borderline and 25% are malignant. These occur in the third fourth and fifth decades of life; malignant cystadenocarcinoma tends to occur more frequently with advancing age.
Ref: Shaw's Textbook of Gynaecology 13th Edition Pg-356
Brenner's Tumor:
They are usually unilateral, 5% are bilateral. The tumors essentially are benign only 5 – 10% are of low malignant potential.

Q. 15. Which one of the following is the most common site of tubal pregnancy in the fallopian tube (UPSC-04)
    (a)   Ampulla
    (b)   Interstitial portion
    (c)   Isthmus
    (d)   Fimbrial portion

Ans. (a)
Note
In a tubal pregnancy, the most frequent implantation site is ampulla, because the plicae are most numerous in this situation, and previous salpingitis is more likely to produce crypts here than elsewhere along the fallopian tube.
Ref: Shaw's Textbook of Gynaecology 13th Edition Pg-362

Q. 16. Which one of the following, causes carcinoma of cervix? (UPSC-04)
    (a)   Herpes simplex type I
    (b)   Pap virus
    (c)   Ebstain bar virus
    (d)   Adeno virus

Ans. (b)
Note
The common causative organism predisposing for Ca cervix are:
a.   Herpes virus type II and
b.   Human papilloma virus types 16, 18, 31 and 33 have been implicated.
Therefore, the most suitable choice from above is (b).
Ref: Shaw's Textbook of Gynaecology 13th Edition Pg-382

Q. 17. Which of the following may be caused in an infant because of the deficiency of folic acid during first trimester of pregnancy? (UPSC-04)
    (a)   Cretinism, CHD, Nephrotic Syndrome
    (b)   Spina bifida, Anencephaly, Encephalocel
    (c)   Diabetes mellitus, Indian childhood cirrhosis, Pancreatitis
    (d)   Cushing syndrome, retinitis pigmentosa, wilson's syndrome

Ans. (b)
Note
Spina bifida (open spine) occurs in about 1,300 babies. Affected babies have varying degrees of paralysis and bladder and bowel problems. Apart from the both genetic and environmental factors insufficient amounts of a vitamin 'Folic acid' is known to play an important role in causation of spina bifida in the first trimester of pregnancy.
The incidence of anencephaly is about 1 in 1000 births.
Ref: Pg-439 – D.C. Dutta 5th Edition

Q. 18. Placenta takes over function of corpus luteum (KPSC/Lect/Phys & Bioch-05)
    (a)   2 weeks
    (b)   12 weeks
    (c)   20 weeks
    (d)   24 weeks

Ans. (b)
Note
Progesterone is a hormone that is produced, and released from the corpus luteum, placenta, and adrenal gland. In females, progesterone prepares the uterus for pregnancy and the breasts for milk production. After ovulation, progesterone blocks proliferation of the endometrium and stimulates the uterus to prepare for implantation of a fertilized egg. Progesterone levels continue to rise in early pregnancy.

Q. 19. Spasmodic dysmenorrhoea is seen in (KPSC/Lect/Phys & Bioch-05)
    (a)   Ovarian tumour
    (b)   DUB
    (c)   Endometriosis
    (d)   Sub mucous fibroid

Ans. (d)

Note
Ovarian tumor
In case of ovarian tumors usually menstrual cycles are not affected. It has no direct relation with dysmenorrhoea as such.
DUB
Abnormal vaginal bleeding pattern are components of anovulationary cycles and they do not cause pain (Dysmenorrhoea). These are not associated with any structural abnormality, diseases in the pelvis or evidence either of general diseases or endocrine disorder.
Endometriosis
It is the occurrence of ectopic endometrial tissue outside the cavity of uterus. It presents as congestive dysmenorrhoea. The pain in this condition begins before the onset of menses and builds up continuously until the flow begins.
Sub mucous fibroid
It causes progressive menorrhagia (profuse menses in terms of either quantity or in duration), or metrorrhagia (intermenstural bleeding). It often results in congestive as well as spasmodic dysmenorrhoea. The pain develops on the first day of menses and lasts for a relatively short time.

Q. 20. Most common cause of post partum endometriosis is (KPSC/Lect/Phys & Bioch-05)
    (a)   E. Coli
    (b)   Gonococcus
    (c)   Streptococcus
    (d)   Proteus

Ans. (c)

Note
Streptococci
Post-partum endometriosis especially after a cesarean section.
Ref: medix.marshall.edu/~lewis42/streptococci

Q. 21. Commonest congenital anomaly of uterus is (KPSC/Lect/Phys & Bioch-05)
    (a)   Uterus bicornous unicolis
    (b)   Uterus unicornous
    (c)   Uterus bicornous bicolis
    (d)   Uterus didelphus

Ans. (b)

Note
Complete failure of development of both the mullerian ducts is only possible with concurrent nondevelopment of the urinary system. As this condition is not compatible with life, only a unilateral development of the Mullerian duct giving rise to the unicornuate uterus is known to occur.
Ref: Shaw's Textbook of Gynaecology 12th Edi- Pg-60

Q. 22. The normal chromosomal pattern in female is (KPSC/Lect/Obs-Gynae-05)
    (a)   46, XX
    (b)   46, XY
    (c)   48, XX
    (d)   48, XY

Ans. (a)

MCQ's in Obstetrics and Gynecology

Human cells contain 23 pairs of chromosomes for a total of 46. There are 22 pairs of autosomes and one pair of sex chromosomes. The sex chromosomes are the X chromosome and the Y chromosome. These chromosomes determine gender.

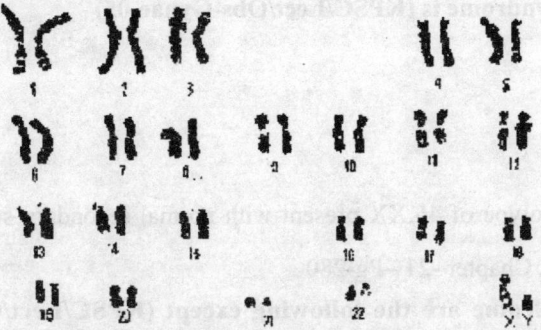

Karyotype of a normal male with 22 pairs of autosomes and one pair of sex chromosomes.
The female has 22 pairs of autosomes ad one pair of sex chromosome XX.

Q. 23. The chromosomal pattern of Turner's syndrome is (KPSC/Lect/Obs-Gynae-05)
    (a)   46, XY
    (b)   46, XX
    (c)   45,X
    (d)   69, XXX

Ans. (c)
Note
A female with Turner's Syndrome lacks one X chromosome, i.e. sex-chromosomes, in place of 46, XX they have 45, X.
This X chromosome carries genes related to the development of ovaries, sex-hormone production, and physical development. Absence of this leads to faulty development of the ovaries and sex-hormone production, that is why the female with turner's syndrome has no menstruation, they cannot get pregnant, do not have normal development of breasts and pubic hair.
Not only this, as the height determination genes is also in the X chromosomes, the lacking X chromosome leads to decreased growth and final height. Approximately 40 % of the Turner girls have a so-called Web-neck. The mental development of Turner girls is within the normal range, but there is a background of the delayed mental maturation process.

Q. 24. Turner's syndrome is characterised by (KPSC/Lect/Obs-Gynae-05)
    (a)   Streak gonad
    (b)   Normal ovary
    (c)   Ovotestis
    (d)   Testis

Ans. (a)
Note
The gonads in case of Turner's syndrome are found to be undifferentiated stroma with absence of sex cells, a mere strip of fibrous tissue attached to the back of broad ligament like a pale strip, the so called "streak" gonad.

Q. 25. The clinical features of Turner's syndrome are the following except (KPSC/Lect/Obs-Gynae-05)
    (a)   Webbed neck
    (b)   Flat chest
    (c)   Cubitus valgus
    (d)   Normal breasts

Ans. (d)

Note
The patient with Turner's syndrome has short stature, muscular trunk, webbed and short neck, cubitus valgus, underdeveloped breasts, scanty or absent pubic and axillary hair.

Q. 26. The chromosomal pattern of Rokitansky syndrome is (KPSC/Lect/Obs-Gynae-05)
    (a)   46,XY
    (b)   46,XX
    (c)   45,X
    (d)   47,XXY

Ans. (b)
Note
Women with simple Mullerian agenesis and a karyotype of 46,XX present with normal secondary sexual character and functional ovaries.
Ref; Shaw's Text Book of Gynaecology 13th Edition, Chapter -21 –Pg-280

Q. 27. The clinical features of Rokitansky syndrome are the following except (KPSC/Lect/Obs-Gynae-05)
    (a)   Primary amenorrhea
    (b)   Well developed secondary sexual characters
    (c)   Absent vagina and uterus
    (d)   Present vagina and uterus

Ans. (d)
Note
The female with Meyer-Rokitansky-Kuster-Hauser Syndrome has primary amenorrhea, absence of vagina and uterus, renal abnormality (One kidney absent) and skeletal abnormality. Secondary sexual characters are normal since the ovaries are functional.

Q. 28. The uterus is developed from (KPSC/Lect/Obs-Gynae-05)
    (a)   The pronephric ducts
    (b)   The mesonephric ducts
    (c)   The mullerian ducts
    (d)   The urogenital sinus

Ans. (c)
Note
In the 7th week of intrauterine life two mullerian ducts develop, grow caudally and fuse in the midline, its middle fused portion forms the uterus and cervix and the caudal part develops into upper three-fourth of vagina.
Ref: Shaw's Text Book of Gynaecology 13th Editon, Chapter -5 –Pg-59

Q. 29. The septate uterus is formed as a result of (KPSC/Lect/Obs-Gynae-05)
    (a)   Fusion of Mullerian ducts,
    (b)   Incomplete fusion of the ducts
    (c)   Non-canalisation of the ducts
    (d)   Non-resorption of the median septum

Ans. (d)
Note
It is one of the Mullerian duct anomalies; septate uterus is formed as a result of failure of disappearance of the intervening septum.
Ref: Shaw's Text Book of Gynaecology 13th Edition, Chapter -5 –Pg-59

Q. 30. The secondary sexual character first to appear is (KPSC/Lect/Obs-Gynae-05)
    (a)   The pubic hair
    (b)   The breasts
    (c)   The axillary hair
    (d)   Any of the above

Ans. (b)

MCQ's in Obstetrics and Gynecology

Note
Changes during puberty in boys and girls:

Stage	Bone age	In boys	In girls
1.	Upto 7.5 Years	Preadolescent stage of stage of childhood	Preadolescent stage
2.	12 years boys and 10.5 years in girls	Genital development begins by enlargement of the testes.	Appearance of 'breast bud' (thelarche).
3.	14 years boys and 11.5 years girls	Pubic and axillary hair begins, penis enlarges.	Pubic and axillary hair begins, (pubarchy) elevation and enlargement of the breasts, gain in height (height spurt)
4.	15.5 years boys and 13 years girls	Further growth of external and internal genitalia occurs with peak gain in height (height spurt)	Projection of areolas, appearance of the menses (menarche)
5.	16.5 years boys and 14 years girls	Adult genitalia with secondary sexual characteristics	Adult genitalia with secondary sexual characteristics

Ref: Textbook of Physiology by Pro. A.K. Jain, Edi 2nd, Pg-758

Q. 31. The usual age of menarche is (KPSC/Lect/Obs-Gynae-05)
    (a)   10 yrs
    (b)   13-14 yrs
    (c)   16-18 yrs
    (d)   20 yrs

Ans. (b)

Note
The usual age of menarche is 12-13 years; however it varies in different races and families.
Ref: Shaw's Text Book of Gynaecology, 13th Edition, Chapter -3 –Physiology-Pg-39

Q. 32. The gonadotropic hormones are secreted by the pituitary (KPSC/Lect/Obs-Gynae/-05)
    (a)   Acidophil cells
    (b)   Basophil cells
    (c)   Chromophobe cells
    (d)   Any of the above

Ans. (b)

Note
The anterior pituitary gland consists of three histologically distinguishable cells:
a. Chromophobe or the parent cell
b. Chromophil cells or the eosinophil (Acidophil) cell or alpha cells
c. Basophil or beta cells.
The chromophil cells secrete the gonadotropins that control the ovarian function and menstrual cycle.
Ref; Shaw's Text Book of Gynaecology, 13th Edition, Chapter 3- Physiology –Pg-34

Q. 33. LH causes (KPSC/Lect/Obs-Gynae-05)
    (a)   Ovarian steroidogenesis
    (b)   Ovulation
    (c)   Luteinisation of granulosa and theca cells
    (d)   All of the above

Ans. (d)

Note
The chromophil cells of the pituitary gland secrete the gonadotropins; FSH, LH and Prolactin.
The LH in conjunction with FSH activates the secretion of estrogen, brings about the maturation of ovum and causes the occurrence of ovulation. Following ovulation, it produces luteinization of the granulosa and the theca cells and initiates progesterone secretion.
Ref: Shaw's Text Book of Gynaecology 13th Edition, Chapter -3-Physiology –Pg-34

Q. 34. Second meiotic division of ovum occurs during (KPSC/Lect/Obs-Gynae-05)
    (a)   Embryonic life
    (b)   Follicular phase
    (c)   Ovulation
    (d)   Fertilization

Ans. (d)

Note
Secondary oocyte completes the second meiotic division only after fertilization by the sperm in fallopian tube and results in formation of two unequal daughter cells. The larger one is called the mature ovum and the smaller one is the second polar body.
Ref: D.C. Dutta Textbook of Obstetrics 5th Edition, Chapter -2 –Pg-17

Q. 35. Normal mature ovum is (KPSC/Lect/Obs-Gynae-05)
    (a)   Diploid
    (b)   Haploid
    (c)   Triploid
    (d)   Tetraploid

Ans. (b)

Note
The mature ovum has haploid number of chromosomes i.e., 23 X the second polar body also has 23, X but with scanty cytoplasm.
Ref: D.C. Dutta Textbook of Obstetrics 5th Edition, Chapter -2 –Pg-17

Q. 36. Oestrogen causes (KPSC/Lect/Obs-Gynae-05)
    (a)   Development of breasts
    (b)   Proliferative changes in the endometrium
    (c)   Deposition of glycogen in the vaginal epithelium
    (d)   All of the above

Ans. (d)

Note
The oestrogen has the following actions:
a. Feminization and secondary sexual characters.
b. Development, vascular and epithelial stimulation of the vulva, vagina, cervix and uterus.
c. It regenerates the endometrium after menses.
d. Stimulates the tubal musculature.
e. Deposition and metabolism of intracellular glycogen in the vaginal epithelium.
Ref: Shaw's Text Book of Gynaecology 13th Edition– Chapter -3 –Physiology-Pg-35

Q. 37. The average duration of menstrual cycle is (KPSC/Lect/Obs-Gynae-05)
    (a) 18 days
    (b) 28 days
    (c) 38 days
    (d) 42 days

Ans. (b)

Note
Menstrual cycle is usually of 28 days, measured by the time between the first day of period and first day of next.
Ref; Shaw's Text Book of Gynaecology 13th Edition, Chapter -3 –Physiology-Pg-46

Q. 38. Ovulation occurs usually (KPSC/Lect/Obs-Gynae-05)
    (a) 14 days prior to the succeeding cycle
    (b) 14 days after the menstruation
    (c) 7 days after the onset period
    (d) at the middle of the cycle

Ans. (a)

Note
Ovulation is estimated to occur 14 days before the first day of succeeding cycle.
Ref: Shaw's Text Book of Gynaecology 13th Edition, Chapter -2 – Hisotlogy-Pg-29

Q. 39. The earliest symptom of pregnancy in a regularly menstruating women is (KPSC/Lect/Obs-Gynae-05)
    (a) Missing the period
    (b) Morning sickness
    (c) Enlargement of abdomen
    (d) Pica

Ans. (a)

Note
Amenorrhea during the reproductive period in an healthy individual having previous regular periods is likely to be due to pregnancy unless proven other wise.
Ref: D.C. Dutta Textbook of Obstetrics, 5th Edition, Chapter – 7- Page – 66

Q. 40. The most sensitive pregnancy test is (KPSC/Lect/Obs-Gynae-05)
    (a) Latex agglutination inhibition test for beta hCG
    (b) Direct latex agglutination test for beta hCG
    (c) Membrane ELISA
    (d) Radio receptor assay

Ans. (d)

Note
Radio receptor assay is the most sensitive pregnancy testing method and can detect presence of HCG in serum as early as 8 to 9 days after ovulation. It is specific to β HCG and does not cross react with LH.
Ref: D.C. Dutta Textbook of Obstetrics 5th Edition – Chapter -7 . Page-70

Q. 41. The best method of diagnosis of viable pregnancy is (KPSC/Lect/Obs-Gynae-05)
    (a) Urine pregnancy test
    (b) Blood beta HCG
    (c) Ultrasonography
    (d) Clinical examination

Ans. (c)

Note
Ultrasound is a safe, non-invasive and cost effective procedure and has several advantages like
a. Accurate determination of gestational stage.
b. Detection of abnormal concepts before clinical manifestation occur.
c. Diagnosis of twins and amniotic fluid index calculations.
d. Placental abnormalities
Ultrasonography is the best method of diagnosis of viable pregnancy, as it permits detail survey of fetal anatomy, placental site. From 28th week onwards the pregnancy is viable.
Ref: D.C. Dutta Text book of Obstetrics 5th Edition, Chapter – 40 – Pg- 686

Q. 42. The precise method of estimation of gestational age during the first trimester is by measuring the (KPSC/Lect/Obs-Gynae-05)
    (a) Gestation sac
    (b) Crown-rump length
    (c) Biparietal diameter
    (d) Femur length

Ans. (b)

Note
For estimation of gestational age following points are noted:
a. In the first trimester, crown rump length.
b. In the second trimester, biparietal diameter and femoral length (BPD and FL).
c. In the third trimester, BPD,FL and abdominal circumference and head circumference (AC and HC)
The estimation of crown-rump length is most precise in the first trimester.
Ref: D.C. Dutta Text book of Obstetrics 5th Edition, Chapter – 7- Pg-77

Q. 43. Conjoined twin may result from (KPSC/Lect/Obs-Gynae-05)
    (a) Division of zygote
    (b) Division of blastocyst
    (c) Division of morula
    (d) Incomplete division of embryonic disc

Ans. (d)

Note
The conjoint (Siamese) twins result when the division occurs after formation of the embryonic disc. These may be of four types:
a. Thoraco-pagus (thoracic cavity is fused)
b. Pyo-pagus (feets are fused)
c. Cranio-pagus (the heads are fused)
d. Ischio-pagus (gluteal regions are fused)
Ref; D.C. Dutta Text book of Obstetrics. 5th Edition Chapter – 16- Pg-216

Q. 44. The diagnostic features of ectopic pregnancy are the following except (KPSC/Lect/Obs-Gynae-05)
    (a) Positive pregnancy test
    (b) Adnexal mass
    (c) Fluid in the Douglas pouch
    (d) Double ring intrauterine sac

Ans. (d)

Note
The diagnostic features of ectopic pregnancy on ultrasonography are:
a. Absence of intrauterine pregnancy with positive pregnancy test.
b. Adnexal mass.
c. Fluid in Pouch of Douglas.
d. Rarely cardiac motion may be seen.
Ref: Text book of Obstetrics by D.C. Dutta, 5th Edition Chapter- 15- Pg-198

Q. 45. The clinical features of threatened abortion include the following except (KPSC/Lect/Obs-Gynae-05)
(a) Vaginal bleeding
(b) Closed cervical os
(c) Size of uterus corresponding the period of amenorrhea
(d) Size of uterus less than the period of amenorrhea

Ans. (d)
Note
It is a clinical entity where the process of abortion has started but hasn't reached the level from where recovery is impossible.
Clinical features:
a. Slight and bright red bleeding
b. Mild backache or abdominal pain
O/E:
External and internal os are closed; uterus and cervix feel soft, uterine size corresponds to the period of amenorrhoea
Ref: Text book of Obstetrics by D.C. Dutta, 5th Edition Chapter- 15- Pg-172

Q. 46. The fetal component of placenta is (KPSC/Lect/Obs-Gynae-05)
(a) Chorion leave
(b) Chorion frondosum
(c) Decidua capsularis
(d) Decidua basalis

Ans. (b)
Note
Maternal component consists of decidua basalis.
The chorion is outermost of the two fetal membranes. It forms finger bud like projections called chorionic villi. The villi overlying the decidua basalis grow and expand to form chorion frondosum. The villi overlying the decidua capsularis are called chorion leave.
Ref: Text book of Obstetrics by D.C. Dutta, 5th Edition Chapter-2- Pg-25

Q. 47. In the intervillous space the maternal blood is separated from the fetal by the following except (KPSC/Lect/Obs-Gynae-05)
(a) The fetal endothelium
(b) The villous connective tissue
(c) The trophoblasts
(d) The maternal endothelium

Ans. (d)
Note
It is bounded on the inner side by chorionic plate and outer side by basal plate.
Ref: Text book of Obstetrics by D.C. Dutta, 5th Edition Chapter- 3 Pg-31

Q. 48. Oxygen is transported to the fetal blood by (KPSC/Lect/Obs-Gynae-05)
(a) Diffusion
(b) Facilitation
(c) Pinocytosis
(d) Active transfer

Ans. (a)

Note
Diffusion
The intake of oxygen and output of carbon dioxide takes place by simple diffusion across the fetal membrane.

Facilitation
Glucose is transported by facilitation diffusion.

Pinocytosis
Droplet transfer virtually intact, across syncytiotrophoblast. Examples; larger molecules.

Active transport
Transport against concentration gradient. Example; Aminoacids, calcium, phosphorus, iron.
Ref: Text book of Obstetrics by D.C. Dutta, 5th Edition Chapter-3 -Pg-35, 36

Q. 49. Routine antenatal check up shall be at an interval of (KPSC/Lect/Obs-Gynae-05)
  (a) 4 weeks till 28 weeks
  (b) 2 weeks till 36 weeks
  (c) 1 week till 40 weeks
  (d) All of the above

Ans. (d)
Note
Checkup is done at interval of 4 weeks upto 28th week of pregnancy, at interval of two weeks upto 36 weeks and thereafter weekly till Expected Date of Delivery (EDD).
Ref: Text book of Obstetrics by D.C. Dutta, 5th Edition Chapter-10-Pg-105

Q. 50. All antenatal women should have their blood tested for (KPSC/Lect/Obs-Gynae-05)
  (a) ABO and Rh group
  (b) STI'S (Sexually transmitted "Infections") Revised as STI'S
  (c) Sugar
  (d) All of the above

Ans. (d)
Note
All antenatal women should have their blood tested for; ABO and Rh group, STD, and sugar.
Ref: Text book of Obstetrics by D.C. Dutta, 5th Edition Chapter-10 -Pg-104

Q. 51. Sonographic features of complete mole are the following except (KPSC/Lect/Obs-Gynae-05)
  (a) Snow storm appearance
  (b) Absent fetal parts
  (c) Absent fetal heart
  (d) Presence of normal placental tissue

Ans. (d)
Note
Features of molar pregnancy are:
  -Vaginal bleeding
  -Abdominal pain
  -Fetal parts not palpable, absence of fetal heart sound, uterus feels doughy.
  -Snow storm appearance in USG.
Ref: Text book of Obstetrics by D.C. Dutta, 5th Edition Chapter-15 -Pg-208-209

Q. 52. Incomplete abortion is diagnosed if (KPSC/Lect/Obs-Gynae-05)
  (a) The cervical os is open
  (b) Products of conception are felt in the uterus
  (c) Uterus is less than the period of amenorrhea
  (d) All of the above are present

Ans. (d)

Note
Incomplete abortion is a clinical entity where the entire product of conception is not expelled; instead a part of it is left inside the cavity.
On examination: Expelled mass is found to be incomplete. (Per Anus Examination): Uterus is smaller than Period of amenorrhea. (Per Veginal Examination): Patulous cervical os often admitting the tip of finger.
Ref: Text book of Obstetrics by D.C. Dutta, 5th Edition Chapter-15 -Pg-175

Q. 53. Incomplete abortion should be (KPSC/Lect/Obs-Gynae-05)
    (a) Observed
    (b) Treated medically
    (c) Completed surgically
    (d) Managed by any of the above method

Ans. (c)
Note
The management of incomplete abortion involves Dilatation & Evacuation under general anesthesia.
Ref: Text book of Obstetrics by D.C. Dutta, 5th Edition Chapter-15 -Pg-175

Q. 54. Normal female pelvis is (KPSC/Lect/Obs-Gynae-05)
    (a) Android
    (b) Anthropoid
    (c) Gynaecoid
    (d) Platypelloid

Ans. (c)
Note
On the basis of shape of the inlet, the female pelvis is divided into four parent types:
a. Gynaecoid (50%) ;Round shaped
b. Anthropoid (25%); Antero-posteriorly oval
c. Android (20%); Triangular
d. Platypelloid (5%); Transversly oval
Ref: Text book of Obstetrics by D.C. Dutta, 5th Edition Chapter-23-Pg-366, 67

Q. 55. The shortest diameter in the plane of least pelvic dimension is (KPSC/Lect/Obs-Gynae-05)
    (a) Transverse
    (b) Anteroposterior
    (c) Posterior sagittal
    (d) Oblique

Ans. (c)
Note
Posterior sagittal (5 cm) it is the distance between sacrum and midpoint of bispinous diameter.
Ref: Text book of Obstetrics by D.C. Dutta, 5th Edition Chapter- 9-Pg-96

Q. 56. Type of pelvis predisposed to occipitoposterior position is (KPSC/Lect/Obs-Gynae-05)
    (a) Gynaecoid
    (b) Anthropoid
    (c) Platypelloid
    (d) Mixed

Ans. (b)
Note
a. Anthropoid pelvis: The shape of the inlet is anterior-posteriorly oval so diameter of engagement is AP and the position is direct occipitopostrior or anterior.
b. Gynaecoid pelvis: The position is occipitolateral or oblique occipitoanterior as the shape is round.
c. Android pelvis: The position is occipitolateral or oblique occipitopostrior.
d. Platypelloid pelvis: The position is occipitolateral.
Ref: Text book of Obstetrics by D.C. Dutta, 5th Edition Chapter-23-Pg-367

Q. 57. Normal presentation is (KPSC/Lect/Obs-Gynae-05)
  (a) Vertex
  (b) Face
  (c) Brow
  (d) Breech
Ans. (a)
The normal labour has vertex presentation.

Q. 58. Engaging diameter of vertex presentation (KPSC/Lect/Obs-Gynae-05)
  (a) Verticomental
  (b) Suboccipito-bregmatic
  (c) Submento-bregmatic
  (d) Basaliac
Ans. (b)
Note
The engaging diameter of head is suboccipito-bregmantic which is 9.5 cm or suboccipito-frontal which is 10 cm.
Ref: Text book of Obstetrics by D.C. Dutta, 5th Edition Chapter-9-Pg-89

Q. 59. Onset of labour is suspected by (KPSC/Lect/Obs-Gynae-05)
  (a) Irregular uterine contractions
  (b) Rupture of membranes
  (c) Vaginal bleeding
  (d) Regular painful uterine contractions
Ans. (c)
Note
The features of true labour pains are:
  -Labour pains: Painful uterine contractions.
  -Show: Expulsion of cervical mucous plug mixed with blood.
  -Dilatatin of internal os: Cervical canal begins to dilate more in the upper part than in the lower.
  -Formation of bag of waters / membrane: With the dilatation of the cervical canal, the lower pole of the fetal membranes becomes unsupported and tends to bulge into the cervical canal. As it contains liquor which has passed below the presenting part, it is called 'bag of waters'. This is almost a certain sign of onset of labour.
Ref: Text book of Obstetrics by D.C. Dutta, 6th Edition Chapter- 12 -Pg-117

Q. 60. Progress of labour is assessed by (KPSC/Lect/Obs-Gynae-05)
  (a) Intensity of uterine contractions
  (b) Dilatation of cervix
  (c) Descent of presenting part
  (d) All of the above
Ans. (d)
Note
The rate of cervical dilatation and descent of presenting part is plotted on a partogram.
Ref: Text book of Obstetrics by D.C. Dutta, 5th Edition Chapter -12- Pg-136-37

Q. 61. First stage of labour lasts from the onset of true labour pains to (KPSC/Lect/Obs-Gynae-05)
  (a) Rupture of membranes
  (b) Expulsion of fetus
  (c) Expulsion of placenta
  (d) Full dilatation of cervix
Ans. (d)

Note
The 1st Stage of labour starts from onset of true labour pains and ends with full dilatation of cervix.
The 2nd Stage of labour starts from full dilatation of cervix to the expulsion of foetus.
The 3rd Stage of labour is from expulsion of fetus to expulsion of placenta and membrane.
The 4th Stage of labour is the stage of observation for at least one hour after expulsion of placenta.
Ref: Text book of Obstetrics by D.C. Dutta, 5th Edition Chapter -12- Pg-122

Q. 62. The last menses period is dated from (KPSC/Lect/Obs-Gynae-05)
    (a)   First day of the last normal period
    (b)   Last day of the last normal period
    (c)   First day of the last bleeding episode
    (d)   Last day of the last bleeding episode

Ans. (a)
Note
The last menses period (LMP) is dated from first day of the last normal period.
Ref: Text book of Obstetrics by D.C. Dutta, 5th Edition Chapter – 7 -Pg-76

Q. 63. Breast examination is done in the (KPSC/Lect/Obs-Gynae-05)
    (a)   Supine position
    (b)   Sitting position
    (c)   Both A and B
    (d)   None of the above

Ans. (c)
Note
The examination of breast is performed mainly in sitting position as this gives more information about lump, level of nipples, and palpation of axillary lymph nodes. It can also be performed in semi-recumbent position and bending forward position.
Ref: A manual of clinical surgery by S. Das chapter – 30, Pg-309

Q. 64. The genital system develops from which embryonic structure (KPSC/Lect/Obs-Gynae-05)
    (a)   Ectoderm
    (b)   Mesoderm
    (c)   Endoderm
    (d)   Embryonic plate

Ans. (d)

Q. 65. Which part of ovary comes to contain the developing follicles (KPSC/Lect/Obs-Gynae-05)
    (a)   Cortex
    (b)   Medulla
    (c)   Both A and B
    (d)   None of these

Ans. (a)
Note
During the reproductive period (i.e., from puberty to menopause) the cortex is studded with numerous follicular structures. These include primordial follicles, graafian follicles, maturing follicles and corpus luteum.
Ref: Text book of Obstetrics by D.C. Dutta, 5th Edition Chapter-1-Pg-9

Q. 66. Which of the following does not form from urogenital sinus? (KPSC/Lect/Obs-Gynae-05)
    (a)   Urethra
    (b)   Hymen
    (c)   Epithelicum of urinary bladder
    (d)   Rectum

Ans. (d)

Note
The cloaca becomes divided by the urorectal septum into a dorsal part that is rectum and ventral part that is urogenital sinus, which forms the labium majus, labia minora, vestibule, urethra, bartholin glands and bladder.
Ref: Text book of Gynaecology By Shaw, 13th Edition, Pg-84

Q. 67. The fallopian tube is derived from (KPSC/Lect/Obs-Gynae-05)
    (a)   Wolffian duct
    (b)   Metanephnric duct
    (c)   Mullerian duct
    (d)   Urogenital sinus

Ans. (c)
Note
The cranial free parts of the Mullerian ducts develop into the fallopian tubes. Ref; Shaw's Textbook of Gynaecology, 13th Edition, Chapter-7-Page 87

Q. 68. Arrest of foetal descent occurs commonly at the plane of (KPSC/Lect/Obs-Gynae-05)
    (a)   Pelvic inlet
    (b)   Greatest dimensions
    (c)   Least dimensions
    (d)   Pelvic outlet

Ans. (c)
Note
The obstetrical outlet is bounded above by the plane of least pelvic dimensions. It extends from lower border of pubic symphysis to the tip of ischial spine and posteriorly to meet the tip of S5.
Ref: Text book of Obstetrics by D.C. Dutta, 5th Edition, Pg-95

Q. 69. The portion of the broad ligament between the ovaries and fallopian tube is (KPSC/Lect/Obs-Gynae-05)
    (a)   Round ligament
    (b)   Ligament of Jocob's
    (c)   Cardinal ligament
    (d)   Mesosalpinx

Ans. (d)

Q. 70. 59 Streak ovary is associated with (KPSC/Lect/Obs-Gynae-05)
    (a)   Klinefelter's syndrome
    (b)   Asherman's syndrome
    (c)   Osteogenisis imperfecta
    (d)   Turner's syndrome

Ans. (d)
Note
The Turner's syndrome is also been called an ovarian or gonadal dysgenesis because on laprotomy the gonads are found to contain undifferentiated stroma with absence of sex cells, a mere strip of fibrous tissue attached to the back of the broad ligament like a pale strip, which is called streak ovary.
Ref: Shaw's Testbook of Gynaecology 13th Edition, Chapter – 8 – Pg-100

Q. 71. The level of the alpha feto protein is normal in amniotic fluid in which of the following condition (KPSC/Lect/Obs-Gynae-05)
    (a)   Spina bifida
    (b)   Anencephaly
    (c)   Esophagal atresia
    (d)   Post maturity

Ans. (c)

Note
The alpha feto protein is elevated in:
- Spina bifida
- Anencephaly
- Duodenal atresia
- Turner's syndrome
- Tetralogy of Fallot

Q. 72. Ptyalism is caused by (KPSC/Lect/Obs-Gynae-05)
(a) Excess production of saliva
(b) Excess production of gastric acid
(c) Inability of the patient to swallow normal amount
(d) Allergic reactions to various food during pregnancy

Ans. Use your discretion
Note
The choices given are the probable definitions of ptyalism and not the causes. Ptyalism denotes 'Excess saliva': excessive production of saliva.

Q. 73. A positive pregnancy test may be associated with (KPSC/Lect/Obs-Gynae-05)
(a) Spontaneous abortion
(b) Intra uterine pregnancy
(c) Ectopic Pregnancy
(d) All of the above

Ans. (d)
Ref; Text book of Obstetrics by D.C. Dutta, 5th Edition, Pg-70

Q. 74. Most common fetal lie found during early pregnancy is (KPSC/Lect/Obs-Gynae-05)
(a) Oblique
(b) Transverse
(c) Vertex
(d) Longitudinal

Ans. (d)
Note
Lie refers to the relationship of the long axis of the fetus to long axis of the centralized uterus or maternal spine. Commonest being longitudinal.
Ref: Text book of Obstetrics by D.C. Dutta, 5th Edition, Pg-78

Q. 75. Older gravidas have an increased incidence of (KPSC/Lect/Obs-Gynae-05)
(a) Uterine inertia
(b) Malpresentation
(c) Hypertension
(d) All of the above

Ans. (d)
Note
Older gravidas have increased incidences of:
- Abortions
- Pre-eclampsia
- Abruptio Placentae
- Uterine fibroid
- Uterine inertia
- Malpresentation
- Medial complications i.e, HT (Hypertension), DM (Diabetes Mellitus), Organic heart lesions.

Ref; Text book of Obstetrics by D.C. Dutta, 5th Edition Pg-263

Q. 76. Meconium aspiration syndrome is associated with (KPSC/Lect/Obs-Gynae-05)
 (a) Prolonged labour
 (b) Post dated pregnancy
 (c) IUGR
 (d) All of the above

Ans. (d)
Note
Meconium aspiration syndrome usually occurs in term or post term babies who are small for gestational age (IUGR-Intra uterine growth retardation).

Q. 77. Mastitis followed by breast abscess is most frequently due to (KPSC/Lect/Obs-Gynae-05)
 (a) Bacterial vaginosis
 (b) Pneumococcus
 (c) Escherichia coli
 (d) Staphylococcus

Ans. (d)
Note
The mastitis is predominantly due to staphylococcus aureus infection. This may come from nasopharynx of the baby.
Ref: Text book of Obstetrics by D.C. Dutta, 5th Edition Pg-475

Q. 78. Most common cause of PPH is (KPSC/Lect/Obs-Gynae-05)
 (a) Uterine laceration
 (b) Uterine atony
 (c) Cervical laceration
 (d) Vaginal laceration

Ans. (b)
Note
PPH is commonly occurs in atonic uterus (80%) this leads to imperfect retraction of uterus and bleeding. It is commonly seen in grand multipara, overdistended uterus as in twins, malnutrition, APH.
Ref: Text book of Obstetrics by D.C. Dutta, 5th Edition, Pg-441, 442

Q. 79. All of the following are factors which predispose to post partum infection except (KPSC/Lect/Obs-Gynae-05)
 (a) Maternal obesity
 (b) Anaemia
 (c) Premature rupture of membranes
 (d) Post dated Pregnancy

Ans. (d)
Note
Post maturity per se does not put the mother at risk.
Ref: Text book of Obstetrics by D.C. Dutta, 5th Edition, Pg-341

Q. 80. Pregnancies with severely affected Rh immunized foetus may be complicated by (KPSC/Lect/Obs-Gynae-05)
 (a) Polyhydramnios
 (b) Fetal hydrops
 (c) Fetal cardiac failure
 (d) All of the above

Ans. (d)

Note
Rh isoimmunization can manifest itself in various ways:
- Hydrops fetalis; there is excessive RBC destruction which leads to adverse effect on fetal heart, brain and liver. There may be presence of poyhydramnios.
- Icterus gravis neonatorum.
- Congenital anaemia of the newborn.

Ref; Text book of Obstetrics by D.C. Dutta, 5th Edition, Pg-354, 355

Q. 81. Complication for an Rh positive fetus with an Rh negative mother will usually first appear in which pregnancy (KPSC/Lect/Obs-Gynae-05)
 (a) First
 (b) Second
 (c) Third
 (d) Fourth

Ans. (b)

Note
The antibodies develop when the Rh positive fetal RBCs enter the maternal blood circulation. Most during the delivery of fist pregnancy. Therefore the complications are unlikely in the first pregnancy.
Ref: Text book of Obstetrics by D.C. Dutta, 5th Edition, Pg-353

Q. 82. Which location of Pleomyoma is most associated with spontaneous abortion? (KPSC/Lect/Obs-Gynae-05)
 (a) Subserosal
 (b) Submucosal
 (c) Intramural
 (d) Pedunculated

Ans. (b)

Note
The uterine fibroid especially of submucous variety might not only be responsible for infertility but also for abortion due to distortion of the uterine cavity and increased uterine irritability.
Ref: Text book of Obstetrics by D.C. Dutta, 5th Edition, Pg-171

Q. 83. Asherman's syndrome is best diagnosed by which of the following (KPSC/Lect/Obs-Gynae-05)
 (a) History
 (b) Physical examination
 (c) Hysteroscopy
 (d) Ultra Sound

Ans. (c)

Note
Uterine synechiae (Asherman's Syndrome) is best diagnosed by: Hysteroscopy – which enables panoramic visualization of the uterine cavity and assessment of the type and extent of synechiae.
Shaw's Text Book of Gynecology 13th Edition- Pg-385

Q. 84. All of the following medical condition are associated with an increased risk of first trimester abortion except (KPSC/Lect/Obs-Gynae-05)
 (a) Diabetes
 (b) Luteal phase inadequacy
 (c) Hyperthyroidism
 (d) Hypothyroidism

Ans. NA

For answer use your discretion
Note
The increased risk of abortion is:
Mid Trimester:

-The maternal factors; Diabetes, Hyperthyroidism, and Hypothyroidism; operate in late abortions (Mid-trimester).

Common causes of 1st trimester abortion are:
- Defective germplasm.
- Hormonal deficiency (poorly controlled DM, presence of thyroid auto-antibodies, PCOD, and inadequate leuteal phase with less production of progesterone).
- Trauma.
- Acute infection.

Ref: D.C. Dutta Textbook of Obstetrics 5th Edition, Pg- 180

Q. 85. The pH of urine in pregnancy as compared with a non pregnant state is (KPSC/Lect/Obs-Gynae-05)
(a) Increased
(b) The same
(c) Decreased
(d) Dependant on gestational age

Ans. (b)

Note
Before and during pregnancy urine pH is same. As the body maintains pH in blood within a range of 7.35 to 7.45. Some foods (such as citrus fruit and dairy products) and medications (such as antacids) can affect urine pH. A high (alkaline) pH can be caused by prolonged vomiting, a kidney disease, some urinary tract infections, and asthma. A low (acidic) pH may be a sign of severe lung disease (emphysema), uncontrolled diabetes, aspirin overdose, prolonged diarrhea, dehydration, starvation, drinking an excessive amount of alcohol.

Q. 86. The risk of congenital rubella syndrome is greatest if infection occurs in (KPSC/Lect/Obs-Gynae-05)
(a) First trimester
(b) Second trimester
(c) Third trimester
(d) Before pregnancy

Ans. (a)

Note
Congenital rubella syndrome occurs in infants born to would be mothers who acquired rubella during the first trimester of pregnancy. The developmental defects include deafness, cataract; microcephaly, mental retardation, congenital heart defects. A miscarriage or stillbirth may occur.

Ref: D.C. Dutta Textbook of Obstetrics 5th Edition, Chapter -19 – Pg – 316

Q. 87. What is the most likely diagnosis of a patient who presents with hypertension in the 12th week of pregnancy? (KPSC/Lect/Obs-Gynae-05)
(a) PET (Pre Eclamptic Toxaemia)
(b) Eclampsia
(c) Chronic hypertension
(d) Hyper thyroidism

Ans. (c)

Note
Pre-eclamptic toxaemia
It is a multi system disorder of unknown etiology characterised by development of hypertension to the extent of 140/90 mm of mercury or more with edema or proteinuria or both induced by pregnancy after the 20th week. (Pg-235)

Eclampsia
Pre-eclampsia when complicated with convulsions and / or coma are called as eclampisa. (Pg- 245)

Chronic hypertension
It is defined as presence of hypertension of any cause antedating or before the 20th week of pregnancy. (Pg-252)

Ref: D.C. Dutta- Textbook of Obstetrics 5th Edition, Pg-234 & 245

From the above points the most obvious choice goes in favour of option- (c).

Q. 88. Intra partum management of twin pregnancy at term is usually determined by (KPSC/Lect/Obs-Gynae-05)
    (a)   Gestational age
    (b)   Presentation of twins
    (c)   Local custom
    (d)   Size of twins

Ans. (b)
Note
The delivery of the first baby is usually conducted on same line as that of a normal delivery. During the delivery of second baby the lie is noted:
a.   If longitudinal low rupture of membrane with oxytocin is used.
b.   If transverse external version is attempted.
Ref: D.C. Dutta; Textbook of Obstetrics 5th Edition Chapter – 16 Pg-221 – 223

Q. 89. Couvelaire uterus is associated with (KPSC/Lect/Obs-Gynae-05)
    (a)   Placenta previa
    (b)   Abruptio placentae
    (c)   Vasapraevia
    (d)   All of the above

Ans. (b)
Note
Couvelaire uterus (Utero-placental apoplexy) this is met with in association with severe form of concealed abruption placentae. This can only be diagnosed on laparotomy.
Ref: D.C. Dutta Textbook of Obstetrics 5th Edition – Pg-269

Q. 90. Which of the following are common to both placenta praevia and abruptio placentae (KPSC/Lect/Obs-Gynae-05)
    (a)   Vaginal bleeding
    (b)   Abdominal discomfort
    (c)   Painful uterine contraction
    (d)   Presence of normal fetal hearts

Ans. (a)
Note
In placenta previa sudden painless causeless and recurrent bleeding is the only symptom. In abruptio placentae, abdominal pain or discomfort is associated with continuous dark coloured blood.
Ref: D. C. Dutta Textbook of Obstetrics 5th Edition – Chapter – 18 Pg-259 and 271

Q. 91. Which of the following sexually transmitted disease is associated with a purulent hemorrhagic secretion (KPSC/Lect/Obs-Gynae-05)
    (a)   Granuloma inguinale
    (b)   Lympho granuloma venerum
    (c)   Chancroid
    (d)   Syphilis

Ans. (c)
Note
Granuloma inguinale
It is a chronic ulcrative granulomatus disease caused by Donovania granulomatis. It is characterised by beefy red granular zone of ulcer which has sharp edges and then inflammatory exudates.
Lympho-granuloma venerum
It is caused by Chlamydia trachomatis. It begins as vesiculo-pustular lesion on the external genitalia which causes ulceration of inguinal lymph node leading to formation of a bubo.
Chancroid

It is an acute STI (Sexually Transmitted Infections) caused by hemophilus ducreyi. It is characterised by painful tender genital ulcer and a heavy foul hemorrhagic discharge.
Ref: T.B. of Gynae by Shwa, 13th Edition – Chapter -11- Pg-140 – 141

Q. 92. Which of the following structures does not provide direct support to the pelvic organs? (KPSC/Lect/Obs-Gynae-05)
    (a)   Pelvic muscles
    (b)   Fascia
    (c)   Pelvic bones
    (d)   Ligaments

Ans. (c)

Q. 93. Small bowel herniation is found in (KPSC/Lect/Obs-Gynae-05)
    (a)   Rectocele
    (b)   Cystocele
    (c)   Urethrocele
    (d)   Enterocele

Ans. (d)
Note
The term enterocele is used to describe prolapse of posterior vaginal wall (Upper part) with pouch of douglas. This protrudes outside vulva and coils of intestine may be palpable in the prolapsed part.
Ref: Text book of Gynaecology by Shaw, 13th Edition Chapter – 25- Pg-322 – 323

Q. 94. Which of the following is not a manifestation of pelvic relaxation (KPSC/Lect/Obs-Gynae-05)
    (a)   Uterine prolapse
    (b)   Procidentia
    (c)   Vault prolapse
    (d)   Uterine retroversion

Ans. (d)
Note
The prolapse of genital tract, urine and fecal incontinence are all related to laxity and atonicity of the muscles of pelvic floor.
Ref: Text book of Gynaecology by Shaw, 13th Edition, Chapter 1- Pg-19

Q. 95. In women, most urinary tract infections happen through (KPSC/Lect/Obs-Gynae-05)
    (a)   Hematogenous spread
    (b)   Lymphatic spread
    (c)   Ascending urethral contamination
    (d)   Retained urine

Ans. (c)
Note
The female urethra is very short and closer to the anal opening. It always contains microorganisms but these are the normal inhabitants. These microorganisms neither do cause urethritis unless the urethral tissue is damaged, nor do these spread upwards to the bladder unless they are transported by catheterization.
Ref: Text book of Gynaecology by Shaw, 13th Edition, Chapter 15- Pg-173

Q. 96. What is the normal effect of progestrone on ureters in pregnancy? (KPSC/Lect/Obs-Gynae-05)
    (a)   There is more dilation of the left ureter than of the right.
    (b)   There is more dilation of the right ureter than the left.
    (c)   Both ureters dilate equally.
    (d)   Both ureters constrict equally.

Ans. (b)

Note
Ureters become atonic due to high progesterone level. Dilatation of the ureter above the pelvic brim with stasis is marked on the right side, especially in primigravida. It is due to dextro-roatation of the uterus pressing the right ureter against the pelvic brim.
Ref: D. C. Dutta Textbook of Obstetrics 5th Edition, Chapter – 5 – Pg- 57

Q. 97. The common cause of fetal tachycardia (KPSC/Lect/Obs-Gynae-05)
- (a) Fetal anaemia
- (b) Maternal anaemia
- (c) Maternal hyperthermia
- (d) Maternal Hypothermia

Ans. (c)
Note
As per the choice given the maternal hyperthermia is commonest cause of fetal tachycardia. However, the other causes of fetal tachycardia are:
-Drug to the mother (Beta- Adrenergic agents)
-Infection both maternal and fetal.
-Anaemia both maternal and fetal
-Fetal distress
Ref: D. C. Dutta Textbook of Obstetrics 5th Edition, Chapter – 38 – Pg- 651

Q. 98. Fetal sleep is associated with what change in fetal heart rate (KPSC/Lect/Obs-Gynae-05)
- (a) Increased
- (b) Unchanged
- (c) Decreased
- (d) Both A and C

Ans. (c)
Note
As the pulse rate falls during sleep in the similar pattern fetal heart rate will be decreased during fetal sleep.

Q. 99. The diagnosis of endometriosis is suspected on the basis of (KPSC/Lect/Obs-Gynae-05)
- (a) Culture and sensitivity
- (b) Histology
- (c) Typical history
- (d) Family history

Ans. (c)
Note
The cytology (Cell study) and histology has no role in diagnosis of endometriosis. However, genetic susceptibility is seen in only 15% of cases. Therefore by exclusion the answer is – (c).
Laparoscopy is gold standard in diagnosis of endometriosis.
Ref: Shaw's TB Gynae , 13th Edition, Chapter – 34 Pg-437

Q. 100. What type of abnormal bleeding is associated with endometriosis? (KPSC/Lect/Obs-Gynae-05)
- (a) Menorrhagia
- (b) Anovulatory bleeding
- (c) Amenorrhea
- (d) Hypermenorrhea metorrhagia

Ans. (a)
Note
Menorrhagia is common with endometriosis, especially in cervical and vaginal lesions.
Ref: Shaw's TB of Gynae 13th Edition, Chapter – 34 – Pg-443

Q. 101. Nipple discharge associated with burning, itching or nipple discomfort in older patients is suggestive of (KPSC/Lect/Obs-Gynae-05)
    (a)   Intra- ductal papilloma
    (b)   Fibroadenoma
    (c)   Ductal ectasia
    (d)   Papillary Carcinoma

Ans. (c)
Note
a. Intraductal papilloma: Majority of patient are in age group of 30 – 50 years and it arises from the lining epithelium of lactiferous ducts.
b. Fibroadenoma: It is seen in young women and presents as a painless and solitary lump in the lower part of breast, discharge is almost unknown. It usually increases in size and becomes painful in premenstrual phase.
c. Ductal ectaisa: There is dialation of the larger periareolar ducts associated with periductal inflammation. The disease appears after menopause and is characterised by a thick creamy or greenish nipple discharge which may cause irritation to the tissues around the ducts.
d. Papillary carcinoma: It is seen in women around 70 years old. It is a small tumor and size is never more than two to three centimeters.
Ref; A Concise Textbook of Surgery By S. Das – Chapter -39

Q. 102. The commonest cause of vulvovaginitis in children is (Kerala MD (Hom)Ent/Paper 2-2001)
    (a)   Gonococcus
    (b)   Trichomoniasis
    (c)   Oxyuriasis
    (d)   Candida

Ans. (c)
Note
Gonococcal vulvovaginitis
It is a disease of child bearing age and the infection is sexually transmited. Oldest known venereal disease. It was described by Hippocrates as 'Strangury' as early as 400 BC. Galen gave it it's present name. The causative organism was detected by Neisser in the nineteenth century who named it Neisseria Gonorrhoea.
Trichomoniasis
It is the disease of child bearing age. The trichomonas vaginalis is found in vagina.
Sings & Symptoms: vaginal discharge is thin creamy or slightly green in colour. Vaginal walls are tender. Discharge causes pruritus and inflammation of the vulva.
Oxyuriasis
A contagious intestinal parasite infestation that occurs commonly in children. It is caused by Entrobius vermicularis (Pinworm) a small whitish worm. It migrages to vagina of young girls and causes vulvovaginitis.
Candida
Candidiasis (moniliasis) is due to a gram positive fungus 'candida albicans'. It flourishes in an acid medium with an abundant supply or carbohydrate. It is therefore common in pregnancy and diabetes. Hormonal contraceptive pills also predispose to monolial vaginitis.
Sign & symptoms
Profuse curdy discharge and intense pruritus. On examination; reddened vaginal wall with profuse watery discharge. Excoriation and inflammation of labia minora and introitus due to scratching. White patches of cheesy material which when removed leave multiple petechial like hemorrhagic areas.
Conclusion
From the above most common cause of vulvovaginitis in children appears to be due to Oxyuriais.

Q. 103. Pregnancy can be first diagnosed by ultrasound at (Kerala MD (Hom)Ent/Paper 2-2001)
    (a)   2 weeks
    (b)   5 weeks
    (c)   12 weeks
    (d)   16 weeks

Ans. (b)

Note
During ultrasonography the characteristic small white gestational ring is evident as early as the 5th week of pregnancy.
Ref; D. C. Dutta Textbook of Obstetrics, 5th Edition Chapter – 7 – Pg- 71

Q. 104. Tuberculosis of genital tract is commonest in (Kerala MD (Hom) Ent/Paper 2-2001)
  (a) Uterus
  (b) Cervix
  (c) Vulva
  (d) Tubes

Ans. (d)
Note
Fallopian tube is the most frequently involved part of genital tract and provides over 90% of all genital tubercular lesions.
Uterus is involved in 70% cases the infection descends from tubes.
Cervix is also involved in tubercular infection however the infection is due to descending type and spreads from fallopian tube.
Vulva and vagina; tuberculosis often appears in the form of shallow ulcer with undermined edges.

Q. 105. The commonest ovarian tumour in a lady aged 20-30 years is (Kerala MD (Hom)Ent/Paper 2-2001)
  (a) Mucinous cystadenoma
  (b) Thecoma
  (c) Dysgerminoma
  (d) Serous cystadenoma

Ans. (a)
Note
The serous cystadenoma are among the most common of cystic ovarian neoplasm accounting for 50% of all ovarian tumors.
Ref: Shaw's TB of Gynae 13th Edition Chapter 28 Pg- 356
Mucious cystadenoma: these occur in women between 30 – 60 Years.

Q. 106. If a pregnant woman at 6 weeks have an ovarian mass 5 x 5 cms and, at 15 weeks have an ovarian mass 2 x 2 cms. The diagnosis is (Kerala MD (Hom)Ent/Paper 2-2001)
  (a) Graffian follicle cyst
  (b) Corpus luteum cyst
  (c) Dermoid cyst
  (d) Luteum of pregnancy

Ans. (b)
Note
Most probably it appears to be corpus luteum cyst.

Q. 107. Longest part of fallopian tube (Kerala MD (Hom)Ent/Paper 2-2001)
  (a) Interstitial
  (b) Isthmal
  (c) Ampullary
  (d) Infundibulum

Ans. (c)
Note
The longest part of fallopian tube is ampullary part (5 cm).
Ref: Shaw's TB of Gynae 13th Edition – Chapter – 1 – Pg 12

Q. 108. Which of the following disease does not transmit through placenta? (Kerala MD (Hom)Ent/ Paper 2-2001)
- (a) Tuberculosis
- (b) Measles
- (c) Syphilis
- (d) Gonorrhea

Ans. (d)
Note

The maternal infections which may be transmitted to the foetus across the so called placental barrier are
- -Viral: Rubella, Chicken pox, measles, mumps, poliomyelitis.
- -Bactria: Treponema pallidium, Tubercular bacillius.
- -Protozoal: Malarial parasite

Ref: D.C. Dutta TB Obs-5th Edition, Chapter – 3- Pg- 36

Q. 109. Common cause of habitual abortion (Kerala MD (Hom)Ent/Paper 2-2001)
- (a) Hormone deficiency
- (b) Fault on ovum
- (c) Sexual transmitted disease
- (d) Uterine abnormalities

Ans. (d)
Note
Mullerian fusion defects such as a double uterus, septate or bicornuate uterus is seen in about 10% cases of recurrent abortions.
Ref: D.C Dutta TB Obs-5th Edition, Chapter – 15 – Pg 181

Q. 110. Metrorrhagia in fibroid indicates (Kerala MD (Hom)Ent/Paper 2-2001)
- (a) Ulceration of submucous fibroid
- (b) Ovarian tumour
- (c) Twisting
- (d) Pregnancy

Ans. (a)
Note
Metrorrhagia is common with submucous fibroid. Other mestrual abnormalities associated with fibroid are menorrhagia, (Due to increased vascularity and endometrial hyperplasia) and polymenorrhea (when PID co-exists with fibroid).
Ref: Shaw's TB Obs-5th Edition, Chapter -27 – Pg 341 – 343

Q. 111. With severe pain and bleeding of 28 weeks of pregnancy, diagnosis is (Kerala MD (Hom)Ent/ Paper 2-2001)
- (a) Premature labour
- (b) Placenta previa
- (c) Accidental hemorrhage
- (d) Threatened abortion

Ans. (c)
Note
Bleeding occurring from or into the genital tract after 28th week of pregnancy is called APH (Ante-Partum Hemorrhage). In a patient with APH with abdominal discomfort or pain the diagnosis is likely to be abruptio placentae or accidental hemorrhage.
Ref: D. C. Dutta TB Obs-5th Edition – Chapter 18 – Pg – 267 and 271

Q. 112. Vaccine contraindicated in pregnancy is (Kerala MD (Hom)Ent/Paper 2-2001)
    (a)   Tuberculin
    (b)   Influenza
    (c)   Typhoid
    (d)   Hepatitis-B

Ans. (c)
Note
Typhoid vaccine injection should not be given to women during pregnancy. Ref: Parks Text Book of Preventive and Social Medicine – Chapter – 5 Section – 2 – Pg 181
All live viral vaccines are dangerous during pregnancy.
Ref: D. C. Dutta; TB Obs-5th Edition, Chapter 33- Pg- 551

Q. 113. The MTP Act was passed in the year
    (a)   1971
    (b)   1973
    (c)   1974
    (d)   1976

Ans. (a)
Note
The MTP act was passed in the year 1971. Deliberate induction of abortion by a registered medical practitioner in the interest of mother's health and life is protected under the MTP Act.
Ref: D.C. Dutta TB Obs-5th Edition Chapter 15 – Pg 185)

Q. 114. Low birth weight baby means weight below
    (a)   2 kg
    (b)   2.3kg
    (c)   2.5 kg
    (d)   2.8 kg

Ans. (c)
Note
The WHO has defined low birth weight baby as one who's birth weight is less than 2.5 Kg irrespective of the gestational age.
Ref: TB Of Obs By D. C.Dutta –5th Edition, Chapter 31 – Pg – 490

Q. 115. Infants born to mother of advanced age have a greater risk of
    (a)   Down's Syndrome
    (b)   Trisomy18
    (c)   Marfan's Syndrome
    (d)   ASD

Ans. (a)
Note
The infants born to mother of advanced age have a greater risk of Down's syndrome.
Ref; D.C. Dutta Obs- 5th Edition Chapter – 22 Pg; 362

Q. 116. The commonest cause of breech presentation is (AIIMS/May2003)
    (a)   Prematurity
    (b)   Hydrocephalus
    (c)   Placenta praevia
    (d)   Polyhydramnios

Ans. (a)
Note
Prematurity is the commonest cause of breech presentation. Smaller size of foetus and comparatively larger volume of amniotic fluid allow the foetus to undergo spontaneous version until the 36th wk.
Ref: Textbook of obstetrics, D.C Dutta, 5th Edition Cp- 25, Pg- 402

Q. 117. According to WHO criteria, the minimum normal sperm count is (AIIMS/May2003)
    (a)   10 million/ml
    (b)   20 million/ml
    (c)   40 million/ml
    (d)   60 million/ml

Ans. (b)
Note
The most important factor is the density of the sperm population and counts below 20 million/ml are associated with infertility.
Ref; Shaw's Textbook of gynecology, 13th Edition, Cp- 17, Pg- 202

Q. 118. In triple screening test for Down's syndrome during pregnancy all of the following are included except (AIIMS/May2003)
    (a)   Serum beta hCG
    (b)   Serum oestradiol
    (c)   Maternal serum alfa fetoprotein
    (d)   Acetylcholinesterase

Ans. (d)
Note
Triple screening is a combined biochemical test, which includes Maternal Serum Alpha Fetoprotein (MSAFP), hCG, & UE3. It is used for detection of Down's syndrome. In an affected pregnancy MSAFP & UE3 tend to be low, while hCG is high.
Ref: Textbook of obstetrics, D.C Dutta, 5th Edition Cp-11, Pg- 112

Q. 119. Periconceptional use of the following agent leads to reduced incidence of neural tube defects (AIIMS/May2003)
    (a)   Folic acid
    (b)   Iron
    (c)   Calcium
    (d)   Vitamin A

Ans. (a)
Note
Folic acid supplementation beginning 1 month before conception to about 12 wks of pregnancy reduces the incidence of neural tube defects (NTD) significantly.
Ref: Textbook of obstetrics, D.C Dutta, 5th Edition Cp-26, Pg- 439

Q. 120. Which statement is true regarding ventose (vaccum extractor)? (AIIMS/May2003)
    (a)   Minor scalp abrasions and subgaleal hematomas in new born are more frequent than forceps.
    (b)   Can be applied when foetal head is above the level of ischial spine.
    (c)   Maternal trauma is more frequent than forceps.
    (d)   Cannot be used when fetal head is not fully rotated.

Ans. (a)
Note
Ventore (Vaccum extractor) is an instrumental device designed to assist delivery by creating a vacuum between it and the fetal scalp.
Advantages:
    -It can be used in incompletely dilated cx, in malrotated occipito-posterior position.
    -It is comfortable to the mother and the chances of injuries are less.
Conditions:
    -The cx should be at least 6 cm dilated.
    -Head should be engaged.
Hazards:
    -Sloughing of scalp.
    -Cephalhematoma.
    -Intracranial hemorrhage.

Ref: Textbook of obstetrics, D.C Dutta, 5th Edition Cp-36, Pg- 620-622

Q. 121. A 21 year old primigravida is admitted at 39 weeks gestation with painless antepartum hemorrhage. On examination uterus is soft non-tender and head engaged. The management for her would be (AIIMS/May2003)
(a) Blood transfusion and sedatives
(b) A speculum examination
(c) Pelvic examination in OT
(d) Tocolytics and sedatives

Ans. (c)
Note
Indications for active interference are:
-Bleeding beyond 37wks of pregnancy
-Patient in labor
-Continuous and moderate bleeding
It includes vaginal examination in OT (Operation Theatre) followed by:
a. Low rupture of membrane
b. C.S. (Cassarean section)
Ref: Textbook of obstetrics, D.C Dutta, 5th Edition Cp-18, Pg-265

Q. 122. The commonest cause of occipito-posterior position of fetal head during labour is (AIIMS/May2003)
(a) Maternal obesity
(b) Deflexion of fetal head
(c) Multiparity
(d) Android pelvis

Ans. (d)
Note
It is a vertex presentation where the occiput is placed posteriorly over the sacro-iliac joint or directly over the sacrum. In >50%, the occipito-posterior position is associated with either an anthropoid or an android pelvis.
Ref: Textbook of obstetrics, D.C Dutta, 5th Edition Cp-25, Pg-390-391

Q. 123. The commonest congenital anomaly seen in pregnancy with diabetes mellitus is (AIIMS/May2003)
(a) Multicystic kidneys
(b) Esophageal atresia
(c) Neural tube defect
(d) Duodenal atresia

Ans. (c)
Note
Fetal hazards noted in D.M. (Diabetes mellitus) are:
-Fetal macrosomia
-Congenital malformation-e.g. Cardiac abnormalities (ASD and VSD), Neural tube defect (anencephaly, spina bifida, microcephaly), caudal regression syndrome
-Birth injuries
-Unexplained fetal death
Ref: Textbook of obstetrics, D.C Dutta, 5th Edition Cp-19, Pg-303-304

Q. 124. A drop in fetal heart rate that typically lasts less than 2 minutes and usually associated with umbilical cord compression is called (AIIMS/May2003)
(a) Early deceleration
(b) Late deceleration
(c) Variable deceleration
(d) Prolonged deceleration

Ans. (c)

Note
Deceleration is the decrease in FHR (Fetal Heart Rate) below the base line by 15beats per min or more.
a. Early deceleration: FHR begins to slow down at the beginning of the uterine contractions, lowest point of the FHR dip coincides with the apex of uterine contraction and FHR returns to normal before the contraction passes off. It is due to head compression.
b. Late deceleration: FHR begins to slow down after the onset of contraction. Lowest point of the dip in FHR occurs after the apex of contraction and FHR returns to normal with in a variable period after the contraction passes off. It is due to chronic placental insufficiency.
c. Variable deceleration: It occurs due to cord compression and may disappear with change in the patient's position.

Ref: Textbook of obstetrics, D.C Dutta, 5th Edition Cp-38, Pg-653-654

Q. 125. A perimenopausal lady with well differentiated adenocarcinoma of uterus has more than half myometrial invasion, vaginal metastasis and inguinal lymph node metastasis. She is staged as (AIIMS/May2003)
  (a) Stage IIIB
  (b) Stage IIIC
  (c) Stage IVA
  (d) Stage IVB

Ans. (d)

Note
A perimenopausal lady with well differentiated adenocarcinoma of uterus has more than half myometrial invasion, vaginal metastasis and inguinal lymph node metastasis.She is staged as stage IVB.
Staging of Endometrial carcinoma:

Stage	Features
IA	Tumor limited to endometrium
IB	Invasion of < ½ myometrium
IC	Invasion of > ½ myometrium
IIA	Endocervicalglandular involvement only
IIB	Cervical stromal invasion
IIIA	Tumor invading serosa or adnexae or positive peritoneal cytology
IIIB	Vaginal metstasis
IIIC	Metastasis to pelvic or para aortic lymph nodes
IVA	Tumor invasion to bladder or bowel mucosa
IVB	Distant metastasis including intra abdominal or inguinal lymph nodes.

Ref: Shaw's Textbook of gynecology, 13th Edition Cp- 29, Pg- 395

Q. 126. With reference to fetal heart rate, a non stress test is considered reactive when (AIIMS/Nov-03)
  (a) Two fetal heart rate accelerations are noted in 20 minutes
  (b) One fetal heart rate acceleration is noted in 20 minutes
  (c) Two fetal heart rate accelerations are noted in 10 minutes
  (d) Three fetal heart rate accelerations are noted in 30 minutes

Ans. (a)

Note
In a non stress test, a continuous electronic monitoring of the fetal heart rate, along with recording of fetal movements is undertaken. There is an observed association of FHR acceleration with fetal movements, which when present indicate a reactive non stress test (NST). A reactive NST is when 2 or more accelerations of >15 beats pm above the base line and longer than 15sec duration occur in 10-20 min observation.
Ref: Textbook of obstetrics, D.C Dutta, 5th Edition Cp-11, Pg-115

Q. 127. The commonest cause of primary amenorrhea is (AIIMS/Nov-03)
    (a)   Genital tuberculosis
    (b)   Ovarian dysgenesis
    (c)   Mullerian duct anomalies
    (d)   Hypothyroidism

Ans. (b)
Note
The most common cause of primary amenorrhoea is ovarian dysgenesis and the second most common cause is Mullerian agenesis.
Ref: Harrison 15th Edition Pg-2162

Q. 128. All of the following are known risk factors for the development of ovarian carcinoma except (AIIMS/Nov-03)
    (a)   Family history of ovarian carcinoma
    (b)   Use of oral pills
    (c)   Use of clomiphene
    (d)   BRCA-1 positive individual

Ans. (b)
Note
a.   Family history of ovarian carcinoma; is a risk factor for ovarian cancer.
b.   Use of oral pills; OCPs is one of the protective factors.
c.   Use of clomiphene; is an ovulation inducing drug and is also a risk factor for ovarian cancer.
d.   BRCA-1 positive individual; One percent malignant ovarian tumours are genetic, and gene BRCA-1 is implicated.

The risk factors associated for the development of ovarian carcinoma are:
    -Low parity, decreased fertility, and delayed child bearing.
    -Familial predisposition (1% of malignant ovarian tumors are genetic and associated with BRCA-1 gene).
    -Increased fat intake and multiple ovulation.
    -Risk increases with age.
    -Mumps prior to menarche.
Protective factors for the development of ovarian carcinoma are:
    -Multiparity, breastfeeding, anovulation, OCPs.
Ref: Shaw's Textbook of gynecology, 13th Edition Cp- 29, Pg- 397

Q. 129. A pregnant woman with fibroid uterus develops acute pain in abdomen with low grade fever and mild leucocytosis at 28 weeks. The most likely diagnosis is (AIIMS/Nov-03)
    (a)   Preterm labour
    (b)   Torsion of fibroid
    (c)   Red degeneration of fibroid
    (d)   Infection in fibroid

Ans. (c)
Note
Red degeneration of the uterine myoma develops most frequently during pregnancy, although it is not rare in cases of painful myomas in women over the age of 40. The myoma becomes tender and tense and causes severe abdominal pain with constitutional upset and fever.
Ref: Shaw's Textbook of gynecology, 13th Edition Cp- 27, Pg- 340

Q. 130. A pregnant woman is found to have excessive accumulation of amniotic fluid. Such polyhdramnios is likely to be associated with all of the following conditions, except (AIIMS/Nov-03)
   (a)   Twinning
   (b)   Microanencephaly
   (c)   Esophageal atresia
   (d)   Bilateral renal agenesis

Ans. (d)
Note
Polyhydramnios is a state where the liquor amnii exceeds 2000 ml.
Causes
   -Fetal anomalies (anencephaly, spina bifida, esophageal or duodenal atresia, facial clefts and neck masses, hydrops fetalis).
   -Placental abnormalities- chorangiocarcinoma of placenta.
   -Multiple pregnancy.
   -Maternal-DM (Diabetes Mellitus), cardiac abnormalities.
Ref: Textbook of obstetrics, D.C Dutta, 5th Edition Cp-16, Pg-218

Q. 131. Use of folic acid to prevent congenital malformation should be best initiated (AIIMS/Nov-03)
   (a)   During 1st trimester of pregnancy
   (b)   During 2nd trimester of pregnancy
   (c)   During 3rd trimester of pregnancy
   (d)   Before conception

Ans. (d)
Note
The neural tube closure occurs approximately 23 days after conception. So folic acid has to be given/ started before conception to prevent it's developmental defect.
Pre-pregnancy folic acid therapy is given when there is any history of neural tube defects in previous birth. Therapy is started 1 month before conception and is continued in the first trimester.
Ref : Textbook of obstetrics, D.C Dutta, 5th Edition Cp-22, Pg-365

Q. 132. Which of the following feature on second trimester ultrasound is not a marker of Down's syndrome (AIIMS/Nov-03)
   (a)   Single umbilical artery
   (b)   Choroid plexus cyst
   (c)   Diaphragmatic hernia
   (d)   Duodenal atresia

Ans. (b)
Note
Choroid plexus cyst is a feature of trisomy 18, 13
Ref: Textbook of obstetrics, D.C Dutta, 5th Edition Cp-40, Pg-687

Q. 133. Which of the following is not associated with chorioamnionitis? (AIIMS/Nov-03)
   (a)   Preterm labour
   (b)   Endometritis
   (c)   Abruptio placentae
   (d)   Placenta accreta

Ans. (d)
Note
Chorioamnionitis is a condition involving the bacterial infection of fetal membranes. It is usually caused by:
   - Preterm rupture of fetal membranes
   -Endometritis
   -Parametritis
   -Herpes Simplex Virus infection
   -Urinary tract infection
   -Vaginitis and cervicitis

-Sexually transmitted diseases that cause pelvic infection and inflammation
-viral infections (e.g., urogenital disease caused by herpes simplex virus)
-Pelvic inflammatory disease

Abruptio placentae
-It is one form of antepartum hemorrhage where the bleeding occurs due to premature separation of normally situated placenta.

Placenta accreta
-It is an extremely rare condition where the placenta is directly anchored, partially or completely to the myometrium.

Q. 134. Apoptosis can occur by change in hormone levels in the ovarian cycle. When there is no fertilization of the ovum, the endometrial cells die because (AIIMS/Nov-03)
- (a) The involution of corpus luteum causes estradiol and progesterone levels to fall dramatically.
- (b) LH (Lautenbing Hormone) levels rise after ovulation.
- (c) Estradiol levels are not involved in the LH surge phenomenon.
- (d) Estradiol inhibits the induction of the progesterone receptor in the endometrium.

Ans. (a)
Note
In the absence of pregnancy both estrogen and progesterone levels decline gradually and the fall in the level of these hormones brings about menstruation.
Ref: Shaw's Textbook of gynecology, 13th Edition Cp- 3, Pg- 45

Q. 135. The use of combined oral contraceptive pill is associated with an increased incidence of (AIIMS/Nov-03)
- (a) Bacterial vaginosis
- (b) Chlamydial endocervicitis
- (c) Vaginal warts
- (d) Genital herpes

Ans. (b)
Note
Oral contraceptives have an increased association with the infection. Chlamydial infection which is common in young, sexually active women. It is often silent, but occasionally there may be vaginal discharge, dysuria, frequency of urination and at times cervicitis.
Ref: Shaw's Textbook of gynecology, 13th Edition Cp- 10, Pg-128

Q. 136. In a young female of reproductive age with regular menstrual cycles of 28 days, ovulation occurs around 14th day of periods. When is first polar body extruded (AIIMS/Nov-03/ Nov-04/ May-05)
- (a) 24 hours prior to ovulation
- (b) Accompanied by ovulation
- (c) 48 hours after the ovulation
- (d) At the time of fertilization

Ans. (b)
Note
Significant changes in oocyte occur just prior to the ovulation (few hours). Cytoplasmic volume is increased along with changes in number and distribution of mitochondria. Completion of arrested 1st meiotic division occurs with extrusion of the 1st polar body, each containing 23X chromosomes.
Ref - Textbook of obstetrics, D.C Dutta, 5th Edition Cp-40, Pg-687

Q. 137. Minimum effective dose of ethinylestradiol in combination oral pills is (AIIMS/May-04)
- (a) 20 μgm
- (b) 35 μgm
- (c) 50 μgm
- (d) 75 μgm

Ans. (a)

Note
Combined oral pill contains a mixture of either ethinyloestradiol in dose of 20-30 µg and orally active progesterone.
Ref: Shaw's Textbook of gynecology, 13th Edition Cp- 18, Pg-226

Q. 138. From which of the following layers the regeneration of endometrium take place (AIIMS/May-04)
    (a)   Zona basalis
    (b)   Zona pellucidum
    (c)   Zona compacta
    (d)   Zona spongiosa

Ans. (a)
Note
Endometrium has:
a. Superficial layer; it is made-up of zona compactum and zona spongiosa, which are supplied by spiral arteries and due to their vasoconstriction, they undergo necrosis and sloughing during the secretory phase.
b. The deep layer is made up of zona basalis and it is supplied by basilar arteries which remain straight during the secretory phase so that the blood supply of this layer is not affected and thus it is not shed and in the proliferative phase, this deep layer causes regeneration of the endometrium.

Q. 139. All of the following pelvic structures support the vagina, except (AIIMS/May-04)
    (a)   Perineal body
    (b)   Pelvic diaphragm
    (c)   Levator ani muscle
    (d)   Infundibulo-pelvic ligament

Ans. (d)
Note
Infundibulo-pelvic ligament – It is a part of broad ligament and it is stretched from lateral pelvic wall to ovary. It has no relation to vagina and it does not support vagina.

Q. 140. All of the following are the indications for myomectomy in a case of fibroid uterus, except (AIIMS/May-04)
    (a)   Associated infertility
    (b)   Recurrent pregnancy loss
    (c)   Pressure symptoms
    (d)   Red degeneration

Ans. (d)
Note
Treatment of red degeneration of fibroid consists of analgesia and sedation. Symptoms usually clear off within 10 days.
Ref: Shaw's Textbook of gynecology, 13th Edition Cp- 20, Pg-327

Q. 141. In which of the following conditions, the medical treatment of ectopic pregnancy is contraindicated (AIIMS/May-04)
    (a)   Sac size is 3 cm
    (b)   Blood in pelvis 70 ml
    (c)   Presence of fetal heart activity
    (d)   Previous ectopic pregnancy

Ans. (c)
Note
Conditions where medical treatment is indicated:
The patient must be hemodynamically stable and tubal diameter should be less than 4 cm without any fetal cardiac activity.
Ref: Textbook of obstetrics, D.C Dutta, 5th Edition Cp-15, Pg-202

Q. 142. Conservative management is contraindicated in a case of placenta previa under the following situations, except (AIIMS/May-04)
- (a) Evidence of fetal distress
- (b) Fetal malformations
- (c) Mother in a hemodynamically unstable condition
- (d) Women in labour

Ans. (c)
Note
The cases selected for conservative management are:
 -Mother in good condition, Hb around 10gm/dl
 -Duration of pregnancy is less than 37 wks
 -FHS (Fetal Heart Sounds) satisfactory
 -Active bleeding absent
Indications for active management are:
 -Recurrence of brisk hemorrhage
 -Pregnancy beyond 37 wks
 -Fetus is dead or congenitally malformed
 -Patient in labor
Ref: Textbook of obstetrics, D.C Dutta, 5th Edition Cp-18, Pg-264-265

Q. 143. A primigravida presents to casualty at 32 weeks gestation with acute pain in abdomen for 2 hours, vaginal, bleeding and decreased fetal movements. She should be managed by (AIIMS/Nov-04)
- (a) Immediate caesarean section
- (b) Immediate induction of labour
- (c) Tocolytic therapy
- (d) Magnesium sulphate therapy

Ans. (b)
Note
Management of APH involves:
a. If patient is in labor: Labor is accelerated by ARM (artificial rupture of membrane) + oxytocin.
b. If patient is not in labor: Pregnancy more than or equal to 38 wks- ARM is done to induce labor
 -Pregnancy less than 38 wks and bleeding continuous then ARM followed by C.S. (Caeserean Section)
 If bleeding stops then patient is put on conservative treatment.
Ref: Textbook of Obstetrics, D.C Dutta, 5th Edition Cp-18, Pg- 273-273

Q. 144. All the following can cause DIC (Desseminated Intravascular coagulation) during pregnancy except (AIIMS/May-05)
- (a) Diabetes mellitus
- (b) Amniotic fluid embolism
- (c) Intrauterine death
- (d) Abruptio placentae

Ans. (a)
Note
The Obstetrical causes of DIC (Disseminated intravascular Coagulation) are:
a. Acute:
 -Abruptio placentae
 - Endotoxaemia; Septic abortion, Chorio-amnionitis, Pyelonephritis in pregnancy.
 -Liquor amnii embolism
 -Severe pre-eclampsia, eclampsia and HELLP Syndrome
 -Instillation of intra-amniotic hypertrtonic saline
 -Dextran infusion
 -Hydatiiform mole
 -Others; Shock, Caeserean section etc
b. Subacute:
 -Prolonged retention of dead fetus in utero.
Ref: Textbook of Obstetrics, D.C Dutta, 5th Edition Pg- 670

Q. 145. Use of oral contraceptives decreases the incidence of all the following except (AIIMS/May-05)
(a) Ectopic pregnancy
(b) Epithelial ovarian malignancy
(c) Hepatic adenoma
(d) Pelvic inflammatory disease

Ans. (c)
Note
Oral contraceptives have been implicated as a cause of benign hepatic adenomas and this risk is related to prolonged use.

Q. 146. The best time to do chorionic villous sampling is (AIIMS/May-05)
(a) Between 6-8 weeks
(b) Between 7-9 weeks
(c) Between 9-11 weeks
(d) Between 11-13 weeks

Ans. (d)
Note
It is performed for prenatal diagnosis of genetic disorders. It is carried out transcervically between 10-12 weeks and trans abdominally from 10 wks to term. A few chorionic villi are collected from chorion frondosum under USG (Ultrasonography) guidance with the help of a long malleable catheter.
Ref - Textbook of Obstetrics, D.C Dutta, 5th Edition Cp-11, Pg- 113

Q. 147. In a young female of reproductive age an absolute contraindication for prescribing oral contraceptive pills is (AIIMS/May-05)
(a) Diabetes
(b) Hypertension
(c) Obesity
(d) Impaired liver function

Ans. (d)
Note
An absolute contraindication for prescribing oral contraceptive pill is impaired liver function.

Q. 148. All of the followings are biochemical markers included for triple test except (AIIMS/May-05)
(a) Alfa fetoprotein (AFP)
(b) Human chorionic gonadotropin (HCG)
(c) Human placental lactogen (HPL)
(d) Unconjugated oestradiol

Ans. (c)
Note
Triple test: It is a combined biochemical test which includes MSAFP, hCG ad UF3 (unconjugated oestradiol). Maternal age in relation to confirm gestation age is also taken into account. It is used for detection of 'Down's Syndrome'. In an affected pregnancy level of MSAFP and UE3 tend to be low while that of hCG is high. It is performed at 15 -18 weeks. It gives a risk ratio and for confirmation aminocentesis has to be done. The result is considered to be screen positive if the risk ratio is 1: 250 or greater.
Ref - Textbook of Obstetrics, D.C Dutta, 5th Edition Pg-112

Q. 149. In a young female of reproductive age with regular menstrual cycles of 28 days ovulation occurs around 14th day of periods. When is the first polar body extruded? (AIIMS/May-05)
(a) 24 hours prior to ovulation
(b) Accompanied by ovulation
(c) 48 hours after the ovulation
(d) At the time of fertilization

Ans. (b)

Note
As the ova is released from ovarian follicle, its nucleus divides by meiosis and a first polar body is expelled from the nucleus of the oocyte.

Q. 150. During laparoscopy the preferred site for obtaining cultures in a patient wtih acute pelvic inflammatory disease is (AIIMS/May-05)
 (a) Endocervix
 (b) Pouch of Douglas
 (c) Endometrium
 (d) Fallopian tubes

Ans. (d)
Note
In acute pelvic inflammatory disease preferred site for obtaining culture is directly from tube.

Q. 151. In the perspective of the busy life schedule in the modern society, the accepted minimum period of sexual cohabitation resulting in no offpsring for a couple to be declared infertile is (AIIMS/May-05)
 (a) One year
 (b) One and a half-year
 (c) Two years
 (d) Three years

Ans. (a)
Note
Infertility implies apparent failure of a couple to conceive. If a couple fails to achieve pregnancy after 1 yr of unprotected and regular intercourse, it is an indication to investigate the couple.
Ref: Shaw's Textbook of gynecology, 13th Edition Cp- 17, Pg-198

Q. 152. Characteristics of an ideal candidate for copper-T insertion include all of the following except (AIIMS/May-05)
 (a) Has borne at least one child
 (b) Is willing to check IUD (Intra Uterine Device) tail
 (c) Has a history of ectopic pregnancy
 (d) Has normal menstrual periods

Ans. (c)
Note
Ideal candidates for IUD are:
 -Multiparous women
 -People with low risk of STD
 -Women in a monogamous relationship
Contraindications:
 -Suspected pregnancy
 -Severe anemia
 -Uncontrolled diabetes
 -PID
 -Heart disease
 -Scarred uterus
 -Fibroid
Family History:
 -H/O Ectopic Pregnancy
 -Menorrhagia & Dysmenorrhea
Ref: Shaw's Textbook of gynecology, 13th Edition Cp- 17, Pg-223

Q. 153. Aspermia is the term used to describe (ALL INDIA-05)
 (a) Absence of semen
 (b) Absence of sperm in ejaculate

(c) Absence of sperm motility
(d) Occurrence of abnormal sperm

Ans. (a)
Note
Aspermia- in absence of semen
Azoospermia-implies no sperm in semen
Asthenospermia-no motile sperm
Necrospermia-dead sperms
Teratospermia-abnormal morphology of sperms
Ref: Shaw's Textbook of gynecology, 13th Edition Cp- 17, Pg-202

Q. 154. Which of the following ultrasound marker is associated with greatest increased risk for trisomy 21 in fetus (ALL INDIA-05)
(a) Echogenic foci in heart
(b) Hyperechogenic bowel
(c) Choroid plexus cysts
(d) Nuchal edema

Ans. (d)
Note
USG markers in case of Trisomy 21 are:
a. Nuchal translucency
b. VSD & ASD
c. Horseshoe kidney, B/L (Bilateral) dilatation of renal pelvis, cystic dysplasia
d. Clinodactyly, short femur, wide gap between 1st and 2nd toes
Ref: Textbook of Obstetrics, D.C Dutta, 5th Edition, Cp-40, Pg- 687

Q. 155. The highest incidence of gestational trophoblastic disease is in (ALL INDIA-05)
(a) Australia
(b) Asia
(c) North America
(d) Western Europe

Ans. (b)
Note
GTD (gestational trophoblastic disease) refers to the spectrum of proliferative abnormalities of the trophoblast associated with pregnancy. It is common in oriental countries: Philippines, China, Indonesia. Highest incidence is in Philippines
Ref - Textbook of Obstetrics, D.C Dutta, 5th Edition Cp-15, Pg-206

Q. 156. The smallest diameter of the true pelvis is (ALL INDIA-05)
(a) Interspinous diameter
(b) Diagonal conjugate
(c) True conjugate
(d) Intertuberous diameter

Ans. (a)
Note
a. Interspinous diameter: It is the distance between the 2 ischial spines (10.5cm).
b. Diagonal conjugate: It is the distance between the lower border of symphysis pubis to the midpoint on sacral promontory (12cm).
c. True conjugate: It is the distance between the midpoints of sacral promontory to upper border of the pubic symphysis (11cm).
d. Intertuberous diameter: It is the distance between the inner borders of the ischial tuberosities (11cm).
Ref: Textbook of Obstetrics, D.C Dutta, 5th Edition, Cp-9, Pg- 93-97

Q. 157. The most common pure germ cell tumor of the ovary is (ALL INDIA-05)
(a) Choriocarcinoma
(b) Dysgerminoma

(c) Embryonal cell tumor
(d) Malignant teratoma

Ans. (b)
Note
The most common ovarian cancers in girls under 20 are germ cell tumors such as dysgerminoma, malignant teratoma and embryonal CA.
Ref: Shaw's Textbook of gynecology, 13th Edition Cp- 28, Pg-356
Dysgerminoma are the most common malignant germ cell tumors, accounting for about 30% to 40% of all ovarian cancers of germ cell origin. The tumor represents only 1% to 3% of all ovarian cancers, but as many as 5% to 10% of ovarian cancers in patients younger than 20 years of age.
Ref: http://www.health.am/cr/more/dysgerminomas/

Q. 158. Infants of diabetic mother are likely to have the following cardiac anomaly (ALL INDIA-05)
(a) Coarctation of aorta
(b) Fallot's tetralogy
(c) Ebstein's anomaly
(d) Transposition of great arteries

Ans. (b)
Note
Timing of diagnosis and description of the principal anomaly in 109 offsprings with major anomaly borne of diabetic mothers is detailed below:

Anomaly	Ante-natally diagnosed	Post-natally diagnosed
Atrioseptal defect	-	2
Hypoplastic left heart	5	-
Ventricular septal defect	1	4
Double inlet left ventricle	1	-
Double outlet right ventricle	2	-
Transposition of great arteries	1	3
Pulmonary artery stenosis	2	2
Pulmonary artery atresia with intact ventricular septum	1	-
Tetralogy of Fallot	3	4

Ref; http://www.bmj.com/cgi/content/full/333/7560/177/TBL6

Q. 159. Which one of the following is the ideal contraceptive for a patient with heart disease (ALL INDIA-05)
(a) IUCD
(b) Depo-provera
(c) Diaphragm
(d) Oral contraceptive pills

Ans. (c)
Note
IUCD, Depo-provera and OCPs are contraindicated in heart diseases, so by elimination (c) is the only option left.
Ref: Shaw's Textbook of gynecology, 13th Edition Cp- 18, Pg-223, 229 and 228 respectively

Q. 160. The karyotype of a patient with androgen insensitivity syndrome is (ALL INDIA-05)
 (a) 46 XX
 (b) 46 XY
 (c) 47 XXY
 (d) 45 XO

Ans. (b)
Note
In women with testicular feminization syndrome or androgen insensitivity syndrome, the phenotype is female and karyotype is 46XY. Gonads are testes but because of androgen insensitivity they present with lack of axillary and pubic hair, absent uterus and upper vagina.
Ref: Shaw's Textbook of gynecology, 13th Edition Cp- 21, Pg-279

Q. 161. The best period of gestation to carry out chorion villous biopsy for prenatal diagnosis is (ALL INDIA-05)
 (a) 8-10 weeks
 (b) 10-12 weeks
 (c) 12-14 weeks
 (d) 14-16 weeks

Ans. (b)
Note
Chorion villous biopsy is performed for prenatal diagnosis of genetic disorders. It is carried out transcervically between 10-12 weeks and trans-abdominally from 10 wks to term. A few chorionic villi are collected from chorion frondosum under USG (Ultrasonography) guidance with the help of a long malleable catheter.
Ref: Textbook of Obstetrics, D.C Dutta, 5th Edition Cp-11, Pg- 113
Also see
Similar to Q 173

Q. 162. Which one of the following biochemical parameters is the most sensitive to detect open spina bifida? (ALL INDIA-05)
 (a) Maternal serum alpha fetoprotein
 (b) Amniotic fluid alpha fetoprotein
 (c) Amniotic fluid acetyl cholin esterase (AChE)
 (d) Amniotic fluid glucohexaminase

Ans. (c)
Note
Amniotic fluid levels of AChE is elevated in most cases of open neural tube defect and has a better diagnostic value than AFP
Ref: Textbook of Obstetrics, D.C Dutta, 5th Edition Cp-11, Pg- 112

Q. 163. Risk of preterm delivery is increased if cervical length is (ALL INDIA-05)
 (a) 25 mm
 (b) 30 mm
 (c) 35 mm
 (d) 40 mm

Ans. (a)
Note
A second-trimester cervical length less than 25 mm was associated with a 75% recurrence of spontaneous preterm birth at less than 35 weeks of gestation.
http://www.greenjournal.org/cgi/content/full/103/3/457

Q. 164. All are the risk factors associated with macrosomia except (ALL INDIA-05)
 (a) Maternal obesity
 (b) Prolonged pregnancy
 (c) Previous large infant
 (d) Short stature

Ans. (d)

Note
Fetal macrosomia or (generalized fetal enlargement): Birth weight of more than 4 kg is considered overweight.
Causes
- Hereditary; parent's constitution
- Poorly controlled DM
- Post maturity
- Multiparity

Ref : Textbook of Obstetrics, D.C Dutta, 5th Edition, Cp-26, Pg- 436

Q. 165. Which of the following statement is incorrect in relation to pregnant women with epilepsy? (ALL INDIA-05)
(a) The rate of congenital malformation is increased in the offspring of women with epilepsy.
(b) Seizure frequency increases in approximately 70% of women.
(c) Breast feeding is safe with most anticonvulsants.
(d) Folic acid supplementation may reduce the risk of neural tube defect.

Ans. (b)
Note
Frequency of convulsions remains unchanged in approximately 50% of patients. Adverse effects on pregnancy are: third trimester bleeding and megaloblastic anemia (which is due to anticoagulant induced folate deficiency), birth defects are increased 2 folds due to folate deficiency. There is no contraindication for breast-feeding.
Ref - Textbook of Obstetrics, D.C Dutta, 5th Edition, Cp-19, Pg- 316

Q. 166. All are the causes of intrauterine growth retardation except (ALL INDIA-05)
(a) Anemia
(b) Pregnancy induced hypertension
(c) Maternal heart disease
(d) Gestational diabetes

Ans. (d)
Note
Causes of fetal growth retardation:
a. Maternal- constitutional, maternal malnutrition, anemia, hypertension, low blood oxygen as in cyanotic heart disease, malabsorption syndrome, UTI (Urinary Treat Infection), smoking, CRF, alcohol
b. Congenital anomalies, chromosomal abnormality, infection (TORCH), parvovirus, multiple pregnancy
c. Placental- pre-eclampsia, hypertension, organic heart disease, placental and cord abnormalities, circumvallate placenta.
d. Unknown

Ref: Textbook of Obstetrics, D.C Dutta, 5th Edition, Cp-31, Pg- 497

Q. 167. In a case of dysgerminoma of ovary one of the following tumor markers is likely to be raised (ALL INDIA-05)
(a) Serum HCG
(b) Serum alpha-fetoprotein
(c) Serum lactic dehydrogenase
(d) Serum inhibin

Ans. (a)
Note
Dysgerminoma comprise 2% of all ovarian CA about 10% are bilateral and 10% of patients have elevated S. HCG level. All dysgerminoma are malignant. Occur commonly in the 2nd to 3rd decade.
Ref: Textbook of pathology by Harsh Mohan, Cp –21 Pg- 734

Q. 168. Use of one of the following vaccination is absolutely contraindicated in pregnancy (ALL INDIA-05)
(a) Hepatitis-B
(b) Cholera
(c) Rabies
(d) Yellow fever

Ans. Use your discretion.

Note
Ans could be either b or d
(b) Although cholera vaccine has not been reported to have any adverse effects on pregnancy, the safety of its use in pregnancy has also not been estimated.
Ref: Park's Textbook of PSM, Cp- 5, section 2, Pg-170
(d) 17D vaccine for yellow fever is a live attenuated virus, although no teratogenic effects have been ascribed to it, yet immunization should be avoided during pregnancy, if there's no risk of exposure.
Ref: Park's Textbook of PSM, Cp- 5, section 2, Pg-217
-All live viral vaccines are contraindicated during pregnancy, as they are potentially dangerous to the fetus.
Ref - Textbook of Obstetrics, D.C Dutta, 5th Edition, Cp-33, Pg-551

Q. 169. The most common cause of secondary amenorrhoea in India is (ALL INDIA-05)
(a) Endometrial tuberculosis
(b) Premature ovarian failure
(c) Polycystic ovarian syndrome
(d) Sheehan's syndrome

Ans. (a)
Note
In about 40% cases of endometrial tuberculosis there is menorrhagia and 10% complain of secondary amenorrhea. If a young woman in her 20s complains of secondary amenorrhea and on examination, if an adnexal swelling is found, the diagnosis of genital TB is considered.
Ref: Shaw's Textbook of gynecology, 13th Edition Cp- 12, Pg-150

Q. 170. The consequences of Rh incompatibility are not serious during first pregnancy because (ALL INDIA-04)
(a) Antibodies are not able to cross placenta.
(b) Antibody titer is very low during primary immune response.
(c) IgG generated is ineffective against foetal red cells.
(d) Massive hemolysis is compensated by increased erythropoiesis.

Ans. (b)
Note
If the fetus is Rh +ve and the mother is Rh –ve. Fetal RBCs enter the maternal circulation and this leads to production of antibodies. This process takes a long time; therefore isoimmunisation in 1st pregnancy is unlikely.
Ref: Textbook of Obstetrics, D.C Dutta, 5th Edition, Cp-22, Pg-353

Q. 171. A 21 year old woman presents with complaints of primary amenorrhea. Her height is 153 cm, weight is 51 kg. She has well developed breasts. She has no pubic or axillary hair and no hirsuitism. Which of the following is the most probable diagnosis? (ALL INDIA-04)
(a) Turner syndrome
(b) Stein-Leventhal syndrome
(c) Premature ovarian failure
(d) Complete androgen insensitivity syndrome

Ans. (d)
Note
A women with testicular feminization syndrome or androgen insensitivity syndrome, the phenotype is female and karyotype is 46XY. Gonads are testes but because of androgen insensitivity they present with lack of axillary and pubic hair, absent uterus and upper vagina. Breast development appears to be normal, these gonads are prone to malignancy and so prophylactic gonadectomy should be done.
Ref: Shaw's Textbook of gynecology, 13th Edition Cp- 21, Pg-279-280

Q. 172. A 28-year old lady has put on weight (10 kg over a period of 3 years), and has oligomenorrhea followed by amenorrhea for 8 months. The blood pressure is 160/100 mm of Hg. Which of the following is the most appropriate investigation? (ALL INDIA-04)
(a) Serum electrolytes
(b) Plasma cortisol

(c) Plasma testosterone and ultrasound evaluation of pelvis
(d) T3, T4 and TSH

Ans. (b)

Note
Most suitable investigation for this case is plasma cortisol. C/F of Cushing's syndrome are- hair thinning, hirsuitism, acne, plethora, cataract, peptic ulcer, hypertension, centripetal obesity, striae, menstrual disturbance, osteoporosis, wasting and weakness of muscles.
Ref: Principles and Practice of medicine –Davidson, Cp- 16, Pg- 723

Q. 173. All of the following conditions are risk factor for urinary tract infections in pregnancy, except (ALL INDIA-04)
(a) Diabetes mellitus
(b) Hypertension
(c) Sickle cell disease
(d) Vesicoureteral reflux

Ans. (b)

Note
Although all pregnant women should be tested for UTIs, those at particularly at high risk are those with the following conditions or situations: Diabetes mellitus, Sickle cell trait and Vesicoureteral reflux (VUR) which is also a source of urinary tract infections. Therefore by elimination the only option left is (b).
Ref: - http://www.umm.edu/patiented/articles/what_risk_factors_urinary_tract_infections__000036_4.htm

Q. 174. Which one of the following perinatal infections has the highest risk of fetal infection in the first trimester? (ALL INDIA-04)
(a) Hepatitis B virus
(b) Syphilis
(c) Toxoplasmosis
(d) Rubella

Ans. (d)

Note

(a) HBV: The risk of transmission in the first trimester is 10% to as high as 90% during the third trimester (Pg 308)

(b) Syphilis: T. pallidum enters the fetal circulation after the 20th wk with disappearance of langerhans layer in villi (Pg 310)

(c) Toxoplasma: Risk of infection of the fetus increases with the duration of pregnancy, being highest (60%) in the third trimester. (Pg 312)

(d) Rubella: Risk of major anomalies is maximum when this infection occurs in the 1st trimester (50%), 2nd (25%), 3rd (10%) month. (Pg 316)

Ref: Textbook of Obstetrics, D.C. Dutta, 5th Edition, Cp-19

Q. 175. All of the following are ultrasonographic fetal growth parameters, except (ALL INDIA-04)
(a) Biparietal diameter
(b) Head cirumference
(c) Transcerebellar diameter
(d) Femur length

Ans. (c)

Note
BPD (biparietal diameter) and FL (femur length) determine the gestational age, AC (abdominal circumference), HC (head circumference) and amniotic fluid volume are used to diagnose IUGR.
Ref: Textbook of Obstetrics, D.C Dutta, 5th Edition, Cp-11, Pg-116, Cp-7, Pg-73

Q. 176. A case of obstructed labour which was delivered by cesarean section complains of cyclical passage of menstrual blood in urine. Which is the most likely site of fistula? (ALL INDIA-04)
  (a) Urethro-vaginal
  (b) Vesico-vaginal
  (c) Vesico-uterine
  (d) Uretero-uterine

Ans. (c)

Note
This is a rare variety of fistula, usually occurring during CS. The patient remains continent and the urine doesn't dribble into the uterine cavity. The patient however complains of cyclical hematuria, because of trickling of menstrual blood in to the bladder through fistula.
Ref: Shaw's Textbook of gynecology, 13th Edition Cp-16, Pg-184

Q. 177. Which of the following is the investigation of choice in a pregnant lady at 18 weeks of pregnancy with past history of delivering a baby with Down's syndrome? (ALL INDIA-04)
  (a) Triple screen test
  (b) Amniocentesis
  (c) Chorionic villous biopsy
  (d) Ultrasonography

Ans. (b)

Note
Indications for amniocentesis are:
  -In cases where open neural tube defects are suspected.
  -For carrying out culture and chromosomal studies under following conditions.
  -Pregnancy above 35 yrs.
  -Previous child with chromosomal abnormalities.
  -Pregnancy in a woman with X linked disorder.
  -Detection of inborn errors of metabolism.
Ref - Textbook of Obstetrics, D.C Dutta, 5th Edition, Cp-11, Pg-112

Q. 178. The most appropriate method for collecting urine for culture in case of vesicovaginal fistula is (ALL INDIA-04)
  (a) Suprapubic needle aspiration
  (b) Midstream clean catch
  (c) Foley's catheter
  (d) Sterile speculum

Ans. (c)

Note
The most appropriate method for collecting urine is by using Foley's catheter.
Ref: Shaw's Textbook of gynecology, 13th Edition Cp-16, Pg-182

Q. 179. Which of the following is the most likely diagnosis in a 27 year old obese woman presenting with oligomenorrhea, infertility and hirsuitism? (ALL INDIA-04)
  (a) Polycystic ovaries
  (b) Endometriosis
  (c) Pelvic inflammatory disease
  (d) Turner's syndrome

Ans. (a)

Note
PCOS or Stein Levanthal Syndrome is characterized by chronic non-ovulation and hyperandrogenemia, associated with a normal or raised estrogen level, raised LH and low FSH/LH ratio. It is often seen in young women who complain of oligomenorrhea, infertility, obesity and hirsuitism.
Ref: Shaw's Textbook of gynecology, 13th Edition Cp-28, Pg-353-354

MCQ's in Obstetrics and Gynecology

Q. 180. Which of the following tests is most sensitive for the detection of iron depletion in pregnancy? (ALL INDIA-04)
- (a) Serum iron
- (b) Serum ferritin
- (c) Serum transferrin
- (d) Serum iron binding capacity

Ans. (b)
Note
Plasma ferritin is a measure of iron stores. It's a very specific test. There is little diurnal variation. Plasma iron and TIBC are measures of availability, hence are affected by many factors. Lower level of transferrin saturation is consistent with iron deficiency but less specific than ferritin measurement. Therefore s. ferritin is best test to confirm iron deficiency
Ref: Principles and Practice of medicine –Davidson, Cp- 19, Pg- 917

Q. 181. A 55 year old lady presenting to out patient department (OPD) with postmenopausal bleeding for 3 months has a 1 × 1 cm nodule on the anterior lip of cervix. The most appropriate investigation to be done subsequently is (ALL INDIA-03)
- (a) Pap smear
- (b) Punch biopsy
- (c) Endocervical curettage
- (d) Colposcopy

Ans. (b)
Note
On speculum examination if a visible growth is seen on cervix then the most appropriate investigation to be done is Punch biopsy.

Q. 182. A primigravida at 37 week of gestation reported to labour room with central placenta praevia with heavy bleeding per vaginum. The fetal heart rate was normal at the time of examination. The best management option for her is (ALL INDIA-03)
- (a) Expectant management
- (b) Caesarean section
- (c) Induction and vaginal delivery
- (d) Induction and forceps delivery

Ans. (b)
Note
CS is indicated in:
  -Placenta praevia especially of type 2 posterior, type 3 and type 4.
  -Severe heavy bleeding or signs of fetal distress.
Ref: Textbook of Obstetrics, D.C Dutta, 5th Edition, Cp-18, Pg-263

Q. 183. All of the following are known risk factors for development of endometrial carcinoma, except (ALL INDIA-03)
- (a) Obesity
- (b) Family history
- (c) Use of Hormone Replacement Therapy
- (d) Early menopause

Ans. (d)
Note
Predisposing factors for development of endometrial CA are:
  -Unsupervised administration of HRT with estrogens alone during menopause.
  -Tamoxifen
  -Obesity, hypertension and DM
  -Infertile women, PCOS
  -Familial predisposition
Ref: Shaw's Textbook of gynecology, 13th Edition Cp-29, Pg-392

Q. 184. Laparotomy performed in a case of ovarian tumor revealed unilateral ovarian tumor with ascites positive for malignant cells and positive pelvic lymph nodes. All other structure were free of disease. What is the stage of the disease? (ALL INDIA-03)
   (a)   Stage II C
   (b)   Stage III A
   (c)   Stage III B
   (d)   Stage III C

Ans. (d)
Note
FIGO Staging of Ovarian Carcinoma:

Stage	Features
Stage I	**Tumor restricted to one or both ovaries**
IA	Tumor restricted to one ovary. No tumour on external surface, capsule intact. No Malignant ascitis.
IB	Tumour limited to ovaries, No tumour on external surface, capsule intact, NO malignant ascitis.
IC	Tumor IA or IB, positive for surface malignant ascites, growth, capsule ruptured, malignant ascites or positive washing
Stage II	**Tumor involves one/both ovaries with pelvic extension.**
IIA	Extension / Metastasis to uterus and / or pelvic extension tubes. No malignant cells in ascites / washing.
IIB	Extension to other pelvic organs. No malignant cells in ascites or washings.
IIC	Tumor IIA or IIB with surface growth, capsule ruptured at /or prior to surgery, malignant ascites or positive washings.
Stage III	**Tumor involves one / Both ovaries, with microscopic implants outside the pelvis, and / or positive nodes (inguinal, retroperitoneal). Tumour limited to true pelvis but with histological evidence of spread to bowel, omentum, and presence of superficial metastases on the liver.**
IIIA	Tumour grossly, limited to the pelvis, nodes negative, but microscopic seeding. Or peritoneum of the abdominal wall.
IIIB	Tumour with abdominal peritoneal implants of less than 2.0 cm size and nodes negative.
IIIC	Abdominal implants of more than 2.0 cm size, and o/or positive nodes.
Stage IV	**Growth involving one or both ovaries with distant metastasis in liver, lungs, and pleura tap fluid for cytology.**

Ref: Shaw's Textbook of gynecology, 13th Edition Cp-29, Pg-402, table

Q. 185. Pure gonadal dysgenesis will be diagnosed in the presence of (ALL INDIA-03)
   (a)   Bilateral streak gonads
   (b)   Bilateral dysgenetic gonads
   (c)   One side streak and other dysgenetic gonads
   (d)   One side streak and other normal looking gonad

Ans. (a)
Note
Streak ovaries, undifferentiated stroma and absence of sex cells characterize -gonadal dysgenesis or Turner's syndrome. The ovaries don't have Graffian follicle so don't produce oestrogen.
Ref: Shaw's Textbook of gynecology, 13th Edition Cp-8, Pg-100

MCQ's in Obstetrics and Gynecology 693

Q. 186. All of the following may be observed in a normal pregnancy except (ALL INDIA-03)
    (a)   Fall in serum iron concentration
    (b)   Increase in serum iron binding capacity
    (c)   Increase in blood viscosity
    (d)   Increase in blood oxygen carrying capacity

Ans. (c)
Note
During pregnancy the RBC volume increases by 20-30% and the plasma volume increases by 50%. The disproportionate increase in plasma and RBC volume produces a state of hemodilution during pregnancy leading to a fall in the plasma viscosity.
Ref - Textbook of Obstetrics, D.C Dutta, 5th Edition, Cp-5, Pg-52

Q. 187. Pyometra is a complication associated with all of the following conditions except (ALL INDIA-03)
    (a)   Carcinoma of the vulva
    (b)   Carcinoma of the cervix
    (c)   Carcinoma of endometrium
    (d)   Pelvic radiotherapy

Ans. (a)
Note
Pyometra is caused by stenosis of cervical canal resulting in collection of pent up discharges from the glands of the endometrium in the uterine cavity and infection. As a result the pus collection causes pyometra. Causes of cervical stenosis are:
    -Ca Cx (Cervix)
    -Amputation of Cx (Cervix)
    -Irradiation
    -Postmenopausal involution of the uterus leading to cervical stenosis
    -Ca endometrium
    -Tubercular endometritis
Ref: Shaw's Textbook of gynecology, 13th Edition Cp-24, Pg-313

Q. 188. A hypertensive pregnant woman at 34 weeks comes with history of pain in abdomen, bleeding per vaginum and loss of fetal movements. On examination the uterus is contracted with increased uterine tone Fetal heart sounds are absent. The most likely diagnosis is (ALL INDIA-03)
    (a)   Placenta praevia
    (b)   Hydramnios
    (c)   Premature labour
    (d)   Abruptio placentae

Ans. (d)
Note
Abruptio placentae is characterized by premature separation of a normally placed placenta. Clinical features are:
    -Acute abdominal pain
    -Continuous discharge of dark blood
    -Severe pallor
    -Tender rigid and tense uterus
    -FHS absent
Ref: Textbook of Obstetrics, D.C Dutta, 5th Edition, Cp-18, Pg-269 and 271

Q. 189. Most common cause of first trimester abortion is (ALL INDIA-03)
    (a)   Chromosomal abnormalities
    (b)   Syphilis
    (c)   Rhesus isoimmunisation
    (d)   Cervical incompetence

Ans. (a)

Note

The commonest cause of 1st trimester abortion is defective germ plasm. Other causes are- hormonal deficiency, acute infection, and trauma.
Ref: Textbook of Obstetrics, D.C Dutta, 5th Edition Cp-15, Pg-172

Q. 190. All of the following are mechanisms of action of emergency contraception except (ALL INDIA-03)
   (a)   Delaying ovulation
   (b)   Inhibiting fertilization
   (c)   Preventing implantation of the fertilized egg
   (d)   Interrupting an early pregnancy

Ans. (d)

Note

Mode of action of emergency contraception methods:
   -Ovulation is prevented or delayed when drug is taken in the beginning of the cycle.
   -Interference with fertilization.
   -Prevention of implantation by rendering the endometrium unfavorable.
   -Interference with the function of corpus luteum.
Ref; Textbook of Obstetrics, D.C Dutta, 5th Edition Cp-35, Pg-588

Q. 191. A 20 year old woman gives a history of sharp pain in the lower abdomen for 2-3 days every month approximately 2 weeks before the menses. The most probable etiology for her pain is (ALL INDIA-03)
   (a)   Endometriosis
   (b)   Dysmenorrhea
   (c)   Pelvic tuberculosis
   (d)   Mittelschmerz

Ans. (d)

Note

Mittelschmerz is a physiological occurrence during the period of ovulation when hormonal changes take place. It is characterized by mid menstrual bleeding, lasting for a few hours and an intermittent cramping pain of short duration.
Ref: Shaw's Textbook of gynecology, 13th Edition Cp-21, Pg-287

Q. 192. A 55-year old woman has recurrent urinary retention after a hysterectomy done for a huge fibroid. The most likely cause is (ALL INDIA-03)
   (a)   Atrophic and stenotic urethra
   (b)   Lumbar disc prolapse
   (c)   Injury to the bladder neck
   (d)   Injury to the hypogastric plexi

Ans. (d)

Note

Radical operations like Wartheim's hysterectomy involve extensive dissection causing denervation of the bladder, leaving the patient with an insensitive bladder, leading to retention of urine. This requires continuous catheterization.
Other causes of post operative retention of urine are:
   -Post-operative edema
   -Pelvic pain
   -Spinal and epidural anesthesia
Ref: Shaw's Textbook of gynecology, 13th Edition Cp-15, Pg-169-170

Q. 193. A 45 year old female is having bilateral ovarian mass, ascites and omental caking on CT scan. There is high possibility that patient is having (ALL INDIA-03)
    (a)   Benign ovarian tumour
    (b)   Malignant epithelial ovarian tumor
    (c)   Dysgerminoma of ovary
    (d)   Lymphoma of ovary

Ans. (b)

Note
Ovarian cancer usually spreads via local shedding into the peritoneal cavity followed by implantation on the peritoneum and via local invasion of bowel and bladder. Tumor cells may also block diaphragmatic lymphatic. The resulting impairment of lymphatic drainage of the peritoneum is thought to play a role in development of ascites in ovarian cancer. Also, transdiaphragmatic spread to the pleura is common.
Ref: http://www.cancer.gov/cancertopics/pdq/treatment/ovarianepithelial/healthprofessional

Q. 194. Complete failure of mullerian duct fusion will result in (ALL INDIA-02)
    (a)   Uterus didelphys
    (b)   Arcuate uterus
    (c)   Subseptate uterus
    (d)   Unicornuate uterus

Ans. (a)

Note
(a)   When the 2 mullerian ducts fail to fuse along the whole of their length, but develop normally and remain separate, the condition is termed as uterus didelphys.
(b)   No deformity as such is present, but instead of the usual dome shaped concavity there's a shallow concave depression.
(c)   Septum is restricted to the body of the uterus.
(d)   Absence of round ligament and fallopian tube on the opposite side. Also associated with abnormalities of the kidney of that side.
Ref: Shaw's Textbook of gynecology, 13th Edition Cp-7, Pg-91

Q. 195. Commonest cause of female pseudohermaphroditism is (ALL INDIA-02)
    (a)   Virlizing ovarian tumor
    (b)   Ovarian dygenesis
    (c)   Exogenous androgen
    (d)   Congenital adrenal hyperplasia

Ans. (d)

Note
Female hermaphroditism is characterized by sex glands of one sex and external genitalia of another sex. It is caused by block in conversion of 17-hydroxyprogesterone to hydrocortisone; therefore the pituitary produces excess of ACTH, which causes adrenal hyperplasia, and excess output of androgens.
Ref: Shaw's Textbook of gynecology, 13th Edition Cp-7, 8, Pg-94, 103

Q. 196. Basanti Devi 45 years old woman, presents with hot flushes after stopping of menstruation. Hot flush can be relieved by administration of following agent (ALL INDIA-02)
    (a)   Ethinyl estradiol
    (b)   Testesterone
    (c)   Fluoxymesterone
    (d)   Danazol

Ans. (a)

Note
Basanti has menopausal complaints especially the hot flushes are due to lack of estrogen. This can be overcome by HRT.

Q. 197. A 25 years old infertile male underwent semen analysis. Results show sperm count 15 million/ml; pH 75; volume 2 ml; no agglutination is seen. Morphology shows 60% normal & 60% motile sperms. Most likely diagnosis is (ALL INDIA-01/02)
    (a)   Normospermia
    (b)   Oligospermia
    (c)   Azoospermia
    (d)   Aspermia

Ans. (b)

Note
A normal semen specimen has following features:
-It should coagulate soon after ejaculation
-Grayish white in color
-Sperm count 60 to120 million/ml
-Morphology 80% or more normal
-Total vol 3 to 5 ml
-Motility-80-90%
Ref: Shaw's Textbook of gynecology, 13th Edition Cp-17, Pg-202

Q. 198. A 28 years old lady, is suspected to have polycystic ovarian disease Sample for testing LH & FSH are best taken on the which days of menstrual cycle (ALL INDIA-02)
    (a)   1-4
    (b)   8-10
    (c)   13-15
    (d)   24-26

Ans. (b)

Note
-PCOS or Stein Leventhal Syndrome is characterized by chronic non-ovulation and hyperandrogenemia, associated with a normal or raised estrogen level, raised LH and low FSH/LH ratio.
Ref: Shaw's Textbook of gynecology, 13th Edition Cp-28, Pg-353
-FSH surge in a normally menstruating woman occurs around the 7th day of menstrual cycle.
Ref: Shaw's Textbook of gynecology, 13th Edition Cp-3, Pg-40

Q. 199. Kamla, a 20 years old young lady, presents with history of hirsutism and amenorrhea with change in voice. To establish a diagnosis you would like to proceed with which of the following tests in blood (ALL INDIA-02)
    (a)   17-OH progesterone
    (b)   DHEA
    (c)   Testosterone
    (d)   LH + FSH estimation

Ans. (c)
Ref: Shaw's Textbook of gynecology, 13th Edition Cp-28, Pg-353

Q. 200. A 35 years old mother of two children is suffering from amenorrhea for last 12 months. She has history of failure of lactation following 2nd delivery but remained asymptomatic thereafter. Skull X-ray shows "empty sella." Most likely diagnosis is (ALL INDIA-02)
    (a)   Menopause
    (b)   Pituitary tumor
    (c)   Sheehan's syndrome
    (d)   Intraductal papilloma of breast

Ans. (c)

Note
Sheehan's syndrome occurs following PPH leading to vascular thrombosis of pituitary vessels, panhypopituitarism, amenorrhea and failure of lactation
Ref: Shaw's Textbook of gynecology, 13th Edition Cp-21, Pg-283

Q. 201. A 35 years old female patient, having children aged 5 and 6 years has history of amenorrhea and galactorrhea. Blood examination reveals increased prolactin. The CT of the head is likely to reveal (ALL INDIA-02)
  (a) Prolactinoma
  (b) Craniopharyngioma
  (c) Sheehan's syndrome
  (d) Pinealoma

Ans. (a)

Note
Prolactin is secreted by α cells of pituitary gland. It's main action is on lactation and has a suppressive effect on H-P-O axis. Therefore a patient who suffers from hyperprolactinemia (as in prolactinoma) may develop amenorrhea or oligomenorrhea due to anovulatory cycles with or without galactorrhea.
Ref: Shaw's Textbook of gynecology, 13th Edition Cp-3, Pg-40

Q. 202. Most common genital prolapse is (ALL INDIA-02)
  (a) Cystocoele
  (b) Procidentia
  (c) Rectocoele
  (d) Enterocoele

Ans. (a)

Note
a. Cytocoele: Prolapse of upper 2/3rds of anterior vaginal wall.
b. Procidentia: Prolapse of whole uterus outside the vulvae, bringing with it both the vaginal walls.
c. Rectocoele: Prolapse of lower 2/3rds of posterior vaginal wall with rectum.
d. Enterocoele: Protrusion of upper posterior vaginal wall with palpation of the coils of intestine.
Ref: Shaw's Textbook of gynecology, 13th Edition Cp-25, Pg-321-322

Q. 203. A 30 years old lady examined for infertility by hysterosalpingography, reveals 'bead-like' fallopian tube & clubbing of ampulla. Most likely cause is (ALL INDIA-02)
  (a) Gonococcus
  (b) Mycoplasma
  (c) Chlamydia
  (d) Mycobacterium tuberculosis

Ans. (d)

Note
Apart from above, other features suggestive of tuberculosis are:
  -A rigid non peristaltic pipe like tube "lead pipe appearance"
  -Beading and variation in filling density
  -Calcification of tube
  -Cornual block
  -Jagged fluffiness of the tubal outline
  -Tobacco pouch and dilated distal ends of tubes
  -Vascular or lymphatic intravasation of the dye
However, in a proven case of genital TB, hysterosalpingography is contraindicated as it may spread the infection.
Ref: Shaw's Textbook of gynecology, 13th Edition Cp-37, Pg-477

Q. 204. All of the following may predispose to endometrial Ca, except (ALL INDIA-02)
  (a) Unopposed estrogen
  (b) Oral contraceptive
  (c) Nulliparity
  (d) Tamoxifen therapy

Ans. (b)

Note
Predisposing factors for endometrial CA are:
- Unsupervised administration of HRT with oestrogens alone during menopause.
- Tamoxifen
- Obesity, hypertension and DM
- Infertile women, PCOS
- Familial predisposition

Ref: Shaw's Textbook of gynecology, 13th Edition Cp-29, Pg-392
Similar to 230

Q. 205. Rokitansky Kustner Hauser syndrome is associated with (ALL INDIA-01)
   (a) Ovarian agenesis
   (b) Absent fallopian tube
   (c) Vaginal atresia
   (d) Bicornuate uterus

Ans. (c)
Note
Vaginal aplasia associated with absence of uterus is seen in Rokitansky-Kustner-Hauser Syndrome.
Ref: Shaw's Textbook of gynecology, 13th Edition Cp-7, Pg-88

Q. 206. A patient of 47 XXY karyotype presents with features of hypogonadism The likely diagnosis is (ALL INDIA-01)
   (a) Turner's syndrome
   (b) Klinefelter's syndrome
   (c) Edward's syndrome
   (d) Down's syndrome

Ans. (b)
Note
Karyotype of patients suffering from Klinefelter's syndrome is 47XY. The patient externally resembles a male, the penis is small or normal, and testes are small but normally placed. Sterility is common, gynecomastia is present. The patient has a high-pitched voice and appearance is eunuchoid and mentally deficient.
Ref: Shaw's Textbook of gynecology, 13th Edition Cp-8, Pg-101

Q. 207. A woman presents with amenorrhea of 6 weeks duration and lump in the right iliac fossa Investigation of choice is (ALL INDIA-01)
   (a) USG abdomen
   (b) Laparoscopy
   (c) CT scan
   (d) Shielded X-ray

Ans. (a)
Note
The female with amenorrhea of 6 weeks duration and lump in right iliac fossa is most probably suggestive of an ectopic gestation.
The choice of investigation which is non-invasive, cost effective and easy to carry out is USG abdomen. It is the first and often the only imaging modality used to demonstrate pelvic anatomy and to document physiological or pathological changes.
Ref: Shaw's Textbook of gynecology, Cp -37, Pg-481

Q. 208. A woman presents with amenorrhea of 2 months duration, lower abdominal pain, facial pallor, fainting and shock. Diagnosis is (ALL INDIA-01)
   (a) Ruptured ovarian cyst
   (b) Ruptured ecotopic pregnancy
   (c) Threatened abortion
   (d) Septic abortion

Ans. (b)

Note
The patient is presenting with classical features such as:
a. Amenorrhea of 2 months duration
b. Lower abdominal pain
c. Facial pallor, fainting and shock

The feataures are pointing to acute abdominal catastrophe. The classical history of amenorrhea of two months duration in a female of child bearing age with above features point to the most probable cause the 'ruptured ectopic pregnancy'. However please remember the classical triads of symptoms of disturbed tubal pregnancy are:
Amenorrhea followed by abdominal pain and appearance of vaginal bleeding.
Ref: Textbook of Obstetrics, D.C.Dutta, 5th Edition Cp-15, Pg-196-198

Q. 209. A young woman with six weeks amenorrhea presents with mass abdomen. USG shows empty uterus. Diagnosis is (ALL INDIA-01)
   (a) Ovarian cyst
   (b) Ectopic pregnancy
   (c) Complete abortion
   (d) None of the above

Ans. (b)

Note
The above features and USG finding are suggestive of ectopic pregnancy. The USG features of ectopic pregnancy are
   -Absence of uterine pregnancy
   -Fluid in POD
   -Adnexal mass separated from the ovary
Ref: Textbook of Obstetrics, D.C.Dutta, 5th Edition Cp-15, Pg-199

Q. 210. Basanti, a 28 years aged female with a history of 6 weeks of amenorrhea, presents with pain in abdomen. USG shows fluid in pouch of Doughlous. Aspiration yields dark colour blood that fails to clot. Most probable diagnosis is (ALL INDIA-01)
   (a) Ruptured ovarian cyst
   (b) Ruptured ectopic pregnancy
   (c) Red degeneration of fibroid
   (d) Pelvic abscess

Ans. (b)

Note
The lead is:
a. Female of 28 years. (Female in reproductive age)
b. H/O six Weeks amenorrhea.
c. C/O pain in abdomen. (Location not specified), associated features of shock are missing.
d. UGC shows fluid in pouch of Doughlous (it does not comment on Uterus; whether pregnancy is there or not. What is state of fallopian tubes, ovaries and other abdominal findings.
e. However the aspiration from pouch of Doughlous yields dark coloured blood that fails to clot – signifies collection of intraperitoneal blood.
Conclusion:
Pain abdomen, with blood in pouch of doughlous in a female of child bearing age with 6 weeks amenorrhea the strongest possibility is of ruptured ectopic pregnancy.

Q. 211. A patient complains of post coital bleed. No growth is seen on per speculum examination. Next step should be (ALL INDIA-01)
   (a) Colposcopic biopsy
   (b) Conization
   (c) Pap smear
   (d) Culdoscopy

Ans. (a)

Note
The post coital bleeding points to a strong possibility of Ca cervix. As on per speculum examination no growth is seen. The colposcopy is next choice, as it facilitates 3 dimensional morphological inspections under binocular vision. It can detect any suspicious lesion and a biopsy can be obtained.

Also see
Pap smear or surface biopsy is a routine test, which can detect other local, inflammatory conditions apart from malignancy and pre-malignant lesions. A positive test requires further investigations like colposcopy, cervical biopsy and fractional curettage.
Ref: Shaw's Textbook of gynecology, Cp-6, Pg-77
Conization or cone biopsy is done when there is discrepancy between cytology and colposcopy.
Ref: Shaw's Textbook of gynecology, Cp-29, Pg-384

Q. 212. A 50 years old woman presents with post coital bleeding. A visible growth on cervix is detected on per speculum examination. Next investigation is (ALL INDIA-01)
- (a) Punch biopsy
- (b) Colposcopic biopsy
- (c) Pap smear
- (d) Cone biopsy

Ans. (a)

Note
When there is a visible growth on cervix per speculum examination the next step is to go for a punch biopsy for further confirmation of diagnosis.

Also see
Indications for cervical punch biopsy:
a. A pap smear indicates significant abnormalities, or
b. When an abnormal area is seen on the cervix during a routine pelvic examination.
Procedure:
First the area is viewed with a colposcope, a small low-power microscope used to magnify the surface of the vagina and cervix (the most accurate method). When an abnormality is located, a sample (biopsy) may be taken using a small biopsy forceps or a large needle. More than one sample may be taken. Cells from the cervical canal may be used as samples as well.
Ref: - http://www.nlm.nih.gov/medlineplus/ency/article/003912.htm

Q. 213. A case of carcinoma cervix is found in altered sensorium and is having hiccoughs. The likely cause is (ALL INDIA-01)
- (a) Septicemia
- (b) Uremia
- (c) Raised ICT
- (d) Intestinal obstruction

Ans. (b)

Note
The presentation is:
a. Known case of CA cervix.
b. O/E: Presents features of altered sensorium.
c. O/E: Hiccoughs.
The most probable cause in present condition appears to be renal complications of Ca cervix leading to renal failure.
"It must be remembered that 70% cases of carcinoma cervix die, not of their primary disease, but of bilateral renal obstruction" as the ureter is particularly subjected to compression in case of Ca cervix or other malignant infiltrations of broad ligament.
Ref: -Shaw's Textbook of gynecology, Cp-15, Pg-177
C/F of uremia:
-Kussmaul respiration, anorexia, nausea, pruritis, hiccough, vomiting, later fits, drowsiness, and coma ensues.

Q. 214. Bilateral ovarian cancer with capsule breached, ascites positive for malignant cells. The stage is: (ALL INDIA-01)
- (a) Stage I
- (b) Stage II
- (c) Stage III
- (d) Stage IV

Ans. (b)

Note
Following are the broad features of different stages of ovarian cancer:

Stage	Features
I	Growth limited to ovaries. Capsule intact. No ascites. The cancer is confined to one or both ovaries. Tumor may be found on the surface of ovary.
II	The cancer involves one or both ovaries with extension into the pelvic region, e.g., capsule ruptured. With ascites. It is found in the uterus, fallopian tubes, bladder sigmoid colon or rectum. Few women are diagnosed at this stage.
III	The cancer has spread beyond the pelvis to the abdominal wall or abdomen, small bowel, lymph nodes or liver surface.
IV	This is the most advanced form of ovarian caner. Stage IV cancers have spread to distant organs such as liver (spread beyond just the surface of liver), spleen or lung.

Ref: http://www.cancerfacts.com/GeneralContent/Ovarian/Gen_Diagnosis.asp?CB=9
Also see
Ref: -Shaw's Textbook of gynecology, Cp-29, Pg-404, Table-29.10

Q. 215. The true statement regarding adenomyosis is
- (a) More common in nullipara
- (b) Surgery only choice of treatment
- (c) Presents with menorrhagia, dysmenorrhea, and an enlarged uterus
- (d) More common in young women

Ans. (c)

Note
Adenomyosis is a condition in which islands of endometrium are found in the wall of the uterus. These women are usually parous, around the age of 40 years; and present with menorrhagia, dysmenorrhea, pelvic discomfort, and dyspareunia.
Treatment consists of:
Diagnostic hysteroscopy and curettage. Since most patients are above the age of 40yrs, total hysterectomy is usually done.
Ref: -Shaw's Textbook of gynecology, Cp-34, Pg-448-449

Q. 216. Primary peritonitis is more common in females because (ALL INDIA-01)
- (a) Ostia of fallopian tubes communicate with abdominal cavity
- (b) Peritoneum overlies the uterus
- (c) Rupture of functional ovarian cysts
- (d) None of the above

Ans. (a)

Note
The primary peritonitis refers to inflammation of peritoneal cavity without a without a documented source of contamination. The fallopian tubes communicate with peritoneal cavity and provide a natural route for spread of infection from female genital tract to the peritoneum.
Ref: A Concise Textbook of Surgery by S. Das, Edi, Cp –51,Pg- 992

Q. 217. False statement regarding HCG is (ALL INDIA-01)
- (a) It is secreted by cytotrophoblasts.
- (b) It acts on same receptor as LH does.
- (c) It has luteotrophic action.
- (d) It is a glycoprotein.

Ans. (a)

Note
HCG is a glycoprotein, secreted by the syncytiotrophoblast of placenta. It has a leutinizing action:
- It stimulates secretion of progesterone.
- Stimulates Leydig cells of the male fetus to produce testosterone.

Ref: Textbook of Obstetrics, D.C.Dutta, 5th Edition Cp-6, Pg-59
Ref: Shaw's Textbook of gynecology, 13th Edition Cp-3, Pg-40

Q. 218. Snow storm appearance on USG is seen in (ALL INDIA-01)
- (a) Hydatidiform mole
- (b) Ectopic pregnancy
- (c) Anencephaly
- (d) None of the above

Ans. (a)

Note
Hydatidiform mole is an abnormal condition of the ovum where there are partly degenerative changes and partly hyperplastic changes in the young chorionic villi.
Ref: Textbook of Obstetrics, D.C.Dutta, 5th Edition Cp-15, Pg-209, Fig: 15.15

Q. 219. All of the following are indications for termination of pregnancy in APH patient except (ALL INDIA-01)
- (a) 37 weeks
- (b) IUD
- (c) Transverse lie
- (d) Continous bleeding

Ans. (c)

Note
Indication for active management of APH:
- Bleeding occurring at 37weeks of pregnancy
- Patient in exsanguinated condition
- Continuous bleeding
- Baby dead or deformed
- Patient in labour

Ref: Textbook of Obstetrics, D.C.Dutta, 5th Edition Cp-18, Pg-265

Q. 220. A lady with 37 weeks pregnancy, presented with bleeding per vagina. Investigation shows severe degree of placenta previa. The treatment is (ALL INDIA-01)
- (a) Immediate CS
- (b) Blood transfusion
- (c) Conservative
- (d) Medical induction of labour

Ans. (a)

Note
Indication for CS in placenta previa are:
- Bleeding beyond 37weeks of pregnancy
- Patient in labour
- Patient in exsanguinated condition
- Continuous bleeding
- Dead or congenitally malformed baby

Ref: Textbook of Obstetrics, D.C.Dutta, 5th Edition Cp-18, Pg-265

Q. 221. A pregnant woman presents with red degeneration of fibroid. Management is (ALL INDIA-01)
(a) Myomectomy
(b) Conservative
(c) Hysterectomy
(d) Termination of pregnancy

Ans. (b)
Note
Red degeneration usually occurs in a large fibroid during 2nd half of pregnancy or puerperium. Cause is vascular in origin. Conservative treatment is given and the symptoms clear off in 10 days.
Ref: Textbook of Obstetrics, D.C.Dutta, 5th Edition Cp-20, Pg-327

Q. 222. An ovarian cyst is detected in a pregnant woman. Management is (ALL INDIA-01)
(a) Immediate removal by laparotomy
(b) Wait and watch
(c) Removal by laparotomy in second trimester
(d) Remove at time of caesarean section

Ans. (c)
Note
If the ovarian tumor is detected during pregnancy the best time for elective operation is between 14th-18th week as the chance of abortion is less and access to pedicle easy. However in case of complication the tumor should be removed irrespective of the period of gestation.
Ref: Textbook of Obstetrics, D.C.Dutta, 5th Edition Cp-20, Pg-329

Q. 223. Most useful investigation in the first trimester to identify risk of fetal malformation in a fetus of a diabetic mother is (ALL INDIA-01)
(a) Glycosylated Hb
(b) Ultrasound
(c) MS-AFP
(d) Amniocentesis

Ans. (a)
Note
Estimation of HbA1c before 14weeks can predict affection of the fetus. Mothers with S. HbA1c of value less than or equal to 8.5% have got least chance of severe fetal malformation. If value is equal to or more than 9.5% the risk of major fetal malformation is high.
Ref: Textbook of Obstetrics, D.C.Dutta, 5th Edition Cp-19, Pg-303

Q. 224. Condition associated with lack of a single pelvic ala is (ALL INDIA-01)
(a) Robert's pelvis
(b) Naegele's pelvis
(c) Rachitic pelvis
(d) Osteomalacia pelvis

Ans. (b)
Note
The condition associated with lack of a single pelvic ala is Naegele's Pelvis.

Also see
a. Robert's pelvis: Ala of both side are absent and sacrum is fused with the innominate bones.
b. Naegele's pelvis: It is a rare type of pelvis and is produced by the arrested development of ala of sacrum
c. Rachitic pelvis: A contracted and deformed pelvis, most commonly a flat pelvis, occurring from rachitic softening of the bones in early life.
d. Osteomalacia pelvis: Occurring primarily in adults that results from a deficiency in vitamin D or calcium. Physical signs include deformities like triradiate pelvis and spinal kyphosis.

Ref: Textbook of Obstetrics, D.C.Dutta, 5th Edition Cp-23, Pg-370
-http://www.biology-online.org/dictionary/Rachitic_pelvis
-http://www.answers.com/main/ntq-tname-osteomalacia-fts_start-

Q. 225. DNA analysis of chorionic villus/amniocentesis is not likely to detect (ALL INDIA-01)
 (a) Tay Sach's disease
 (b) Hemophilia A
 (c) Sickle cell disease
 (d) Duchenne muscular dystrophy

Ans. (a)

Note
Amniocentesis is done:
 -To estimate AFP in liqor amnii where open neural tube is suspected.
 -Detection of inborn errors of metabolism.
 -Pregnancy in a woman with X linked disorders.
 -Previous child with chromosomal abnormalities.
Ref: Textbook of Obstetrics, D.C.Dutta, 5th Edition Cp-11, Pg-112

Q. 226. A woman has had 2 previous anencephalic babies, risk of having a third one is (ALL INDIA-01)
 (a) 0%
 (b) 10%
 (c) 25%
 (d) 50%

Ans. (b)

Note
The recurrence risk of incidence of anenephaly is 5% after first affected child and after second affected child it is 10%. Ref; Nelson.

Q. 227. MTP is done upto how many weeks
 (a) 28
 (b) 7
 (c) 14
 (d) 10

Ans. (c)

Note
MTP is permitted upto 20 weeks of pregnancy.
Ref: -Textbook of Obstetrics, D.C.Dutta, 5th Edition Cp-15, Pg-186

Q. 228. Cervical fibroid is commonly present with (UPSC-06)
 (a) Menorrhagia
 (b) Retention of urine
 (c) Abdominal mass
 (d) Mass from vagina

Ans. (b)

Note
Cervical fibroids are relatively uncommon, accounting for 2% of uterine leiomyomat. They arise in the cervix and are usually single.
Cervical leiomyoma tend to distort and elongate the cervical canal, and push the uterus upwards. Large tumours may cause elongation and distortion of the urethra, resulting in urinary retention.

Q. 229. Tuberculosis of genital organs is more frequently seen in (UPSC-06)
- (a) Fallopian tube
- (b) Ovary
- (c) Uterus
- (d) Cervix

Ans. (a)

Note
Fallopian tube is the most frequently involved part of the genital tract and provides over 90% of all genital TB cases. Various types of tubercular salpingitis are: -tuberculous endosalpingitis, tuberculous exosalpingitis, interstitial tuberculous salpingitis.

Q. 230. Which part of the fallopian tube is the most common site for ectopic pregnancy? (UPSC-06)
- (a) Isthmic
- (b) Fimbrial
- (c) Interstitial
- (d) Ampullary

Ans. (d)

Note
The most common site of ectopic gestation is ampula of the fallopian tube.
Ref: Textbook of Obstetrics, D.C.Dutta, 5th Edition Cp-15, Pg-191, Table

Q. 231. Which one of the following is/are responsible for proliferative phase of the menstrual cycle?
- (a) Estrogen only
- (b) Estrogen and progesterone
- (c) Progesteron only
- (d) HCG

Ans. (a)

Note
The phase of the menstrual cycle which starts when regeneration of menstruating endometrium is complete and lasts until the 14th day of a 28 days cycle is referred to as the 'Proliferative' or 'Estrogenic Phase.
Ref: Shaw's Textbook of gynecology, 13th Edition Cp-2, Pg-31

Q. 232. Low Backache and pain in lower abdomen in a patient of dysmenorrhea are present in (UPSC-06)
- (a) GIT
- (b) GUT
- (c) Reproductive organs
- (d) Surgical scars of abdomen

Ans. (c)

Note
'Low Backache' as a referred pain phenomenon and pain in lower abdomen in a patient of dysmenorrhoea are commonly associated with 'Reproductive organs' as such.

Q. 233. Blood stain discharge from the nipple is typical of (UPSC-06)
- (a) Intraductal papiloma
- (b) Fibroadenoma
- (c) Filarial mastitis
- (d) Paget's disease of nipple

Ans. (a)

Note
Blood stained discharge from the nipples is usually seen in papilloma of duct and ductal carcinoma. Very rarely though it may be seen in pregnancy due to physiological epithelial hyperplasia. In which case it is B/L (Bilateral).
Ref: -A concise text book of surgery, S. Das, Cp-39, Pg-704

Q. 234. Where are intramural fibroids present? (UPSC-06)
  (a) Within the walls of uterus
  (b) In cervix
  (c) Outward of uterine surface
  (d) In the interior of the uterine cavity

Ans. (a)
Note
Intramural fibroids remain within the myometrial walls and grow symmetrically. If the tumor grows outwards towards the peritoneal surface it is termed as a subserous fibroid. If it is forced by uterine contractions into the cavity it is called submucous fibroid.
Ref: Shaw's Textbook of gynecology, 13th Edition Cp-27, Pg-338

Q. 235. Menopausal hot flushes are due to (KPSC-Lect/Physio-Bio/05)
  (a) Decreased estrogen
  (b) Decreased progesterone
  (c) LH surge
  (d) FSH surge

Ans. (a)
Note
During menopause withdrawal of estrogen causes hot flushes and it is not due to low progesterone, LH surge or FSH surge. That is why the medical treatment involving hormone replacement therapy works by restoring the estrogen that nature has taken away.

Bibliography

Books
Shaw's Textbook of Gynecology
A Concise Text Book of Surgery, S. Das
Textbook of Obstetrics, D.C.Dutta

Websites
www.similima.com
www.fleshandbones.com

Chapter 11
PRACTICE OF MEDICINE

Q. 1. A male aged 50 years presents with flu-like symptoms and complains of malaise and tiredness. He also complains of bleeding gums, epistaxis and mouth ulcers. On examination, liver and spleen are found enlarged. Total leucocyte count is 1,00,000/ cu mm. Bone-marrow is hyper-cellular with blast-cells more than 30% and with the presence of Auer rods in the blast-cells. The most likely diagnosis is (UPSC-02)
(a) Acute Myeloblastic Leukemia
(b) Chronic Myeloid Leukemia
(c) Acute Lymphoblastic Leukemia
(d) Chronic Lymphatic Leukemia

Ans. (a)
Note
The most likely diagnosis is 'Acute Myeloblastic Leukemia'.
Also see
In AML, bone marrow consists of at least 30% of blast cells. Myeloblast shows presence of rod like cytoplasmic inclusions called Auer rods which represents abnormal derivatives of primary azurophilic granules.
Ref: Harsh Mohan Text Book of Pathology 5th Ed. Pg-279,288

Extended information
Presence of Auer rods is usually seen in Acute Myelocytic Leukemia, however in the above clinical presentation the peripheral blood smear showing a 'Auer rod' in the blast cell is suggestive of choice of (a).
Ref: Davidson 20th Ed.

Q. 2. A 27-year old man consults you with a 3 month history of diarrhea. Now he has developed right upper abdominal pain and high fever with chill. On enquiry he also complains of pain in his right shoulder. The clinical diagnosis in this case is (UPSC-02)
(a) Ameobic Hepatitis
(b) Koch's abdomen
(c) Malaria
(d) AIDS

Ans. (a)
Note
The clinical diagnosis in this case is 'Ameobic Hepatitis'.
Also see
The h/o diarrhea is most commonly due to ameobiasis and in this case it appears to be that infection has reached to liver and resulted in ameobic liver abscess. The abscess is usually found in right hepatic lobe. The high fever with chill is characteristic of pyogenic infection. Here the pain appears due to stretching of liver capsule and is referred to the right shoulder, all above constellation of symptoms are in favour of liver pathology that is more in consistent of 'Ameobic hepatitis'.
Ref: Davidson 20th Ed.

Extended information
Ameobic abscess develops after an attack of ameobic dysentery.
In ameobic hepatitis fever may shoot upto 39° C and it is usually accompanied by chills and sweating. Pain is usually felt over right intercostal space. There may be slight bulging and pitting edema. Superior surface abscess may cause pain referred to right shoulder.
Ref. Textbook of Surgery S. Das 3rd Ed. Pg-869

Q. 3. A 65-years old woman presents with tremors of hands especially on rest. She complains of slowness in her daily activities and drooling of saliva. She cannot perform fine movements and often has difficulty in writing. On examination: Fixity of facial expression with poor modulation (UPSC-02)
- (a) Wilson's disease
- (b) Parkinson's disease
- (c) Huntington's disease
- (d) Alzheimer's disease

Ans. (b)

Note
The above clinical features are in favour of 'Parkinson's disease'.
Parkinson's disease
Slowly progressive degenerative condition of extrapyramidal system, resulting in disturbance of motor function and characterised by slowing of body movements, muscular rigidity, tremors and postural disturbances.
Ref: Davidson 20th Ed, Box-26.86.

Also see
James Parkinson first described, in 1817, the classical manifestations of this syndrome in a paper entitled 'Essay on Shaking Palsy'.
Characteristics of Parkinson's disease:
- Resting tremors (pill rolling tremors)
- Rigidity, akinesia and postural disturbances
- Face is expressionless (mask like)
- Generalized slowness of motor activity
- Hand becomes smaller (micrographia)
- Increased salivation

Ref: API, 7th Ed.Pg-835

Extended information
Wilson's disease
Genetic disorder of copper metabolism resulting in hepato-lenticular degeneration and accumulation of copper in basal ganglia and liver, and characterised by increasing muscular rigidity, tremor, mental disturbances, Kayser-Fleisher ring and cirrhosis. However the age of onset in this case should be early as compared to the case of Parkinson's disease.

Huntington's chorea (Chorea Major)
Hereditary disorder resulting in degeneration of forebrain and caudate nucleus, and characterised by widespread spontaneous jerky, involuntary quasi-purposeful movements, emotional liability, dysarthria and unsteadiness of gait.

Alzheimer's disease
Pre-senile dementia due to diffuse cortical atrophy, and characterised by gradual memory impairment, decreased ability to think and concentrate, and personality deterioration.

Just Note
Alzheimer's disease was named after German neuropathologist, Alois Alzheimer, who described it in 1906. He described that nerve cells in the brain die prematurely and the brain shrivels like a dried walnut.

Q. 4. Match list –I (Homeopathic medicine) with List – II (Diagnosis) and select the correct answer using the codes given below the lists (UPSC-02)

List I (Homeopathic Medicine)	List II (Diagnosis)
A. Parotidinum	1. Quinsy
B. Pertussin	2. Puerperal fever
C. Pyrogenium	3. Whooping cough
D. Baryta carbonica	4. Mumps

Code:

	A	B	C	D
(a)	4	3	2	1
(b)	4	3	1	2
(c)	3	4	2	1
(d)	3	4	1	2

Ans. (a)

Note
The suitable correalation is as under:

List I (Homeopathic Medicine)	List II (Diagnosis)
A. Parotidinum	4. Mumps
B. Pertussin	3. Whooping cough
C. Pyrogenium	2. Puerperal fever
D. Baryta carbonica	1. Quinsy

Q. 5. In a suspected case of "Acute infective Appendicitis" which one of the following investigations will confirm the diagnosis? (UPSC-02)
  (a) Ultrasonography
  (b) Skiagram
  (c) Barium meal follow through
  (d) Total leucocytic count

Ans. (a)

Note
In a suspected case of "Acute infective appendicitis" ultrasonography is the choice of investigation.

Also see
Acute appendicitis
Examination of the abdomen usually reveals tenderness in the right iliac fossa with guarding due to localized peritonitis. There may be a tender mass in the right iliac fossa. Laboratory tests are unhelpful except that the white cell count may be raised. An ultrasound scan is accurate for the detection of an inflamed appendix and will also indicate an appendix mass or other localized lesion.
Ref: Kumar and Clark, 6th Ed. Page-342

Extended information
Diagnosis is based primarily on clinical grounds and may also be established by the ultrasonic demonstration of an enlarged and thick-walled appendix. Ultrasound is most useful to exclude ovarian cysts, ectopic pregnancy, or tubo-ovarian abscess.

Q. 6. Match List –I (Radiological findings) with the List- II (Type of calculi) and select the correct answer using the codes given below the lists (UPSC-02)

List I (Radiological findings)	List II (Type of Calculi)
A. Radio-opaque, spiky	1. Staghorn stone
B. Radio-opaque and soft like bee wax	2. Urate stone
C. Dirty white, hard, smooth surface and opaque	3. Oxalate stone
D. Non-opaque and smooth surface	4. Cystine stone

Code

	A	B	C	D
(a)	3	4	1	2
(b)	2	1	4	3
(c)	3	1	4	3
(d)	2	4	1	3

Ans. (a)
Note
The correct sequence as under:

List I (Radiological findings)	List II (Type of Calculi)
A. Radio opaque, spiky	3. Oxalate stone
B. Radio opaque and soft like bee wax	4. Cystine stone
C. Dirty white, hard, smooth surface and opaque	1. Staghorn stone
D. Non-opaque and smooth surface	2. Urate stone

Also see
Oxalate stones
They are usually single and extremely hard. It is dark in colour. It is spiky being covered with sharp projections which cause bleeding. Due to high calcium content it casts a shadow radiologically.
Urate stones
They are rare and not visible on x-ray i.e. not radio-opaque. These are usually multiple and faceted, are moderately hard. Their colour varies from yellow to dark brown. The surface of these stone is smooth.
Cystine calculi
It is an amino-acid rich in sulphur. They are usually multiple, are soft and yellow or pink in colour. Pure cystine calculi are not radio-opaque but as they contain sulphur they are usually radio-opaque.
Staghorn calculi
It is a type of secondary stone. Majority of these are composed of ammonium magnesium phosphate known as triple phosphate. Such calculi is usually smooth soft and friable. It is usually dirty white in colour. Such stones enlarge rapidly and gradually fill up pelvis and renal calyces to take up the shape of staghorn calculus.
Ref. Textbook of surgery S. Das 3rd Ed. Pg-1167, 168

Q. 7. Lumbar puncture is considered in the following cases (UPSC-02)
  (a) Bacterial meningitis
  (b) Brain abscess
  (c) Multiple sclerosis
  (d) Syphilis

Ans. (a)
Note
Lumbar puncture is considered in bacterial meningitis.
Also see
Lumbar puncture is indicated in investigations of infections (e.g. meningitis, encephalitis), subarachnoid hemorrhage, inflammatory conditions (e.g. multiple sclerosis, sarcoidosis and cerebral lupus) and some neurological malignancies (e.g. carcinomatous meningitis, lymphoma and leukemia) and to measure CSF

pressure e.g in idiopathic intra-cranial hypertension. In multiple sclerosis MRI is the most sensitive technique for imaging lesion in both brain and spinal cord.
Ref. Davidson, 19th Ed. Pg-1116, 1170

Extended information
Bacterial meningitis
Lumbar puncture is best considered in cases of 'Meningitis', where is is a therapeutic as well as a diagnostic tool.

Brain abscess
However, in case of brain abscess with elevated CSF pressure, lumbar puncture will potentially prove fatal as cerebellar or tentorial herniation may follow LP. This possibility one should keep in mind while dealing with all patients with focal neurologic findings, altered mental status, or papilledema. If at all CSF examination is required in such cases, it is wise to first obtain a neuroimaging scan to exclude a mass lesion. Meningitis is an exception to this rule, where immediate CSF examination is indicated.
Brain abscess is better diagnosed on Cranial CT or MRI of head shows the abscess and its exact location.

Multiple sclerosis
In case of multiple sclerosis the head MRI is more suitable for diagnosis as it will show scarring or a lesion.

Syphilis
In case of syphilis lumbar puncure has no value. However, The CSF-VDRL test is used to diagnose neurosyphilis.

Q. 8. Most diagnostic feature of duodenal ulcer is (UPSC-02)
(a) Constant deformity of the cap
(b) Fleeting filling of the cap
(c) Ulcer crater
(d) Increased peristaltic activity of stomach

Ans. (c)
Note
Most diagnostic feature of duodenal ulcer is 'Ulcer crater'.

Also see
- On barium meal X-ray, a normal duodenal bulb is rounded and full.
- In case of ulcer disease there is irritability and the bulb becomes difficult to be filled with contrast material.
- Demonstration of ulcer crater itself is the positive evidence of active ulcer.
Ref: Textbook of Surgery S. Das 3rd Ed. Pg-825

Extended information
To rule out the peptic ulcer barium studies of the proximal gastrointestinal tract are still common. As sensitivity of older single-contrast barium meals for detecting a duodenal ulcer is as high as 80%. Sensitivity for detection is decreased in small ulcers (05 cm), presence of previous scarring, or in postoperative patients. A duodenal ulcer appears as a well-demarcated crater, most often seen in the bulb.

Q. 9. Match the list –I 'P' wave abnormalities with List –II 'Conditions', and select the correct answer using the codes given below the list (UPSC-02)

List I (P wave abnormality)	List II (Condition)
A. Absent P wave	1. Left atrial enlargement
B. Tall and peaked P wave	2. Dextrocardia
C. Inverted P wave in lead I	3. Right atrial enlargement
D. Wide and notched P wave	4. Atrial fibrillation

Code

	A	B	C	D
(a)	2	1	4	3
(b)	4	3	2	1
(c)	2	3	4	1
(d)	4	1	2	3

Ans. (b)

Note
The correct sequence:

List I (P wave abnormality)	List II (Condition)
A. Absent P wave	4. Atrial fibrillation
B. Tall and peaked P wave	3. Right atrial enlargement
C. Inverted P wave in lead I	2. Dextrocardia
D. Wide and notched P wave	1. Left atrial enlargement

Ref: P.J. Mehta's Practical Medicine, 16th Ed. Pg-315

Q. 10. Match List-I (Characteristic Temperature Patterns) with List-II (Disease Conditions and select the correct answer using the codes given below the lists (UPSC-02)

List-I (Characteristic Temperature Patterns)	List-II (Disease Conditions)
A. Saddle back	1. Typhoid 2nd week temperature
B. Step Ladder	2. Hodgkin's disease
C. Pel-Ebstein fever	3. Typhoid 1st week
D. Continuous fever	4. Dengue fever

Code

	A	B	C	D
(a)	4	1	2	3
(b)	2	3	4	1
(c)	4	3	2	1
(d)	2	1	4	3

Ans. (c)

Note
The correct sequence:

List-I (Characteristic Temperature Patterns)	List-II (Disease Conditions)
A. Saddle Back	4. Dengue Fever
B. Step Ladder	3. Typhoid 1st week
C. Pel-Ebstein Fever	2. Hodgkin's Disease
D. Continuous Fever	1. Typhoid 2nd week temperature

Also see
Step-ladder fever
In case of Typhoid fever Step-ladder pattern in the first week, but it may be remittent type also.
Continuous fever
The temperature remains above normal throughout the day and does not fluctuate more than 1°C in 24 hours. e.g. typhoid second week, UTI, lobar pneumonia, infective endocarditis.
Pel-Ebstein fever
There is an irregular alteration of recurrent bouts of fever and afebrile period. The temperature may take 3 days to rise and remain high for 3 days and followed by apyrexia for 9 days. Seen in Hodgkin's lymphoma.
Saddle back fever
It is seen in case of dengue; it disappears after few days of onset and returns after few days.
Ref: P.J. Mehta's Practical Medicine, 16th Ed. Pg-32, 81, 304

Q. 11. A 28-year old female consults you with 6 weeks history of numbness and paraesthesia in her hands and feet associated with diplopia and blurred vision in her right eye. These symptoms resolve with the treatment of few weeks. What is the clinical diagnosis?
 (a) Hysteria
 (b) Multiple sclerosis
 (c) Guillain-Barre Syndrome
 (d) Brain tumour

Ans. (b)
Note
The clinical diagnosis is 'Multiple Sclerosis'.
Also see
Hysteria
For hysteria there has to be premorbid personality and past history of similar complaints.
Multipe sclerosis
The features point to lesions in CNS which has more than one location. The diplopia is classical all the complaints resolved with within few weeks time, points to natural recovery which is very common in MS.
Gullain Barre Syndrome
Acute infective polyneuropathy resulting in rapid, progressive, bilaterally symmetrical sensory-motor disturbances and characterised by rapidly spreading paralysis of muscles of limbs, trunk and face, with tendency to bulbar and respiratory paralysis.
Brain tumor
SOL, which result in raised intracranial pressure, and characterised by headache, vomiting, and progressive focal neurological deficit depending on the site of involvement.

Extended information
Multiple sclerosis: Commonest age of onset is between 20-45 years, a diagnosis before puberty or after 60 years is rare. It is more common in women. It is relapsing and remitting type. The symptoms are:
-Optic neuropathy: blurring of vision in one eye develops over hours or days, varying between a "looking throw frosted glass" sensation to severe unilateral vision loss but rarely complete blindness.
 -Diplopia
 -Vertigo

- Facial numbness
- Dysarthria
- Dysphagia
- Spastic paresis developing over days or weeks
- Trigeminal neuralgia

Ref: Kumar and Clark, 6th Ed. Pg-1234

Q. 12. Match List-I (Clinical Sign) With List-II (Diseases) and select the correct answer using the codes given below the lists (UPSC-02)

List-I (Clinical Sign)	List-II (Diseases)
A. Osler's Node	1. CA Stomach
B. Haberden's Node	2. Rheumatoid arthritis
C. Haygarth's Node (Fusiform swelling of proximal interphalangeal Joint)	3. Osteo-arthritis
D. Virchow's Node	4. Subacute bacterial endocarditis

Code

	A	B	C	D
(a)	1	2	3	4
(b)	4	3	2	1
(c)	1	3	2	4
(d)	4	2	3	1

Ans. (b)

Note
The correct sequence is as under:

List-I (Clinical Sign)	List-II (Diseases)
A. Osler's Node	4. Subacute bacterial endocarditis
B. Haberden's Node	3. Osteo-arthritis
C. Haygarth's Node (Fusiform swelling of proximal interphalangeal Joint)	2. Rheumatoid arthritis
D. Virchow's Node	1. CA Stomach

Q. 13. Match List – I (Character of sputum) with List-II (Diagnostic value); and select the correct answer using the codes given below the list (UPSC-02)

List I (Abnormality)	List II (Condition)
A. Green and yellow sputum	1. Bronchiectasis
B. Rusty sputum	2. Left ventricular failure
C. Large amount, purulent and offensive sputum	3. Bacterial infection
D. Pink and frothy sputum	4. Lobar pneumonia (Pneumococcal)

Code

	A	B	C	D
(a)	3	4	1	2
(b)	3	4	1	2
(c)	3	4	2	1
(d)	4	3	2	1

Ans. (b)
Note
The correct sequence is as under:

List I (Abnormality)	List II (Condition)
A. Green and yellow sputum	3. Bacterial infection
B. Rusty sputum	4. Lobar pneumonia (Pneumococcal)
C. Large amount, purulent and offensive sputum	1. Bronchiectasis
D. Pink and frothy sputum	2. Left ventricular failure

Q. 14. Generalised edema can not be caused by (UPSC-02)
    (a) Nephrotic syndrome
    (b) Cirrhosis of liver
    (c) Starvation
    (d) Hyperthyroidism

Ans. (d)
Note
Generalised edema can not be caused by 'Hyperthyroidism'.
Also see
Hyperthyroidism
It is characterized by polyphagia, diarrhea, excessive sweating, weight loss, palpitations. Signs are: tremors, hyperkinesia, widened palpebral fissures, tachycardia. The hyperthyroidism does not case generalized edema.
Ref: Family practice notebook.com

Extended information
Nephrotic syndrome
The features of nephriotic syndrome include: edema, hypoalbuminemia, hyperalbuminuria, hypertension, hyperlipidemia, and renal insufficiency. Generalised edema is common feature in nephrotic syndrome.
Ref: Family practice notebook.com
Cirrhosis of liver
In a case of cirrhosis of liver, causes portal hypertension resulting in ascitis.
However, the generalized edema can be a late finding as liver functional is deteriorating and can not produce albumin, hypoalbuminemia develops with predisposes for generalized edema.
Starvation

In case of starvation apart from fat is mobilized from the subcutaneous reserve and muscle mass breaks down for energy. Associated with vitamin deficiency often resulting in anemia, beriberi, pellagra and scurvy. These diseases collectively may cause diarrhea, skin rash, generalized edema and heart failure.
Ref: From Wikipedia

Q. 15. The peripheral blood field in iron deficiency anemia is (UPSC-02)
    (a)   Hyperchromic macrocytic
    (b)   Normochromic normocytic
    (c)   Hypochromic microcytic
    (d)   Normochromic microcytic

Ans. (c)
Note
The peripheral blood field in iron deficiency anemia is consistent with 'hypochromic microcytic' features.
Also see
Peripheral smear in case of iron deficiency shows:
    -Hypochromia
    -Microcytosis
    -Anisocytosis
    -Poikilocytosis
In severe iron deficiency, the red blood cells are smaller than normal, and their central area of pallor (Hypochromia) is extended therefore cells appear to have thin rim of hemoglobin.

Q. 16. A male patient aged 50 years was suffering from severe pain in bones blood examination revealed hemoglobin 7.8g/dl and ESR 140 mm in first hour. Bone marrow examination showed the presence of plenty of plasma cells arranged in sheets. The most likely diagnosis was (UPSC-02)
    (a)   Hypoplastic anemia
    (b)   Osteoporosis
    (c)   Multiple myeloma
    (d)   Secondary deposits in bones

Ans. (c)
Note
The most likely diagnosis is 'multiple myeloma'.
Also see
Above clinical presentation is consistent of:
    -Bone pains
    -Anemia
    -High ESR
    -Bone marrow shows plenty of plasma cells

Extended information
The features are consitent with 'multiple myeloma' which has following presentation:
    -Bone pains which involve spine and ribs < movement / activity.
    -Anemia; which results from replacement of normal bone marrow by infiltrating tumor cells.
    -Increased risk of infection due to immune deficiency.
    -Renal failure due to hypercalcemia due to breakdown of bone and also due to tubular damage form excretion of light chains also called 'Bence Jones Proteins'.
    -Neurological symptoms: Common ones are weakness, confusion and fatigue due to hypercalcemia. Headache, cord compression may lead to bladder bowl disturbances. Infiltration of peripheral nerves by amyloid may cause carpal tunnel syndrome.
Diagnosis:
    -By presence of 'Bence Jones Protein in urine.
    -Bone marrow biopsy: shows plasma cells.
    -X-Ray shows lytic bone lesions with compression fractures.
Multiple myeloma
It is a neoplastic proliferation of plasma cells in bone marrow associated with painful swelling of bones and joints, and Bence Jones proteinuria.

Mnemonic for Multiple myeloma
"CRAB":
- C: Calcium (Raised)
- R: Renal Failure
- A: Anemia
- B: Bone pains / lesions

Q. 17. Which one of the following clinical features is not a feature of Plummer Vinson's syndrome? (UPSC-02)
   (a) Clubbing of fingers
   (b) Glossitis
   (c) Iron deficiency anemia
   (d) Dysphagia

Ans. (a)

Note
Clubbing of fingers is not a feature of 'Plummer Vinson's syndrome'.

Also see
Plummer Vinson's syndrome
Its features are:
- Atrophy of oral mucosa
- Spoon shaped fingers
- Brittle nails
- Long standing anemia
- Cervical dysphagia
- Fibrous web partially obstructing the esophageal lumen at its upper end a few millimeters below the cricopharyngeal muscle.

Ref: Textbook of Surgery, S.Das 3rd Ed. Pg-805

Extended information
Plummer Vinson's syndrome; (sideropenic dysphagia; Paterson-Kelly syndrome)- It is a conditions linked to severe, long term iron deficiency anemia; resulting in glossitis and swallowing difficulty (dysphagia) caused by 'webs' of tissue that grows in the esophagus.
The clubbing is not associated with above; rather koilonychias may be a feature.

Q. 18. Korsakoff's Psychosis is associated with (UPSC-02)
   (a) Schizophrenia
   (b) General paralysis of insane
   (c) Thiamin deficiency
   (d) Bi-polar mental illness

Ans. (c)

Note
Korsakoff's psychosis is associated with thiamin deficiency.

Also see
Korsakoff's psychosis (amnesic-confabulatory syndrome)
It is a degenerative brain disorder caused by the lack of thiamine (vitamin B1) in the brain.
There are six major symptoms of Korsakoff's syndrome:
- Anterograde amnesia
- Retrograde amnesia, severe memory loss.
- Confabulation, that is, invented memories which are then taken as true due to gaps in memory sometimes associated with blackouts.
- Meager content in conversation.
- Lack of insight
- Apathy - The patients lose interest in things quickly and generally appear indifferent to change.

Signs:
- Ataxia
- Tremors
- Paralysis of muscles controlling the eye
- Coma

Korsakoff's psychosis: it is often sequelae of Wernicke encephalopathy. Patient is although alert but retrograde or antigrade amnesia is charecteristic feature.
Ref: API, 7th Ed.Pg-849

Q. 19. Increased level of serum amylase is of great importance in (UPSC-02)
    (a) Acute pancreatitis
    (b) Chronic hepatitis
    (c) Toxemia of pregnancy
    (d) Parotitis

Ans. (a)

Note
Increased level of serum amylase is of great importance in 'Acute pancreatitis'.

Also see
Elevated serum amylase is well established feature of acute pancreatitis. The higher the serum amylase level higher is the probability of acute pancreatitis. Normal serum amylase level is 80-150 somogyi units. <400 units is suggestive of acute pancreatitis.
Ref: Textbook of Surgery S. Das 3rd Ed. Pg- 943

Extended information
Increased level of serum amylase is found in:
- Salivary trauma (including anaesthetic intubation).
- Mumps due to inflammation of the salivary glands.
- Pancreatitis because of damage to the cells that produce amylase.
- Renal failure due to reduced excretion

Q. 20. Match list – I (Type of hemorrhage) with the list-II (Characteristic) and select the correct answer using the codes given below the lists; (UPSC-02)

List I (Type of Hemorrhage)	List II (Characteristic)
A. Petechiae	1. Hemorrhage large enough to produce elevation
B. Purpura	2. Hemorrhage more than 5 mm in diameter
C. Echymosis	3. Hemorrhage 2-3 mm in diameter
D. Hematoma	4. Hemorrhage less than 1 mm in diameter

Code

	A	B	C	D
(a)	3	4	1	2
(b)	4	3	2	1
(c)	3	4	2	1
(d)	4	3	1	2

Ans. (b)

Note
Following is the correct sequence:

List I (Type of Hemorrhage)	List II (Characteristic)
A. Petechiae	4. Hemorrhage less than 1 mm in diameter
B. Purpura	3. Hemorrhage 2-3 mm in diameter
C. Echymosis	2. Hemorrhage more than 5 mm in diameter
D. Hematoma	1. Hemorrhage large enough to produce elevation

Ref: P.J. Mehta's Practical Medicine, 16th Ed. Pg-26

Q. 21. Which one of the following is the treatment of choice for recurrent/ sub-acute appendicitis? (UPSC-04)
 (a) Belladonna
 (b) Rhus toxicodendron
 (c) Lycopodium clavatum
 (d) Iris tenax

Ans. (d)
Note
In a case of recurrent / sub-acute appendicitis is Iris tenax.
Also see
Dr. George Wigg of Portland, Oregon proved Iris tenax in the later part of 1885 (Med. Adv. xvii. 235, Amer. Hom, April 1888, H.W., xxxv. 364). He published the proving under the name of Iris minor. This, as Heath has shown, is a local name only, its true botanical name being Iris tenax.
Abdomen
Fearful pain in ileo-cecal region. Pressure in ileo-cecal region causes deathly sensation at stomach pit.
Clincial Indication: Appendicitis.
Ref: Clarke's materia medica.

Q. 22. Which of the following medicines should be prescribed to a female-21 years of age, newly married, has burning micturition and has to sit for a long period to pass urine with marked irritation at the genitals? (UPSC-04)
 (a) Cantharis vesicatoria
 (b) Staphysagria
 (c) Nitricum acidum
 (d) Sulphur

Ans. (b)
The staphysagria is the best indicatied remdey, from the above listed medicines.
Also see
The above clinical presentation points the diagnosis of 'honeymoon cystitis'. For which the Staph. is important medicine.
Extended information:
The honeymoon cystitis is the term for a urinary tract infection that can occur as a result of irritation and bruising from frequent, strenuous and prolonged sexual intercourse. The condition more often affects women, during honeymoon.
The staphysagria is the on the following grounds:
Remedy profile
Nervous affections with marked irritability, diseases of the genitourinary tract and skin, most frequently give symptoms calling for this drug.
Precipitating cause
Sphincters lacerated or stretched.

Bad effects of onanism, sexual excesses
Sign/Symptoms of honeymoon cystitis
Urging to urinate has to sit at urinal for hours; in young married women; after coition; after difficult labor; burning in urethra when not urinating.
Ref: Allen's Key Notes

Q. 23. Match List-I (Orgasnisms) with List-II (Type of cell they affect) and select the correct answer using the codes given below the lists (UPSC-04)

List-I Orgasnisms	List-II (Type of cell they affect)
A. Plasmodium vivax and ovale	1. All the cells except non nucleated erythrocytes
B. Trophozoites of toxoplasma gondii	2. Immature erythrocytes
C. Plasmodium falciparum	3. Only senescent erythrocytes
D. Plasmodium malarie	4. Prefers younger erythrocytes but invades red cells of all ages

Code

	A	B	C	D
(a)	4	3	2	1
(b)	2	3	4	1
(c)	4	1	2	3
(d)	2	1	4	3

Ans. (d)

Note Following is the correct secquence:

List-I Orgasnisms	List-II (Type of cell they affect)
A. Plasmodium vivax and ovale	2. Immature erythrocytes
B. Trophozoites of toxoplasma gondii	1. All the cells except non nucleated erythrocytes
C. Plasmodium falciparum	4. Prefers younger erythrocytes but invades red cells of all ages
D. Plasmodium malarie	3. Only senescent erythrocytes

Also see
Plasmodium vivax
- It shows a greater tendency to invade younger blood cells (which are usually of greater diameter) and reticulocytes than mature erythrocytes.

Plasmodium falciparum
- Shows special affinity for any particular type of RBC but invades both the reticulocytes and erythrocytes (young and old).

Plasmodium malariae

-Shows special affinity to invade mature and old erythrocytes (less than 1 % of red cells are infected)
Ref: Parasitology by K.D. Chatterjee, 12th Ed. Pg- 77, 79, 81

Q. 24. Pulsus alternans, clinically encountered as alternate large and small pulse without any change or rhythm is suggestive of (UPSC-04)
    (a)   Left ventricular failure
    (b)   Right ventricular failure
    (c)   Respiratory failure
    (d)   Congestive cardiac failure

Ans. (a)
Note
Pulsus alternans is suggestive of 'left ventricular failure'.
Also see
Pulsus alternans
Left ventricular failure alters the contractile force of heart which may cause alternate large and small pulse without any change.
Ref: P.J. Mehta's Practical Medicine, 16th Ed. Pg-157

Extended information
Pulsus alternans may be detected by sphygmomanometer and in more severe instances by palpation, and is observed most commonly in patients with cardiomyopathy or hypertensive or ischemic heart disease.
Ref: Chapter 225 Physical findings, Harrison 15th Edition

Q. 25. What is the most common cause of transmission of leprosy? (UPSC-04)
    (a)   Skin to skin contact
    (b)   Insect vectors
    (c)   Through fomites
    (d)   Droplet infection

Ans. (d)
Note
The most common cause of transmission of leprosy is 'droplet infection'.
Also see
Skin-to-skin contact
It is generally not considered an important route of transmission.
Insect vetror
Evidence for insect vectors of leprosy includes the demonstration that bedbugs and mosquitoes in the vicinity of leprosaria regularly harbor M. leprae and that experimentally infected mosquitoes can transmit infection to mice.
Droplet infection
A sneeze from lepromatous patient may contain >10^{10} AFB. Furthermore, both IgA antibody to M. leprae and genes of M. leprae demonstrable by polymerase chain reaction (PCR) have been found in the nose of individuals without signs of leprosy from endemic areas and in 19% of occupational contacts of lepromatous patients. Therefore the spread of leprosy is by prolonged contact and droplet infectiton. Most infectious being the lepromatous leprosy.
Ref: Harrison 15th Edition

Extended information
Mode of transmission of leprosy:
Droplet infection:
There is more and more evidence that leprosy may be transmitted via aerosol cantaining M.leprae. With the realization of the importance of the nose as the portal of exit, there has been increased emphasis on the respiratory tract as the portal of entry.
Contact transmission:
This contact may be direct skin to skin or indirect, e.g. contact with soil and fomites.

Other routes:
- Via breast milk from lepromatous mother
- By insect vector or
- By tattoing needle

Ref: Park & Park 18th Ed. Pg-255

Q. 26. Colicky nature of pain around umbilicus and marked tenderness in right illiac fossa, accompained or followed by nausea, vomiting, anorexia, pyrexia with constipation are the diagnostic features of (UPSC-04)
(a) Acute peritonitis
(b) Acute appendicitis
(c) Acute regional ileitis
(d) Acute cholecystitis

Ans. (b)

Note
The above features are diagnostic of 'Acute appendicitis'.

Also see
Clinical features of acute appendicitis:
- Pain: Initially it is diffuse and dull and is situated in the umbilical or lower epigastric region. There is intermittent cramping, and gradualy the pain localizes in the right lower quadrant. It takes about 1-12 hours for such localization.
- Anorexia
- Nausea: Vomiting is variable. Children and teenagers frequently vomit but the vomiting may be entirely absent in adult. Vomiting appears after the onset of pain.
- Many patients give history of constipation before the onset of abdominal pain.
- Temperature: Temperature elevation is usually restricted to 99^0 to 100^0F.

Ref. Textbook of surgery S. Das 3rd Ed. Pg-1005

Q. 27. Consider the following statements. The papillary thyroid carcinoma is characterised by (UPSC-04)
1. Slow growing
2. Common lymph node spread
3. Being multicentric
4. Metastasis to bone in early stages

Which of the statement given above are correct?
(a) 1, 2 and 3
(b) 2, 3 and 4
(c) 1, 2 and 4
(d) 1, 3 and 4

Ans. (a)

Note
The papillary thyroid carcinoma is characterized by 1, 2 and 3 of above.

Also see
Papillary thyroid carcinoma:
- It is the slowest growing among the malignant tumour of thyroid.
- Multicentricity of the primary tumour is the most important feature of this cancer.
- They tend to invade lymphatics and spread to the normal surrounding thyroid tissue.

Ref: Textbook of Surgery S. Das 3rd Ed. Pg-662

Q. 28. Consider the following features (UPSC2004)
1. Bossing of head
2. Retarded growth
3. Late milestones
4. X-ray of wrist joint

Which of these features is/are helpful in confirming the rickets?
    (a)   1 and 2
    (b)   1 and 3
    (c)   2 and 3
    (d)   1 and 4

Ans. (d)
Note
The features diagnostic of rickets are 1 and 4.

Also see
From features given above most important ones for the diagnosis of rickets are:
1. Bossing of head; head apparently larger than normal in horizontal diameters; forehead prominent (fronal bossing). Occiput an dault flattened out, anterior fontanelle larger than normal and closing delayed, posterior portion of skull, in the first year may have demonstratble softening on pressure (ping-pong resilience, cranio-tabes).
2. X-Ray
    a. Fraying and cupping of distal ends of radius and ulna are the earliest change.
    b. Diminution in density of bone shaft.
    c. Increased distance between distal end of bones of forearm and metacarpal bones because of non calcification of large rachitic metaphysic.

Ref: Golwalla 15th Ed Pg-596

Extended information
Early signs of rickets are:
    a. Restlessness and irritability
    b. Sweating of head
    c. Head rolling
    d. Craniotabes (posterior prortion of skull, in the first year may show thin, soft membranous spots called craniotabes)
    e. Enlargement of epiphyses at the wrists
    f. Delayed dentition

Ref: Medicine for Students By A.F. Golwalla 10th Ed, Pg-766

Q. 29. Which one of the following is not a feature of nephrotic syndrome? (UPSC-04)
    (a)   Albuminuria
    (b)   Hyperlipidemia
    (c)   Edema
    (d)   Increased urine output

Ans. (d)
Note
From above 'Increased urine output' is not a feature of nephrotic syndrome.

Also see
Nephrotic syndrome is a group of diseases having different pathogenesis and characterized by clinical findings of massive proteinuria, hypoalbuminemia, edema, hyperlipidaemia, lipiduria and hypercoagulability.
Ref: Textbook of Pathology- Harsh Mohan short handbook, Pg no 488,489

Q. 30. A man about 59 suffering from polyuria, polyphagia, polydipsia and progressive emaciation visits his physician for a proper diagnosis. Which of he following is most likely diagnosis? (UPSC-04)
    (a)   Prostatic hypertrophy with malignancy
    (b)   Diabetes insipidus
    (c)   Diabetes mellitus
    (d)   Diabetic acidosis

Ans. (c)
Note
The above clinical presentation is in favour of 'Diabetes mellitus' (NIDDM).

Also see
a. *Prostatic hypertrophy*
It should present with urgency, frequency and precipitancy of micturation, without polydipsia, associated malignancy will present with loss of appetite and unexplained fever and general weakness.
b. *Diabetes insipidus*
It has presentation of polydipsia and polyuria and general weakness.
c. *Diabetes mellitus*
The symptoms favouring diagnosis of Type II diabetes are; elderly man of 59 years (age is in accordance with -Adult onset diabetes) c/o polyphagia, polydipsia and progressive emaciation – are classical presentation of DM.
d. *Diabetic acidosis*
It is common in Type I DM and associated with kussumaul respiration.

Q. 31. Which one of the following is the cause of sudden loss of vision in a patient with diabetic retinopathy? (UPSC-04)
   (a) Cataract
   (b) Glaucoma
   (c) Vitreous hemorrhage
   (d) Papilledema

Ans. (c)
Note
Sudden loss of vision in a patient with diabetic retinopathy is usually due to 'Viterous hemorrhage'.
Also see
Diabetic retinopathy is one of the leading causes of blindness. Patients with diabetes are prone to develop cataracts and glaucoma, but diabetic retinopathy is the main threat to vision. Diabetes affects the blood circulation of the retina.
The initial phase of the disease is known as background diabetic retinopathy. In this phase, the arteries in the retina become weakened and leak, forming small, dot-like hemorrhages. These leaking vessels often lead to swelling or edema in the retina and decreased vision.
The next stage is proliferative diabetic retinopathy. In this stage, circulation problems cause areas of the retina to become oxygen-deprived or ischemic. New, fragile, vessels develop as the circulatory system attempts to maintain adequate oxygen levels within the retina. This is called neovascularization. However, these delicate vessels bleed easily. Blood may leak into the retina and vitreous, causing spots or floaters, along with decreased vision.

Extended information
Many patients, after years of diabetes, have non-proliferative or background retinopathy.
It in itself does not cause visual loss.
If it does not progress, it is of minimal clinical significance in peripheral visual field.
Proliferative retinopathy is much more threatening.
It leads to visual loss and blindness.
Ophthalmoscopic findings:
Non-proliferative or background retinopathy:
    -Venous dilatation
    -Microaneurysms
    -Superficial flame hemorrhages
    -Deep dot-blot hemorrhages
Hard exudates:
    -Characteristic of diabetic retinopathy
    -Result from leakage of plasma from abnormal retinal capillaries
    -Overlie areas of neuronal degeneration
Pre-proliferative retinopathy:
    -Cotton wool spots (soft exudates)
    -Represent arteriolar occlusions
    -Seen in rapidly advancing retinopathy
    -Usually in association with uncontrolled hypertension

-Venous abnormalities (loops, bendings)
-Arterial abnormalities (segmental narrowing or occlusion)

Proliferative retinopathy:
-Neovascularisation
-Pre-retinal hemorrhage
-Vitreous hemorrhage
-Retinal detachment
-Exudative maculopathy
-Macular edema

To prevent the complications of diabetic retinopathy control of diabetes and associated high blood pressure is the aim of treatment. However, such treatment usually does not reverse the existing damage but may show the progress of the disease. Laser surgery may be indicated to control scar tissue or bleeding. Vitrectomy is suggested in cases of hemorrhage into the vitreous with or without retinal detachment.

Q. 32. Atherosclerosis is inversely proportional to (UPSC-04)
     (a) LDL level
     (b) VLDL level
     (c) Chylo-micron level
     (d) HDL level

Ans. (d)

Note
The Atherosclerosis is inversely proportional to HDL level.

Also see
Atherosclerosis is the primary cause of cardiovascular disease, and the risk for atherosclerosis is inversely proportional to circulating levels of high-density lipoprotein (HDL) cholesterol.

Extended information
HDL is protective 'good cholesterol' against atherosclerosis.
Ref: Harsh Mohan Handbook of Pathology, 5th Ed. Pg-187
Circulating levels of HDL cholesterol are inversely related to the risk of atherosclerosis, and therapeutic increases in HDL reduce the incidence of cardiovascular events.
The risk of cardiovascular disease from atherosclerosis is inversely proportional to serum levels of HDL and the major HDL apolipoprotein apoAI.
1. In fact, low HDL levels predict an increased risk of coronary artery disease independently of LDL levels, and 60–70% of major cardiovascular events cannot be prevented with current approaches focused on LDL, such as statin therapy.
2. In addition, low HDL levels are particularly common in males with early-onset atherosclerosis.
3. Based on these observations, prevention trials have been performed with agents such as niacin and fibrates, which raise HDL, and they indicate that modest increases in HDL independently yield a significant reduction in cardiovascular events.
4. Thus, there is compelling evidence that HDL is not solely a marker of lower risk of cardiovascular disease but instead is a mediator of vascular health.

Ref: http://www.pubmedcentral.nih.gov/articlerender.fcgi?artid=338271

Q. 33. Consider the following features (UPSC-04)
     1. Severe vertigo
     2. Engorged pulsating neck vein
     3. Unconsciousness
     4. Enlarged tender liver
     5. Pedal edema

     Which of the above features are helpful for the confirmation of CCF:
     (a) 1 and 4
     (b) 2, 4 and 5
     (c) 1 and 3
     (d) 1, 2, 3, 4 and 5

Ans. (b)

Note
The features 2, 4 and 5 listed above are helpful for the confirmation of CCF.
Also see
The congestive cardiac failure is characterized by (2). Raised JVP (Engorged pulsating neck vein), (5). Soft tender enlarged liver (Enlarged tender liver) and (5). Pedal edema.
Ref: Kumar and Clark 6th Ed, Pg -788

Q. 34. Match List -1 (wave in an ECG) with List – II (normal values) and select the correct answer using the codes give below the list (UPSC-04)

List – I	List-II
A. Normal Septal Q wave	1. 004 – 10 Second
B. PR Interval	2. < 002 Second
C. QRS Interval	3. 012 – 020 Second
D. Normal R in V1	4. < 04 Mv

Code

(a)	A	B	C	D
	4	1	3	2
(b)	A	B	C	D
	2	3	1	4
I	A	B	C	D
	4	3	1	2
(d)	A	B	C	D
	2	1	3	4

Ans. (b)
Note
Following is the correct sequence:

List I (Waves in an ECG)	List-II (Normal Values)
A. Normal Septal Q waves	2. < 002 Second
B. PR Interval	3. 012 - 020 Second
C. QRS Interval	1. 004 – 010 Second
D. Normal R in V1	4. < 04 Mv

Q. 35. Skin Pigmentation is found in (UPSC-04)
    (a) Addison's disease
    (b) Cushing disease
    (c) Conn's Syndrome
    (d) Andro-genital Syndrome

Ans. (a)
Note
Skin pigmentation is found in 'Addison's disease'
Also see
Addison's disease
It is the adrenocortical insufficiency caused by gradual adrenal destruction is characterized by an insidious onset of fatigability, weakness, anorexia, nausea and vomiting, weight loss, characteristic cutaneous and mucosal pigmentation, hypotension, and occasionally hypoglycemia.

Extended information
Cushing's syndrome (Hypercortisolism or Hyperadrenocorticism)
It is an endocrine disorder caused by high levels of cortisol in the blood.
Causes:
Primary pituitary adenoma, primary adrenal hyperplasia or neoplasia, ectopic ACTH production (e.g., from a small cell lung cancer).
Sign & Symptoms:
Rapid weight gain, (central obesity), "moon face", excess sweating, telangiectasia, thinning of the skin, easy bruising. Purple or red striae on the trunk, buttocks, arms, proximal muscle weakness and hirsutism (facial male-pattern hair growth). Insomnia, impotence, amenorrhea and infertility. Psychological disturbances, euphoria / psychosis. Depression and anxiety are also common. Persistent hypertension, insulin resistance leading to hyperglycemia, hyperpigmentation, impaired wound healing and osteoporosis.
Ref: http://en.wikipedia.org/wiki/Cushing's_syndrome

Conn's syndrome (aldosterone-producing adrenal adenoma)
Constitution is characterized by the overproduction of the mineralocorticoid hormone aldosterone by the adrenal glands. Aldosterone causes sodium and water retention and potassium excretion in the kidneys, leading to arterial hypertension.
Sign & Symptoms: Hypersecretion of aldosterone increases the renal distal tubular exchange of intratubular sodium for secreted potassium and hydrogen ions, with progressive depletion of body potassium and development of hypokalemia. Most patients have diastolic hypertension, which may be very severe, and headaches. The hypertension is probably due to the increased sodium reabsorption and extracellular volume expansion. *Potassium depletion* is responsible for the muscle weakness and fatigue and is due to the effect of potassium depletion on the muscle cell membrane. The polyuria results from impairment of urinary concentrating ability and is often associated with polydipsia.
Ref: http://en.wikipedia.org/wiki/Conn_syndrome

Androgenital syndrome
A genetic disorder present at birth characterised by a deficiency of the hormones aldosterone and cortisol and an overproduction of male sex hormones (androgens). In males this may manifest as enlarged penis, small testes and early development of masculine characteristics. In females features include ambiguous genitalia, failure to menstruate, deep voice and excessive hair.
Ref: http://www.medicineword.com/androgenital+syndrome.shtml

Q. 36. In electrocardiogram, which limb is used as an earth complexion? (UPSC-04)
  (a) Left Leg
  (b) Right Leg
  (c) Right Arm
  (d) Left Arm

Ans. (b)
Note
In electrocardiogram right leg is used as an earth complexion.
Also see
The Earth lead is attached to the right leg. The right leg electrode functions as a ground.
Ref: Harrison 16th Editon pg-1313

Q. 37. Consider the following (UPSC-04)
  1. Calcitonin
  2. Oxytocin
  3. Vasopressin
  4. Prolacatin
  Which of the hormones given above are released by pituitary gland?
  (a) and 3
  (b) 1 and 3
  (c) 1, 2 and 4
  (d) 2, 3 and 4

Ans. (d)

Note
Of the above 2: Oxytocin, 3: Vasopression and 4: Prolactin are released by pituitary gland.
Also see
Oxytocin
It is released from the posterior pituitary. Oxytocin; effects contraction of smooth muscles of uterus after childbirth and of lactating mammary glands.
Vasopressin
It is secreted from posterior pitutitary. It constricts smooth muscles of blood vessels, raises arterial blood pressure.
Prolactin
It is secrecrted from anterior pituitary. It is a lactogenic hormone is necessary for the initiation of milk production.
Ref: Harrison 15th Edition, Section 1 – Endocrinology.

Extended information
Calcitonin
This hormone is secrected from thyroid. It is of limited physiological significance in humans. Its medical significance however is because of its role as a tumor marker in sporadic and hereditary cases of medullary carcinoma and its medical use as an adjunctive treatment in severe hypercalcemia and in Paget's disease of bone.
Ref: Harrison 15th Edition, Section 2- Disorders of bone and mineral metabolism.

Q. 38. Hepatitis B is caused by (UPSC-04)
    (a)   RNA Virus
    (b)   DNA Virus
    (c)   Mycoplasma
    (d)   Rickettsia

Ans. (b)
Note
Hepatitis B is caused by DNA Virus.
Also see
The hepatitis B virus belongs to a family of DNA viruses called Hepadnaviridae. These viruses primarily infect liver cells. The name of the family comes from Hepa, meaning liver; DNA, referring to deoxyribonucleic acid, the virus' genetic material; and viridae, meaning virus.
Ref: http://www.stanford.edu/group/virus/hepadna/2004tansilvis/Intro.htm

Q. 39. Aschoff giant cells are found in (UPSC-04)
    (a)   Rheumatoid arthritis
    (b)   Rheumatic fever
    (c)   Hodgkins disease
    (d)   Sarcoidosis

Ans. (b)
Note
Aschoff giant cells are found in rheumatic fever.
Also see
Rheumatic fever affects all the heart tissue (rheumatic pancarditis). From all the pathological changes, only the granulomas, called Aschoff granulomas, are pathognomonic, often located perivascularly. In the centre, fibrinoid necrosis is visible. It is encompassed by lymphocytes, plasma cells, fibroblasts and individual neutrophils. Also mononuclear Anitschkow's cells (histiocytes) and characteristic Aschoff giant cells are present (these latter represent multinucleated macrophages). Anitschkow's cells appear like an owl's eye and have abundant pale eosinophilic cytoplasm with a characteristic "caterpillar" or lacy nucleole in the bright nucleus. They are often arranged in a palisade around the center. Aschoff cells have a single or multiple bean-shaped nuclei. Peripherally, fibroblasts and sclerotic fibrous tissue can be seen. The granuloma sometimes immediately borders partially fragmented muscle fibers. Ultimately, Rheumatic heart disease results in a "fish mouth" appearing stenosis of the mitral valve, causing left atrial dilation, right ventricular hypertrophy, and mural thrombi. Patients are predisposed endocarditis and CHF.
Ref: http://en.wikipedia.org/wiki/Granuloma

Q. 40. Which of the following enzyme is deficient in diabetes mellitus? (UPSC-04)
    (a) Glyco-kinase
    (b) Insulin
    (c) Hexokinase
    (d) Phosphorylase

Ans. (b)
Note
Out of the above enzymes 'insulin' is deficient in diabetes mellitus.
Also see
Insulin is a hormone. Insulin is secreted from the islet cells of pancreas. Carbohydrates (or sugars) are absorbed from the intestines into the bloodstream after a meal. Insulin is then secreted by the pancreas in response to this detected increase in blood sugar. Most cells of the body have insulin receptors which bind the insulin which is in the circulation. When a cell has insulin attached to its surface, the cell activates other receptors designed to absorb glucose (sugar) from the blood stream into the inside of the cell.
Without insulin, carbohydrates can not be utilized for energy produciton and a state of starvation occurs, since cells cannot access the calories contained in the glucose without the action of insulin.

Extended information
Type 1 Diabetes
In such patients there absolute lack of insulin, therefore they cannot sustain without insulin injections.
Type 2 Diabetes
In this more commonly, patients develop insulin resistance, rather than a true deficiency of insulin. In such case, the levels of insulin in the blood are similar or even a little higher than in normal, non-diabetic individuals. However, many cells of Type 2 diabetics respond sluggishly to the insulin they make and therefore their cells cannot absorb the sugar molecules well. This leads to blood sugar levels which run higher than normal. Occasionally Type 2 diabetics will need insulin injections but most of the time other methods of treatment will be effective.

Q. 41. For the diagnosis of Hodgkin's Lymphoma, during histological examination one should confirm the presence of (UPSC-04)
    (a) Reed-Sternberg Cells
    (b) Lymphocytes
    (c) Shikata Cells
    (d) Macropolycytes

Ans. (a)
Note
For the diagnosis of Hodgkin's lymphoma, during histological examination one should confirm the presence of Reed-Sternberg cells.
Also see
Reed-Sternberg cell is a large cell with a bi-lobed nucleus and prominent nucleoli, histologically; these are the diagnostic of Hodgkin's lymphoma.

Q. 42. On which one of the following does the erythrocyte sedimentation rate depend? (UPSC-04)
    (a) Fibrogen content of the blood
    (b) Prothrombin content of blood
    (c) Quantity of cellular element of the blood
    (d) Platelet count

Ans. (a)
Note
From the above listed choices the ESR depends on 'Fibrogen content of blood'.
Also see
A raised ESR reflects an increase in the plasma concentration of large proteins such as fibrinogen and immunoglobins. These proteins cause rouleaux formation, when cells clump together like a stack of coins, and therefore fall more rapidly.

Ref: Kumar and Clark 6th Ed. Pg-421
Factor which affects the ESR is viscosity of blood: the ESR is reduced when viscosity is more.
Ref: Sembulingam 2nd Ed. Pg- 58

Extended information
The test measures the distance that erythrocytes have fallen after one hour in a vertical column of anticoagulated blood under the influence of gravity. The basic factor influencing the ESR is the amount of fibrinogen in the blood as it directly correlates with the ESR. The most satisfactory method of performing the test was introduced by Westergren in 1921

Q. 43. Match List-1 (Causative Factors) with List –II (Disease Produced) and select the correct answer using the codes given below in the lists (UPSC-04)

List-I (Causative Factor)	List-II (Disease Produced)
A. Entamoeba histolytica	1. Syphilis
B. Leishmania donovani	2. Ankylstomiasis
C. Treponema pallidum	3. Amoebiasis
D. Hookworm	4. Kala azar

Codes

	A	B	C	D
(a)	3	4	1	2
(b)	1	2	3	4
(c)	3	2	1	4
(d)	1	4	3	2

Ans. (a)
Note
The following is the correct sequence:

List-I (Causative Factor)	List-II (Disease Produced)
A. Entamoeba histolytica	3. Amoebiasis
B. Leishmania donovani	4. Kala azar
C. Treponema pallidum	1. Syphilis
D. Hookworm	2. Ankylostomiasis

Q. 44. Koplik's Spots are pathognomonic of (UPSC-04)
    (a) Chicken pox
    (b) Dengue
    (c) Measles
    (d) Addison's Disease

Ans. (c)
Note
Koplik's spots are pathognomonic of 'Measles'.

Also see
Koplik's spots are seen in measles these appear in the buccal mucosa against upper 2nd molar tooth 72 hours before the measles rash.

Q. 45. Eosinophilia is not a characteristic feature of (UPSC-04)
    (a)   Hodgkins lymphoma
    (b)   Mycosis fungoides
    (c)   Rheumatoid arthritis
    (d)   Steroid therapy

Ans. (d)
Note
Eosinophilia is not a characteristic feature of 'Steroid therapy'.
Also see
Eosinophilia occurs in collagen vascular disease (e.g rheumatoid arthritis, eosinophilic fascitis, allergic angitis) and malignancies (e.g Hodgkin's disease, mycosis fungoides)
Ref: Harrison's 16th Ed. Pg-356

Extended information
Eosinophilia refers to conditions in which abnormally high amounts of eosinophils in blood.
Causes:
Its commonest causes are:
    -Allergic diseases: Asthma, hay fever.
    -Parasitic infection
Rarer causes include:
    - Lung diseases, eg Loeffler's syndrome
    - Vasculitis (inflammation of blood vessels), eg Churg-Strauss syndrome
    - Some tumours, eg lymphoma
    - Liver cirrhosis
    - Some antibody deficiencies; not typically AIDS
    - Other rarer skin diseases, eg dermatitis herpetiformis
    - Unknown causes, labelled hypereosinophilic syndrome
Current allopathic treatment:
    -Treatment for hypereosinophilic syndrome is oral corticosteroid therapy.
Conclusion:
    -If some other medical condition is being treated with steroid therapy the patient will not present with eosinophilia as a characteristic feature.
Ref: http://www.netdoctor.co.uk/diseases/facts/eosinophilia.htm

Q. 46. Of the below which spreads through the lymphatics? (KPSC-R/E-05)
    (a)   Leiomyoma
    (b)   Carcinoma
    (c)   Sarcoma
    (d)   Rhabdomyoma

Ans. (b)
Note
From choice givren above 'carcinoma' spreads through lymphatics.
Also see
Lymphatic spread- In general, carcinomas metastasized by lymphatic route while sarcomas favour hematogenous route. However, sarcomas can also spread by lymphatic pathway. Blood-borne metastasis is the common route for sarcomas but certain carcinomas also frequently metastasized by this mode, especially those of lungs, breast, kidney, thyroid, liver, prostate and ovary.
Ref: Harsh Mohan's Short Handbook of pathology, 5th edn Pg-137

Extended information
Leiomyoma
It is a benign smooth muscle neoplasm that is not premalignant. However they can occur in any organ, but the most commonly occur in the uterus and esophagus. They do not metastasis through blood or lymphatics.
Carcinoma
The carcinoma is any cancer that arises from epithelial cells. It is malignant and invades surrounding tissues and organs, and spread (metstasis) through lymphatics to distant sites.
Sarcoma
The sarcoma is a cancer of connective or supportive tissue i.e., bones, cartilage, fat, muscle, blood vessel. Sarcomas spread through the blood, often to the lung, liver, and brain.
Ref: http://orthopedics.about.com/cs/tumors/g/sarcoma.htm
Rhabdomyoma
Rhabdomyomas muscle tumors occur most often in cardiac muscle.Rhabdomyomas are non-cancerous; they do not metastasize. The symptoms associated withy these tumors are dependent on their location, number and size. Large tumors within the heart may obstruct the cardiac valves or great vessels that enter the heart.

Q. 47. To which disease in the below serum glutamic oxaloautic transaminase level is studied? (KPSC-R/E-05)
    (a)   Hepato cellular damage
    (b)   Renal glomerular damage
    (c)   Enlarged prostate
    (d)   Bronchiectasis

Ans. (a)
Note
Out of the above conditions only cases of 'Hepatocellular damage' result in raised level of 'Serum glutamic oxaloacetic transaminase' (SGOT).
Also see
Aspartate amino transferase (AST) is primarily a mitochondrial enzyme (80%; 20% in cytoplasm) and is also present in heart, muscle, kidney, brain. High levels are seen in hepatic necrosis, myocardial infarction, muscle injury and congestive cardiac failure.Pg.352-353, Kumar and Clark, 6th Ed. Pg- 352, 353

Extended information
SGOT is also called aspartate aminotransferase (AST). It is an enzyme normally present in liver and heart cells. SGOT is released into blood when the liver or heart is damaged. The blood SGOT levels are thus elevated with liver damage i.e. from viral hepatitis or with an injury to heart muscle'i.e. Myocardial infarction. Some medications can also raise SGOT levels.
Ref: http://www.medterms.com/script/main/art.asp?articlekey=6315

Q. 48. Of the below which is pterygium? (KPSC-R/E-05)
    (a)   Pigments present in the retina
    (b)   Pigments present in the conjunctiva
    (c)   Twitching of the eyelid
    (d)   Blood vessels are growing in the outer canthus

Ans. Use your discretion
Note
None of the choices given above qualifies to represent 'pterygium'.
Also see
It is a triangular fold of tissue that grows from the nasal side of conjunctiva onto the cornea of the eye. The cause is unknown, but it may be the result of exposure to ultraviolet light. Risk factors are exposure to sunny, dusty, sandy, or windblown areas. It is rare in children.
Ref: http://en.wikipedia.org/wiki/Pterygium_(conjunctiva)

Q. 49. Of these which is Tennis Elbow? (KPSC-R/E-05)
    (a)   Tenderness on the lateral epicondyle of the humerus
    (b)   Tenderness on the medial epicondyle of the humerus

(c) Swelling of the elbow joint
(d) Atrophy of the muscles attached to the lateral epicondyle of the humerus

Ans. (a)
Note
Of the above given choices 'Tenderness on the lateral epicondyle of humerus' suggest the diagnosis of 'Tennis Elbow'.
Also see
Tennis elbow (Lateral epicondylitis)
Tendonitis at the pont of insertion over lateral epicondyle. It is characterised by pain and tenderness over lateral epicondyle of humerus. The pain is aggravated by active dorsiflexion of the wrist. It is cause by repeated movement involving extensors muscles at the wrist.
Ref: Kumar and Clark, 6th Ed. Pg-538

Q. 50. Of the below which method is useful to stain mycobacterium tuberculosis? (KPSC-R/E-05)
(a) Ziehl-neelsen's method
(b) Gram's method
(c) Albert's stain
(d) Fleming's method

Ans. (a)
Note
Fom the above 'Ziehl-neelsen's method' is useful to stain mycobacterium tuberculosis.
Also see
M. tuberculosis hominis is a slender rod like bacillus and can be demonstrated by acid fast (ziehl-neelson) staining.
Ref.: Harsh Mohan Handbook of Pathology, 5th Ed. Pg-102

Q. 51. Of these which test is done to diagnose tubercular infection? (KPSC-R/E-05)
(a) Casoni's test
(b) Frei test
(c) Mantoux test
(d) Dick test

Ans. (c)
Note
From the above suggestions 'Montoux test' is done to diagnose tubercular infection.
Also see
Mantoux test is used for diagnosis of tubercular infection:
 -0.1 ml of 1:1000 strength PPD (Purified Protein Derivative) (equivalent to 10 tuberculin units) is injected intradermally.
 -The induration (not the erythema) is measured after 72 hours. The test is positive if the induration is 10mm or more in diameter.
Ref: Kumar and Clark, 6th Edition Pg-934

Extended information
Casoni's Test
The Casoni's test is an immediate hypersensitivity test originally introduced by Casoni in 1911. The antigen is hydatid fluid collected from animal or human cysts and sterilized by Seitz or membrane filtration. 0.2 ml of the antigen is injected intradermally on one arm and an equal volume of saline as control on the other arm. In positive cases a large wheal, about 5 cm in diameter, with multiple pseudopodial projections appears within 20-30 minutes at the test site and fades in an hour. The test is very sensitive, but false positive reactions may appear in a number of other conditions. The test itself can sensitize the patient or result in anaphylaxis in an already sensitized patient and is no longer recommended as a diagnostic procedure.
Frei test
A skin test for venereal lymphogranuloma that uses antigen prepared from chlamydiae grown in the yolk sac of a chick embryo.
Mantoux test

A skin test for tuberculosis. Tuberculin is a glycerine extract of the tubercule bacilli. Purified Protein Derivative (PPD) tuberculin is a precipitate of non-species-specific molecules obtained from filtrates of sterilized, concentrated cultures. It was announced in 1890 by Robert Koch. The test is named after Charles Mantoux, a French physician who developed on the work of Koch and Clemens Von Pirquet to created this test in 1907.

Dick test

Test for determining immunity or susceptibility to scarlet fever in which scarlet fever toxin is injected into the skin, susceptibility being characterized by redness at the injection area. Etymology: From the name of the US inventor of the test, George Frederick Dick

Q. 52. Which is the varicose ulcer? (KPSC-R/E-05)
    (a) Ulcer in the neck, axilla
    (b) Ulcer in the upper part of the face
    (c) Ulcer on the medial malleolus of lower limb
    (d) Ulcer in glans penis

Ans. (c)

Note
Vericose ulcer is 'ulcer on the medial mallelous of lower limb'.

Also see
Varicose ulcers are mostly found on or near the medial malleolus.
Ref. Textbook of Surgery S.Das 3rd Ed. Pg-206

Extended information
Venous ulcer- stasis occurs through incompetent perforators veins through which the high deep venous pressure is transmitted to the superficial veins. The location of these perforating veins determines the prediction of ulcer formation extending from the malleoli upto the lower half of the leg
Text book of surgery. S. Das, 3rd Ed. Pg- 209
Varicose veins are dilated, tortuous superficial veins that result from defective structure and function of the valves of the saphenous veins. Symptoms consist of a dull ache or pressure sensation in the legs after prolonged standing; it is relieved with leg elevation. The legs feel heavy, and mild ankle edema develops occasionally. Extensive venous varicosities may cause skin ulcerations near the ankle.

Q. 53. Pain worse after use. The joint feels stiff after rest and it hurts the patient to get going. The joint may give way or locked, crepitus is felt. X-ray shows diminution of joint space of the below in which condition these clinical points are elicited? (KPSC-R/E-05)
    (a) Tuberculosis of the knee
    (b) Osteoarthritis of the knee
    (c) Acute pyogenic arthritis
    (d) Osteochondroitis

Ans. (b)

Note
Above clinical presentation is in favouir of 'Osteoarthritis'.

Also see
Clinical features of OA:
    -Pain: pain in or around the involved joint is the cardinal symptom.
    -Initially pain is aggravated by joint used and relieved by rest.
    -In advance cases pain becomes persistent.
    -Morning stiffness: usually last 5 minutes.
    -Crepitation is observed in knee join in 90% patients.
    -X-ray shows joint space narrowing in early stages.
Ref: API 7th Ed. Pg-1152, 1153

Extended information
Tubercular arthritis
Chronic, progressive, potentially crippling tubercular infection, commonly affecting synovial joints and intervertebral joints of thoracic and lumbar spine.
Osteoarthritis

Non-inflammatory degenerative disorder of synovial joints, and characterised by wear and tear of articular surfaces and new bone formation at joint margins.
Acute Pyogenic arthritis
Acute infection of joint with pyogenic bacteria characterised by red, swollen, tender joint and high fever.
Osteochondroitis
Probably the term 'chondrosis' should be used instead of 'chondritis', as 'itis' means 'inflamed', and cartilage softens and degenerates under stress rather than becoming 'inflamed'. Chondrosis just implies that there is an abnormal process going on in the joint cartilage.

Q. 54. Of the below which organism is having terminal spore? (KPSC-R/E-05)
- (a) Streptococcus
- (b) Pneumococcus
- (c) Anthrax bacillus
- (d) Tetanus bacillus

Ans. (d)
Note
Out of above 'Tetanus bacillus' is having terminal spore.
Also see
Clostridium tetani is a gram positive anaerobic rod with terminal round spore giving rise to a typical drum stick appearance.
Ref: Textbook of surgery S.Das 3rd Ed. Pg-133

Extended information

Clostridium tetani is a bacterium of the genus Clostridium. It is found in nature as spores in soil or parasitising the gastrointestinal tracts of animals, and causes serious toxicity in humans. Like other Clostridium species, it is gram-positive, and its appearance on a gram stain is said to resemble tennis rackets or drumsticks. Terminal spore: An endospore located at the end of the cell.

Q. 55. Of the below who is with glycosuria-closely related to diet, who becomes sugar free with slight restriction (KPSC-R/E-05)
- (a) Potential diabetes
- (b) Renal glycosuria
- (c) Pregnancy glycosuria
- (d) Emotional glycosuria

Ans. (a)
Note
Out of above 'Potential diabetes' is the one whose glycosuria is related to diet, and becomes sugar free with slight restriction.
Also see
Glycosuria: (glycose, older variant of glucose + uria)
The presence of glucose in the urine, especially excretion of an abnormally large amount in the urine, such as more than 1 g in 24 hours. Called also dextrosuria and glycosuria.

Extended information
Potential diabetes
Before one develops Type-II Diabetes, they almost always have an asymptomatic state called "pre-diabetes." or "potential diabetes", also known as "impaired glucose tolerance". Pre-diabetes is a term that refers to who has blood glucose levels that are higher than normal, but are not high enough to be classified as diabetes.
Fasting blood sugar
Blood sample after eight hours or overnight fasting, having a blood sugar level lower than 100 milligrams per deciliter (mg/dL) is normal. A blood sugar level from 100 to 125 mg/dL is considered prediabetes. This is referred to as impaired fasting glucose (IFG). A blood sugar level of 126 mg/dL or higher may indicate diabetes.
Post prandial sugar
After eight hours or overnight fasting 70 gm sugary solution is taken by mouth, and blood sugar level is

measured after two hours. A blood sugar level less than 140 mg/dL is normal. A blood sugar level from 140 to 199 mg/dL is considered prediabetes. This is sometimes referred to as impaired glucose tolerance (IGT). A blood sugar level of 200 mg/dL or higher may indicate diabetes.

Renal glycosuria
Glycosuria occurring when there is only the normal amount of sugar in the blood, due to inability of the renal tubules to reabsorb glucose completely. Called also nondiabetic or normoglycemic glycosuria and renal diabetes.

Pregnancy glycosuria
Glycosuria is common during pregnancy due to lowering of the renal threshold for glucose excretion.
There is a diurnal variation in glycosuria: being least evident in the morning and most evident after meals. Females who develop diabetes during pregnancy are said to have gestational diabetes. Some will remain diabetic after delivery of the fetus while others will revert to apparent normality.

Reference
Diabetes UK. Recommendations for the management of pregnant women with diabetes (including gestational diabetes). 2003

Emotional glycosuria
Glycosuria induced by violent emotion.

Q. 56. In which condition cardiac-enzymes raised? (KPSC-R/E-05)
    (a)   Endocarditis
    (b)   Angina pectoris
    (c)   Myocardial infarction
    (d)   Left ventricular hypertrophy

Ans. (c)

Note
In case of 'Myocardial infarction' cardiac enzymes are raised.
Acute myocardial infarction causes necrosis of myocardial cells which releases certain enzymes in the blood:
    -SGOT starts to rise with in a few hours reaching a peak at 24 hours and declining over the next 48-72 hours.
    -Serum creatinine phosphokinase (CPK) rises immediately and reaches peak with in 18-24 hours.
    -CPK-MB is more specific for cardiac tissue and its levels are related to the extent of myocardial infarction.

Ref: API, 7th Ed. Pg-442

Also see
Cardiac enzymes are raised in acute myocardial infarction:
a.   CPK
    -Starts to rise at 4 - 6 hours of myocardial infarction.
    -Peaks about 12 hours.
    -Becomes normal at 48-72 hours.
b.   AST
    -Starts to rise after 12 hours of myocardial infarction.
    -Peaks about 24 hours.
    -Comes to normal on 4th or 5th day.
c.   LDH
    -Starts to rise after 12 hours of myocardial infarction.
    -Peaks on 3rd day.
    -Becomes normal on 7th day.

Q. 57. In which "Statut dysfunction in absence of demonstrable organic pathology? (KPSC-R/E-05)
    (a)   Cholera
    (b)   Dysentery
    (c)   Irritable bowel syndrome
    (d)   Diveritcolitis coli

Ans. (c)

Note
Out of the above 'Irritable bowel syndrome' is the 'gut dysfunction in absence of demonstrable organic pathology.
Also see
Irritable bowel syndrome is a condition characterised by signs and symptoms suggestive of gastro-intestinal dysfunction without any organic lesion, but dependent on disturbed colonic motility.

Extended information
Manning's criteria for diagnosis of IBS:
- Pain eased after bowel movement
- Loose stools at onset of pain
- More frequent bowel movements at onset of pain
- Abdominal distention
- Mucous per rectum
- Feeling of incomplete emptying

Ref: API 7th Ed.Pg-560

Q. 58. In which "pea soup diarrhea is noted? (KPSC-R/E-05)
 (a) Cholera
 (b) Typhoid
 (c) Rheumatic fever
 (d) Pyelitis

Ans. (b)
Note
In 'Typhoid' case 'pea soup diarrhea is noted'.
Also see
In typhoid there may be marked constipation, especially in early stage or there is "pea soup" diarrhea.
Ref: Park & Park, 18th Ed. Pg-188

Extended information
A clinical manifestation of typhoid includes fever, typhoid facies (early flushed cheeks with bright eyes and listless expression) towards the end of first week with a dull and a heavy look when the disease is established. Abdominal tenderness and splenomegaly occur in majority of patients. Rose spots are very characteristic and consist of variable number of rose coloured spots appearing on seventh to tenth day starting from abdomen. Other signs include furred tongue, loose and pale stools (Pea soup stool), ronchi, epistaxis, tremor, ataxic gait, cardiac signs, jaundice and meningism.
Ref: API, 7th Ed. Pg-51

Q. 59. Which is intermediate host for Tenia saginata? (KPSC-R/E-05)
 (a) Man
 (b) Cattle
 (c) Cat
 (d) Dog

Ans. (b)
Note
Cattle is the intermediate host for Tenia saginata.
Also see
T. Saginata passes its life cycle in two hosts:
 -The definitive host: man, harbours the adult worm.
 -The intermediate host: cattle (cow or buffalow), harbours the larval stage.
Ref: Parasitology by K.D. Chatterjee, 12th Ed. Pg-117

Extended information
Tenia saginata life cycle
The life cycle of Tenia saginata- Humans are the only definitive host for T.S. and cannot act as intermediate host. Cattle and the other herbivores become infected by ingesting vegetation contaminated with eggs (or

proglottids).In the animal's intestine, the eggs release the oncosphere, which evaginates, invades the intestinal wall and migrates to the striated muscles,where it developes into a cysticercus. The cysticercus can survive for several years in animal. Humans become infected by ingesting raw or undercooked infected meat. In the human intestine, the cysticercus develops over 2 months into an adult tapeworm, which can survive for more than 30 years.
Ref: API, 7th Ed. Pg-123

Q. 60. Which is caused by Echinococcus granulosus? (KPSC-R/E-05)
    (a)   Polycystic ovary
    (b)   Hydatid cyst
    (c)   Hepatitis infective
    (d)   Cystic lung

Ans. (b)

Note
Hydatid cyst disese is caused by Echinococcus granulosus.

Also see
When the embryo of echinococcus granulosus settles, it forms a hydatid cyst, the younger larva being transformed into a hollow bladder.
Ref: Parasitology by K.D. Chatterjee, 12th Ed. Pg-122.

Extended information
Echinococcus granulosus (Dog tapeworm / Hydatid cyst):
Adult worm develops in small intestine of dog (definitive host) and eggs are passed in feces. Intermediate hosts, like sheep, ingest eggs, which pass from stomach to liver, lung, brain to form hydatid cyst. On eating infected sheep meat dog gets worm and cycle is completed. Accidentally while handling dog, humans ingest eggs and develop cysts in brain, liver, lung.

Q. 61. Of the below which is fat soluble vitamin? (KPSC-R/E-05)
    (a)   Thiamine
    (b)   Riboflavine
    (c)   Pyridoxine
    (d)   Vitamin E

Ans. (d)

Note
Out of the above 'vitamin E' is fat soluble vitamin.

Also see
Thiamin (Viamin B1): It is a water soluble vitamin.
Beriberi is caused by deficiency of thiamine (vitamin B1) and is characterised by polyneuropathy (dry beri beri) and a high cardiac output state (wet beri beri).
Riboflavin (Vitamin B2): It is a water soluble vitamin.
Ariboflavinosis [Vitamin B2 deficiency] is characterised by cheilosis, angular stomatitis, glossitis and corneal vascularisation.
Pyridoxine (B6): It is a water soluble vitamin.
It plays an important role in metabolism of amino-acids, fats and carbohydrates. Pyridoxine deficiency is associated with peripheral neuritis.
The Vitamin E is a fat soluble vitamin.
Vitamin E-It is the generic name for a group of closely related and naturally occuring fat soluble compounds Tocopherols.
Ref. Park's textbook of PSM 18th Ed. Pg-445

Extended information
The mechanism of action of vitamin E in humans is unclear. It is commonly thought to function as an antioxidant, protecting membranes and other cellular structures from attacks of free radicals. Therefore it plays a role in protection against cancer, coronay artery disease and cataract.

Q. 62. Which is causing quartan disease? (KPSC-R/E-05)
    (a)   Plasmodium vivax
    (b)   Lymphangitis
    (c)   Plasmodium ovale
    (d)   Neuritis

Ans. Use your discretion
Note
Plasmodium malaria causes quartan malaria.
Also see
Types of Malaria:
Benign tertian malaria: (Paroxysm after 48 hours):
    -Caused by P. vivax and P. ovale commonest in India.
Benign quartan malaria: (Paroxysm after 72 hours):
    -Caused by P. malariae rare in India.
Malignant malaria: (Periodicity not marked / Hyperpyraxia).
    -Caused by P. falciparum.
Ref: Parasitology by K.D. Chatterjee, 12th Ed. Pg-87

Q. 63. The skin lesion Oriental sore is caused by? (KPSC-R/E-05)
    (a)   Leishmania tropica
    (b)   Plasmodium falciparum
    (c)   Flaviviridae
    (d)   Plasmodium malariae

Ans. (a)
Note
Skin lesion Oriental sore is caused by Leishmania tropica.
Also see
Infection with Leishmania tropica produces a cutaneous lesion called oriental sore or Delhi boil.
Ref: Parasitology by K.D. Chatterjee, 12th Ed. Pg-66

Extended information
Delhi Boil
Infection with Leishmania tropica produces a cutaneous lesion called Oriental sore or Delhi boil. It is transmitted by Phlebotomus sergenti in India, Iraq, Iran. The lesion begins as a raised nodule about one inch in diameter in majority of cases it ulcerates, having a clean cut margin with a raised indurated edge, surrounded by red areola.

Q. 64. Which is the infecting agent of ankylostoma duodenale? (KPSC-R/E-05)
    (a)   Filariform larva
    (b)   Mosquito bite
    (c)   Inhalation of dust
    (d)   Bite of sand fly

Ans. (a)
Note
Filariform larva is the infecting agent of ankylostoma duodenale.
Also see
The rhabditiform larva of ankylostoma duodenale hatches out in the soil in about 48 hours. It moulds twice on 3rd and 5th day and than develops into filariform larva, the infective stage of parasite.
Ref: Parasitology by K.D. Chatterjee, 12th Ed. Pg-172.

Extended information
Ankylostoma duodenale
Disease caused by hookworm living in the small intestine and clinically characterized by anemia, edema, debility and prostration. The adult hookworms produce thousands of eggs daily. The eggs are deposited with feces in soil, where rhabditiform larvae hatch and develop over a 1-week period into infectious *filariform*

larvae. Infective larvae penetrate the skin and reach the lungs by way of the bloodstream. There they invade alveoli and ascend the airways before being swallowed and reaching the small intestine.
Ref: Harrison 15th Edition

Q. 65. Which type displays the female sex characters? (KPSC-R/E-05)
      (a)   Anthropoid pelvis
      (b)   Gynaecoid pe'vis
      (c)   Platy pelloid type
      (d)   None of the above

Ans. (b)
Note
The gynaecoid type pelvix displays the perfect female sex characters.
Also see
The gynaecoid pelvis
It is the "perfect" female pelvis. The key feature is that the inlet is almost circular the transverse diameter is the greatest diameter of the inlet.
The android pelvis
It has a heart-shaped inlet with the sacral promontory jutting in. If the heart shape is too pronounced, this may cause difficulty in childbirth.
The anthropoid pelvis
It (so-called because this shape is seen in anthropoid apes) is somewhat oval, with the anteroposterior diameter being the greatest diameter of the inlet.
The platypelloid (meaning a flat pelvis)
It has a transverse diameter (inlet) much greater than the anteroposterior diameter. The last two types do not necessarily cause difficulty in childbirth unless exaggerated.

Q. 66. Of the below which is responsible for infantile convulsion? (KPSC-R/E-05)
      (a)   Asphyxia neonatorum
      (b)   Icterus neonatorum
      (c)   Ophthalmia neonatorum
      (d)   Patent foramen ovale

Ans. (a)
Note
The 'Asphyxia neonatorum is mostly responsible for infantile convulsions.
Also see
Asphyxia neonatorum
It has been linked to low birth weight, late deliveries, and flattening or twisting of the umbilical cord during labor. Smoking during pregnancy is also considered a risk factor for asphyxia because it tends to produce low birth-weight babies.
Asphyxia requires emergency treatment, preferably in a hospital. Brain damage can result if the infant doesn't start breathing within about five minutes. Death can result if the asphyxiation lasts over 10 minutes. Asphyxia can also lead to seizures, especially if the baby requires intubation and has a low Apgar score five minutes after birth, and if the blood from the cutting of the umbilical cord has a high acid content. In older preterm infants (32-36 weeks), asphyxia has been linked to lung and kidney damage as well as brain damage.
Icterus neonatorum
A mild temporary jaundice in newborn infants caused mainly by functional immaturity of the liver.
Ophthalmia neonatorum
Ophthalmia neonatorum is a form of bacterial conjunctivitis contracted by newborns during delivery. The baby's eyes are contaminated during passage through the birth canal from a mother infected with either Neisseria gonorrheae or Chlamydia trachomatis.
Patent Foramen ovale
Fetuses have a normal opening between the left and right atria (upper chambers) of the heart. If this opening fails to close naturally soon after the baby is born, the condition is called patent foramen ovale (PFO).

Q. 67. Which of the following can be used as a screening test for hemophilia? (KPSC-Lect/Physio-Bio/05)
 (a) Clotting time
 (b) Bleeding time
 (c) Prothrombin time
 (d) Partial thromboplastin time

Ans. (d)

Note
The 'Partial thromboplasin time' can be used as screening test for hemophilia.

Also see
In Hemophilia-Laboratory test of coagulation will show a normal prothrombin time (PT) and abnormal activated partial thromboplastin time.
Ref: API, 7th Ed. Pg-969
The screening laboratory test including platelet count and morphology, bleeding time, PT, APTT and Factor XIII assay.
Ref: API 7th Ed. Pg-696.

Extended information
Hemophilia A is a hereditary coagulation disorder occurring due to deficiency or reduced activity of factor VIII (Anti-Hemophilic factor). The disorder is inherited as a sex – (X) linked recessive trait and therefore manifests in males, while females are usually the carriers.

Laboratory test	Factor / Function Measures	Associated disorders
1. Bleeding Time: (Normal < 8 min)	Platelet function, vascular integrity.	1. Qualitative disorders of platelets 2. Von Willebrand's Disease 3. Quantitative disorders of platelets 4. Acquired vascular disorders
2. Platelet Count: (N: 150 – 400 x 10^9/L)	Quantification of platelets	(a) Thrombocytopenia (b) Thrombocytosis
3. Prothrombin Time: (N:12 – 15 Sec.)	Evaluation of extrinsic and common pathway (Deficiency of factors I, II, V, VII and X)	(a) Oral anticoagulant therapy (b) DIC (c) Liver disease
4. Partial Thromboplastin Time: (N: 30 – 40 Sec.)	Evaluation of intrinsic and common pathway (Deficiency of factors I, II, V, VIII, IX, X, XI and XII	(a) Parenteral heparin therapy (b) DIC (c) Liver disease

Q. 68. Following are features of hyperthyroidism except (KPSC-Lect/Physio-Bio/05)
 (a) Tachycardia
 (b) Exophthalmos
 (c) Increased appetite
 (d) Cold intolerence

Ans. (d)

Note
All of the above are the features of hyperthyroidism except 'cold intolerance'.

Also see
Hyperthyroidism
In hyperthyroidism there is usually a gradual onset of symptoms and signs. Weight loss in face of increased appetite, irritability, palpitations, increased sweating, tremors, dyspnea (due to respiratory muscle weakness or cardiac failure), frequency of stools (occasionally diarrhea) and heat intolerance are the common presentation.
Ref: API, 7th Ed. Pg-1054

Q. 69. Spasticity indicates (KPSC-Lect/Physio-Bio/05)
- (a) Cerebellar disease
- (b) Autonomic imbalance
- (c) Lower motor neuron injury
- (d) Upper motor neuron injury

Ans. (d)
Note
Spasticity indicates 'Upper motor neuron injury / lesion'.
Also see
Cerebellar lesions
These are characaterised by hypotonia, pendular DTR's, ataxic gait / drunken gait, inco-ordination, past pointing, nystagmus and scanning speech.
Autonomic imbalance
It involves disorder of sympathetic and parasympathetic activity like vasomotor disturbances.

Lower motor neuron injury
This results in flassid paralytic state which is like post polio paralytic state.

Upper motor neuron injury
As the joint is passively flexed or extended, there is increased resistance to begin with, but as the movement is continued, the resistance disappears suddenly (clasp-knife spasticity). It is more marked in one direction than in the other.
Spasticity indicates the lesion involving plyramidal tract or corticospinal tract. UMN injury is characterized by spasticity / hypertonia, extensor plantar, hyperactive DTR's.

Also see
Differential/diagnosis of motor deficit:

Clinical Sign	Upper motor (pyramidal) lesion	Lower motor lesion	Extra pyramidal lesion	Cerebellar lession
Power	Weak	Weak	No Weakness	No Weakness
Wasting	No	Yes	None	None
Fasciculation	No	Yes	None	None
Tone	Increase (Spastic)	Decreased (Flaccid)	Rigidity (cogwheel)	Normal / Reduced
Contractures	Not Marked	Marked	None	None
Reflexes	Increased	Reduced / absent	Normal	Pendular
Plantar	Extensor	Flexor	Flexor	Flexor
Coordination	Reduced by weakness	Reduced by weakness	Normal (but slowed)	Impaired

Ref: Davidson, 20th Edition Table: 26.33 (Modified)

Also see

Features	LMN	UMN
Muscle tone	Hypotonia	Spasticity / clasp knife
Wasting	Wasting marked	Disuse atrophy
DTR's	Depressed or absent reflexes	Exaggerated reflexes + clonnus
Plantar	Absent / Lost	Extensor plantars
Abdominal reflex	Present	Absent

Ref: API, 7th Ed. Pg-733

Q. 70. Mean arterial pressure refers to (KPSC-Lect/Physio-Bio/05)
- (a) Systolic pressure + Diastolic pressure/2
- (b) Diastolic pressure/2
- (c) Systolic pressure + Pulse pressure/2
- (d) Diastolic pressure + Pulse pressure/3

Ans. (d)

Note
Mean arterial pressure refers to 'diastolic pressure + pulse pressure /3'.

Also see
The Mean Arterial Pressure (MAP)
It is a normal average bood pressure in an individual. It is defined as 'the average arterial pressure during a single cardiac cycle'.

Estimation
At normal resting heart rates MAP can be measured by:
MAP = DP + PP/3
(DP= Diastolic Pressure, SP= Systolic pressure, PP= Pulse pressure.)

Cinical Significance
Mean arterial pressure above 60 mm Hg is enough to sustain the organs of of the average person under normal conditions. If the MAP falls below for a longer time the end organs will not get the enough blood and ischemia will result.
Ref: Textbook of Physiology, Vol-1, By A. K. jain, Pg-343

Q. 71. In Addison's disease, the followings are seen except (KPSC-Lect/Physio-Bio/05)
- (a) Hyponatremia
- (b) Hypokalemia
- (c) Hypoglycemia
- (d) Low blood pressure

Ans. (b)

Note
In Addison's disease, all of the above are seen except 'Hyperkalemia'.

Also see
In Addison's disease hyponatremia, hypoglycemia, low blood pressure is seen along with hyperkalemia and not hypokalemia.
The investigations in case of Addison's disease show:
ACTH and renin levels: raised.
Sodium level: low.
Due to cortisol deficiency.
Potassium level: raised.
Due to aldosterone deficiency.

Calcium level: raised.
Due to dehydration and increased gastrointestinal calcium absorption.
Chloride level: low.
Urea and creatine level: raised.
Due to dehydration.
Sugar level: low.
Due to cortisol deficiency.
Ref: Kumar & Clark, 6th Ed. Pg-1083

Extended information
Addison's disease
It was very first time described by Thomas Addison in 1855, even before anything was known about function of adrenal cortex. His original classical description remains unaltered to date.
Primary adrenocortical insufficiency due to bilateral adrenal destruction or inability of adrenal gland to produce adequate amounts of cortical steroids, resulting in failure of adrenocortical function, and characterised by asthenia, hypotension, easy fatiguability, anorexia, frequent episodes of nausea, vomiting, wasting, and pigmentation of skin and mucous membranes.

Q. 72. An important factor in Kwashiorkor is (KPSC-Lect/Physio-Bio/05)
    (a)   Mineral deficiency
    (b)   Protein deficiency
    (c)   Vitamin deficiency
    (d)   None of them

Ans. (b)
Note
An important factor in Kwashiorkor is 'Protein deficiency'.
Also see
Kwashiokar-It is one of the most important florid forms of PEM occurring mostly in children between the age of 1 and 3 years when they are completely weaned.
Ref: API, 7th Ed. Pg-231
The essential feature is deficiency of protein with relatively adequate energy intake. It is severe form of protein calorie malnutrition with edema. The word 'Kwashiorkor' comes from Ghana and means 'the neglected one.'

Q. 73. Diagnostic test of secondary syphilis is (KPSC-Lect/Physio-Bio/05)
    (a)   VDRL
    (b)   TPHA
    (c)   Wassermann
    (d)   Kahn

Ans. (b)
Note
Diagnostic test of secondary syphilis is 'TPHA'.
Also see
VDRL
A blood test for syphilis (VDRL stands for Venereal Disease Research Laboratory) that detects an antibody that is present in the bloodstream when a patient has syphilis.
A negative (nonreactive) VDRL is compatible with a person not having syphilis, but in the early stages of the disease, the VDRL often gives false negative results. Conversely, a false positive VDRL can be encountered in infectious mononucleosis, lupus, antiphospholipid antibody syndrome, hepatitis A, leprosy, malaria and, occasionally pregnancy.
TPHA
Treponema pallidum haemagglutination test is more sensitive than the VDRL.
Wassermann Test
The Wassermann test is a complement-fixation (Complement system) antibody test for syphilis, named after the bacteriologist August Von Wassermann.
The reaction is not actually specific to syphilis and will produce a positive reaction to other diseases, including

malaria, tuberculosis, and numerous other diseases. It is possible for an infected individual to produce no reaction and for a successfully treated individual to continue to produce a reaction (called Wassermann fast or fixed).

Kahn Test
The fist flocculation test used widely was the tube flocculation test of Kahn. The Kahn test has been replaced by the simpler and more rapid VDRL test.

Q. 74. Salk vaccine is a (KPSC-Lect/Physio-Bio/05)
    (a)   Killed vaccine
    (b)   Live vaccine
    (c)   Live attenuated vaccine
    (d)   Toxoid

Ans. (a)
Note
Salk vaccine is a 'killed vaccine'.

Also see
The Salk vaccine is inactivated virus, the vaccine is safe for those with compromised (weakened) immune systems it is given in two intramuscular injections spaced one month apart and requires boosters every 5 years.
Salk vaccine or inactivated polio vaccine -this vaccine contains all the three types of polio virus inactivated by formalin. It contains 20, 2 and 4 D antigen units of type 1, 2 and 3 respectively.
Ref: Park & Park, 18th Ed. Pg-164

Q. 75. Egg contains all the vitamins except (KPSC-Lect/Physio-Bio/05)
    (a)   Vitamin B
    (b)   Vitamin D
    (c)   Vitamin C
    (d)   Vitamin E

Ans. (c)
Note
Egg contains all the vitamins except 'Vitiamin C'.

Also see
Eggs are one of nature's most perfectly balanced foods, containing all the protein, vitamins (except vitamin C) and minerals essential for good health.
Egg contains all the nutrients except carbohydrates and vitamin C.
Ref: Park and Park, 18th Ed.Pg-456

Q. 76. LD bodies are seen in (KPSC-Lect/Physio-Bio/05)
    (a)   Salmonellosis
    (b)   Leprosy
    (c)   Guinea worm infestation
    (d)   Leishmaniasis

Ans. (d)
Note
LD bodies are seen in 'Leishmaniasis'.

Also see
It is a protozoal infection cuased by Leishmania Donovani and characterised by chronic irregular fever, pigmentation, progressive wasting, hepato-splenomegaly, anemia and leucopenia.
For the diagnosis of Leishmaniasis, the tissue demonstration of Leishmania Donovani bodies remains the method of choice.
    -Bone marrow:
        Positive for L.D. bodies.
    -Splenic puncture:
        Positive for L.D. bodies.

Extended information
Leishmaniasis- Parasitological diagnosis. The demonstration of the parasite LD bodies in the aspirates of the spleen, liver, bone marrow, lymphnodes or in the skin. Skin is the only way to confirm Kala azar or cutaneous Leishmaniasis conclusively. The parasite must be isolated in culture to confirm the identity of the parasite.
Ref: Park and Park, 18th Ed.Pg-246

Q. 77. Commonest cause of sudden death is (KPSC-Lect/Physio-Bio/05)
- (a) Ventricular fibrillation
- (b) Cerebro vascular accident
- (c) Ventricular asystole
- (d) Acute renal failure

Ans. (a)
Note
Commonest cause of sudden death is 'ventricular fibrillation'.

Also see
Venrticualr fibrillation
The commonest cuse of sudden death is due to myocardial ischemia / MI resulting in ventricular fibrillation.
Ref: Davidson 19th Ed. Pg-403
CVA
It is ischemia of CNS due to blockage of a blood vessel in supplying to CNS.

Ventricular asystole
This occurs when there is no electicial activity of the ventricles and is usually due to the failure of the conducting tissue or massive ventricular damage complicationg myocardial infarction.

Acute renal failure
Condition is characterised by rapid deterioration of kidneys ability to excrete wastes, concentrate unrine and conserve electrolytes, associated with oliguria, proteinuria, hematuria and uremia.

Q. 78. Positive benedict test is not with the following, except (KPSC-Lect/Physio-Bio/05)
- (a) Salicylates
- (b) Glucose
- (c) Vitamin C
- (d) Cholesterol

Ans. (b)
Note
Positive benedict test is with 'glucose' only.

Also see
Benedict's reagent can be used to test for the presence of glucose in urine. Glucose found to be present in urine is an indication of diabetes.
Procedure
5.0ml of Benedict's qualitative solution is mixed with 0.5ml of urine and the mixture is put in a boiling water bath for 5 minutes. The results are recorded thus:

Observation	Interpretation
No precipitate	—
Green	A trace
Yellow	+
Orange	++
Red	+++

Once sugar is detected in urine, further tests have to be undergone in order to ascertain which sugar is present. Only glucose is indicative of diabetes.

Refer: Textbook of Biochemistry, by S.P. Singh 4th Ed. Pg-386

Q. 79. Commonest site of cerebral embolism is (KPSC-Lect/Physio-Bio/05)
    (a)   Anterior cerebral artery
    (b)   Middle cerebral artery
    (c)   Posterior cerebral artery
    (d)   Posterior communicating artery

Ans. (b)
Note
Commonest site of cerebral embolism is 'middle cerebral artery'.

Also see
Cerebral embolism
25% of all systemic emboli reach the brain and 60% of them lodge in middle cerebral arterial territory.
Ref: API, 7th Ed. Pg. 803.

Q. 80. Oedipus complex has been described by (KPSC-Lect/Physio-Bio/05)
    (a)   Plato
    (b)   Socrates
    (c)   Freud
    (d)   Huxley

Ans. (c)
Note
Oedipus complex has been described by 'Freud'.

Also see
Freud believed that the genitals become the major focus of sexual excitement in the phallic stage. It is also at this time that he felt children develop sensual feeling towards the parent of opposite sex. Freud called these thoughts and feelings in boys the Oedipus complex after the mythical story of Oedipus, who unknowingly killed his father and married his mother.
Ref: Psychology by Morgan Pg. 581

Extended information
According to Freud, the observed difference between male and female genitalia may lead to childhood fantasy that the female genitalia result from loss of penis. The boy then develops castration complex, fearing castration at the hands of his father in retaliation for his desire to replace his father in his mother's affection. This leads to envious and aggressive feelings toward the father [the Oedipus complex; after the main character in Sophocles tragedy Oedipus Rex, who killed his father and married his mother without knowing the identity of either] this is resolved by identification with the parent of the same sex. A similar complex seen in the girl is called the Electra complex.

Q. 81. Radio-femoral delay occurs in (KPSC-PM/05)
    (a)   Coarctation of aorta
    (b)   ASD
    (c)   VSD
    (d)   PDA

Ans. (a)
Note
Radio-femoral delay occurs in 'Coarctation of aorta'.

Also see
Radiofemoral delay
The radial and femoral pulses are palpated simultaneously. An appreciable delay in the femoral pulse is suggestive of coarctation of the aorta. Coarctation of the aorta may lead to hypertension in the circulatory system serving the head and upper limbs.
In coarctation of aorta the femoral pulses are weak, and delayed in comparison with radial pulse.
Ref: Davidson 19th Ed, Pg-471

Q. 82. Eisenmongers Syndrome occurs in (KPSC-PM/05)
    (a)   PDA
    (b)   Heart failure
    (c)   MS
    (d)   AS

Ans. (a)

Note
Eisenmongers Syndrome occurs in 'PDA'.

Also see
A PDA is a persistent connection between the aorta and pulmonary artery. This connection would normally close shortly after birth. Eisenmenger's syndrome in rare instances may develop when in due course of time Pulmonary hypertension supervenes resulting in reversal of the shunt. The blood initially which was shunted from (Left to right) aorta high pressure ingredient to the pulmonary trunk (low pressure ingredient) is reversed (Right to left) resulting in deoxygenated blood reaching from pulmonty trunk to aorta ensuing in differential cyanosis (The lower extremities are cyanosed and upper extremities have normal pink color due to oxygenated unmixed blood supply).

Exrtended information
Eisenmenger's syndrome- In PDA if pulmonary vascular resistance increases, pulmonary artery pressure rises and may continue to do so until it equals or exceeds aortic pressure. The shunt through the defect may then reverse, causing central cyanosis, which may be more apparent in the feet and toes than in the upper part of the body. The murmur becomes quieter, may be confined to systole or may disappear. The ECG shows evidence of right ventricular hypertrophy.
Ref: Davidson 19th Ed, Pg-471

Q. 83. 'a' wave in the JVP corresponds to (KPSC-PM/05)
    (a)   Ventricular contraction
    (b)   Ventricular filling
    (c)   Atrial filling
    (d)   Atrial contraction

Ans. (d)

Note
'a' wave in JVP corresponds to 'atrial contraction'.

Also see
The positive 'a' wave is caused by the right atrial pressure transmitted to the jugular veins during right atrial systole, the 'a' wave peaks just before or during the first heart sound (S1) and before the onset of ventricular ejection (carotid pulse upstroke).

Extended information
Jugular veins usually depict three positive waves (a, c, v). The 'a' wave is due to atrial systole, 'c' wave is due to ballooning of tricuspid valve into the right atrium during systole, it is also due to transmitted carotid pulse, the 'v' wave that follows the 'x' descent is the wave of venous filling of the right atrium during ventricular systole.
Ref: API,7th Ed. Pg-361

Q. 84. Malignant hypertension occurs in (KPSC-PM/05)
    (a)   Diabetes mellitus
    (b)   Heart disease
    (c)   Renal disease
    (d)   None of above

Ans. (c)

Note
Malignant hypertension occurs in 'Renal disease'.

MCQ's in Practice of Medicine

Also see
Malignant hypertension is marked and rapid increase of blood pressure 200/140 mm Hg or more and the patient have pappilledema, retinal hemorrhages and hypertensive encephalopathy.
Ref: Harsh Mohan's textbook of pathology, short handbook, 5th Ed. Pg-510
Causes of Malignant hypertension are:
Renal diseases:
-Renal vascular disease
-Parenchymal renal disease, particularly glomerulonephritis
-Polycystic kidney disease
Ref: Davidson's 19th Ed. Pg-390

Extended information
Malignant hypertension affects about 1% of people with high blood pressure. It is more common in younger adult men. It also occurs in women with toxemia of pregnancy, and persons with kidney disorders or collagen vascular disorders.
Ref: http://www.nlm.nih.gov/medlineplus/ency/article/000491.htm

Q. 85. Specific enzyme detected in blood in Acute MI is (KPSC-PM/05)
    (a)   CPK-MB
    (b)   SGOT
    (c)   SGPT
    (d)   Aldosterone

Ans. (a)
Note
Specific enzyme detected in blood in Acute MI is 'CPK-MB'.

Also see
Creatine Phosphokinase - CPK-MB an enzyme is high in heart, 3 to 6 hours after myocardial infarction CPK-MB levels rise in blood and peaks at 12 to 24 hours and returns to normal 48 hours after infarcion. It does not rise with chest pain caused by angina, pulmonary embolism, or congestive cardiac failure.
The CPK isoenzyme, CPK-MB is more specific for cardiac tissue: its levels have been related to the extent of myocardial infarction.
Ref: API, 7th Ed. Pg-442

Q. 86. In respiratory distress syndrome of new born (RDS) (KPSC-PM/05)
    (a)   Cilia is devoid
    (b)   Mucous is collected
    (c)   Surfactant in alveoli is reduced
    (d)   None of above

Ans. (c)
Note
In respiratory distress syndrome of new born (RDS) 'surfactant in alveoli is reduced'.

Also see
Neonatal respiratory distress syndrome: entry of air into alveoli is essential for formation of neonatal RDS, i.e. dead born infants do not develop neonatal RDS. The basic defect in neonatal RDS is the deficiency of pulmonary surfactant, normally synthesized by Type-2 alveolar cells.
Ref: Harsh Mohan's textbook of pathology, short handbook, 5th Ed. Pg-331

Extended information
Respiratory distress syndrome
The disease is caused by a lack of lung surfactant, a chemical that normally appears in mature lungs. Surfactant keeps the air sacs from collapsing and allows them to inflate with air more easily.
In respiratory distress syndrome, the air sacs collapse and prevent the child from breathing properly. Symptoms usually appear shortly after birth and become progressively more severe.
Risk factors are prematurity, diabetes in the mother, and stress during delivery that produces acidosis in the newborn at birth.
Pathophysiology:

The development of RDS starts with damage to the alveolar epithelium and vascular endothelium resulting in increased permeability to plasma and inflammatory cells into the interstitium and alveolar space. Damage to the surfactant-producing Type II cells and the presence of protein-rich fluid in the alveolar space disrupts the production and function of pulmonary surfactant leading to microatelectasis and impaired gas exchange.
Clincial Features:
RDS is characterized by rapid breathing, nasal flaring, grunting noise with each breath, and blue around lips and nail beds, which indicates a lack of oxygen. Symptoms usually appear shortly after birth and become more severe over time.
Ref: http://en.wikipedia.org/wiki/Infant_respiratory_distress_syndrome#Prevention

Q. 87. Chronic Cor-pulmonale means (KPSC-PM/05)
    (a)   Heart failure
    (b)   Respiratory failure
    (c)   Heart disease secondary to lung disease
    (d)   Primary heart disease

Ans. (c)
Note
Chronic Cor-pulmonale means 'heart disease secondary to lung disease'.

Also see
Cor-pulmonale is a term used to describe the pathologic effects of lung disinfection on the right side of the heart. Pulmonary hypertension is the link between the two and common threat in all diseases of the lung is increased right ventricular after load. It is a form of secondary heart disease.
Ref: API,7th Ed. Pg-487

Extended information
Features of Cor-pulmonale are:
Cor pulmonale is characterized by; breathlessness, cough, hemoptysis, hyperresonance to percussion, diminished breath sounds, wheezing, distant heart sounds, cyanosis, distended neck veins, peripheral edema. Signs of RVH and Congestive heart failure.
Ref: http://en.wikipedia.org/wiki/Cor_pulmonale

Q. 88. If the unconscious patient is un-arousable by all external stimuli it is in (KPSC-PM/05)
    (a)   Stupor
    (b)   Deep sleep
    (c)   Dead
    (d)   Coma

Ans. (d)
Note
If the unconscious patient is un-arousable by all external stimuli it is in 'coma'.

Also see
Coma is the most severe state of impaired consciousness. It is a state of unarousable psychological unresponsiveness in which the subjects lie with eye closed. They show no psychologically understandable response to external stimulus or inner needs.
Ref: API,7th Ed. Pg-759

Extended information
Coma (from the Greek word koma, meaning deep sleep):
It is a profound state of unconsciousness. A comatose patient cannot be awakened, fails to respond normally to pain or light, does not have sleep-wake cycles, and does not take voluntary actions. Coma may result from a variety of conditions, including intoxication, metabolic abnormalities, central nervous system diseases, acute neurologic injuries such as stroke, and hypoxia.
Ref: http://en.wikipedia.org/wiki/Coma

Q. 89. Koilonychia is seen in (KPSC-PM/05)
    (a)   Vit C deficiency
    (b)   Malignancy

(c) Folic acid deficiency
(d) Iron deficiency anemia

Ans. (d)

Note

Koilonychia is seen in 'Iron deficiency anemia'.

Also see

Koilonychia (concave or spoon shaped nails) the nails are spoon shaped, the nail plate itself may be thinned, thickened or normal. In India iron deficiency anemia is a common cause but others can be cardiological, endocrinal or occupational causes.
Ref: API, 7th Ed. Pg-1322

Koilonychia

It is an abnormal shape of the fingernail where the nail has raised ridges and is thin and concave. This disorder is associated with iron deficiency anemia.
Ref: http://en.wikipedia.org/wiki/Koilonychia

Q. 90. For psoriasis palmaris important medicine is (KPSC-PM/05)
(a) Sulphur
(b) Arsenicum-iodatum
(c) Selenium
(d) Lycopodium clavatum

Ans. Use your discretion

Note

For psoriasis palmaris important medicine are 'Lyco and Phos' as per the Knerr repertory and on referring material medica of Boericke we find an indirect freference for selenium. Therefore there is not a unanimous reference in favour of a single remedy from above.

Also see

The choice of the most important medicine is from above is debatable.

Exended information

However, following are the reference from different Repertories:
Chapter Extremities- Eruption; Hand; Palm; Psoriasis: Aur, Calc, *Clem*, Crot-h, Graph, Hep, Kali-s, *Lyc*, *Merc*, *Mur-ac*, *Nat-s.*, Petr, PHOS, *Psor*, Sars, *Sel*, Sil, Sul-ac, *Sulph*.
Ref: kent Repertory
Chapter- Upper Extremity- Symptom/Rubric: Psoriasis palmaris affecting whole palm- Skookum Chuck.
Ref: Repertory - Gentry
Chapter; Upper Extremiety – Symptom / Rubric – Psoriasis palmamaris affecting whole palm itching and burning so that it was impossible to do any work; thick scales: Petr.
Ref: Repertory- Gentry
Chapter; Upper Limb – Symptom; Hand; Eruption; Psoriasis, affecting whole palm; *Petr*.
Ref: Repertory- Knerr
Repertory- Knerr-Chapter; Upper Limb – Symptom; Hand; Eruption; Psoriasis, on palms; **Lyco**.
Ref: Repertory- Knerr
Chapter; Upper Limb – Symptom; Hand; Eruption; Psoriasis, syphilitic, on palms; **Phos**.
Ref: Repertory- Knerr
Palms; Psoriasis: Petr, Phos, Sel.
Ref: Repertory- Phatak

See Materia Medica

Selenium: Skin; dry, scaly eruption in palms, with itching.
Ref: Boericke's materia medica

Q. 91. Stimulates the growth of epithelium on ulcerated surfaces and found useful in gastric and duodenal ulcer (KPSC-PM/05)
(a) Symphytum
(b) Sulphur
(c) Calcarea carbonica
(d) Arnica montana

Ans. (a)

Note
To stimulates the growth of epithelium on ulcerated surfaces 'symphytum is found useful in gastric and duodenal ulcer.

Also see
Symphytum
The root contains a crystalline solid that stimulates the growth of epithelium on ulcerated surfaces. It may be administered internally in the treatment of gastric and duodenal ulcers. Also in gastralgia, and externally in pruritus ani.
Ref: Boericke's materia medica

Q. 92. Faeco-oral route of spread of infection is found in (KPSC-PM/05)
    (a)   Hepatitis-B
    (b)   Hepatitis-C
    (c)   Hepatitis-D
    (d)   Hepatitis-E

Ans. (d)
Note
Faeco-oral route of spread of infection is found in 'hepatitis E'.
Also see
Hepatitis E

It is a liver disease caused by the hepatitis E virus (HEV). Transmission is faeco-oral route in most of the same way as hepatitis A virus. In India most of the epidemics of jaundice are due to 'hepatitis E'.
Ref: API, 7th Ed. Pg-596

Q. 93. Clinical finding not associated with typhoid fever (KPSC-PM/05)
    (a)   Splenomegaly
    (b)   Rose-spots
    (c)   Erythema marginatum
    (d)   Abdominal distention

Ans. (c)
Note
Clinical finding not associated with typhoid fever is 'erythema maraginatum'.
Also see

'Erythema marginatum' is the clinical finding not associated with typhoid fever; however, it is seen in patients with rheumatic fever, primarily on the trunk. Lesions are pink-red in color, flat to mildly elevated, and transient.
Ref: Harrison 15th Edition, Section 9- Alternations in skin.

Extended information
The classical symptoms associated with typhoid are:
Gradual onset of fever showing step ladder pattern, headache, abdominal discomfort, nausea, vomiting, constipation, diarrhea, cough, malaise, anorexia, and nose bleeds.
Classical signs include fever, typhoid facies towards the end of first week with dull and heavy look. Abdominal tenderness and splenomegaly occur in majority.
Rose spots appear on the 7th to 10th day starting from abdomen.
Signs of enteric fever includes furred tongue, loose and pale stools (pea soup stools).
Ref: API, 7th Ed. Pg-50-51

Q. 94. Bradycardia is seen in the following situations except (KPSC-PM/05)
    (a)   Hyperthyroidism
    (b)   Obstructive jaundice
    (c)   Hypothyroidism
    (d)   Complete heart block

Ans. (a)

Note
Bradycardia is seen all of above situations except 'Hyperthyroidism'.
Also see
Bradycardia:
- Pulse rate < 60 / min
Causes:
1. Physiological: Atheletes, Sleep
2. Pathological: Severe Hypoxia, Hypothermia, Sick sinus syndrome, Myxedema, Obstructive jaundice, Acute inferior wall infarction, Raised ICT, IIIO heart blocks, drugs (beta blockers, Verapamil, diltiazen, digoxin).
Ref: http://www.tnhealth.org/facts/bradycardia.htm

Q. 95. What is wrong about Kwashiorkor? (KPSC-PM/05)
    (a)   Severe wasting
    (b)   Generelised edemas
    (c)   Low serum albumin
    (d)   Moon face

Ans. (c)
Note
The 'low serum albumin is main feature of kwashiorkor'.
Also see
PEM-has two severe forms, Kwashiorkor and marasmus. Features of Kwashiorkor include:
    -Edema
    -Moon face: cheeks may be swollen with fluid or fatty tissue.
    -Growth retardation
    -Child is irritable
    -Hair looses its healthy sheen and becomes silkier and thinner
    -Dermatosis
    -Respiratory tract infections, diarrhea or dysentery
    -Serum albumin is < 3gms/dl
Ref: API, 7th Ed. Pg-231,232

Extended information
The basic fault with Kwashiorkor is low seum albumion, which secondarily manifests in sign & symptoms which are listed above.
Kwashiorkor occurs most commonly in areas of famine, limited food supply, and low levels of education, which can lead to inadequate knowledge of proper diet.
Early symptoms of any type of malnutrition are very general and include fatigue, irritability, and lethargy. As protein deprivation continues, growth failure, loss of muscle mass, generalized swelling (edema), and decreased immunity occur.

Q. 96. All are features of vitamin A deficiency except (KPSC-PM/05)
    (a)   Xerophthalmia
    (b)   Osteomalacia
    (c)   Follicular hyperkeratosis
    (d)   Keratomalacia

Ans. (b)
Note
All of the above fecataures of vit 'A' deficiencyt except 'osteomalacia'.
Also see
Osteomalacia
When the newly formed bone of the growth plate does not mineralize, the growth plate becomes thick, wide and irregular. This results in the clinical diagnosis of rickets, and is seen only in children because adults no longer have growth plates. When the remodeled bone does not mineralize, osteomalacia occurs, and this happens in all ages.
Ref: http://courses.washington.edu/bonephys/hypercalU/opmal2.html

Extended information
Osteomalacia is 'adult rickets' and is due to vitamin D deficiency.
However, conditions that may lead to osteomalacia include inadequate dietary intake of vitamin D, inadequate exposure to sunlight (ultraviolet radiation), which produces vitamin D in the body and malabsorption of vitamin D by the intestines.
Features of vitamin A deficiency are as under:
- Night blindness
- Bitots spots
- Conjuctival xerosis
- Keratomalacia
- Follicular keratosis

Ref: API, 7th Ed.Pg-240

Q. 97. Continuous murmur is heard in (KPSC-PM/05)
- (a) Atrial septal defect
- (b) Ventricular septal defect
- (c) Fallot's tetralogy
- (d) Patent-ductus arteriosus

Ans. (d)
Note
Continuous murmur is heard in 'PDA'.
Also see
Patent ductus arteriosus (PDA) is a condition where a temporary blood vessel near an unborn baby's heart, the ductus arteriosus, fails to close after birth. (The blood vessel normally closes after birth because it is no longer needed). The word "patent" means open.
A stethoscope examination (auscultation) of the heart usually reveals a loud, continuous murmur (the sound of the blood rushing across the hole).
Continuous murmurs are audible uninterrupted throughout the cardiac cycle. The blood flow is in the same direction throughout. They are caused by flow of blood from high to low pressure areas, e.g. in patent ductus arteriosus.
Ref: API, 7th Ed. Pg-364

Q. 98. The part of electrocardiogram that corresponds with ventricular depolarisation is (KPSC-PM/05)
- (a) P wave
- (b) QRS complex
- (c) PR interval
- (d) ST-segment

Ans. (b)
Note
The part of electrocardiogram that corresponds with ventricular depolarisation is 'QRS Complex'
Also see
QRS complex is the deflection produced by ventricular depolarization.
Ref: API, 7th Ed. Pg-366

Extended information
Depolarization of the heart is the initiating event for cardiac contraction. The electric currents that spread through the heart are produced by three components: cardiac pacemaker cells, specialized conduction tissue, and the heart muscle itself. The ECG, however, records only the depolarization (stimulation) and repolarization (recovery) potentials generated by the atrial and ventricular myocardium. The part of electro cardiogram that corresponds with ventricular depolarisation is 'QRS' complex.

Q. 99. The parameter is Liver function Test that is suggestive of acute parenchymal liver damage is (KPSC-PM/05)
- (a) Decreased serum albumin
- (b) Increased alkaline phosphatase

(c) Increased SGPT
(d) Increased acid phosphatase

Ans. (c)
Note
The parameter is liver function test that is suggestive of acute parenchymal liver damage is 'SGPT'.
Also see

Serum aminotransferases includes SGOT and SGPT. They are elevated in most liver disorders. Highest elevations are found in conditions causing extensive hepatic necrosis such as severe acute viral hepatitis, toxic hepatitis or prolonged circulatory collapse. Lesser elevations are found in mild acute viral hepatitis, diffuse and focal liver disease like chronic active hepatitis, cirrhosis and hepatic metastasis.
SGPT elevation is more specific for liver damage then SGOT.
Ref: API, 7th Ed. Pg-585

Q. 100. Massive splenomegaly can be caused by all of the following except (KPSC-PM/05)
(a) Typhoid fever
(b) Chronic myeloid leukemia
(c) Kala azar
(d) Chronic malaria

Ans. (a)
Note
Massive splenomegaly can be caused by all of the following except 'Typhoid fever'.
Also see
Degree of splenomegaly varies with the disease:
Mild enlargement (upto 5cm):
 -Occurs in congestive heart failure, acute malaria, typhoid fever, bacterial endocarditis, SLE, RA, thalassaemia minor.
Moderate enlargement (upto umbilicus):
 -Occurs in hepatitis, cirrhosis, lymphomas, infectious mononucleosis, hemolytic anemia, splenic abscesses and amyloidosis.
Massive enlargement (below umbilicus):
 -Occurs in CML, myeloid metaplasia with myelofibrosis, storage diseases, thalassemia major, chronic malaria, leishmaniasis (kala azar) and portal vein obstruction.
Ref: Pathology by Harsh Mohan, 2nd Ed, Pg-325,326

Q. 101. What is not true regarding peripheral cyanosis? (KPSC-PM/05)
(a) It is produced by increased extraction of oxygen from the stagnant blood by the tissues.
(b) The extremities are blue and warm.
(c) The earlobes and tip of nose are usually cyanosed.
(d) It is usually associated with hypotension.

Ans. (b)
Note
Not true regarding peripheral cyanosis is that the 'extremities are blue and warm'.
Also see
In case of peripheral cynosis the extremities are blue and cold. Therefore the statement given at (b) is not rue.
Ref: Kumar and Clark, clinical medicine, 6th Ed.-735

Extended information
Cyanosis
It is the bluish discolouration of the skin and mucous membrane due to the presence of reduced hemoglobin exceeding 5g % in the circulation. Therefore in gross anemia, when hemoglobin is less than 5g %, no cyanosis occurs.
Cynosis can be of following type:
a. Central cyanosis:

It is seen at the tip of nose, lips, tip of tongue. With central cyanosis extremities are warm to touch.
Causes:
> Cardiovascular
> -Congenital cyanotic heart diseases, Left ventricular failure, Congestive cardiac failure.
> Respiratory
> -Pulmonary edema, emphysema, cor-pulmonale, status asthmaticus, pleural effusion, asphyxia neonatorum, pulmonary infarction, spontaneous pneumothorax, polycythemia vera, bulbar paralysis.

b. Peripheral cyanosis:
It is seen in the extremities and they are cold to touch.
Causes:
> -Raynaud's disease, scleroderma, buerger's disease.

Ref: An Introduciton to Case Taking for Homeopaths (Under Print)

Q. 102. Commonest cause of community acquired pneumonia is (KPSC-PM/05)
- (a) Streptococcus pneumoniae
- (b) Staphylococcus aureus
- (c) Hemophilus influenzes
- (d) Klebsiella pneumoniae

Ans. (a)
Note
The commonest cause of community acquired pneumonia is 'Streptococcus pneumoniae'
Also see
Common organisms of community acquired pneumonia:
> -Streptococcus pneumoniae (frequency-30%)
> -Chlamydia pneumoniae (10%)
> -Mycoplasma pneumoniae '(9%)
> -Legionella pneumoniae (5%)

Ref: Davidson 19th Ed, Pg-527

Extended information
Pneumonia is an infection of the lung parenchyma. Community-acquired pneumonia refers to pneumonia acquired outside of hospitals or extended-care facilities. Streptococcus pneumoniae remains the most commonly identified pathogen in community-acquired pneumonia.

Q. 103. Predisposition to bronchogenie carcinoma is seen with (KPSC-PM/05)
- (a) Silicosis
- (b) Byssinosis
- (c) Coal worker's pneumoconiosis
- (d) Asbestosis

Ans. (d)
Note
Asbestos exposure is a recognized risk factor for the development of a number of respiratory diseases including carcinoma of lung and larynx.
Ref: Davidson, 19th Ed. Pg-558

Also See
Silicosis
It is a fibrotic lung disease caused by inhalation of silica.
It predisposes to:
> -Increased incidence of tuberculosis
> -Progressive fibrosis
> -Emphysema
> -Cor-pulmonale.

Byssinosis
It is an occupational disease of lungs caused by allergic reaction (Occupaional asthma) to the cotton fibers produced while processing the cotton.

It predisposes to:
- Chronic bronchitis and emphysema

Coal workers pneumoconiosis
It is a lung disease caused by inhalation of coal dust for prolonged period.
It Predisposes to:
- Cor-pulmonale
- Pulomnary tuberculosis.

Asbestosis
It is a lung disease caused by inhaling asbestos fibers.
It Predisposes to:
- Bronchogenic carcinoma

Ref: Kumar and Clark 6th Ed, Pg-946

Q. 104. Tension Pneumothorax causes all the following clinical signs, except (KPSC-PM/05)
(a) Severs dyspnea
(b) Displacement of mediastinum
(c) Increased vocal resonance
(d) Hyper resonant percussion note

Ans. (c)
Note
Tension pneumothorax causes; severe dyspnea, displacement of mediastinum, hyperresonant percussion note and decreased vocal resonance. Therefore the (c) Increased vocal resonsnce is not corrent sign. As the air is not a good conductor of sound.

Also see
Pneumothorax causes mediastinal displacement towards the opposite side, and results in rapidly progressive breathlessness associated with marked tachycardia, hypotension and cyanosis.
Ref: Davidson 19th Ed, Pg-571

Q. 105. Which of the following "statements is not true of Type 1 Diabetes mellitus"? (KPSC-PM/05)
(a) They are usually obese
(b) Absolute insulin deficiency
(c) Polyuria, polydipsia and nocturia are frequent
(d) More prone for keto acidosis

Ans. (a)
Note
All of the above statements are in favour of Type I Diabetes mellitus except (a) they are usually obese. Type II Diabetes / Adult onset diabetes is associated with obesity. The obesity is a risk factor for Type II DM.

Also see
Type I diabetes
Type 1 diabetes mellitus is characterized by loss of the insulin-producing beta cells of the islets of Langerhans in the pancreas, leading to a deficiency of insulin. It is also called as "juvenile diabetes" because it represents a majority of cases of diabetes affecting children.

Type II diabetes
Type 2 diabetes mellitus is due to insulin resistance or reduced insulin sensitivity, combined with reduced insulin secretion.
Central obesity (fat concentrated around the waist in relation to abdominal organs, but not subcutaneous fat) is known to predispose individuals for insulin resistance. Abdominal fat is especially active hormonally, secreting a group of hormones called adipokines that may possibly impair glucose tolerance. Obesity is found in approximately 55% of patients diagnosed with type 2 diabetes. Other factors include ageing and family history (type 2 is much more common in those with close relatives who have had it).
Ref: http://en.wikipedia.org/wiki/Diabetes_mellitus

Q. 106. Thyrotoxicosis is characterised by the following features, except (KPSC-PM/05)
(a) Tachycardia
(b) Constipation

(c) Tremor
(d) Weight loss

Ans. (b)

Note
The features given above - tachycardia, tremor and weight loss point to thyrotoxicosis except constipation.

Also see
Features of hypothyroidism are: slow, dry hair, thick skin, deep voice, weight gain, cold intolerance, bradycardia and constipation.
Ref: Kumar & Clark, 6th Ed. Pg-1072

Extended information
Other features of hypothyroidism include: sluggishness, cold sensitivity, depression, forgetfulness, dry hair, dry skin, weight gain.

Q. 107. Hypertension is a feature of all the following except (KPSC-PM/05)
(a) Renal artery stenosis
(b) Pheochromocytoma
(c) Addison's disease
(d) Cushing's syndrome

Ans. (c)

Note
Hypertension is a feature of all above except 'Addison's disease'. Rather, Hypotension is a feature of 'Addison's disease'.

Also see
Features of Addison's disease are:
 -Muscle weakness
 -Loss of appetite, loss of weight
 -Nausea, diarrhea, or vomiting
 -Hypotension; worse when standing (orthostatic hypotension)
 -Hyperpigmentation; cutaneous and oral mucosa.
 -Mentally: irritable, depression.
 -Desire: craving for salt and salty foods
 -Menses: becomes irregular or cease
 -Axillary or pubic hypotrichosis.
Investigation:
 -Hypoglycemia (low blood sugar)
 -Hyponatraemia (low blood sodium levels)
 -Hyperkalemia (Raised blood potassium levels)
 -TLC; Increased number of eosinophils
Ref: http://en.wikipedia.org/wiki/Addison's_disease

Q. 108. Trousseau's sign is characteristic of (KPSC-PM/05)
(a) Hyperthyroidism
(b) Hypothyroidism
(c) Tetanus
(d) Tetany

Ans. (d)

Note
Trousseau's sign is characteristic of latent 'Tetany'.

Also see
Tetany is a medical sign, the involuntary contraction of muscles.
Cause:
Low serum calcium, uderfunction of the parathyroid gland can lead to tetany.
Low levels of carbon dioxide causes tetany as seen in cases of hyperventilation syndrome of anxious patients.

Extended information
Trousseau's sign is named on 'Armand Trousseau' (October 14, 1801 — June 27, 1867) French physician who first described the Trousseau sign.
Procedure:
Place blood pressure cuff is placed around the arm and inflated to a pressure above the systolic blood pressure and held in place for 3 minutes. If carpal spasm occurs, manifested as flexion at the wrist and metacarpophalangeal joints, extension of the distal interphalangeal and proximal interphalangeal joints, and adduction of the thumb and fingers, the sign is said to be positive and the patient likely has hypocalcemia.
Value:
This sign may become positive (in case of latent tetany) before other gross manifestations of hypocalcemia such as hyperreflexia and tetany, but is generally believed to be less sensitive than the Chvostek sign for hypocalcemia.
Ref: http://en.wikipedia.org/wiki/Trousseau_sign_of_latent_tetany

Extended information
Clinical features of hypoparathyroidism:
- Paraesthesiae, circumoral numbness, cramps and anxiety
- Tetany
- Chvostek's sign: gentle tapping over facial nerve causes twitching of ipsilateral facial muscles.
- Trousseau's sign: inflation of sphygmomanometer cuff above systolic pressure for 3 min induces tetanic spasm.

Ref: Kumar & Clark, 6th Ed. Pg-1095

Q. 109. Ptosis is caused by paralysis of (KPSC-PM/05)
    (a) III Cranial Nerve
    (b) IV Cranial Nerve
    (c) V Cranial Nerve
    (d) VI Cranial Nerve

Ans. (a)
Note
Ptosis is caused by paralysis of III cranial nerve the 'Occulomotor'.

Also see
In 3rd nerve palsy ptosis is usually complete, extraocular muscle palsy (eye 'down and out') and depending on site of lesion, other cranial nerve lesion palsies (e.g. 4, 5, 6) or contralateral upper motor neuron signs.
Ref: Davidson's, 19th Ed. Pg-1156
However review the following:
a. The III cranial nerve is Occulomotor; it supplies to levator palpabrae superioris, rectus medialis, rectus superioris, rectus inferioris, and inferior oblique. Third cranial nerve paralysis is associated double vision and drooping of eyelid (Ptosis).
b. The IV cranial nerve is Trochlear and supplies to superior oblique.
c. The V cranial nerve is Trigeminal and is predominantly sensory to face having three divisions ophthalmic, maxillary, mandibuar, and has a small motor part.
d. The VI cranial nerve is abducent and supplies rectus latralis.
Ref: Anatomy by Chaurisia Vol III

Extended Information
Ptosis is an abnormally low position (drooping) of the upper eyelid.
Causes:
Ptosis occurs when the muscles that raise the eyelid (levator and müller's muscles) are not strong enough to do so properly. It can affect one eye or both eyes and is more common in the elderly, as muscles in the eyelids may begin to deteriorate. One can, however, be born with ptosis, congenital ptosis. Congenital ptosis is not hereditary. Causes of congenital ptosis remain unknown. Ptosis may be caused by damage/trauma to the muscle which raises the eyelid, or damage to the nerve (3rd cranial nerve (oculomotor nerve)) which controls this muscle. Such damage could be a sign or symptom of an underlying disease such as diabetes mellitus, a brain tumor, and diseases which may cause weakness in muscles or nerve damage, such as myaesthenia gravis.
Classification:
Depending upon the cause it can be classified into:
    - Neurogenic ptosis which includes IIIrd cranial nerve palsy, Horner's Syndrome, Marcus Gunn jaw winking syndrome, IIIrd cranial nerve misdirection.

Homeopathically: Causticum
- Myogenic ptosis which includes myasthenia gravis, myotonic dystrophy, ocular myopathy, simple congenital ptosis, blepharophimosis syndrome

Homeopathically: Gelsemium (myasthemic cause)
- Aponeurotic ptosis which may be involutional or post-operative.

Homeopathically: Causticum, Silicea (Stricture) Thiosinaminum (Stricutre)
- Mechanical ptosis which occurs due to edema or tumors of the upper lid.
- Neurotoxic ptosis which is a classic symptom of envenomation by cobras or kraits. Neurotoxic ptosis is a precursor to respiratory failure and eventual suffocation caused by complete paralysis of the thoracic diaphragm. *Urgent medical intervention is therefore required.*

Ref: http://en.wikipedia.org/wiki/Ptosis_ (eyelid)

Q. 110. Short-shuffling gait is characteristic of (KPSC-PM/05)
(a) Parkinsonism
(b) Cerebellar dysfunction
(c) Sensory ataxia
(d) Proximal myopathy

Ans. (a)

Note
Short-shuffling gait is characteristic of Parkinsonism.

Also see

Parkinsonism
It has characteristic short 'shuffling gait'.

Cerebellar dysfunction
Is characterized by typical 'drunken gait'.

Sensoty ataxia (Tabes dorsalis)
Has typical 'thumping gait'/ 'high stepping gait'.

Proximal myopahty
Is having a characteristic 'duck gait' / 'waddling gait'.

Q. 111. All are characteristic features of hemolysis, except (KPSC-PM/05)
(a) Reticulocytosis
(b) Indirect hyperbilirubinemia
(c) Absent urobilinogers in urine
(d) Polychromasia

Ans. (c)

Note
All are characteristic features of hemolysis, except 'absent urobilinogen in urine'.

Also see
All above are the characteristic features of hemolysis except 'Absent urobilinogen in urine' as absence of urobilinogen is not found in case of hemolysis or hemolytic anemia.

Reticulocytosis
Reticulocytosis is a condition where there is an increase in reticulocytes. It is commonly seen in anemia. A reticulocyte is an immature red blood cell that appears especially during regeneration of lost blood.

Causes of unconjugated (Indirect) hyperbilirubinemia
Increased production of bilirubin (hemolytic anemias, shortened red cell life due to immaturity or transfused cells, increased enterohepatic circulation, infection)

Absence of urobilinogen in urine
It indicates the obstructive jaundice. When the bile salts reach the intestine via the common bile duct, the bilirubin is acted on by bacteria to form chemical compounds called urobilinogens. Most of the urobilinogen is excreted in the feces; some is reabsorbed and goes through the liver again and a small amount is excreted in the urine. Urobilinogen gives feces their dark color. An absence of bilirubin in the intestine, such as may occur with bile duct obstruction, blocks the conversion of bilirubin to urobilinogen, resulting in clay-colored stools.

Polychromasia
New red cells contain RNA, which they lose after 1-2 days in the circulation. Enumerating reticulocytes therefore gives a measure of marrow red cell production. The RNA can only be seen in a specially-stained

blood film, as a 'reticulum' (hence the name). On the regular blood film, reticulocytes have a greyish tinge, which is known as 'polychromasia'.

Q. 112. Spasticity is a feature of (KPSC-PM/05)
    (a) Pyramidal lesion
    (b) Extra pyramidal lesion
    (c) Cerebellar lesion
    (d) LMN lesion

Ans. (a)

Note
Spasticity is a feature of 'pyramidal lesion'.

Also see
Spasticity (clasp knife) is a feature of pyramidal lesion, it affects the anti-gravity muscles.
Ref: API, 7th Ed. Pg-732
Features of Pyramidal lesions:
    -Muscle tone is raised -The spasticity is a feature of pyramidal lesion. It affects antigravity muscles.
    -DTR's are increased.
    -Plantar is Extensor.
Features of Extra pyramidal lesion:
    -Tremors (Pil rolling as in parkinson's disease), choreoform movements; as in chorea, and athetosis.
    -Cog-wheel rigidity.
Features of cerebellar lesion:
    -Intention tremors, nystagmus, dysdidocokinesia, past pointing, incoordinaion.
Features of Lower motor neuron lesion:
    -Loss of tone in muscles and flaccidity.
    -Loss of DTR's
    -Plantar is lost.

Q. 113. Which of the following is not a feature of Systemic Lupus Erythematosus? (KPSC-PM/05)
    (a) Malar Rash
    (b) Leucocytosis
    (c) Serositis
    (d) Anti-DNA antibodies

Ans. (b)

Note
All of above are features of SLE, except 'Leucocytosis' i.e. Malar rash, Serositis and anti-DNA antibodies are features of Systemic Lupus Erythmatosis.

Also see
Classical features of SLE are:
    -Malar rash
    -Discoid lupus
    -Photosensitivity
    -Arthritis
    -Serositis
    -Renal: proteinuria
    -Neurological: seizures, psychosis
    -Hematological: hemolytic anemia, leucopenia, lymphopenia, thrombocytopenia
    -Immunologic feature: Anti-DNA antibody
Ref: API, 7th Ed. Pg-1174

Extended information
A useful mnemonic for SLE is:

'SOAP BRAIN MD'
    -**S**erositis
    -**O**ral ulcers
    -**A**rthritis

-**P**hotosensitivity
-**B**lood Changes
-**R**enal involvement (proteinuria or casts)
-**A**NA positive
-**I**mmunological changes
-**N**eurological signs (seizures, frank psychosis)
-**M**alar Rash
-**D**iscoid Rash

Q. 114. A 22 year old primi gravida on her 7th day of full term normal delivery, developed headache, vomiting, convulsion and weakness both legs. The most likely diagnosis is (KPSC-PM/05)
(a) Thrombosis of the middle cerebral artery
(b) Intracranial hemorrhage
(c) Brain abscess
(d) Superior sagital sinus thrombosis

Ans. (d)
Note
Above clinical presentation suggests to the diagnosis of 'Superior sagital sinus thrombosis.
Also see
Clinical features of superior sagital sinus are:
-Headache, papilledema, seizures
-May involve veins of both hemispheres, causing advancing motor and sensory focal deficits
Ref: Davidson's 19th Ed. Pg- 1168

Extended information
The fearures of superior sagital sinus thrombosis are:
Headache, vomiting, convulsions and weakness of both lower legs suggest central nervous system insult. The cause is acute and it is involving both lower limbs – the lesions that can cause this type of functional motor loss, is situated in relation to super sagittal sinus at vertex and that is precentral gyrus (upper part which is related to motor activity of lower limbs) is situated. Therefore, thrombosis of superior sagittal sinus is only possibility.

Q. 115. HBsAG is found to be associated with (KPSC-PM/05)
(a) Polymyositis
(b) Rheumatoid arthritis
(c) Polyarteritis nodosa
(d) SLE

Ans. (c)
Note
HBsAG is found to be associated with 'Polyarteritis nodosa'.
Also see
Hepatitis B is a risk factor, and the incidence of PAN is ten times higher in the unit population of Alaska, where hepatitis B infection is endemic.
Ref Davidson's 19th Ed. Pg-1042
PAN may be associated with drug abuse and hepatitis B infection.
Ref: Kumar and Clark 6th Ed. Pg-635
HBsAg: Hepatitis B surface antigen is a marker of infecticvity. Its presence indicates either acute or chronic HBV infection. There is a well established association between infection with both hepatitis B and C viruses and Polyarteritis nodosa, although not all patients are infected with one of these viruses.
Ref: Cecil, 6th Ed, Pg-769

Q. 116. HemophiIia-A is (KPSC-PM/05)
(a) X linked dominant
(b) Mucosal bleeding is a common presentation
(c) Due to factor IX deficiency
(d) Manifested only in males

Ans. (d)

Note
Hemophilia-A is manifested only in males.
Also see
In haemophilia A, the level of factor VIII is reduced. It is inherited as an X-linked disorder. If a female carrier has a son, he has 50% chance of having hemophilia and a daughter has a 50% chance of being a carrier. All daughters of men with hemophilia are carriers and sons are normal.
Ref: Kumar & Clark, 6th Ed. Pg-472

Extended information
Haemophilia A is a X-linked, recessively inherited bleeding disorder which results from deficiency of procoagulant factor VIII (FVIII). Affected males suffer from joint and muscle bleeds and easy bruising, the severity of which is closely correlated with the level of activity of coagulation factor VIII (FVIII:C) in their blood.

Among the genes and chromosomes we inherit from our parents are two sex chromosomes, labeled X and Y. Females inherit two X chromosomes, one from the mother and one from the father. Males inherit one X chromosome from the mother and one Y chromosome from the father. If a person inherits only X chromosomes that have the hemophilia gene, then that person will have hemophilia.

Q. 117. Features of cushing's syndrome include the following, except (KPSC-PM/05)
(a) Centripetal obesity
(b) Hypotension
(c) Striae
(d) Osteoporosis

Ans. (b)
Note
Cushing's syndrome includes the all of the above, except 'hypotension'.
Also see
Clinical features of Cushing's syndrome:
Symptoms:
-Depression
-Insomnia
-Amenorrhea / oligomenorrhea
-Poor libido
-Hair growth
-Polyuria / polydipsia
-Psychosis
Signs:
-Moon face
-Plethora
-Thin skin, bruising
-Hypertension
-Osteoporosis
-Striae (purple or red)
-Proximal myopathy
-Buffalo hump
-Hirsutism, acne
-Central obesity
Ref: Kumar and Clark, 6th Ed. Pg-1085

Q. 118. Murphy's sign is characteristic of (KPSC-PM/05)
(a) Acute pancreatitis
(b) Intestinal obstruction
(c) Acute cholecystitis
(d) Acute pericarditis

Ans. (c)
Note
Murphy's sign is characteristically encountered in acute cholecystitis.

Also see
Feataures of acute cholecystitis:
Patient complains of acute pain during deep inspiration with inspiratory arrest when tender inflamed gallbladder comes down and touches the palpating fingers.
Ref: S.Das, 3rd Ed. Pg-902

Extended information
Positive Murlphy's sign is a characteristic of acute cholecystitis.
Technique:
a. Maneuver: deep subcostal palpation on inspitration.
b. Positive: worsened pain and inspiratory arrest.
Suggests:
   -Acute cholecystitis.

Q. 119. Non pulsatile distended neck viens are likely to be due to (KPSC-PM/05)
   (a)   Congestive heart failure
   (b)   Portal hypertension
   (c)   Pericardial effusion
   (d)   Mediastinal obstruction

Ans. (d)
Note
The most likely cause of non-pulsatile distended neck veins from choice given above is 'Meidiastinal obstruction'. Leading to 'Superior vena cava syndrome'

Also see
Superior vena cava syndrome':
Superior vena cava is the big vein that drains the head and neck and both upper extremities. When this vein gets blocked it can result in superior vena cava syndrome.
Common causes:
Lung cancer extending into the vein, invasion/involvement from lymphoma, breast cancer, thrombosis, thyroid cancer, thymus gland tumor.
Sign & Symtoms:
Facial swelling, facial edema, neck edema, facial plethora and cyanosis, prominent neck veins, prominent chest veins, shortness of breath, cough, tachypnea, Horner's syndrome, feeling of fullness in eyes and ear.
Ref: www.diseasesdatabase.

Q. 120. Koilonychia is seen in (KPSC-PM/05)
   (a)   Wilson's Disease
   (b)   Iron deficiency anemia
   (c)   Hemochromatosin
   (d)   Megaloblastic anemia

Ans. (b)
Note
Koilonychia (concave or spoon shaped nails):
The nails are spoon shaped; the nail plate itself may be thinned, thickened or normal. In India, iron deficiency anemia is a common cause.
Ref: API, 7th Ed. Pg-1322

Also see
Koilonychia is seen in iron deficiency anemia is present when the hemoglobin level is less than 6 gm% for a longer period of time as a full growth of nail take place in 6 months.

Q. 121. Pyogenic Meningitis in Pre-School Children—the commonest organism is (KPSC-PM/05)
   (a)   Hemophilus influenza
   (b)   Group B streptococci
   (c)   Neisseria meningitidis
   (d)   E Coli

Ans. (c)

Note
Pyogenic meningitis in Pre-School Children—the commonest organism is Neisseria meningitidis.

Also see
Hemophilus influenza B (Hib) is a bacteria. It is not related to "Influenza" (the flu). Before the widespread use of the Hib vaccine, this was the most common bacterial meningitis in children between two months and five years.
Neisseria meningitidis:
"Neisseria meningitidis", also known as "Meningococcal meningitis", is one of the most common causes of bacterial meningitis. Meningitis is inflammation of the membranes, called meninges, covering the brain and spinal cord. It has a high mortality rate if it goes untreated; death can occur within a few hours of onset. Mostly adults are infected.

Q. 122. Haematemesis is commonly caused by all of the following except (KPSC-PM/05)
  (a) Duodenal ulcer
  (b) Carcinoma of stomach
  (c) Liver abscess
  (d) Erosive gastritis

Ans. (c)
Note
Haematemesis is common in all of above except 'Liver abscess'.

Also see
Causes of haematemesis:
    -Prolonged and vigorous retching causing tear in blood vessels of the throat or the esophagus, resulting in streaks of blood in the vomit.
    -Bleeding ulcer located in the stomach, duodenum, or esophagus
    -Erosion of esophagus or stomach
    -Bleeding esophageal varices
    -Tumors / cancer of the stomach or esophagus
    -Esophagitis
    -Gastritis
    -Ingested blood i.e. swallowed after a nosebleed)
Ref: http://www.nlm.nih.gov/medlineplus/ency/article/003118.htm

Q. 123. Incubation period of chicken pox is (KPSC-PM/05)
  (a) 7 days
  (b) 14 days
  (c) 21 days
  (d) 28 days

Ans. (b)
Note
The incubation period for chicken pox is usually 14 to 16 days, although extremes as wide as 7 – 21 days have been preported.
Ref: Park and Park, 18th Ed, P-123

Q. 124. Features of increased intra-cranial tension include all of the following except (KPSC-PM/05)
  (a) Headache
  (b) Vomiting
  (c) Hypertension
  (d) Tachycardia

Ans. (d)
Note
Features of increased 'Intra-cranial tension' include all of the following except 'tachycardia'.

Also see
Clinical features of raised intracranial pressure:
    -Severe headache
    -Vomiting: projectile

-Papiledema
-Bradycardia
-Hypertension
-Respiratory irregularities
-Pupillary dilatation

Ref: API, 7th Ed. Pg-755

Extended information
Bradycardia (rate less than 60 beats per minute):
Physiological:
In athletes.
Pathological:
Relative bradycardia (rate not proportionate to the raised temperature):
-Typhoid first week,
-Meningitis,
-Dengue,
-Influenza.
Endocrinal: myxedema.
Obstructive jaundice.
Increased intracranial tension.
Cardiac arrhythmias: heart block.

Q. 125. Lumbar puncture is contraindicated in (KPSC-PM/05)
(a) Meningitis
(b) Subarachnoid hemorrhage
(c) Guillain Barre syndrome
(d) Raised intracranial tension

Ans. (d)
Note
Lumbar puncture is contraindicated in case of raised intracranial pressure (brain tumor) due to the possibility of herniation of brain stem.
Also see
However, in case of meningitis, subsarachnoid hemorrhoage and Guillain Barre syndrome it is an exception and provides very useful diagnostic information.

Q. 126. Hyperpigmentation is not a feature of (KPSC-PM/05)
(a) Pheochromocytoma
(b) Hemochromatosis
(c) Addison's diseases
(d) Nelson's syndrome

Ans. (a)
Note
The hyperpigmentation is not a feature of 'Pheochromocytoma'.
Also see
Pheochromocytoma
Pheochronocytoma usually has 3 classic symptoms; headache, sweating, and heart palpitations (a fast heart beat).
Hemochromatosis
A darkish colour to the skin (hence its called as 'Bronze diabetes' when it was first described by Armand Trousseau in 1865)
Addison's disease
Addison's disease is characterised by lethargy, weakness, nausea, vomiting, and weight loss, pigmentation of skin and mucous membrane.
Nelson's syndrome
It is characterised by hyperpigmentation, headaches, vision impairment, and the cessation of menstrual periods in women.
Pituitary-dependent hypersecretion of ACTH results in two clinical conditions that are of particular interest to the neurosurgeon:

(a) Cushing's disease and Nelson's syndrome. Cushing's disease is the hypersecretion of ACTH by a pituitary source, usually a pituitary adenoma that causes bilateral adrenal cortical hyperplasia and consequent hypercortisolism.
(b) Nelson's syndrome, which some patients develop after undergoing adrenalectomy for the treatment of Cushing's disease, is the hypersecretion of ACTH by a pituitary adenoma that results in cutaneous hyperpigmentation.

Ref: www.peacehealth.org/kbase/nord/nord484.htm

Q. 127. Death during first hour of acute myocardial infarction is mostly caused by (KPSC-PM/05)
    (a) Pulmonary edema
    (b) Arrhythmias
    (c) Papillary muscle-rupture
    (d) Thromboembolism

Ans. (b)

Note
Death during first hour of acaute myocardial infarctrion is mostly caused by arrhythmias.

Also see
60 percent of deaths associated with acute MI occurred within the first hour and were particularly related to ventricular arrhythmia.

Ref: Clinical features and treatment of ventricular arrhythmias during acute myocardial infarction by Philip J Podrid, MD, Leonard I Ganz, MD , Morton F Arnsdorf, MD, MACC

Q. 128. Flag sign is characteristic to (KPSC-PM/05)
    (a) Psoriasis
    (b) Leprosy
    (c) Kwashiorkor
    (d) Malnutrition

Ans. (c)

Note
Flag sign is a characateristic feature of Kwashiorkor.

Also see

Features	
Kwashiorkor	**Marasmus**
Definition	
- Protein deficiency with sufficient calorie intake	- Starvation in infants with overall lack of calories
Clinical features	
- Occurs in children between 6 month and 3 years of age	- Common in infants under one year of age
- Growth failure	- Growth failure
- Wasting of muscles but preserved adipose tissue	- Wasting of all tissues including muscles and adipose tissues
- Edema localised or generalized present	- Edema absent
- Enlarged fatty liver	- No hepatic enlargement
- Flag sign; alternate bands of light (depigmented) and dark (Pigmented) hairs	- Monkey like face, protubernet abdomen, thin limbs
- Enlarged fatty liver	- No fatty liver
Investigations	
Hb; Low (Anemia Present)	Hb; Low (Anemia Present)
Serum Proteins low	Serum Proteins low

Ref: Text book of pathology 4th edition By Harshmohan Pg-227

Q. 129. Bitot's spots seen in (KPSC-PM/05)
    (a)   Vit 'A' Deficiency
    (b)   Vit 'C' Deficiency
    (c)   Both A and B
    (d)   None of above

Ans. (a)
Note
Bitot's spots are seen in deficiency of vitamin A. they are triangular, pearly white or yellowish, foamy spots on the bulbar conjuctiva on either side of cornea.
Ref: Park & Park, 18th Ed. Pg-443

Also see
Vit 'A' deficiency
An early symptom of vitamin A deficiency is night blindness. The sclera and cornea may become dry – the condition called xerophthalmia. Xerophthalmia is particularly common among children with inadequate intake of vitamin A. Bitot's spots also seen in the sclera of the eyes. The dry cornea ulcerates, and leads to blindness. Vitamin A deficiency is a common cause of blindness in developing countries.

Q. 130. Anti-Sterility vitamin is (KPSC-PM/05)
    (a)   Vit B
    (b)   Vit C
    (c)   Vit D
    (d)   Vit E

Ans. (d)
Note
Anti sterility Vitamin is 'E'.

Also see
Vitamin E is the official designation for alpha tocopherol, a fat-soluble nutrient found in the diet in varying amounts.

Extended information

History: "anti-sterility factor" described in 1911; isolated in 1936; identified in 1938; recognized as essential for humans in 1968; deficiency syndrome described in 1977.
Food source:
Fish, shellfish, fresh meat, grains, eggs, chicken, liver, and garlic.
Function:
Acts as an antioxidant, stimulates antibody formation in response to vaccines. It protects against the toxic effects of heavy metals and other substabnces. Effects fertility in males by improving production of sperms and their motility.

Q. 131. The function of selenium is (KPSC-PM/05)
    (a)   An enzyme
    (b)   To increase sperm motility
    (c)   Both A and B
    (d)   None of above

Ans. (c)
Note
The function of selenium is both (a) an enzyme and (b) to increase sperm motility.

Also see
Selenium is a component of several enzymes; it is closely related to vitamin 'E'. It is required for sperm motility and may reduce the risk of miscarriage.
Ref: API, 7th Ed. Pg-244

Extended information
Selenium
Selenium was an essential component of the glutathione peroxidase enzyme system. The importance of selenium in the human diet was discovered in 1979.

Q. 132. In diphtheria sudden death occurs due to (KPSC-PM/05)
    (a)   Tachycardia
    (b)   Atrial fibrillation
    (c)   Ventricular fibrillation
    (d)   None of above

Ans. (c)
Note
In diphtheria sudden death occurs due to ventricular fibrillation.
Also see
Approximately two-thirds of patients develop myocarditis-inflammation and weakness of the cardiac muscle-one to two weeks after the illness begins. A third to one half of these patients are so severely affected that they develop cardiac dysfunction, arrhythmias, and heart failure. About three-quarters of patients develop toxin-mediated paralysis or weakness. These symptoms occur two to eight weeks following onset and, fortunately, resolve completely in most instances.

Q. 133. Complication of cholera is (KPSC-PM/05)
    (a)   Hypokalemia
    (b)   Fever
    (c)   Dehydration
    (d)   None of above

Ans. (c)
Note
Complication of cholera is 'dehydration'.
Also see
The complication of cholera is dehydration; therefore, treatment typically consists of aggressive rehydration and replacement of electrolytes, since the death rate is generally high due to the serious dehydration caused by the illness.

Extended information
The patient passes into the stage of collapse because of dehydration. Classical signs of dehydration are:
    -Sunken eyes
    -Hollow cheeks
    -Scaphoid abdomen
    -Subnormal temperature
    -Washerman's hand and feet
    -Absent pulse and unrecordable blood pressure
    -Loss of skin elasticity
    -Shallow and quick respiration
    -Oliguria
    -Death occurs due to dehydration and acidosis resulting from diarrhea.
Ref: Park and Park 18th Ed.Pg-178

Q. 134. Kaposi's sarcoma is associated with (KPSC-PM/05)
    (a)   Lymphoma
    (b)   Hepatoma
    (c)   AIDS
    (d)   None of above

Ans. (c)
Note
Kaposi's sarcoma is associated with AIDS.
Also see
AIDS is the end stage of HIV infection. A number of opportunist infections commonly occur at this stage or cancers that occur in people with otherwise unexplained defects in immunity. Death is due to uncontrolled or untreatable infection. Tuberculosis and Kaposi sarcoma are usually seen relatively early. Kaposi sarcoma is a tumor featuring reddish brown or purplish plaques or nodules on the skin and mucus membrane. With

HIV infection it affects a wider range and both sexes and is charecterised by lesion in the mouth and gut; or lesions are generalized.
Ref: Park and Park 18th Ed.Pg-276

Q. 135. Kala-azar is caused by (KPSC-PM/05)
  (a) Leishmania
  (b) Streptococci
  (c) E Coli
  (d) Leishmania donovani

Ans. (d)
Note
Kala-Azar is caused by Leismania donovani.

Also see

Leishmaniasis are a group of protozoal diseases caused by parasites of the genus Leishmania. They are responsible for various syndromes in humans- kala azar or visceral leishmaniasis, cutaneous leishmaniasis, mucocutaneous leishmaniasis.
Ref: Park and Park 18th Ed. Pg-245

Q. 136. Kussmaul's respiration occurs in (KPSC-PM/05)
  (a) Respiratory failure
  (b) Metabolic acidosis
  (c) Cardiac failure
  (d) Head injury

Ans. (b)
Note
Kussmaul's respiration occurs in 'metabolic acidosis'.

Also see
Severe metabolic acidosis is clinically manifest as hyperventilation (kussmaul's respiration), respiratory distress and fatigue, reduced cardiac output and arterial blood pressure, and cardiac dysrhythmias. Patients are frequently confused or drowsy.
Ref: Davidson's 19th Ed. Pg-291

Q. 137. Leukoplakia is a (KPSC-PM/05)
  (a) Vit deficiency
  (b) Thickened mucous membrane
  (c) Cancerous condition
  (d) Pre-cancerous condition

Ans. (d)
Note
Leukoplakia is a 'Pre-cancerous condition'.

Also see
The practical importance of leukoplakia is the danger of its developing into carcinoma. It is considered to be a premalignant or pre-cancerous condition.
Leukoplakia is a slowly progressive hyperkeratosis. There is proliferation and heaping up of the cornified epithelium with the formation of milk white patches. This condition may occur anywhere in the mouth, but most commonly seen on the tongue, in this case the tongue looks as if it has been smeared with white paint. Leukoplakia is now more often involving the lips and occasionally the cheek, gums, and palate.
Ref: S. Das, 3rd Ed. Pg-583

Extended information
People with leukoplakia are typically middle-aged and older adults; men are more likely than women to develop the disease. The risk is much higher in smokers and users of smokeless tobacco than in people who do not use tobacco products of any kind. Betel nut chewers are also at high risk.

Q. 138. Duodenal ulcer is more common in Blood Group (KPSC-PM/05)
    (a)   AB
    (b)   O
    (c)   A
    (d)   B

Ans. (b)

Note
Duodenal ulcer is more common in Blood Group 'O'.

Also see
Person of blood group 'O' who do not posses AB antigen are peculiarly apt to develop duodenal ulcers.
Ref: S Das, 3rd Ed. Pg-820

Q. 139. Virchow's node is present in (KPSC-PM/05)
    (a)   Carcinoma of stomach
    (b)   Hepatoma
    (c)   Renal cell carcinoma
    (d)   Tuberculosis

Ans. (a)

Note
Virchow's node is present in 'Carcinoma of stomach'.

Also see
Carcinoma of stomach patient presents with distant metastasis like Krukenberg's tumor, enlargement of virchow's lymph nodes in the left supraclavicular fossa (Troisier's sign).
Ref: S Das, 3rd Ed. Pg-856

Extended information
Virchow's node
A firm and palpable enlargement of left supraclavicular lymph node. They are metastases usually indicative of primary carcinoma of thoracic or abdominal organs, most commonly visceral cancer.

Q. 140. Cullen's sign is a feature of (KPSC-PM/05)
    (a)   Hepatitis
    (b)   Chronic pancreatitis
    (c)   Acute pancreatitis
    (d)   None of above

Ans. (c)

Note
Cullen's sign is a feature of 'acute pancreatitis'.

Also see
Cullen's sign
It is the discolouration of skin around the umbilicus. Discolouration of the skin is a characteristic finding of acute pancreatitis. Such discolouration of skin varies from slate blue to mottled yellowish brown colour due to ecchymosis and extravasated blood.
Ref: S. Das 3rd Ed. Pg-943

Extended Informaiton / Reading
Cullen's Sign (Description):
Bluish discoloration of the periumbilical skin (periumbilical cyanosis and grid cyanosis) due to subcutaneous intraperitoneal hemorrhage. This may be caused by ruptured ectopic pregnancy, or acute pancreatitis.

Q. 141. Acute complication of Diabetes is (KPSC-PM/05)
    (a)   Coma
    (b)   Blindness
    (c)   Diabetic keto acidosis and coma
    (d)   Heart failure

Ans. (c)

Note
Acute complication of Diabetes is 'Diabetic keto-acidosis and coma'.

Also see
Acute complication of diabetes is diabetic ketoacidosis which is one of the most serious acute metabolic complications of DM.
Ref: API, 7th Ed. Pg-1113

Extended information
Diabetes is a chronic disease with many complications. Short-term and long-term complications, as well as co-existing diseases, are a constant threat. Both type 1 and type 2 diabetes may develop the same complications, but symptoms of the complications in people with type 2 may be the first signs of diabetes.
Ref: kidshealth.org/parent/diabetes
Acute Glycemic Complications:
Diabetic Ketoacidosis
Diabetic ketoacidosis (DKA) is characterized by absolute insulin deficiency, increase hepatic glucose production, decrease peripheral glucose utilization, release of fatty acids from fat cells and production of ketones by the liver. These changes cause hyperglycemia, osmotic diuresis, volume depletion, and acidosis.
S/S:
- Altered mental status
- Fatigue
- Weight loss
- Blurred vision
- Thirst
- Excessive urination
- Enuresis
- Abdominal pain
- Nausea or vomiting

Disgnosis:
Glucose / ketone urine dipstick may give guiding information about the presence of diabetes or DKA.

Q. 142. Proximal inter phalangeal joints are affected in (KPSC-PM/05)
    (a)   Rheumatic Fever
    (b)   Rheumatoid Artritis
    (c)   Psoriatic Arthritis
    (d)   Osteoarthritis

Ans. (b)
Note
The proximal interphalangeal joints are affected in Rheumatoid Arthtiris.

Also see
Rheumatoid Arthritis
Articular manifestation of RA – Joints involved is MCPJ, Proximal interphalangeal hoint (PIPJ), Wrist, Knee.
Distal IP jt is spared.
Ref: API, 7th Ed. Pg-1161

Extended Information / reading
Rheumatic Fever
Joints affected are; Big joints, shifting in nature.
Psoriatic Arthritis
Joints affected are Distal inter phalangeal joints.
Osteoarthritis
It is a non-inflammaory degenerative disorder. Joints affected are major weight bearing / over used joints like knee, hip. However, the distal interphalangeal joints are also involved and show bony prominences at articular margins called as 'Haberden's Node' especially found in females.
Ref: Handbook of clinical Rheumatology By Dr Chauhan and Meeta Gupta.

Q. 143. Erythematous, Photo sensitive, Butterfly Rash affecting the cheeks and nose are diagnostic to: (KPSC-PM/2005)
    (a)   RA
    (b)   OA
    (c)   SLE
    (d)   None of the above

Ans. (c)
Note
Erythematous, Photo sensitive, Butterfly Rash affecting the cheeks and nose are diagnostic to 'SLE'.
Also see
Skin affection in SLE – in 75% of cases- erethema, in a butterfly distribution in the cheeks of the face and across the bridge of nose is characteristic.
Ref: Kumar & Clark, 6th Ed. Pg-578

Q. 144. Permanent dialatation and distortion of bronchi is called (KPSC-PM/05) 2005
    (a)   Emphysema
    (b)   Bronchitis
    (c)   Fibrosis of Lung
    (d)   Bronchiectasis

Ans. (d)
Note
Permanent dialatation and distortion of bronchi is called 'Bronchiectasis'.
Also see
Bronchiectasis:
It is a localized irreversible dilatation and distortion of bronchi. The disease runs a chronic course, characterized by repeated bronchial infection and hemoptysis.
Ref: API, 7th Ed. Pg-305

Q. 145. Clubbing of the fingers is seen in (KPSC-PM/2005)
    (a)   Tuberculosis
    (b)   Lung abscess
    (c)   Chronic bronchitis
    (d)   Pneumothorax

Ans. (b)
Note
Clubbing of the fingers is seen in 'Lung abscess'.
Also see
Clubbing is associated with:
 Pulomnary causes:
    - Lung cancer
    - Interstitial lung disease
    - Tuberculosis
    - Suppurative lung disease: lung abscess, empyema, bronchiectasis
    - Pulmonary hypertension
Cardiac causes:
    - Congenital cyanotic heart disease (most common cardiac cause)
    - Subacute bacterial endocarditis
Gastrointestinal causes:
    - Crohn's disease and ulcerative colitis
Liver diseases:
    - Cirrhosis
Miscellaneous:
    - Familial

Extended information
Hippocrates has document clubbing as a sign of disease, therefore clubbing is also known as Hippocratic fingers.
Test for clubbing (Schamroth's test or Schamroth's Window test):
When distal phalanges of corresponding fingers of opposite hands are directly apposed (placed against each other back to back), a small diamond-shaped "window" is normally apparent between the nailbeds. If this window is obliterated, the test is positive and clubbing is present.
Pathophysiology of clubbing:
The mechanism of clubbing is not well understood.
Ref: From Wikipedia

Q. 146. Gross enlargement of spleen occurs in (KPSC-PM/2005)
    (a)   Chronic Myeloid Leukemia
    (b)   Chronic Lymphatic Leukemia
    (c)   Acute Lymphatic Leukemia
    (d)   Anemia

Ans. (a)
Note
Gross enlargement of spleen occurs in 'Chronic Myloid Leukemia'.
Also see
Massive enlargement of spleen (below umbilicus) occurs in chonic myeloid leukaemia, myeloid metaplasia with myelofibrosis, storage diseases, thalassemia major chronic malaria leishmaniasis and portal vein obstruction.
Ref: Pathology by Harsh Mohan, 2nd Ed. Pg-326

Q. 147. Painless asymmetrical circumscribed enlargement of lymphnodes of rubbery consistency is seen in (KPSC-PM/2005)
    (a)   Lymphoma
    (b)   Tuberculosis
    (c)   Malignancy
    (d)   Hodgkin's Lymphoma

Ans. (d)
Note
Painless asymmetrical circumscribed enlargement of lymphnodes of rubbery consistency is seen in 'Hodgkin's disease'.
Also see
In Hodgkin's disease the usual presentation is with painless lymphadenopathy, commonly in cervical region and they have a typical rubbery consistency.
Ref: API, 7th Ed. Pg-1002.

Q. 148. Severe bleeding occurs when the platelet falls below (KPSC-PM/2005)
    (a)   1 lakh/cmm
    (b)   50,000 per cmm
    (c)   20,000 per cmm
    (d)   15 lakhs/cmm

Ans. (c)
Note
Severe bleeding occurs when the platelet falls below '20,000 per cmm'.
Also see
It is life threatening if platelet count is below 10000 to 25000/cu/mm.
Ref: API, 7th Ed. Pg-973

Extended information
    -Surgical bleeding due solely to thrombocytopenia occurs when platelets < 50,000/μL.
    -The spontaneous bleeding occurs when platelets < 10,000/μL.

-Thrombocytopenic patients can develop "dry" bleeding, i.e. petechiae and ecchymoses only. They do not develop fatal hemorrhage, unless they first have extensive mucosal bleeding, or "wet" bleeding.
-Therefore, in those with no bleeding or only "dry" bleeding, the threshold for transfusion should be between 5,000 to 10,000/μL. A more conservative threshold of 20,000/μL should be used in those with a fever or other risk factors for bleeding.
Ref: http://en.wikipedia.org/wiki/Plateletpheresis

Q. 149. Presence of RBC cast in urine is indicative of (KPSC-PM/2005)
(a) Acute glomerulonephritis
(b) Acute pyelonephritis
(c) Nephrotic Syndrome
(d) Renal failure

Ans. (a)
Note
Presence of RBC cast in urine is indicative of 'Acute glomerulonephritis'.
Also see
Acute glomerulonephritis presents with Acute Nephritic Syndrome having sudden and abrupt onset following an episode of sore throat 1-2 weeks prior to the development of symptoms. The features include microscopic or intermittent hematuria, red cell casts, mild non selective proteinuria (less than 3 gm/ 24 hr), hypertension, periorbital edema and variably oliguria.
Ref: Pathology by Harsh Mohan, 2nd Ed. Pg-494

Q. 150. The commonest cause of intracranial hemorrhage is (KPSC-PM/2005)
(a) Rupture of aneurysm
(b) Diabetes Mellitus
(c) Hypertension
(d) Trauma

Ans. (a)
Note
The commonest cause of intracranial hemorrhage is 'Rupture of aneurysm'.
Also see
Rupture of cerebral aneurysm is the commonest cause of subarachnoid hemorrhage.
Ref: API, 7th Ed. Pg-1251

Q. 151. Verruca vulgaris is caused by (KPSC-PM/2005)
(a) RNA virus
(b) DNA virus
(c) Both A and B
(d) Papilloma virus

Ans. (b)
Note
Verruca vulgaris is caused by 'DNA virus'.
Also see
Common Warts (Verruca vulgaris) is caused by various types of human papilloma virus (HPV) which are DNA viruses.
Ref: API, 7th Ed. Pg-1305, 1306.

Extended information
Verruca vulgaris is common wart. It can occur at any age, but are more frequently seen in children. Warts commonly seen on the fingers and hands, but they can grow anywhere on the skin and are transmitted by casual skin-to-skin contact.

Q. 152. The commonest form of MND is (KPSC-PM/2005)
    (a) Amyotrophic lateral sclerosis
    (b) Western pacific form
    (c) Progressive bulbar palsy
    (d) Primary lateral sclerosis

Ans. (a)

Note
The commonest form of MND is 'Amyotrophic lateral sclerosis'.

Also see
Amyotrophic lateral sclerosis and other motor neuron diseases- amyotrophic lateral sclerosis (ALS) is the most common form of progressive motor neuron disease.
Ref: Harrison vol-2, 16th Ed. Pg-2424

Extended Information
MND is a neurological disease that affects the neurones (nerves) that provide the stimulus to our muscles through which we move, breathe, eat and drink. The disease is given different names depending upon how the symptoms present themselves. All forms of the disease are ultimately fatal.
The three main forms are: amyotrophic lateral sclerosis (ALS), progressive muscular atrophy (PMA) and progressive bulbar palsy (PBP).
When the upper motor neurones alone are affected the disease has two names: if limb involvement is predominant the disease is called progressive lateral sclerosis; if brain stem involvement is predominant the disease is called progressive pseudobulbar palsy. When lower motor neurones alone are affected the disease is called progressive muscular atrophy. When both upper and lower motor neurones are involved the disease is called amyotrophic lateral sclerosis. This is the commonest form.

Q. 153. Bell's Palsy is a (KPSC-PM/2005)
    (a) UMN type of facial palsy
    (b) LMN type of facial palsy
    (c) Both UMN and LMN type
    (d) None of above

Ans. (b)

Note
'Bell's Palsy" is a lower motor neuron type of facial palsy.

Also see
'Bell's palsy is lower motor neuron facial palsy. In which both upper and lower part of face is paralised.
Ref: Davidson's 19th Ed. Pg-1183

Q. 154. Common psycho-somatic respiratory disorder is (KPSC-PM/2005)
    (a) Bronchitis
    (b) Emphysema
    (c) Bronchial asthma
    (d) Pneumonia

Ans. (c)

Note
Common psycho-somatic respiratory disorder is 'Bronchial Asthma'.

Extended information
Psychosomatic medicine is an interdisciplinary medical field. Now a day's psychosomatic illness are referred as psychophysiologic illness. This group includes disease conditions where psychological processes operate as a major factor affecting medical outcome.
The psychosomatic syndromes are classified as neurotic, stress-related and somatoform disorders by the World Health Organization in the International Statistical Classification of Diseases and Related Health Problems. Psychosomatic medicine integrates interdisciplinary evaluation and management involving diverse specialties, i.e. psychiatry, psychology, neurology; surgery; gynecology; pain management; pediatrics; dermatology; and psychoneuroimmunology.

Many illnesses previously been labeled as 'hysterical' or 'psychosomatic', for example asthma, allergies, false pregnancy, coeliac disease, peptic ulcers and migraines.
Ref: en.wikipedia.org/wiki/Psychosomatic_illness - 44k

Q. 155. Which of the following is a cause of bilateral lower motor neuron facial palsy? (K/MD/Ent-II/2001)
- (a) Mumps
- (b) Leprosy
- (c) Tabes dorsalis
- (d) Sarcoidosis

Ans. (b)
Note
Lelprosy is a common cause of bilateral lower motor neuron facial palsy.
Also see
Bilateral VII weakness
    -Definition: 2nd facial nerve paresis occuring within 30 days of 1st
    -Frequency: 0.3% to 2% of patients with facial paralysis
VII nerve lesions
    -Guillain Barré
    -Leprosy
    Other peripheral causes
    -Motor neuron disorders
    -Myasthenia gravis
    -Myopathies
Ref: http://www.neuro.wustl.edu/neuromuscular/nanatomy/vii.htm

Q. 156. If husband is sex linked recessive and wife is normal which of the following will suffer from the disease? (K/MD/Ent-II/2001)
- (a) Daughters
- (b) Grand daughters
- (c) Daughter's son
- (d) Son's daughter

Ans. (d)
Note
If husband is sex linked recessive and wife is normal then 'son's daughter' will suffer from the disease
Also see

X-linked recessive (XLR) vary from mild to severe. The genotype is 46 XY or 46XX, where X is the recessive gene. Usually males are affeced, and usually female suffers only when she is homozygous for the recessive allele. An affected male does not transmits the disorder to any of the sons, but the abnormal gene is transmitted to all his daughters (who may be carriers if the mother is normal) a carrier female transmits the disease to half her sons or half of her daughters.
Example
For an X-linked recessive disorder:
If only the father caries the recessive gene, all of his daughters will be carriers and all of his sons will be normal.
In the next generation:
The mother is carrier (one abnormal X but no disease) and father is normal, if it is assumed that 4 children are produced (2 boys and 2 girls), the statistical expectation is for:
    -1 boy normal
    -1 boy with disease
    -1 girl normal
    -1 girl carrier without disease
The X-Linked recessive disorders are:
    -Hemophilia, G6PD deficiency, Duchenne Muscular Dystrophy, Fabry's disease, Colour blindness, Lesch Hyhan Syndrome.

Q. 157. The commonest cause of Cushing's syndrome is (K/MD/Ent-II/2001)
 (a) Steroids
 (b) Adrenal tumour
 (c) Bilateral adrenal hyperplasia
 (d) Tuberculosis

Ans. (a)

Note
The commonest cause of Cushing's syndrome is 'Steroid'.

Also see
Causes:
Commonest cause of Cushing's syndrome is exogenous administration of glucocorticoid.
ACTH dependent causes:
Autonomous ACTH secretion by pituitary corticotroph tumours. These are usually microadenomas (less than 1 cm in diameter) and account for 80% of ACTH dependent causes of Cushing's Syndrome.

Extended information
Pseudo-Cushing's syndrome
Depression and Pseudo-Cushing's Syndrome:
About 80% of patients with severe depression have abnormally regulated cortisol secretion which is mediated by increased hypothalamic secretion of CRH. The hormonal abnormalities disappear with the remission of depression.
Alcohol and Pseudo-Cushing's Syndrome:
Chronic alcoholism is also an uncommon cause of Pseudo-Cushing's Syndrome. The mechanism of hormonal abnormality is either increased CRH secretion or impaired hepatic metabolism of cortisol. Hormonal abnormalities disappear rapidly during abstinence from alcohol.
Ref: BMJ. Web Ref: http://student.bmj.com/issues/00/04/education/100.php

Q. 158. In Nephrotic Syndrome, levels of following serum proteins decreases (K/MD/Ent-II/2001)
 (a) Albumin
 (b) Transferrin
 (c) Fibrinogin
 (d) Ceruloplasmin

Ans. (a)

Note
In nephrotic syndrome levels of serum protein decreases is 'albumin'.

Also see
Nephorotic syndrome is characterized by proteinuria (>3.5g/day), hypoalbuminemia, hyperlipidemia and edema.

Extended information
In case of nephrotic syndrome level of following are as:
a. Albumin: is the most abundant blood plasma protein and is produced in the liver and forms a large proportion of all plasma protein. Hypoalbuminaemia is caused by liver disease, nephrotic syndrome, burns, protein-losing enteropathy, malabsorption, malnutrition and malignancy. High albumin is either caused by dehydration or artefact. (Ref: Wikipedia)

b. Transferrin: A deficiency is associated with Atransferrinemia. Atransferrinemia is an autosomal recessive metabolic disorder in which there is absence of transferrin, a plasma protein that transports iron through the blood.

c. Fibrinogin: Increases (hyperfibrinogenaemia – results in increased coronary and thrombotic risk, which may be inhanced by high lipoprotein)
(Ref: Euaropean journal of clinical investigation)
(Net ref: http://student.bmj.com/issues/00/04/education/100.php)

d. Ceruloplasmin: it is synthesized in liver and contains copper in its structure. Levels are decreased in patients with hepatic diseases due to reduced synthesizing capabilities i.e., in Wilson's disease, and copper deficiency. (Ref: wikipedia)

Q. 159. Hypokalemia occurs in (K/MD/Ent-II/2001)
  (a) Meningitis
  (b) Hepatitis
  (c) Osteomylitis
  (d) Bronchiectasis

Ans. (a)
Note
From the choice given above chances of 'Hypokalemia' are more in case of Meningitis.
Also see
More commonly, however, hypokalemia occurs due to excessive loss of potassium, often associated with excess water loss, which "flushes" potassium out of the body. Typically, this is a consequence of vomiting and diarrhea, but may also occur with excessive sweating in athletes. Therefore if severe vomiting takes place in a case of meningitis may lead to the hypokalemia.
However, the vomiting is also a common symptom of acute hepatitis but the vomiting is not so severe.

Q. 160. Common presentation of primary hyperparathyroidism is (K/MD/Ent-II/2001)
  (a) Gallstone
  (b) Abdominal pain
  (c) Recurrent abortion
  (d) Subtle neurological and psychiatric symptoms

Ans. (b)
Note
Common presentation of primary hyperparathyroidism is 'abdominal pain'.
Also see
Patients with hyperparathyroidism may have a chronic or non-specific history. Their symptoms are brought to mind by the Adage / Mnemonic: 'bones, stones and abdominal organs'
Ref: Davidson, 19th Ed. Pg. 716
Additional Information
The common presentation of hyperparathyroidism is abdominal pain. The majority of patients with hyperparathyroidism are asymptomatic. Manifestations of hyperparathyroidism usually involve the kidney (stones) and the skeletal system (bone pain due to fibrous tissue replacement, termed osteitis fibrosa cystica).

If symptomatic, hyperparathyroidism can be classically remembered by the rhyme "moans" (myalgia), "groans" (abdominal pain), "stones" (kidney), "bones" (bone pain), and "psychiatric overtones" (confusion, altered mental state, lethargy, fatigue).
Other symptoms include: headaches, sleep disorders, memory problems, gastroesophageal reflux, and decreased sex drive, thinning hair, hypertension, and heart palpitations.
Hyperparathyroidism is caused by overactive parathyroid glands. Overactive parathyroid glands produce too much parathyroid hormone, which in turn stimulate increased levels of calcium in the blood stream.
The excess calcium released by the bones leads to osteoporosis and osteomalacia (both bone-weakening diseases). Other results of hyperparathyroidism are kidney stones, because of high levels of calcium excreted into the urine by the kidneys.

Q. 161. Earliest sensation lost in diabetic neuropathy (K/MD/Ent-II/2001)
  (a) Weakness of small muscles of hand
  (b) Temperature
  (c) Pain
  (d) Vibration

Ans. (c)
Note
The earliest sensation lost in diabetic neuropathy is 'Pain'.
Also see
In diabetic neuropathy, sensory abnormalities dominate the clinical presentation. Symptoms include paraesthesia in the feet and rarely in the hands, pain in the lower limbs, burning sensation in sole of feet, cutaneous

hyperaesthesia and an abnormal gait often associated with sense of numbness in the feet.
Ref: Davidson's 19th Ed. Pg-675

Q. 162. Region of spine most commonly affected in rheumatoid arthritis (K/MD/Ent-II/2001)
    (a)   Cervical
    (b)   Thoracic
    (c)   Lumbar
    (d)   Sacral

Ans. (a)

Note
The region of spine most commonly affected in Rheumatoid arthritis is 'cervical spine'.

Also see
In articular manifestations of RA, cervical spine may be involved particularly in juvenile chronic arthritis. In Indian adults it is relatively uncommon. Significant C1-C2 instability may occur.
Ref: API, 7th Ed. Pg-1162

Extended information
The histological changes noted classically in rheumatoid arthritis are similar or identical to those of ankylosing spondylitis. However, the general pattern of distribution of these changes is usually quite distinct from that of ankylosing spondylitis. For example, rheumatoid arthritis predominantly involves the cervical spine, with apophyseal joint erosion and malalingment, intervertebral disc space narrowing with endplate sclerosis and without osteophytes, and with multiple subluxations, especially at the atlanto-axial junction. Abnormalities of the thoracolumbar spine and sacroiliac joints are infrequent and less prominent than those of ankylosing spondylitis.

Q. 163. Vit-B deficiency causes (K/MD/Ent-II/2001)
    (a)   Hemorrhage
    (b)   CNS affections
    (c)   Fits
    (d)   Depression

Ans. (b)

Note
Vit-B deficiency causes 'CNS affections'.

Also see
Vitamin B1 (Thiamin) causes:
Wernick's Encephalopathy; causes confusion.
Korsakoff's Syndrome; Examples: forgetfulness and confabulation.
Wet Beriberi (peripheral neuritis)
B3 (Niacin) deficiency:
It prevents pellagara. Which is characterized by diarrhea, dermatitis and dementia.
Ref: Park and Park, 18th Ed.Pg-446
B 6 deficiency:
Pyritoxine deficiency is associated with peripheral neuritis.
B 12 deficinecy:
Subacute combined degeneration
From above it becomes clear that the vitamin B deficiency results in most of CNS affections. (CNS includes Brain and Spinal cord)

Q. 164. Diagnostic of fresh M I (K/MD/Ent-II/2001)
    (a)   P- waves
    (b)   S-T depression
    (c)   S-T elevation
    (d)   U- waves

Ans. (c)

Note
ECG diagnostic feature of fresh M I is ST elevation.
Also see
Electrocardiographic changes in myocardial infarction are ST elevation and according to the leads involved, location of MI is suggested as under:
- In V1 to V4: anterior wall MI
- In L1, aVL V5, V6: lateral wall MI
- In L2, L3, aVF: inferior MI

Ref: API, 7th Ed. Pg-442

Q. 165. Irradiation causes (K/MD/Ent-II/2001)
 (a) Osteosarcoma
 (b) Paget's disease of breast
 (c) Paget's disease of skin
 (d) Ewing 's Tumour

Ans. (a)
Note
Irradiation causes 'Osteosarcoma'.
Ref: Textbook of Surgery by S.Das, 3rd Ed. Pg-.437
Also see
Osteosarcoma
It has been demonstrated that there is an increased risk of osteosarcoma in adults who had survived nuclear accidents, received radiation therapy, or received cyclophosphamide chemotherapy for acute lymphoblastic leukemia as children. In the elderly, osteosarcoma is found in increased incidence in patients with Paget's disease. Contrary to popular belief, osteosarcoma is not caused by a traumatic injury.
Pagets disease of breast
Paget's disease of the breast is generally associated with an underlying breast cancer. It is generally seen in females between the ages of 40 and 80 years. Cases in men have been identified, but they are extremely rare.
Paget's disease of the breast may also be called Mammary Paget's Disease (MPD).
Paget's disease of skin
There is a much rarer form of this disease called Extramammary Paget's Disease (EMPD). MPD affects the breast nipple and is also called Paget's disease of the nipple. EMPD can affect the skin of the external genital tissues in both women and men, as well as the skin of the eyelids and external ear canal. MPD is believed to develop from a tumor growth within the milk ducts of the breast. EMPD may represent a spreading (metastasis) of MPD to other parts of the body.
Causes and symptoms:
The cause of Paget's disease of the breast is unknown, but it is usually associated with an underlying cancer of the breast.
Ewing's Tumor
Ewing's sarcoma is a highly malignant tumor that is a type of peripheral primitive neuroectodermal tumor (PNET). Ewing's sarcoma is found in the lower extremity more than the upper extremity, but any long tubular bone may be affected. The most common sites are the metaphysis and diaphysis of the femur followed by the tibia and humerus. Ewing's sarcoma is most common in the first and second decade.

Q. 166. Egg shell - calcification of hilar lymphnodes is characteristically seen in (K/MD/Ent-II/2001)
 (a) Tuberculosis
 (b) Sarcoidosis
 (c) Teratoma
 (d) Silicosis

Ans. (d)
Note
Egg shell - calcification of hilar lymphnodes is characteristically seen in 'silicosis'.

Also see
Diagnosis of silicosis is based on history of exposure to free silica and a roentgenographic pattern, hilar adenopathy with egg-shell calcification, progressive massive fibrosis.
Ref: API, 7th Ed. Pg-329

Q. 167. In a case of suspected left pleural effusion, X-Ray chest should be done in (K/MD/Ent-II/2001)
(a) Left lateral position
(b) Left lateral decubitus position
(c) Right lateral decubitus position
(d) A P view supine

Ans. (b)
Note
In a case of suspected left pleural effusion, X-Ray chest should be done in left lateral decubitus position.
Also see
In small pleural effusion, lateral decubitus X-ray should be taken with patient lying on the affected side.
Ref: API, 7th Ed. Pg-342

Q. 168. The commonest symptom of foreign body in bronchus a child is (K/MD/Ent-II/2001)
(a) Cough
(b) Vomiting
(c) Dyspnea
(d) Wheezing

Ans. (a)
Note
The commonest symptom of foreign body in bronchus a child is 'cough'.
Also see
Bronchial foreign bodies typically present with cough, unilateral wheezing, and decreased breath sounds, but only 65% of patients present with this classic triad.
Extended information
Aspiration foreign body natural history has 3 stages:
1. Choking/coughing/gagging
2. Asymptomatic interval (up to ½ cases diagnosed beyond 1 week)
3. Complications: cough, hemoptysis, pneumonia, lung abscess, fever, malaise
Workup: I/E CXR, lateral decubitus
Ref: www.utmb.edu/otoref/grnds/Stridor-2003-1231/Stridor-slides-2003-1231.ppt

Q. 169. The commonest symptom of nasopharyngeal carcinoma (Fossa of Rosenmuller) is (K/MD/Ent-II/2001)
(a) Epistaxis
(b) Hoarseness
(c) Nasal block
(d) Deafness

Ans. (a)
Note
The commonest symptom of naso-pharyngeal carcinoma is 'epistaxis'.
Also see
Nasopharyngeal carcinoma produces few symptoms in its early stages; as a result cases are detected at a advanced stage. When tumor expands from its site of origin in the lateral wall of the nasopharynx, it may obstruct the nasal passages and cause nasal discharge or nosebleed. Obstruction of the auditory tubes may cause chronic ear infections, and patients may experience referred pain to the ear.
Ref: http://en.wikipedia.org/wiki/Nasopharyngeal_carcinoma

Q. 170. The commonest cause of epistaxis in an elderly is (K/MD/Ent-II/2001)
- (a) Nasopharyngeal carcinoma
- (b) Trauma
- (c) Hypertension
- (d) Antro-choanal polyp

Ans. (b)

Note
The most common cause of epistaxis in an elderly is 'trauma'.

Also see
Trauma, commonly caused by nose picking, is the most common local etiology. Promonged epistaxis in the elderly that is difficult to control with direct pressure is commonly secondary to atherosclerosis and anticoagulant therapy.
Ref: Geriatic Emergency Medicine by Stephen Meldon
Ref: http://books.google.com/books

Q. 171. In a 4 year old with ASOM, commonest organism is (K/MD/Ent-II/2001)
- (a) Pneumococcus
- (b) Staphylococcus
- (c) Streptococcus
- (d) H. Influenza

Ans. (c)

Note
In a 4 year old with ASOM, commonest organism is 'Streptococcus'.

Also see
Acute otitis media is an acute inflammation of the middle ear cavity. It is a common condition, occurring most frequently in children, and is often bilateral. Acute otitis media has a peak incidence of between 6 months and 3 years.
In acute suppurative otitis media, Streptococcus pneumoniae causes more than half the cases at all ages. Hemophilus influenzae is mainly a pathogen of infancy, accounting for about one-third of the cases. viruses, mycoplasma - seldom isolated

Q. 172. Which of the following is characteristic of T B Otitis Media? (K/MD/Ent-II/2001)
- (a) Multiple perforations
- (b) Large central perforation
- (c) Marginal perforation
- (d) Attic perforation

Ans. (a)

Note
Characteristic of T B Otitis Media is 'Multiple Perforations'.

Also see
T B Otitis Media
It is most often secondary to pulmonary tuberculosis; infection reaches the middle ear through Eustachian tube. Sometimes it is blood borne from tubercular focus in the lungs, tonsils, cervical or mesenteric lymph nodes. The disease is mostly seen in children and young adults.
The perforations; typically these are 2 or 3 in number seen in pars tensa and form a classical sign of disease. At times these may coalesce into a single large perforation.
Ref; Disease of Ear Nose and throat by P. L Dhingra First edition, Tubercular otitis media.Pg-94.

OPHTHALMOLOGY

Q. 173. The earliest change noticed in hypertensive retinopathy is (K/MD/Ent-II/2001)
 (a) Hard exudates
 (b) Arterial spasm
 (c) Venus spasm
 (d) Soft exudate

Ans. (b)
Note
The earliest change noticed in hypertensive retinopathy is 'Arterial spasm'.
Also see
Keith-Wagner-Barker classification of the hypertensive retinopathic changes in the fundus:
Grade I (mild / borderline hypertension):
 -Reversible state of arterial spasm.
Grade II (moderate / sustained hypertension):
 -Irreversible state of retinal arteriosclerosis.
Grade III (accelerated hypertension):
 -Leakage of blood due to increased capillary permeability and local ischaemia as a result of the vascular damage caused by severe hypertension.
Grade IV (malignant hypertension):
 -Grade III changes, plus
 -Edema of the optic disc (Papilloedema).
(Grade III and Grade IV changes are almost indistinguishable and are therefore considered under one group).

Q. 174. Most toxic intra ocular foreign body is (K/MD/Ent-II/2001)
 (a) Iron
 (b) Copper
 (c) Lead
 (d) Glass

Ans. (a)
Note
Most toxic intra ocular foreign body is 'Iron'.
Also see
Among intra-ocular foreign bodies, those of iron are most numerous as a result of industrial accidnents. The retention of an iron foreign body in the eye almost always results in progressive iron deposition throughout the eye, inducing degeneration of retina, cartaract formation and secondary glaucoma in the late stage.

Q. 175. 23 Sub-conjunctival hemorrhage maybe seen in (K/MD/Ent-II/2001)
 (a) Rabies
 (b) Measles
 (c) Mumps
 (d) Pertusis

Ans. (d)
Note
Sub-conjunctival hemorrhage maybe seen in 'pertusis'.
Also see
In case of whooping cough (Pertusis) the violence of the paroxysms of cough may precipitate sub-conjuctival hemorrhages, epistaxis, haemoptysis and punctuate cerebral hemorrhages which may cause convulsions and coma.
Ref: Park & Park, 18th Ed. Pg-137

Q. 176. Normal size of optic disc is (K/MD/Ent-II/2001)
    (a)   2.5 mm
    (b)   2.0 mm
    (c)   1.5 mm
    (d)   1.0 mm

Ans. (c)
Note
The normal diameter of optic disc is 1.5 mm.
Also see
There are about one million nerve fibers in the 1.5 mm size optic disc.

Q. 177. Impaired colour vision is seen in (K/MD/Ent-II/2001)
    (a)   Papilledema
    (b)   Papillitis
    (c)   Toxic Amblyopia
    (d)   Eales disease

Ans. (c)
Note
Impaired colour vision is seen in 'Toxic Amblyopia'.
Also see
a. *Papilledema (or papilloedema)*
It is optic disc swelling that is caused by increased intracranial pressure. The swelling is usually bilateral and can occur over a period of hours to weeks. Persistent and extensive optic nerve head swelling, or optic disc edema, can lead to loss of these fibers and *permanent visual impairment.*
b. *Papillitis*
It is also known as optic neuritis, is characterized by inflammation and deterioration of optic disc. Individuals with papillitis experience loss of vision in one eye that may occur within several hours of onset. The severity of visual impairment may vary from case to case, ranging *from slight visual deficiency to complete loss of light perception.* In addition, affected individuals experience a reduction in color perception.
c. *Toxic Amblyopia*
It is caused by agents such as lead, quinine, salicylates, cyanide intoxication due to tobacco, ethambutanol, rifampicin and methanol.
Tobacco Amblyopia is characterised by a central loss of vision for colours, in the order, green, green and red, and in extreme cases, white. Optic atrophy results in severe cases. In quinine amblyopia, the retinal vessels also become constricted and the peripheral vision is reduced. Methanol poisoning is accompanied by acidosis.
d. *Eales Disease*
Itis an idiopathic obliterative vasculopathy that usually involves the peripheral retina of young adults. In 1880, Henry Eales first described it in healthy young men with abnormal retinal veins and recurrent vitreal hemorrhages.
Clinical findings are characterized by avascular areas in the retina periphery.
Usually, *vision is suddenly blurred* because the clear jelly that fills the eyeball behind the lens of the eye seeps out (vitreous hemorrhaging)

Q. 178. The local anaesthesia is contra indicated in (K/MD/Ent-II/2001)
    (a)   Diabetic gangrene of foot
    (b)   Hemophilia
    (c)   Intermittent claudication
    (d)   All of the above

Ans. (d)
Note
The local anesthesia is contra indicated in 'all of above'.
Also see
Contraindications of local anaesthesia:

a. Known allergy to local anesthetics
b. Pronounced bradycardia, grade II, III AV block.
c. Severe hypotension
d. Angina pectoris
e. Arteriosclerosis
f. Injection into an inflamed / infected area
g. Considerable impaired blood coagulation.

Q. 179. Colour of oxygen cylinder is (K/MD/Ent-II/2001)
  (a) Blue
  (b) Black & White
  (c) Grey
  (d) Orange

Ans. (b)
Note
Medical oxygen cylinders can be identified using the following features:
 -Black cylinder with white collar

Q. 180. Erosive arthritis is seen in all except (K/MD/Ent-II/2001)
  (a) Gout
  (b) Osteo arthritis
  (c) SLE
  (d) Hyperparathyroidism

Ans. (d)
Note
Erosive arthritis is seen in all Gout, SLE, and OA except hyperparathyroidism.
Also see
Erosive osteoarthritis is considered a subtype of generalized osteoarthritis. Erosive osteoarthritis is sometimes referred to as inflammatory osteoarthritis, which seems like a contradictory term to many who believe osteoarthritis is not associated with inflammation.
Hyperparathyroidism:

S/S of primary hyperparathyroidism are those of hypercalcemia. These are remembered by mnemonic "stones, bones, abdominal groans and psychic moans".
 -"Stones": refers to kidney stone formation.
 -"Bones" : refers to bone-related complications are osteitis fibrosa cystica, osteoporosis, osteomalacia, and arthritis.
 -Abdominal groans" refers to GIT complaints - constipation, indigestion, nausea and vomiting. Hypercalcemia can lead to peptic ulcers and acute pancreatitis.
 -"Psychic moans" refers to complaints of CNS which include lethargy, fatigue, depression, memory loss, psychosis, ataxia, delirium, and coma.
Others:
These include proximal muscle weakness, itching, and band keratopathy of the eyes.

Q. 181. In gout the crystals are (K/MD/Ent-II/2001)
  (a) Calcium pyrophosphate
  (b) Monosodium urate
  (c) Monopotassium urate
  (d) Double phosphate

Ans. (b)
Note
In gout the crystals are of 'monosodium urate'.
Also see
In gout the crystals are of monosodium urate. These are needle shaped. The main environmental factors leading to hyperuricaemia in western society are alcohol in young men and diuretics in the elderly.
Ref: API, 7th Ed. Pg-1157

Q. 182. Angular kyphosis is most commonly produced by (K/MD/Ent-II/2001)
 (a) Rickets
 (b) Senile osteoporosis
 (c) TB of spine
 (d) Hyperparathyroidism

Ans. (c)
Note
Angular kyphosis is most commonly produced by 'TB Spine'.
Also see
X-ray changes in Pott's spine include erosion of vertebral bodies, narrowing of intervertebral disc space, anterior wedging and lateral collapse of the vertebral body and kyphosis.
Ref: API, 7th Ed. Pg-1196

Extended information
An abrupt alteration in the normally smooth thoracic curvature is called angular kyphosis. It is accompanied by an unusually prominent spinous process called a gibbus.
Angular kyphosis is often due to tuberculosis of spine.

Q. 183. Commonest site of prolapsed intervertebral disc is in between (K/MD/Ent-II/2001)
 (a) C5-C6
 (b) C7-T1
 (c) T12 – L1
 (d) L4-L5 & L5—S1

Ans. (d)
Note
Commonest site of prolapsed intervertebral disc is in between 'L4-L5 & L5-S1.
Also see
Sites of prolapse of intervertebral disc:
 -Lumbosacral region-above and below the L5 vetebra, i.e.L4/5 and L5/S1. 80% of disc prolapse occurs in this region.
 -Lower cervical region- above and below C6 vertebra. 19% of disc prolapse occurs in this region.
 -Dorsal region- constitutes 1% of disc prolapses.
Ref: Textbook of surgery by S. Das, 3rd Ed.'Pg-509

Extended information
The commonest site of prolapsed intervertebra disc is in between L4-L5 & L5-S1. As this joints are most weight bearing as well as having most of the mobility which leads to more wear and tear.

Q. 184. Plaster of paris chemically is (K/MD/Ent-II/2001)
 (a) Calcium sulphate
 (b) Calcium phosphate
 (c) Hydrated calcium sulphate
 (d) Hemi hydrated calcium sulphate

Ans. (d)
Note
Plaster of paris. Synonyms: Calcium sulphate hemihydrate; dried calcium sulphate; Gypsum hemihydrate; Hemihydrate gypsum.

Q. 185. Tetanus neonatorum is best prevented by giving injection 'Tetanus Toxide' to (K/MD/Ent-II/2001)
 (a) Fetus after birth
 (b) Mother in 1st trimester
 (c) Mother in 2 & 3 trimester
 (d) Fetus at 3 month of age

Ans. (c)

Note
Tetanus neonatorum is best prevented by giving injection Tetanus Toxide to 'Mother in 2 & 3 trimester'.
Also see
According to the national immunization schedule:
a. Unimmunized pregnant women; Neonatal tetanus can be prevented by giving two doses of tetanus toxide. First as early as possible during pregnancy and second at least a month later and at least three weeks before delivery. These doses may be given between 16 – 36 weeks of pregnancy, allowing an interval of 1 – 2 months between the two doses.
b. In previously immunized pregnant women, a booster dose is considered sufficient. There is no need for a booster at every consecutive pregnancy.
Ref: Park and Park, 16th Ed, Pg- 238.

Q. 186. 37 Which of the following is true about Iron deficiency anemia? (K/MD/Ent-II/2001)

Total Iron Binding Capacity (TIBC)	Serum Iron
(a) Decreased	Decreased
(b) Increased	Increased
(c) Increased	Decreased
(d) Decreased	Increased

Ans. (c)
Note
Total Iron Biding Capacity increased and Serum iron decreased in case of iron deficiency anemia.
Also see
Biochemical findings in Iron- deficiency anemia:
    -Serum iron level is low
    -Total iron binding capacity (TIBC) is high
    -Serum ferritin is very low
    -Red cell protoporphyrin is very low
Ref: Pathology by Harsh Mohan, 5th Ed. Pg-258

Q. 187. The most common complication of mumps in children (K/MD/Ent-II/2001)
    (a) Appendicitis
    (b) Pancreatitis
    (c) Aseptic meningitis
    (d) Orchitis

Ans. (d)
Note
The most common complication of mumps in children is 'orchitis'.
Also see
Mumps complications; though frequent are not serious. These includes orchitis, ovaritis, pancreaitis, meningoencephalatis, and myocardtis.
Ref: Park & Park, 18th Ed. P-130

Q. 188. In a newborn, liver is 1 cm enlarged. The child has (K/MD/Ent-II/2001)
    (a) Hemolytic disease
    (b) Malaria
    (c) Nutritional cirrhosis
    (d) Normal development

Ans. (d)
Note
In a newborn, Liver is 1 cm enlarged. The child has 'normal development'.

Also see
In normal children liver is palpable 1 cm below the costal margin and in infants it may be felt upto 2cm below the rib margin.
Ref: O.P. Ghai, 4th Ed. Pg-207
Throughout infancy and childhood the liver is normally remains palpable upto 1.5 cm below right costal margin, in mid-clavicular line.
Ref: Principles of pediatrics by Dr. Tirthankar Datta 1st Edition.

Q. 189. Hemolytic disease in new born is seen if Rh factor in (K/MD/Ent-II/2001)

	MOTHER	FETUS
(a)	Positive	Negative
(b)	Negative	Positive
(c)	Positive	Positive
(d)	Negative	Negative

Ans. (b)
Note
Hemolytic disease in new born is seen if Rh factor in Mother is negative and Fetus is positive.
Also see
Erythroblastosis fetalis occurs if the fetus is Rh+ve and Mother is Rh –ve. Some of the fetal red cells cross the placenta and enter the maternal circulation where they act as foreign antigen and the production of Rh antibodies.
The Rh antibodies are of two main types:
a. The strong or saline antibodies.
b. The weak or albumin antibodies.
The weak or albumin antibodies are small 75 gamma globulins which cross the placental barrier and pass back into the fetal circulation. When this happens, the RBC of fetus are destoryed leading to hemolysis.

Q. 190. Poor prognostic feature in schizophrenia (K/MD/Ent-II/2001)
    (a) Family history of schizophrenia
    (b) Late onset
    (c) Affective symptoms
    (d) Severe precipitating cause

Ans. (a)
Note
Poor prognostic feature in schizophrenia is 'F/H of Schizophrenia'.
Also see
The poor prognostic features of schizophrenia are:
    -Younger patient
    -Single, separated, widowed, dioverced
    -Disease of longer duration
    -Family history of schizophrenia
    -Social isolation
    -Poor work record
    -Poor psycho-sexual adjustment
    -Previous psychiatric history
    -No obvious precipitation cause
    -Gradual onset
    -No affective symptoms
    -Paranoid symptoms
    -Loss of initiative in life
    -Presence of 'soft' neurological sings
    -Predominant negative symptoms
    -Delayed treateament
Ref: Golwala.

Extended information
Poor prognostic factors in schizophrenia
- Insidious onset
- Onset < 20years of age
- Absence of stressor
- Poor premorbid adjustment
- Absence of depression
- Chronic course
- Family history of schizophrenia
- Past history of schizophrenia
- Male sex
- Thin physic
- Poor social support or unmarried
- Flat or blunted affect
- Absence of proper treatment of poor response to treatment
- Long term hospitalization
- Evidence of ventricular enlargement on cranial CT scan

Pg 63, Neeraj Ahuja, 5th edition

Q. 191. False perception without stimulus is (K/MD/Ent-II/2001)
(a) Illusion
(b) Delusion
(c) Hallucination
(d) Deja Vu

Ans. (c)
Note
False perception without stimulus is 'Hallucination'.

Also see
Hallucination (perception without stimulation); are usually experienced as originating in the outside world or within one own body but not within the mind as through imagination.
Ref: API, 7th Ed. Pg-1378

Extended information
Hallucination
A hallucination is a false perception occurring without any identifiable external stimulus and indicates an abnormality in perception. The false perceptions can occur in any of the five sensory modalities. Therefore, a hallucination essentially is seeing, hearing, tasting, feeling, or smelling something that is not there. The false perceptions are not accounted for by the person's religious or cultural background, and the person experiencing hallucinations may or may not have insight into them. Therefore, some people experiencing hallucinations may be aware that the perceptions are false, whereas others may truly believe that what they are seeing, hearing, tasting, feeling, or smelling is real. In cases when the person truly believes the hallucination is real, the individual may also have a delusional interpretation of the hallucination.

Q. 192. Alcohol dependence is best indicated by (K/MD/Ent-II/2001)
(a) Early morning drinking
(b) Physical complications
(c) Withdrawal symptoms
(d) Increased consumption

Ans. (c)
Note
Alcohol dependence is best indicated by 'withdrawal symptoms'.

Also see
In the diagnosis of alcohol dependence a special emphasis is palced on evidence of tolerance and / or withdrawal, condition referred to as dependence with the physiological componant and which is associated with the more severe clinical course.
Ref: Harrison's Principles of Internal Medicine VOl. II 15th Ed, – Pg-2564

Extended information
Alcohol withdrawal states -

Withdrawal (6-8 hrs after last drink, lasting a week to 10 days):
- Tremors
- Sweating
- Nausea or vomiting
- Tachycardia or Hypertension
- Anxiety
- Motor restlessness
- Insomnia
- Weakness and malaise
- Headache
Can be complicated by:
- Seizures
- Transient hallucinations
Delirium Tremens:
- Withdrawal symptoms
- Confusion
- Disorientation
- Agitation
- Visual auditory and tactile hallucinations
Wernicke's Encephalopathy:
- Confusion
- Ataxia
- Ophthalmoplegia
Korsakoff Syndrome:
- Recent memory deficits
- New learning problems
- Apathy

Ref: API 7th Ed. Pg-1390

Q. 193. In Lithium toxicity, following organs are affected except (K/MD/Ent-II/2001)
   (a) Kidney
   (b) Liver
   (c) Brain
   (d) Heart

Ans. (b)

Note
In Lithium toxicity, following organs are affected except 'liver'.

Also see
The common side effects of lithium toxicity are listed below:
- Neurological – tremor, muscular weakness, cog wheel rigidity, seizures, neurotoxicity.
- Renal – polyurea, polydipsia, tubular changes, nephrogenic diabetes insipidus, nephrotic syndrome.
- CVS – the effects on heart are similar to those of hypokalemia. The commonest ECG change is T wave depression.
- Endocrine - goiter, hypothyroidism, abnormal thyroid function, weight gain.
- GIT- nausea, vomiting, diarrhea, metallic taste, and abdominal pain.
- Skin- acneform eruptions, popular eruptions, and exacerbation of psoriasis.

Ref: Neeraj Ahuja, 5th Ed. Pg-195-96

Extended information
Lithium toxicity
"Lithium carbonate may provide relief from acute episodes of mania or depression and can help prevent them from recurring. Lithium is often helpful in treating manic episodes that are not mixed with any depressive mood. Long-term use of lithium has been shown to reduce the risk of suicide related to bipolar disorder."
"High blood levels of lithium carbonate can be life-threatening. People who take lithium carbonate need to have their blood checked regularly about every two weeks to measure the amount of the drug in their blood. Your doctor will need to periodically test the function of your kidneys and thyroid gland if you are taking lithium. Sometimes other medications cause higher- or lower-than-expected amounts of lithium carbonate in a person's blood. People who take lithium carbonate need to tell their health professional if they take other medications.

The following adverse effects have been reported usually related to serum lithium concentrations:

Gastrointestinal:
Anorexia, nausea, vomiting, diarrhea, thirst, dryness of the mouth, metallic taste, abdominal pain, weight gain or loss.

Neurological:
General muscle weakness, ataxia, tremor, muscle hyperirritability, (fasciculation, twitchings, especially of facial muscles and clonic movements of the limbs), choreoathetotic movement, hyperactive deep tendon reflexes.

CNS:
Anesthesia of the skin, slurred speech, blurring of vision, blackout spells, headache, seizures, cranial nerve involvement, psychomotor retardation, somnolence, toxic confusional states, restlessness, stupor, coma, acute dystonia. EEG changes recorded consisted of diffuse slowing, widening of the frequency spectrum, potentiation and disorganization of background rhythm. Sensitivity to hyperventilation and paroxysmal bilateral synchronous delta activity have also been described.

Cardiovascular:
Arrhythmia, hypotension, ECG changes consisting of flattening or inversion of T waves, peripheral circulatory failure, cardiac collapse.

Genitourinary:
Albuminuria, oliguria, polyuria, glycosuria.

Allergic:
Allergic vasculitis.

Dermatological:
Dryness and thinning of the hair, leg ulcers, skin rash, pruritis

Hematological:
Anemia, leucopenia, (low white blood cell count) leucocytosis (High white blood cell count).

Metabolic:
Transient hyperglycemia, slight elevation of plasma magnesium, goiter formation. Hypercalcemia, associated with lithium induced hyperparathyroidism, has also been reported.

Miscellaneous:
General fatigue, dehydration, peripheral edema.

Q. 194. Acrodermatitis is seen due to the deficiency of (K/MD/Ent-II/2001)
(a) Zinc
(b) Copper
(c) Iron
(d) Pyridoxine

Ans. (a)

Note
Acrodermatitis is seen due to the deficiency of 'Zinc'.

Also see
Acrodermatitis
This is a genetically- determined autosomal recessive condition due to impaired absorption of zinc characterized by the triad of dermatitis, diarrhea and alopecia.
Ref: API, 7th Ed. Pg-1336

Extended information
Zinc deficiency
The first signs of zinc deficiency are impairment of taste, a poor immune response and skin problems. Other symptoms of zinc deficiency can include hair loss, diarrhea, fatigue, delayed wound healing, and decreased growth rate and mental development in infants. It is thought that zinc supplementation can help skin conditions such as acne and eczema, prostate problems, anorexia nervosa, alcoholics and those suffering from trauma or post-surgery.

Copper deficiency
Symptoms of copper deficiency include fatigue, bleeding under the skin, damage to blood vessels, and an enlarged heart. Anemia is common, and the number of white blood cells is decreased.

Iron deficiency
It leads to Iron deficiency anemia.

Pyridoxine deficinecy
Pyridoxine deficiency is associated with peripheral neuritis.

Q. 195. Pityriasis versicolor is caused by (K/MD/Ent-II/2001)
(a) Epidermophyton
(b) Malassezia furfur
(c) Fungus
(d) Trichophyton

Ans. (b)

Note
This Pityriasis versicolor is caused by an overgrowth of the yeast fungus called Pityrosporum orbiculare (Malassezia furfur).

Also see
Pityrosporum
This yeast occurs as a part of normal flora of human skin. Colonization is prominent in scalp, flexures, and upper trunk. The two morphological variants called P. ovale and P. orbicular and the mycelial form of this yeast is called Malassezia furfur. Pityrosporum can over grow in some individuals and has been implicated in three dermatosis:
1. Pityrisis versicolor
2. Seborrheic eczema
3. Pityrosporum folliculitis
Ref: Kumar & Clark, 6th Ed. Pg- 1324

Q. 196. Incubation period of syphilis is (K/MD/Ent-II/2001)
(a) 2 - 7 days
(b) 15 - 20 days
(c) 9 - 90 days
(d) 2 - 6 weeks

Ans. (c)

Note
Incubation period of syphilis is 9-90 days.

Also see
Primary syphilis- the incubation period is usually between 14 and 28 days with a range of 9 - 90 days
Ref: Davidson's 19th Ed. Pg- 97

Q. 197. Umbilicated white pearly papule is seen in (K/MD/Ent-II/2001)
- (a) Chicken pox
- (b) Small pox
- (c) Herpes Zoster
- (d) Molluscum contagiosum

Ans. (d)

Note
Umbilicated white pearly papule is seen in 'Molluscum contagiosum'.

Also see
Molluscum Contagiosum - infection by molluscum contagiosum virus, both sexual and non sexual, produces flesh-coloured umblicated hemispherical papules usually upto 5mm in diameter after an incubation period of 3-12weeks.
Ref: Davidson's 19th Ed. Pg-106

Q. 198. A patient with single hypopigmented anesthetic patch with satellite lesions on fore arm, most likely diagnosis is (K/MD/Ent-II/2001)
- (a) Tuberculoid leprosy
- (b) Indeterminate leprosy
- (c) Neuritic leprosy
- (d) Lepromatous leprosy

Ans. (a)

Note
A single anesthetic patch with satellite lesion of forearm the most likely diagnosis is tuberculoid leprosy.

Also see
Borderline tuberculine leprosy
Satellite lesions; has featurtes of sharply defined hypopigmented area having loss of sensation, hair loss, neural involvement less localized, lepromin test positive.
Ref: Color Atlas of Dermatology, by Bhutani Ist Ed. Pg-31

Extended information
Tuberculoid leprosy- a localized disease that occurs in individuals with a high degree of cell mediated immunity. The T cell response to an antigen releases interferons which activates macrophages to destroy the bacilli but associated with destruction of tissue.
Clinical Features - the characteristic, usually single, skin lesion is a hypopigmented, anesthetic patch with thickened, clearly demarcated edges, central healing and atrophy.
Ref: Kumar & Clark, 6th Ed. Pg- 80

Q. 199. To differentiate the cause of splenomegaly - best is (K/MD/Ent-II/2001)
- (a) Bone marrow
- (b) Splenic pulp smear
- (c) Spleno portography
- (d) Peripheral smear

Ans. (d)

Note
To differentiate the cause of splenomegaly - best is peripheral smear.

Also see
Laboratory investigations in a patient with spleenomegaly depend upon suspected aetiology.Full blood count (hemoglobin, red blood cell indices, total white cell count, platelet count), reticulocyte count, blood film examination is mandatory in all cases.
Ref: API, 7th Ed. Pg-929

Extended information
Bone Marrow:
Useful in diagnosis of hematological malignancy including leukaemia, myeloproliferative disorders, lymphoma, myeloma, kala-azar.
Splenic pulps smear:
For obtaining smear of spleen tissue if other methods are negative or questionable; Lymph-sarcoma, Hodgkin's disease, etc.
Spleno-portography:
Useful in diagnosis of vascular cause.
Peripheral smear:
For diagnosis of malaria, leukaemia, polycythemia, infectious mononucleosis, hereditary spherocytosis.

Q. 200. Useful test for diagnosis of primary hypothyroidism (K/MD/Ent-II/2001)
    (a)   TSH
    (b)   T3 T4
    (c)   Biopsy
    (d)   Scan

Ans. (a)
Note
Useful test for diagnosis of primary hypothyroidism is assay of serum TSH. It provides an exquisitely sensitive marker of primary hypothyroidism.
Also see
Serum TSH is the investigation of choice; a high TSH level confirms primary hypothyroidism. A low free T4 level confirms hypothyroid state (and is also essential to exclude TSH deficiency if clinical hypothyroidism is strongly suspected and TSH is normal or low.)
Ref: Kumar & Clark, 6th Ed. Pg-1072

Q. 201. Best artery for coronary angiography (K/MD/Ent-II/2001)
    (a)   Brachial
    (b)   Femoral
    (c)   Carotid
    (d)   Axillary

Ans. (b)
Note
Best artery for coronary angiography is femoral artery.
Also see
Catheter angiography is indicated in the evaluation of patients with vascular pathology particularly of small intracranial vessels. Patient undergoing angiography should be well hydrated before and after the procedure. Since the femoral route is used most commonly, the femoral artery must be compressed after the procedure to prevent a hematoma from developing. The puncture site and distal pulses should be evaluated carefully after the procedure; complications can include thigh hematoma or lower extremity emboli.
Ref: Harrison, 16th Ed. Pg-2356

Extended information
The test is done on an outpatient basis. The patient is mildly sedated but awake during the procedure. A local anesthetic is used to numb the area (usually the right groin). Soft plastic tubes ("catheters") are inserted into the artery and then advanced under X-ray guidance. The dye is injected into the heart chambers and coronaries and pictures are taken from different angles. This is the best test available to find and visualize the blockages.

Q. 202. Painless swelling below hyoid bone - most common diagnosis is (K/MD/Ent-II/2001)
    (a)   Thyroglossal cyst
    (b)   Ectopic thyroid
    (c)   Lymph node
    (d)   Brachial cyst

Ans. (a)

Note
Painless swelling below hyoid bone - most common diagnosis is 'Thyroglossal cyst'.
Also see
The thyroglossal cyst is mainly diagnosed by its characteristic position. It being a cyst of thyroglossal tract, it is mainly a midline structure. The commonest position is the sub-hyoid (just below the hyoid bone) and next common is the suprahyoid (just above the hyoid bone) position. The cyst is essentially midline in position in these two places. It may be seen at the level of the thyroid cartilage, when it is shifted to the left and must be differentiated from cervical lymph node enlargement. The least common position is at the level of the cricoid cartilage when it may mimic an adenoma of the isthmus of the thyroid.
Ref: Clinical Surgery S. Das, 6th Ed. Pg-296

Q. 203. Most common site of metastasis from cancer kidney is (K/MD/Ent-II/2001)
    (a)   Bone
    (b)   Liver
    (c)   Brain
    (d)   Lungs

Ans. (d)
Note
Most common site of metastasis from cancer kidney is lungs.
Also see

The first symptom is usually blood in the urine. Sometimes both kidneys are involved. The cancer spreads easily, most often to the lungs and other organs. About one-third of patients have spreading (metastasis) at the time of diagnosis.
Renal cell carcinoma-Mode of spread:
Due to numerous large thin walled blood vessels which are present in the tumour, blood spread is by far the most important. In no other carcinoma it is seen at such a great degree. Blood spread occurs in two ways- Embolism and Permeation.
In embolism pieces of growth become detached and are swept into the venous circulation to become first arrested in the lungs. In the lungs the metastasis produces 'Canon-ball' deposits which are revealed in the X-ray as round opaque metastasis in lungs and later on further small pieces may enter into arterial circulation and may be deposited in the bones.
Ref: Textbook of surgery S DAS 3rd Ed. Pg-1187

Q. 204. Most common symptom of cancer bladder (K/MD/Ent-II/2001)
    (a)   Hematuria
    (b)   Urinary incontinence
    (c)   Pain
    (d)   Fever

Ans. (a)
Note
Most common symptom of cancer bladder is hematuria.
Also see

The earliest and most common symptom of CA bladder is painless hematuria. Hematuria is usually intermittent as with all tumours of urinary tract. Bleeding may be mild or severe, transient or prolonged. Bleeding may occur once or twice and then it may stop to start again after many months to cause concern. Bleeding may be so profuse as to cause clot retention. Occasionally it may require emergency admission and blood transfusion immediately.
Ref: Textbook of Surgery S. Das 3rd Ed. Pg-1217

Q. 205. Commonest cause of cerebral infarction (K/MD/Ent-II/2001)
    (a)   Thrombosis
    (b)   Embolism
    (c)   Arteritis
    (d)   Cysticercosis

Ans. (a)

Note
Commonest cause of cerebral infarction is thrombosis.

Also see
A common cause of stroke is atherosclerosis. (See stroke secondary to atherosclerosis.) Fatty deposits and blood platelets collect on the wall of the arteries, forming plaques. Over time, the plaques slowly begin to block the flow of blood. The plaque itself may block the artery enough to cause a stroke.

Extended information
Cerebral infarction is mostly due to thromboembolic disease secondary to atherosclerosis in the major extracranial arteries (carotid artery and aortic arch). About 20% of infarctions are consequent upon embolism from the heart, and a further 20% are due to occlusion of the small lenticulostriate perforating vessels by intrinsic disease (lipohyalinosis), producing so called' lacunar' infarctions.
Ref: Davidson, 19th Ed. Pg-1160

Q. 206. Commonest cause of adrenal insufficiency in India is (K/MD/Ent-II/2001)
(a) T B
(b) Auto immune
(c) Steroid withdrawal
(d) Surgery

Ans. (a)

Note
Commonest cause of adrenal insufficiency in India is T.B.

Also see
Addison's disease –It results from progressive destruction of adrenal glands. Before the symptoms and signs of Addison's disease become apparent, 90% of gland is destroyed. The commonest cause in underdeveloped countries is Tuberculosis. However, in developed countries, the most common cause is autoimmune destruction of the adrenal cortex.
Ref: API, 7th Ed. Pg-1073

Q. 207. Bleeding per rectum is present in following except (K/MD/Ent-II/2001)
(a) Ulcerative colitis
(b) Meckel's diverticulum
(c) Rectal carcinoma
(d) Sigmoid valvulus

Ans. (d)

Note
Bleeding per rectum is present in following except 'Sigmoid valvulus'.

Also see
A. Local causes:
  1. Anal causes: Hemorrhoides, Anal fissure, Mucosal prolapse, Ulceration (Crohn's, disease), Carcinoma & Fistula -in –ano.
  2. Perianal causes: Prolapsed rectum and piles, Ruptured perianal hematoma, Ruptured Anorectal abscess, Injury, Condylomata, Carcinoma and Skin excoriation.
  3. Colorectal causes: Diverticular disease, Various types of polyps, Villous adenoma, Carcinoma, Ulcerative colitis, Angiodysplasia, Inflammatory bowel disease, Endometriosis, Crohn's disease, Hemangioma.
  4. Small intestine causes: Intussusception, Crohn's disease, Meckle's diverticulum, Tumours.
B. General causes: Blood dyscrasias, Drugs, Liver failure, Renal failure
Ref: Textbook of Surgery S. Das 3rd Ed. Pg-1080

Extended information
Whereas patients with sigmoid volvulus more typically have the picture of colonic obstruction in which marked distention predominates, with relatively less pain.

Q. 208. Which hernia is least likely to strangulate? (K/MD/Ent-II/2001)
(a) Direct inguinal hernia
(b) Indirect inguinal hernia
(c) Femoral hernia
(d) Umbilical hernia

Ans. (d)

Note

Hernia is least likely to strangulate is 'Umbilical Hernia'.

Also see

Umbilical hernia: This is a hernia through a weak umbilical scar, may be following neonatal sepsis. The hernia is usually symptomless and increase in size during crying. Small hernia is spherical in shape but when they increase in size they tend to assume a conical shape. Strangulation is extremely rare in this type of hernia.
Ref: Textbook of surgery S. Das 3rd Ed. Pg-1115

Extended information

A strangulated hernia is a surgical emergency. Even if strangulation is only suspected, medical advice should be sought without delay. If strangulation is not relieved urgently, so that blood circulation is restored, the loop of bowel will die and become gangrenous. This can cause life-threatening blood poisoning (septicemia). The three commonest types of hernia to strangulate are, in order of frequency:
- Femoral hernias
- Indirect inguinal hernias
- Umbilical hernias.

Q. 209. False about filaria is (K/MD/Ent-II/2001)
(a) Man is intermediate host.
(b) Adult worms are found in lymphatics of man.
(c) Culex is a vector.
(d) Life span of microfilaria is not exactly known.

Ans. (a)

Note

False about Filaria is 'Man is intermediate host'. However, the true is man is the 'definite host'.

Also see

Filaria man is the definitive host and mosquito is the intermediate host of bancroftian and brugian filiriasis. The adult worms are usually found in the lymphatic system of man. The life span of the MF is not exactly known. Culex, Anopheles, Aedes serves as vecors for W.bancrofti.
Ref: Park & Park, 18th Ed. Pg-212, 213

Q. 210. In case of Cholera true is (K/MD/Ent-II/2001)
(a) Cholera toxin acts on GM, receptor
(b) Mortality is more with El Tor
(c) Activates cycle AMP
(d) Is neurotoxic

Ans. (c)

Note

In a case of cholera ture is 'Activates cycle AMP'

Also see

The E1 Tor biotype which are known for their hemolytic property, lost this property as pandemic progress.
Toxin production: the vibrio multiply in the lumen of small intestine and produce exotoxin.
This toxin produces diarrhea through its effect on adenylate cyclase-cyclic AMP system of mucosal cell of small intestine. The exotoxin has no effect on any other tissue except intestinal epithelial cells.
Cases range from inapparent infection to severe ones. In choler E1 Tor, most infections are mild and asymptomatic.
Ref: Park and Park, 18th Ed. Pg-177

Q. 211. Gonococcus does not cause involvement of (K/MD/Ent-II/2001)
(a) Epidydimis
(b) Testis
(c) Prostate
(d) Ant-urethra

Ans. (b)

Note
Gonococcus does not cause involvement of testis.

Also see
Uncomplicated gonoccocal infection in the males results in acute anterior urethritis with symptoms of dysuria and urethral discharge often of a purulent nature. Complications may result from spread of the infection to cause epididymitis, chronic prostatitis, balanitis, and posterior urethritis.
Ref: API, 7th Ed. Pg-36

Extended information
Gonorrhea is an infectious disease. It causes following complications:
a. Tysonitis: Inflammation of the glands on either side of the frenulum.
b. Littritis: Inflammation of littris glands.
c. Cowperitis: Bulbo-urethral glands ae enlarged, discovered when investigating a chronic discharge.
d. Prostatitis: May be acute, subacute or chronic
e. Vesiculiotis: The seminal vesicles are not palpable normally but when infected a small mass will be palpable just above the prostate.
f. Epididymo-orchitis.
g. Cystitis.
h. Utethral stricute- rare now a days. However, it is due to fibrosis of the uretheral mucous membrane - commonly occurs at the bulbo urethra.
Ref: Medicine form Students by Golwalla 10th Ed, Pg-878

Q. 212. True about lepra bacilli are (K/MD/Ent-II/2001)
(a) Anti leprosy vaccine gives life long protection.
(b) INH inhibits their growth.
(c) Incubation period is 3-4 months.
(d) Microbacterium leprae can be grown in foot pad of mice.

Ans. (d)

Note
True about lepra bacilli is 'Microbacterium leprae can be grown in the foot pad of mice'.

Also see
a. Vaccination at birth with Bacille Calmette-Guerin (BCG) has proved variably effective in preventing leprosy, ranging from totally ineffective to 80% efficacious.
b. The Dapsone is bateriostatic. (Not INH). The WHO recommends that paucibacillary adults be treated with 100 mg of dapsone daily and 600 mg of rifampin monthly (supervised) for 6 months. Multibacillary adults should be treated with 100 mg of dapsone plus 50 mg of clofazimine daily (unsupervised) and with 600 mg of rifampin plus 300 mg of clofazimine monthly (supervised). Originally, the WHO recommended that lepromatous patients be treated for 2 years or until smears became negative (generally in 5 years); subsequently, the acceptable course was reduced to 1 year a change that remains controversial in the absence of clinical trials.
c. Because leprosy transmission appears to require close prolonged household contact, hospitalized patients need not be isolated. The incubation period prior to manifestation of clinical disease can vary between 2 and 40 years, although it is generally 5 to 7 years in duration.
d. Lepra bacilli was the first bacterium to be etiologically associated with human disease, yet till now *M. leprae* has not been cultivated on artificial medium or tissue culture. The multiplication of *M. leprae* in mouse footpads has provided a means to evaluate antimicrobial agents. *M. leprae* grows best in cooler tissues (the skin, peripheral nerves, anterior chamber of the eye, upper respiratory tract, and testes), sparing warmer areas of the skin (the axilla, groin, scalp, and midline of the back).
Ref: Harrison's 16th Ed. Pg- 966, 967, 970, 971

Q. 213. Immunoglobulin which crosses placental barrier is (K/MD/Ent-II/2001)
- (a) IgG
- (b) IgM
- (c) IgD
- (d) IgE

Ans. (a)

Note
Immunoglobulin which crosses placental barrier is IgG.

Also see
IgG is the most abundant immunoglobin in serum, present as monomer IgG is the antibody of secondary response, and has high antigen affinity. It is the only antibody to cross the placenta in significant quantities, thereby providing protection to the fetus in its first weeks of life before its own immune system has developed.
Ref: Kumar and Clark 6th Ed. Pg-207

Extended information
IgG is a monomeric immunoglobulin, built of two heavy chains γ and two light chains. Each molecule has two antigen binding sites. It can bind to many kinds of pathogens, for example viruses, bacteria, and fungi, and protects the body against them by complement activation (classic pathway), opsonization for phagocytosis and neutralisation of their toxins. There are 4 subclasses: IgG1 (66%), IgG2 (23%), IgG3 (7%) and IgG4 (4%). -IgG1, IgG3 and IgG4 cross the placenta easily. -IgG3 is the most effective complement activator, followed by IgG1 and then IgG2. IgG4 does not activate complement. - IgG1 and IgG3 bind with high affinity to Fc receptors on phagocytic cells. IgG4 has intermediate affinity and IgG2 affinity is extremely low.

Q. 214. For HTLV-III infection (AIDS) - the most specific test is (K/MD/Ent-II/2001)
- (a) ELISA test
- (b) Manospot test
- (c) Western blot test
- (d) Virus culture

Ans. (c)

Note
For HTLV-III infection (AIDS) - the most specific test is 'Western Blot Test'.

Also see
To ensure accuracy, two different tests are commonly applied. At first a sensitive test is done to detect HIV-antibdies (ELISA), while a second confirmatory test (Western Blot) is used to find out any false positive results.
Pg- 263 Park and Park

Additional information
HTLV-III: The human T-lymphotropic virus type III. An absolute term for the human immunodeficiency virus or HIV.

Q. 215. Negri bodies are most often found in (K/MD/Ent-II/2001)
- (a) Midbrain
- (b) Hippocampus
- (c) Basal ganglia
- (d) Frontal cortex

Ans. (b)

Note
Negri bodies are most often found in Hippocampus.

Also see
The most characteristic pathologic finding of rabies in the CNS is the formation of cytoplasmic inclusions called Negri bodies within neurons. Negri bodies are distributed throughout the brain, *particularly in Ammon's horn*, the cerebral cortex, the brainstem, the hypothalamus, the Purkinje cells of the cerebellum, and the dorsal spinal ganglia. Negri bodies are not demonstrated in at least 20% of cases of rabies, and their absence from brain material does not rule out the diagnosis.
Ref: Harrison- 16th Ed. Pg-1157

Extended information
Ammon's horn is an alternative name for the hippocampus, a brain region involved in learning and memory; although most neuroscientists now use the latter term. Unfortunately, different scientists used the term in different ways-some used it to refer to the entire hippocampus, while others excluded the dentate gyrus from the definition.
Ref: everything2.com/index.pl?node_id=1034012 - 18k

Q. 216. Epidemiologic study of Hepatitis-B (K/MD/Ent-II/2001)
(a) HBs Ag is used
(b) IgG and HBc
(c) HBcAg
(d) HBeAg

Ans. (a)

Note
In epidemiologic study of Hepatitis-B 'HBsAg' is used.

Also see
Epidemiology: Studying the distribution of disease in human population. Hepatitis B virus has a surface antigen also known as 'Australia antigen' (HBsAg). It is the first to be detected. It appears in the serum during the incubation period before biochemical evidence of liver damage or the onset of jaundice. It persists durig acute illness and is usually cleared from the blood stream during convalescence.
Ref: Park and Park, 18th Ed. Pg-167

Q. 217. Adult hemoglobin consists of chains (MD (Hom) Ent / Paper -1 /2001)
(a) 2a+2B
(b) 2B+2Y
(c) 2a+2Z
(d) 2a+2Y

Ans. (a)
Adult hemoglobin consists of chains 2a+2B.

Also see
Globin is a protein built from four polypeptide chains, two 'alpha' and two "beta' chains. Therefore the normal adult hemoglobin HbA(A2 B2).
Ref: Textbook of Physiology by A.K. Jain Pg- 51 Edition

Q. 218. The encephalopathy commonly seen in chronic alcoholics is (MD-Hom/Ent-I/2001)
(a) Reye's Syndrome
(b) Multicystic encephalopathy
(c) Wernike's encephalopathy
(d) Spongiform encephalopathy

Ans. (c)

Note
The encephalopathy commonly seen in chronic alcoholics is 'Wernicke's encephalopathy'.

Also see
'Wernicke's encepalopathy' is caused by malnutrition especially lack of Vitamin B1 (Thiamine) which commonly accompanies habitual alcohol use or alcoholism.

Extended information
In the western world alcohol dependent patients and those with severe acute illness receiving high carbohydrate infusions with out vitamins are the only major groups to suffer from thiamine deficiency. Rarely do they develop wet beri beri, which must be distinguished from alcoholic cardiomyopathy. More usually, however, thiamine deficiency presents with polyneuropathy or with the wernicke-korsakoff syndrome.
Ref: Kumar and Clark, 6th Ed. Pg-245

Q. 219. The hepatocytes formed only in the carriers of chronic Hepatitis B are (MD-Hom/Ent-I/2001)
 (a) Tombstone cells
 (b) Councilman bodies
 (c) Ground glass cells
 (d) Kupffer cells

Ans. (c)

Note
The hepatocytes formed only in the carriers of chronic Hepatitis B are 'Ground glass cells'.

Also see
Cases of chronic hepatitis B shows scattered ground glass hepatocytes indicative of abundance of HBs Ag in the cytoplasm.
Ref: Harsh Mohan, 2nd Ed. Pg-450

Extended information
Acute Viral Hepatitis: The pathologic changes are the same for Hepatitis A; B; and C. There is hepatocyte injury with swelling also called "ballooning" degeneration), necrosis with formation of Acidophil (Councilman) bodies, disarray of the hepatic lobules, Kupfer cell hyperplasia, and inflammatory cells in portal areas (lymphocytes, eosinophils, and neutrophils).
"Ground glass hepatocytes" (GGHs) are the historic hallmarks for the hepatocytes in the late and non-replicative stages of hepatitis B virus (HBV) infection.

Q. 220. The eggs of Schistosoma mansoni are characterised by (MD-Hom/Ent-I/2001)
 (a) Lateral spine
 (b) Terminal spine
 (c) Lateral knob
 (d) None of the above

Ans. (a)

Note
The eggs of Schistosoma mansoni are characterised by 'lateral spine'.

Also see
Egg of S. masoni is 150 by 60 micrometer, and has a lateral spine.
Ref: Parasitology by K.D.Chaterjee, 12th Ed.Pg-138, Table differentiating features of schistosomes

Extended information
The schistosome egg differs from those of related digenean parasites in that they are non-operculate, and have terminal or *lateral spines*. The egg shells are sclero-proteic, being lined on the inside by a vitelline membrane adhering to the shell by means of two (or sometimes more) vacuoles which press on the developing larvae anteriorly and posteriorly.

Q. 221. The only nematode having a free living life cycle along with parasitic life cycle is (MD-Hom/Ent-I/2001)
 (a) Nector americanus
 (b) Strongyloides stercoralis
 (c) Dracunculus medinensis
 (d) Trichinella spirates

Ans. (b)

Note
The only nematode having a free living life cycle along with parasitic life cycle is 'Strongyloides stercoralis'.

Also see
Strongyloides require no intermediate host. The worm passes its life cycle in one host and unlike other nematodes, a change of host is not essential as it undergoes a hyperinfective form of development.
Ref: Parasitology by K. D. Chaterjee, 12th Ed. Pg- 168

Extended information

a. *Nector americanus*
One of the two hookworm species (A. duodenale and N. americanus):
One-fourth of the world's population is infected with one of the two hookworm species (A. duodenale and N. americanus). Most infected individuals are asymptomatic. Hookworm disease develops from a combination of factors a heavy worm burden, a prolonged duration of infection, and an inadequate iron intake and results in iron-deficiency anemia and, on occasion, hypoproteinemia.

b. *Strongyloides stercoralis (Threadworms)*
Threadworm infection is caused by *Strongyloides stercoralis*, a roundworm that lives in soil and can survive there for several generations. Mature threadworms may grow as long as 1–2 in (2.5–5 cm). The larvae have two stages in their life cycle: a rod-shaped (rhabdoid) first stage, which is not infective; and a threadlike (filariform) stage, in which the larvae can penetrate intact human skin and internal tissues. Threadworms are unique among human parasites in having both free-living and parasitic forms. In the *free-living life cycle*, some rhabdoid larvae develop into adult worms that live in contaminated soil and produce eggs that hatch into new rhabdoid larvae. The adult worms may live as long as five years.

c. *Dracunculus medinensis (Guinea worm)*
Dracunculiasis, caused by Dracunculus medinensis, is a parasitic infection whose incidence has declined dramatically because of global eradication efforts. Humans acquire this infection when they ingest water containing infective larvae derived from Cyclops, a crustacean that is the intermediate host. Larvae penetrate the stomach or intestinal wall, mate, and mature. The adult male probably dies; the female Dracunculus develops over a year and migrates to subcutaneous tissues, usually in the lower extremity. As the thin female Dracunculus, ranging in length from 300 cm to 1 m, approaches the skin, a blister forms that, over days, breaks down and forms an ulcer. When the blister opens, large numbers of motile, rhabditiform larvae can be released into stagnant water; ingestion by Cyclops completes the life cycle.

d. *Trichinella spirartes*
Trichina is the common name for species of roundworm of the phylum Nematoda. The species Trichinella spiralis is an important parasite, occurring in rats, pigs, and man, and is responsible for the disease trichinosis.
Maturity
The small adult worms mature in the intestine of an intermediate host such as a pig. Each adult female produces batches of up to 1,500 live larvae, which bore through the intestinal wall, enter the blood and lymphatic system, and are carried to striated muscle tissue. Once in the muscle, they encyst, or become enclosed in a capsule.
Larvae encysted in the muscles remain viable for some time. When the muscle tissue is eaten by a human, the cysts are digested in the stomach; the released larvae migrate to the intestine to begin a new life cycle. Female trichina worms live about six weeks and in that time may release 15,000 larvae. The migration and encystment of larvae can cause fever, pain, and even death. Encysted larvae in pork are destroyed by thorough cooking or long periods of low-temperature storage. Trichina are classified in the phylum Nematoda.

Q. 222. Pernicious malaria is caused by (MD-Hom/Ent-I/2001)
    (a) Plasmodium ovale
    (b) Plasmodium falciparum
    (c) Plasmodium malariae
    (d) Plasmodium vivax

Ans. (b)
Note
Pernicious malaria is caused by 'Plasmodium falciparum'.
Also see
Following are the types of Malaria:
Benign tertian malaria:
    Paroxysm after 48 hours.
    Caused by P. vivax and P. ovale.

Commonest in India.
Benign quartan malaria:
  Paroxysm after 72 hours.
  Caused by P. malariae.
  Rare in India.
Malignant malaria:
  Periodicity not marked.
  Caused by P. falciparum.

Extended information
Severe (Pernicious) malaria: about 1% of patients with plasmodium falciparum infection may develop more severe manifestation culminating in failure of various organ systems. This does not occur with P.vivax infection because the vivax parasite undergoes their entire erythrocytic lifecycle in circulating RBCs. The infected cells develop small protrusions on their cell membrane which serve to attach to the capillary endothelium. The parasite probably gets some nutrition frpm the endothelium and mature into schizonts, and merozoites. This results in microcirculatory obstruction. Moreover, unlike P.vivax which infect only young RBCs, P.falciparum can infect RBCs of all ages, producing heavier parasitaemia.
Ref: API, 7th Ed. Pg-105

Q. 223. 50% of the gastric carcinomas arise from (MD-Hom/Ent-I/2001)
  (a) Cardiac end of the stomach
  (b) Lesser curvature
  (c) Antrum
  (d) Greater curvature

Ans. (c)
Note
The majority of gasctic carcinomas arsis form 'antrum'.
Also see
Gastric carcinoma site- gastric adenocarcinoma mostly develops from the mucosal cells anywhere within the stomach although the majority develop in pyloric and antric region particularly along the lesser curvature. So the most common site is pyloric and antral regions. Next common is along the lesser curvature.
Ref: Textbook of Surgery, S. Das.3rd Ed. Pg- 853

Q. 224. The intradermal test diagnostic of Echinococcus granulosis is (MD-Hom/Ent-I/2001)
  (a) Casoni's test
  (b) Leishmanin test
  (c) Sabinfeidman dye test
  (d) Bentonite test

Ans. (a)
Note
The intradermal test diagnostic of Echinococcus granulosis is 'Casoni's test'.
Also see
The diagnosis of hydatid cyst is made by peripheral blood eosinophilia, radiologic examination and serological test such as indirect hemagglutination test and casoni skin test.
Ref: Textbook of pathology by Harsh Mohan, 4th Ed., Ch- 17 – GIT, Pg- 598

Q. 225. Meleyney's ulcer is caused by (MD-Hom/Ent-I/2001)
  (a) Wet gangrene
  (b) Dry gangrene
  (c) Synergistic gangrene
  (d) Gas gangrene

Ans. (c)
Note
Meleyney's ulcer is caused by 'synergistic gangrene'.
Also see
Meleney's gangrene; a postoperative gangrene with a chronic enlarging ulcer due to infection.

Extended information
Gangrene
It is a form of tissue death or necrosis, commonly involving an extremity and due to insufficient blood supply.

Wet Gangrene
Wet gangrene occurs when blood supply to the organ is blocked and bacterial contamination occurs i.e., in intestines.

Dry Gangrene
Dry gangrene or senile gangrene is usually caused by progressive atherosclerosis and involves small portions of extremities, such as fingers and goes. It has a sharp inflammatory border marks the edge of the adjacent viable tissue.

Synergistic gangrene
Meleney's gangrene; a postoperative gangrene with a chronic enlarging ulcer due to infection with microaerophilic streptococcus and staphylococcus aureus.

Gas gangrene
Gas gangrene (myonecrosis) is a type of moist gangrene that is commonly caused by bacterial infection with Clostridium welchii, Cl. perfringes, Cl. septicum, Cl. novyi, Cl. histolyticum, Cl. sporogenes, or other species that are capable of thriving under conditions where there is little oxygen (anaerobic). Once present in tissue, these bacteria produce gasses and poisonous toxins as they grow.

Q. 226. The purple discolouration which develops in the dependent parts of a dead body is called (MD-Hom/Ent-I/2001)
- (a) Postmortem clotting
- (b) Livor mortis
- (c) Algar mortis
- (d) Rigor mortis

Ans. (b)
Note
The purple discolouration which develops in the dependent parts of a dead body is called 'livor mortis'.
Also see
Post mortem hypostasis- This is bluish purple or purplish red discolouration which appears under the skin in most superficial layers of dermis of the dependent parts of body after death, due to capillovenous distention. It is called post mortem staining, subcutaneous hypostasis, livor mortis, cadaveric lividity, suggilation, vibices and darkening of death.
Ref: Nararyan Reddy, 19th Ed. Pg-128
Livor Mortis
The reddish-blue discoloration of the cadaver that occurs in the dependent portions of the body due to gradual gravitational flow of unclotted blood.

Q. 227. Lines of zahnare seen in (MD-Hom/Ent-I/2001)
- (a) Ischeniia
- (b) Thrombosis
- (c) Embolism
- (d) Fibroids

Ans. (b)
Note
Line of zahnare seen in 'Thrombosis'.
Also see
Grossly thrombi may be of various shapes, size and composition depending upon the site of origin. Arterial thrombi tend to be white and mural while the venous thrombi are red and occlusive. Mixed or laminated thrombi are also common and consist of alternate white and red layers called lines of Zahn. Red thrombis are soft, red and gelatinous whereas white thrombi are white and pale.
Ref: Harshmohan, 4th Ed. Pg-100

Q. 228. Wilson's disease is caused by accumulation in the body of (MD-Hom/Ent-I/2001)
    (a)   Iron
    (b)   Magnesium
    (c)   Calcium
    (d)   Copper

Ans. (d)
Note
Wilson's disease is caused by accumulation in the body of 'Copper'.

Also see

Wilson's disease is a very rare inborn error of copper metabolism that results in copper deposition in various organs, including liver, the basal ganglia of the brain and the cornea. It is potentially treatable and all young patients with liver disease must be screened for this condition.
Ref: Kumar and Clark 6th Ed. Pg-387

Extended information
Wilson's disese (Hepatolenticular degeneration) is a disease of copper toxicosis inherited as autosomal recessive trait.

Q. 229. Inhalation of dust, dander, pollen molds initiates the formation of (MD-Hom/Ent-I/2001)
    (a)   １gM
    (b)   IgA
    (c)   IgE
    (d)   IgG

Ans. (c)
Note
Inhalation of dust, dander, pollen molds initiates the formation of 'IgE'.

Also see
IgM
IgM antibodies appear early in the course of an infection and usually do not reappear after further exposure. IgM antibodies do not pass across the human placenta. These are the first to appear in an immune response (primary antibody response) and is the initial type of the antibody made by neonates. IgM is an important component of immune complexes in autoimmune disease i.e., IgM antibodies against IgG molecules (Rheumatoid factor) are present in high titer in rheumatoid arthritis and other collagen disordrs and some infectious disease like Subacute Bacterial Endocarditis.
Ref: Harrison Ed-16th –Pg-1922
IgA

IgA is secreted in tears, saliva, nasal scerections gastrointestinal tract fluid and human milk in the form of secretory IgA ((sIgA). IgA fixes compliment via the alternative compliment pathway and has potent antiviral activity in humans by prevention of virus binding to respiratory and gastrointestinal epithelial cells.
Ref: Harrison Ed-16th –Pg-1922
IgE
IgE, that can specifically recognise an "allergen" (a protein, such as dust mite, grass or ragweed pollen, etc.) has a unique long-lived interaction with its high affinity receptor, so that basophils and mast cells, capable of mediating inflammatory reactions, become "primed", ready to release chemicals like histamine, leucotrienes and certain interleukins, which cause many of the symptoms we associate with allergy, such as airway constriction in asthma, local inflammation in eczema, increased mucous secretion in allergic rhinitis and increased vascular permeability, ostensibly to allow other immune cells to gain access to tissues, but which can lead to a potentially fatal drop in blood pressure as in anaphylaxis.
Ref: Harrison Ed-15th
IgG
IgG is a monomeric immunoglobulin, built of two heavy chains γ and two light chains. Each molecule has two antigen binding sites. This is the most abundant immunoglobulin and is approximately equally distributed in blood and in tissue liquids. This is the only isotype that can pass through the placenta, thereby providing

protection to the fetus in its first weeks of life before its own immune system has developed. It can bind to many kinds of pathogens, for example viruses, bacteria, and fungi, and protects the body against them by complement activation (classic pathway), opsonization for phagocytosis and neutralisation of their toxins.
Ref: Harrison Ed-15th

Q. 230. Post-pneumonic fibrosis is called (MD-Hom/Ent-I/2001)
(a) Caranification
(b) Hepatization
(c) Consolidation
(d) Legionnaires disease

Ans. (a)
Note
Post-pneumonic fibrosis is called 'Caranificaiton'.

Also see
Organisation in pneumonia: In about 3 % of cases, resolution of the exudates does not occur instead it is organized. There is ingrowth of fibroblast from the alveolar septa resulting in fibrosed, tough, airless leathery lung tissue. This type of post pneumonic fibrosis is called carnification.
Ref: Harshmohan, 4th Ed. Pg-442

Q. 231. Chronic bacterial pneumonia can occur as a result of (MD-Hom/Ent-I/2001)
(a) A sequele to acute pneumonia
(b) Prolonged smoking
(c) In a part of lung caused by bronchogenic carcinoma
(d) All of the above

Ans. (d)
Note
Chronic bacterial pneumonia can occur as a result of 'All of above'.

Also see
Prolonged smoking, alcohol and corticosteroid therapy impares the ciliary and immune functions. Other risk factors include old age, recent influenzeal infection, pre-existing lung disease.

Extended information
Precipitating factors of Pneumonia:
   -Strep.pneumoniae- often follows viral infection with influenza or -parainfluenza.
   -Hospitalized "ill" patients-often infected with gram negative organism.
   -Cigarette smoking (the strongest independent risk factor for invasive pneumococcal disease).
   -Alcohol excess
   -Bronchiectasis
   -Bronchial obstruction (e.g. carcinoma-occassionally associated with infection with "non-pathogenic" organisms)
   -Immunosupression
   -Intravenous drug abuse
   -Inhalation from esophageal obstruction.
Ref: Kumar and Clark 6th Ed. Pg-923

Q. 232. The disease occurring in cotton workers is (MD-Hom/Ent-I/2001)
(a) Berryliosis
(b) Pneumoconiosis
(c) Byssinosis
(d) Brucellosis

Ans. (c)
Note
The disease occurring in cotton workers is 'byssinosis'.

Also see
Byssinosis is due to inhalation of cotton fibre dust over long period of time. The symptoms are chronic cough and progressive dyspnea, ending in chronic bronchitis and emphysema.
Park & Park, 18th Ed. Pg- 609

Extended information
Cottton dust (Byssinosis) exposures can causes occupational asthma. It results in pronounced obstructive patterns of pulmonary dysfunction that may be reversible. Measurement of change in forced expiratory volume (FEV1) before and after a working shift can be used to detect an acute inflammatory or bronchoconstrictive response. An acute decrement of FEV1 over the first work shift of the week is a characteristic feature of cotton textile workers with byssinosis

Q. 233. The following dietary factors are responsible for carcinoma stomach except (MD-Hom/Ent-I/2001)
    (a)   Nitrates
    (b)   Nitrites
    (c)   Nitro-carbons
    (d)   Poly cyclic hydrocarbons

Ans. (c)
The all of above responsible for ca stomach except 'Nitro-carbons'.
Note
Role of diet in gastric carcinoma: Population consuming certain food stuff have high risk of developing gastric cancer, e.g. ingestion of smoked foods, high intake of salt, pickled raw vegetables, high intake of carcinogens as nitrates in food and drinking water, nitrites as preservatives for certain meats etc. tobacco smoke, tobacco juice and consumption of alcohol.
Ref: Shortbook of Pathology by Harshmohan. Pg- 402
The process of smoking meat and fish adds carcinogens and carcinogenic hydrocarbons to these foods.
Ref: Textbook of Surgery, S. Das.3rd Ed. Pg- 852
Diet rich in salted, smoked or pickled foods and the consumption of nitrites and nitrates are associated the cancer risk. Carcinogenic N-nitroso-compounds are formed from nitrates by the action of nitrite reducing bacteria which colonized the achlorhydric stomach.
Ref: Devidson's Edition 18th Pg-639

Q. 234. A malignant tumour arising from extreme apex of a lung (MD-Hom/Ent-I/2001)
    (a)   Pancoast tumour
    (b)   Wilm's tumour
    (c)   Salivary tumour
    (d)   Blastoma

Ans. (a)
Note
A malignant tumour arising from extreme apex of a lung is 'Pancoast tumor'.
Also see
Pancoast tumor
The pancoast tumour is a tumor of the pulmonary apex. The growing tumor causes disruption of the sympathetic ganglion due to pressure on it.
Pancoast tumors are named for Henry Pancoast, a US radiologist, who described them in 1924 and 1932.
Ref: Davison's Pg- 360

Q. 235. River blindness is caused by (MD-Hom/Ent-I/2001)
    (a)   Brugia timori
    (b)   Loa ba
    (c)   Onchocerca volvulus
    (d)   Mansonella Ozzardi

Ans. (c)

Note
River blindness is caused by 'Onchocerca volvulus'.

Also see
O.volvulus: Ocular lesions are seen in persons with nodules on head and face, they result from presence of microfilaria which may be found moving about in substantia propria of cornea and the anterior chamber. The clinical manifestation consists of simple conjunctivitis, round small opacities and pannus in the anterior quadrant of cornea. Later there may be iridocyclitis, secondary glaucoma and pappilitis eventually leading to blindness.
Ref: Parasitology by K. D. Chaterjee, 12th Ed. Pg-200-201

Extended information
Filariasis causative agents
Filariasis is caused by nematodes (roundworms) that inhabit the lymphatics and subcutaneous tissues. Eight main species infect humans. Three of these are responsible for most of the morbidity due to filariasis: Wuchereria bancrofti and Brugia malayi cause lymphatic filariasis, and Onchocerca volvulus causes onchocerciasis (river blindness). The other five species are Loa loa, Mansonella perstans, M. streptocerca, M. ozzardi, and Brugia timori. (The last species also causes lymphatic filariasis.)

Q. 236. A brisk, acute inflammatory reaction which develops within few minutes after an injection of antigen into the skin of an animal is (MD-Hom/Ent-I/2001)
    (a)   Tuberculin reaction
    (b)   Arthus reaction
    (c)   Contact sensitivity
    (d)   Cytotoxic reaction

Ans. (b)
Note
A brisk, acute inflammatory reaction which develops within few minutes after an injection of antigen into the skin of an animal is 'Arathus reaction'.

Also see
Arthus reaction is a localized inflammatory reaction, usually an immune complex vasculitis of skin, often individual with circulating antibody. Large immune-complexes are formed due to excess of antibodies, which precipitate locally in the vessel wall causing fibrinoid necrosis. Example of local immune complex disease is as under:
-Injection of anti-tetanus serum
-Farmers lung in which there is allergic alveolitis in response to bacterial antigen from mouldy hay.
Ref: Harsh Mohan, 4th Ed. Pg 59

Extended information
The arthus reaction involves the in situ formation of antigen/antibody complexes after the intradermal injection of an antigen. If the animal/patient was previously sensitized (has circulating antibody), an arthus reaction occurs. This manifests as local vasculitis due to deposition of immune complexes in dermal blood vessels.

Q. 237. Down's syndrome is associated with (MD-Hom/Ent-I/2001)
    (a)   Trisomy 21
    (b)   Mother aged 30-45 years
    (c)   Mangoloid face
    (d)   All of the above

Ans. (d)
Note
Down's syndrome is associated with; Trisomy 21, Mother aged 30 – 45 Years, and Mangoloid face. It included all above.

Also see
Down's syndrome is caused by an extra chromosome 21. Down's children have a characteristic appearance; head may be smaller than normal, flattened nose, protruding tonguem upward slanting eyes (Mongolian slant). The inner corner of eyes may have a rounded fold of skin (epicanthal fold) rather than coming to a point.

Hands are short and broad with short fingers and often have a single palmar crease (simian crease). Average metnal age is 8 year old.

Mother's who became pregnant after 30 years are also at increased risk for having a child with Down's syndrome.

Q. 238. The cells in the most of chronic lymphogenous leukemia are (MD-Hom/Ent-I/2001)
- (a) Lymphoblasts
- (b) Lymphocytes
- (c) Palger-Huet Phenomenon
- (d) T-cells

Ans. (d)

Note
The cells in the most of chronic lymphogenous leukemia are 'lymphocytes'.

Also see
Lab findings of CLL:
Blood picture:
1. Anemia: mild to moderate, normocytic normochromic.
2. White blood cells: Typically there is marked leucocytosis but less than that seen in CML. Usually more than 90% of leucocytes are small mature leucocytes. Smear cells are present.
3. Platelet count: normal or moderately reduced.

Bone marrow examination:
1. Increased lymphocyte count (25-95%).
2. Reduced myeloid precursors.
3. Reduced erythroid precursors.

Ref: Harsh Mohan, 2nd Ed. Pg-291

Extended information
Chronic lymphocytic leukemia is charactrised by persistence presence of lymphocytosis more than 10×10^9/liter and lymphoid infiltration of the bone marrow of atleast 40%.

Investigation:
Peripheral blood shows: Lymphocytosis wih or without anemia or thrombocytopenia. Chronic Lymphatic Leukaemia-lymphocytes are small clumped chromatin; larger nucleoated cells (e.g. prolymphocytes) may be seen, but comprise less than 10% in typical Chronic Lymphatic Lekemia.

Ref; Medicine for Students by Golowalla, 20th Edition. Chronic lymphocytic leukemia pg-364.

Q. 239. Humoral immunity is mediated by (MD-Hom/Ent-I/2001)
- (a) T Lymphocytes
- (b) B Lymphocytes
- (c) Kupffer cells
- (d) Monocytes

Ans. (b)

Note
Humoral immunity is mediated by 'B-Lymphocytes'.

Also see
Humoral immunity comes from the B-cells (bone marrow derived lymphocytes) which proliferate and manufacture specific antibodies after antigen presentation by macrophages. The antibodies are localized in the immunoglobulin fraction of the serum. Immunoglobulins are divided into 5 main classes: IgG, IgA, IgM, IgE, IgD.

Ref: Park and Park, 18th Ed. Pg- 94

Extended information
B-cells are responsible for humoral immunity. They arise from a separate population of stem cells of the bone marrow than that which gives rise to T-cells. These cells undergo multiplication and processing in lymphoid tissue elsewhere than in the thymus gland.

B-cells, like T-cells, have surface receptors which enable them to recognise the appropriate antigen, but do not themselves interact to neutralise or destroy the antigen. On recognition of the antigen they take up residence in secondary lymphoid tissue and proliferate to form daughter lymphocytes, processed in the same way as themselves. These B-cells then develop into short-lived plasma cells.

The plasma cells produce antibodies and release them into the circulation at the lymph nodes.

Some of the activated B-cells do not become plasma cells instead they turn into memory cells which continue to produce small amounts of the antibody long after the infection has been overcome.

Q. 240. The malignant pustule with vesiculation, white cell infiltration and necrosis is usually produced by (MD-Hom/Ent-I/2001)
- (a) Adeno virus
- (b) Leishmania donovani
- (c) Anthrax bacillus
- (d) Pasterella tulerensis

Ans. (c)

Note
The malignant pustule with vesiculation, white cell infiltration and necrosis is usually produced by 'Anthrax bacillus'.

Also see
The cutaneous lesion in anthrax is most often found on exposed areas of skin. A small red macule develops within days after inoculation of B. anthracis spores into skin. During the next week, the lesion typically progresses through papular and vesicular or pustular stages to the formation of an ulcer with a blackened necrotic eschar surrounded by a highly characteristic expanding zone of brawny edema.

Harrison's 15th Edition. Section 5. Diseases caused y Gram Positive bacteria – 141- Diphtheria, other corynebacterial infections and anthrax.

Q. 241. Which of the following may be found in a patient with pulmonary infarction? (MD-Hom/Ent-I/2001)
- (a) Dyspnea
- (b) Pain in breathing
- (c) Hemoptysis
- (d) All of the above

Ans. (d)

Note
Dyspnea, pain in breathing, and hemoptysis all are found in a patient with pulmonary infarction.

Also see
Clinical features of pulmonary embolism are variable and at times not specific. Dyspnea may be the only symptom; unexplained dyspnea should always raise the suspicion of pulmonary embolism. Pleuritic chest pain and hemoptysis indicate pulmonary infarction and their onset may be delayed for a day or more after the initial presentation.

Ref: API, 7th Ed. Pg-338-339

Extended information
Pulmonary infarction usually results form pulmonary emboli caused by clots from right side from heart, amniotic fluid, or clots originating from Deep Vein Thrombosis. CF include; Cough with bloody sputum, Dyspnea (shortness of breath), chest pain; charcter sharp, stabbing worse by breathing.

Q. 242. Gastrin is produced primarily in (MD-Hom/Ent-I/2001)
- (a) Antrum
- (b) Pylorus
- (c) Pancreas
- (d) Liver

Ans. (a)

Note
Gastrin is produced primarily in 'Antrum'.

Also see
The hormone gastrin is produced by G cells in the antrum.
Davidsons 20th Ed, Pg-853
Gastrin is produced by cells called G cells in the lateral walls of the glands in the antral portion of the gastric mucosa
Ref: Ganong, 21st edition
The pyloric gland also secrets the hormone gastrin which plays a key role in gastric secretion.
Ref: Physiology by Guyton, 10th Ed. Pg. 744.

Q. 243. The following may be common manifestation of mumps (MD-Hom/Ent-I/2001)
    (a)   Orchitis
    (b)   Pancreatitis
    (c)   Parotitis
    (d)   All of the above

Ans. (c)
Note
The following may be common manifestation of mumps is 'parotitis'.
Also see
Clinical features of mumps: Mumps is a generalized virus infection, charecterised by pain and swelling in either one or both the parotid glands, but may involve the sub-lingual and submandibular glands.
Complications of mumps are orchitis, ovaritis, pancreatitis, meningo-encephalitis and myocarditis.
Pg 130, K. Park, 18th edition
Clinical features of mumps:
Mumps is a generalized virus infection, charecterised by pain and swelling in either one or both the parotid glands, but may involve the sub-lingual and submandibular glands.
Complications of mumps are orchitis, ovaritis, pancreatitis, meningo-encephalitis and myocarditis.
Ref: park and Park 18th Ed. Pg-130

Extended information
Mumps is an acute contagious (spreads through droplet infection) paramyxovirus disease characterised by parotitis, however other organs may become imvolved include testis (orchitis), CNS, the pancreas (Pancreatitis), and the breast. Most vulnerable age is 2 to 12 years. Incubation period is 12 – 24 days.

Q. 244. Pulmonary emboli most commonly originate from (MD-Hom/Ent-I/2001)
    (a)   The right heart
    (b)   Superficial veins of the lower extremity
    (c)   Deep leg veins of the lower extremity
    (d)   Pelvic veins

Ans. (c)
Note
Pulmonary emboli most commonly originate from 'Deep veins of leg'.
Also see
Venous thrombo-embolism:
    -Thrombi in the veins of lower legs are the most common cause of venous emboli
    -Thrombi in pelvic veins
    -Thrombi in the veins of upper limbs
    -Thrombosis in cavernous sinus of veins
    -Thrombi in the right side of heart
Ref: Short Handbook of Pathology, Harsh Mohan, 2nd Ed. Pg-79

Extended information
The most significant lessons about PE are those obtained from a careful study of the autopsy literature. Deep vein thrombosis (DVT) and PE are much more common than usually realized. Most patients with DVT develop PE and the majority of cases are unrecognized clinically. Untreated, approximately one third of

patients who survive an initial PE, die of a future embolic episode. This is true whether the initial embolism is small or large.
Ref: www.emedicine.com/emerg/topic490.htm - 143k

Q. 245. The most common cause of death in cirrhosis is (MD-Hom/Ent-I/2001)
    (a)   Hemorrhage
    (b)   Renal failure
    (c)   Liver failure
    (d)   Septicemia

Ans. (c)
Note
The most common cause of death in cirrhosis is 'Liver failure'.

Also see
Cirrhosis, especially in advanced cases, can cause profound abnormalities in the brain. In cirrhosis, some blood leaving the gut bypasses the liver as blood flow through the liver is decreased. Metabolism of components absorbed in the gut can also be decreased as liver cell function deteriorates. Both of these derangements can lead to hepatic encephalopathy as toxic metabolites, normally removed from the blood by the liver, can reach the brain. In its early stages, subtle mental changes such as poor concentration or the inability to construct simple objects occurs. In severe cases, hepatic encephalopathy can lead to stupor, coma, brain swelling and death.

Q. 246. The excretion of uric acid is impaired by (MD-Hom/Ent-I/2001)
    (a)   Morphin
    (b)   Nicotine
    (c)   Alcohol
    (d)   None of the above

Ans. (c)
Note
The excretion of uric acid is impaired by 'Alcohol'.

Also see
Alcohol may induce increased lipogenesis and cholesterol synthesis from acetyl coenzyme A. The increased NADH/NAD+ ratio also cause an increased lactate/pyruvate ratio that results in hyperlacticidaemia which inturn decrease the capacity of kidney to excrete uric acid.
Ref: Biochemistry by S P Singh, Pg-421
Iatrogenic cause:
For example, the following types of medicines can lead to hyperuricemia because they reduce the body's ability to remove uric acid:
Diuretics:
Which are taken to eliminate excess fluid from the body in conditions like hypertension, edema, and heart disease, and which decrease the amount of uric acid passed in the urine.
Salicylates:
These are anti-inflammatory medicines made from salicylic acid, such as aspirin.
Niacin:
The vitamin niacin, also called nicotinic acid.
Cyclosporine:
A medicine used to suppress the body's immune system (the system that protects the body from infection and disease) and control the body's rejection of transplanted organs.
Levodopa:
A medicine used to support communication along nerve pathways in the treatment of Parkinson's disease.
Alcohol:
The evidence linking alcohol and gout is not extensive, but is persuasive, especially when allied with several hundred years' of experience. Men with gout are probably best advised to refrain from alcohol.

Q. 247. The most common organism in burn sepsis is (MD-Hom/Ent-I/2001)
    (a)   Streptococcus
    (b)   Staphylococcus

(c) Proteins
(d) Pseudomonas

Ans. (d)
Note
The most common organism in burn sepsis is 'Psedudomonas'.

Also see
Pseudomonas found to be predominantly grown organism in positive blood cultures of burn patients followed by Klebsiella and Staphylococci.
Ref: Bombay hospital Journal – Original / Research.
Ref: www.bhj.org/journal/2005_4703_july/html/original_eval_230.htm - 19k

Q. 248. Organisms that may cause crepitant cellulitis include all except (MD-Hom/Ent-I/2001)
(a) Clostridia
(b) Bacteroides
(c) Staphylococcus
(d) Anerobic streptococcus

Ans. (c)
Note
Organisms that may cause crepitant cellulitis include all except 'Staphylococcus'.

Also see
Cellulitis is caused by S. aureus, but β-hemolytic streptococci are more common agents of this disease. Secondary infection of surgical and traumatic wounds is more likely to be staphylococcal in etiology than is cellulitis arising from minor or inapparent breaks in the skin, and empiric treatment directed against both S. aureus and streptococci is reasonable in these settings.

Q. 249. Amoebic ulceration is most commonly noted in (MD-Hom/Ent-I/2001)
(a) Ileum
(b) Caecum
(c) Appendix
(d) Ascending colon

Ans. (b)
Note
Amoebic ulceration is most commonly noted in 'caecum'.

Also see
Some trophozoids invade the bowel and cause ulceration, mainly in the caecum, and ascending colon; then in the rectum and sigmoid.
Ref: Park and Park Ed- 18th, Pg-193

Q. 250. A commonly observed complication of botulism is (MD-Hom/Ent-I/2001)
(a) Massive hematemesis
(b) Respiratory failure
(c) Convulsions
(d) Tetany

Ans. (b)
Note
A commonly observed complication of botulism is 'Respiratory failure'.

Also see
Botulism is frequently fatal, death occurring 4-8 days later due to respiratory or cardiac failure.
Ref: Park and Park Ed- 18th, Pg-191

Extended information
Botulism is a rare, paralytic illness caused by a toxin, botulin. Causative organism is 'Clostridium botulinum'. The toxin 'botulin' acts by blocking nerve function and leads to respiratory and musculoskeletal paralysis. Respiratory failure is the most serious complication and, generally, the cause of death.

Q. 251. The most important factor in preventing tetanus is (MD-Hom/Ent-I/2001)
    (a)   Tetanus antitoxin
    (b)   Tetanus toxoid
    (c)   Previous immunization
    (d)   Proper initial wound care

Ans. (c)
Note
The most important factor in preventing tetanus is 'Previouis immunization'.
Also see
For prevention of tetanus following are the recommendations:

Immunization status	Wounds less than 6 hours old, clean, non-penetrating and with negligible tissue damage	Other type of wounds
a. Complete course of tetanus toxoid (TT) or a booster dose within the past five years.	Nothing required	Nothing required.
b. Complete course of TT or a booster dose more than 5 years ago but less than 10 years.	TT one dose	TT one dose.
c. Complete course of TT or a booster dose more than 10 years ago.	TT one dose	TT one dose + Human tetanus globulin.
d. Had not completed course of TT or immunization status known.	TT complete course	TT complete course + Human tetanus globulin.

Ref: Park and Park 16th Ed, P- 238
Immunization against tetanus is recommended for all infants 6 to 8 weeks of age and older, all children, and all adults. Immunization against tetanus consists first of a series of either 3 or 4 injections, depending on which type of tetanus toxoid you receive. In addition, it is very important that you get a booster injection every 10 years for the rest of your life. Also, if you get a wound that is unclean or hard to clean, you may need an emergency booster injection if it has been more than 5 years since your last booster.

Q. 252. Cyclodevelopmental parasite (MD-Hom/Ent-I/2001)
    (a)   Micro filarial
    (b)   Flavi virus
    (c)   P. vivax
    (d)   S.Japonicum

Ans. (a)
Note
Cyclodevelopmental parasite is 'Micro filaria'.
Also see

Cyclodevelopmental Transmission
The parasite undergoes cyclical changes within the vector but does not multiply, i.e., there are only developmental changes of the parasite without multiplication. The term usually relates to the development of a parasite in its intermediate host.

Filaria transmission
Filaria is usually acquired in childhood.

The disease may then take years to manifest. The person may just remain an asymptomatic carrier. The filarial worms remain dormant in the lymph nodes, and come out into the blood periodically around midnight. This is the time the culex mosquito also looking for a blood meal.

Once the filarial worm enters the mosquito, it begins to develop into the form infective to humans. This process takes between seven to 21 days. It eventually settles in the mosquito's salivary glands.
Once this has occurred, the next person to get bitten gets a dose of infective micro filarial larvae.
Ref: A bite of filaria - Newindpress.com

Extended information
Biological transmission (Obligatory, part of the pathogen life cycle):
Pathogens transmitted by this type of transmission require incubation period. The transmitted pathogens may change morphologically as well as physiologically and may be transmitted from the mouth parts or from the anus.

In biological transmission, four patterns have been described:
1. Propagative:
   The pathogen multiplies with no apparent morphological change as in flea (plague) and Culex (rift valley)
2. Cyclopropagative:
   The pathogen multiplies and morphologically changes during incubation period in the arthropods as in Anopheles (malaria), Sandfly (Leishmania) and tsetse fly (Trypanosomes)
3. Cyclodevelopment:
   The pathogen will change morphologically without multiplication as in Culex (filariasis)
4. Transovarian:
   The pathogen passes from the female adult to the progeny through the egg as in ticks and mites.
Ref:www.drfalbraikan.com/Introductionmuscaglossinaandsimulium.htm - 69k

Q. 253. Food poisoning is caused by (MD-Hom/Ent-I/2001)
    (a)   V. Cholerae type 139
    (b)   S. para typhi A
    (c)   Cl. perfringens
    (d)   Staph epidermis

Ans. (c)
Note
Food poisoning is caused by 'Cl. perfringens'.
Also see

Food poisoning is caused by Cl.perfringes. the organism has been found in faeces of humans and animals, and in soil, water and air.
Ref: Park & Park, 18th Ed.- Cl. perfringens Food poinoning, Pg-191
Additional information
Some strains of C. perfringens produce toxins which cause food poisoning if ingested, with poorly prepared meat and poultry the main culprits in harboring the bacterium. The clostridial enterotoxin mediating the disease is often heat-resistant and can be detected in contaminated food and feces. Incubation period is 8 - 16 hours after ingestion of contaminated food. Manifestions typically include abdominal cramping and diarrhea - vomiting and fever are unusual. The whole course usually resolves within 24 hours.
Ref: Clostridium perfringens - Wikipedia, the free encyclopedia
Further reading:
Clostridium perfringens is a Gram-positive bacterial pathogen that has the capability of forming an endospore. The dormant spores can change to potentially harmful vegetative cells if exposed to cooking temperatures and allowed to stand at temperature between 41°F and 120°F, especially in the temperature range from 70°F and 120°F. Cl. perfringens vegetative cells are killed in foods when the foods are cooked at 140°F or above. However, spores may still be present after cooking. Spores can survive the cooking process. Cl. perfringens can only thrive in conditions of very little or no oxygen: that is, it is an anerobic organism. Cl. perfringens will not grow at refrigeration or freezing temperatures.
Populations most at risk for Cl. perfringens foodborne illness:

Hospitals, nursing homes, prisons, school cafeterias are places that pose the highest risk of an outbreak of foodborne illness due to Cl. perfringens. In these locations, foods are cooked but may not be kept at safe, adequate temperatures, prior to serving. Although present in small numbers in (raw) foods, improper storage and handling of these foods allows the pathogen to grow to large, harmful numbers.

Q. 254. Vitamin-D is not present in (MD-Hom/Ent-I/2001)
    (a)   Cod liver oil
    (b)   Fish fat
    (c)   Milk
    (d)   **Egg**

Ans. (c)
Note
Vitamin-D is not present in 'Milk'.
Also see
Sources of Vitamin-D:
    -Sunlight
    -Foods: vitamin D is seen in foods of animal origin. Liver, egg yolk, butter and cheese and some species of fish contain usual amounts. Fish liver oils are the richest source os vitamin-D. Human milk has considerable amounts of water-soluble Vitamin-D sulphate.
Ref: Park and Park, 18th Ed. Pg-444

Extended information
Cod liver oil:
An excellent source of vitamin A and vitamin D, it is also a good source of omega-3 fatty acids.
Fatty fish:
Fatty fish, such as salmon and mackerel, contain large amounts of vitamin D.
Milk:
Milk from all lactating animals including human breast milk, contain very little vitamin D.
Egg:
Egg, whole; vitamin D is found in egg yolk.

Q. 255. Normal iron requirement during pregnancy (MD-Hom/Ent-I/2001)
    (a)   20 mg
    (b)   40 mg
    (c)   80 mg
    (d)   100 mg

Ans. (b)
Note
Normal iron requirement during pregnancy is '40 mg'.
Also see

The RDA (Recommended Daily Allowance) table no 31 suggests Iron requirement during pregnancy is 38 mg daily. Which points to the correct answer as (b)
Ref: Park and Park 16th Edition, Pg-428

Q. 256. Additional calories required during lactation (MD-Hom/Ent-I/2001)
    (a)   450
    (b)   550
    (c)   650
    (d)   750

Ans. (b)
Note
Additional calories required during lactation is '550'.
Also see
The standereded in India are those recommended by the Indian Cuncil of Meidcal Research and energy requirement suggested for lactating mother, during first 6 months are additional 550 Kal/Kg/day and for next

6 – 12 months 400 kcal/kg/day.
Ref: Park and Park, 16th Edition Table 24, Pg-425

Q. 257. Most common source of Lenolic Acid (MD-Hom/Ent-I/2001)
  (a) Mustard oil
  (b) Sunflower oil
  (c) Groundnut oil
  (d) Safflower oil

Ans. (d)

Note
Most common source of Lenolic Acid is 'safflower oil'.

Also see
Linoleic acid is a polyunsaturated fatty acid used in the biosynthesis of prostaglandins and cell membranes and in other natural oils. These oils include vegetable oil, especially safflower oil.

Extended information
Essential fatty acid are those that cannot be synthesized by humans. They can be derived only from food. The most important EFA is Linoleic acid, which servers as a basis for the production of other essentiaol fatty acids (Lenolenic acid and Arachidonic acids). All polyunsaturated fatty acids are not essential fatty acids. Linoleic acid is abanduntly found in vegetable oil. Dietary sources of essential fatty acid are:

Essential Fatty Acids	Dietary Source	Per cent content
Linoleic acid:		
	-Safflower oil	73
	-Corn oil	57
	-Sunflower oil	56
	-Soyabean oil	51
	-Sesame oil	40
	-Groundnut oil	39
	-Mustard oil	15
	-Palm oil	9
	-Coconut oil	2

Ref: Park and Park, Ed -18th, Pg-440

Q. 258. Following are good sources of Vitamin-B12 except (MD-Hom/Ent-I/2001)
  (a) Soyabean
  (b) Liver
  (c) Fish
  (d) Meat

Ans. (a)

Note
Following are good sources of Vitamin-B12 except 'Soyabean'.

Also see
Vitamin B12 is found in food derived from animals including dairy products. Good sources are liver, kidney, meat, fish, eggs, milk, and cheese. It is not found in foods of vegetable origin.
Ref: Park and Park, 18th Edition, Pg-447

Q. 259. In Japanese encephalitis following are true except (MD-Hom/Ent-I/2001)
  (a) Mortality 10%
  (b) Tritaeneorhyrichus most important vector in South India.
  (c) I P 5-15 days.
  (d) Vaccination of population at risk recommended.

Ans. (a)

Note
In Japanese encephalitis all above are true except 'Mortality 10%.
Also see
a. Mortlity / Case fatality rate varies between 20 – 40% but, it may reach 58% and over. The average period between the onset of illness and death is about 9 days.
b. Notably C. Tritaeneorhyrichus has been implicated as the most important vactor in South India. These mosquitoes breed in irrigated rice fields, shallow ditches and pools.
c. Incubation period in man, following mosquito bite is not exactly known. Probably it varies from 5 – 15 days.
d. Vaccination of population at risk is recommended.
Ref: Park & Park 16th Edition Pg- 216

Q. 260. Immunity develops — after Japanese Encephalitis vaccination (MD-Hom/Ent-I/2001)
    (a) 7 days
    (b) 15 days
    (c) 30 days
    (d) 60 days

Ans. (c)
Note
Immunity develops '30 days' after Japanese Encephalitis vaccination.
Also see
A killed 'mouse – brain' caccine is available for primary immunization of JE, 2 doses of 1 ml each (0.5 ml for children under the age of 3 years) should be administered subcutaneously at an interval of 7 -14 day. A booster injection of 1 ml should be given after a few months (before 1 year) in order to develop full protection. Protective immunity develops in about a month's time after the second dose.
Ref: Park & Park, 16th Edition, Pg- 216

Q. 261. In a suspected case of Polio following are done except (MD-Hom/Ent-I/2001)
    (a) Isolation
    (b) Notification
    (c) Immunization
    (d) Chemotherapy

Ans. (c)
Note
Suspected case of Polio is put in isolation, notified, and given symptomatic medication except injections and is not to be immunized.
Also see
If the suspected case comes out to be the case of 'polio' he will be developing the natural resistance. However, in the area were the case is reported needs mopping up exercise.
Additional information
The contraindications for the administration of OPV are actue infectioius disease, fevers, diarrhea and dysentery. Patient suffering from leukemias and malignancy and those receving coritcosteorids may not be given OPV.
Ref: Park and Park, 18th Ed, Pg- 165

Q. 262. Daily requirement of calcium in pregnancy is (MD-Hom/Ent-I/2001)
    (a) 50mg
    (b) 100mg
    (c) 500mg
    (d) 1000 mg

Ans. (d)
Note
Daily equirement of calcium in pregnancy is 1000 mg.
Ref: Park and Park Table 31- Pg 428 – Edition 16th

Q. 263. A child develops food poisoning 16-18 hours after consuming ice-cream, the most probable causative organism in this case is (MD-Hom/Ent-I/2001)
   (a) Staphylococcus aureus
   (b) Salmonella typhimurium
   (c) Clostridium perfringes
   (d) Clostridium botulinum

Ans. (b)
Note
Child develops food poisoning 16-18 hours after consuming ice-cream, the most probable causative organism in this case is 'S. Typhimurium.'
Also see
Food poisoning is caused by:
a. Styphylococcus aureus; Incubation period; 1-6 hours (Short incubation period is due to preformed toxins). Food involved is salads, custered, milk and milk productes. Milk and milk products can get comtaminated with staphylococcus either during handling or cows suffering from mastitis. The toxins are formed at optimum temperature of 35 – 37 degree C. are relatively heat stable and resist boiling for 30 minutes or more.
b. Salmonella (Typhimurium) typhi: Source; through contaminated meat, milk and milk products, sausages, custard, egg and egg products. Incubation period is 12- 24 hours. Mechanism of food poisoning: organism on ingestion reaches intestine and give rise to acute enteritis and colitis.
c. Clostridium perfringes; Source; Human and animal faeces – through soil water and air. Spread: ingestion of meat, meat dishes and poultry. Incubation period; 6 to 24 hours. Usual H/O – Cookded food not consumed within 24 hours allowed to cool slowly at room temperature and heated immediately prior to serving.
d. Clostridium botulium: Source; canned preserved food; canned vegetables, smoked of pickled fish, home made cheese. Incuabtion period; 12 – 36 hours. Mechanism: the toxin 'preformed' in the food act on parasympathetic nervous system and include: dysphagia, dysarthria, diplopia, ptosis, blurring of vision and muscle weakness.
Ref: Park and Park 16th Editon, Pg-178,79

Q. 264. Jaggery is rich in (MD-Hom/Ent-I/2001)
   (a) Vitamin-B2
   (b) Iron
   (c) Niacin
   (d) Vitamin-C

Ans. (b)
Note
Jaggery is rich in Iron.
Also see
Foods containing iron are liver, meat, poulty and fish. Those of vegetable origin are cereals, green leafy vegetables, legumes, nuts, jaggery and dry fruits.
Ref: Park and Park, 18th Ed. Pg-449

Extended information
For a vegetarian, sources of iron are green leafy vegetables, dry fruits and jaggery.
Ref: API Text Book of Medicine, Ed-6th, Pg-859

Q. 265. Man is intermediate host for (MD-Hom/Ent-I/2001)
   (a) Enterobiasis
   (b) Schistosoma haematobium
   (c) Echinococcus granulosus
   (d) Taenia saginata

Ans. (c)
Note
Man is intermediate host for 'Echinococcus'.

MCQ's in Practice of Medicine 821

Also see
Basically, it is a 'dog-sheep' cycle with man as an accidental intermediate host for echinococcus.
Park and Park 16th edition Pg 230
Life cycle of Echinococcus granulosus includes canines and felines as the definitive host and a variety of herbivores and humans as the intermediate host.
Ref: API, 7th Ed. Pg- 125

Q. 266. Breast feeding is contra-indicated, if mother receiving (MD-Hom/Ent-I/2001)
  (a) Saline
  (b) Broad spectrum antibiotics
  (c) Anti thyroid drugs
  (d) Streptomycine

Ans. (c)
Note
Breast feeding is contra-indicated, if mother receiving 'Antithyroid drugs'.
Also see
If mother is receiving:
a. Saline: is not a contraindication for breast feeding.
b. Broad spectrum antibiotics: not a contraindication for breast feeding.
c. Anti-thyroid drugs: should not nurse their babies.
d. Streptomycine: caustion safety not established.

Extended information
The patient of thyroid disorder should be under constant review and the drugs may be discontinued 4 weeks before the expected date of delivery to avoid fetal hypothyroidism at the time of maximum brain development.
Ref: API, 7th Ed. Pg-1458

Q. 267. Noise induced hearing loss affects frequency of (MD-Hom/Ent-I/2001)
  (a) 1000 Hz
  (b) 2000 Hz
  (c) 3000 Hz
  (d) 4000 Hz

Ans. (d)
Note
Noise induced hearing loss affects frequency of '4000 Hz and above'.
Also see
Auditory effects of noise exposure:
Temporary hearing loss occurs in frequency range between 4000 – 6000 Hz. Repeated or continuous exposure to noise around 100 decibels may result in a permanent hearing loss. Exposure to noise above 160 decibels may rupture the tympanic membrane and cause permanent loss of hearing.
Ref: Park and Park 18th Ed, Pg-551

Q. 268. Ringer lactate solution contains following electrolytes (MD-Hom/Ent-I/2001)
  (a) Na+ and Cl
  (b) Na+ K+ and Cl
  (c) Na + K + Cl and Ca
  (d) Na + K + and HCO

Ans. (d)
Note
Ringer lactate solution contains 'Na+ K and HCO'.
Also see
The Ringer lactate solution is also known as Hartmann's solution for injection. It is best commercially available solution. It supplies adequate concentrations of Na and K and lactate yields bicarbonates for correction of the acidosis. It can be used to correct dehydration due to acute diarrheas of all causes.
Ref: Park and Park 16th Ed, Pg-169, Park and Park 18th Ed. Pg-181

Q. 269. Adult hemoglobin consists of chains (MD-Hom/Ent-I/2001)
    (a)   2a+2B
    (b)   2B+2Y
    (c)   2a+2Z
    (d)   2a+2Y

Ans. (a)

Note
Adult hemoglobin consists of chains '2a+2B'.

Also see
Hemoglobin synthesis: In normal post natal life the globin part of normal hemoglobin is made up of two alpha chains and two beta chains containing 141 ammino acids and 146 ammino acids in each respectively. This is HbA 1.
Ref: API, 7th Ed. Pg- 920

Q. 270. In which of the following hemoglobin is abnormal? (MD-Hom/Ent-I/2001)
    (a)   Sickle cell anemia
    (b)   Pernicious anemia
    (c)   G-6 P-D deficiency
    (d)   Hereditary spherocytosis

Ans. (a)

Note
Out of listed above the hemoglobin is abnormal in 'Sickle cell anemia'.

Also see
Abnormal hemoglobins occur in:
a.   Globin chain production (e.g. thalassaemia)
b.   Structure of the globin chain (e.g. sickle cell disease)
c.   Combined defects of globin chain production and structure, e.g. sickle cell β-thalassaemia
Ref: Clincial Medicine by Kumar and Clark 6th Ed, Pg-439

Extended information
Sickle cell anemia is an autosomal recessive disorder in which an abnormal hemoglobin leads to chronic hemolytic anemia with a variety of clinical consequences. The disorder is a classical example of disease caused by a point mutation in DNA.
Ref: Park and Park, 18th Ed. Pg- 626

Q. 271. Liver does not synthesise (MD-Hom/Ent-I/2001)
    (a)   Gamma globulin
    (b)   Albumin
    (c)   Prothrombin
    (d)   Fibrinogen

Ans. (a)

Note
Liver does not synthesize 'Gamma globulin'.

Also see

Serum proteins; the plasma proteins (albumin, fibrinogen, alpha-antitripsin, haptoglobin, ceruloplasmin, transferring and prothrombin)are produced by the hepatocytes.
Ref: API, 7th Ed. Pg- 585

Extended information
Gamma globulin
Gamma globulin a group of globulin proteins in human blood plasma, including most antibodies. These antibody substances are produced as a protective reaction of the body's immune system.

272. Membrane integrity of RBC is due to (MD-Hom/Ent-I/2001)
    (a)   P Protein
    (b)   Spectrin

(c) Ankyrin
(d) Glycophorin

Ans. (b)
Note
Membrane integrity of RBC is due to 'Spectrin'.
Also see
RBC caontains hemoglobin which takes pink colour with leishman's stain. The cell membrane contains circular pores which are concerned with ingress or egress of water and electrolytes. Below the cell membrane is a contractile layer of lipoprotein-"spectrin", which is arranged in a fibrillar manner. It maintains shape and flexibility of RBC membrane and also contains specific blood group substances, the antigens.
Ref: Textbook of Physiology, A.K.Jain, Pg-57

Q. 273. Essential features of nephrotic syndrome includes all except
(a) Increased urinary excretion
(b) Hypoalbuminemia
(c) Peripheral edema
(d) Decreased serum cholesterol

Ans. (d)
Note
Essential features of nephrotic syndrome includes all except 'Decreased serum cholesterol'.
Also see
Nephrotic syndrome is characterized by:
Massive proteniuria (> 3.5 g/day), hypoalbumaemia, oedema, and hyperlipidaemia.
Ref: Clincial medicine by Kumar and Clark 6th Ed, Pg-620

Extended information
Hyperlipidemia is a frequent accompaniment of nephrotic syndrome. It is hypothesized that the liver faced with the stress of massive protein synthesis in response to heavy urinary protein loss, also causes increased synthesis of lipoproteins. There are increased blood levels of total lipids, cholesterol, triglycerides, VLDL and LDL but decrease in HDL. Low blood level of HDL is partly due to its loss in the urine.
Ref: Textbook of Pathology, Harshmohan, 4th Ed. Pg- 645

Q. 274. Immune complexes located within the basement membrane would most likely be found in a patient with
(a) Acute glomerulonephritis
(b) Membranous GN
(c) Type 1 Membrano-proliferative GN {MPGN}d) Type-2 MPGN
(d) All of the above

Ans. (d)
Note
Immune complexes located within the basement membrane would most likely be found in a patient with 'all of above'.
Also see
Immune complex GN is observed in following human disease:
1. Primary GN, e.g. acute diffuse proliferative GN, Membranous GN, Membrano-proliferative GN, IgA nephropathy and some cases of RPGN and focal GN.
2. Systemic diseases e.g. glomerular disease in SLE, Malaria, syphilis, hepatitis, henoch schonlein purpura and idiopathic mixed cryoglobulinaemia.
Ref: Short handbook of Harsh Mohan, 2nd Ed. Pg-491

Q. 275. Highly selective proteinuria contains
(a) Fibrinogen and albumin
(b) Transferin
(c) Transferrin and fibrinogen
(d) Fibrinogen

Ans. (a)

Note
Highly selective proteinuria contains 'albumin'.

Also see
A highly selective proteinuria consists mostly of loss of low molecular weight protein. In nephrotic syndrome proteinuria mostly consists of loss of albumin in the urine.
Ref: Short handbook of pathology by Harsh Mohan, 5th Ed. Pg-448.

Q. 276. Edward syndrome is due to
    (a)   Chromosome 18 anomaly
    (b)   Chromosome 13 anomaly
    (c)   Chromosome 11 anomaly
    (d)   Chromosome & anomaly

Ans. (a)

Note
Edward syndrome is due to 'Chromosome 18 anomaly'.

Also see
Edwards' syndrome has characteristic skull and occiput, frequent malformations of heart, kidney and other organs (Trisomy 18 (47, XY,+18)
Ref: Davidson 20th Ed, Pg-47.
Edward's syndrome(Trisomy 18):
    -Has chromosome karyotype 47+18
    -Incidence: 1:3000
    -Clinical feature: low set ears, micrognathia,, rocker-bottom feet, learning difficulties.
    -Rarely survive for more than a few weeks.
Ref: Kumar and Clark, 6th Ed. Pg-175

Extended information
Trisomy 18 or Edwards Syndrome (named after John H. Edwards who first described the syndrome in 1960) is a genetic disorder.

Q. 277. Turner's syndrome is
    (a)   XO
    (b)   XXY
    (c)   XXX
    (d)   XXO

Ans. (a)

Note
Turner's syndrome is 'XO'.

Also see
Turner's syndrome encompasses chromosomal abnormalities, of which monosomy X, is the most common. It occurs in 1 out of every 2,500 female births.
Instead of the normal XX sex chromosomes for a female, only one X chromosome is present and fully functional. This is called 45, X or 45, X0.
Clinical features:

Infantilism, primary amenorrhea, short stature, webbed neck, cubitus valgus, normal IQ.
Ref: Kumar and Clark, 6th Ed. Pg-175
45, XO- Turner's syndrome (short stature, webbed neck, primary amenorrhoea.
Ref: Davidson 20th Ed, Pg-47

Q. 278. Ulcerative colitis is characterized by all except
    (a)   Crypt abscess
    (b)   Sub mucosal inflammation
    (c)   Pseudo polyps seen
    (d)   Fistula formation

Ans. (d)

Note
Ulcerative colitis is characterized by all except 'Fistula formation'.

Also see
Microscopically, the earliest lesions in ulcerative colitis starts in the bases of the crypts of lieberkuhn, where neutrophils pass between the lining cells to accumulate inside the crypt lumen forming *"crypt abscess"* along with eosinophils, serum and RBCs.
These crypt abscesses ultimately rupture through the mucosal surface forming tiny ulcers or may rupture into the *submucosa*. In between these ulcers, normal mucosa becomes inflamed and edematous with proliferation of granulation tissue. This is known as *pseudopolyp*.
Ref: Textbook of Surgery by S. Das 3Rd Ed. Pg-1017

Q. 279. M4 stage of AML is called as (IHMA-MEE-II)
(a) Acute myelomonoblastic leukemia
(b) Acute monoblastic leukemia
(c) Myelomonocytic leukemia
(d) Monocytic leukemia

Ans. (a)
Note
The M4 stage of AML is called as 'Acute myelomonoblastic leukemia'.

Also see
FAB class M4 of acute leukaemia:
  -Acute myelomonocytic leukaemia
  -Incidence: 30% cases
  -Morphology: mature cells of both myeloid and monocytic series in peripheral blood; myeloid cells resemble M2 (AML with maturation)
  -Cytochemistry: myeloperoxidase ++, non-specific estrase +
Ref: Short Handbook of Pathology, by Harsh Mohan, 2nd Ed. Pg-140

Q. 280. Cerebellar ataxia is characterized by all except (IHMA-MEE-II)
(a) Resting tremor
(b) Dysdiadochokinesis
(c) Ataxia
(d) Hypotonia

Ans. (a)
Note
Cerebellar ataxia is characterized by all of the above except 'Resting tremor'.

Aslo see
Cerebellar limb ataxia is characterized by dysmetria (irregular error's im amplitude and course of movements), inention tremors, dysdiadochokinesia an excessive rebound of outstretchred arm against a resistance that is suddenly removed.
Ref: Harrison 16th Ed, Pg-140

Extended information
In place of 'Resting tremor' which are encountered in disordedr of subcortical nuclei i,e. parkinson's disease, the cerebellar ataxia is has charactereristic 'Intention tremor'.

Q. 281. The mosquito, which transmits classical dengue fever (IHMA-MEE-II)
(a) Anophelus
(b) Culex
(c) Stephansi
(d) Aedes aegypticus

Ans. (d)
Note
The mosquito, which transmits classical dengue fever, is 'Aedes aegypticus'.

Also see
Apart from dengue the aedes aegypti also transmits (Yellow fever, but strangely it is not in India),

Chikungunya.

Extended information
Dengue fever is a self limiting disease and represents the majority of cases of dengue infection. A prevalence of aedes aegypti and aedes albopictus together with circulation of dengue virus of more than one type in any particular area tends to be associated with outbreak of DHF/DSS
Aedes aegypti breeds in clean water such as water found in discarded tins, broken bottles, fire buckes, flower pots. It do not fly long distance and remain within 100 mt. it bits during daytime and takes vertical flight upto 2 ½ feet.
Ref: Park and Park 18th Ed, Pg-198

Q. 282. Unit of absorbed dose of radiation is (IHMA-MEE-II)
    (a)   rad
    (b)   rem
    (c)   rot
    (d)   roentgen

Ans. (a)
Note
Unit of absorbed dose of radiation is 'rad'.

Also see
The rad is the unit of absorbed dose of radiation. It is the amount of radioactive energy absorbed per gram of tissue or any material. One mrad – 0.001 rad.

Q. 283. Defect most commonly occurring in congenital rubella (IHMA-MEE-II)
    (a)   Deafness
    (b)   Cataract
    (c)   Microcephaly
    (d)   All the Above

Ans. (d)
Note
Defect most commonly occurring in congenital rubella are 'All of the above'.

Also see
Rubella infection inhibits cell division, and this is probably the reason for congenital malformation and low birth weight. The most common congenital defects are:
    -Deafness
    -Cardiac malformations
    -Cataract
    -Other resulting defects include glaucoma, retinopathy, microcephalus, cerebral palsy, IUGR, hepatosplenomegaly, mental and motor retardation.
These defects occurring singly or in combination have become known as congenital rubella syndrome.
However, if the infection is severe spontaneous abortion and stillbirth may occur or the infant may develop multiple defects such as the classical triad of patent ductus arteriosis, cataract and deafness.
Ref: Park and Park 18th Ed, Pg-128, 29

Q. 284. Pleomorphic rash is a feature of
    (a)   Small pox
    (b)   Chicken pox
    (c)   Erythyma infectiosum
    (d)   Erythyma Subitium

Ans. (b)
Note
Pleomorphic rash is a feature of 'Chicken pox'.

Also see
The characteristic rash 'Pleomorphism' i.e. all stages of the rash (Papules, vesicles, and crust) may be seen simultaneously at one time and in the same area, is a feature of chickenpox. This is due to rash appearing in successive crops for 4-5 days in the same area.

Ref: Park and Park 18th Ed, Pg-123

Q. 285. Most virulent form of Shigellosis is caused by
    (a)   Sh. dysenteriae
    (b)   Sh. sonnei
    (c)   Sh. flexneri
    (d)   Sh. boydii

Ans. (a)

Note
Most virulent form of Shigellosis is caused by 'Sh. dysenteriae'.

Also see
Bacillary dysentery (shigellosis): The organism Shigella dysenteriae type I remains the most virulent of the shigella and it was probably the cause of much of the severe dysentery that ravages during wars, famines and natural calamities.
Ref: API, 7th Ed. Pg- 54

Extended information
The shigella infection is a classical cause of bacillary dysentery. Four species in decreasing order of severity of disease they give rise to are:
a.   Sh. dysenteriae
b.   Sh. flexneri
c.   Sh. boydii
d.   Sh. sonnei

Q. 286. Bitot's spots are seen in deficiency of
    (a)   Thiamine
    (b)   Niacin
    (c)   Pyridoxine
    (d)   Riboflavin

Ans. Use your discretion

Note
Bitot's spots are seen in deficiency of 'vit A'

Also Note
Thiamin
Thiamine (vitamin B1) is a vitamin used by the body to break down sugars in the diet. The medication helps correct nerve and heart problems that occur when a person's diet does not contain enough thiamine.
Niacin
Niacin or Nicotinc acid (also known as vitamin B-3) is found in dairy products, poultry, fish, lean meats, nuts, and eggs. Legumes and enriched breads and cereals also supply some niacin.
Pyridoxine
Pyridoxine (vitamin B 6) is necessary for normal breakdown of proteins, carbohydrates, and fats.
Riboflavin
Riboflavin (vitamin B-2) works with the other B vitamins. It is important for body growth and red blood cell production and helps in releasing energy from carbohydrates.

Extended information
Vitamin A deficiency shows following ocular manifestations:
    -Night blindness
    -Conjuctival xerosis
    -Bitot's spots
    -Corneal xerosis
    -Keratomalacia
Ref Park and Park, 18th Ed. Pg- 443

Q. 287. Earliest change in diabetic retinopathy is
    (a)   Hard exudate
    (b)   Soft exudate

(c) Dot hemorrhage
(d) Microaneurism

Ans. (d)

Note
Earliest change in diabetic retinopathy is 'Microaneurism'.

Also see
Diabetic retinopathy is classified into two stages:
a. Nonproliferative:
   Nonproliferative diabetic retinopathy usually appears late in the first decade or early in the second decade of the disease and is marked by retinal vascular *microaneurysms*, blot hemorrhages, and cotton wool spots. Mild nonproliferative retinopathy progresses to more extensive disease, characterized by changes in venous vessel caliber, intraretinal microvascular abnormalities, and more numerous microaneurysms and hemorrhages.
b. Proliferative:
   The appearance of neovascularization in response to retinal hypoxia is the hallmark of proliferative diabetic retinopathy. These newly formed vessels may appear at the optic nerve and/or macula and rupture easily, leading to vitreous hemorrhage, fibrosis, and ultimately retinal detachment.
Ref: Harrison's 16th Edition.Pg-2163

Q. 288. Blue sclera is seen in
    (a) Alkaptonuria
    (b) Osteogenesis imperfecta
    (c) Ehler-Danlos syndrome
    (d) Kawasaki Syndrome

Ans. (b)

Note
Blue sclera is seen in 'Osteogenesis Imperfecta'.

Also see
This is an inherited serious bone disorder and usually seen at birth. Infants may have multiple fractures which result in shortened arms and legs. Mild cases may not be detected until later in life.
Usual clinical features include:
    -Multiple fractures, blue sclera, deafness, high pitched voice, deformities of long bones, joint hyper-extensibility, pectus deformity, dental abnormality, thin skin and generally normal intelligence.
Ref: API Text Book of Medicine 6th Ed, Pg-1102
Clinical features of osteogenesis imperfecta: The patient are of short stature with limb deformities. There is usually a broad skull which shows wormian bones on X-ray. Other features are blue sclera, scoliosis, oteosclerosis and ligament laxity.
Refr: Textbook of Surgery, S. Das 3rd Ed. Pg-423

Q. 289. Smoking most commonly causes
    (a) CA Lung
    (b) Thrombo angiitis obliterans
    (c) Chronic bronchitis
    (d) Myocardial ischaemia

Ans. (c)

Note
Smoking most commonly causes 'chronic bronchitis'.

Also see
Smoking causes all of above. However, early and direct complains to develop is Ch. bronchitis, emphysema, corpulmonale and particularly lung cancer, throat cancer, and mouth cancer which hardly ever affects the non smoker. Smoking also predisposes to HT, atherosclerosis, coronary artery disease, CVA, as well as precipitates Thromboangitis obliterans (Buerger's disease).
Ref: www.netdoctor.co.uk/health

MCQ's in Practice of Medicine   829

Extended information
Chronic bronchitis etiopathogenesis: The two most important etiological factors responsible for majority of cases of chronic bronchitis are cigarette smoking and atmospheric pollution. Other contributory factors are occupation, infection, familial and genetic factors.
Ref: Textbook of Pathology, Harsh Mohan, 4th Ed. Pg- 447-448

Q. 290. Commonest site of multiple myeloma is
- (a) Long bones
- (b) Skull
- (c) Rib
- (d) Vertebrae

Ans. (b)
Note
The most common site of multiple myeloma is 'Skull bone'.
Also see
Most commonly bones affected in multiple myeloma are those with red marrow i.e. skull, spine, ribs and pelvis, but later long bones of limbs are also involved.
Ref: Textbook of Pathology, Harsh Mohan, 4th Ed. Pg- 422

Q. 291. Fish head appearance of the vertebral bodies is seen in? (IHMA-MEE-II)
- (a) Paget's disease
- (b) Rickets
- (c) Osteomalacia
- (d) Osteoporosis

Ans. (d)
Note
Fish head appearance of the vertebral bodies is seen in 'Osteoporosis'.
Also see
In osteoporosis vertebrae are mostly affected where the vertebral bodies become biconcave due to indentation of the intervertebral disc, as the bone becomes soft. This gives the typical appearance of fish head.
Ref: Textbook of surgery S Das 3rd Ed. Pg-429

Q. 292. Commonest recurrent dislocation is seen with (IHMA-MEE-II)
- (a) Shoulder
- (b) Patella
- (c) Elbow
- (d) Hip

Ans. (a)
Commonest recurrent dislocation is deen with 'Shoulder joint'.
Also see
Most common joint to undergo recurrent dislocation is shoulder joint.
Ref: Anatomy by Vishram singh, 2nd Ed. Pg -99

Q. 293. Which hallucination is characteristic of alcoholism?
- (a) Visual
- (b) Tactile
- (c) Auditory
- (d) Gustatory

Ans. (c)
Note
In alcoholism the acute hallucinations are 'Auditory hallucinations'.
Also see
Alcoholic hallucinosis is characterised by the presence of hallucinations (usually auditory) during abstinence, following regular alcohol intake.
Ref: Textbook of Psychiatry by Niraj Ahuja, 5th Ed. Pg- 40

Q. 294. Most characteristic of Korsakoffs psychosis is
   (a)   Visual hallucination
   (b)   Peripheral neuropathy
   (c)   Long-term memory loss
   (d)   Confusion

Ans. (c)

Note
Most characteristic of Korsakoffs psychosis is 'Long-term memory loss'.

Also see
Clinically, Korsakoff's psychosis presents as an amnestic syndrome, characterized by gross memory disturbances with confabulation.
Ref: Textbook of Psychiatry by Niraj Ahuja, 5th Ed. Pg- 41

Extended information
Korsakoff's syndrome (Korsakoff's psychosis, amnesic-confabulatory syndrome), is a continuum of Wernicke's encephalopathy, though a recognised episode of Wernicke's is not always obvious. Individuals diagnosed with Korsakoff's syndrome usually have symptoms of severe anterograde and retrograde amnesia, as well as confabulation. The syndrome is named for Sergei Korsakoff, the neuropsychiatrist who popularized the theory.
These symptoms are caused by damage to mammillary bodies and other brain regions due to deficiency of thiamine (Vitamin B1). This is most often caused by chronic alcoholism.

Q. 295. Dementia is produced by deficiency of which vitamin?
   (a)   A
   (b)   D
   (c)   Pyridoxine
   (d)   Niacin

Ans. (d)

Note
Dementia is produced by vitamin 'niacin deficiency'.

Also see
Niacin deficiency results in pellagra which is charecterised by three D's- Diarrhea, Dementia and Dermatitis.
Per: Park and Park, 18th Ed. Pg- 446

Extended information
Nicotinic acid was first discovered from the oxidation of nicotine. When the properties of nicotinic acid were discovered, it was thought prudent to choose a name to dissociate it from nicotine and to avoid the idea that either smoking provided vitamins or that wholesome food contained a poison. The resulting name 'niacin' was derived from nicotinic acid + vitamin. Vitamin B3 is also referred to as "vitamin PP", a name derived from the obsolete term "pellagra-preventing factor."

Q. 296. Neurotransmitter which is found in increased quantities in schizophrenia is
   (a)   Noradrenalin
   (b)   Serotonin
   (c)   Dopamine
   (d)   GABA

Ans. (c)

Note
Neurotransmitter which is found in increased quantities in schizophrenia is 'Dopamine'.

Also see
The most widely accepted explanation for the biochemical pathophysiology of schizophrenia was the dopamine hypothesis, which suggests that the disorder is primarily caused by a functional hyperactivity in the amine system.
Ref: API, 7th Ed. Pg-1378

Extended information
Disruption to the dopamine system has also been strongly linked to psychosis and schizophrenia. Dopamine neurons in the mesolimbic pathway are particularly associated with these conditions. This is partly due to the discovery of a class of drugs called the phenothiazines (which block D2 dopamine receptors) that can reduce psychotic symptoms, and partly due to the finding that drugs such as amphetamine and cocaine (which is known to greatly increase dopamine levels) can cause psychosis. Because of this, most modern antipsychotic medication is designed to block dopamine function to varying degrees.

Q. 297. Nasal allergy is most often due to
(a) Dust
(b) Pollen grain
(c) Animal dandies
(d) Smoke

Ans. (b)
Note
Nasal allergy is most often due to 'Pollen grain'.
Also see
Allergic rhinitis is due to an immediate hypersensitivity reaction in the nasal mucosa. The antigens concerned in the seasonal form of disorder are pollens from grasses, flowers, weeds or trees.
Ref: Davidson's 19th Ed. Pg-566

Extended information
Allergic rhinitis, or hay fever, frequently include nasal congestion, a clear runny nose, sneezing, nose and eye itching, and tearing eyes. Post nasal dripping of clear mucous frequently causes a cough.
Allergic rhinitis is caused by pollens. Commonly, allergic rhinitis is a result of an allergic person coming in contact several times with pollens from plants. Many trees, grasses, and weeds produce extremely small, light, dry protein particles called pollen.

Q. 298. Commonest symptom of laryngeal CA (IHMA-MEE-II)
(a) Hoarseness of voice
(b) Cough
(c) Dyspnea
(d) Hemoptysis

Ans. (a)
Note
Commonest symptom of laryngeal CA is 'Hoarseness of voice'.
Also see
Symptoms of laryngeal carcinoma: Hoarseness of voice is an early sign because lesions of cord affect its vibratory capacity. It is because of this that glottic cancer is detected early.
Ref: ENT by P.L. Dhingra. Pg- 372

Extended information
In a vast majority of cases, laryngeal carcinoma originates in the glottic region. Free edge and upper surface of vocal cord in its anterior and middle third is the most frequent site.
Signs and symptoms are:
-Hoarseness of voice is an early sign because lesions of vocal cord affect its vibratory capacity. Increase in size of the growth with accompanying edema or cord fixation may cause stridor and laryngeal obstruction.
Ref: Diseases of Ear Nose & Throat by P.L. Dhingra, Ch 62, Pg 371-372

Q. 299. Rhinosporidosis is due to
(a) Protozoa
(b) Bacteria
(c) Fungus
(d) Virus

Ans. (c)
Note
Rhinosporidosis is due to 'Fungus'.

Also see
Rhinosporidium is a fungus-like organism, not yet cultured, that causes rhinosporidiosis. Pedunculated nasal masses that grow over months or years cause obstruction and a foul odor and must be surgically excised.
Ref; Harrison - Sectiono 4. Disorders of eyes, ears, nse and throat. 30 Infection of the upper respiratory tract

Q. 300. Sub mucous resection is done in
 (a) Tonsillitis
 (b) Nasal polyp
 (c) DNS
 (d) Adenoid

Ans. (c)

Note
Sub mucous resection is done in 'DNS'.

Also see
Deviated nasal septum can involve any age and sex. Males are affected more than females. It causes; nasal obstruction, headache, sinusitis, epistaxis, external deformity. If deflected nasal septum causes mechanical nasal obstruction than it is treated with Submucous Resection (SMR) operation.
Ref; Diseases of Earm Nose, and Throat by P. L. Dhingra.

Q. 301. The presence of Keyser-Fleischer ring is pathognomonic of
 (a) HTN
 (b) Lew's syndrome
 (c) Wilson's disease
 (d) Hemochromatosis

Ans. (c)

Note
The presence of Keyser-Fleischer ring is pathognomonic of 'Wilson's disease'.

Also see
Kayser-Fleischer ring: It is a grey-green or golden brown colour in cornea in the form of a ring, it is seen in hepatolenticular degeneration (Wilson's disease) and is due to deposition of copper.

Extended information
Wilson's disease is charecterised by cirrhosis of liver, degeneration of basal ganglia and development of pigmented ring at periphery of cornea (kayser-fleisher ring).
Ref: API, 7th Ed. Pg-266

Q. 302. Roth's spot's are seen in
 (a) Diabetes
 (b) Chonoretinitis
 (c) Bacterial endocarditis
 (d) HTN

Ans. (c)

Note
Roth's spot's are seen in 'Bacterial Endocarditis'.

Also see
White centered retinal hemorrhages (Roth's spots) are pathognomonic for subacute bacterial endocarditis, but they also appear in leukemia, diabetes.
Ref; Harrison's 15th Edition. Section 4. Disorders of eyes
Roth's spots are retinal hemorrhages which are oval or flame shaped with a pale centre, are seen in infective endocarditis.
Ref: API, 7th Ed. Pg- 427

Q. 303. Deficiency of which vitamin is not seen in newborn
 (a) E
 (b) D
 (c) C
 (d) K

Ans. (a)

Note
Deficiency of vitamin E is not seen in newborn.

Q. 304. A wide and fixed split second heart sound occurs in
    (a)   Mitral stenosis
    (b)   ASD
    (c)   VSD
    (d)   Coarctation of aorta

Ans. (b)
Note
A wide and fixed split second heart sound occurs in ASD.
Also see
In ASD, the second heart sound is widely split and fixed with accentuated pulmonary component.
Ref: API, 7th Ed. Pg- 466

Q. 305. Delayed dentition is most characteristic of
    (a)   Cretinism
    (b)   Mongolism
    (c)   Acromegaly
    (d)   Malnutrition

Ans. (a)
Note
Delayed dentition is most characteristic of 'cretinism'.
Also see
Delayed tooth eruptions, receding chin and a protruding tongue are occasional features of cretinism and hypopituitarism.
Ref: Harrison's 16th Ed., Pg-194

Q. 306. In an infant with ASOM, the infecting organism is likely to be
    (a)   Pneumococcus
    (b)   H. Influenza
    (c)   Streptococcus
    (d)   Staphylococcus

Ans. (c)
Note
In an infant with ASOM, the infecting organism is likely to be Streptococcus pneumoniae.
Also see
In ASOM, most common organisms in infants and young children are Streptococcus pneumoniae (30%), Haemophilus influenzae (20%), and Morexella catarrhalis(12%)
Ref: ENT by P.L.Dhingra Pg-81,

Q. 307. Most common complication of measles in children is
    (a)   ASOM
    (b)   Broncho pneumonia
    (c)   Orchitis
    (d)   Meningitis

Ans. (a)
Note
Most common complication of measles in children is ASOM.
Also see
In young children, otitis media is the most common complication of measles.
Ref: Harrison's 16th edition, Pg- 1149.

Q. 308. In bronchial asthma, there is constriction of
    (a) Large airway
    (b) Medium airway
    (c) Terminal bronchiole
    (d) Respiratory bronchioles

Ans. (c)
Note
In bronchial asthma, there is constriction of 'terminal bronchiole'.

Q. 309. Chancroid is caused by
    (a) H. ducreyi
    (b) H. vaginalis
    (c) Treponema pallidum
    (d) Treponema pertinuae

Ans. (a)
Note
Chancroid is caused by H. ducreyi'.
Also see
Chancroid is a sexually transmitted disease and is caused by Hemophilus ducreyi a short gram negative bacillus. Incubation priod is 3-10 days. Genital lesions; includes single or multiple painful ulcers with ragged undermined edges. Inguinal Lymph nodes involved in 50% cases; it is tender, usually unilateral, matted, sdherent unilocular, suppurative bubo.
Ref: Davidson 20th Ed.
Causative organism of chancroid is Hemophilus ducreyi. It forms multiple painful ulcers which are tender, bleeding.

Ref: Skin diseases and sexually transmitted infections, by Dr. Uday Khopkar, Pg- 280

Q. 310. Pitting of nails is seen in
    (a) Lichen planus
    (b) Psoriasis
    (c) Pemphigus
    (d) Leprosy

Ans. (b)
Note
Pitting of nails is seen in psoriasis.
Ref: Davidson 20th Ed. Fig-27.25
Also see
Nail psoriasis: Nails are involved secondary to affection of nail matrix or nail bed. Numerous pits in the nail plate and subungual hyperkeratosis are the commonest manifestations of nail psoriasis.

Ref: Skin diseases and sexually transmitted infections, by Dr. Uday khopkar, Pg -128

Q. 311. Fir - tree appearance is seen in
    (a) Pityriasis rosea
    (b) Psoriasis
    (c) Measles
    (d) Secondary syphilis

Ans. (a)
Note
Fir - tree appearance is seen in 'Pityriasis rosea'.
Also see
In case of pityriasis rosea rash often preceded by herald patch; oval to round plaques with trailing scale; most often affects the trunk, and eruptions line on skin folds give 'fir- tree' like appearance; generally sapres palms and soles. Ref: Robin's table 56-2. Papulosquamous disorders 15th Edition

In pityriasis rosea there is a single large lesion to precede the generalized eruption by 2-5 days. Lesions begin as macules and progress to form papules that keep on expanding at the periphery and clear in the centre, thereby resulting in annular plaques. Fine scales can be seen attached to inner border of the ring shaped lesion forming a "collarette". Oval lesions arranged symmetrically along the ribs give rise to a "fir tree or Christmas tree" pattern.

Ref: Skin diseases and sexually transmitted infections, by Dr. Uday Khopkar Pg-131

Q. 312. Necrobiosis lipoidica is most marked on
- (a) Forearms
- (b) Face
- (c) Front of legs
- (d) Back of legs

Ans. (c)

Note
Necrobiosis lipoidica is most marked on 'Front of legs'.

Also see
Yellow lesions: Several systemic disorders are characterised by yellow colored cutaneus papules or plaques- hyperlipidaemia (xanthomas), gout (tophi), diabetes (necrobiosis lipoidica).

Lesions of necrobiosis lipoidica are found primarily on the shins (90%) and patient can have diabetes mellitus or develop it subsequently. Characteristic finding include a central yellow color, atrophy (transparency), telangiectasias, and an erythmatous border.
Ref: Robins Chapter 57 Skin manifestations of internal disease 15th Edition
Necrobiosis lipoidica (a patch of spreading erythema over the shin which become yellowish and atrophic in the centre and may ulcerate)
Ref: Kumar and Clark, 6th Ed. Pg-1345

Q. 313. A flat discolouration in skin of 1cm is called
- (a) Plaque
- (b) Macule
- (c) Papule
- (d) Wheal

Ans. (b)

Note
A flat discolouration in skin of 1cm is called 'macule'.

Also see
A flat, colored lesion, <2 cm in diameter, not raised above the surface of surrounding skin is called 'Macule".
Ref: Robins Table 55.1 Description of Primary Skin Lesions 15th Edition
Macule is flat, circumscribed non-palpable lesions.
Ref: Kumar and Clark, 6th Ed. Pg-1318

Q. 314. Torre's inclusion body is found in (IHMA-MEE-II)
- (a) Yellow fever
- (b) Dengue
- (c) KFD
- (d) Wiel's disease

Ans. (a)

Note
Torre's inclusion body is found in 'yellow fever'.

Also see
In yellow fever, in liver, acute mid zonal necrosis leads to deposits of hyaline called councilman's bodies and intra nuclear eosinophilic inclusions called torre's bodies.
Ref: Kumar and Clark, 6th Ed. Pg- 61

Q. 315. Sonogyi phenomena is (IHMA-MEE-II)
 (a) Hypoglycemia followed by hyperglycemia
 (b) Hyperglycemia followed by hypoglycemia
 (c) Glycosuria with normal blood sugar
 (d) Reactive hyperglycemia

Ans. (a)
Note
Sonogyi phenomena is 'Hypoglycemia followed by hyperglycemia'.
Also see
Somogyi effect: Hyperglycemia develops after an episode of insulin induced hypoglycemia. Usually this occurs over-night when fasting blood glucose tends to be high and worsens after the preceding night time insulin dose is increased.
Ref: API, 7th Ed. Pg- 1112

Q. 316. Satellite lesions is seen in (IHMA-MEE-II)
 (a) Borderline leprosy
 (b) Tuberculoid leprosy
 (c) Lepromatous leprosy
 (d) Intermediate leprosy

Ans. (b)
Satellite lesion is seen in 'Tuberculoid leprosy'.
Also see
In borderline tuberculoid leprosy usually large satellite lesions are seen.
Ref: API, 7th Ed. Pg-1358

Q. 317. Icterus is most marked in sclera because
 (a) High content of collagen
 (b) High content of elastin
 (c) It is white
 (d) It is exposed to sunlight

Ans. (b)
Note
Icterus is most marked in sclera because ' high content of elastin'.
Also see
Slight increases in serum bilirubin are best detected by examining the sclerae which have a particular affinity for bilirubin due to their high elastin content. The presence of scleral icterus indicates a serum bilirubin of at least 3.0 mg/dL.
Ref: Harrison Vol –I 16th Ed. Pg-436

Q. 318. Which vitamin prevents development of pernicious anemia, but doesn't protect against CNS manifestation?
 (a) Pyridoxine
 (b) B12
 (c) Biotin
 (d) Folic acid

Ans. (d)
Note
'Folic acid' prevents development of pernicious anemia, but doesn't protect against CNS manifestation.
Also see
Both the vitamins B 12 and folic acid deficiency causes megaloblastic anemia. The clinical features of cobalamine deficiency (B 12) involve the blood, gastrointestinal tract and nervous system. However, in contrast to B12 (Cobalamine) deficiency, the neurological abnormalities do not occur in folic acid deficiency.

MCQ's in Practice of Medicine

Q. 319. Enzyme raised within hours of MI and lasting 2-3 days is
    (a)   LDH
    (b)   CPK
    (c)   AST
    (d)   ALT

Ans. (b)
Note
Enzyme raised within hours of Ml and lasting 2-3 days is ' CPK'.
Also see
CPK starts to rise at 4-6 hours, peak at about 12 hours and falls to normal within 48-72 hours.
Ref. Davidson's 19th Ed. Pg-436

Extended information
Changes in plasma enzyme concentrations after myocardial infarction:
LDH:
    -Starts to rise after 12 hours of myocardial infarction.
    -Peaks on 3rd day.
    -Becomes normal on 7th day.
CPK:
    -Starts to rise at 4 - 6 hours of myocardial infarction.
    -Peaks about 12 hours.
    -Becomes normal at 48-72 hours.
AST:
    -Starts to rise after 12 hours of myocardial infarction.
    -Peaks about 24 hours.
    -Comes to normal on 4th or 5th day.

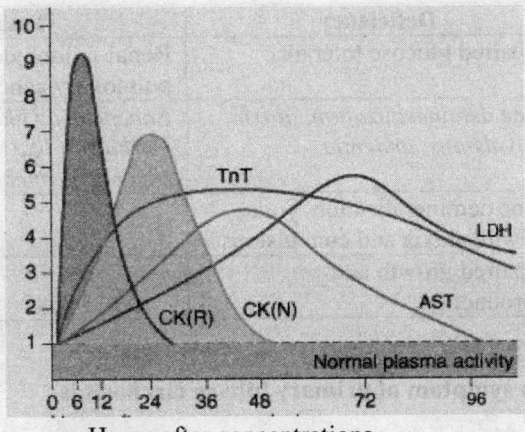

Hours after concentrations

Changes in plasma enzyme concentrations after myocardial infarction. Creatine kinase (CK) and troponin T (TnT) are the first to rise, followed by aspartate aminotransferase (AST) and then lactate (hydroxybutyrate) dehydrogenase (LDH). In patients treated with a thrombolytic agent, reperfusion is usually accompanied by a rapid rise in plasma creatine kinase (curve CK (R)) due to a washout effect; if there is no reperfusion, the rise is less rapid but the area under the curve is often greater (curve CK (N)).

The most important biochemical markers used diagnosis of MI are creatine kinase (CK), a more sensitive and cardiospecific isoform of this enzyme (CK-MB), and the cardiospecific proteins, troponins T and I. The troponins are also released, to a minor degree, in unstable angina with minimal myocardial damage. Serial (usually daily) estimations are particularly helpful because it is the change in plasma concentrations of these markers that is of diagnostic value.
Ref: Davidsons 20th Ed.

Q. 320. Most common cardiac involvement in RA
    (a)   Pancarditis
    (b)   Pericarditis
    (c)   Myocarditis
    (d)   Endocarditis

Ans. (a)
Note
Most common cardiac involvement in RA 'Pancarditis'.
Also see
Clinically apparent heart diseases atributred to the rheumatoid process is rare, but evidence of asymptomaic pericarditis is found at autopsy in 50% of cases.
Ref: Harrison's 15th Ed.
Cardiac manifestations in RA includes pericarditis, myocarditis, endocarditis, conduction defects, coronary vasculitis, granulomatous aortitis.
Ref. Davidson's 19th Ed. Pg-1005

Q. 321. Parkinsonism may occur due to chronic exposure to
    (a)   Chromium
    (b)   Manganese
    (c)   Molybdenum
    (d)   Nickel

Ans. (b)
Note
Parkinsonism may occur due to chronic exposure to 'Manganese'.
Also see

Element	Deficiency	Toxicity
Chromium	Impaired glucose tolerance	Renal failure, dermatitis, pulmonary cancer
Magnanese	*Bone demineralization, ataxia, convulsions, anaemia*	*Encephalitis like syndrome, Parkinson like syndrome, psychosis, pneumconiosis*
Molybdenum	Bone demineralization, poor growth, ataxia and convulsions	-
Nickel	Impaired growth and reproduction.	-

Ref. Harrison's 16th Ed., Pg- 2414.

Q. 322. The most common symptom of primary biliary cirrhosis is
    (a)   Pain abdomen
    (b)   Fever
    (c)   Weakness
    (d)   Pruritis

Ans. (d)
Note
The most common symptom of primary biliary cirrhosis is 'Pruritus'.
Also see
Clinical features of primary biliary cirrhosis:
    -Lethargy and fatigue
    -Arthralgia
    -Pruritus
    -Jaundice

-Diarrhea
-Bone pains and fractures
Ref: Davidson's 19th edition. Pg.873

Extended information
Many patients of PBC are asymptomatic and the disease is initially detected on the basis of elevated serum alkaline phosphatase level during routine screening. Among the patients with asymptomatic disease 90% are females in the age group of 35 – 60 years. The earliest symptom is pruritus, which may be either generalized or limited initially to the palms and soles. In addition fatigue is commonly a prominent early symptom. After several months or years jaundice and gradual darkening of exposed areas of skin (melanosis) may ensue.
Ref: Harrison's

Q. 323. Kimmelstein-Wilson lesions are specific for
(a) Type I DM (IDDM)
(b) Type II DM (NIDDM)
(c) MODY (Matury Onset Diabetes of Young)
(d) DIDMOAD

Ans. (a)
Note
Kimmelstein-Wilson lesions are specific for 'Type I DM (IDDM)'
Also see
Kimmelstein-Wilsons lesions or intercapillary glomerulosclerosis. These lesions are specific for juvenile-onset diabetes or islet cell antibody positive diabetes mellitus.
Ref: TB of Pathology by Harsh Mohan, 4th Edition Pg- 662
DIDMOAD (Wolfran syndrome) is diabetes associated genetic syndrome – Diabetes insipidus, diabetes mellitus, optic atrophy, nerve deafness, lipoatrophy, muscular dystrophies.
Ref: Clinical Medicine By Kumar & Clark 6th Ed, Pg-1090

Q. 324. Most common cranial nerve involved in opthalmoplegic migraine
(a) 2nd Cranial Nerve
(b) 3rd Cranial Nerve
(c) 5th Creanial Nerve
(d) Ophthalmic Branch of Trigeminal Nerve

Ans. (b)
Note
Most common cranial nerve involved in ophthalmoplegic migraine '3rd cranial nerve'.
Also see
Ophthalmoplegic migraine: Headache is commonly around the eyes and is accompanied by weakness of movements of one eye due to involvement of 3rd Cranial Nerve, which may outlast the headache by some days. Children are more commonly affected.

Extended information
Ophthalmoplegic Migraine: This is a third nerve or exceptionally a 6th nerve palsy with migraine and difficult to diagnose without investigation to exclude other conditions.
Ref: Kumar and Clark, 6th Ed. Pg-1248

Q. 325. Whiplash injury refers to that involving
(a) Spine
(b) Long bones
(c) Skull
(d) Ribcage

Ans. (a)
Note
Whiplash injury refers to that involving 'spine'.

Also see
Whiplash injury is due to a violent acceleration or deceleration force applied to the passenger, usually front seat occupant. There is acute hyperflexion and than a reactionary hyperextension. In either cases this violent extension flexion movement can cause dislocation of upper cervical spine, or less commonly a fracture dislocation in the lower part of spine at about C5-C6.
Pg, 234, Textbook of forensic medicine by Narayan Reddy, 19th edition.

Extended information
The name or denomination Whiplash injury derives from the etiopathogenic description of the sudden sharp whipping movement of the head and neck, produced at the moment of a traffic accident, particularly subsequent to collisions from the rear, head-on or side collisions. In the case of a head-on collision, a forward displacement of the body is produced as a result of the inertia provoking tension upon the safety belt together with a neck hyperflexion followed by a hyperextension of it, thus producing "the whiplash". In the case of a collision from the rear, the mechanism is inverted, first hyperextension followed by hyper flexion of the neck.
Ref: -http://www.vertigo-dizziness.com/english/whiplash_injury.html

Q. 326. About neutrophils all are incorrect except
(a) 10-20% of all leucocytes
(b) Phagocytosis
(c) Antibody formation
(d) Increase in chronic infections

Ans. (b)
Note
About neutrophils all are incorrect except 'phagocytosis'.
Also see
The normal functions of neutrophils are:
1. Phagocytosis
2. Chemotaxis
3. Killing
Ref: Short Handbook of Pathology by Harsh Mohan, 2nd Ed. Pg 281

Q. 327. In leprosy nerve involved is
(a) Ulnar nerve
(b) Median
(c) Radial
(d) Axillary

Ans. (a)
Note
In leprosy nerve involved is 'Ulnar nerve'.
Also see
In tuberculoid leprosy there is ulnar paralysis which results in claw hand, foot drop on account of lateral popliteal nerve involvement and facial nerve palsy.
Ref: API, 7th Ed. Pg-1358
Tuberculoid leprosy associated with peripheral-nerve enlargement. Common to get involved nerves are those which are subcutaneously placed. The most commonly involved nerves therefore are ulnar, posterior auricular and common peroneal. Deep nerves which are covered witht muscles are protected form trauma and exposure to cold by body heat and those which are exposed to cold and frequently traumatized are easy to be affected with leprosy.

Q. 328. Hypertrophic pulmonary osteoarthropathy is due to
(a) Oat cell carcinoma
(b) Squamous cell carinoma
(c) Adenocarcinoma
(d) Adenosqumous

Ans. (c)
Note
Hypertrophic pulmonary osteoarthropathy is due to 'Adenocarcinoma'.

Also see
Hypertrophic pulmonary osteoarthropathy in 1 to 10% of cases (usually adenocarcinomas) with periostitis and clubbing giving pain, tenderness, and swelling over the affected bones and a positive bone scan.
Ref; 88. Neoplasms of lung. Harrison.

Q. 329. Stricture of gut is caused by
    (a)   Typhoid
    (b)   Tuberculosis
    (c)   Crohn's disease
    (d)   Ulcerative colitis

Ans. (b)

Note
Stricture of gut is caused by 'Tuberculosis'.

Also see
Typhoid
An infectious disease caused by salmonella typhi and paratyphi. Common complications in 3rd week being intestinal perforation and hemorrhage.
Tuberculosis
In case of tuberculous enteritis common presentation is pain right lower abdomen, constipation weight loss and subacute intestinal obstruction due to stricture at ileum.
Colonic tuberculosis can take several forms, with the most common being segmental ulcers and colitis, inflammatory strictures and hypertrophic lesions resembling polyps and masses.
Ref: API, 7th Ed. Pg-563
Crohn's disease
Active CD is characterized by focal inflammation and formation of fistula tracts, which resolve by fibrosis and stricturing of the bowel. The bowel wall thickens and becomes narrowed and fibrotic, leading to chronic, recurrent bowel obstructions.
Ulcerative colitis
UC is a mucosal disease that usually involves the rectum and extends proximally to involve all or part of the colon. Approximately 40 to 50% of patients have disease limited to the rectum and rectosigmoid, 30 to 40% have disease extending beyond the sigmoid but not involving the whole colon, and 20% have a total colitis.

Extended information
The stricture can occur in tuberculosis and Crohn's disease. However, tuberculosis is more common in India.

Q. 330. Which of the following markers in the blood is the most reliable indicator of recent hepatitis B infection? (AIIMS/May2003)
    (a)   HBs Ag
    (b)   IgG anti-HBs
    (c)   IgM anti-HBc
    (d)   IgM anti-HBe

Ans. (a)

Note
The HBs Ag of the above markers in the blood is the most reliable indicator of recent hepatitis B infection.

Also see
Diagnosis of HBV infection is based on estimating various antigens and antibodies in the sera and demonstration of HBV DNA in the sera or liver tissue. Presence of HBsAg (Australia antigen) in the blood suggests that patient is infected with HBV. Presence of HBeAg in the blood suggests active viral replication. IgM anti-HBc antibodies indicate acute infection. Anti- HBc IgG antibodies remain in the blood lifelong after exposure to HBV.
Ref: API, 7th Ed. Pg-598
The surface antigen is the first to be detected. It appears in the serum during the incubation period before biochemical evidence of liver damage or the onset of jaundice. It persists during acute illness, and is usually cleared from the blood stream during convalescence. This may take 4 to 6 months the next to appear are the 'e' antigen and DNA polymerase. All these three marakeers precede the onset of disease. The 'e' antigen (HBeAg) is a marker of virus replication and, therefore, a marker of infectivity. Detected within 3 – 5 days following

the appearance of the surface antigen, it persists for 2 to 6 weeks. In acrriers, the 'e' antigen may persist for years without sero-conversion. The presence of 'e' antigben indicates that the patient is higly infectious. The sero-convursion of 'e' antigen into 'e' antaibody is considered a good prognostic feature.
Ref: Park & Park, 18th Ed, Pg-170

Patterns of Principal HBV Serological Markers in Acute and Chronic Hepatitis		
	Acute	Chronic
HBsAg	Positive, disappears on recovery	Positive, persists
Anti-HBs	Appears on recovery	Usually negative
IgM Anti-HBc	Positive, high titer-acute HBV infection. Lower titer-Chronic HBV infections, Absent-chronic HBV infection.	Low or negative
IgG Anti-HBc	Negative	Positive (Past exposure)
HBeAg	Positive - Continued infectious state (replicative state) acute or chronic HBV infection.	Positive in carriers
Anti-HBe	When present, it is a good sign (Convalescence)	Negative
HBV DNA	Positive, disappears on recovery	Positive in case of continued infectious state.

Ref: Adapted from; API Textbook of Medicine, 7th Ed, Pg-599

Table 10.11 Interpretation of main investigations used in the serological diagnosis of hepatitis B Virus infection

Interpretation	HBsAg	Anti-HBc IgM	Anti-HBc IgG	Anti-HBs
Incubation period	+	+	-	-
Acute hepatitis				
Early	+	+	-	-
Established	+	+	+	-
Established (occasional)	-	+	+	-
Convalescence				
(3-6 months)	-	±	+	±
(6-9 months)	-	-	±	+
Post infection				
> 1 year	-	-	+	+
Uncertain	-	-	+	-
Chronic infection				
Usual	+	-	+	-
Occasional	-	-	+	-
Immunisation without infection				
-Very variable				

+ – positive; - – negative; ± – present at how titre or absent. (HBsAg = surface antigen; anti-HBc – antibody to core antigen, anti-HBs – antibody to surface antigen

Ref: Davidson 18th Ed, Pg-712

Q. 331. Which of the following is the most common central nervous system parasitic infection? (AIIMS/May2003)
    (a) Echinococcosis
    (b) Sparganosis
    (c) Paragonimiasis
    (d) Neurocysticercosis

Ans. (d)

Note
'Neurocysticercosis' from above is the most common central nervous system parasitic infection.
In endemic areas, as many as 4% of population is known to be affected with neurocysticercosis.
Ref: API, 7th Ed. Pg-124

Also see
Echinococcosis
It is a infection of humans caused by larval stage of Echinococcus granulosus. The definitive hosts are dogs that pass eggs in their feces. Cysts develop in the intermediate hosts – sheep, cattle, humans, goats, camels and horses for E. granulosus. After the humans ingest the eggs embryos escape from the eggs, penetrate the intestinal mucosa enter the portal circulation, and are carried to various organs, most commonly the liver and lungs. Larvae develop into fluid filled Unilocular hydatid cysts.

Sparganosis
Humans can be infected by the sparganum, or plerocrocoid larva, of a diphylllobothrid tapeworm of the genus Spirometra. Infection is acquired by consumption of water containing infected Cyclops. The worm migrates slowly in tissues, and infection commonly presents as a subcutaneous swelling. Periorbital tissues can be involved, and ocular sparganosis may destroy the eyes. Surgical excision is used to treat localized sparganosis.
Ref: Harrison 15th Edition Section 18 Helminthic Infections 223. Cestodes

Paragonimiasis
Humans acquire lung fluke Paragonimus westernani infection by ingesting infective metacercariae encysted in the muscles and viscera of crayfish and freshwater crabs. Onces the organism reach theduodenum, they excyst, penetrate the gut wall, and travel through the peritoneal cavity, diaphragm, and pleural space to reach the lungs. Mature flukes are found in the bronchioles surrounded by cystic lesions. Parasite eggs are either expectorated with sputum or swallowed and passed to the outside environment with feces. The lifecycle is completed in snails and freshwater crustacean.

Neurocysticercosis
The pork tapeworm T. Solium can cause two distinct forms of infection. The form that develops depends on whether humans are infected with adult tapeworms in the intestine or with larval forms in the tissues (Cysticercosis) humans are definitive hosts for T. Solium; pigs are usually intermediate hosts. Infection that causes human cysticercosis follows the ingestion of T. Solium eggs usually from fecally contaminated food. Autoinfection may ccur if an individual with an egg-producing tapeworm ingests eggs derived from his or her own feces.
Ref: Harrison 15th Edition Section 18 Helminthic Infections 223. Cestodes

Q. 332. The severity of mitral stenosis is clinically best decided by (AIIMS/May2003)
    (a) Length of diastolic murmur
    (b) Intensity of diastolic murmur
    (c) Loudness of first heart sound
    (d) Split of second heart sound

Ans. (a)

Note
The severity of mitral stenosis is clinically best decided by 'Length of diastolic murmur'.

Also see
In mitral stenosis murmur is typically a low frequency, low pitched, rumbling murmur of varying duration. The duration of the murmur is a useful auscultatory hallmark of the severity of stenotic lesion, with severe stenosis (mitral valve area <1cm^2) the murmur is characteristically long, loud and present throughout diastole with presystolic crescendo component marching into the loud first heart sound.
Ref: API, 7th Ed. Pg-411

In general, the duration of diastolic murmur correlates with the severity of the mitral stenosis. In patients with sinus rhythm, the murmur becomes accentuated during atrial systole, as atrial contraction re-elevates the rate of blood flow across the narrowed orifice.

Q. 333. A young female presents with history of dyspnea on exertion. On examination, she has wide, fixed split S2 with ejection systolic murmur (III/VI) in left second intercostal space. Her EKG shows left axis deviation. The most probable diagnosis is (AIIMS/May2003)
- (a) Total anomalous pulmonary venous drainge
- (b) Tricuspid atresia
- (c) Ostium primum atrial septal defect
- (d) Ventricular septal defect with pulmonary arterial hypertension

Ans. (c)

Note
The most probable diagnosis is 'Atrial Septal Defect'.

Also see
In ASD, the first heart sound is normal or accentuated due to large tricuspid closure and the second heart sound is widely split and fixed with accentuated pulmonary component.

Extended information
Features are in favor of ASD.

Features	Interpretation	Comments
DOE	Cardiac dyspnoea	
Wide fixed split of S2	Prolonged emptying time of Right ventricle.	
Ejection systolic murmur III/VI in left second intercostal spae.	Pulmonary Artery Hypertension	
EKG shows Left axis deviation	Right ventricular hypertrophy	Anticlockwise rotation

Q. 334. The severity of mitral regurgitation is decided by all of the following clinical findings except (AIIMS/May2003)
- (a) Presence of mid-diastolic murmur across mitral valve
- (b) Wide split second heart sound
- (c) Presence of left ventricular S3 gallop
- (d) Intensity of systolic murmur across mitral valve

Ans. (a)

Note
The severity of mitral regurgitation is decided by all of the above clinical findings except 'Presence of mid-diastolic murmur across mitral valve'.

Also see
The presence of mid- diastolic murmur has no significance in case of intensity of mitral regurgitation as it is only heared in MR with MS. However a systolic murmur of at least grade III/VI intensity is most characteristic auscultatory finding in severe MR.

Q. 335. Which of the following is not a usual feature of right middle cerebral artery territory infarct? (AIIMS/May2003)
- (a) Aphasia
- (b) Hemiparesis
- (c) Facial weakness
- (d) Dysarthria

Ans. (a)

Note
'Aphasia' from above is not a usual feature of right middle cerebral artery territory infarct.

Also see
Aphasia
Aphasia is loss of the ability to produce and/or comprehend language. It is not due to deficits in sensory, intellect, or psychiatric functioning or muscle weakness.
Cause:
Aphasias is caused by damage to Broca's area. Broca's area is the language centres of the brain and is situated in the left cerebral hemisphere, which controls right side of body. Common causes of damage to broca's area are; stroke (involveing Lt. Middle Cerebral Artery), trauma. When sudden in origin. Slowly developing aphasia may occur in brain tumor or progressive neurological disease. It is usually associated with right hemiplagia as left sided cerebral hemisphere controls the right side of body.
Global Aphasia; speech output is nonfluent, and comprehension of spoken language is severely impaired. Naming, repetition, reading, and writing are also impaired. This syndrome represents the combined dysfunction of Broca's and Wernicke's areas and usually results from strokes that involve the entire middle cerebral artery distribution in the left hemisphere.
Ref: Harrison's Section 3 – Nervous system dysfunction 25 Aphasia the other focal cerebral disorders.

Hemiparesis
Hemiparesis in case of right middle cerebral artery will result in Left hemiparesis, however, it will not be associated with aphasia, rather patient will retain his ability to speak and understand.

Facial Weakness
In case of Right Middle Cerebral artery involvement upper motor neuron type left sided facial palsy will be a encountered.

Dysarthria
Dysarthria is a motor speech disorder due to some lesion in the nerves which loses effective control over, tongue, throat, lips or lungs. It is associated with dysphagia. The cranial nerves whicbh have a control over these muscles are; facial nerve (VII), the glossopharyngeal nerve (IX), the vagus nerve (X), and the hypoglossal nerve (XII).
Causes:

Dysarthria can be due to stroke, Amyotrophic Lateral Sclerosis, Parkinson's disease, Cranial nerve lesions, cerebral palsy. Dysarthria can also be present in some cases of 'Transient Ischaemic Attack' which is an early warning sign of stroke.

Q. 336. The risk of developing infective endocarditis is the least in a patient with (AIIMS/May2003)
    (a)   Small ventricular septal defect
    (b)   Severe aortic regurgitation
    (c)   Severe mitral regurgitation
    (d)   Large atrial septal defect

Ans. (d)

Note
The risk of developing infective endocarditis is the least in a patient with 'Large atrial septal defect'.

Also see
Endocarditis takes place where the endothelium is damaged by high pressure jet of blood i.e., ventricular septal defect, persistent ductus arteriosus, or regurgitant mitral or aortic valves. Or on damaged valves. Endocardial damage leads to deposition of platelets and fibrin which are colonized by blood borne organisms.
Ref: Davidsons 20th Ed.
Small ventricular defects require no specific treatment apart from endocarditis prophylaxis.
Ref: Davidsons 20th Ed. Pg-294
A small ventricular septal defect may never cause any problems. Larger defect however predisposes to increased risk of endocarditis.
Ref: MayoClinic.com
In case of Large ASD the risk of infective endocarditis is quite low as the pressure difference is less so risk is less, unless the defect is complicated by valvular regurgitation.

Q. 337. The following statements regarding turner's syndrome are true except (AIIMS/May2003)
    (a)   Occurence of turner's syndrome is influenced by maternal age
    (b)   Most patients have primary amenorrhea
    (c)   Most patients have short stature
    (d)   Edema of hands and feet is an important feature during infancy

Ans. (a)
Note
All of the above statements regarding turner's syndrome are true except 'occurrence of turner's syndrome is influenced by maternal age'.
Also see
Features of turner's syndrome:
    -Lymhedema of dorsum of hand and feet, loose skin folds in the nape of neck
    -Short stature, short neck, with webbing and low posterior hairline
    -Prominent narrow and high arched palate, small mandible and epicanthal folds
    -Chest is broad, shield like with widely spaced hypoplastic nipples
    -At puberty sexual maturation fails to occur
Ref: O P Ghai, Pg- 416

Extended information
Turner's syndrome is not related to mother's age. The patient has chromatin negative buccal smear and 46 X configuration.
Features of turner's syndrome include:
    -Short in height
    -Lack of sexual development
    -Webbed neck
    -Low hairline at the back of the neck
    -Drooping of the eyelids
    -Ears are set lower on the sides of the head than usual.
There are a number of other problems like:
    -Kidney problems
    -HT
    -Heart problems
    -Overweight
    -Hearing difficulties
    -Diabetes, cataracts
    -Thyroid problems
Ref: Net

Q. 338. Atrial fibrillation may occur in all of the following conditions, except (AIIMS/May2003)
    (a)   Mitral stenosis
    (b)   Hypothyroidism
    (c)   Dilated cardiomyopathy
    (d)   Mitral regurgitation

Ans. (b)
Note
Atrial fibrillation may occur in all of the following conditions, except 'Hypothyroidism'
Also see
The common causes of atrial fibrillation are:
a.   CAD, and Acute MI
b.   Valvular Heart Disease (Especially rheumatic mitral valve disease)
c.   Idiopathic (Lone atrial fibrillation)
d.   Hypertension
e.   Thyrotoxicosis
f.   Sinoatrial disease
g.   Alcohol

h. Congenital Heart Disease
i. Pulmonary embolism
j. Pericardial diseases
k. Pneumonia
Ref: Davidson's Principle and Practice of Medicine 18th Edition, Pg-562

Q. 339. Which of the following conditions is associated with Coombs' positive hemolytic anemia (AIIMS/May2003)
    (a) Thrombotic thrombocytopenic purpura
    (b) Progressive systemic sclerosis
    (c) Systemic lupus erythematosus
    (d) Polyarteritis nodosa

Ans. (c)
Note
'SLE' from the above conditions is associated with Coombs' positive hemolytic anemia.
Also see
Systemic lupus erythematosus (SLE) is a disease of unknown etiology in which tissues and cells are damaged by pathogenic autoantibodies and immune complexes. Ninety percent of cases are in women, usually of child-bearing age. Anemia of chronic disease occurs in most patients when SLE is active. Hemolysis occurs in a small proportion of those with positive Coombs' tests.

Q. 340. Which of the following is the most common tumor associated with type I neurofibromatosis? (AIIMS/May2003)
    (a) Optic nerve glioma
    (b) Meningioma
    (c) Acoustic Schwannoma
    (d) Low grade astrocytoma

Ans. (a)
Note
Most common tumor associated with type I neurofibromatosis is 'Optic Glioma'.
Also see
Neurofibromatosis Type 1 (Von Recklinghausen's Disease is an Autosomal dominant disorder. Gene involved = 17, gene product = Neurofibromin.
Criteria for diagnosis of neurofibromatosis type 1 (any two of the following seven):
1. Neurofibromas (one plexiform neuroma; or two +)
2. Cafe au lait spots (six or more measuring at least 1.5 cm in greatest dimension)
3. Frekling in axilliary or inguinal areas
4. Two or more iris hamartomas (Lisch nodules)
5. Optic Glioma
6. Sphenoid dysplasia or thinning of cortex of long bones.
7. Immediate Relative with Neurofibromatosis Type 1

Q. 341. Ophthalmoplegic migraine means (AIIMS/May2003)
    (a) When headache is followed by complete paralysis of the III and VI nerve on the same side as the hemicrania.
    (b) When the headache is followed by partial paralysis of the III nerve on the same side as the hemicrania without any scotoma.
    (c) Headache associated with III, IV and VI nerve paralysis.
    (d) Headache associated with optic neuritis.

Ans. (c)
Note
Ophthalmoplegic migraine means 'Headache associated with III, IV and VI nerve paralysis'
Also see
'In ophthalmoplegic migraine headache occurs in conjunction with diplopia. As the intensity of an ipsilateral severe headache subsides after a day or more, paresis of 1 or more of cranial nerves III, IV, and VI occurs.

The third cranial nerve is affected in about 80% of cases, initially with ptosis and then oculomotor paresis, which is usually complete but may be partial.

Q. 342. After a minor head injury a young patient was unable to close his left eye and had drooling of saliva from left angle of mouth. He is suffering from (AIIMS/May2003)
- (a) VII nerve injury
- (b) V nerve injury
- (c) III nerve injury
- (d) Combined VII and III nerve injury

Ans. (a)

Note
After a minor head injury a young patient was unable to close his left eye and had drooling of saliva from left angle of mouth. He is suffering from 'VII Cranial Nerve (Facial) injury'.

Also see
Clinical presentation after 'Minor head Injury"
 -Left sided complaints.
 -Inability to close left eye
 -Drooling from left angle of mouth

Anamnesis:
 -Muscles around the eyes and moth are involved.
 -It points to the upper and lower part of facial muscle involvement.
 -Facial muscles are suppled by facial nerve.
 -Trigeminal the Vth cranial nerve is sensory and motor to muscles of mastication which are spared in this case.
 -Occulomotor (3rd CN) is motor to extrinsic and intrinsic muscles (except; Superior obloque, lateral racatus,) which are spared.

Inference:
 -It points to the facial nerve (7th CN) paralysis, as facial nerve is motor to the sphincter of eye and oral orifice.
 -As upper and lower parts of face, both are involved – it points to LMN type paralysis.
 -The most probable site of facial nerve involvement could be at the exit of facial canal.

Conclusion:
 -He is suffering from LMN paralysis due to injury to left VII Cranal nerve.

Q. 343. "Sleep apnea", is defined as a temporary pause in breathing during sleep lasting at least (AIIMS/May2003)
- (a) 40 seconds
- (b) 30 seconds
- (c) 20 seconds
- (d) 10 seconds

Ans. (d)

Note
"Sleep apnea", is defined as a temporary pause in breathing during sleep lasting at least '10 seconds'.

Also see
Sleep apnea is defined as an intermittent cessation of airflow at the nose and mouth during sleep. By convention, apneas of at least 10 second duration have been considered important, but in most patients the apneas are 20 to 30 seconds in duration and may be as long as 2 to 3 min.
Ref: Harrison, Sleep apnea

Q. 344. A 45 years old hypertensive male presented with sudden onset severe headache, vomiting and neck stiffness. On examination he didn't have any focal neurological deficit His CT scan showed blood in the Sylvain fissure. The probable diagnosis is (AIIMS/May2003)
- (a) Meningitis
- (b) Ruptured aneurysm
- (c) Hypertensive bleed
- (d) Stroke

Ans. (b)

Note
The probable diagnosis for the above clinical presentation is 'Ruptured aneurysm'.

Also see
The salient features of above case include:
Subject is Male, 45 years of age, onset is sudden, C/O: Severe headache, vomiting and neck stinness. H/O: HT. O/E: No neurological deficit. On/In: CT shows blood in Syvian fissure.
These features are consistent with Ruptured aneurysm.

Extended information
a. *Meningitis*
It mainly in childrens or young adults. Nisseria meningitides is most common cause of bacterial meningitis. Headache, drowsiness, fever, neck stiffness are presenting complaints. Later patient may become comatose. CSF examination is diagnostic.

b. *Ruptured aneurysm*
An aneurysm is an abnormal widening or ballooning of a section of a blood vessel.
Cause:
The majority of intracranial aneurysms are congenital or berry aneurysms which occur at the bifurcations of medium-sized arteries at the base of the brain. The incidence of congenital aneurysms in the general population is about 1-2%.

Arteriosclerotic aneurysms usually have a fusiform shape; traumatic, mycotic and neoplastic aneurysms are much less common and occur in smaller distal vessels.

In cases of subarachnoid hemorrhages, the most common aneurysms are posterior communicating (38%), anterior communicating (36%), and middle cerebral (21%). These three locations account for 95% of all ruptured aneurysms. The basilar artery accounts for only 2.8% and posterior fossa aneurysms are even less common.

Symptoms of ruptured aneurysm may include:
- Sudden severe headache
- Headaches with nausea or vomiting
- Stiff neck
- Muscle weakness, depends on the location of bleed
- Numbness in any part of the body
- Vision disturbances; diplopia / loss of vision
- Eyelid drooping
- Seizures
- Speech impairment

Investigations:
CT patterns of ruptured aneurysm:
- An anterior communicating aneurysm is suggested by blood in the cisterna lamina terminalis, anterior pericallosal cistern, and interhemispheric fissure.
- Localizing posterior communicating artery aneurysms is more difficult because the blood is usually diffuse within the cisterns.
- Rupture of a middle cerebral aneurysm is characterized by blood in the sylvian fissure and a hematoma in the temporal lobe.

Ref: Subarachnoid Hemorrhage and Intracranial Aneurysms by John R. Hesselink, MD, FACR ttp://spinwarp.ucsd.edu/NeuroWeb/Text/br-730.htm

c. *Hypertensive bleed*
The most common sites of hypertensive bleed are the basal ganglia (Putamen, thalamus, and adjacent deep white matter), deep cerebellum, and pons. However, the putamen is the most common site for hypertensive hemorrhage.

d. *Stroke*
Srokes may be **ischemic** (lack of blood flow), or hemorrhagic (leakage of blood into the brain). The featues depends on the cause and location of stroke in CNS.

Remember:
Sudden severe generalized headache associated with vomiting with absence of focal neurological symptoms is hallmark of aneurismal rupture.
Ref: Harrison. Cerebrovascular diseases – Intracranial haemorrhage.

Q. 345. Which test is performed to detect reversible myocardial ischemia? (AIIMS/May2003)
    (a)   Coronary angiography
    (b)   MUGA scan
    (c)   Thallium scan
    (d)   Resting echocardiography

Ans. (c)

Note
'Thallium scan' is performed to detect reversible myocardial ischemia.

Also see
Thallium scan

It involves obtaining scintiscans of the myocardium at rest and during stress after intravenous venous administration of thallium 201 (201TI). A pefrfusion defect presen during stress but not at rest provides evidence of reversible myocardial ischemia. But a persistent perfusion defect found to be present in both the phases of study is indicative of irreversible myocardial ischemia i.e., previous myocardial infarction.
Ref: Davidson Pg-250

Extended information
Coronary angiography
    -Detects and evaluates site, nature and severity of coronary artery stenoses in coronary artery disease.
MUGA scan
Multiple Gated (MUGA) Blood Pool Scan:
    -Technetium can be tagged to the albumin or to the red cells
    -This permits equilibrium studies in which all the cardiac chambers are visualised simultaneously.
Utility:
    -Detects abnormal myocardial **contraction**
    -Evaluates ventricular function.
Myocardial thallium perfusion scan:
    -Radioactive tracer Thallium 201 is injected intravenously, which accumulates in myocardium with adequate perfusion.
Utility:
    -Distinguishes between ischemic and non-ischemic, or between normal and infarcted myocardium.
Resting echocardiography
    -Sensitive and more accurate investigation than the ECG to assess left ventricular size and wall thickness.
    -Provides an independent measure of severity in mild to moderate hypertension, even in the early stage.
    -Useful in the assessment of patients with borderline hypertension or who are suspected to have white coat hypertension, where, the finding of the left ventricular hypertrophy may indicate that the blood pressure level is more sustained.
    -Also useful in the follow up of patients who have enlargement of the left ventricle to see whether hypertrophy regresses as the blood pressure is controlled.
    -Ultrasound echocardiography provides accurate measurements of:
    -Size, arrangement and movement of cardiac chambers.
Colour Doppler echocardiography provides information about:
    -Velocity and direction of blood flow within heart and great vessels.

Q. 346. Kenny packs were used in the treatment of (AIIMS/May2003)
    (a)   Poliomyelitis
    (b)   Muscular dystrophy
    (c)   Polyneuropathies
    (d)   Nerve injury

Ans. (a)
Note
Kenny packs were used in the treatment of 'Poliomyelitis'.

Also see
In case of acute polio, the Kenny approach for the pain was to apply hot packs and stretch all of the two-joint muscle groups. The Kenny Packs were hot, wool cloth packs.

Q. 347. The level of alpha fetoprotein is raised in all of the following except (AIIMS/May2003)
- (a) Cirrohosis of liver
- (b) Hepatocellular carcinoma
- (c) Yolk sac tumor
- (d) Dysgerminoma

Ans. (d)

Note
The level of alpha fetoprotein is raised in all of the above except 'Dysgerminoma'.

Also see
The level of AFP is increased in hepatocellular carcinoma, non-seminomatous germ cell tumour of testis, dysgerminoma.
Ref: Handbook of Pathology by Harsh Mohan, Pg-163, 564
The raised levels of AFP may indicate:
- Cancer testes, ovaries, biliary tract, stomach or pancreas.
- Cirrhosis of liver
- Liver cancer
- Malignant teratoma
- Recovery from hepatitis

During pregnancy raised level of AFP may indicate:
- Foetal defects; spina bifida, anencephaly, tetralogy of Fallot, Turner's syndrome.

Q. 348. A hypertensive individual had a sudden headache and became unconscious within a few minutes. On regaining consciousness, there was complete flaccid hemiplegia with no involvement of upper face, absence of tendon reflexes and a positive Babinski sign. Which one of the following arteries could have ruptured? (AIIMS/Nov2003)
- (a) Lateral striate branch of middle cerebral
- (b) Medial striate branch of anterior cerebral
- (c) Posterolateral branch of posterior cerebral
- (d) Posterior choroidal branch of posterior cerebral

Ans. (a)

Note
The above clinical presentation is consistent with the 'acute stroke / hypertensive (small) hemorrhage in the territory of lateral striate branch of middle cerebral artery'.

Also see
The hemiplagia suggested above is:
- Flaccid hemiplagia
- No involvement of upper face
- Absences of tendon jerks
- Positive babinski's sign

The above features indicates the 'acute hemiplegic state', that's why the presentation is of 'flasscid' in presentation. However the positive Babinksi's' suggest that the true natute of the paralysis is 'upper motor neuron' type. Again the examination shows no involvement of upper part of face, this is also in favour of hemiplagia. The upper part of face is not involved as it has ipsilateral as well as contralateral supply and the fibers which are snapped in the internal capsule are compromised with the contralateral supply. Therefore the lesion is in the internal capsule. The internal capsule is supplied with striate branches of anterior, middle and posterior cerebral arteries. The most common artery to bleed is hubener's artery.

Extended information
Middle cerebral arteries provide most of the blood supply to the corpus striatum. The striatas, which are arterial branches of the middle cerebral arteries, are known as the arteries of stroke as they are the main source of blood for the internal capsule. A rupture of the lenticulo-striate artery results in bleeding usually in the region of the internal capsule (Steadman, 1997). When one of these arteries is damaged, the bottleneck of fibers

within the internal capsule, including the pyramidal tract, can be affected, causing many disabilities. The striatas have relatively thin walls and pressure within them is high. For this reason, they are more vulnerable to hemorrhages than to blockages.

Q. 349. History of dislike for sweet food items is typically present in (AIIMS/Nov2003)
- (a) Diabetes mellitus
- (b) Glycogen storage disease
- (c) Hereditary fructose intolerance
- (d) Galactosemia

Ans. (c)
Note
History of dislike for sweet food items is typically present in 'Hereditary fructose intolerance'.
Also see
Patients with hereditary fructose intolerance are healthy and asymptomatic until fructose or sucrose (table sugar) is ingested (usually from fruit, fruit juice, or sweetened cereal).

C/F: Include jaundice, hepatomegaly, vomiting, lethargy, irritability, and convulsions. Lab / findings include prolonged clotting time, hypoalbuminemia, elevation of bilirubin and transaminases, and proximal renal tubular dysfunction. If the disease is not diagnosed and intake of the noxious sugar persists, hypoglycemic episodes recur, and liver and kidney failure progress, eventually leading to death.
Ref: Harrison, Glycogen Storage Disease

Q. 350. Acute intravascular hemolysis can be caused by infection due to all of the following organisms except (AIIMS/Nov2003)
- (a) Clostridium tetani
- (b) Bartonella bacilliformis
- (c) Plasmodium falciparum
- (d) Babesia microti

Ans. (a)
Note
Acute intravascular hemolysis can be caused by infection due to all of the following organisms except 'Clostridium tetani'.
Also see
The clostridium tetani do not cause intravascular hemolysis. It causes 'Tetanus' which is a neurologic disorder, characterized by increased muscle tone and spasms, that is caused by tetanospasmin, a powerful protein toxin elaborated by Clostridium tetani. Tetanus occurs in several clinical forms, including generalized, neonatal, and localized disease.
Ref: Harrison, See tetanus

Q. 351. A 45 year old coalmine worker presents with cutaneous nodules, joint pain and occasional cough with dyspnea. His chest radiograph shows multiple small (1-4 cm) nodules in bilateral lung fields. Some of the nodules show cavitation and specks of calcification. Most likely these features are diagnostic of (AIIMS/Nov2003)
- (a) Sjogren's syndrome
- (b) Caplan's syndrome
- (c) Silicosis
- (d) Wegener's granulomatosis

Ans. (b)
Note
Most likely these features are diagnostic of 'Caplan's syndrome'.
Also see
Rheumatoid pneumoconiosis (Caplan's syndrome)
The development of rheumatoid arthritis in a few cases of coal workers pneumoconiosis, silicosis or asbestosis is termed rheumatoid pneumoconiosis or Caplan's syndrome.

Chest radiograph:
The lungs have rounded, firm nodules with central necrosis, cavitation or calcification.

Clinical features:
Simple coal workers pneumoconiosis is a mild form of disease characterized by chronic cough with black expectoration. The radiological findings of nodularities in the lungs appear after working for several years in coal mines. Progressive massive fibrosis is however a serious disabling condition is manifested by progressive dyspnoea and chronic cough with jet black sputum.
Ref: Textbook of Pathology Harsh Mohan's 5th Ed. Pg-348

Extended information
Sjogern's syndrome
Sjogren's syndrome is a chronic, inflammatory, autoimmune disorder characterized by dry mouth (xerostomia) and dry eye (keratoconjuctivitis sicca).

Silicosis
Disease is now becoming rare due to raised industrial hygiene. Inhalation of fine silicone dust is most fibrogenic and disease progresses even when exposure to dust ceases. The radiological features include; enlarged hilar shadow with 'egg-shell' calcification in the hilar lymph nodes is distinctive feature.
Ref: Davidson, Pg-373

Wegener's granuloma
Wegener's granulomatosis is a form of vasculitis that affects the lungs, kidneys and other organs. Due to its end-organ damage, it can be a serious disease.
Clinical features:
Initial s/s are non-specific in nature however rhinitis is mosly the first symptom in majority.
Nose: pain, stuffiness, nosebleeds, rhinitis, crusting, saddle-nose deformity due to a perforated septum.
Eyes: pseudotumours, scleritis, conjunctivitis, uveitis, episcleritis.
Lungs: pulmonary nodules (referred to as "coin lesions"), infiltrates (often interpreted as pneumonia), cavitary lesions, hemoptysis.
Kidney: rapidly progressive segmental necrotising glomerulonephritis.
Arthritis: Pain or swelling as rheumatoid arthritis.
Skin: nodules on the elbow, purpura.

Q. 352. A 35 year old non-smoker presents with 2 episodes of mild hemoptysis. There is no history of fever or any constitutional symptoms. A plain x-ray of chest is found to be normal. Which one of the following should be the next step in the diagnostic evaluation of this patient? (AIIMS/Nov2003)
    (a) Bronchography
    (b) High-resolution computed tomography
    (c) Contrast-enhanced computed tomography
    (d) Fiberoptic bronchoscopy

Ans. (d)
Note
The next step in the diagnostic evaluation of this patient is 'Fiberoptic Bronchoscopy'.

Also see
The bronchoscope may provide the opportunity for treatment as well as diagnosis.

Q. 353. A 55 year old man, a chronic smoker is brought to emergency with history of polyuria, polydipsia, nausea and altered sensorium for last two days. He had been diagnosed as having squamous cell carcinoma of lung two months prior to this. On examination, he was lethargic and confused. An ECG was normal except for a narrowed QT interval. Which one of the following is the most likely metabolic abnormality? (AIIMS/Nov2003)
    (a) Hypernatremia
    (b) Hypercalcemia
    (c) Hypokalemia
    (d) Hyponatremia

Ans. (b)

Note
The most likely metabolic abnormality 'Hypercalcemia'.

Also see
Hypercalcemia of malignancy, the most common paraneoplastic endocrine syndrome, is responsible for approximately 40% of all hypercalcemia. Hypercalcemia with cancer is classified as humoral hypercalcemia of malignancy (HHM), which is caused by circulating hormones.
The cancers associated with HHM are non-small cell lung cancer and cancers of the breast, kidney, head and neck, and bladder. HHM is particularly common in patients with cancers of squamous cell histology.
C/F: Includes malaise, fatigue, confusion, anorexia, bone pain, polyuria, polydipsia, weakness, constipation, nausea, and vomiting. Neurologic symptoms and signs in profound hypercalcemia (>3.5 mmol/L) include confusion, lethargy, coma, and death.
(Harrison; neoplastic disorders)

Q. 354. In stable angina (AIIMS/Nov2003)
    (a)   CK-MB is elevated
    (b)   Troponin I is elevated
    (c)   Myoglobin is elevated
    (d)   The levels of cardiac markers remain unchanged

Ans. (d)
Note
In stable angina 'the levels of cardiac markers remain unchanged'.
Also see

The stable angina pectoris is an episodic clinical syndrome due to transient myocardial ischaemia.
The levels of cardiac markers remain unchanged in stable angina pectoris.
In the absence of above diagnosis of stable angina can be arrived at by lab tests as under:
a.   Urine examination; for evidence of diabetes mellitus and renal disease since both these conditions accelerate atherosclerosis.
b.   Thyroid profile for Myxoedema or Thyrotoxicosis.
c.   Lipid profile to assess the risk factors for atherosclerosis.
d.   X-Ray chest to find cardiac enlargement, ventricular aneurysm, or features of heart failure.
e.   ECG to evaluate the T-wave and ST segment changes suggestive of IHD.
f.   Stress ECG.
g.   Angiography
Ref: Harrison. IHD

Q. 355. A 45 year old hypertensive male patient presented in the casualty with two hours history of sudden onset of severe headache associated with nausea and vomiting. On clinical examination the patient had necks stiffness and right sided ptosis. Rest of the neurological examination was normal. What is the clinical diagnosis? (AIIMS/Nov2003)
    (a)   Hypertensive brain hemorrhage
    (b)   Migraine
    (c)   Aneurysmal subarachnoid hemorrhage
    (d)   Arteriovenous malformation hemorrhage

Ans. (c)
Note
The above features are in favour of clinical diagnosis of 'Aneurysmal subarachnoid hemorrhage'.
Also see
Aneurysms
    -Majority of intracranial aneurysms are saccular (berry) aneurysms. Saccular aneurysms occur at bifurcation of arteries forming circle of Willis. Rupture commonly occurs in association with activities that increase BP.
Clinical features:
    -Headache (85-95%). Sudden and intense
    -Orbital pain, diplopia, ptosis, visual loss, fits, motor or sensory deficit, dysphasia, dizziness.
    -Pain radiating into the occipital or cervical region

- Nuchal rigidity and other signs of meningism
- Photophobia, nausea, vomiting, lethargy or altered mentation
- Variable conscious level.
- Motor or sensory deficits, hyper-reflexia, visual field deficits
- III nerve palsy associated with PCA aneurysms, less frequently may be seen in association with other aneurysms

Investigations:
CT: Will demonstrate subarachnoid blood in 85% of patients scanned within 48 h of bleed.
Also see Harrison 16th Ed, Pg-2388

Q. 356. Early diagnosis of acute hepatitis-B infection is made by (AIIMS/Nov2003)
    (a)   Presence of HbeAg in serum
    (b)   Presence of IgM anti-HBc in serum
    (c)   Presence of HbsAg in serum
    (d)   Presence of IgG anti-HBc in serum

Ans. (c)

Note
The early diagnosis is made by presence of HbsAg in serum.

Also see

Test	Result	Interpretation	Vaccination
HBs Ag anti-HBc anti-HBs	Negative Negative Negative	Susceptible	Vaccinate if indicated
HBs Ag anti-HBc anti-HBs	Negative Negative Positive with ≥ 10 mIU/mL*	Immune due to vaccination	No vaccination necessary
HBs Ag anti-HBc anti-HBs	Positive Positive Positive	Immune due to natural infection	No vaccination necessary
HBs Ag anti-HBc IgM anti-HBc Anti-HBs	Positive Positive Positive Negative	Acutely infected	No vaccination necessary
HBs Ag anti-HBc IgM anti-HBc Anti-HBs	Positive Positive Positive Negative	Chronically infected	No vaccination necessary (may need treatment)
HBs Ag anti-HBc anti-HBs	Negative Positive Negative	Four interpretations possible*	Use clinical judgement

*Positive vaccination testing. When it is recommended, should be performed 1 – 2 months after the last dose of vaccine. Infants born to HBsAg – Positive mothers should be tested 3-9 months after the last dose.
1. May be recovering from acute HBV infections.
2. May be distantly immune, but test may not be sensitive enough to detect a low level of anti-HBs in serum.
3. May be susceptible with a false positive anti-HBc.
4. May be chronically infected and have an undetectable level of HBs Ag present in the serum.

Q. 357. A 22 years old male patient presents with a complaints of severe itching and white scaly lesions in the groin for past month. Which of the following is most likely to be the causative agent? (AIIMS/Nov2003)
(a) Trichophyton rubrum
(b) Candida albicans
(c) Candida glabrata
(d) Malassezia furfur

Ans. (a)
Note
Above clinical presentation point to the clinical diagnosis of 'Trichophytom rubrum'.
Also see
Tinea cruris, commonly referred to as "jock itch," involves the medial aspect of the upper thighs (groin). Unlike yeast infections, tinea cruris generally does not involve the scrotum or the penis. This dermatophyte infection occurs more often in men than in women and rarely affects children. The causative agent is Tricophytom rubrum.

Q. 358. A 16 year old student reported for the evaluation of multiple hypopigmented macules on the trunk and limbs. All of the following tests are useful in making a diagnosis of leprosy, except (AIIMS/Nov2003)
(a) Sensation testing
(b) Lepromin test
(c) Slit smears
(d) Skin biopsy

Ans. (b)
Note
All of the above tests are useful in making a diagnosis of leprosy, except 'Lepromin test'.
Also see
In case of leprosy especially the lepromatous type there will be negative result. In some cases of tuberculoid leprosy cases it may be positive. This test is used primarily as a research tool and only helps in the classification of leprosy. It should not be used to establish a diagnosis of leprosy

Q. 359. A 24 year old man had multiple, small hypopigmented macules on the upper chest and back for the last three months. The macules were circular, arranged around follicles and many had coalesced to form large sheets. The surface of the macules showed fine scaling. He had similar lesions one year ago which subsided with treatment. The most appropriate investigation to confirm the diagnosis is (AIIMS/Nov2003)
(a) Potassium hydroxide preparation of scales
(b) Slit skin smear from discrete macules
(c) Tzanck test
(d) Skin biopsy of coalesced macules

Ans. (a)
Note
The most appropriate investigation to confirm the diagnosis is 'Potassium hydroxide preparation of scales'.
Also see
Malassezia furfur is part of the normal flora of the human skin but can cause tinea (pityriasis) versicolor or catheter-acquired sepsis. Tinea versicolor appears as asymptomatic, well-delineated, hyperpigmented or hypopigmented macules centered on the upper trunk and upper arms. Confluent lesions may cover large areas, making the border difficult to find. A fine "branny" scale or folliculitis is sometimes visible. When examined microscopically by KOH mount, skin sections are seen to contain characteristic round and elongated cells. On inspection with Wood's light, lesions either do not fluoresce or appear yellow-green.

Therefore the answer is (a)
Ref: Harrison, Section 15 Funus andalgal infections. 208 Miscellaneous mycoses and algal infections.

Q. 360. A 22 year old woman developed small itchy wheals after physical exertion, walking in the sun, eating hot spicy food and when she was angry. The most likely diagnosis is (AIIMS/Nov2003)
- (a) Chronic idiopathic utricaria
- (b) Heat urticaria
- (c) Solar urticaria
- (d) Cholinergic urticaria

Ans. (d)
Note
The most likely diagnosis is 'Cholinergic uriticaria'.

Also see
Cholinergic urticaria is precipitated by heat, exercise, or emotion and is characterized by small wheals with relatively large flares. They are occasionally associated with wheezing.

Q. 361. A 45 year old male had multiple hypoesthetic mildly erythematous large plaques with elevated margins on trunk and extremities. His ulnar and lateral popliteal nerves on both sides were enlarged. The most probable diagnosis is (AIIMS/Nov2003)
- (a) Lepromatous leprosy
- (b) Borderline leprosy
- (c) Borderline tuberculoid leprosy
- (d) Borderline lepromatous leprosy

Ans. (d)
Note
The most probable dignosis for the above clinical presentation is 'borderline tubercular leprosy'.

Also see

Cl. Features	Tuberculoid	B. Tuberculoid	B. lepromatous	Borderline	Lepromatous
a. Infiltrated lesions	Defined plaques, irregular plaques, healing centres	Polymorphic partially raised edges, satellites	Papules, nodules, punched - out centres	Diffuse thickening	Diffuse thickening
b. Macular lesions	Single, small	Several, any size	Multiple, all sizes, bizarre	Innumerable, small	Innumerable, confluent
c. Peripheral nerve lesions	Solitary enlarged nerve	Irregular enlargement of several large nerves, asymmetrical pattern	Many nervs involved, symmetrical pattern	Late neural thickening, asymmetrical anesthesia and paresis	Slow, symmetrical 'glove and stocking' anesthesia.

Medicine for Students By Golwalla 20th Edition.

Q. 362. All of the following conditions are known to cause diabetes insipidus except (AIIMS/May2004)
- (a) Multiple sclerosis
- (b) Head injury
- (c) Histiocytosis
- (d) Viral encephalitis

Ans. (a)
Note
All of the above can cause 'diabetes insipidus' except, 'multiple scleroris'.

Also see
Causes of pituitary diabetes insipidus:
Acquired:
   -Head trauma
Neoplasm:
Primary:
   -Craniopharyngioma, -Pituitary adenoma (suprasellar),
   -Dysgerminoma

Secondary:
    -Metastatic (Lung, Breast), Hematologic (Lymphoma, Leukemia)
Granulomas:
    -Neurosarcoid
    -Histiocytosis
    -Xanthoma disseminatum
Infectious:
    -Chronic meningitis
    -Viral encephalitis
    -Toxoplasmosis
Inflammatory:
    -Lymphotic infundibuloneurohypophysitis
    -Wegeners granulomatosis
    -Lupus erythematosus
    -Scleroderma
Chemical toxins:
    -Tetrodotoxin
    -Snake venom
Vascular:

    -She hans syndrome
    -Aneurism (Internal carotid)
    -Aortocoronary bypass
    -Hypoxic encephalopathy
Pregnancy (vasopressinase)
Idiopathic
Congenital malformations:
    -Septoopic dysplasia
    -Midline craniofacial defects
    -Holoprosencephaly
    -Hypogensis, ectopia of pituitary
Genetic:
    -Autosomal dominant (AVP-neurophysin gene)
    -Autosomal recessive (AVP-neurophysin gene)
    -Autosomal recessive –Wolfram (4p-WFS 1 gene)
    -X-linked recessive (Xq28)
    -Deletion chromosome7q
Ref: Harrison -Table 329-1.

Q. 363. Raised serum amylase levels are used to diagnose (AIIMS/May2004)
    (a)   Autoimmune disease
    (b)   Degenerative diseases
    (c)   Acute cholecystitis
    (d)   Acute pancreatitis
Ans. (d)
Note
Raised serum amylase levels are used to diagnose 'acute pancreatitis'.
Also see
Increased plasma levels are found in:
Salivary trauma (including anaesthetic intubation).
Mumps — due to inflammation of the salivary glands.
Pancreatitis — because of damage to the cells that produce amylase.
Renal Failaure — due to reduced excretion .
Total amylase readings of over 10x the upper limit of normal (ULN) are suggestive of pancreatitis 5-10x times the ULN may indicate ileus or duodenal disease or renal failure, and lower elevations are commonly found in salivary gland disease

MCQ's in Practice of Medicine

Q. 364. Which of the following lesions is associated with HIV infection (AIIMS/May2004)
  (a) Hairy leukoplakia
  (b) Erythroplakia
  (c) Oral lichen planus
  (d) Bullous pemphigoid

Ans. (a)

Note
Lesion from associated with HIV infection is 'Hairy leukoplakia'.

Also see
"Hairy" leukoplakia of mouth is an unusual form of leukoplakia that is only seen in AIDS, ARC and HIV positive individuals. It consists of fuzzy (Hairy) white patches on the tongue and less frequently elsewhere in the mouth. It may resemble thrush, a candida infection which, in adults, is also commonly associated with HIV and AIDS. Hairy leukoplakia may be one of the first signs of infection with HIV. (Encyclopedia)

Q. 365. A 59-year-old male came with Hb 18.0 gm/dl on three occasions. The resident doctor wants to exclude polycythemia vera. Which of the following is the most relevant investigation? (AIIMS/May2004)
  (a) Hematocrit
  (b) Total leukocyte count
  (c) Red cell mass
  (d) Reticulocyte count

Ans. (c)

Note
Most relevant investigation to rule out polycythemia vera is 'red cell mass'.
Red cell mass. Other names; MCH (Mean Corpuscular Hemoglobin) MCHC (Mean corpuscular Hemoglobin Concentration); MCV (Mean Corpuscular Volume)
The MCV, MCH, MCHC reflect the size and hemoglobin content of individual red blood cells.

Q. 366. A 25-year-old man presented with fever and cough for two months. CT chest showed bilateral upper lobe fibrosis and mediastinal enlarged necrotic nodes with peripheral rim enhancement. What is the most likely diagnosis? (AIIMS/May2004)
  (a) Sarcoidosis
  (b) Tuberculosis
  (c) Lymphoma
  (d) Silicosis

Ans. (b)

Note
The most likely diagnosis is 'Tuberculosis'.

Also see
The CT findings mediastinal enlarged necrotic nodes and peripheral rim enhancement suggests active tubercular infection.

Extended information
A study reference:
In 49 patients with mediastinal tuberculous lymphadenitis, CT findings of nodes with central low attenuation and peripheral rim enhancement suggested active disease. Low-attenuation areas within the nodes had pathologic correspondence to areas of caseation necrosis and may be a reliable indicator for disease activity.

Q. 367. Which one of the following statements is wrong regarding adult polycystic kidney disease? (AIIMS/May2004)
  (a) Kidneys are enlarged in size
  (b) The presentation is unilateral
  (c) Intracranial aneurysms may be associated
  (d) Typically manifests in the 3rd decade

Ans. (b)

Note
The wrong statement from above regarding adult polycystic kidney disease is 'The presentation is unilateral'.

Also see
Polycystic kidney disease (PKD) is a genetic disorder characterized by the growth of numerous cysts in the kidneys. The cysts are filled with fluid. PKD cysts can slowly replace much of the mass of the kidneys, in both the kidneys reducing kidney function and leading to kidney failure.

Q. 368. Most common cause of subarachnoid hemorrhage is (AIIMS/May2004)
- (a) Hypertension
- (b) Aneurysm
- (c) Arterio-venous malformation
- (d) Bleeding disorders

Ans. (b)

Note
Most common cause of subarachnoid hemorrhage is 'aneurysm'.

Also see
Subarachnoid hemorrhage occurs when there is bleeding into the space between the brain and the arachnoid membrane This commonly occurs from a ruptured cerebral aneurysm.

Extended information
Spontaneous SAH is most often due to rupture of cerebral aneurysms (85%), weaknesses in the wall of the arteries of the brain that enlarge.

Classification
There are several grading scales available for subarachnoid hemorrhage. Three specialized scores are in use.

Hunt and Hess scale
The first scale of severity, described by Hunt and Hess in 1968:
Grade 1:
  -Asymptomatic; or minimal headache and slight nuchal rigidity. Approximate survival rate 70%.
Grade 2:
  -Moderate to severe headache; nuchal rigidity; no neurologic deficit except cranial nerve palsy. 60%.
Grade 3:
  -Drowsy; minimal neurologic deficit. 50%.
Grade 4:
  -Stuporous; moderate to severe hemiparesis; possibly early decerebrate rigidity and vegetative disturbances. 20%.
Grade 5:
  -Deep coma; decerebrate rigidity; moribund. 10%.

Fisher grade
The fisher grade classifies the appearance of subarachnoid hemorrhage on CT scan:
Grade 1= No hemorrhage evident
Grade 2= Subarachnoid hemorrhage less than 1 mm thick
Grade 3= Subarachnoid hemorrhage more than 1 mm thick
Grade 4= Subarachnoid hemorrhage of any thickness with intra-ventricular hemorrhage (IVH) or parenchymal extension
World Federation of Neurosurgeons classification:[8]
Class 1 - GCS (Glasgow Coma Scale)15
Class 2 - GCS 13-14 without focal neurological deficit
Class 3 - GCS 13-14 with focal neurological deficit
Class 4 - GCS 7-12 with or without focal neurological deficit
Class 5 - GCS <7 with or without focal neurological deficit
Ref: http://en.wikipedia.org/wiki/Subarachnoid_hemorrhage

Q. 369. Subdural hematoma most commonly results from (AIIMS/May2004)
- (a) Rupture of intracranial aneurysm
- (b) Rupture of cerebral AV malformation

(c) Injury to cortical bridging veins
(d) Hemophilia

Ans. (c)

Note
Subdural hematoma most commonly results from Injury to bridging veins.

Also see
An SDH is the most common type of intracranial mass lesion, occurring in about a third of those with severe head injuries (Glasgow Coma Scale [GCS] score less than 9).

Q. 370. A 30-year-old male patient presents with complaints of weakness in right upper and both lower limbs for last 4 months. He developed digital infarcts involving 2nd and 3rd fingers on right side and 5th finger on left side. On examination, BP was 160/140 mmHg, all peripheral pulses were palpable and there was asymmetrical neuropathy. Investigations showed Hb 12 gm%, TLC 12,000 per cumm, platelets 4,30,000 and ESR 49 mm. Urine examination showed proteinuria and RBC 10-15/hpf with no casts. What is the most likely diagnosis? (AIIMS/May2004)
(a) Polyarteritis nodosa
(b) Systemic lupus erythematosus
(c) Wegener's granulomatosis
(d) Mixed cryoglobulinemia

Ans. (a)

Note
The most likely diagnosis is 'Polyarteritis Nodosa'.

Also see
Polyarteritis nodosa is a rare autoimmune disease featuring spontaneous vasculitis. Because arteries are involved, the disease can affect any organ of the body. The most common areas of involvement include the muscles, joints, intestines (bowels), nerves, kidneys, and skin. Poor function or pain in any of these organs can be a symptom. Poor blood supply to the organs can cause local tissue death.

The present problem points to polyarteritis nodosa as the diagnosis is supported by investigations that indicate elevation of ESR. The white blood cell count and platelet count are elevated, while the red blood count is decreased although mildly. Urine show protein and red blood cells in the urine. The patient has weakness in right upper and both lower limbs for 4 months and he developed digital infarcts involving 2nd and 3rd finger on right side and 5th finger on the left side.

Q. 371. A 23-year-old college student has asymptomatic and hyperpigmented macules on both palms for three weeks. The most appropriate diagnostic test is (AIIMS/May2004)
(a) Venereal Diseases Research Laboratory (VDRL) test
(b) Skin biopsy
(c) Serum cortisol levels
(d) Assay for arsenic in hair, skin and nails

Ans. (a)

Note
The most appropriate diagnostic test is VDRL test.

Also see
As the patient is 23 year old college student and presented with hyperpigmented macular asymptomatic lesions the best thing is to rule out the syphilis as this could be the secondary presentation of syphilis. Therefore the veneral disease research laboratory test is suggested.

Q. 372. A 42-year-old engineer developed redness of the glans and radial fissuring of the prepuce 2 weeks ago. A potassium hydroxide preparation of scrapings from the glans. showed pseudohyphae and buds. Which one of the following systemic illness should he be screened for? (AIIMS/May2004)
(a) Pulmonary tuberculosis
(b) Diabetes mellitus
(c) Systemic candidiasis
(d) Chronic renal failure

Ans. (b)

Note
From above given choice the most important disease to be screed for is diabetes mellitus.
Also see
The history and clinical appearance are consistent with balanitis and prosthetitis. KOH preparation of scrapings from glans reveals pseudohyphae and budding yeast. The most probable systemic cause in this patient is diabetes mellitus which is acting as a predisposing cause for genital candidiasis.

Q. 373. All of the following are the electrocardiographic features of hyperkalemia, except (AIIMS/May2004)
    (a)   Prolonged PR interval
    (b)   Prolonged QT interval
    (c)   Sine wave patterns
    (d)   Loss of P waves

Ans. (b)
Note
All of above are the ECG features of hyperkalemia, except 'Prolonged QT interval.
Also see
Certain life-threatening electrolyte disturbances may be diagnosed initially and monitored from the ECG. *Hyperkalemia* produces a sequence of changes usually beginning with narrowing and peaking (tenting) of the T waves. Further elevation of extracellular K^+ leads to AV conduction disturbances, diminution in P-wave amplitude, and widening of the QRS interval. Severe hyperkalemia eventually causes cardiac arrest with a slow sinusoidal type of mechanism ("sine-wave" pattern) followed by asystole.

Q. 374. Which one of the following cardiac lesions is at highest risk of occurrence of infective endocarditis? (AIIMS/May2004)
    (a)   Atrial septal defect
    (b)   Mitral valve prolapse without regurgitation
    (c)   Valvular aortic regurgitation
    (d)   Mitral stenosis

Ans. (c)
Note
Amongest the above, highest risk for occuurance of infective endocarditis is in case of 'Valvular aortic regurgitaion'.
Also see
Infective endocarditis

Relatively high risk	Intermediate risk	Low risk
Prosthetic heart valve	MVP	ASD
Aortic valve disease	MS	Atherosclerotic plaques
MR + Stenosis	Tricuspid valve disease	Syphilitic Aortitis
Previous Infective Endocarditis	Pulmonary valve disease	Cardiac pacemakers
Congenital heart disease: PDA, VSD, Coarctation of Aorta, Marfan's syndrome, Cyanotic congenital heart disease	Asymmetrical septal hypertrophy	Surgically corrected cardiac lesions (wihout prosthetic implant)
	Calcified aortic sclerosis	Valve bearing conduits, or indwelling plastic catheters for hydrocephalus in children
	Non-valvular intracardial prosthetic implant	Postmyocardial infarction thrombi, atrial thrombi and ventricular aneurysms

Ref; Medicine for Students by Golwalla 20th Edition.

Q. 375. The most common cause of sporadic viral encephalitis is (AIIMS/May2004)
- (a) Japanese B encephalitis
- (b) Herpes simplex encephalitis
- (c) Human immunodeficiency virus encephalitis
- (d) Rubeola encephalitis

Ans. (b)
Note
The most common cause of sporadic viral encephalitis is 'Herpes simplex encephalitis'.
Also see

Arthropod-borne viral encephalitis is responsible for most epidemic viral encephalitis. The viruses live in animal hosts and mosquitos that transmit the disease. The most common form of non-epidemic or sporadic encephalitis is caused by the herpes simplex virus, type 1 (HSV-1) and has a high rate of death.

Q. 376. All of the following are features of juvenile myoclonic epilepsy, except (AIIMS/May2004)
- (a) Myoclonus on awakening
- (b) Generalized tonic-clonic seizures
- (c) Automatism
- (d) Absence seizures

Ans. (c)
Note
All of the above are the features of juvenile myoclonic epilepsy, except 'Automatism'.
Also see
Juvenile myoclonic epilepsy (JME)
It is a generalized seizure disorder of unknown cause that appears in early adolescence and is usually characterized by *bilateral myoclonic jerks* that may be single or repetitive. The *myoclonic seizures are most frequent in the morning after awakening* and can be provoked by sleep deprivation. Consciousness is preserved unless the myoclonus is especially severe. Many patients also experience *generalized tonic-clonic seizures*, and up to one-third have *absence seizures*. The condition is otherwise benign, and although complete remission is uncommon, the seizures respond well to appropriate anticonvulsant medication. There is often a family history of epilepsy, and genetic linkage studies suggest a polygenic cause.
Ref; Harrison 360 Seizures and epilepsy.
Automatisms

Automatisms are involuntary, automatic behaviors that have a wide range of manifestations. Automatisms may consist of very basic behaviors such as chewing, lip smacking, swallowing, or "picking" movements of the hands, or more elaborate behaviors such as a display of emotion or running. The patient is typically confused following the seizure, and the transition to full recovery of consciousness may range from seconds up to an hour.
Ref; Harrison 360 Seizures and epilepsy.

Q. 377. All of the following statements about Creutzfeldt-Jakob disease are true, except (AIIMS/May 04)
- (a) It is a neurodegenerative disease.
- (b) It is caused by infectious proteins.
- (c) Myoclonus is rarely seen.
- (d) Brain biopsy is specific for diagnosis.

Ans. (c)
Note
All of the above statements about Creutzfeldt-Jakob disease are true, except 'Myoclonus is rarely seen'.
Also see
Creutzfeldt-Jakob disease (CJD):
It is a degenerative disease of the central nervous system (CNS) that is caused by infectious proteins called *prions*. CJD typically presents with dementia and myoclonus, is relentlessly progressive, and usually results in death within a year of onset.
Ref; Harrison 15th Edition 375 Prion Diseases.

Q. 378. Which one of the following is not a prion associated disease? (AIIMS/Nov2004)
  (a) Scrapie
  (b) Kuru
  (c) Creutzfeldt-Jakob disease
  (d) Alzheimer's disease

Ans. (d)
Note
The 'Alzheimer's disease' listed above is not a prion associated disease.
Also see
Prion diseases

Prion is Proteinaceous infectious particles that lack nucleic acid. They can cause scrapie in animals and related neurodegenerative disease of humans which includes - Creutzfeldt-Jakob disease (CJD) and Kuru. "Scrapie agent" is a synonym.
Ref: Harrison 15th Edition
Kuru
Kuru of the 'Fore people' (host) of New Guinea is thought to have resulted from the consumption of brains from dead relatives during ritualistic cannibalism.
Alzheimer's disease
It is the most common cause of dementia, pathologically there is gross, diffuse atrophy of the cerebral cortex with secondary enlargement of the ventricular system. The most important risk factors for AD are old age and a positive family history.

Q. 379. Which of the following is the most common extrarenal involvement in autosomal dominant polycystic kidney disease? (AIIMS/Nov2004)
  (a) Mitral valve prolapse
  (b) Hepatic cysts
  (c) Splenic cysts
  (d) Colonic diverticulosis

Ans. (d)
Note
The 'colonic diverticulosis' of above given choice is most common extrarenal involvement in autosomal dominant polycystic kidney disease.
Also see
The extrarenal manifestation of autosomal dominant polycystic kidney disease includes; *Hepatic cysts occur in 50 to 70% of patients. Cysts are generally asymptomatic, and liver function is normal. Cyst formation has also been observed in the spleen, pancreas, and ovaries.* Intracranial aneurysms are present in 5 to 10% of asymptomatic patients. **Colonic diverticular disease is the most common extrarenal abnormality.** *Mitral valve prolapse is found in 25% of patients, and the prevalence of aortic and tricuspid valve insufficiency is increased.*

Q. 380. A 27 year old man is noted to have blood pressure of 170/100 mm Hg. He has prominent aortic ejection click and murmurs heard over, the ribs on both sides anteriorly and over the back posteriorly. In addition, the pulses in the lower extremities are feeble and he complains of mild claudication with exertion. The most likely diagnosis is (AIIMS/Nov2004)
  (a) Atrial septal defect
  (b) Aortic stenosis
  (c) Coarctation of aorta
  (d) Cardiomyopathy

Ans. (c)
Note
The most likely diagnosis is 'Coarctation of aorta'.
Also see
The above clinical presentation has following important features:
  -High B.P., in upper upper limbs
  -Prominent aortic ejection click

- Murmur over the anterior and back of the chest
- Feeble pulse in lower extremities
- Intetrmittent claudicaiton in lower limbs with exertion

All above features are in favour of 'Coractation of Aorta'

Q. 381. A 30 year old male patient presents with urethritis. All of the following can be the causative agent except (AIIMS/Nov2004)
- (a) Neisseria gonorrheae
- (b) Chlamydia trachomatis
- (c) Trichomonas vaginalis
- (d) Hemophilus ducreyi

Ans. (d)

Note
All of the following can be the causative agent except *Hemophilus ducreyi.*

Also see

Hemophilus ducreyi is the etiologic agent of chancroid, a sexually transmitted disease characterized by genital ulceration and inguinal adenitis.

Q. 382. Ebstein barr virus is associated with (AIIMS/Nov2004)
- (a) Carcinoma larynx
- (b) Carcinoma bladder
- (c) Carcinoma nasopharynx
- (d) Carcinoma maxilla

Ans. (c)

Note
Ebstin Barr virus is associated with 'Carcinoma nasopharynx'.

Also see
The strongest evidence linking EBV and cancer formation is found in Burkitt's lymphoma and nasopharyngeal carcinoma.

Extended information
Burkitt's lymphoma is a type of Non-Hodgkin's lymphoma and is most common in equatorial Africa and is co-existent with the presence of malaria. Malaria infection causes reduced immune surveillance of EBV immortalised B cells, so allowing their proliferation. This proliferation increases the chance of a mutation to occur. Repeated mutations can lead to the B cells escaping the body's cell-cyle control, so allowing the cells to proliferate unchecked, resulting in the formation of Burkitt's lymphoma. Burkitt's lymphoma commonly affects the jaw bone, forming a huge tumour mass. It responds quickly to chemotherapy treatment, namely cyclophosphamide, but recurrence is common.

Other B cell lymphomas arise in immunocompromised patients such as those with AIDS or who have undergone organ transplantation with associated immunosuppression. Smooth muscle tumors are also associated with the virus in maligent patients.

Nasopharyngeal carcinoma is a cancer found in the upper respiratory tract, most commonly in the nasopharynx, and is linked to the EBV virus. It is found predominantly in Southern China and Africa, due to both genetic and environmental factors. It is much more common in people of Chinese ancestry (genetic), but is also linked to the Chinese diet of a high amount of smoked fish, which contain nitrosamines, well known carcinogens (environmental).

Q. 383. The most common causative organism for lobar pneumonia is (AIIMS/Nov2004)
- (a) Staphylococcus aureus
- (b) Streptococcus pyogenes
- (c) Streptococcus pneumoniae
- (d) Hemophilus influenzae

Ans. (c)

Note
The most common causative organism for lobar pneumonia from the choice given above is 'Streptococcus pneumoniae'.

Also see
The pneumonic process may involve primarily the interstitium or the alveoli. Involvement of an entire lobe is called **lobar pneumonia**. Common pulmonary pathogens in the nasopharynx include *Streptococcus pneumoniae*, *S. pyogenes*, *Mycoplasma pneumoniae*, *Hemophilus influenzae*, and *Moraxella catarrhalis*. Aspiration of these pathogens is the most common mechanism for the production of pneumonia. About 50% of healthy adults aspirate oropharyngeal secretions into the lower respiratory tract during sleep.

Q. 384. All of the following statements are true regarding central nervous system infections, except (AIIMS/Nov2004)
- (a) Measles virus is the causative agent for subacute sclerosing panencephalitis (SSPE).
- (b) Cytomegalovirus causes bilateral temporal lobe hemorrhagic infarction.
- (c) Prions infection causes spongiform encephalopathy.
- (d) JC virus is the causative agent for progressive multifocal leukoencephalopathy.

Ans. (b)
Note
All of above are true except 'Cytomegaloviurs causes bilateral temporal lobe hemorrhagic infarction'.
Also see
Congenital CMV Infection
Infections range from asymptomatic to severe clinical form. Seen in infants born to mothers who develop primary infections during pregnancy. Petechiae, hepatosplenomegaly, and jaundice are the most common presenting features. Microcephaly with or without cerebral calcifications, intrauterine growth retardation, and prematurity is common. Inguinal hernias and chorioretinitis are less common. Laboratory abnormalities include elevated alanine aminotransferase levels, thrombocytopenia, conjugated hyperbilirubinemia, hemolysis, and elevated cerebrospinal fluid protein levels.
JC virus
A human papilloma virus that is the etiologic agent of *progressive multifocal leukoencephalopathy* (PML), is an important opportunistic pathogen in patients with AIDS.

Q. 385. All of the following diseases cause massive splenomegaly except (AIIMS/Nov2004)
- (a) Malaria
- (b) Kala azar
- (c) Lymphoblastic leukaemia
- (d) Idiopathic myelofibrosis

Ans. (c)
Note
All of the following diseases cause massive splenomegaly except 'Lymphoblastic leukaemia'.
Also see
Acute lymphoblastic leukemia causes hepatospleomegly but not the huge one.

Extended information
Causes of splenomegaly:

Massive splenomegaly	Moderate Splenomegaly	Slight Splenomegaly
Chronic granulocytic leukemia	Hodgkins disease	All infections
Hairy cell leukemia	Leukemia	Cirulatory causes
Lymphocytic lymphoma	Polycythemia	Inflammatory and collegen disorders
Malaria	Portal hypertension	
Kala azar	Chronic hemolytic anemia	
Bilharziasis	Tuberculosis	
Myelofibrosis	Storage diseases	

Medicine for Students by Golwalla 20th Edition. Pg -380.

Q. 386. Which one of the following organs. should always be imaged in a suspected case of bronchogenic carcinoma? (AIIMS/Nov2004)
- (a) Adrenals
- (b) Kidneys
- (c) Spleen
- (d) Pancreas

Ans. (a)
Note
The 'Adrenals' should be imaged in a suspected case of 'Bronchogenic carcinoma'.
Also see
Paraneoplastic syndromes of lung cancer, which are numerous, are extrapulmonary, remote effects of tumors.
The onset of Cushing's syndrome may be sudden particularly in patients with Ca lung because such tumors may produce large amouts of ACTH.
Ref: Harrison 18th Edition Cushig's syndrome

Q. 387. A middle aged man presents with progessive atrophy and weakness of hands and forearms. On examination he is found to have slight spasticity of the legs, generalized hyper-reflexia and increased signal in the cortico-spinal tracts on T2 weighted MRI. The most likely diagnosis is (AIIMS/Nov2004)
- (a) Multiple sclerosis
- (b) Amyotrophic lateral sclerosis
- (c) Subacute combined degeneration
- (d) Progressive spinal muscular atrophy

Ans. (b)
Note
The above clinical feataures are in favour of 'Amyotrophic lateral Sclerosis'.
Also see
The features of generalized hypereflexia and progressive atrophy and weakness of hands and forearms in a middle aged man go in favor of amyotrophic lateral sclerosis.

Q. 388. Which of the following is generally not seen in idiopathic thrombocytopenic purpura (TIP)? (AIIMS/Nov2004)
- (a) More common in females
- (b) Petechiae, ecchymosis and bleeding
- (c) Palpable splenomegaly
- (d) Increased megakaryocytes in bone marrow

Ans. (c)
Note
'Palpable splenomegaly' is not seen in idiopathic thrombocytopenic purpura'.
Also see
The above features of ITP include; more commonly affects the females, petechiae, ecchymosis and epistaxis (bleeding) and bone marrow revelas an obvious increase in megakaryocytes.
(However, no clear cut evidence of spleenomegaly is given in Harrison and Davidson)

Q. 389. A 62 year old diabetic female patient presented with history of progressive right-sided weakness of one month duration. The patient was also having speech difficulty. Fundus examination showed papilledema. Two months ago, she also had a fall in her bathroom and struck her head against a wall. The most likely clinical diagnosis is (AIIMS/Nov2004)
- (a) Alzheimer's disease
- (b) Left parietal glioma
- (c) Left MCA territory stroke
- (d) Left chronic subdural hematoma

Ans. (d)

Note
The above clinical features are more in favour of 'Left chronic subdural hematoma'.

Also see
The female in present clinical presentation is a known diabetic which is a strong predisposing factor for atherosclerosis and it can lead to CVA which should be sudden in onset. However, she is presening with progressive weakness in right side along with difficulty in speech. This points to left cerebral lesion. The fundus examination reveals papilledema which suggests some space occupying lesion. The H/O fall in bathroom two months back and fundus showing papilledema with progressive weakness on the right side with involvement of speech points to left parital subdural hematoma could be the most logical cause.

Q. 390. Ramkali bai, a 35 year old female presented with one year history of menstrual irregularity and galactorrhea. She also had off-and-on headache. Her examination revealed bitemporal superior quadrantanopia. Her fundus examination showed primary optic atrophy. Which of the following is the most likely diagnosis in this case? (AIIMS/Nov2004)
(a) Craniopharyngioma
(b) Pituitary macroadenoma
(c) Ophthalmic ICA aneurysm
(d) Chiasmal glioma

Ans. (b)
Note
The most likely diagnosis in this case is 'Pituitary macroadenoma'.

Also see
The above clinical presentation of one year H/O Menstrual irregularity, Headache, galactorrhea and fundus showing primary optic atrophy along with bitemporal superior quadratanopia is suggestive of space occupying lesion specifically in the vicininity of optic chiasma. Pituitary dysfunction is suggested by galactorrhea and menstrual irregularity. Therefore the most probable cause here is Pituitary macroadenoma -(b).

Q. 391. A young female patient with long history of sinusitis presented with frequent fever along with personality changes and headache of recent origin. The fundus examination revealed papilledema. The most likely diagnosis is (AIIMS/Nov2004)
(a) Frontal lobe abscess
(b) Meningitis
(c) Encephalitis
(d) Frontal bone osteomyelitis

Ans. (a)
Note
The most likely diagnosis for above clinical presentation is 'Frontal lobe abscess'.

Also see
The above clinical presentation is in favor of complication of frontal sinusitis, the sinus is opened and dischged into anterior cranial foss causing frontal lobe abscess.

Q. 392. The most common side-effect of chemotherapy administration is (AIIMS/May2005)
(a) Nausea
(b) Alopecia
(c) Myelosuppression
(d) Renal distinction

Ans. (a)
Note
Most common side effect of chemotherapy is 'Nausea'.

Also see
The most common side effect of chemotherapy administration is nausea, with or without vomiting.
Ref: Harrison 15th Edition, Section 1, Neoplastic disorders

MCQ's in Practice of Medicine   869

Q. 393. All of the following conditions are observed in gout, except
    (a)   Uric acid nephrolithiasis
    (b)   Deficiency of enzyme xanthine oxidase
    (c)   Increase in serum urate concentration
    (d)   Renal disease involving interstitial tissues

Ans. (b)
Note
All of above conditions are observed in gout, except 'Deficiency of enzyme xanthine oxidase'.
Also see
All of the following conditions are found in gout i.e.,
a.   Uric acid nephrolithiasis. Uric acid urolithiasis is common in the presence of excessive production and excretion of urate. Overproduction of urate and persistently acid urine
b.   Xanthine oxidase deficiency is an autosomal recessive trait, and causes xanthinuria.
c.   Increase in serum urate concentration precipitates active inflammatory gouty arthritis by urate deposition in synovial tissue.
d.   Renal disease involving interstitial tissue; as prolonged hyperuricemia may deposit uric acid in the renal intersitium, and in the renal tubules causing renal failure or nephrolithiasis.
From above it is clear that the deficiency of enzyme xanthine oxidase is not related to gout.

Extended information
A competitive inhibitor of xanthin oxidase has been developed to control gout by prevenying the formation of urates so that excess purines are excreted as hypoxanthin and xanthin.
Ref: Biochemistry by S.P. Singh 4th Ed. Pg-106

Q. 394. The most common site of intestinal obstruction in gallstone ileus is (AIIMS/May2005)
    (a)   Duodenum
    (b)   Jejunum
    (c)   Ileum
    (d)   Sigmoid colon

Ans. (c)
Note
The most common site of intestinal obstruction in gallstone ileus is 'Ileum'.
Also see
Spontaneous internal biliary fistulae are uncommon and are usually discovered at cholecystectomy when a communication between the gallbladder and the duodenum. This usually results when a stone has ulcerated into the duodenum and disappeared in the faeces. There are no specific symptoms to suggest that this has happened, except when a large stone escapes and impacts in the terminal ileum, giving rise to gallstone ileus.

Q. 395. Which one of the following is not a feature of multiple myeloma? (AIIMS/May2005)
    (a)   Hypercalcemia
    (b)   Anemia
    (c)   Hyperviscosity
    (d)   Elevated alkaline phosphatase

Ans. (d)
Note
From above 'elelvated alkaline phosphate' is not a feture of multiple myeloma.
Also see
The feataures of multiple myeloma are:
a.   Hypercalcemia,
b.   Anemia, usually improves when the disease responds to treatment,
c.   Hyperviscosity syndrome which includes; lethargy, confusion, loss of vision, coma.
d.   Levels of serum alkaline phosphatase are normal even when there is extensive bone involvement because of the absence of osteoblastic activity.
In case of multiple myeloma there is absence of osteoblastic activity therefore, the alkaline phosphatase is in the normal range. Elevated alkaline phosphatase is not a feature of multiple myeloma.

Q. 396. Which one of the following diseases is an autosomal dominant disorder? (AIIMS/May2005)
    (a)   Hemochromatosis
    (b)   Phenylketonuria
    (c)   Maturity onset diabetes of the young
    (d)   Glucose-6-phosphate dehydrogenase deficiency

Ans. (c)
Note
From above the 'Maturity onset diabetes of the young' is an autosomal dominant disorder.
Also see
a.   Hemochromatosis is most often caused by inheritance of a mutant HFE gene.
b.   Phenylketonuria; is transmitted as autosomal recessive trait.
c.   Maturity onset diabetes of the young (MODY) is a subtype of DM characterised by autosomal dominant inheritance, early onset of hyperglycemia, and impairment in insulin secretion.
d.   Glucose – 6-phosphate dehydrogenase deficiency; is a X liked genetic disorder.

Therefore the choice (c) Maturity onset diabetes of youg is autosomal dominant disorder is correct answer.

Q. 397. Alpha-fetoprotein in maternal serum and / or amniotic fluid is increased in all except (AIIMS/May2005)
    (a)   Fetal neural tube defects
    (b)   Down's syndrome
    (c)   Anencephaly
    (d)   Encephalocele

Ans. (b)
Note
Alpha-fetoprotein in maternal serum and / or amniotic fluid is increased in all of above except 'Down's syndrome'.
Also see
The alpha feto protein (AFP) is an oncofetal protein produced by fetal yolk sac and fetal liver. Maternal serum alpha feto protein (MSA FP) level reaches a peak around 32 weeks. MSA FP levels are elevated in:
a.   Fetal neural tube defects
b.   Anencephaly
c.   Encephalocele
d.   Multiple pregnancy
e.   IUFD (Intra Uterine Fetal Death)
f.   Renal anamolies etc.
Whereas low levels of MSAFP are seen in; Chromosomal trisomies (Down's syndrome)
Ref: Textbook of Obstetrics by Dutta 5th Edition, Pg-112

Q. 398. A 10-year-old school girl has recurrent episodes of boils on the scalp. The boils subside with antibiotic therapy but recur after some time. The most likely cause of the recurrences is (AIIMS/May2005)
    (a)   Primary immunodeficiency syndrome
    (b)   Juvenile diabetes mellitus
    (c)   Pediculosis capitis
    (d)   HIV infection

Ans. (c)
Note
The most likely cause of the recurrence of boils in above case is 'Pediculosis capitis'.
Also see
The presenting features are recurrent boils on the scalp. In case of IDDM the other features could have present like weight loss, polydipsia, polyuria, polyphagia etc. In immune deficiency other infections like chest infection could have been there. HIV infection should have some predisposing cause like H/O blood transfusion. The child is a school going girl, who is at very high risk for pediculosis capitis only – which is not properly investigated and treated – i.e. personal hygiene. Therefore, most **suitable choice heare** appears to be (c).

Extended information
In Pediculosis capitis, itching of scalp could be mild to severe. Resultant scratching cause secondary pyoderma. If neglected for long, the infestation causes matting of hair because of exudates and pus condition.
Ref: API 7th Ed. Pg-1309

Q. 399. All of the following are features of absence seizures except (AIIMS/May2005)
    (a)   Usually seen in childhood
    (b)   3-Hz spike wave in EEG
    (c)   Postictal confusion
    (d)   Precipitation by hyperventilation

Ans. (c)
Note
All of above are the features of absence seizure except 'Postictal confusion'.
Also see
Absence Seizures (Petit Mal Epilepsy)
a.   Usually *begins in childhood* ages 4 to 8 years.
b.   The *electrophysiologic hallmark* of typical absence seizures is a generalized, symmetric, *3-Hz spike-and-wave discharge* that begins and ends suddenly on a normal EEG background.
c.   The seizure typically lasts for only seconds, consciousness returns as suddenly as it was lost, and there is '*no postictal confusion*'.
d.   The EEG often shows many more periods of abnormal cortical activity than were suspected clinically. *Hyperventilation tends to provoke* these electrographic discharges and even the seizures themselves and is routinely used when recording the EEG

Therefore the most subtable choice of answer is (c).

Q. 400. All of the following statements about HRT (hormone replacement therapy) are true except (AIIMS/May2005)
    (a)   It increases the risk of coronary artery disease.
    (b)   It increases bone mineral density.
    (c)   It increases the risk of breast cancer.
    (d)   It increases the risk of endometrial cancer.

Ans. (a)
Note
All of above about HRT are true except that 'it increases the riks of coronary artery disease'.
Also see
The benefits of HRT are:
    -Hot flushes are relieved.
    -Osteoporosis; HRT maintains the bone mass.
    -Prevents colonic cancer
Doubtful benefits of HRT:
    -Prevention of dementia
Evils of HRT:
    -Coronay heart disease
    -Breast cancer
    -Cholecystitis
    -Thrombotic events
    -Strokes

Extended information
The HERS, a recent clinical trial of HRT for the *secondary* prevention of IHD, showed no noteworthy difference in cardiovascular events with HRT. Indeed, in the HRT group, there was about a 50% increase in cardiovascular events in the first year of the trial. The Women's Health Initiative is investigating directly the impact of various HRT modalities as a *primary* prevention of IHD risk. Until further data are available, caution should be exercised in prescribing HRT to women with a history of IHD, or for cardioprotection alone.
Ref: Harrison 15th Edition, Women's Halth.

In hormone replacement therapy—there is:
- Symptomatic improvement in most menopausal symptoms
- Protection against fracture of wrist, spine and hip, secondary to osteoporosis
- A significant reduction in the risk of large bowel cancer
- A significant increase in the risk of breast cancer
- A significant increase in the risk of endometrial cancer
- A significant increase in the risk of ischaemic heart disease and stroke

Ref: Kumar and Clarke, 6th Ed. Pg-1052

Q. 401. In which of the following arthritis erosions are not seen? (AIIMS/May2005)
- (a) Rheumatoid arthritis
- (b) Systemic lupus erythematosus (SLE)
- (c) Psoriasis
- (d) Gout

Ans. (b)

Note
Out of above arthritic conditions erosions are not seen in 'SLE'.

Also see
Erosion of articular cartilage is common to RA, Psoriasis and Gout. However, Arthritis erosions are rare in case of SLE.
Ref: Harrison 15th Edition SLE.

Q. 402. Flapping tremors are seen in the following conditions except (AIIMS/May2005)
- (a) Uremic encephalopathy
- (b) Parkinsonism
- (c) Hepatic encephalopathy
- (d) Carbon dioxide narcosis

Ans. (b)

Note
Flapping tremors are seen all of above except, 'Parkinsonism'.

Also see
The Parkinson's disease the typical tremors are of 'pill rolling' type.

Q. 403. Which one of the following is not feature of irritable bowel syndrome? (AIIMS/May2005)
- (a) Abdominal pain
- (b) Constipation
- (c) Rectal bleeding
- (d) Bloating

Ans. (c)

Note
'Rectal bleeding' is not a feature of IBS from above given choices.

Also see
The rectal bleeding is not a feature of IBS, since it is a functional disorder of GIT motility.
Stool may be accompanied by passage of large amounts of mucous; hence, the term *mucous colitis* has been used to describe **IBS**. This is a misnomer, since inflammation is not present. Bleeding is not a feature of **IBS** unless hemorrhoids are present, and malabsorption or weight loss does not occur.
Ref: Harrison 15th Edition, IBS.

Q. 404. In which of the following conditions of malabsorption, an intestinal biopsy is diagnostic? (AIIMS/May2005)
- (a) Celiac disease
- (b) Tropical sprue
- (c) Whipple's disease
- (d) Lactose intolerance

Ans. (c)

MCQ's in Practice of Medicine

Note
From above 'whipple's disease' is diagnosed on intestinal biopsy.

Also see
Whipple's disease
It is a chronic multisystem disease caused by bacteria 'Tropheryma whippelii' and characterised by diarrhea, steatorrhea, weight loss, arthralgia, CNS and cardiac problems.

The diagnosis is suggested by obtaining tissue biopsies from the small intestine and/or other organs that may be involved (e.g., liver, lymph nodes, heart, eyes, central nervous system, or synovial membranes). The presence of PAS- (Periodic acid Schiff) positive macrophages containing the characteristic small (0.25 x 1 to 2 um) bacilli is suggestive of this diagnosis.
Ref: Harrison 15th Edition, Disorders of absorption.

Q. 405. Which one of the following is not a non-metastatic complication of malignancies? (AIIMS/May2005)
- (a) Cushing's syndrome
- (b) Cerebral cortical degeneration
- (c) Cerebellar degeneration
- (d) Polymyositis

Ans. (b)

Note
The 'cerebral cortical degeneration' from above is not a non-metastatic complication of malignancies.

Also see
About 90% of Paraneoplastic Cerebellar Degeneration occurs with Small Cell Lung Cancer, Hodgkin's lymphoma, or breast or ovarian cancer. Patients usually present with the subacute onset of a pancerebellar disorder consisting of nystagmus, oculomotor ataxia.
Ref: Harrison 15th Edition, Naraneoplastic Neurological syndromes

Q. 406. Complications of lobar pneumonia do not include (AIIMS/May2005)
- (a) Lung abscess
- (b) Amyloidosis
- (c) Suppurative arthritis
- (d) Infective endocarditis

Ans. (b)

Note
Compliations of lobar pneumonia do not include 'amyloidosis'.

Also see
Reactive systemic amyloidosis is associated with chronic infections, long standing inflammatory diseases - RA and malignant neoplasms e.g., myeloma.
Ref; Medicine for Students, 20th Edition by Golwalla. Amyloidosis.

Q. 407. Hemolytic anemia may be characterized by all of the following except (AIIMS/May2005)
- (a) Hyperbilirubinemia
- (b) Reticulocytosis
- (c) Hemoglobinuria
- (d) Increased plasma haptoglobin level

Ans. (d)

Note
Hemolytic anemia may be characterized by all of the above except 'Increased plasma haptoglobin level'.

Also see
During acute hemolysis, a rapid drop in hematocrit is accompanied by a rise in plasma hemoglobin and unconjugated bilirubin and a decrease in plasma haptoglobin.
Ref; Harrison's 15th edition. Section 2- Disorders of hematopoiesis, 108. Hemolytic anemias and acute blood loss.

Q. 408. Which of the following is the most common type of pituitary adenoma? (AIIMS/May2005)
    (a)   Thyrotropinoma
    (b)   Gonadotropinoma
    (c)   Prolactinoma
    (d)   Corticotropinoma

Ans. (c)
Note
From the choice given above 'Prolactinoma' is the most common type of pituitary adenoma.
Also see
Prolactinoma (lactotroph adenomas) account for about half of all functioning pituitary tumors.
Ref: Harrison 15th Edition Disorders of the anterior pituitary and hypothalamus.

Q. 409. Which is the most common site of metastatic disease? (AIIMS/May2005)
    (a)   Lung
    (b)   Bone
    (c)   Liver
    (d)   Brain

Ans. (c)
Note
'Liver' is the most common site of metastatic disease.
Also see
Metastatatis to liver is very common from malignant diseases. The liver is exceptionally susceptible to invasion by tumor cells. Its size, high rate of blood flow, double perfusion by the hepatic artery and portal vein, and its Kupffer cell filtration function combine to make it the next most common site of metastases after the lymph node.

Q. 410. Which of the following infestation leads to malabsorption?
    (a)   Giardia lamblia
    (b)   Ascaris lumbricoides
    (c)   Vecator americanus
    (d)   Ancylostoma duodenale

Ans. (a)
Note
'Giardia lamblia' infestation from above leads to malabsorption.
Also see
Giardia; causes digestive disturbances with passage of sprue like stools in children.
(Sprue: condition is characterized by imability to absorb fat, glucose, calcium and present with morning diarrhea, bulky gaseous stools, sore tongue, megalocytic anemia and wasging)
Ref: Medicine for Students By Golwalla 10th Ed, Pg-752

Q. 411. All of the following can cause osteoporosis except
    (a)   Hyperparathyroidism
    (b)   Steroid use
    (c)   Fluorosis
    (d)   Thyrotoxicosis

Ans. (c)
Note
All of above can cause osteoporosis except 'Fluorosis'.
Also see
Causes of osteoporosis
Endocrine diseases:
    -Hyperparathyroidism, Hyperthyroidism, Cushing's syndrome.
Inflammatory diseases:
    -Inflammatory bowel disease, Rheumatoid arthritis, Ankylosing spondylitis

Gastrointestinal diseases:
   -Malabsorption, Chronic liver disease
Miscellaneous:
   -Myeloma, Gaucher's disease, Immobilisation.
Drugs:
   -Corticosteriods.
Ref: Davidson 20th Ed, Pg-1123

Q. 412. All of the following are the causes of relative polycythemia except
   (a)   Dehydration
   (b)   Dengue haemorrhagic fever
   (c)   Gaisbock's syndrome
   (d)   High altitude

Ans. (d)
Note
All of the above are the causes of relative polycythemia except 'high altitude'
Also see
Polycythemia refers to any increase in circulating red blood cells above normal.
Polycythemia is has abnormally high Hb i.e., - 17g/dl for men and 15 g/dl for women. Hematocrit levels > 50% in men or > 45% in women may be abnormal. Hematocrit > 60% in men and > 55% in women are almost invariably associated with increased red cell mass.
Relative (Spurious) polycythemia:
Relative polycythemia is only apparent or relative because of a decrease in plama volume.
Causes of relative polycythemia are:
   -Dehydration; diarrhoea causing decrease in plasma volume
   -Burn
   -Gailbock's Syndrome
The secondary causes are associated with increase in Erythropoietin levels:
   -Living at high altitude
   -CO poisoning
   -Lung disease
   -Heavy smoking
   -Cardiovascular disease (Right to left shunt)

Extended information
Gaisbock's syndrome
Condition was originally thought to be stress incuded. The red cell volume is normal, but as the result of a decreased plasma volume, there is a relative polycythaemia. 'Relative' polycythemia is more common than PV and occurs in middle aged men, particularly in smokers who are obese and hypertensive. The condition may present with cardiovascular problems such as myocardial or cerebral inshaemia.
Ref: Clincial Medicine By Kumar and Clarke, 6th Ed, Pg-453, 455
Dengue hemorrhagic fever
The clinical criteria for diagnosis are as follows: (1) fever; (2) hemorrhagic manifestations, including at least a positive tourniquet test result and a major or minor bleeding phenomenon; (3) hepatic enlargement; (4) shock (high pulse rate and narrowing of the pulse pressure to 20 mm Hg or less, or hypotension). The laboratory criteria include (5) thrombocytopenia (â 100,000/mm3), and (6) hemoconcentration (hematocrit increase ô 20%). Thrombocytopenia with concurrent high hematocrit levels differentiates DHF from classic DF.
Ref: http://www.bhj.org/journal/2001_4303_july01/review_380.htm

Q. 413. All of the following may cause ST segment elevation on EKG, except
   (a)   Early repolarization variant
   (b)   Constrictive pericarditis
   (c)   Ventricular aneurysm
   (d)   Prinzmetal angina

Ans. (b)
Note
All of above may cause ST segment elevation on EKG except, 'Constrictive pericarditis'

Also see
ECG features in case of constrictive pericarditis are:
- Low voltage QRS complexes
- Flat or inverted T waves
- Slurred QRS complexes
- Bifid P waves

Q. 414. Cluster headache is characterized by all except
(a) Affects predominantly females
(b) Unilateral headache
(c) Onset typically in 20-50 years of life
(d) Associated with conjunctival congestion

Ans. (a)
Note
Cluster headache is characterized by all of above except that it affects 'predominantly females'.
Also see
Cluster headache: It is a devastating painful headache, mainly affecting men. It is considerably less common than migraine and generally begins in second or third decade. The pain is accompanied by lachrimation, rhinorrhea or miosis.
Ref API 7th Ed. Pg-752
Review of the choice give above:
a. The statemet that it affects predominantly females is – incorrect. Men are affected seven to eight times more often than women.
b. Headache is unilateral and usually affects the same side for subsequent months; it is ture.
c. Onset typically in 20 – 50 years of life is ture.
d. It is associated with homolateral lacarimatioon, reddening of the eye, nasal stuffiness, lid ptosis, and nausea.

Cluster headache is also known as Raeder's syndrome, histamine cephalalgia, and sphenopalatine neuralgia. Alcohol provokes attacks in about 70% of patients but ceases to be provocative when the bout remits, this on-off vulnerability to alcohol is pathognomonic of 'cluster headache'.
Ref: Harrison's 15th Edition. Headache including Migraine and Cluster Headache..

Q. 415. The most sensitive test for the diagnosis of myasthenia gravis is
(a) Elevated serum ACh-receptor binding antibodies.
(b) Repetitive nerve stimulation test.
(c) Positive edrophonium test.
(d) Measurement of jitter by single fibre electromyography.

Ans. (a)
Note
The most sensitive test for the diagnosis of myasthenic gravis is 'Elevated serum ACh-recepteror binding antibodies'.
Also see
Acetylcholine (ACh) receptor antibodies: the demonstration in serum of anbtibodies against ACh receptiors is a sensitive diagnostic test. Patients with pure ocular myasthemia may not show ACh receptor antibodies in their serum. False positive results are very rate.
Ref: Ref: API Test Book ofg medicine, 6th Ed, Pg- 849

Extended information
Antiacetylcholine receptor Antibody
As noted above, anti-AChR antibodies are detectable in the serum of approximately 80? of all myasthenic patients, but in only about 50? of patients with weakness confined to the ocular muscles. The presence of anti-AChR antibodies is virtually diagnostic of MG, but a negative test does not exclude the disease. The measured level of anti-AChR antibody does not correspond well with the severity of MG in different patients. However, in an individual patient, a treatment-induced fall in the antibody level often correlates with clinical improvement.

Q. 416. Vitamin B12 deficiency can give rise to all of the following, except
  (a) Myelopathy
  (b) Optic atrophy
  (c) Peripheral neuropathy
  (d) Myopathy

Ans. (d)

Note
Vitamin B12 deficiency can give rise to all of the following, except 'Myopathy'.

Also see
Vitamin B 12 (Cynocobalamin) is a water soluble vitamin. Its deficiency causes megaloblastic anemia, fatigue and loss of sensation in limbs. Prolonged deficiency leads to degeneration of nervous system.
Ref: Park and Park 15th Ed, Pg-448

Q. 417. EEG is usually abnormal in all of the following except
  (a) Subacute sclerosing panencephalitis
  (b) Locked-in state
  (c) Creutzfeldt-Jackob disease
  (d) Hepatic encephalopathy

Ans. (b)

Note
EEG is usually abnormal in all of above except 'Locked-in state'.

Also see
Recognizable slow wave EEG abnormalities appear in encephalitis, prion (Creutzfeldt-Jakob) disease and metabolic states (e.g. hypoglycemia and hepatic coma).
Ref: Kumar and Clark 6th Ed. Pg-1203

Locked-in state
Condition is characterised as pseudocoma in which an awake patient has no ability to speak or move his legs, face, so as to indicate that he or she is awake, but vertical eye movements and lid elevation remain unimpaired. Thus in a "locked-in" state of preserved consciousness with quadriplegia and cranial nerve signs suggest complete pontine and lower midbrain infarction. The usual cause is infarction of the ventral pons, which contains all descending corticospinal and corticobulbar fibers.
EEG is normal in Locked in state.
Ref: Harrison's 15th Edition. Nervous system dysfunction.

Q. 418. Which of the following is not a neuroparasite?
  (a) Tenia solium
  (b) Acanthamoea
  (c) Naegleria
  (d) Trichinella spiralis

Ans. (d)

Note
'Trichinella spiralis' from the above is not a neuroparasite

Also see
Trichinella spiralis is a tissue roundworm. Distribution; worldwide. Intermediate host (Transmission); Swine / humans. Definitive Hosts; Swine /humans. Parasitic stage; Larva. Diagnosis; Muscle biopsy.
Ref: Harrison's 15th Edition. Section -16. 211. Laboratory diagnosis of parasitic infections.

Q. 419. Which of the following is a cause of reversible dementia?
  (a) Subacute combined degeneration
  (b) Picks disease
  (c) Creutzfeld-Jakob disease
  (d) Alzheimer's disease

Ans. (a)

Note
From above given causes 'Subacute combined degeneration' is reversible dementia.

Also see
Response to the treatment of subacute combined degeneration in early stages usually results in complete recovery.

Extended information
Causes of dementia

Reversible causes	Irreversible causes	Psychiatric disorders
-Hypothyroidism	-Alzheimer's	-Depression
-Thiamine deficiency	-Frontotemporal dementia	-Schizophrenia
-Vit-B-12 Deficiency	(Pick's Disease)	-Conversion Reaction
-Normal Pressure	-Huntington's	
Hydrocephalus	-Dementia with Lewy bodies	
-Chroncin infection	-Multi-infract	
-Brain tumor	-Leukoencephalopathies	
-Drug intoxication	-Parkinson's	

Ref: Ref: Harrison, 16th Ed, Pg-2396

Q. 420. All of the following CSF findings are present in tuberculous meningitis, except
    (a)   Raised protein levels
    (b)   Low chloride levels
    (c)   Cob-web formation
    (d)   Raised sugar levels

Ans. (d)
Note
All of the above CSF findings are present in tuberculous meningitis, except 'raised sugar levels'.
Also see
There is a rise in protein and a marked fall in glucose.
Ref: Davidson's 20th Ed, Pg-1228

Q. 421. Which one of the following serum levels would help in distinguishing an acute liver disease from chronic liver disease?
    (a)   Aminotransaminase
    (b)   Alkaline phosphatase
    (c)   Bilirubin
    (d)   Albumin

Ans. (d)
Note
Serum 'albumin' levels would help in distinguishing an acute liver disease from chronic liver disease.
Also see
The half life of albumin is about 22 days and hence, in acute liver injury, levels are normal, whereas in chronic liver disease it is low.
Ref: API Text Book of Medicine 6th Ed, Pg-560

Extended information
In case of acute liver diseases the aminotransaminase and bilirubin level are raised. However, in chornic liver disease the serum levels of albumin will be low. Because albumin is synthesized in by the liver, decreased serum albumin may result from liver disease. It can also result from kidney disease, which allows albumin to escape in the urine. Decreased albumin may also be explained by malnutrition or a low protein diet.

Q. 422. Paralysis of 3rd, 4th 6th nerves with involvement of ophthalmic division of 5th nerve, localizes the lesion to
- (a) Cavernous sinus
- (b) Apex of orbit
- (c) Brainstem
- (d) Base of skull

Ans. (a)

Note
The lesion is localized in 'Cavernous sinus'.

Also see
All these nerve pass through the cavernous sinus.
The cavernous sinus syndrome is a distinctive and frequently life-threatening disorder. It often presents as orbital or facial pain; orbital swelling and chemosis due to occlusion of ophthalmic veins; fever; occulomotor neuropaphty affecting the third, fourth, land sixth cranial nerves; and trigeminal neuropathy affecting the ophthalmic (V1) and occasionally the maxillary (V2) division of trigeminal nerve.
Ref: Harrison, 16th Ed, Pg-2438

Q. 423. Which one of the following is the most common location of hypertensive bleed in the brain?
- (a) Putamen/external capsule
- (b) Pons
- (c) Ventricles
- (d) Lobar white matter

Ans. (a)

Note
The most common location of hypertensive bleed in the brain is 'putamen / external capsule'.

Also see
The putamen is the most common site for hypertensive hemorrhage, and the adjacent internal capsule is invariably damaged. It results in contralateral hemiparesis. If the hemorrhages are large, drowsiness is followed by stupor as the hematoma compress brainstem. Coma ensues, accompanied by deep, intermittent respiration. Harrisons 15th Edition. Section 2- Diseases of central nervous system 361- Cerebrovascular diseases – Intracranial hemorrhage.

Q. 424. In which of the following diseases, the overall survival is increased by screening procedure?
- (a) Prostate cancer
- (b) Lung cancer
- (c) Colon cancer
- (d) Ovarian cancer

Ans. (c)

Note
In 'colon cancer' the overall survival is increased by screening procedure.

Also see
Screening means detecting disease early in asymptomatic stage with the aim of decreasing morbidity and mortality. Screening for **cancer** is possible as modern technology has come up with number of diagnostic tests and procedures that are safe, quick, and inexpensive. While screening can potentially save lives, and has been shown clearly to do so in the case of breast, cervical, and colon cancer.

Prostate Cancer
The most common prostate cancer screening modalities are digital rectal examination and assays for serum prostate-specific antigen (PSA). No well designed trial has demonstrated the true benefit of prostate cancer screening and treatment, but trials are in progress.

Lung Cancer
For lung cancer screening, chest radiographs and sputum cytology have been evaluated as methods for lung cancer screening. No reduction in lung cancer mortality has been found in these studies, although all the controlled trials performed have had low statistical power. Even screening of high-risk subjects (smokers) has not been proved to be beneficial. Spiral computed tomography (CT) can diagnose lung cancers at early stages; however, false-positive rates are high.

Colorectal Cancers
Two case-control studies suggest that regular screening of people over 50 with sigmoidoscopy decreases mortality.
Ovarian Cancer

Adnexal palpation, transvaginal ultrasound, and serum CA-125 determination have been considered for ovarian cancer screening. Adnexal palpation is too insensitive to detect ovarian cancer at an early enough stage to affect mortality substantially.
Ref: Section 1 – Neoplastic disorders 80. Prevention and early detection of cancer. Harrison's Principles of internal Medicine – 15th Edition.

Q. 425. Fordyce's (spots) granules in oral cavity arise from
    (a)   Mucous glands
    (b)   Sebaceous glands
    (c)   Taste buds
    (d)   Minor salivary glands

Ans. (b)
Note
Fordyce's (spots) granules in oral cavity arise from 'Sebaceous glands'.
Also see
Fordyce's spots (ectopic sebaceous glands), which have no erythematous halos and are found in the mouth of healthy individuals.
Harrison's 15th Edition. Section 2- Alterations in body temperature. 18. Fever and Rash.
Fordyce's disease: It is aggregation of small yellowish spots just beneath mucosal surface at buccal and labial mucosa, no symptoms, due to hyperplasia of sebaceous glands. Prognosis; remains without apparent change indefinitely.
Harrison's 15th Edition. Table 31-2 Pigmented lesions of oral mucosa.

Q. 426. Epstein Barr (EB) virus has been implicated in the following malignancies, except
    (a)   Hodgkin's disease
    (b)   Non-Hodgkin's lymphoma
    (c)   Nasopharyngeal carcinoma
    (d)   Multiple myeloma

Ans. (d)
Note
Epstein Barr (EB) virus has been implicated in the above malignancies, except 'Multiple myeloma'.
Also see
EBV is associated with following malignancies:
    -Burkitt's lymphoma
    -Anaplastic nasoparyngeal carcinoma
    -Hodgkin's disease (Especially mixed cellular type)
    -Tonsillar carcinoma
    -T cell lymphoma
    -Thymoma
    -Gastric carcinoma
Ref: Epstein Barr Virus Infections. Clincial manifestations. Harrison's Principles of Internal Medicine -15th Edition.
Multiple myeloma
Cause of multiple myeloma is not known. Myeloma has been seen more commonly than expected among farmers, wood workers, leather workers and those exposed to petroleum products.
Myeloma occurred with increased frequenct in tose exposed to the radiation of nuclear warheads in World War II after a 20 year latency.
Ref: Plasma cell disorders. Harrison's Principles of Internal Medicine -15th Edition.
Non-Hodgkins lymphoma
The neoplastic diseae clearly seen with an increased frequency in patients ith HIV infction are Kaposi's sarcoma and non-Hodgkin's lymphoma.

Ref: AIDS and related clinical manifestations.
Ref: Harrison's Principles of Internal Medicine -15th Edition.

Q. 427. HbA1c level in blood explains
(a) Acute rise of sugar
(b) Long term status of blood sugar
(c) Hepatorenal syndrome
(d) Chronic pancreatitis

Ans. (b)

Note
HbA1c level in blood explains 'Long term status of blood sugar'.

Also see
Hb A1c (GHb, glycohemoglobin, Diabetic control index, Hemoglobin-glycosylated)
It is a blood test that measures the amount of glycosylated hemoglobin.
Value:
The HbA1c is is performed to measure blood sugar control in individuals with diabetes mellitus.
Normal value:
Glycosylated hemoglobin is 2.2 to 4.4% of total Hb is normal.
Abnormal results mean:
Inadequate regulation of blood glucose levels over a period of weeks to monts (poorly controlled diabetes mellitus).

Extended information
Glycosylated haemoglobin:
This test provides a long term index of glucose control. This test is based on the following rationale: glucose in the blood is complexed to certain fraction of hemoglobin to an extent proportional to the blood glucose concentrtation. The percentage of such glycosylated hemoglobin reflects the mean blood glucose levels during the red cell life – time i.e. about the previous 2-3 months.
Ref: Park and Park 18th Ed, Pg-315

Q. 428. The most common histologic type of thyroid cancer is
(a) Medullary type
(b) Follicular type
(c) Papillary type
(d) Anaplastic type

Ans. (c)

Note
The most common histologic type of thyroid cancer is 'papillaty type'.

Also see
The papillary carcinoma of thyroid is the most common cancer of thyroid gland. About 75-85% cancers diagnosed in US are papillary carcinoma. It is more common in women than in men.

Cell Type	Frequency	Behaviour	Spread	Prognosis
Papillary	70%	Occurs in young	Local, sometimes lung/bone secondaries	Good, especially in young
Follicular	20%	More common in females	Metastases to lung/bone	Good if respectable
Anaplastic	<5%	Aggrresive	Locally invasive	Very poor
Lymphoma	2%	Variable		Sometimes responsive to radiotherapy
Medullary cell	5%	Often familial	Local and Metastases	Poor, but indolent course

Ref: Clinical Medicine by Kumar and Clark 6th Ed, Pg-1080

Q. 429. Persistent vomiting most likely causes
  (a) Hyperkalaemia
  (b) Acidic urine excretion
  (c) Hypochloremia
  (d) Hyperventilation

Ans. (c)

Note
Persistent vomiting most likely causes 'hypochloremia'.

Also see
Metabolic alkalosis occurs as a result of net gain of [HCO_3^-] or loss of nonvolatile acid (usually HCl by vomiting) from the extracellular fluid. Since it is unusual for alkali to be added to the body, the disorder involves a generative stage, in which the loss of acid usually causes alkalosis, and a maintenance stage, in which the kidneys fail to compensate by excreting HCO_3^- because of volume contraction, a low GFR, or depletion of Cl^- or K^+.
Persistent vomiting (pyloric obstruction or conitious gastric aspiration) causes loss of chlorides with accelerated loss of sodium and biocarbonate in urine and increased renal excretion of potassium.
Ref: Text Book of Surgery by S. Das 4th Ed, Pg-32

Q. 430. In which of the following a 'Coeur en Sabot' shape of the heart is seen?
  (a) Tricuspid atresia
  (b) Ventricular septal defect
  (c) Transposition of great arteries
  (d) Fallot's Tetralogy

Ans. (d)

Note
From above in 'Fallot's Tetralogy' the 'Coeur en Sabot' shape of heart is seen.

Also see
Tetralogy of fallot is a congenital cyanotic cardiac disease. The four component of Fallot's Tetralogy are:
  -High large ventricular septal defect
  -Overriding aorta
  -Right ventricular hypertrophy
  -Pulomnary stenosis
The X-Ray reveals: A 'Coeur en sabot' (boot shaped heart; appearance of heart due to lifting of apex of the heart above diaphragm from right ventricular hypertrophy seen in 10% cases) with:
  -Right ventricular hypertrophy
  -Deep Pulmonary bay due to hypoplastic pulmonary artery/ Concavity in the region of the pulmonary conus.
  -The pulmonary vascular markings are typically diminished.
  -Aortic arch and knob may be on the right side.
The radiological examination characteristically reveals a boot shaped heart (Coeur en sabot) with prominence of the right ventricle and a concavity in the region of pulmonary conus.
Ref: Harrison 16th Ed, Pg-1389

Q. 431. In Budd Chiari syndrome, the site of venous thrombosis is
  (a) Infrahepatic inferior vena cava
  (b) Infrarenal inferior vena cava
  (c) Hepatic veins
  (d) Portal vein

Ans. (c)

Note
In Budd- Chiari syndrome, the site of venous thrombosis is 'hepatic veins'.

Also see
Budd-Chiari syndrome
It results from occlusion of the hepatic veins. Condition is characterised by grossly enlarged and tender liver

and ascites. Fatures of CCF are absent. The most common causes of thrombosis of the hepatic veins are; polycythemia rubra vera, myeloproliferative syndromes, oral contraceptive use. It may also result from invasion of the inferior vena cava by tumor, such as renal cell or hepatocellular carcinoma. Idiopathic membranous obstruction of the inferior vena cava is the most common cause of this syndrome in Japan. Hepatic venography or liver biopsy showing centrilobular congestion and sinusoidal dilatation in the absence of right-sided heart failure confirms diagnosis of Budd-Chiari syndrome.

Harrison's Principle of Internal Medicine – 15th Edition. Liver and biliary tract disease.

Q. 432. Polycystic disease of the kidney may have cysts in all of the following organs, except
- (a) Lung
- (b) Liver
- (c) Pancreas
- (d) Spleen

Ans. (a)

Note
Polycystic disease of the kidney may have cysts in all of the following organs, except 'Lung'.

Also see
Autosomal Dominant Polycystic Kidney Disease (ADPKD) or Adult type polycystic kidney disease is characterised by multiple bilateral cysts that cause enlargement of kidney causing reduced functioning of renal tissue due to pressure effect.

It is associated with:
- Cysts in liver, spleen, pancreas
- Saccular aneurysms
- Colonic diverticulosis especially cerebral
- Colonic diverticulosis
- CVS; Aortic root dilatation, AR, MR, Mitral valve prolapse
- Others; Hereditary spherocytosis, myotonic dystrophy

Ref; Polycystic Disease of Kidneys-Page 614-Medicine for Students by Golwalla – 12th Edition.

Q. 433. Kinky-hair disease is a disorder where an affected child has peculiar white stubby hair, does not grow, brain degeneration is seen and dies by age of two years. Mrs A is hesitant about having children because her two sisters had sons who had died from kinky hair disease. Her mother's brother also died of the same condition. Which of the following is the possible mode of inheritance in her family?
- (a) X-linked recessive
- (b) X-linked dominant
- (c) Autosomal recessive
- (d) Autosomal dominant

Ans. (a)

Note
From above the 'X-linked recessive' mode of inheritance.

Also see
Menkes kinky hair syndrome is an X-linked recessive metabolic disturbance of copper metabolism characterized by mental retardation, hypocupremia, and decreased circulating ceruloplasmin. It is caused by mutations in a copper-transporting *ATP7A* gene. Children with this disease often die within 5 years due to dissecting aneurysms or cardiac rupture.

Disorder:
- Menkes disease

Substance involved:
- Copper

Tissue Manifesting Transport Defect:
- Most tissues except liver

Proposed Molecular Basis of defect:
- Copper-transporting ATPase (ATP7A)

Major Clinical Manifestations:

-Severe mental retardation, pili torti (kinky hair), typical facies, arterial tortuosity, excess wormian bones, thermal instability.

Mode of inheritance:
  -X-linked recessive

Ref; Harrison's Principles of Internal Medicine – 15th Edition. Disorders of endocrinology and etabolism.

Q. 434. The occurrence of hyperthyroidism following administration of supplemental iodine to subjects with endemic iodine deficiency goiter is known as
  (a) Jod-Basedow effect
  (b) Wolff-Chaikoff effect
  (c) Thyrotoxicosis factitia
  (d) De Quervain's Thyroiditis

Ans. (a)

Note
The condition is known as 'Jad-Besedow effect'.

Also see
In cases of nontoxic multinodular goiter iodine containing substances should be avoided because of the risk of inducing the Jod Basedow effect, characterised by enhanced thyroid hormone production by autonomous nodules.
Ref; Harrison's 15th Edition. Disorders of thyroid gland.

Q. 435. In hematuria of glomerular origin the urine is characterized by the presence of all the following except
  (a) Red cell casts
  (b) Acanthocytes
  (c) Crenated red cells
  (d) Dysmorphic red cells

Ans. (b)

Note
In hematuria of glomerular origin the urine is characterized by the presence of all of the above except 'acanthocytes'.

Also see
Acanthocytes; Spur cells or acanthocytes (Spur cell anemia) are recognized as distorted red blood cells containing several irregularly distributed thorn like projections. It occurs in severe liver diseases.

Extended information
Presence of red cells confirms the presence of blood in the urine and with phase-contrast dicroscope, dysmorphic appearance of RBC's, which suggests glomerular aetiolgoy, can be appreciated.
Ref: API, 6th Ed, Pg-625
Rapidly progressive glomerulonephritis; Hematuria, microscopic or gross, and RBC casts are always present. Telescopic sediment may be present.
Ref: API, 6th Ed, Pg-630

Q. 436. A middle aged man presents with paresthesia of hands and feet. Examination reveals presence of Mees' lines in the nails and rain drop pigmentation in the hands. The most likely causative toxin for the above mentioned symptoms is
  (a) Lead
  (b) Arsenic
  (c) Thallium
  (d) Mercury

Ans. (b)

Note
The most likely causative toxin for the above mention symptoms is 'arsenic'.

Also see
In cases of chronic arsenic poisoning, the onset of symptoms takes palce about 2 – 8 weeks. The findings include, skin and nail changes, such as hyperkeratosis, hyperpigmentation, exfoliative dermatitis and Mees

lines (transverse white striae of the fingernails) sensory and motor polyneuritis manifesting as numbness and tingling in a 'stocking –glove' distribution, distal weakness and quadriplegia. The epidemiological studies have linked chronic consumption of water containing arsenic.

Extended information
Arsenic (herbilside; insecticide) poisoning; skin changes, Mees' lines in nails; painful; systemic effects.
Ref: Harrison, 16th Ed, Pg-2505

Q. 437. All of the following can cause neuropathies with predominant motor involvement, except
    (a)   Acute inflammatory demyelinating polyneuropathy
    (b)   Acute intermittent porphyria
    (c)   Lead intoxication
    (d)   Arsenic intoxication

Ans. (d)
Note
All of above can cause neuropathies with predominant motor incvolvement except 'arsenic intoxicaiton'.
Also see
Aresnic intoxication leads to sensorty motor involvement.
Acute intermittent porphyria
The peripheral neuropathy is due to axonal degeneration and primarily affects motor neurons. Motor neuropathy affects the proximal muscles (shoulders and arms). Sensory changes such as paresthesia and loss of sensation are less prominent. Progressive muscular weakness can lead to respiratory and bulbar paralysis.
Lead intoxication
The lead poisoning is characterized by abdominal pain, headache, irritability, joint pain, fatigue, anemia, peripheral motor neuropathy, and deficits in short-term memory and the ability to concentrate.
Acute inflammatory demyelinating polyneuropathy (GBS)
It involves rapidly evolving paralysis with areflexia.
Ref: Harrison Ed 16th, Pg-2503, Table 363 -3 -4

Q. 438. An HIV positive patient complains of visual disturbances. Fundal examination shows bilateral retinal exudates and perivascular hemorrahges. Which of the following viruses are most likely to be responsible for this retinitis
    (a)   Herpes simplex virus
    (b)   Human herpes virus 8
    (c)   Cytomegalovirus
    (d)   Epstein-Barr(EB) virus

Ans. (c)
Note
From above viruses are most likely to be responsible for this retinitis is 'Cytomegalovirus'.
Also see
The above retitins findings are in tune with the cytomegalovirus.
Ref; Harrison's 15th Edition. Atlas of Fundoscopic findings, IV-2 Cytomegalovirus.

Q. 439. Which of the following viruses is not a common cause of viral encephalitis?
    (a)   Herpes simplex virus type 2
    (b)   Japanese encephalitis virus
    (c)   Nipah virus
    (d)   Cytomegalovirus

Ans. (c)
Note
From above viruses 'Nipah virus' is not a common cause of viral encephalitis.
Also see
New causes of viral encephalitis are constantly appearing and in this line the Nipah Virus is a new virus to cause recent outbreak of encephalitis in Malaysia.
Ref; Harrison's. 15th Edition. Viral meningitis and encephalitis.

Q. 440. All of the following infections are often associated with acute intravascular hemolysis except
(a) Clostridium tetani
(b) Bartonella bacilliformis
(c) Plasmodium falciparum
(d) Babesia microti

Ans. (a)

Note
All of the above infections are often associated with acute intravascular hemolysis except 'Clostridium tetani'.

Also see
Red cells injured directly by various infections. The most common infection causing hemolysis is malaria. Other infections that lead to hemolytic anemia are infections by protozoa babesia, trypanosomiasis, and visceral leishmaniasis. A severe acute hemolytic anemia is produced in bartonellosis, caused by bacillus Bartonella bacilliformis. Profound fatal hemolytic anemia can occur in clostridial sepsis with severe intravascular erythrocyte destruction. Hemolytic anemia may occur with bacterial septicaemia caused by gram positive or nevgative organisms and is especially common in children.
Ref: API textbook of Medicine, 7th Ed, Pg-946
The clostridium tetani do not cause intravascular hemolysis. It causes 'Tetanus' which is a neurological disorder, characterized by increased muscle tone and spasms, which is caused by tetanospasmin, a powerful protein toxin produced by Clostridium tetani. Tetanus occurs in several clinical forms, including generalized, neonatal and localized disease.
Ref: Harrison.

Q. 441. All of the following are the electrocardiographic features of severe hyperkalemia except
(a) Peaked T waves
(b) Presence of U waves
(c) Sine wave pattern
(d) Loss of P waves

Ans. (b)

Note
All of the above are the electrocardiographic features of severe hyperkalemia except 'Presence of U waves'.

Also see
The earliest electrocardiographic changes include increased T-wave amplitude, or *peaked T waves*. More severe degrees of hyperkalemia result in a *prolonged PR interval and QRS duration*, atrioventricular conduction delay, and *loss of P waves. Progressive widening of the QRS complex and merging with the T wave produces a 'sinewave pattern'.* The terminal event is usually *ventricular fibrillation or asystole.*
Fig 12.9 Progressive ECG changes with increasing hyperkalemia.
Ref: Clincial Medicine by Kumar Clark 6th Ed, Pg-709

Q. 442. Commonest cause of sporadic encephalitis is
(a) Japanese B Virus
(b) Herpes Simplex Virus
(c) Human Immunodeficiency Virus
(d) Rubeola Virus

Ans. (b)

Note
Commonest cause of sporadic encephalitis is 'Herpes Simplex Virus'.

Also see
HSV accounts for sporadic cases of viral encephalitis. Cases are distributed throughout the year, and the age distribution appears to be biphasic, with peaks at 5 to 30 and > 50 years of age.
Harrison's 15th Edition. Herpes simplex viruses Epidemiology.

Q. 443. Raised serum level of lipoprotein is a predictor of
  (a) Cirrhosis of liver
  (b) Rheumatic arthritis
  (c) Atherosclerosis
  (d) Cervical cancer

Ans. (c)
Note
Raised serum level of lipoprotein is a predictor of ' Atherosclerosis'.
Also see
High serum cholesteriol, especially when associated with a low value of htihg density lipoproteins (HDL), is strongly associated with coronary atheroma. The raised serum lipoproteins are a high risk factor for atherosclerosis.
Ref: Kumar & Clarke, 6th Ed, Pg-801

Q. 444. Which one of the following conditions may lead to exudative pleural effusion?
  (a) Cirrhosis
  (b) Nephrotic syndrome
  (c) Congestive heart failure
  (d) Bronchogenic carcinoma

Ans. (d)
Note
From the conditions given above 'the Bronchogenic carcinoma' may lead to exudative pleural effusion.
Also see
An exudative pleural effusion occurs when local factors that influence the formation and absorption of pleural fluid are altered. The leading causes of exudative pleural effusions are bacterial pneumonia, malignancy, viral infection, and pulmonary embolism.
Ref: Harrison 16th Ed, Pg-1566
The cirrhosis, nephrotic syndrome and CCF can cause transudate; however, the bronchogenic carcinoma will be responsible for exudative pleural effusion.
A prospective study of 76 consecutive patients over the age of 40 years, with exudative pleural effusion, was undertaken to determine the common causes of such a clinical condition. Malignant pleural effusions were the most common in this series, found in 49 patients (64.47%), all but one being metastatic from elsewhere. Forty were secondary to a carcinoma of the bronchus, 3 from carcinoma of the breast, 1 each from carcinoma of the ovary, esophagus, and larynx; lymphoma accounted for the remaining 2. Infective causes accounted for 24 of the effusions (31.57%). Of the infections, tuberculosis was the most common, accounting for 17 of the 24. Other infective causes included bacterial empyemas in 4, ruptured amoebic liver abscess in 2, and actinomycosis in 1. Pancreatitis, pulmonary thromboembolism, and a post-cardiotomy syndrome were diagnosed in 1 patient each, while the diagnosis remained unknown in the remaining 5 patients. In 2 patients the diagnosis was made on autopsy.
Ref: Prabhudesai PP, Mahashur AA, Mehta N, Ajay R
Dept of Chest Medicine, KEM Hospital, Parel, Bombay, Maharashtra

Q. 445. A 60 year old man is diagnosed to be suffering from Legionnaire's disease after he returns home from attending a convention. He could have acquired it
  (a) From a person suffering from the infection while travelling in the aeroplane.
  (b) From a chronic carrier in the convention center.
  (c) From inhalation of the aerosol in the air-conditioned room at convention center.
  (d) By sharing an infected towel with a fellow delegate at the convention.

Ans. (c)
Note
He could have acquired it 'From inhalation of the aerosol in the air-conditioned room at convention center'.
Also see
Three epidemiological patterns of this disease are recognized:
a. Outbreaks among previously fit individuals staying in hotels, institutions or hospitals where the shower facilities of cooling systems have been contaminated with the organism.

b. Sporadic cases where the source of infection is unknown, most cases involve middle aged and elderly men who are smokers, but it is also seen in children.
c. Outbreaks occurring in immunocompromised patietnts, e.g. on corticosteroid therapy.
Ref: Clincial Medicine by Kumar and Clarke, 6th Ed, Pg-925

Extended information:
Leigonnaire's disease is an acute respiratory infection (pneumonia) caused by bacteria Legionella pneumophilis.
The bacteria has been found in water delivery systems and can survive in the warm, moist, air conditioning systems of large buildings including hospitals. The infection is transimmited through the respirtory route. Persons to person spread have not been proven.

Q. 446. The earliest immunoglobulin to be synthesized by the fetus is
    (a)   IgA
    (b)   IgG
    (c)   IgE
    (d)   IgM

Ans. (d)
Note
The earliest immunoglobulin to be synthesized by the fetus is 'IgM'.

See Q.No 274

Q. 447. The following are true regarding Lyme's disease, except
    (a)   It is transmitted by Ixodes tick.
    (b)   Erythema chronicum migran.
    (c)   Borrelia recurrentis is the etiological agent.
    (d)   Rodents act as natural hosts.

Ans. (c)
Note
All above are true regarding Lyme's disease, except that 'Borrelia recurrentis is the etiological agent'.
Also see
a. Is correct
b. Is Correct
c. Is incorrect as the causative agent is Borrelia burgdorferi.
d. Is correct.
Therefore the choice of answer is (c).
Ref: Harrison 15th Ed.

Q. 448. A couple, with a family history of beta thalassemia major in a distant relative, has come for counseling. The husband has HbA2 of 48% and the wife has HbA2 of 2.3%. The risk of having a child with beta thalassemia major is
    (a)   50%
    (b)   25%
    (c)   5%
    (d)   0%

Ans. (d)
Note
The risk of having a child with beta thalassemia major is '0%'.
Also see
Thalassemia is autosomal recessive, wife level of HbA 2 is normal (1-3% CMDT or HPIM 1.5-3.2 %). Husband has thalessemia.Children born can at most be carriers.
Ref: Clinical medicine By Kumar & Clarke, 6th Ed, Pg-440

Q. 449. A 2 month old baby with acute icteric viral hepatitis like illness slips into encephalopathy after 48 hours. The mother is a known hepatitis B carrier. Mother's hepatitis B virus serological profile is most likely to be
   (a)   HBsAg positive only
   (b)   HBsAg and HBeAg positive
   (c)   HBsAg and HBe antibody positive
   (d)   HBV DNA positive

Ans. (b)
Note
Mother's hepatitis B virus serological profile is most likely to be 'HBsAg and HBeAg positive'
Also see
HBs Ag carrier mothers who are HBeAg-positive alsomst invariably (>90%) transmit hepatitis B infection to their offspring, whereas HBsAg carrier mother witgh antiHBe rearely (10 to 15%) infect their offspring.
Ref: Harrison 16th Ed, Pg-1823

Q. 450. A 7 year old girl from Bihar presented with three episodes of massive hematemesis and melena. There is no history of jaundice. On examination, she had a large spleen, non-palpable liver and mild ascites. Portal vein was not visualised on ultrasonography. Liver function tests were normal and endoscopy revealed esophageal varices. The most likely diagnosis is
   (a)   Kala azar with portal hypertension
   (b)   Portal hypertension of unknown etiology
   (c)   Chronic liver disease with portal hypertension
   (d)   Portal hypertension due to extrahepatic obstruction

Ans. (d)
Note
The most likely diagnosis is 'Portal hypertension due to extrahepathic obstruction'.
Also see
The reference of Bihar is a distractor; it does not qualify for Kala azar infection. Child do not show any liver enlargement, Moreover, Kala azar is ont only cause of liver / splenic enlargement. The point of significance is that portal vein is not visualized on U/S it points to reduced blood flow across portal vein and prompts to the possibility of extra hepatic obstruction; which can explain mild ascites and splenomegaly and esophageal varices in this case.
Portal vein occlusion mayt result in massive hematemesis from gastroesophageal varices, but ascites us usually found only when cirrhosis is present.
Ref: Harrison, 16th Ed, Pg-1836

Q. 451. A 40 year old male had undergone splenectomy 20 years ago Peripheral blood smear examination would show the presence of
   (a)   Dohle bodies
   (b)   Hypersegmented neutrophils
   (c)   Spherocytes
   (d)   Howell-Jolly bodies

Ans. (d)
Note
Peripheral blood smear examination would show the presence of 'howell-Jolly bodies'
Also see
Asplenic patients should have a blood smear examined to confirm the presence of Howell-Jolly bodies indicating the absence of splenic function.
Effects of splenectomy
Splenectomy in a normal individual is followed by significant hematological alterations. Induction of similar hematological effects is made use in the treatment of certain pathological conditions.
i.   Red Cells: There is appearance of tareget cells in the blood film. Howell-Jolly bodies are present in the red cells as they are no longer cleared by the spleen. Osmotic fragility test shows increased resistance to hemolysis. Thre may be appearance of normoblasts.

ii. White cells: Thre is leucocytosis reaching its peak in 1 – 2 days after splenectomy. There is a shift to left of the myeloid cells with appearance of some myelocytes.
iii. Platelets: Within hours after splenectomy, thre is rise in platelet count up to 3-4 times.
Ref: Patholgoy Quick Review and MCQs, based on Harsh Mohan's Textbook of pathology, 5th Ed, Pg-326

Q. 452. Which of the heart valve is most likely to be involved by infective endocarditis following a septic abortion?
    (a)   Aortic valve
    (b)   Tricuspid valve
    (c)   Pulmonary valve
    (d)   Mitral valve

Ans. (b)
Note
Heart valve is most likely to be 'involved by infective endocarditis following a septic abortion 'tricuspid valve'
Also see
Damaged vascular endothelium promotes platelet and fibrin deposition which allow organism to adhere and grow. Abnormal vascular entothelium can be the result of valcular lesions, which create areas of non-laminer blood glow, or jet lesions resulting from ventricular septal defects or a patent ductus arteriosus. Infective endocarditis is less likely to develop where the hemodynamic disturbance is minimal (i.e. low pressure systems). Hence it is more common in ventricular septal defects than atrial septal defects. Aortic and mitral valves are athe commonest valves to be affected. Right sided endocarditis is typically related to intravenous drug use, although the exact pathological mechanism is that underline this association are not fully known.
Ref: Clincial Medicine By Kumar & Clarke, 6th Ed, Pg-828

Q. 453. Which of the following statements represent most correct interpretation from the ECG wave form given below?
    (a)   X-originated from an atrial ectopic focus
    (b)   X reset the cardiac rhythm
    (c)   Both heart sounds would have been present at X beat
    (d)   The path of spread of excitation was normal

Ans. (c)
Note
In the above ECG tracing X-originated from an atrial ectopic focus.
Also see
The X –complex pointed in the ECG is represents ventricular ectopic.
Choice (a) is incorrect as the ventricular ectopic arises from ventricle and not from atrial ectopic focus.
Choice (b) is incorrect as before and after the ectopic X there is no change in the rhythm.
Choice (c) is correct.
Choice (d) is incorrect as if the path of spread of excitation was noprmal than X complex in the ECG could have a Normal QRS morphology.
Refer: Shamroth.

Q. 454. A 60 year old male presented to the emergency with breathlessness, facial swelling and dilated veins on the chest wall. The most common cause is
    (a)   Thymoma
    (b)   Lung cancer
    (c)   Hodgkin's lymphoma
    (d)   Superior vena caval obstruction

Ans. (b)
Note
The most common cause for above condition is 'Lung cancer'
Also see
This man of 60 years who is having breathlessness, facial swelling and dilated veins on the chest wall suggests the superior vena caval obstruction. However the cause of this could be lung cancer, having secondaries in the mediatimum. Therefore, the choice of (b) is appropriate.

Extended information
Bronchial carcinoma can also directly invade the phrenic nerve, causing paralysis of the ipsilateral hemidiaphragm. It can involve the esophagus, producing progressive dysphagia, and the pericardium, producing pericardial effusion and malignant dysrhythmias. *Superior vena caval obstruction* causes early morning headache, facial congestion and edema involving the upper limbs; the jugular veins are distended, as are the veins on the chest that form a collateral circulation with veins arising from the abdomen.
Ref: Kumar and Clark 6th Ed, Pg-948

455. All of the following conditions may predispose to pulmonary embolism except
(a) Protein S deficiency
(b) Malignancy
(c) Obesity
(d) Progesterone therapy

Ans. (d)
Note
All of above can predispose for pulmonary emobilism except 'Progesterone therapy'.
Also see
Risk Factors for Thromboembolism:
   -Patient
   -Age
   -Obesity
   -Immobility
   -Pregnancy/puerperium
   -High dose oestrogen therapy
   -Prev. DVT/PE
   -Thrombophilia
   -Trauma or surgery, esp. pelvis, hip, lower limb.
   -Malignancy, esp. pelvic, abdominal metastatic.
   -Heart failure
   -Recent M I
   -Lower limb paralysis
   -Infection
   -Inflammatory bowel disease
   -Nephrotic syndrome
   -Polycythemia
   -Paraproteinemia
   -Paroxysmal nocturnal hemoglobinuria
   -Behcet's disease
   -Homocystinemia
Ref: http://www.gp-training.net/protocol/cardiovascular/dvt.htm

Extended information
Progesterone only contraceptive pill with this there. There is no need to stop these preparations prior to elective surgery.
Ref: http://www.gp-training.net/protocol/cardiovascular/dvt.htm
May predispose to pulmonary embolism predisposing factors for DVT:
Venosus stasis:
-Immobility (Bed rest, surgery, lomb paralysis), low cardiac output, varicose veins.
Venous injury:
   -Trauma, intravenous canaulation.
Increased coagulability:
   -Malignant disease, drugs (e.g. oestrogens, oral contraceptives), dehydration, polycythemia, nephritic syndrome, ulcerative colitis, lupus anticoagulant.
Inherited coagulation defects:
   -Antithrombin-III, Protein C, Protein S deficiency, factor V Leiden mutation.
Increased age.
Ref: API Textbook of Mediicne 7th Ed, Pg-337

Q. 456. An early systolic murmur may be caused by all of the following except
(a) Small ventricular septal defect
(b) Papillary muscle dysfunction
(c) Tricuspid regurgitation
(d) Aortic stenosis

Ans. (b)
Note
An early systolic murmur may be caused by all of the above except 'Papillary muscle dysfunction'.
Also see
Small ventricular septal defect
Presents loud pansystolic murmur and thrill maximum in 4th left ICS.
Ref: Harrison 16th Ed, Pg- 1310
Papillary muscle dysfunction (Mitral regurgititon)
Late systolic murmur; these are related to papillary muscle dysfunction caused by infarction or ischemia of these muscles or to their distortion by left ventricular dilatation.
Ref: Harrison 16th Ed, Pg- 1310
Tricuspid regurgitation
Pansystoic murmur in tricuspid area that increases with inspiration or exercise.
Ref: Medicine for students, By Golwalla. 20th Ed. Tricuspid regurgitation.
Aortic stenosis
In aortic area ejection systolic murmur beginning slightly after the first sound, rising to a peak in midsystole and tapering off before the second sound. Ejection systolic click may precede the murmur in many cases. It is caused by sudden tension of a pliable dome-shaped stenotic valve at the time of its opening. Disappears with calcification of the valve.
Ref: Medicine for students, By Golwalla. 20th Ed. Aortic stenosis.

Q. 457. The most common cause of tricuspid regurgitation is secondary to
(a) Rheumatic heart disease
(b) Dilatation of right ventricle
(c) Coronary artery disease
(d) Endocarditis due to intravenous drug abuse

Ans. (b)
Note
The most common cause of tricuspid regurgitation is secondary to 'Dilatation of the right ventricle'
Also see
Most commonly, tricuspid regurgitation is functional and secondary to marked dilatation of the right ventricle and the tricuspid annulus.
Ref: Harrison 15th Edition Valvular heart disease.

Q. 458. Absence seizures are characterized on EEG by
(a) 3 Hz spike & wave
(b) 1-2 Hz spike & wave
(c) Generalized polyspikes
(d) Hypsarrythmia

Ans. (a)
Note
Absence seizures are characterized on EEG by '3 Hz spike & wave'.
Also see
The electrophysiologic characteristic of typical absence seizures is a generalized, symmetric, 3-Hz spike-and-wave discharge that begins and ends suddenly on a normal EEG background.
Ref: Harrison 15th Edition Seizures and epilepsy.

Q. 459. All of the following heart sounds occur shortly after S2 except
(a) Opening snap
(b) Pericardial knock

(c) Ejection click
(d) Tumor plop

Ans. (c)
Note
All of the above heart sounds occur shortly after S2 except 'Ejection click'.
Also see
A pulmonary or aortic ejection sound occurs shortly after S1.
Ref: Fig 4.4 Page Cecil 6th Ed, Pg-41.

Extended information
A "tumor plop" (a sound related to movement of the tumor).

Q. 460. The most frequent cause of recurrent genital ulceration in a sexually active male is
(a) Herpes genitalis
(b) Aphthous ulcer
(c) Syphilis
(d) Chancroid

Ans. (a)
Note
The most frequent cause of recurrent genital ulceration in a sexually active male is 'Herpes genitalis'.
Also see
Herpes genitalis is caused by HSV-2 and is sexually transmitted. In males it presents as grouped vesicles on the glans or prepuce. Recurrent herpes on the penis is common.
Ref: Medicine for Students by Golwalla, 20th Edition, Pg-884.

Q. 461. The most effective drug against M leprae is
(a) Dapsone
(b) Rifampicin
(c) Clofazimine
(d) Prothionamide

Ans. (b)
Note
The most effective drug against M leprae is 'Rifampicin'.
Also see
Dapsone; inhibits bacterial folic acid synthesis. It is now considered the second drug of choice (after rifampin).
Rifampin; is considered the most active agent for the treatment of leprosy.
Clofazimine; is weakly bactericidal against *M. leprae*.
Prothionamide; may be used in place of rifampin, but they are considered less effective.
Ref: Harrison 15th Edition, Drug Information for the health care professional.

Q. 462. A 30-year old HIV positive patient presents with fever, dyspnea and non-productive cough, patient is cyanosed. His chest X-ray reveals bilateral, symmetrical interstitial infiltrates. The most likely diagnosis is
(a) Tuberculosis
(b) Cryptococcosis
(c) Pneunocystis carinii pneumonia
(d) Toxoplasmosis

Ans. (c)
Note
The most likely diagnosis is 'Pneumocystis carinii pneumonia'.
Also see
Pneumocystis carinii is an opportunistic pathogen whose natural habitat is the lung. The organism is an important cause of pneumonia in the compromised host.

In HIV subject most common pulmonary disease is pneumocystis carinii pneumonia. Physical findings include tachypnea, tachycardia, and cyanosis, but lung auscultation reveals few abnormalities. The classic findings on chest radiography consist of bilateral diffuse infiltrates beginning in the perihilar regions, but various atypical manifestations (nodular densities, cavitary lesions) have also been reported.
Ref: Harrison 15th Edition, Pneumocystis carinii infection. Pg-1194-95

Q. 463. Extensive pleural thickening and calcification especially involving the diaphragmatic pleura are classical features of
- (a) Coal worker's pneumoconiosis
- (b) Asbestosis
- (c) Silicosis
- (d) Siderosis

Ans. (b)
Note
Extensive pleural thickening and calcification especially involving the diaphragmatic pleura are classical features of 'Asbestosis'.

Also see
Asbestosis has peculiar radiological findings:
The CXR in case of asbestos past exposure is indicated by pleural plaques, which are characterized by either thickening or calcification along the parietal pleura, particularly along the lower lung fields, the diaphragm, and the cardiac border.
Ref: Harrison 15th Edition, Environmental Lung diseases Pg-1522

Q. 464. Commonest presentation of neurocysticercosis is
- (a) Seizures
- (b) Focal neurological deficits
- (c) Dementia
- (d) Radiculopathy

Ans. (a)
Note
Commonest presentation of neurocysticercosis is 'seizures'.

Also see
More common neurological manifestation are:
-Seizure associated with inflammation surrounding cysticerci in the brain parenchyma. These seizures may be generalized, focal, or Jacksonian.
Ref: Harrison, 16th Ed, Pg- 273
Neurocysticecosis can cause epilepsy.
Ref: Medicine for Students by Golwalla 10th Ed. Pg-750

Q. 465. A 60-year old man with diabetes mellitus presents with painless, swollen right ankle joint. Radiograph of the ankle shows destroyed joint with large number of loose bodies. The most probable diagnosis is
- (a) Charcot's joint
- (b) Clutton's joint
- (c) Osteoarthritis
- (d) Rheumatoid arthritis

Ans. (a)
Note
The most probable diagnosis is 'Charcot's joint'.

Also see
Charcot's joint
Charcot's joint are a feature of tabes dorsalis. (Pg-855). Loss of protective function leads to deranged joints (Charcot's Joints). Davidson Pg-1105
Diabetic neuropathy can lead to structural damage and it includes; ulcer, osteomyelitis, Charcot joint. Davidson Pg-503.

Ref: Davidson's Principles and Practice of Medicine.
Charcot's joint: Tabes dorsalis, syringomyelia and peripheral neuritis are the common causes.
Ref: A Manual of Clinical Surgery by S. Das 6th Ed, Pg-166
Clutton's joint
Congenital syphilis can be associated with painful para-articular swelling due to epiphyseal involvement soon after birth, or painless effusions (Cultton's joint) of knees in adolescents.
Ref: Davidson Pg- 655

Q. 466. Most suitable radioisotope of iodine for treating hyperthyroidism is
    (a)   Iodine-123
    (b)   Iodine-125
    (c)   Iodine-131
    (d)   Iodine-132

Ans. (c)
Note
Most suitable radioisotope of iodine for treating hyperthyroidism is 'Iodine-131'.
Also see
Internal radiotherapy is by administering or planting a small radiation source, usually a gamma or beta emitter, in the target area. Iodine-131 is commonly used to treat thyroid cancer, probably the most successful kind of cancer treatment. It is also used to treat non-malignant thyroid disorders.
The hyperthyroidism of Graves's disease is treated by reducing thyroid hormone synthesis, using antithyroid drugs, or by reducing the amount of thyroid tissue with radioiodine (^{131}I) treatment or by subtotal thyroidectomy.
Ref: Harrison, 16th Ed, Pg- 2115

Q. 467. All of the following statements are correct about potassium balance, except
    (a)   Most of potassium is intracellular.
    (b)   Three quarter of the total body potassium is found in skeletal muscle.
    (c)   Intracellular potassium is released into extra-cellular space in response to severe injury.
    (d)   Acidosis leads to movement of potassium from extracellular to intracellular fluid compartment.

Ans. (d)
Note
All of the above statements are correct about potassium balance, except option '(d)'.
Also see
The converse, movement of K^+ into cells, may be seen with metabolic alkalosis.
Ref: Harrison 15th Edition, 49 Fluid and Electrolyte disturbances.

Q. 468. Hypocalcemia is characterized by all of the following features except
    (a)   Numbness and tingling of circumoral region
    (b)   Hyperactive tendon reflexes
    (c)   Shortening of Q-T interval in ECG
    (d)   Carpopedal spasm

Ans. (c)
Note
Hypocalcemia is characterized by all of the following features except 'Shortening of Q-T inverval in ECG'.
Also see
The QT interval on the electrocardiogram is prolonged, in contrast to its shortening with hypercalcemia.
Ref: Harrison 15th Edition, Section 2 Disorders of Bone and Mineral Metabolism.

Q. 469. All of the following are risk factors for deep vein thrombosis (DVT) except
    (a)   Duration of surgery more than thirty minutes
    (b)   Obesity
    (c)   Age less than forty years
    (d)   Use of the oestrogen-progesterone contraceptive pills

Ans. (c)

Note
All of the above are risk factors for deep vein thrombosis (DVT) except 'age less than forty years'.
Also see
The risk factors for deep vein thrombosis are all of above except (c).
Factors predisposing to venous thrombosis are:
Patient factors:
- Varicose veins
- Previous deep venous thrombosis
- Oral contraceptives
- Pregnancy / puerperium
- Dehydration
- Immobility

Surgical Condition:
- Surgery especially if > 30 minutes duration, abdominal or pelvic orthropaedic to lower limb

Medical condition:
- Myocardial infarction / Heart failure
- Inflammatory bowel disease
- Malignancy
- Nephrotic syndrome
- Bethcat's syndrome
- Homocystinemia

Hematological disorders:
- Primary proliferative polycythemia
- Essential thrombocythemia
- Myelofibrosis
- Paroxysmal nocturnal hemoglobinuria

Deficiency of anticoagulants:
- Antithrombin
- Protein C
- Protein S
- Factor II or V Leiden

Antiphospholipid antibody:
- Lupus anticoagulant
- Anticardiolipin antibody

Ref: Davidson 16th Ed, Pg-795, Kumar and Clark 6th Ed – Pg-477

Q. 470. A labourer involved with repair-work of sewers was admitted with fever, jaundice and renal failure. The most appropriate test to diagnose the infection in this patient is
    (a)   Weil Felix test
    (b)   Paul Bunnel test
    (c)   Microscopic agglutination test
    (d)   Micro immunofluorescence test

Ans. (c)
Note
The most appropriate test to diagnose the infection in this patient is 'microscopic agglutination test'.
Also see
Leptospirosis is a zoonosis that especially rats. Transmission of leptospires may follow direct contact with urine, blood, or tissue from an infected animal or exposure to a contaminated environment; human-to-human transmission is rare. The most severe form of leptospirosis (Weil's syndrome), is characterized by jaundice, renal dysfunction, hemorrhagic diathesis, and high mortality.
A definite diagnosis of leptospirosis is based either on isolation of the organism from the patient or on seroconversion or a rise in antibody titer in the microscopic agglutination test (MAT).
Ref: Harrison 16th Ed, Pg-990

Q. 471. Gluten sensitive enteropathy is most strongly associated with
    (a)   HLA-DQ2
    (b)   HLA-DR4
    (c)   HLA-DQ3
    (d)   Blood group 'B'

Ans. (a)
Note
Gluten sensitive enteropathy is most strongly associated with 'HLA-DQ3.

Also see
Genetic factor(s) also appear to be involved in celiac sprue; about 95% of patients with celiac sprue express the HLA-DQ2 allele.
Ref: Harrison, 16th Ed, Pg-314

Q. 472. Most sensitive and specific test for diagnosis of iron deficiency is
    (a)   Serum iron levels
    (b)   Serum ferritin levels
    (c)   Serum transferrin receptor population
    (d)   Transferrin saturation

Ans. (b)
Note
Most sensitive and specific test for diagnosis of iron deficiency is 'Serum ferritin levels'.

Also see
The serum ferritin is used to evaluate total-body iron stores. Adult males have serum ferritin levels that average about 100 ug/L, corresponding to iron stores of about 1 g. Adult females have lower serum ferritin levels averaging 30 ug/L, reflecting lower iron stores. A serum ferritin level of 10 to 15 ug/L represents depletion of body iron stores.
Ref: Harrison, 15th Edition, Iron deficiency anemia
Three stages of Iron deficiency have been described.
a.   First stage characterised by decreased storage of iron without any other detectable abnormalities.
b.   An intermediate stage of 'Latent iron deficinecy' that is iron stores are exhausted, but anemia has not occurred as yet. Its recognition depends upon measurement of serum ferritin levels. The percentage saturation of transferring falls from a normal value of 30% to less than 15%. This is the most widely prevalent stage in India.
c.   The third stage is that of overt iron deficicncy when thre is a decrease in the concentration of circulating hemoglobin due to impaired hemoglobin synthesis.
    The end result of iron deficiency is nutritional anemia which is not a disease intitiy. It is rather syndrome cause by malnutrition.
Ref: Park and Park 16th Ed. Pg-416-17.

Q. 473. Exercise testing is absolutely contraindicated in which one of the following
    (a)   One week following myocardial infarction
    (b)   Unstable angina
    (c)   Aortic stenosis
    (d)   Peripheral vascular disease

Ans. (b)
Note
Exercise testing is absolutely contraindicated in 'Unstable angina' out of the above.

Also see
The patients who are suitable candidates for revascularization should undergo an exercise tolerance test approximately 4 weeks after the infarct; this will help to idendtify those individuals with significant residual myocardial ischaemia and require further investigation.
Ref: Davidson 18th Ed, Pg-265

Q. 474. A nineteen year old female with short stature, wide spread nipples and primary amenorrhea most likely has a karyotype of
  (a) 47, XX+18
  (b) 46, XXY
  (c) 47, XXY
  (d) 45 X

Ans. (d)
Note
Most likely has a karyotype is '45 X'.

Also see
A female with short stature, wide spread nipples and primary amenorrhea most likely has a karyotype of 45X (Turner's syndrome).
Ref: Harrison's 16th Ed, Pg-2215

Q. 475. A 23-year old woman has experienced episodes of myalgias, pleural effusion, pericarditis and arthralgias without joint deformity over course of several years. The best laboratory screening test to diagnose her disease would be
  (a) D4 lymphocyte count
  (b) Erythrocyte sedimentation rate
  (c) Antinuclear antibody
  (d) Assay for thyroid hormones

Ans. (c)
Note
The best laboratory screening test to diagnose her disease would be 'Antinuclear antibody'.

Also see
Above symptoms do not correspond to AIDS – CD4 count is useless.
ESR shows only organic pathology that is already there.
Antinuclear antibody is important and best screening test for SLE and ther features of above clinical conditions could be due to SLE.
Ref: Harrison 16th Ed, Pg-1961
Assay for Thyroid harmone is also un-ecessary as clinical features given above are not in favour of hypo or hyperthyroidism.

Q. 476. A 5-year old boy is detected to be HBsAg positive on two separate occasions during a screening program for hepatitis B. He is otherwise asymptomatic. Child was given 3 doses of recombinant hepatitis B vaccine at the age of one year. His mother was treated for chronic hepatitis B infection around the same time. The next relevant step for further investigating the child would be to
  (a) Obtain HBe Ag and anti-HBe antibodies
  (b) Obtain anti-HBs levels
  (c) Repeat HBsAg
  (d) Repeat another course of hepatitis B vaccine

Ans. (a)
Note
The next relevant step for further investigationng the child would be 'Obtaining HBe Ag and Anti HBe antibodies'.

Also see
HbsAg positive serum containing HBeAg is more likely to be highly infectious and to be associated with the presence of hepatitis B virions (and detectable HBV DNA,) than HBeAg negative or anti-HBe-positive serum. For example, HBsAg carrier mothers who are HBeAg-positive alsomst invariably (>90%) transmit hepatitis B infection to their offspring, whereas HBsAg carrier mothers with anti-HBe rarely (10 to 15%) infect their offspring. The aim is to know whether the child is carrier / chronically affected.
Early during the course of acute hepataitis B, HBeAg appears transiently; its disappearance may be a harbinger of clinical improvement and resolution of infection. Persistence of HBeAg in serum beyond the first 3 months of acute infection may be predictive of development of chronic infection, and the presence of HbeAg during chronic hepatitis B is associated with ongoing viral replication, infectiontivity, and inflammatory liver injury.
Ref: Harrison 16th Ed, Pg-1823

Q. 477. Which of the following hepatitis viruses have significant perinatal transmission?
  (a) Hepatitis E virus
  (b) Hepatitis C virus
  (c) Hepatitis B virus
  (d) Hepatitis A virus

Ans. (c)
Note
'Hepatitis B virus' hepatitis viruses have significant perinatal transmission.
Also see
Mode of transmission
HBV is transmitted by the blood-borne route in recipients of infected blood and blood products, intravenous drug abusers, hemodialysis patients, sexual transmission, percutaneous exposure like needle stick injuries, shared razor blades, tattooing, acupuncture, shared tooth brushes and maternal to fetal transmission. In India 60% of infections are acquired horizontally, while 20% of infections results from mother to child vertical transmission.
Ref: API Textbook of Medicine 7th Ed, Pg-597

Q. 478. Osler's nodes are typically seen in which one of the following?
  (a) Chronic candida endocarditis
  (b) Acute staphylococcal endocarditis
  (c) Pseudomonas endocarditis
  (d) Libman sack's endocarditis

Ans. (b)
Note
The osler's nodes are typically seen in acute staphylococcal endocarditis.
Also see
Osler's nodes are painful, tender, pea-sized erythmatous nodules in the pulp of fingers which trend to occur in crops and are indicators either of embolism to distal digital arteries or an immunological phenomenon.
Ref: API Textbook of Medicine 7th Ed,Pg-427

Q. 479. Thiamine deficiency is known to occur in all of the following except
  (a) Food faddist
  (b) Homocystinemia
  (c) Chronic alcoholic
  (d) Chronic heart failure patients on diuretics

Ans. (b)
Note
Thiamine deficiency is known to occur in all of the following except 'Homocystinemia'.
Also see
Elevated plasma levels of homocysteine have been assorated with increased cardiovascular risk, independent of known risk factors, in several epidemiological studies. Even modest elevations of homocysteine may lead to significant increases in risk. One important determinant of plasma homocysteine levels is B-vitamin status; suboptimal intake or impaired absorption offolate, vitamin B6, or vitamin B12 can lead to increases in homocysteine.
Harrison 16th Ed, Pg-2334

Q. 480. Radiation exposure during infancy has been linked to which one of the following carcinoma?
  (a) Breast
  (b) Melanoma
  (c) Thyroid
  (d) Lung

Ans. (c)
Note
Radiation exposure to head and neck in child hood is a risk factor for thyroid cancer.
Ref: Harrison 15th Edition, Disorders of the thyroid gland.

Q. 481. Following are the features of corticospinal involvement except
    (a) Cog-wheel rigidity
    (b) Spasticity
    (c) Plantar extensor response
    (d) Exaggerated deep tendon reflexes

Ans. (a)
Note
Following are the features of corticospinal involvement except 'Cog-wheel rigidity'.
Also see
The pyramidal tract lesions are b, c, and d. the Cog-wheel rigidity is the feature of extrapyramidal involvement.
Evidence of upper motor neuron lesions are:
    -Increased tone of spastic type
    -Exaggerated tendon reflexes
    -An extensor planter response
    -Loss of fine finger / toe movements
    -Loss of abdominal reglexes
    -No muscle wasting
    -Normal electrical excitability of muscle
Ref: Kumar and Clark 6th Ed, Pg-1192

Q. 482. The most common mode of inheritance of congenital heart disease is (ALL INDIA/02)
    (a) Autosomal dominant
    (b) Autosomal recessive
    (c) Sex linked dominant
    (d) Multifactorial

Ans. (d)
Note
The most common mode of inheritance of congenital heart disease is 'Multifactorial'.
Also see
The overall congenital heart disease (CHD) is 1 per 100 live births; it is more common in premature babies as there is a high rate of patency of ductus arteriousus and a four times higher prevalence of ventricular sepatal defect..
The aetiologgical mechanisms included:
a. Primary genetic factors 8%
b. Primary environmental factors 2%
c. Multifactorial inheritance 90%
Multifactorial genetic and environmental factor account for the majority of cases.
Ref: API Textbook of Medicine 7th Ed, Pg-465

Q. 483. Which one of the following is an autosomal dominant disorder? (ALL INDIA/02)
    (a) Cystic fibrosis
    (b) Hereditary spherocytosis
    (c) Sickle cell anemia
    (d) G-6-PD deficiency

Ans. (b)
Note
From above the 'Hereditary spherocytosis' is an autossomal dominant disorder'.
Also see
Autosomal diseases are inherited through the non-sex chromosomes (pairs 1 through 22). Dominant inheritance occurs when an abnormal gene from one parent is capable of causing disease even though the matching gene from the other parent is normal. The abnormal gene dominates the outcome of the gene pair.
Chances of inheriting a trait for an autosomal dominant disorder:
If one parent has an abnormal gene and the other parent a normal gene, there is a 50% chance each child will inherit the abnormal gene, and therefore the dominant trait.

If it is assumed that 4 children are produced from a couple in which one parent has an abnormal gene for a dominant disease, the statistical expectation is for:
- 2 children normal
- 2 children with the disease

It means that EACH child has a 50:50 chance of inheriting the disorder. Children who do not inherit the abnormal gene will not develop or pass on the disease.

Autosomal dominant diseases are:
Hereditary sphrecytosis, Familial hypercholesterolemia, Huntington's disease, Marfan's syndrome, Neurofibromatosis, Tuberous sclerosis, Von Hipple-Lindau Syndrome, Autosomal Dominat Polycystic Kidney Disease.

Hereditary Spherocytosis:
Hereditary spherocytosis is a common type of hereditary hemolytic anemia of autosomal dominanct inheritance in which the red cell membrane is abnormal.

Ref: Pathology Quick Review and MCQ's Based on TB of Pathology by Harsh Mohan, 5th Ed, Pg-270

Q. 484. Which type diabetes is HLA associated? (ALL INDIA/02)
(a) Type I diabetes
(b) Tyep II diabetes
(c) Malnutrition related type dibetes
(d) Pregnancy related type diabetes

Ans. (a)

Note
'Type I diabetes' is HLA associated diabetes.

Also see
Type I diabetes (IDDM) are either HLA DR3 or HLA DR4. No HLA association is seen with Type II diabetes (NIDDM). During the 1970s investiogations revealed some links between bearing so certain human leucocyte antigens (HLA) and incidnecne of type I DM

Ref: API Textbook of Medicine 7th Ed, Pgf-1100

Q. 485. All of the following are sexually transmitted, except (ALL INDIA/02)
(a) Candida albicans
(b) Echionococcus
(c) Molluscum contagiosum
(d) Group B streptococcus

Ans. (b)

Note
Echinococcus granulosus spreasds by orofecal route.

Also see
The classificatuion of sexually transmitted disease agents:
1. **Bacterial agents**
   a. Neisseria gonorrheae
   b. Chlamydia trachomatis
   c. Treponema pallidum
   d. Hemophilus ducreyi
   e. Mycoplasma hominis
   f. Ureaplasma urelyticum
   g. Calymmatobacterium granulosatis
   h. Shigella spp.
   i. Campylobacteter app
   j. Group B streptococcus
   k. Bacterial vaginosis – associated organism
2. **Viral agents**
   a. Human (alpha) herpes virus 1 or 2 (Herpes simplex virus)
   b. Human (beta) herpes virus 5 (formerly cytomegalo virus)
   c. Hepatitis virus B
   d. Human papilloma virus

    e. Molluscus contagiosum virus
    f. Human immunodeficiency virus
3. **Protozoal agents**
    a. Entamoeba histolytica
    b. Giardia lambia
    c. Trichomonas vaginalis
4. **Fungal agents**
    a. Candida albicans
    b. Ectoparasite
    c. Phthirus pubis
    d. Sarcoptes scabiei

Ref: Preventive and social Medicine by Park and Park 18th Ed, Pg-265

Q. 486. All of the following infections may be transmitted via blood transfusion, except (ALL INDIA/02)
(a) Parvo B19
(b) Dengue virus
(c) Cytomegalovirus
(d) Hepatitis G virus

Ans. (b)
Note
All of the above infections may be transmitted via blood transfusion, except 'Dengue virus'.
Also see
Arboviruses are a group of viruses transmitted by arthropods to vertebrate hosts. This host might be a human or a lower animal. Virus replication takes plce in the artherpod vector which is a mosquito, tick, sand fly or midge. The vertebrate host becomes viremic following a bite and then in turns capable of passing on the infection to a second biting arthropod. Therefore, the denguevirus is not transmitted via blood transfusion.
Ref: API Terxtbook of Medicine 7th Ed, Pg-99

Q. 487. Hypoglycemia is a recognized feature of all of the following conditions except (ALL INDIA/02)
(a) Uremia
(b) Acromegaly
(c) Addison's disease
(d) Hepatocellular failure

Ans. (b)
Note
Hypoglycemia is a recognized feature of all of the following conditions except 'Acromegaly'.
Also see
Acromegaly is associated with hyperglycaemia (diabetes mellitus).
Ref: API Terxtbook of Medicine 7th Ed, Pg-1099

Q. 488. All of the following feature may be seen in thrombotic thrombocytopenic purpura, except (ALL INDIA/02)
(a) Fever
(b) Hemolysis
(c) Hypertension
(d) Low platelet count

Ans. (c)
Note
All of the above feature may be seen in thrombotic thrombocytopenic purpura, except 'Hypertension'.
Also see
Thrombotic thrombocytopenic purpura is a disorder of vessel wall characterised by lesions in arteriolar walls in various organs. Features of thrombotic thrombocytopenic purpura include thrombocytopenia, hemolytic anemia, fever, renal failure, fluctuating levels of consciousness.
Classical pentad of TTP consists of hemolytic anemia with fragmentation of erythrocytes and signs of intravascular

hemolysis, thrombocytopenia, diffuse and non-focal neurological findings, decreased renal function and fever.
Ref: Harrison 16th Ed, Pg-678

Q. 489. The following laboratory determinants is abnormally prolonged in ITP (ALL INDIA/02)
(a) APTT
(b) Prothrombin time
(c) Bleeding time
(d) Clotting time

Ans. (c)

Note
From above laboratory determinants 'Bleeding time' is abnormally prolonged in ITP.

Also see
The function of platelets is best evidenced by the bleeding time. As the platelets are affected in all types of thrombocytopenia, the bleeding time is also altered.
Prothormbin Time, APTT (Activated Partial Thromboplastin Time), and clotting time are associated with disorders of coagulation.
Bleeding time (BT) is a measure of interaction of platelets with the blood vessel wall. A prolonged bleeding time is seen in thrombocytopenia.
Ref: API Textbook of Medicine 7th Ed, Pg-926
In ITP, platelet survival studies reveal markedly reduced platelet life span, sometimes less than one hour as against normal life span of 7-10 days.
Ref: Pathology quick review and MCQs, based on harshmohan's textbook of pathology.

Q. 490. Hypergastrinemia with hypochlorhydria is seen in (ALL INDIA/02)
(a) Zollinger-Ellison syndrome
(b) VIPoma
(c) Pernicious anemia
(d) Glucagonoma

Ans. (c)

Note
Hypergastrinemia wiht hypochlorhydria is seen in pernicious anemia.

Also see
In pernicious anemia, lab examination shows hypergastrinemia and pentagastrin-fast achlorhydria.
Ref: Harrison 16th Ed, Pg-604

Q. 491. All of the following phases of the jugular venous pulse and their causes are correctly matched, except (ALL INDIA/02)
(a) 'c'wave – onset of atrial systole
(b) 'a-x' descent – atrial relaxation
(c) 'v-y' descent – emptying of blood from right atrium into right ventricle
(d) 'y-a' ascent – filling of the right atrium from the vena cava

Ans. (a)

Note
All of the above phases of the jugular venous pulse and their causes are correctly matched, except '(a)'.

Also see
The *c* wave, often observed in the JVP, is a positive wave produced by the buldging of the tricuspid valve into the right atrium during right ventricular isovolumetric systole and by the impact of the carotid artery adjacent to the jugular vein.
Ref: Harrison 16th Ed, Pg-1306

Q. 492. Which of the following is the correct statement regarding findings in JVP? (ALL INDIA/02)
(a) Cannon wave: Complete heart block
(b) Slow v-y descent: Tricuspid regurgitation
(c) Giant c wave: Tricuspid stenosis
(d) Increased JVP with prominent pulsations:SVC obstruction

Ans. (a)

Note
From above the correct statement regarding findings in JVP is 'cannon wave: complete heart block'.

Also see
"Cannon" *a* wave may occur regularly(as during junctional rhythm) or irregularly (as in atrioventricular dissociation with ventricular tachycardia or *complete heart block)*.
Ref: Harrison 16th Ed, Pg-1306

Q. 493. All of the following are clinical features of myxoma, except (ALL INDIA/02)
    (a)   Fever
    (b)   Clubbing
    (c)   Hypertension
    (d)   Embolic phenomenon

Ans. (c)
Note
All of the above are clinical features of myxoma, except 'hypertension'.

Also see
Constitutional manifestations are weight loss, fever, fatigue, anemia, joint pains and rash. Elevation of ESR and serum globulins, leucocytosis, thrombocytopenia and clubbing also occurs. Embolic phenomenon is also seen in the systemic arterial circulation.
Ref: API Textbook of Medicine 7th Ed, Pg-495

Q. 494. Renal vein thrombosis is most commonly associated with (ALL INDIA/02)
    (a)   Diabetic nephropathy
    (b)   Membranous glomerulonephritis
    (c)   Minimal change disease
    (d)   Membranoproliferative glomerulonephritis

Ans. (b)
Note
Renal vein thrombosis is most commonly associated with 'Membranous glomerulonephritis'.

Also see
Renal vein thrombosis is common in pregnant women, users of oral contraceptives, subjects with nephrotic syndrome, or dehydrated infants. Nephrotic syndrome accompanying membranous glomerulopathy and certain carcinomas seems to predispose to the development of RVT, which occurs in 10 to 50% of patients with these disorders.
Harrisons 15t Edition. Disorders of the kidney and urinary tracat.
Membranous glomerulonephritis is the commonest glomerular disease associated with hypercoaguable state and renal vein thrombosis.
Ref: API Textbook of Medicine 7th Ed, Pg-666

Q. 495. Characteristic of Henoch-Schonlein purpura is (ALL INDIA/02)
    (a)   Blood in stool
    (b)   Thrombocytopenia
    (c)   Intracranial hemorrhage
    (d)   Susceptibility to infection

Ans. (a)
Note
Characteristic of Henoch-Schonlein purpura is 'Blood in stool'.

Also see
Henoch Schonlein purpura is a systemic vasculitic syndrome involving small and medium sized vessels and presents as under:
    -Skin; purpuric skin lesions
    -Joint; arthralgia
    -GIT; colic, malena, hematemesis
    -Renal; proteinuria, microsopic hematuria

Extended information
Gastro-intestinal involvement in Henoch-Schonlein purpura is charecterised by colicky abdominal pain usually associated wioth nausea, vomiting, diarrhea or constipation and is frequently accompanied by passage of blood and mucous per rectum.
Ref: Harrison 16th Ed, Pg-2010

Q. 496. Renal osteodystropy differs from nutritional and genetic forms of oesteomalacia in having (ALL INDIA/02)
    (a)   Hypocalcemia
    (b)   Hypercalcemia
    (c)   Hypophosphatemia
    (d)   Hyerphosphatemia

Ans. (d)
Note
Renal osteodystropy differs from nutritional and genetic forms of osteomalacia in having 'hyperphosphatemia'.

Also see
As renal failure advances the decrease in functional renal mass and hyperphosphatemia results in decrease 1-α hydroxylase activity, thus decreasing production of 1, 25-$(OH)_2D_3$.
Ref: API Textbook of Medicine 7th Ed, Pg. 697

Q. 497. A patient with nephrotic syndrome on long- standing corticosteroid therapy may develop all the following except (ALL INDIA/02)
    (a)   Hyperglycemia
    (b)   Hypertophy of muscle
    (c)   Neuropsychiatric symptoms
    (d)   Suppression of the pituitary adrenal axis

Ans. (b)
Note
A patient with nephrotic syndrome on long- standing corticosteroid therapy may develop all the following except 'hypertrophy of muscle'.

Also see
Iatrogenic Cushing's syndrome
Prolonged therapeutic uses of glucocorticids or ACTH may result in Cushing's syndrome which causes severe osteoporosis, proximal myopathy & muscle wasting.
Ref: Harshmohan's Handbook of Pathology, 5th Ed; Pg 604,
Ref: API 7th Ed; Pg 1071.

Q. 498. A 40 years old man presented with repeated episodes of bronchospasm and hemoptysis. Chest X-ray revealed perihilar bronchiectasis. The most likely diagnosis is (ALL INDIA/02)
    (a)   Sarcoidosis
    (b)   Idiopathic pulmonary fiborsis
    (c)   Extrinsic allergic alveolitis
    (d)   Bronchopulmonary aspergillosis

Ans. (d)
Note
Repeated episodes of bronchospasm, hemoptysis, and cental bronchiectasis are suggestive of Broncho-pulmonary aspergillosis.

Also see
Allergic broncopulmonary aspergillosis occurs in patients with pre-existing asthma or cystic fibrosis & causes intermittent episodes of wheezing, pulmonary infiltrates from transient bronchial plugging, sputum and blood eosinophilia, low grade fever brownish thick greenish flecks in sputum .some patients with repeated exacerbations develop central bronchiectasis and progressive loss of pulmonary function.
Ref: Harrison 16th Ed. Pg- 1188

Q. 499. Which of the following is characteristically not associated with the development of interstitial lung disease? (ALL INDIA/02)
(a) Coal dust
(b) Sulphur dioxide
(c) Thermophilic actenomycetes
(d) Tobacco smoke

Ans. (d)

Note
All above can be associated ith the development of interstitial lung disease except; Tobacco smoke'.

Also see
Dangers of cigarette smoking:
General:
    Lung cancer
    COPD
    Oesophagus CA
    Ischemic heart disease
    Peripheral vascular disease
    Blood cancer
    Abnormal spermatozoa
    Memory problems.
Maternal:
    Low birth wt. baby
    Neonatal mortality
    Increase in asthma
Passive smoking:
    Risk of athma, pneumonia & bronchitis in infants of smoking parents.
    Increase in cough & breath lessness in smokers & nonsmokers with COPD & asthma.
    Increased cancer risk.
    Atmospheric air pollution due to burning of coal for energy & heat has been characteristic of urban living in developed countries from two centuries it consists black smoke (coal burning) & SO_2.

Ref: Kumar & Clarke, Ed; 6th. Table No.14.6, Pg -893

Q. 500. A 35 years old man was found +ve for HBsAg and HBeAg, accidentally during screening of blood donation. On laboratory examination SGOT and SGPT are normal. What should you do next? (ALL INDIA/02)
(a) Liver biopsy
(b) Interferon therapy
(c) Observation
(d) HBV-DNA estimation

Ans. (d)

Note
HBV-DNA estimation is next investition which point to HBV replication.

Also see
Detection of HBV-DNA by molecular hybradisation using the southern blot technique is the most effective index of hepatitis B infection. It is present in pre-symptomatic phase & transiently during early acute stage.
Ref: Handbook of Harsh Mohan's Pathology 5th Ed. Pg-446

Q. 501. A 25 years women presents with bloody diarrhea and is diagnosed as a case of ulcerative colitis. Which of the following condition is not associated? (ALL INDIA/02)
(a) Sclerosing cholengitis
(b) Iritis
(c) Ankylosing spondylitis
(d) Pancreatitis

Ans. (d)

Note
The pancreatitis is not associated with ulcerative colitis as extra-intestinal disease.
Also see
The extra-intestinal diseases associated with ulcerative colitis can be autoimmune hepatitis, Primary Sclerosing Cholengitis, Cholangiocarcinoma, Gallstones, Amyloidosis, oxalate calculi, Iritis, Episcleritis, Anklosig Spondylitis.
Ref: Davidsnon's 20th Ed. Pg-914, Fig-22.53

Q. 502. Investigation of choice for invasive amebiasis is (ALL INDIA/02)
    (a)   Indirect hemagglutination
    (b)   ELISA
    (c)   Counter immune electrophoresis
    (d)   Microscopy

Ans. (b)
Note
Investigation of choice for invasive amebiasis is 'ELISA'.
Also see
Now a days Serology is an important addition for diagnosis of invasive amebiasis. ELISAs are available, and the results of these tests are positive in more than 90% of patients with colitis, amebomas, or liver abscess. Positive results in association with the corresponding clinical syndrome suggest active disease because serologic findings usually revert to negative within 6 to 12 months.
Ref: Harrisons 15th Editon, Protozoal infections.

Q. 503. A 20 years young man presents with exertional dyspnea, headache, and giddiness. On examination, there is hypertension and LVH. X-ray picture shows notching of the anterior ends of the ribs. The most likely diagnosis is (ALL INDIA/02)
    (a)   Pheochromocytoma
    (b)   Carcinoid syndrome
    (c)   Coarctation of the aorta
    (d)   Superior mediastinal syndrome

Ans. (c)
Note
The most like diagnosis is with above clincail features is 'Coarctation of aorta'.
Also see
Notching of the ribs, an important radiographic sign, is due to erosion by dilated collateral vessels, in case of Coarctation of aorta.
Ref: Harrisons 15th Edition, Congenital heart diseases.

Q. 504. Rheumatoid factor in rheumatoid arthritis is important because (ALL INDIA/02)
    (a)   RA factor is associated with bad prognosis.
    (b)   Absent RA factor rules out the diagnosis of rheumatoid arthritis.
    (c)   It is very common in childhood-rheumatoid arthritis.
    (d)   It correlates with disease activity.

Ans. (d)
Note
Rheumatoid factor in rheumatoid arthritis is important because is 'correlates with disease activity'.
Also see
RA factor is associated with bad prognosis. It is seen that aggressive disease is largely restricted to those patients with high titers of rheumatoid factor. By contrast, elderly patients who develop RA without elevated titers of rheumatoid factor (seronegative disease) generally have less severe, often self-limited disease.
Ref: Harrisons 15th Edition, Rheumatoid arthtitis.

Q. 505. Conn's syndrome is associated with all except (ALL INDIA/02)
    (a)   Hypertension
    (b)   Hypernatremia

(c) Hypokalemia
(d) Edema

Ans. (d)

Note
Conn's syndrome is associated with all of the abvoe except 'edema'.

Also see
Conn's Syndrome: Hypersecretion of aldosterone increases the renal distal tubular exchange of intratubular sodium for secreted potassium and hydrogen ions, with progressive depletion of body potassium and development of hypokalemia. Most patients have diastolic hypertension, which may be very severe, and headaches. The hypertension is probably due to the increased sodium reabsorption and extracellular volume expansion. *Potassium depletion* is responsible for the muscle weakness and fatigue and is due to the effect of potassium depletion on the muscle cell membrane. The polyuria results from impairment of urinary concentrating ability and is often associated with polydipsia.
Harrison; 15th Edition, Section 1 Endocrinology. 331. Disorders of adrenal cortex

Q. 506. The triad originally described by Zollinger-Ellison syndrome is characterized by (ALL INDIA/02)
    (a) Peptic ulceration, gastric hypersecretion, non beta cell tumour
    (b) Peptic ulceration, gastric hypersecretion, beta cell tumour
    (c) Peptic ulceration, achlorhydria, non beta cell tumour
    (d) Peptic ulceration, achlorhydria, beta cell tumour

Ans. (a)

Note
The triad originally described by Zollinger-Ellison syndrome is characterized by '(a)'.

Also see
Severe peptic ulcer diathesis secondary to gastric acid hypersecretion due to unregulated gastrin release from a non-Beta cell endocrine tumor (gastrinoma) defines the components of the ZES.
Ref: Harrison, 15th Edition,285 Peptic ulcer disease and related disorders.

Q. 507. All of the following are features of pheochromocytoma except (ALL INDIA/02)
    (a) Hypertensive paroxysm
    (b) Headache
    (c) Orthostatic hypotension
    (d) Wheezing

Ans. (d)

Note
All of the following are features of pheochromocytoma except 'wheezing'.

Also see
Most patients come to medical attention as a result of hypertensive crisis, paroxysmal symptoms suggestive of anxiety attacks, or hypertension which is associated with headaches, excessive sweating, and/or palpitations. Orthostatic hypotension is a consequence of diminished plasma volume and blunted sympathetic reflexes.
Ref: Harrison, 332 Pheochromocytoma.
Paroxysmal sustained hypertension is the commonest presenting feature other symptoms are abdominal and chest pain headache sweating palpitation gastrointestinal symptoms weakness, visual disturbances, orthostatic hypotension or increased pressure response to anesthesia may occur.
Ref: API 7th Ed, Pg-1077

Q. 508. A 60 years old man presents with nonproductive cough for 4 weeks. He has grade III clubbing, and a lesion in the apical lobe on X-ray. Most likely diagnosis here is (ALL INDIA/01)
    (a) Small cell CA
    (b) Non-small cell CA
    (c) Fungal infection
    (d) Tuberculosis

Ans. (b)

Note
Most likely diagnosis here is for above featuer is 'Non-small cell CA.

Also see
The incidence of CA lungs increases between 55 and 65years. 90% pateitns with lung cancers of all histologic types are cigarette smokers. Particularly with the non small cell cardinomas of lung has associated clubbing. In the given clinical situation the non productive cough and clubbing with associated radiographic finding of lesion in the apical lobe points to 'non-small cell cancers'. However, this presentation of localized lesion may be cured with either surgery or radiotherapy. Non-small cell cancers do not respond as well to chemotherapy as small cell cancers.
Ref: Harrison 15th Edition, Neoplasm of lung.

Q. 509. A 60 years old man is suspected of having bronchogenic CA, TB has been ruled out in this patient, what should be the next investigation? (ALL INDIA/01)
    (a)   CT guided FNAC
    (b)   Bronchoscopy and biopsy
    (c)   Sputum cytology
    (d)   X-ray chest

Ans. (b)
Note
The next investigation in above situation is 'Bronchoscopy and biopsy'.

Also see
As the signs, symptoms, or screening studies hint at lung cancer, a tissue diagnosis is must. The tumor tissue may be obtained by a bronchial or transbronchial biopsy during fiberoptic bronchoscopy.
Ref: Harrison 15th Edition, Neoplasm of lung.

Q. 510. A man presents with fever, weight loss and cough. Mantoux reads an induration of 17 × 19 mm; sputum cytology is negative for AFB. Most likely diagnosis is (ALL INDIA/01)
    (a)   Pulmonary tuberculosis
    (b)   Fungal infection
    (c)   Viral infection
    (d)   Pneumonia

Ans. (a)
Note
With above features the most likely diagnosis is 'Pulmonary tuberculosis'.

Also see
All the feature in given clinical situation points to pulmonary tuberculosis. However, negative cytology for AFB do not rule out the possibility of tuberculosis.

Extended information
In some cases culture will be negative but a clinical diagnosis of tuberculosis will be supported by positive PPD skin test & a compatible clinical & radiographic response to treatment.
Ref: Harrison, 16th Ed, Pg-961

Q. 511. A 26 years old asymptomatic woman is found to have arrhythmias and a systolic murmur associated with midsystolic clicks. Which investigation would you use? (ALL INDIA/01)
    (a)   Electrophysiological testing
    (b)   CT scan
    (c)   Echocardiography
    (d)   Angiography

Ans. (c)
Note
With above features the most likely investigation suggested is 'Echocardiography'.

Also see
The above clinical situation points to:
    -Pt is young female of 26 years of age

-Asymptomatic
-Pulse shows arrhythmias
Auscultaroty findings are:
-Systolic murmur associated with midsystolic clicks.
Above features points to the diagnosis of 'mirtal valve prolapse'.

Extended information
Mitral valve prolapse; as it is more common in females, common age is 14 – 30 years. Most patients remain asymptomatic. Arrhythmias occur mostly due to ventricular premature contractuions or paroxysmal or supraventricular tachycardia. On auscultation the most important finding is mid or late systolic click and followed by high pitched systolic crescendo-decrescendo murmur, which heard best at apex.
Investigations:
ECG; may be nowmal, however it may show biphasic or inverted T in lead II, III, and aVF, associated with supraventricular or ventricular premature contractions.
Echocardiography; it is the investigation of choice. It effectively poits to abnormal position and prolapse of the mitral valve leaflets.
Ref: Harrison 15th Edition, Mitral valve prolapse.
Mitral valve prolapse is more common in females. The patient presents with atypical chest pain of variable duration palpitation shortness of breath & fatigue there is no paroxysmal nocturnal dyspnea. The hallmark of is mid systolic click with late systolic murmur.
Ref: API 7th Ed, Pg- 422

Q. 512. A patient complains of intermittent claudication, dizziness and headache. Most likely cardiac lesion is (ALL INDIA/01)
   (a)   TOF
   (b)   ASD
   (c)   PDA
   (d)   Coarctation of aorta

Ans. (d)
Note
With above clinical presentation the most likely associated cardiac lesion is 'Coarctation of aorta'.
Also see
The above clinical presentation is maked with:
-Intermittent claudication
-Dizziness
-Headache
The symptoms point to Coarction of aorta:
-It is twice more common in males than females
-May remain asymptomatic
-Symptoms include; headache, epistaxis, cold extremities, and claudication
On examination:
-Hypertension in upper extremities and diminished pulsations in femoral arteries
Investigation:
-ECG; shows LVH
-CXR; shows a dilated left subclavian artery and a dilated ascending aorta. Notching of the ribs is an important radiographic sign and is due to dilated collateral vessels.
Ref: Harrison 15th Edition, Congenital aortic stenosis.
Ref: Harrison 16th Edition, Pg- 1387

Q. 513. All of the following are true about ASD except (ALL INDIA/01)
   (a)   Right atrial hypertrophy
   (b)   Left atrial hypertrophy
   (c)   Right ventricular hypertrophy
   (d)   Pulmonary hypertension

Ans. (b)

Note
All of the above are true about ASD except 'left atrial hypertrophy'.

Also see
Since the normal right ventricle is more compliant than the left, a large volume of blood shunts through the defect from the left to the right atrium and then to the right ventricle and pulmonary arteries. As a result there is gradual enlargement of the right side of the heart and of the pulmonary arteries. Pulmonary hypertension.
Ref; Davidson's 20th ED. Pg-638

Extended information
The effects of ASD are produced due to left to right shunt at atrial level with increased pulmonary flow. These effects are:
a. Volume hypertrophy of right atrium and right ventricle.
b. Focal or diffused endocardial hypertrophy of the right atrium and right ventricles.
c. Volume atrophy of the left atrium and left ventricle.
d. Small sized mitral and aortic orifices.
Ref: Harsh Mohan's Pocket book of Pathology, 2nd Ed. Pg- 212

Q. 514. Mitral valve vegetations do not usually embolise to (ALL INDIA/01)
  (a) Lung
  (b) Liver
  (c) Spleen
  (d) Brain

Ans. (a)
Note
Mitral valve vegetations do not usually embolise to 'Lung'.

Also see
As the blood passes through LA to LV and then in systemic circulation, therefore lungs are spared.

Extended information
Mural thrombi in the left atrium or the left ventricle, vegetations on the mitral or aortic valves, prosthetic heart valves and cardiomyopathy usually progress to systemic circulation.
Ref: Harsh Mohan's Pocket book of Pathology 2nd Ed. Pg-78

Q. 515. Kussmaul's sign is not seen in (ALL INDIA/01)
  (a) Restrictive cardiomyopathy
  (b) Constrictive pericarditis
  (c) Cardiac tamponade
  (d) RV infarct

Ans. (c)
Note
Kussmaul's sign is not seen in 'Cardiac temponade'.

Also see
Kussmaul's sign an increase rather than the normal decrease in the CVP during inspiration is most often caused by severe right-sided heart failure; it is a frequent finding in patients with constrictive pericarditis or right ventricular infarction.
Also see
Ref: Harrison 16th Ed Pg-1416

Q. 516. A patient presents with engorged neck veins, BP 80/50 mmHg and pulse rate of 100/min following blunt trauma to the chest. Diagnosis is (ALL INDIA/01)
  (a) Pneumothorax
  (b) Right ventricular failure
  (c) Cardiac tamponade
  (d) Hemothorax

Ans. (c)
Note
The diagnosis in above clinical presentation is 'Cardiac temponade'.

Also see
The present clinical presentation has - H/O blunt trauma to the chest which is followed by engorged neck veins, BP 80/50mm Hg, and tachycardia, it indicats a falling arterial pressure, and features are more in tune with cardiac tamponade.

Extended information
The classic findings of falling arterial pressure, rising venous pressure, and faint heart sounds usually occur only with severe, acute tamponade, as occurs with cardiac trauma or rupture. Tamponade may also develop more slowly, and under these circumstances the clinical manifestations may resemble those of heart failure, including dyspnea, orthopnea, hepatic engorgement, and jugular venous hypertension. A high index of suspicion for cardiac tamponade is required, since, in many instances, no obvious cause for pericardial disease is apparent.
Harrison, 15th Edition, 239 Pericardial diseases.

Q. 517. A patient being investigated for anemia has a dry marrow tap; peripheral smear reveals tear drop cells. Most likely diagnosis is (ALL INDIA/01)
    (a)   Leukemia
    (b)   Lymphoma
    (c)   Myelofibrosis
    (d)   Polycythemia rubra vera

Ans. (c)
Note
The above clinical featues and presence of tear drop cells in peripheral smear suggest for myelofibrosis as most suitable choice.
Ref: Harrison; 15th Ed, Section 2 Disorders of hematopoiesis.

Also see
Lab findings of Myelofibrosis are:
    -Mild anemia is usual except in cases where features of polycythemia vera are coexistent.
    -Peripheral blood smears show bizarre red cell shapes, tear drop poikilocytes, basophilic stippling, nucleated red cells, immature leucocytes (i.e. leucoerythroblastic reaction), basophilia and giant platelet forms.
Ref: Harshmohans Pocket book of Pathology 2nd Ed, Pg-292.

Q. 518. A young patient presents with jaundice. Total bilirubin is 21 mg%, direct is 9.6 mg%, alkaline phosphatase is 84 KA units. Diagnosis is
    (a)   Hemolytic jaundice
    (b)   Viral hepatitis
    (c)   Chronic active hepatitis
    (d)   Obstructive jaundice

Ans. (d)
Note
The above presensation clinically suggestes the obstructive jaundice.

Also see
The seum alkaline phosphatse is high (Normal; 3 – 13 KAU) which suggests obstructive cause. Other features in favour are; total bilirubin is 21 mg% which is high as well as direct bilirubin (conjugated) 9.6 mg%.
In case of hemolytic jaundice the unconjugated bilirubin is high.
Alkaline phosphatase increased in hepato-biliary disease (highest in biliary obstruction), bone disease, pregnancy.
Ref: Harsh Mohan's Pocket book of Pathology 2nd Ed. Pg-434.

Q. 519. A young male with gallbladder stones shows the following test results; serum bilirubin 25 mg%, Hb 6 g%, urine test positive for urobilinogen. Diagnosis is
    (a)   Hemolytic jaundice
    (b)   Obstructive jaundice
    (c)   Hepatocellular jaundice
    (d)   Protoporphyria

Ans. (a)

Note
With above clinical featues dignosis is 'hemolytic jaundice'

Also see
Present clinical presentation is in favor of hemolytic jaundice; as the patient is very young with low Hb% and gall stone. He is probably suffering from some hemolytic disease and prolonged haemolysis results in precipitation of bilirubin salts within the gall bladder to form gallstones in which bilirubin is major content. The diagnosis of hemolytic jaundice is further strengthen by the the urine test which is positive for urobilinogen. Urinary urobilinogen excretion normaly does not exceed 4 mg/d. in presence of hemolysis, which increases the amount of bilirubin entering the gut and hence the amount of urobilinogen formed and reabsorbed leading to rise in plasma urobilinogen and same is excreatd in urine.
Ref: Harrison, 15th Ed, Section 2 – liver and biliary tract disease, 294. Bilirubin metabolism and the hyperbilirubinemia.

Extended information
Hyperbilirubinemia develops when the capacity of liver to conjugate large amount of bilirubin is exceeded. Bile pigment being unconjugated type is absent from urine (acholuric jaundice). There is a dark brown colour of stool due to excessive faecal excretion of bile pigment and increased urinary excretion of urobilinogen.
Ref: Harsh Mohan's Pocket book of Pathology 2nd Ed, Pg-435

Q. 520. Urine analysis shows RBC casts. Likely source is
    (a) Kidney
    (b) Ureter
    (c) ladder
    (d) Urethra

Ans. (a)
Note
Urine analysis shows RBC casts. Likely source is 'Kidney'.

Also see
The finding of **RBC casts** in interstitial nephritis has been reported but should prompt a search for glomerular diseases. It is an indication for early renal biopsy as the pathological pattern has important implications for diagnosis, prognosis, and treatment from allopathic point of view.
Harrison, 15th Edition, Section 7- Alterations in renal and urinary tract functiono. 47. Azotemia and Urinary abnormalities.
Symptomatic hematuria with proteinuria with/without BP and or RBC casts, dysmorphic red cells is seen in glomerular disease.
Ref: API, 7th Ed, Pg-659

Q. 521. A patient's CSF report reads as follows: sugar 40 mg%, protein 150 mg%, chloride 550 mg%; lymphocytosis present. The picture is suggestive of
    (a) Fungal meningitis
    (b) Viral meningitis
    (c) TB meningitis
    (d) Leukemia

Ans. (c)
Note
The aboe featues are suggestive of 'TB meningitis'

Also see
The CSF findings suggested as Sugar; 40 mg% is low (Normal 50 -80 mg/100ml), Proteins; 150 mg% Increased (Normal 15 -45 mg/dl), Chloride; 550mg%, Low (Normal 700 -750 mg/dl). Cells; Lymphocytosis present this picture is suggestive of TB Meningitis.
Ref: Golwalla 12th Edition

Q. 522. Lacunar infarcts are caused by
    (a) Lipohyalinosis of penetrating arteries
    (b) Middle carotid artery involvement

(c) Emboli to anterior circulation
(d) None of the above

Ans. (a)
Note
Lacunar infarcts are caused by 'Lipohyalinosis of penetrating arteries'.
Also see
The term *lacunar infarction* refers to infarction following atherothrombotic or lipohyalinotic occlusion of one of the small, penetrating branches of the circle of Willis, middle cerebral artery stem, or vertebral and basilar arteries.
C/F: Common lacunar syndromes are:
(1) Pure motor hemiparesis from an infarct in the internal capsule.
(2) Pure sensory stroke from an infarct in the ventrolateral thalamus.
(3) Ataxic hemiparesis from an infarct in the base of the pons.
(4) Dysarthria and a clumsy hand due to infarction in the base of the pons / genu of the internal capsule.
(5) Pure motor hemiparesis with "motor (Broca's) aphasia" due to thrombotic occlusion of a lenticulostriate branch supplying the genu and anterior limb of the internal capsule.
Harrison- 15th Edition, Section 2 –Diseases of Central Nervus System, 361 – Cerebrovascular diseases.

Q. 523. Dinesh, a 56 years aged man presents with complaints of slowness of movements, postural instability, tremors, rigidity and memory loss. Most likely diagnosis is
(a) Multi-infarct dementia
(b) Alzheimer's disease
(c) Parkinsonism
(d) None of the above

Ans. (c)
Note
The above clinical features are in favour for the diagnosis of 'Parkinsonism'.
Also see
Parkinsonism
It is a slowly progressive degenerative condition of extrapyramidal system, resulting in disturbance of motor function and characterised by slowing of body movements, muscular rigidity, tremors and postural disturbances. *James Parkinson first described, in 1817, the classical manifestations of this syndrome in a paper entitled 'Essay on Shaking Palsy'.*

Q. 524. All of the following may be seen in Wilson's disease except
(a) Cerebellar ataxia
(b) Peripheral neuropathy
(c) Dysphagia
(d) Chorea

Ans. (b)
Note
All of the above are seen in Wilson's disease except 'peripheral neuropathy'.
Also see
Wilson's disease is an inherited disorder of copper metabolism. Impairment of excretion of hepatic copper results in toxic accumulation of the metal in liver, brain, and other organs.
Clinical features:
  -Kayser Fleischer ring
  -Cirrhosis of liver
  -Neurological manifestations include resting and intention tremors, spasticity, rigidity, chorea, drooling, dysphagia, and dysarthria. However, sensory changes never occur, except for headache.
  -Psychiatric disturbances include; Schizophrenia, manic-depressive psychoses, and classic neuroses may take place but the commonest disturbances are bizarre behavioral patterns that defy classification.
Harrison 15th Edition – Section 3- Disorders of interediaty metabolism. 348 – Wilson's disease.

MCQ's in Practice of Medicine

Q. 525. An elderly man presents with features of dementia, ataxia, difficulty in downward gaze and a history of frequent falls. Likely diagnosis is
    (a) Parkinson disease
    (b) Progressive supranuclear gaze palsy
    (c) Alzheimer's disease
    (d) None of the above

Ans. (b)
Note
Most likely diagnosis for the above clinical features is 'Progressive supranuclear gaze palsy'.
Also see
Progressive supranuclear palsy is a dementing illness associated with parkinsonian features of rigidity, bradykinesia, and postural instability. Resting tremor is often absent, there is a vertical gaze palsy, and patients are resistant to treatment with L-dopa.
Harrison's 15th Edition; Section 3- Nervous system dysfunction 26 Memory loss and dementia.

Q. 526. A chromosomal anomaly associated with Alzheimer's dementia is
    (a) Trisomy 18
    (b) Patau syndrome
    (c) Trisomy 21
    (d) Turner syndrome

Ans. (c)
Note
A chromosomal anomaly associated with Alzheimer's dementia is 'Trisomy 21'.
Also see
Adults with trisomy 21 (Down's syndrome) consistently develop the typical neuropathologic hallmarks of Alzheimer's dementia, if they survive beyond age 40. Many also develop a progressive dementia superimposed on their baseline mental retardation.
Ref; Harrison's 15th Edition.
Ref: Cecil Essentials of Medicine, 6th Ed, Pg-983.

Q. 527. All are true about Huntington's disease, except
    (a) Chorea
    (b) Depression, apathy
    (c) Progressive dementia
    (d) Cog-wheel rigidity

Ans. (d)
Note
All of the above are true about Huntington's disease, except 'Cog-Wheel rigidity'.
Also see
The classic triad of Parkinson's disease consists of *bradykinesia*, the *resting tremor*, and *cogwheel rigidity*.
'Cog-Wheel rigidity'
Rigidity is characteristic of extrapyramidal disease. At times it resembles a lever engaging on the teeth of a cogwheel (cogwheel rigidity). It can be enhanced by asking the patient to contract another muscle, e.g. to clench the fist, or to move the hand up and down on the opposite side (Jendrassik manoeuvre). When rigidity is discovered, especially in association with rest tremor, the examiner should consider the diagnosis of parkinsonism
Ref: Hutchinson's Clincial Methods 20th Ed. Pg-314
Huntington's disease
It is a genetic, autosomal dominant, degenerative brain disorder. The clinical hallmarks of the disease are *chorea* and behavioral disturbance. Onset is usually in the fourth or fifth decade. The movement disorder is slowly progressive & eventually disabling. Memory impaired occurs late, but *attention, judgment, awareness, and executive functions develop at an early stage. Depression, apathy*, social withdrawal is common. Delusions and obsessive-compulsive behavior may occur.
Huntington's disease is charecterised by: *chorea*, behavioural disturbances, *dementia*.
Ref: API 7th Ed, Pg-839.

Q. 528. A 30-year-old male complains of loss of erection; he has low testosterone and high prolactin level in blood. What is the likely diagnosis?
(a) Pituitary adenoma
(b) Testicular failure
(c) Craniopharyngioma
(d) Cushing's syndrome

Ans. (a)

Note
In the above clinical situation the most likely diagnosis is 'Pituitary adenoma'.

Also see
The above features can be caused by pituitary adenoma, resuting in hyperprolectinemia. The cardinal male features are; decreased libido, erectile impotency, reduced shaving frequency and lethargy, galactorrhea, and hypogonadiam.
Ref: Davidson 18th Ed. Pg-551.
Harrison's 15th Edition - Table 328-5. Classificatio by Pituitry adenomas.

At present, classification of pituitary tumors is based on plasma hormone levels or immunohistochemical staining:

Type of adenoma	Secretion	Staining	Pathology
Corticotrophic adenomas	secrete adrenocorticotrophic hormone (ACTH) and pro-opiomelanocortin (POMC)	basophilic	Cushing's disease
Somatotrophic adenomas	secrete growth hormone (GH)	acidophilic	acromegaly (gigantism)
Thyrotrophic adenomas (rare)	secrete thyroid stimulating hormone (TSH)	basophilic	occasionally hyperthyroidism usually doesn't cause symptoms
Gonadotrophic adenomas	secrete luteinizing hormone (LH), follicle stimulating hormone (FSH) and their subunits	basophilic	usually doesn't cause symptoms
Lactotroph adenomas or prolactinomas (most common)	secrete prolactin	acidophilic	galactorrhea, hypogonadism, amenorrhea, infertility, and impotence
Null cell adenomas	do not secrete hormones	may stain positive for synaptophysin	

Ref: http://en.wikipedia.org/wiki/Pituitary_adenoma

Q. 529. A woman has bilateral headache that worsens with emotional stress. She has two children, both doing badly in school. Diagnosis is
    (a)   Migraine
    (b)   Cluster headache
    (c)   Tension headache
    (d)   Trigeminal neuralgia

Ans. (c)
Note
The diagnosis for the above clinical presentation is 'tension headache'.
Also see
Tension headache is a chronic head pain characterized by bilateral tight, bandlike uneasiness. The pain develops slowly, fluctuates in severity, and continues for many days. The anxiety, depression or emotional stress commonly co-exists with this. Exertion do not < the headache. Tension-type headache is common in all age groups, and females tend to predominate. Here the cause of tension appears to be two children who are not doing well in school.
Harrison's 15th Edition. Section -1. Pain 15. Headache, including migraine and cluster headache.

Q. 530. A female aged 30 years, presents with episodic throbbing headache for past 4 years with nausea and vomiting. Most likely diagnosis is
    (a)   Migraine
    (b)   Cluster headache
    (c)   Angle closure glaucoma
    (d)   Temporal arteritis

Ans. (a)
Note
The most likely diagnosis for the above presentation is 'Migraine'.
Also see
Migraine is a benign and recurring syndrome of headache, nausea, vomiting, and/or other symptoms of neurologic dysfunction in varying admixtures. It is the most common cause of vascular headache, afflicts approximately 15% of women and 6% of men.
Migrain is a syndrome of episodic recurrent headaches, more often unilateral, which is associated with nausea vomiting, photophobia or phonophobia. It is more common in women than in men (2 to 3:1) and a family history is present in more than 60% of cases.
Ref: API 7th Ed,. Pg-750

Q. 531. A young basketball player with height 188 cm and arm span 197 cm has a diastolic murmur best heard in second right intercostal space. Likely cause of murmur is
    (a)   AS
    (b)   Coarctation of aorta
    (c)   AR
    (d)   MR

Ans. (c)
Note
The likely cause of murmur is 'AR'.
Also see
The features of the young basketball player points to Marfan syndrome. It is a hereditary disorder of connective tissue which affects both sexes. They have cardiovascular involvement; dilation of aorta, dissecting aneurysm, aortic imcompetence. The diastolic murmur in the right second intercostal space points to aortic incompetence.

Extended information
Individuals with Marfan's syndrome are tall with long slender limbs, arm span is more than the height, musles are underdeveloped and hypotonic and the body lacks subcutaneous fat. Cardio-vascular manifestations are aortic regurgitation, floppy mitral valve with mitral regurgitation, CCF and rupture of aorta.
Ref : API 7th Ed, Pg-1198.

Q. 532. A patient presents with arthritis, hyperpigmentation of skin and hypogonadism. Likely diagnosis is:
    (a)   Hemochromatosis
    (b)   Ectopic ACTH secreting tumor of lung
    (c)   Wilson's disease
    (d)   Rheumatoid arthritis

Ans. (a)
Note
The most likely diagnosis for above presentation is 'hemochromatosis'.
Also see
Hemochromatosis is disorder leading to inappropriate increase in intestinal iron absorption whih is deposited in excessive amounts in parenchymal cells with eventual tissue damage and impaired function of organs, especially the liver, pancreas, heart, joints, and pituitary, leading to fibrosis and organ failure. Cirrhosis of the liver, diabetes mellitus, arthritis, cardiomyopathy, and hypogonadotrophic hypogonadism, hyperpigmentation are common manifestations.
Harrison's 15th Edition. Section 3. Disorders of intermediaty metabolism – 345. Hemochromatosis.

Q. 533. In myasthenia gravis, correct statement regarding thymectomy is (ALL INDIA/01)
    (a)   Should be done in all cases
    (b)   Should be done in cases with ocular involvement only
    (c)   Not required if controlled by medical management
    (d)   Should be done only in cases that are associated with thymoma

Ans. (a)
Note
In myasthenia gravis, thymectomy should be done in all cases.
Also see
The available evidence suggests that up to 85% of patients experience improvement after thymectomy. The improvement is delayed for months to years. However, the advantage of thymectomy is that it offers the possibility of long-term benefit, in some cases diminishing or eliminating the need for continuing medical treatment. In view of these potential benefits, thymectomy should be carried out in all patients with Myasthenia Gravis who are between the ages of puberty and at least 55 years.
Harrison's 15th Edition. Section 3. Disorders of Nerve and Muscle – 380. Myasthenia Gravis and other diseases of the Neuromuscular junction

Q. 534. The following group of tests should be done to optimise graft uptake in bone marrow transplant
    (a)   Blood grouping
    (b)   HLA matching
    (c)   Culture for infection
    (d)   All of the above

Ans. (b)
Note
The 'HLA' matching should be done to optimize graft uptake in bone marrow transplant.
Also see
In bone marrow transplant, the level of HLA matching is much more critical than for solid organ graft because of the risk of graft versus host disease, where T-cells in the stem cell graft react against allogenic host HLA molecules expressed in tissues.
Ref : API 7th Ed, Pg-207

Q. 535. A 45 years male presents with hypertension. He has sudden abnormal flinging movements in right upper and lower limbs. Most likely site of hemorrhage is
    (a)   Substantia nigra
    (b)   Caudate nuclei
    (c)   Pons
    (d)   Subthalamic nuclei

Ans. (d)

Note
The most likely site of bleeding is 'subthalamic nuclei'.

Also see
The lesion in subthalamic nucleus will cause contralateral hemiballismus.
Ref: Harrison 15th Edition, Cerebrovascular diseases.
Hemiballismus commonly follows a stroke involving contralateral subthalamic nucleus. The movement is confined to one side of the body.
Ref: API 7th Ed, Pg-839.

Q. 536. IPPV (Intermittent Positive Pressure Ventilation) can cause (ALL INDIA/01)
  (a) Barotrauma
  (b) Pleural effusion
  (c) Increased venous return
  (d) None of the above

Ans. (a)

Note
IPPV (Intermittent Positive Pressure Ventilation) can cause 'Barotrauma'.

Also see
Positive-pressure mechanical ventilation has direct and indirect effects on several organ systems. Pulmonary complications include Barotrauma - which occurs when high pressures (i.e., > 50 cmH2O) disrupt lung tissue, and clinically presents itself as; interstitial emphysema, pneumomediastinum, subcutaneous emphysema, or pneumothorax.
Ref: Harrison 15th Edition, Diseases of the Respiratory system
Ventilator associated lung injury: extreme overdistention of lungs during mechanical ventilation with high tidal volume and PEEP can rupture alveoli and cause air to dissect centrally along the perivascular sheath. This barotraumas may be complicated by pneumo-mediastinum, subcutaneous emphysema, pneumo-peritoneum, pneumothorax and intra-abdominal air.
Ref: Kumar and Clark, Clinical Medicine, 6th Ed, Pg-984

UPSC-06

Q. 537. Toxic Shock syndrome is caused by which one of the following? (UPSC-06)
  (a) Staphylococci
  (b) Pneumococci
  (c) Streptococci
  (d) Pseudomonas

Ans. (a)

Note
Toxic shock syndrome is caused by 'Staphylococci'.

Also see
Toxic Shock Syndrome
TSS is due to TSST-1 and enterotoxin-β produced by staphylococci. Toxic shock syndrome is characterized by high fever, myalgia with gastro-intestinal disturbance like vomiting, diarrhea and hypovolemia.
Ref. API, 7th Ed, Pg-31

Extended information
The Toxic Shock Syndrome (TSS) is caused by a toxin produced by Staphylococcus aureus. It is most common in menstruating women using highly absorbent tampons and occurs within 5 days of the onset of a menstrual period. The syndrome has also been seen in children, infants, and men, skin wounds or infections caused by Staphylococcus aureus elsewhere in the body.

Q. 538. Consider the following statements (UPSC-06)

Babinki's sign is positive in a case of:
1. Upper motor neuron lesion
2. Lower motor neuron lesion

Which of the statements given above is/ are correct?
(a) 1 Only
(b) 2 Only
(c) Both 1 and 2
(d) Neither 1 nor 2

Ans. (a)

Note
From above the 'Babinki's sign is positive in cases of' correctly corroborates with '1. Upper Motor Neuron Lesion'.

Also see
In case of LMN lesions the planter is lost and Babinki's sign (Extensor planter) is positive in UMN lesion.

Extended information
An extension of the great toe, sometimes with fanning of the other toes, in response to stroking of the sole of the foot. It is a normal reflex in infants, but is associated with a disturbance of the pyramidal tract in children and adults. Also called Babinski's sign, toe reflex.

A lower motor neuron lesion (such as destruction of cell bodies or transection of axons in a ventral root or peripheral nerve) causes flaccid paralysis, loss of the stretch reflex, and considerable atrophy.

(The poliomyelitis virus kills motor neuron cell bodies. In ALS - (short for amyotrophic lateral sclerosis, also called Lou Gehrig's disease from a sportsman who died from it) - death of motor neurons occurs more slowly than in polio but is progressive and relentless. Axonal transection may result from physical injury to a nerve or from general or localized diseases, of which diabetic neuropathy and the Guillaine-Barre syndrome, an autoimmune disease, are common examples.)

The major descending pathways are the vestibulospinal, reticulospinal, and corticospinal (pyramidal) tracts. The first of these is largely concerned with postural adjustments, and the last with voluntary movements. Most corticospinal fibers decussate at the caudal end of the medulla.

Also see

Features:	UMN Cortico-spinal or (Pyramidal)	LMN (Ant. Horn cells & Peripheral nerves)	Sub-cortical Lesions (Extra-Pyramidal	Cerebellar Ataxia
Presentation	Spasticity	Flaccidity	Rigidity	Low tone
Muscle affected	Antigravity muscles	Antagonists and agonists both	Antagonists and agonists both	Antagonists and agonists both
Nature	Clasp knife	Lead pipe and cog wheel	Lead pipe and cog wheel	Ataxia / Incoordination
Accompanying sign	Hyperreflexia babinski response positive, clonus	Tremors, bradikinesia	Tremors, bradikinesia	Pendullar jerks Nystagmus, Past pointing, intention tremors

Q. 539. Consider the following (UPSC-06)
1. Amenorrhea
2. Menorrhagia
3. Polymenrrhea

Which of he above is / are commonly seen in a woman with Cushing's syndrome?
- (a) 1 Only
- (b) 1 and 2
- (c) 2 and 3
- (d) 3 only

Ans. (a)

Note
From the listed above the only 1 is encountered in a woman with Cushing's syndrome.

Also see
In Cushing's syndrome; acne, hirsutism, oligomenorrhea and amenorrhea are common presentation in women.
Ref: API, 7th Ed, Pg-1071

Extended information
Cushing's disease was first described by Cushing Harvey Williams (1869-1939). It is due to hyperactivity of the cortex of the adrenal glands and affects women more than men. The symptoms include obesity (moonface, an accumulation of fat at the back of the neck called buffalo hump, and abdominal protrusion), Abdominal fat accumulation can be significant and can also be associated with vertical purplish striations (stretch marks), thin arm and leg, hypertension, hirsutism, and easy bruisability. Symptoms usually include fatigue, weakness, depression, mood swings, increased thirst and urination, and lack of menstrual periods in women.

Q. 540. What is the most common site of Kaposi's sarcoma in AIDS? (UPSC-06)
- (a) Lymph nodes
- (b) Stomach
- (c) Liver
- (d) Skin

Ans. (d)

Note
The most common site of Kaposi's sarcoma in AIDS is 'skin'.

Also see
In Kaposi's sarcoma lesions are wide spread and often affect the skin, bowel, oral cavity and lungs.
Ref. Kumar and Clark, 6th Ed. Pg-1353

Extended information
Before the AIDS epidemic Kaposi's sarcoma was seen primarily in elderly Italian and Jewish men In AIDS, the disease is caused by immune suppression. If often involves skin, lungs, gastrointestinal tract. The tumors consist of bluish red or purple nodules made-up of vascular tissue.

Symptoms:
- Bluish red macule or papules
- Bleeding in GIT lesions
- Bloody sputum with pulmonary lesions

Test:
- Skin lesions biopsy showing Kaposi's sarcoma
- Endoscopy showing Kaposi's lesions

Q. 541. A tuberculosis patient could be infectious when he has (UPSC-06)
- (a) TB Meningitis
- (b) TB lymph node
- (c) Pott's Disease
- (d) Pulmonary TB

Ans. (d)

Note
A tuberculos patient is infectious when he has 'Pulmonary tuberculosis'.

Also see
Tuberculosis is transmitted mainly by droplet infection and droplet nuclei generated by sputum-positive patients with pulmonary tuberculosis.
Ref. Park & Park, 18th Ed, Pg-150.

Extended information
In cases of T.B meningitis, Pott's disease and TB lymph node the bacteria remains isolated. So these types of tubercular infections are non-infectious.

Q. 542. Consider the following (UPSC-06)
1. Pain colicy in nature in right hypochondrium
2. On examination; Murphy's sign is positive
3. Vomiting with severe pain on eating fatty food
4. Burning micturition

Which of the above features is the diagnostic for cholelithiasis?
- (a) 1, 2 and 4
- (b) 4 only
- (c) 3 only
- (d) 1, 2 and 3

Ans. (d)

Note
The features from above diagnostic of cholelithiasis are (d) 1, 2 and 3.

Also see
Features of cholelithiasis:
The most common presenting symptom is upper abdominal pain which is generally localized to the right upper quadrant or epigastrium. Anorexia, nausea and vomiting and positive murphy's sign may be detected
Ref: API, 7th Ed, Pg-644, 645

Extended information
Pain in the right upper quadrant which is precipitated after eating fatty food (Fatty food reflexly initiates contraction of gall bladder so the bile is poured for facilitating the digestion of fat), it triggers the colic due to presence of gall stone. The colic is associated with nausea and vomiting. The typical biliary colic begins suddenly and may persist for 30 min to few hours. It frequently radiated to interscapular area, right scapula or right shoulder. Gallstones when obstruct cystic duct may cause acute inflammation of gallbladder. Mechanism for gallbladder inflammation includes:
  -Mechanical cause:
Increased intraluminal pressure and distention with resulting ischemia of gall bladder mucosa and wall.
  -Chemical cause:
Release of lysolecithin and other local tissue factors.
  -Bacterial cause:
The organisms includes; E. Coli, Klebsiella spp, Streptococcus etc
In cases of gall stone which is usually associated with acute cholecystitis presents with 'positive Murphy's sign'. Here the burning micturition is put up as a distracter. Therefore, the correct answer appears to be (d).
Ref: Harrison's 5th Ed. Gallstones, and Chronic Cholecystitis.

Q. 543. Consider the following (UPSC-06)
1. Unsteady gait
2. Disturbed coordination of volitional movement
3. Rigidity
4. Tremor at rest

Which of the features given above are associated with cerebellar lesion?
- (a) 1 and 2
- (b) 1 and 3
- (c) 2 and 3
- (d) 3 and 4

Ans. (a)

Note
The features given above (a) 1. Unsteady gait and 2. disturbed coordination of volitional movement are associated with cerebellar lesion.
Aso see:
The ataxia and in-coordination in volitional movements are the only features are given above which point to 'Cerebellar ataxia'. Hypotonia is associated with cerebellar ataxia. Rigidity and Tremor at rest is associated with Lesions of subcortical nuclei – i.e., and are the classical features 'Parkinson's disease'.

Extended information
Features of cerebellar lesion:
- Gait becomes broad and ataxic-patient falters towards the lesion
- Movement is imprecise in direction, in force and in distance (dysmetria)
- Nystagmus
- Dysarthria
- Intention tremors

Ref: Kumar and Clark, 6th Ed Pg-1195

Q. 544. Consider the following (UPSC-06)
1. Severe pain in chest left side with sweating
2. Anxiety with increased palpitation
3. Severe headache
4. ECG showing changes in ST segment

Which of the above features is/ are suggestive of myocardial infarction?
- (a) 1, 2 and 3
- (b) 1, 2 and 4
- (c) 2 and 4 only
- (d) 3 only

Ans. (b)

Note
The most suitable features out of above suggestive for acute myocardial infarction is (c) which includes; 2. Anxiety with palpitation and 4. ECG showing changes in ST segment

Also see
Discussion
1. Severe pain in chest left side with sweating:
   A non specific symptom in reference to acute MI, the classical pain occurs in substernal region and it is associated with sweating.
2. Anxety with increased palpitation:
   Anxiety is a symptom encountered in acute MI however, the palpitation is more of a subjective symptom and could be felt due to irregular heart action of ventricular ectopics. The majority of pateitns who suffer from MI die within 1st hour due to ventricular fibrilaiton.
3. Severe headache:
   This symptom is directly or indirectly not related to acute MI. However the patient who may have taken 'sorbitrate' may have this feature.
4. ECG showing ST segment canges:
   The above features take place within hours of MI and the ST elevation is diagnostic feature for acute MI.

Q. 545. Which one of the following conditions is present in "Ludwig's angina"? (UPSC-06)
- (a) Angina pain felt abut the left hand
- (b) Form of cellulites starts in the submandibular region and spreads to the floor of the mouth
- (c) Rigidity of the lower limbs
- (d) Bleeding from the mouth

Ans. (b)

Note
The condition present in 'ludwig's angina' consist of 'cellulitis, starts in the submandibular region and spreads to the floor of the mouth'.

Also see
Ludwig's angina:
It is described as a clinical entity characterized by a brawny swelling of the submandibular region combined with inflammatory edema of mouth.
Clinical course-unless the infection is controlled, cellulites may extend down the neck beneath the deep facial layers to involve the larynx causing glottic edema.
Bailey and Love's Short Practice of Surgery, 24th Ed, Pg-773

Extended information
Other names of 'Ludwig's angina' are – Neck abscess, sublingual infection, neck infection; submandibular space infection; cellulites, neck.
It is defined as 'an acute bacterial infection of the mouth and throat with swelling that may block the airway. Ludwig's angina is most common infection of neck and surrounding areas. It is a type of cellulites that involves inflammation of the tissues of the neck, jaw, and below he tongue It often occurs following infection of the roots of the teeth ie, tooth abscess or after oral trauma. Swelling of the tissues occurs rapidly and may block the airways.

Q. 546. Consider the following (UPSC-06)
1. Proteinuria
2. Hypoproteinemia
3. Generalised edema

Nephrotic syndrome is characterised by which of the above?
(a) 1 and 2 only
(b) 2 and 3 only
(c) 1 and 3 only
(d) 1, 2 and 3

Ans. (d)
Note
Nephrotic syndrome is characterised by (d) 1. Proteinuria, 2. Hypoproteinemia and 3. Generalised edema.
Also see
Nephrotic syndrome is charecterised by massive proteinuria (urinary protein excretion $>3.5gm/1.73m^2/24h$ in adults or $>40mg/m^2/h$ in children), hypoalbuminemia, edema, hyperlipidemia and lipiduria.
Ref. API 7th Ed, Pg-664, 645

Q. 547. Consider the following (UPSC-06)
1. Wilson's disease
2. Diabetes mellitus
3. Whipple's Disease
4. Retinitis pigmentosa

Chromosomal localization is known in which of the above disorders?
(a) 1,2 and 3
(b) 1,2 and 4
(c) 1,3 and 4
(d) 2,3 and 4

Ans. (b)
Note
The Chromosomal localization is known in 1, 2, and 4 of above.
Also see
Wilson's disease
It is an autosomal recessive disorder with a molecular defect within a copper-transporting ATPase encoded by a gene located on chromosome.
Ref: Kumar and Clark, 6th Ed, Pg387
Diabetes mellitus
HLA genes on chromosome 6 are highly polymorphic and modulate the immune defence system of the body. More than 90% of the patients with Type-I Diabetes carry HLA-DR3-DQ2, HLA-DR4-DQ8 or both.
Ref: Kumar and Clark, 6th Ed, Pg-1105

Whipple's Disease
Whipple's disease is caused by bacteria named 'Tropheryma whippelii'. It can affect any system of the body, but occurs most often in the small intestine.
Symptoms include diarrhea, intestinal bleeding, abdominal pain, loss of appetite, weight loss, fatigue, and weakness. Arthritis and fever often occur several years before intestinal symptoms develop. Diagnosis is based on symptoms and biopsy of tissue from the small intestine or other organs that are affected.
Ref: http://digestive.niddk.nih.gov/ddiseases/pubs/whipple

Retinitis pigmentosa:
It is an X linked syndrome. Gene product- retinitis pigmentosa GTPase regulator.
Ref: Kumar and Clark, 6th Ed, Pg-184

Q. 548. Consider following (UPSC-06)
1. Pulmonary stenosis
2. Overriding of the ventricular septal defect by aorta
3. Ventricular septal defect
4. Right ventricular hypertrophy

Which of the above is/are the features of Tetralogy of Fallot?
(a) 1 only
(b) 1 and 2 only
(c) 3 and 4 only
(d) 1, 2, 3 and 4

Ans. (d)
Note
The (d) 1, 2, 3, and 4 are the features of Tetralogy of fallot.
Also see
The Fallot's tetralogy is classified as a congenital cyanotic heart disease consisting of 4 abnormalities which are listed as above 1, 2, 3, and 4.
Ref: Kumar and Clark, 6th Ed, Pg-838

Q. 549. A 48 year old male who is known to be HIV positive has been admitted with high fever, headache, vomiting and drowsiness for the past seven days. The following tests were advised (UPSC-06)
1. CT of head
2. CSF serology
3. Indian ink preparation of CSF

Which of the above investigations would be helpful in establishing the etiological diagnosis?
(a) 1 and 2 only
(b) 2 and 3 only
(c) 1 and 3 only
(d) 1, 2, and 3

Ans. (b)
Note
The 2. CSF serology and 3. Indian ink preparation of CSF would be helpful in establishing the aetiological diagnosis in above situation.
Discussion
- Pt is known case of AIDS
- Presenting complains are; high fever, headache, vomiting and drowsiness, since last seven days – these point to menintis.
- People with AIDS, are especially susceptible to disseminated cryptococcosis. Cryptococcal meningitis
Diagnosis of cryptococcal meningitis will depend on:
- Indian ink preparation of CSF – is a specific for cryptococcus infection.
- SCF serology will be able to differentiate with other similar offending organism – TB, Toxoplasmosis.

Q. 550. Which one of the following diseases has the characteristic features of 'breathlessness (Pulmonary Congestion), fatigue, edema, ascitis (Right sided Heart Failure), hemoptysis, and signs of mitral facies, mid-diastolic murmur and pulmonary hypertension? (UPSC-06)
1. Tricuspid regurgitation
2. Mitral stenosis
3. Mitral regurgitation
4. Atrial Fibrillation

Ans. (b)
Note
The above clinical features point to the diagnosis of 'Mitral Stenosis'.

Also see
Mitral stenosis results in hemodynamic disturbance leading to pulmonary venous congestion, pulmonary hypertension and progressively severe dyspnea. A cough productive of blood tinged frothy sputum, occasionally frank hemoptysis may develop. Pulmonary hypertension eventually leads to right heart failure and its symptoms are weakness, fatigue and abdominal and lower limb swellings.

Mitral facis is a bilateral cyanotic or dusky pink discoloration over the upper cheeks due to arterio-venous anastomosis and vascular stasis.

Auscultation reveals opening snap due to increased left atrial pressure and is followed by low pitched rumbling with diastolic murmur best heard with the bell of the stethoscope at the apex with the patient lying on the left side.
Ref: Kumar and Clark, 6th Ed, Pg-818
The signs of Mitral stenosis include:
 -Mitral facies
 -On / Auscultation; Loud 1st Heart Sound, Opening Snap Mid-diastolic Murmur
 -Signs of raised pulmonary capillary pressure; cripitations, pulmonary edema, effusions
 -Signs of pulmonary hypertension; Right ventricular heave, Loud P2
Ref: Davidson's 18th Ed

Q. 551. Which one of the following types of disorders is Myasthenia gravis? (UPSC-06)
(a) Heredity disorder
(b) Autoimmune disorder
(c) Involuntary muscle disorder
(d) Metabolic disorder

Ans. (b)
Note
Myasthenia gravis is an auto-immune disorder.

Also see
Myasthenia gravis is a autoimmune disorder It is characterised by chronic weakness of voluntary muscles, which improves with rest and worsens with activity.

Extended information
Myasthenia gravis is an immunologically mediated disorder effecting neuromuscular transmission characterized by fluctuating weakness of voluntary muscles worsened by repetitive use with a tendency of recovery after a period of inactivity and with anticholinesterase drugs.
Ref: API, 7th Ed. Pg- 912
There is an increased incidence of other autoimmune disease as the disease is linked with certain HLA halotypes (B8 and DRw3).
Ref: Davidson, 19th Ed. Pg-1184

Q. 552. 40 Year old woman complaints of breathlessness and pain in chest on exertion, better by rest. Heaviness of feet by the evening. On examination, face has patches of dark pigmentation, conjunctivae pale, nails flattened and lusterless. All the complaints are getting progressively worse for last few months. If you are allowed only one investigation to clinch the diagnosis, which one of the following would you choose? (UPSC-06)
(a) X-Ray Chest
(b) U/S abdomen

(c) ECG
(d) Hemogram

Ans. (d)

Note

The most important choice of investigation in above clinical situtaiton is 'Hemogram'.

Also see

The formulation of the case is as under:
-Age: 40 years
-Sex: Female
-P/C:
Breathlessness
Pain in chest worse on exertion better by rest
Heaviness of feet in the eveing
-O/E:
Face: has dark pigmentation
Conjunctiva: pale
Nails: Flattended and lusterless
-Course: Progressively worse for last few months
-Anamnesis:
A female in the productive age nearing the menopause presenting with gross features of anemia having no Personal / Past / Family H/O Hypertension, Dyslipidemia, CAD or renal disease and obesity. The presenting features are consistent with progressive anaemia and the best investigation to propose in above situation is 'hemogram'.

Extended information

There are many clues suggestive for investigating the –Hemogram:
(a) The female who is 40 years of age is in the reproductive age group and at the point of menopause; may have irregular menstruation.
(b) Females in the Joint family do eat in the last and may not get the sufficient nutrition and develop the nutritional anemia.
(c) Her symptoms are breathlessness and pain in chest on exertion; these are more likely due to anemia – rather than due to hypertension and Coronary artery disease as in pre-menopausal female –estrogen' provides a natural protection against CAD and HT.
(d) On examination her face has dark pigmentation – these are usually due to iron deficiency anemia
(e) Conjunctiva is pale – as pallor is a common featues of anemia.
(f) Flattening of nails – The Koilonychia usually takes six months time to develop – however, the flattening is the onset of process of developing koilonychias- it is a strong suggestion for iron deficiency anemia
(f) Her complaints are progressively getting worse for last few months – suggests the progressive worsening of anemia.

Q. 553. 'The Trigger Zones' are the localized (UPSC-06)
(a) Hypo-aesthetic spots on the face, gums or tongue
(b) Hyper-aesthetic spots on the face, gums or tongue
(c) Slimy spots o the face, gums or tongue
(d) Black spots on the face, gums or tongue

Ans. (b)

Note

The 'Trigger Zones' are the localized 'Hyper-aesthetic spots on the face, gums or tongue'.

Also see

The 'Trigger Zone' is a specific area that, when stimulated by touch, pain, or pressure, excites an attack of neurologic pain.
Stimulation of the face, lips, or gums, such as talking, eating, shaving, tooth-brushing, touch, or even a current of air, may trigger the severe knifelike or shocklike pain of trigeminal neuralgia, often described as excruciating. Trigger zones may be a few square millimeters in size, or large and diffuse. The pain usually starts in the

trigger zone, but may start elsewhere. Approximately 17% of patients experience dull, aching pain for days to years before the onset of paroxysmal pain; this has been termed pretrigeminal neuralgia.
Relief of the pain following injection of a local anaesthetic into these trigger points supports the diagnosis.
Ref: Harrison, 16th Ed, Pg-75

Q. 554. Which one of the following is not in the characteristic triad of manifestations in Reiter's Syndrome? (UPSC-06)
    (a) Conjunctivitis
    (b) Tonsillitis
    (c) Arthritis
    (d) Urethritis

Ans. (b)
Note
Characteristic triad of manifestations in Reiter's Syndrome include; Conjunctivitis, Arthritis and Urethritis.
Also see
Triad of Reiter's syndrome is characterized by:
The classic triad of RS presents of: Arthritis, Urethritis and Conjunctivitis.
Ref: API, 7th Ed, Pg-168

Q. 555. Korsakoff's psychosis occurs in the deficiency of which one of the following? (UPSC-06)
    (a) Thiamin
    (b) Thyroxin
    (c) Pyridoxine
    (d) Vitamin K

Ans. (a)
Note
Korsakoff's psychosis occurs in the deficiency of 'Thiamin' (Tamin B1).
Also see
It is also known as; Alcoholic encephalopathy; Korsakoff's psychosis - It is a brain disorder involving loss of specific brain function due to thiamine deficiency. It results in impairment of memory and intellect – cognitive skills such as problem soling or learning, along with multiple symptoms of nerve damage. The most distinguishing symptom is confabulation (Fabrication) where the person makes up detailed believable stories about experiences or situation to cover the gaps in memory.

Extended information
Thiamine deficiency leads to polyneuropathy, cardiac failure, and an amnestic syndrome called 'Wernicke-Korsakoff Sycosis' caused due to the ischemic damage in the brainstem and its connections.
It consists of:
    -Nystagmus- Bilateral lateral rectus palsies, conjugate gaze palsies, fixed pupils
    -Ataxia-broad based gait, cerebellar signs and vestibular paralysis
    -Cognitive changes-amnestic syndrome, restlessness, stupor and coma
    -Hypotermia and hypertension-due to hypothalamic involvement
Ref: Kumar and Clark, 6th Ed, Pg-1263

Q. 556. Consider the following (UPSC-06)
    1. Goiter
    2. Fine tremors on extending the hands
    3. Bradycardia
    4. Exophthalmos

Which of the above are the features pertaining to Grave's Disease?
    (a) 1 and 2 Only
    (b) 1 and 3 only
    (c) 1, 2 and 4
    (d) 2 and 4 only

Ans. (c)

Note
From above the features pertaining to Grave's disease are 1. Goiter, 2. Fine tremors on externding hands and 4. Exophthalmos.

Also see
The Grave's disease (Basedow's disease) is associated with over activity of thyroid gland. It is characterised by Goiter (Enlarged thyroid gland) Exophthalmos, Tachycardia and fine Tremors of hands.
Ref: Kumar and Clark, 6th Ed, Pg-1074

Q. 557. Which one of the following eruptive fevers exhibits pleomorpism? (UPSC-06)
    (a)   Small pox
    (b)   Measles
    (c)   Chicken pox
    (d)   Allergic rash with pyrexia

Ans. (c)
Note
From above 'chicken pox' is the eruptive fever which exhibits pleomorpism.

Also see
Pleomorphic; different stages of the rash evident at one given time, because rash appears in successive corps i.e., Chicken pox.

Extended information
The features of chickenpox are:
The rash is symmetrical. It first appears on the trunk (where it is abundant), then on the face, arms and legs (where it is less abundant). All the stages of rash (papules, vesicles and crusts) may be seen simultaneously at one time, in the same area. This is due to the rash appearing in successive crops for 4-5 days in the same area. This phenomenon is called pleomorphism.
Ref: Park and Park, 18th Ed. Pg-123

Q. 558. Consider the following statements (UPSC-06)
Obesity is an important factor associated with:
1. Insulin dependant diabetes mellitus
2. Non-insulin dependant diabetes mellitus

Which of the statements given above is / are correct?
    (a)   1 Only
    (b)   2 Only
    (c)   Both 1 and 2
    (d)   Neither 1 nor 2

Ans. (b)
Note
Obesity is an important factor associated with Non-insulin dependent diabetes mellitus.

Also see
Obesity is most important predisposing factor in type II Diabetes (Adult onset DM) or Non Insulin Dependent Diabetes Mellitus (NIDDM).

Extended information
Patients with Type II Diabetes have Insulin Resistance (usually relative rather than absolute insulin deficiency). They do not need insulin treatment for their survival. Most patients with this form of diabetes are obese and obesity itself causes insulin resistance. Even those who are not obese by traditional criteria have an increased percentage of body fat predominantly in the abdominal region.
Ref: API, 7th Ed Pg-1105

Q. 559. The commonest site of an amebic lesion in the bowel is (UPSC-06)
    (a)   Rectum
    (b)   Sigmoid colon
    (c)   Ascending colon
    (d)   Transverse colon

Ans. (b)

Note
The commonest site of an amebic lesion in the bowel is 'Caecum'.

Also see
The trophozoits invade the colon wall and typical flask like ulcers. The site of involvement in order of frequency is caecum, ascending colon, rectum, sigmoid colon, appendix and terminal ilum.
Ref: Textbook of medicine By Panda, First Ed, Pg-145
Amebiasis is characterized by varying degree of ulceration of colonic mucosa. Focal lesions are seen in caecum and ascending colon .The other sites affected are recto-sigmoid region, sigmoid colon, appendix and terminal ileum in order of frequency.
Ref: API, 7th Ed, Pg-08

Extended information
Trophozoites attach to colonic mucous and epithelial cells by a galactose-inhibitable lectin. The earliest intestinal lesions are microulcerations of the mucosa of the cecum, sigmoid colon, or rectum that release erythrocytes, inflammatory cells, and epithelial cells. Proctoscopy reveals small ulcers with heaped up margins and normal intervening mucosa. Submucosal extension of ulcerations under viable-appearing surface mucosa causes the classic "flask-shaped" ulcer containing trophozoites at the margins of dead and viable tissues.
Ref: Harrison 15th Edition
The parasite may invade the mucous membrane of the large bowel producing lesions, maximal in the caecum but found as far down as the anal canal.
Ref: Davidson's Principles and PLracticce of Medicine 19th Ed, Pg-45
The trophozoits in the intestine colonise in the caecum and large bowel.
Ref: Pathology Quick Review and MCQs based on Harsh Hohan's Textbook of Pahtolgoy 5th Ed, Pg-128
Trophozoites dwell in the lcolon where they multiply and encyst. These colonize the large intestine, some trophozoits invade the bowel and cause ulceration, mainly in the caecum and ascending colon; then in the rectum and sigmoid.
Ref: Park's Textbook of Preventive and Social Medicine, 18th Ed, Pg-193

Q. 560. Osler's nodes are a clinical feature of (UPSC-06)
    (a)   Osteoarthritis
    (b)   Rheumatoid arthritis
    (c)   Leprosy
    (d)   Infective endocarditis

Ans. (d)

Note
Osler's nodes are a clinical feature of 'infective endocarditis'.

Also see
Osler's nodes
These are clinical noncardiac manifestation of subacute endocarditis. These are painful tender swellings at the fingertips that are probably the product of vasculitis; they are rare.
Ref: Davidson's Principles and PLracticce of Medicine 19th Ed, Pg-464

Extended information
Heberden's Nodes
These are typically seen in middle aged women and affected joints develop posterolateral swellings each side of the extensor tendon. They slowly enlarge and harden to become 'haberden's node' at distal interphalangeal joints. A similar swellings at proximal interphalangeal joint is known as 'Bouchard's node'.
Ref: Davidson's Principles and PLracticce of Medicine 19th Ed, Pg-999
Rheumatoid nodes
These are seen in case of rheumatoid arthritis. , the 'rheumatic nodes are seen on the subcutaneously over the bony prominences, usually at he site of pressure or friction, usually at the extensor surfaces of forearm, sacrum, Achilles tendons and toes. They may get complicated by ulceration and secondary infection.
Ref: Davidson's Principles and PLracticce of Medicine 19th Ed, Pg-1005
Leprosy
In case of lepromatous leprosy common skin lesions are papules, nodules or diffuse infiltration of skin.
Ref: Davidson's Principles and PLracticce of Medicine 19th Ed, Pg-88

Q. 561. Match List I with List II and select the correct answer using the code given below the lists (UPSC-06)

List- I (Disease)	List-II (Type of Anaemia)
A. Iron deficiency anemia	1. Macrocytic Normochromic
B. Pernicious anemia	2. Macrocytic hypohromic
C. Aplastic anemia	3. Normocytic Normochromic

Code:

	A	B	C
(a)	2	1	3
(b)	3	2	1
(c)	3	1	2
(d)	1	2	3

Ans. Use your discretion

Note
Appearnlty a Typhographic mistake for Iron deficiency anemia – there has to be choice of Mircrocytic hypochromic than:
The following choice takes palce

List- I (Disease)	List-II (Type of Anaemia)
A. Iron deficiency anemia	1. Macrocytic hypochromic
B. Pernicious anemia	2. Macrocytic Normochromic
C. Aplastic anemia	3. Normocytic Normochromic

Extended information
Anemia
The scehemes for the investigation of anemias are often based on the size f the red cells, which are most accurately indicvated by the Mean Cell Volume (MCV) in the FBC (Full Blood Count):
- A normal MCV (Normocytic anaemia) suggests either acute blood loss or the anemia of chronic disease
- A low MCV (Microcytic anaemia) suggests iron deficiney or thalassaemia
- A high MCV (Macrocytic anaemia) suggests vitamin B12 or folate deficiency.

Ref: Davidnson's Principles and Practice of Medicine, 19th Ed, Pg-904

Microcytic Anemia
A form of hypochromic microcytic anemia due to the dietary lack of iron or to a loss of iron from chronic bleeding.
Iron deficiency anemia is the most common type of anemia overall, and it is often hypochromic microcytic iron deficiency anemia is caused when the dietary intake or absorption of iron is insufficient. Iron is an essential part of hemoglobin, and low iron levels result in decreased incorporation of hemoglobin into red blood cells. The principal cause of iron deficiency anemia in premenopausal women is blood lost during menses. Iron deficiency is the most prevalent deficiency state on a worldwide basis. Iron found in animal meats are more easily absorbed by the body than iron found in non-meat sources. In countries where meat consumption is not as common, iron deficiency anemia is six to eight times more prevalent than in Europe. A characteristic of iron deficiency is angular chelitis, which is an abnormal fissuring of corners of the mouth.

Macrocytic anemia
Anemia in which the average size of the red blood cells in circulation is greater than normal. Megaloblastic anemia occurs due to deficiency of vitamin B12 and Folic acid.

Pernicious anemina is anautoimmune condition directed against the parietal cells of the stomach. Parietal cells produce intrinsic factor, required to absorb vitamin B12 from food. Therefore, the destruction of the parietal cells causes a lack of intrinsic factor, leading to poor absorption of vitamin B12
    -Alcoholism
    -Iatrogenic; Drugs like Methotrexate, zidvudine inhibit DNA replication. This is the most common etiology in nonalcoholic patients.
Macrocytic anemia can be further divided into "megaloblastic anemia" or "non-megaloblastic macrocytic anemia". The cause of megaloblastic anemia is primarily a failure of DNA synthesis with preserved RNA synthesis, which result in restricted cell division of the progenitor cells. The megaloblastic anemias often present with neutrophil hypersegmentation (6-10 lobes). The non-megaloblastic macrocytic anemias have different etiologies (ie there is unimpaired DNA synthesis,) which occur, for example in alcoholism.

The treatment for vitamin B12-deficient macrocytic and pernicious anemias was first devised by William Murphy who bled dogs to make them anemic and then fed them various substances to see what (if anything) would make them healthy again. He discovered that ingesting large amounts of liver seemed to cure the disease.

Normocytic anemia:
    -Acute lood loss Anemia of chronic disease
    -Aplastic anemia (bone marrow failure)

Remember:
    -Iron deficiency anemia is -Microcytic Hypochromic
    -Pernicious anemia (Megaloblastic) – Macrocytic Hypochromic
    -Aplastic anemia – Normocytic Normocronic

Summary

Type	Normochromic	Hypochromic
Normocytic	(1) After acute haemorrhage (2) All haemolytic anaemias except Thalassaemia (3) Aplastic anaemia	After chronic haemorrhage
Macrocytic	All megaloblastic anaemias due to deficiency of Vit.B12;Folic acid or intrinsic factor	Secondary to liver disease
Microcytic	Chronic infections	(1) Iron deficiency anaemia (2) Thalassaemia

Textbook of Physiology, A.K. Jain Pg-66

562. Match List I with List II and select the correct answer using the code given below the lists (UPSC-06)

List- I (Test)	List-II (Disease Condition)
A. Casoni's Test	1. Kala Azar
B. Weilfelix Reaction	2. Rickettsial Infection
C. Ascoti's Test	3. Plague
D. Paul Bunnel Test	4. Infectious Mononucleosis

Code

	A	B	C	D
(a)				
(b)				
(c)				
(d)				

Ans. Use your discretion
Note
The correct answer is as under

List- I (Test)	List-II (Disease Condition)
A. Casoni's Test	4. Hydatid Cyst / Kala Azar
B. Weilfelix Reaction	3. Rickettsial Infection
C. Ascoti's Test	1. Plague
D. Paul Bunnel Test	2. Infectious Mononucleosis

Please remember that the 'Casoni's test is for 'hydatid diseases' rather than for Kala azar.

Also see
Casoni's Test (reaction)
It is an immediate hypersensitivity skin test for diagnosis of Hydatid cyst. An intradermal injection of a fresh hydatid fluid produces within half an hour, in all positive cases, a large wheal (5cm in diameter) with multiple pseudopodia; it fades in an hour. Normal saline is injected in other arm for control. Hydatid fluid from human cases or animals is used as antigen.
Ref: Parasitology, K.D.Chatterjee, 12th Ed, Pg- 127
Weil-felix Reaction
The weil-felix reaction is the non-specific agglutination of the somatic antigens of non-motile Proteus species by the patient's serum. A four fold rise in titre is diagnostic.
Ref: Davidson, 19th Ed, Pg-64
Paul-Bunnel Test
The heterophil antibodies, which are present in during the acute illness and during convalescence, agglutinate erythrocytes of other species, for e.g., sheep and horse. The antibody which has a specific absorption pattern is detected by classical Paul-Bunnel tritration.
Pg.16, Davidson, 19th Edition

Q. 563. Assertive and Reasoning type question
Assertion (A): The pathognomonic symptom of cholera is copious rice water stools
Reason (R): The pathogenesis of cholera is the inhibition of absorption fluids in the small intestine
Code:
(a) Both A and R are individually true and R is the correct explanation of A.
(b) Both A and R are individually true but R is **not** the correct explanation of A
(c) A is true but R is false
(d) A is false but R is true

Ans. (c)
Note
The A is correct
The B is incorrect as it predominantly caused intestine to lose the fluids in lumen however, the intestine at the same time cannot absorb the fluids.
Therefore A is correct and B is not truly correct.
The answer become –c

Also see
There is a dual effect on two different intestinal ion-transport sites. In the villus cell, the absorption of sodium chloride via the neutral sodium chloride co-transport system is inhibited. In the crypt cells the increased intracellular cAMP results in active stimulation of chloride secretion. The net effect is the rapid outpouring of isotonic fluid into the intestinal lumen at a rate that exceeds the absorptive capacity of the colon resulting in intra-luminal loss of isotonic fluid.
Ref: API, 7th Ed, Pg-56.

Q. 564. Consider the following features (UPSC-06)
1. Massive proteinuria
2. Oligouria

3. Hypoalbuminemia
4. Hematuria

Which of the above are the features consistent with Nephrotic syndrome?
(a) 1 and 2
(b) 1 and 3
(c) 2 and 3
(d) 2 and 4

Ans. (c)

Note
The above features consistent with Nephrotic syndrome are 2. Massive proteinuria and 3. Hypoalbuminemia.

Also see
Nephrotic syndrome is characterized by proteinuria >3.0 to 3.5 g per 24 h, hypoalbuminemia, edema, hyperlipidemia, lipiduria, and hypercoagulability.
Ref: Harrison 15th Ed.

Q. 565. Consider the following: (UPSC-06)
1. Pericardial effusion
2. Menorrhagia
3. Delayed ankle relaxation
4. Tachycardia during sleep
5. Heat intolerance

Which of above are the features for confirmation of hyperthyroidism?
(a) 1, 2 and 3
(b) 2, 4 and 5 Only
(c) 2, 3, 4 and 5
(d) 4 and 5 Only

Ans. (d)

Note
Features given above which are confirmatory of hyperthyroidism are 4 and 5 only.

Also see
The above symptoms in reference to the hyper and Hypo-thyroidism are as under:

Features	Hypothyroidism	Hyperthyroidism
1. Pericardial effusion	Present	NA
2. Menorrhagia	Present	NA
3. Delayed ankle relaxation	Present	NA
4. Tachycardia during sleep	NA	Yes+++
5. Heat intolerance	NA	Yes+++

Extended information
1. *Pericardial effusion*
   Associated with hypothyroidism.
   Other causes are:
   Viral pericarditis, Bacterical (Tubercular) pericarditis, SLE, Post myocardial infarction pericarditis, renal failure (Uremic pericarditis).
2. *Menorrhagia*
   Asscisted with hypothyroidism.
   Other causes are:
3. Delayed ankle relaxation
4. Tachycardia during sleep
5. Heat intolerance
   In case of hyperthyroidism tachycardia during sleep and heat intolerance is very specific features.
Ref: API 7th Ed, Pg-1054

Q. 566. Among the following, the most common cause of maternal death in septic abortion is (UPSC-06)
    (a)   Endotoxic septic shock
    (b)   Uterine perforation
    (c)   Tetanus
    (d)   Renal failure

Ans. (d)
Note
Among the above, the most common cause of maternal death in septic abortion is 'Renal failure'.
Also see
In case of septic shock – hypotension will be a strong presenting feature – results in – renal damage, which is irreversible – therefore, the cause of death in such a case would be 'Renal failure'

Q. 567. The complaints of a patient suffering from diabetes include (UPSC-06)
    (a)   Retinopathy
    (b)   Neuropahty only
    (c)   Gangrene of feet only
    (d)   All of above

Ans. (d)
Note
The patient suffering from diabetes includes 'all of above'.
Also see
The patient suffering from diabetes commnly develops follwing:
a.   Diabetic retinopathy
b.   Diabetic neuropathy
c.   Diabetic foot which includes gangrene of feet
Diabetic retinopathy, nephropathy and neuropathy tend to manifest 10-20 years after diagnosis of diabetes in young patients. With diabetes amputation of foot for gangrene is 50 times as likely. Diabetes can damage peripheral nervous tissue in a number of ways.
Ref: Kumar and Clark, 6th Ed, Pg- 1123, 1124, 1128

PSYCHIATRY

Q. 568. A patient with pneumonia for 5 days is admitted to the hospital. He suddenly ceases to recognize the doctor and staff, thinks that he is in jail and complains of scorpions attacking him. He is in altered sensorium. This condition is
    (a)   Acute delirium
    (b)   Acute dementia
    (c)   Acute schizophrenia
    (d)   Acute paranoia

Ans. (a)
Note
Delirium is characterized by acute clouding of consciousness, disturbed orientation, impaired perception, concentration, disordered thinking, and poor comprehension. It is a reversible state.
Acute organic brain syndrome is known as "Delirium". Celsus coined this word in the first century A.D. It is reversible and most commonly encountered condition.
Predominant Miasm:
It is an acute state under the domain of acute miasm.
In present case the cause is infection (Pneumonia).

Also see

FEATURES	DELIRIUM
Onset	Usually acute
Course	Usually recover in one week
Clinical Features:	
-Consciousness	Clouded
-Orientation	Grossly disturbed
-Memory	Immediate retention and recall disturbed

Ref. A short book of psychiatry, by Niraj Ahuja, 5th Ed, Pg-23.

Q. 569. A person missing from home, is found wandering purposefully. He is well groomed, and denies of having any amnesia. Most likely diagnosis is
- (a) Dissociative fugue
- (b) Dissociative amnesia
- (c) Schizophrenia
- (d) Dementia

Ans. (a)

Note
Most likely diagnosis is 'dissociative fugue'.

Also see
Dissociative fugue state

Features are:
- Sudden change in state of consciousness.
- Patient may appear quite normal to his casual observer.
- Forgets his name and past history.
- Assumes false name and identity.
- Performs complicated activities.
- May travel over long distances.

Fugues of short duration:
- Wanders aimlessly.
- Is highly emotional, agitated, confused.

Fugues of long duration:
- Travels far away.
- Appears self possessed.
- Lives in every way like normal person except that he is not where he should be.

On termination of fugue:
- He is aware of his identity with full memory of past life.
- Complete amnesia for fugue period.

Extended information
In *dissociative fugue*, patients not only loose their memory but wander away from their usual surroundings, and when found deny all memories of their where-abouts during this wandering. The differential diagnosis of fugue state includes post-ictal automatism, depressive illness and alcohol abuse.
Ref: Kumar and Clark, Clinical Medicine, 6th Ed, Pg-1286

Q.570. Babu, a 40 years aged male complains of sudden onset palpitations and apprehension. He is sweating for the last 10 minutes and fears of impending death. Diagnosis is
- (a) Hysteria
- (b) Cystic fibrosis
- (c) Panic attack
- (d) Generalized anxiety disorder

Ans. (c)

Note
Diagnosis is 'Panic attack'.

Also see
Panic attack
Sudden, paroxysmal, unpredictable attacks of severe anxiety that are usually accompanied by severe physical symptoms.
Onset: is sudden
During attack: intense fear, apprehension, fear of impending death.
Duration: reaches peak within minutes. Lasts for several minutes to 2 hours.
After attack: feels agitated and fatigued for several hours.
In-between the attacks patient is free of anxiety: however, secondary avoidance behaviour may be prominent.

Extended information
Panic attacks are usually associated with an automatic disturbance such as tachycardia, sweating and pilo-erection.
Ref: Kumar and Clark, Clinical Medicine, 6th Ed, Pg-1226.

Q. 571. A lady, while driving a car meets with an accident. She was admitted in an ICU for 6 months. After being discharged, she often gets up in night and feels terrified. She is afraid to sit in a car again. The diagnosis is
    (a)   Panic disorder
    (b)   Phobia
    (c)   Conversion disorder
    (d)   Post traumatic stress disorder

Ans. (d)
Note
The diagnosis for above presentation is 'Post Traumatic Stress Disorder'.

Also see
Post traumatic stress disorder is a delayed and protracted response to stressful event or situation of exceptionally threatening or catastrophic nature outside the range of everyday human experience, which is likely to cause pervasive distress in almost anyone.

Ref: Kumar and Clark, Clinical Medicine, 6th Ed, Pg-1300.

Extended information
Mnemonics for PTSD
'IRAN PTSD':
I - Intrusive
R - Recollections
A - Autonomic features
N - Numbing
P - Post trauma
T - Temporal link
S - Stimulus avoidance
D - Detachment/ Depression

Q. 572. A patient present with waxy flexibility, negativitism and rigidity. Diagnosis is
    (a)   Catatonic schizophrenia
    (b)   Paranoid schizophrenia
    (c)   Hebephrenic schizophrenia
    (d)   Simple schizophrenia

Ans. (a)
Note
The diagnosis for the above presentation is 'catatonic schizophrenia'.

Also see
Criterion for catatonic schizophrenia:
- Motoric immobility as evident by catalepsy or stupor
- Excessive motor activity
- Extreme negativism or mutism
- Echolalia or echopraxia

Ref: API 7th Ed, Pg-1380.

Extended information
People who have schizophrenia have lost touch with reality. Following are the main features:
a. Delusions: Bizarre, false beliefs.
b. Hallucination; Unreal perceptions could be auditory, visual, olfactory and tactile.
c. Disorganized thinking / Speech: Abnormal thoughts measured by disorganized speech.
d. Negative symptoms: The absence of normal behaviour.
e. Catatonia: Immobility and 'waxy flexibility'.

When people show any of these five symptoms, they are considered to be in the "active phase" of the disorder. Time and again schizophrenics have milder symptoms before and after the active phase.

The three main types of schizophrenia are:
1. Disorganized Schizophrenia (previously called "hebephrenic schizophrenia"): Lack of emotion, disorganized speech.
2. Catatonic Schizophrenia: Waxy flexibility, reduced movement, rigid posture, sometimes too much movement.
3. Paranoid Schizophrenia: Strong paranoid delusions or hallucinations.

Catatonic Schizophrenia
Catatonia is a negative symptom where people become fixed in a single position for a long period of time. "Waxy flexibility" describes how a person's arms will remain frozen in a particular position if they are moved by someone else.
Ref: from web –www.schizophrenia.com

Q. 573. Chandu, age 32 presents with abdominal pain and vomiting. He also complains of some psychiatric symptoms and visual hallucinations. Most likely diagnosis is
    (a) Intermittent porphyria
    (b) Hypothyroidism
    (c) Hyperthyroidism
    (d) Hysteria

Ans. (a)

Note
Most likely diagnosis for Chandu's problem is 'intermittent porphyria'.

Also see
Intermittent porphyria is an autosomal dominant condition resulting from half-normal level of HMB synthesis activity. Activation of disease is related to environmental or hormonal factors, such as drugs, diet and steroid hormones. Abdominal pain most common symptom, abdominal tenderness, fever and leucocytosis are usually absent or mild. Nausea, vomiting, constipation, tachycardia, hypertension, mental symptoms, pain in limbs, head, neck, or chest, muscle weakness, sensory loss, dysuria and urinary retention are characteristic.
Ref; Harrison, 15th Edition, Section 3- Disorders of intermediary metabolism 346. The porphyrias.
Ref: Harrison, 16th Ed, Pg-2305

Q. 574. Basanti 27 years aged, female thinks her nose is ugly; her idea is fixed and not shared by anyone else. Whenever she goes out of home, she hides her face with a cloth. She visits a Surgeon Next step would be
    (a) Investigate and then operate
    (b) Refer to psychiatrist
    (c) Reassure the patient
    (d) Immediate operation

Ans. (b)

Note
The next step in case of Basanti is to 'Refer to psychiatrist'.

Also see
Basanti has 'fixed idea' that her nose is ugly. Which is not shared by anyone else it prompts that this false belief is not well received by her socio-cultural and educational background. She is having a delusional disorder. There is no requirement of investigation. The best course of action is to refer to psychiatrist.
(Homeopathically the – suggested drug is – Thuja.)

Q. 575. The treatment of choice in attention deficit hyperactivity disorder who can not control dancing while listening music is
    (a)   Tarentula Group
    (b)   Cina
    (c)   Bufo rana
    (d)   Chamomilla

Ans. (a)
Note
The selection of remedy from the above for ADHD who can not control dancing while listening music is 'Tarentula group'.

Also see
The tarentula group (Spider / Arachnida) includes following:
1. Aranea diadema
2. Aranea ixobola
3. Aranea scinencia
4. Aranerum tela (cobweb)
5. Latrodactus heseltii
6. Latrodactus katipo
7. Latrodactus mactans
8. Mygale lasiodora
9. Tarentula cubensis
10. Tarentula hispania
11. Theridion curassavicum

Extended information
Its main features as under:
a. Onset of complaints: Sudden.
b. Trembing twitching. Chorea / involuntary movements.
c. Instability: Of action, purpose, wisdom.
d. Periodicity: Symptoms recur periodically. Same hour; Aranea, 21st day; Tarent.
e. Restlessness: Changes place, cannot remain in one position.
f. < Brighrt objects, Touch, Noice, Light, Cotion, after or durng menses.
g. > Music, Rubbing, Smoking
h. Desires: Alcohol, Ashes, Bananas (Theridion), Cold drinks, seasoned food, raw food, Tobacco.
i. Aversion: Bread, Meat, Chocolate.
j. A/F; contradition.

Q. 576. Yawning is a common feature of
    (a)   Alcohol withdrawal
    (b)   Cocaine withdrawal
    (c)   Cannabis withdrawal
    (d)   Opioid withdrawal

Ans. (d)
Note
Yawning is a common feature of 'opioid withdrawal'.

Also see
Opiate withdrawal syndrome:

12-16 hours after last dose of opiate:
- Yawning
- Rhinorrhea
- Lachrymation
- Pupilary dilatation
- Sweating
- Pilo-erection
- Restlessness

24-72 hours after last dose of opiate:
- Muscle twitching
- Aches and pains
- Abdominal cramps
- Vomiting
- Diarrhea
- Hypertension
- Insomnia
- Anorexia
- Agitation
- Profuse sweating
- Weight loss

Ref: Kumar and Clark, Clinical Medicine, 6th d, Pg-1306

Q. 577. False sense of perception without any external object or stimulus is known as
    (a)   Illusions
    (b)   Impulse
    (c)   Hallucination
    (d)   Phobia

Ans. (c)

Note
False sense of perception without any external object or stimulus is known as 'hallucinaitons'.

Also see
Hallucinations (perception without stimulation) are usually experienced as originating in the outside world, or within one's own body but not within the mind as through imagination.
Ref : API 7th Ed, Pg-1378

Q. 578. The following is a Schneider's first rank symptom
    (a)   Persecutory delusion
    (b)   Voices commenting on actions
    (c)   Delusion of guilt
    (d)   Incoherence

Ans. (b)

Note
The following is a Schneider's first rank symptom 'voice commenting on acitons'.

Also see
Schneider's first rank symptoms:
1. Hallucinations:
   - Audible thoughts: voices speaking out thoughts aloud or thought echo.
   - Voices heard arguing: Two or more hallucinatory voices discussing the subject in third person.
   - Voices commenting on one's action.
2. Thought alienation phenomenon:
   - Thought withdrawal
   - Thought insertion
   - Thought broadcasting
3. Passivity phenomenon
4. Delusional perception

Ref: A Short book of Psychiatry by Niraj Ahuja, 5th Ed, Pg-56.

Extended information
Mnemonics for remembering Schneiderian first rank symptoms is as easy as:
'ABCD':
A- Auditory hallucinations - 3rd person/echo-de-la-pensé
B- Broadcasting of thoughts/ insertion/withdrawal
C- Control experiences/ passivity phenomena
D- Delusional perception

Q. 579. A 30-year old male with history of alcohol abuse for 15 years is brought to the hospital emergency with complaints of fearfulness, mis-recognition, talking to self, aggressive behavior, tremulousness and seeing snakes and reptiles that are not visible to others around him. There is history of drinking alcohol two days prior to the onset of the present complaints. He is most likely suffering from
   (a)   Delirium tremens
   (b)   Alcoholic hallucinosis
   (c)   Schizophrenia
   (d)   Seizure disorder

Ans. (a)
Note
He is most likely suffering from 'Delirium tremens'.
Also see
Delirium tremens is the most serious withdrawal state and occurs 2-3 days after alcohol cessation. Patients are disorientated, agitated and have a marked tremor and visual hallucinations (e.g. insects or small animals coming menacingly towards them). Signs include seating, tachycardia, tachypnea and pyrexia.
Ref: Kumar and Clark, Clinical Medicine, 6th Ed, Pg-1304

Extended information
Alcohol withdrawal syndrome (Delirium Tremens)
Onset:
     -Acute, after alcoholic debauch or withdrawal.
     -(Patients are often hospitalized for different reasons).
Symptoms:
     -Aversion to food. Nausea, Retching.
     -Fear. Irritability. Restlessness. Prolonged insomnia.
     -Nocturnal anxiety. Night mares.
     -Terrifying dreams. Clouding of consciousness.
     -Impairment of recent memory.
Illusions:
     -Figures on wall appear menacing animate objects.
     -Ink spots appear insects, which patient attempts to seize and destroy.
Hallucinations:
     -Small animals, e.g. mice, rat, insects (zoopsia).
     -Feels insects on his skin.
     -Delusions.

Q. 580. A 25 year old university student had a fight with the neighboring boy. On the next day while out, he started feeling that two men in police uniform were observing his movements. When he reached home in the evening he was frightened. He expressed that police was after him and would arrest him. His symptoms represent
   (a)   Delusion of persecution
   (b)   Ideas of reference
   (c)   Passivity
   (d)   Thought insertion

Ans. (a)
Note
His symptoms represent 'Delusion of persecution'.

Also see
This student is presenting with disturbed thinking, which is delusion of persecution: Suspicion that others are trying to harm / kill / poison him. Such a feature point strongly to the possibility of - Paranoid schizophrenia.

Extended information
Paranoid schizophrenia: Preoccupation with one or more delusion persecutory: being persecuted by friends, neighbours or spouses; being followed, monitored or spied on by government.
Ref: API 7th Ed, Pg-1380

Q. 581. A 40-year old male is admitted with complaints of abdominal pain and headache. General physical examination revealed six scars on the abdomen from previous surgeries. He seems to maintain a sick role and seeks attention from the nurses. He demands multiple diagnostic tests including a liver biopsy. The treating team failed to diagnose any major physical illness in the patient. His mental status examination did not reveal any major psychopathology. One of the treating staff recognized him to have appeared in several other hospital with abdominal pain and some other vague complaints. He is most likely suffering from
  (a) Schizophrenia
  (b) Malingering
  (c) Somatisation disorder
  (d) Factitious disorder

Ans. (d)
Note
He is most likely suffering from 'Factitious disorder'.

Also see
Factitious Disorders
Extreme form of abnormal illness behaviour characterized by conscious, consistent, deliberate, repeated and superstitious feigning or fabrication of physical or psychological symptoms to simulate disease, in absence of distinct psychiatric or physical disorder. Commonest presentation among factitious disorders is that of Munchausen's Syndrome.

Extended information
Munchausen's Syndrome
Term Munchausen's syndrome was coined by Asher in 1951, named after German Baron Karl Freidrich Von Munchausen.
Munchausen served as Calvary officer in Russian army, and was legendary for his inventive lying. He was well known for wandering about from town to town telling extravagant war stories.

People with Munchausen syndrome may pose symptoms in a variety of ways. These include (1) Total fabrication; such as falsely claiming to be HIV-positive; (2) Simulation; such as mimicking a seizure; (3) illness aggravation; such as manipulating a wound so it will not heal.

Factitious disorder (Munchausen syndrome) also known as hospital addiction, patients repeatedly simulate or fake disease for the sole purpose of obtaining medical attention. There is no other recognizable motive. It can present with predominantly physical signs and symptoms or psychological signs and symptoms.

Ref: API 7th Ed, Pg-389

Q. 582. A 23-year-old engineering student is brought by his family to the hospital with history of gradual onset of suspiciousness, muttering and smiling without clear reason, decreased socialization, violent outbursts, and lack of interest in studies for 8 months. Mental status examination revealed a blunt effect, thought broadcast, a relatively preserved cognition, impaired judgement and insight. He is most likely to be suffering from
  (a) Delusional disorder
  (b) Depression
  (c) Schizophrenia
  (d) Anxiety disorder

Ans. (c)

MCQ's in Practice of Medicine

Note
This young student is presenting with the feature of schizophrenia.
Ref: API 7th Ed, Pg- 1379-1380

Also see
In brief the feature schizophrenia is as under:

Clinical features of Schizophrenia		
Aspects	Features	
1.	At Perceptive level:	
	a.	Breakdown in perceptual selectivity
	b.	Hallucinations
2.	At Cognition / Thought level:	
	a.	Formal thought disorder
	b.	Delusions
	c.	Impaired judgement and reality testing
	d.	Confused state of self
3.	Affect / Emotional level:	
	a.	Prodromal anxiety and depression
	b.	Inappropriate affect
	c.	Flattened affect and impoverished affect
	d.	Post-psychotic depression
4.	Interpersonal adjustment:	
	a.	Poor school / work performance
	b.	Withdrawal from peer relationships
	c.	Deterioration in family relationship
5.	Behaviour:	
	a.	Prodromal sleep disturbances
	b.	Prodromal impulsiveness
	c.	Prodromal repetitive compulsive behaviour
	d.	Impaired goal directed behaviour
	e.	Catatonia, negativism, and mutation

Q. 583. Many of our bad habits of day to day life can be removed by
(a) Positive conditioning
(b) Biofeedback
(c) Negative conditioning
(d) Generalization

Ans. (a)

Note
Many of the habits of day to day life can be removed by 'Positive conditioning'.

Also see
The common methods for augmenting and adaptive behaviour are:
Positive reinforcement here the desirable behaviour is reinforced by a reward, material or symbolic.

Ref: A Short Textbook of Psychiatry by Neeraj Ahuja.5th Ed, Pg-221

Extended information
Positive Conditioning
The positive (reinforcement) conditioning is more acceptable procedure which can be undertaken in day to day activity and without any special need of settings.
In this the desirable behaviour is reinforced by a reward. The reward could be in the form of material or symbolic.

Biofeedback
The biofeedback technique utilizes our innate potential to influence the autonomic functions of our body by sheer force of will.

Special electronic instruments are used, which provide immediate feedback to the patient in respect of his physiological activities, which the human mind is not aware of. Sensors present in these machines record muscle contractions, skin temperature, heart rate, blood pressure which increases under stress. Once 'feedback' is received, the individual can recognise and control the stress response.

Biofeedback is found to be effective in treatment of enuresis, migraine, tension headache, essential hypertension, cardiac arrhythmias and uncontrolled generalized tonic clonic seizures.

Negative (reinforcement) Conditioning
Here, on performance of the desirable behaviour, punishment can be avoided.

Q. 584. A 30 year old unmarried woman of average socio-economic background believes that her boss is in secretly love with her. She rings him up at odd hours and writes love letters to him despite his serious warnings not to do so. She holds this belief despite contradiction from her family members and his denial. However, she is able to manage her daily activities as before. She is most likely to be suffering from
   (a) Depression
   (b) Schizophrenia
   (c) Delusional disorder
   (d) No psychiatric ailment

Ans. (c)
Note
This lady is presenting with delusional fixed idea, and the most appropriate choice is (c).

Q. 585. A 35 year old male, with pre-morbid anxious traits and heavy smoker, believes that he has been suffering from 'lung carcinoma' for a year. No significant clinical finding is detected on examination and relevant investigations. He continues to stick to his belief despite evidence to the contrary. In the process, he has spent a huge amount of money, time and energy in getting himself unduly investigated. He is most likely suffering from
   (a) Carcinoma lung
   (b) Delusional disorder
   (c) Hypochondriacal disorder
   (d) Malingering

Ans. (c)
Note
The most likely diagnosis form above is 'Hypochondriacal diorder'.

Also see
The above case has following features:
   -Age 35 years
   -Sex: M
   -Pedrsonality trait: Pre-morbid anxious personality traits
   -Addiction: Heavy smoker
   -Current thought content:
    Believes that he has been suffering from 'lung carcinoma' for a year.
   -Medical Examination: Shows no significant findings.
   -Investigations: No supporting Investigative findings.
   -Has spent a huge amount of money, time and energy in investigations.

Conclusion:
The features points to disturbed thought content. However, his main complaint is that he has (some incurable disease) lung cancer. This fits in to the diagnosis of hypochondical disorder / delusion.

Extended information
The current psychiatric diagnostic manual (DSM-IV), indicates the following diagnostic criteria:
1. Preoccupation with fears of having, or the idea that one has, a serious disease based on the person's misinterpretation of bodily symptoms.

2. The preoccupation persists despite appropriate medical evaluation and reassurance.
3. The belief criterion A is not of delusional intensity (as in Delusional Disorder, somatic Type) and is not restricted to a circumscribed concern about appearance (as in Body Dysmorphic Disorder).
4. The preoccupation causes clinically significant distress or impairment in social, occupational, or other important areas of functioning.
5. The duration of the disturbance is at least 6 months.
6. The preoccupation is not better accounted for by Generalized Anxiety Disorder, Obsessive-Compulsive Disorder, Panic Disorder, a Major Depressive Episode, Separation Anxiety, or another Somatoform Disorder..

Ref: http://www.bio-behavioral.com/hypochondriasis.asp

Q. 586. A 14 year old boy has difficulty in expressing himself in writing, and makes frequent spelling mistakes. He passes his examinations with poor marks. However, his mathematical ability and social adjustment are appropriate for his age. Which of the following is the most likely diagnosis?
   (a) Mental retardation
   (b) Lack of interest in studies
   (c) Specific learning disability
   (d) Examination phobia

Ans. (c)
Note
Most likely diagnosis for above clinical presentation is 'Speicific learning disability'.
Also see

The clinical presentation above is pointing to a specific learning disability in writing where he is making frequent spelling istkes.
The common inability in functioning well at school is due to:
Specific learning disability:
Dyslexia (specific reading disability).
Dyscalculia (difficulty with mathematics).
Dysgraphia (difficulty with writing).

Q. 587. A 35 year old man with an obsessive-compulsive personality disorder is likely to exhibit all of the following features, except
   (a) Perfectionism interfering with performance
   (b) Compulsive checking behaviour
   (c) Preoccupation with rule
   (d) Indecisiveness

Ans. (d)
Note
A patient of OCD is likely to exibit all of above except 'Indecisiveness'.
Also see
Individual with this disorder is preoccupied with details and lose the sense of overall goals. They are strict, perfectionistic, overconscious, and inflexible. They are also obsessed with work and productivity and are hesitant to delegate tasks to others.
Mnemonics for Obsessive Compulsive (Anakastic) Personality disorder:

'PREOCCUPIED'
   -Preoccupied with details and rules
   -Rigid and Stubborn
   -Excessively concerned with productivity
   -Overconsciencious and scrupulous
   -Conventionalist & pedantic
   -Cautious and doubting
   -Urges others to submit to their wishes
   -Perfectionist
   -Inhibited due to perfectionism

- Eager to save money
- Discarding of things difficult

Q. 588. Exercise is also prescribed as an adjuvant treatment for depression Most probably it acts by
    (a) Increasing pulse pressure
    (b) Improving hemodynamics
    (c) Raising endorphin levels
    (d) Inducing good sleep

Ans. (c)
Note
Exercise most probably helps treating depression by raising endorphin levels.

Also see
Exercise when prescribed as an adjuvant treatment for depresson most probably it acts by raising endorphin levels. Endorphins are bodies natural pain-killers and can provide relief from some aches and pains, release muscle tension, help you sleep better, and reduce levels of the stress hormone cortisol. It also increases body temperature, which may have calming effects. All of these changes in your mind and body can improve such symptoms as sadness, anxiety, irritability, stress, fatigue, anger, self-doubt and hopelessness. However, 80% depression sufferers have insomnia, in such a case exercise regulaes sleep patterns.

Q. 589. A 16-years-old male is found to have a mental age of 9 years on IQ testing. He has (AIIMS-May 05)
    (a) Mild mental retardation
    (b) Moderate mental retardation
    (c) Severe mental retardation
    (d) Profound mental retardation

Ans. (a)
Note
Intelligent Quotient = Mental Age / Cronological age x 100

Therefore in this case IQ = 9/16x100 = 56.2
See Following Table:

S. No	Mental Retardatioon Level	I.Q. Range
1	Mild	50 – 70
2	Moderate	35 – 49
3	Severe	20 – 34
4	Profound	Less than 20

Therefore the above case falls into the category of Mild metal retardation.

Q. 590. A 50-year-old male present with a 3-year history of irritability, low mood, lack of interest in surroundings and general dissatisfaction with everything. There is no significant disruption in his sleep or appetite. He is likely to be suffering from
    (a) Major depression
    (b) Non psychiatric disorder
    (c) Dysthymia
    (d) Chronic fatigue syndrome

Ans. (c)
Note
He is likely to be suffering from dysthymia.

Also see
Dysthymia is more mild depression that lasts intermittently for two years or more & is characterized by tiredness & low mood, lack of pleasure, low self esteem, & a feeling of discouragement. The mood relapses & remits, with several weeks of feeling well, soon followed longer periods being unwell. It can be punctuated by depressive episodes of severity called double depression.

Ref: Kumar & Clarke 6th Ed, Pg-1289

Q. 591. A 25-year-old woman complains of intense depressed mood for 6 months with inability to enjoy previously pleasurable activities. This symptom is known as (AIIMS-May 05)
    (a)   Anhedonia
    (b)   Avolition
    (c)   Apathy
    (d)   Amotivation

Ans. (a)

Note
The above features are in favour of 'Anhedonia'.

Also see
The inability to enjoy previously pleasurable activities is 'Anhedonia'. Subjects with 'anhedonia' have inability to experience or imagine pleasant emotions. They have little or no response to emotionally charged external events.

Extended information
Disorders of affect
These include apathy, emotional blunting, emotional shallowness, anhedonia (incapability of experiencing pleasure) & inappropriate emotional response (emotional response inappropriate to thought).
Ref: Neeraj Ahuja 5th Ed, Pg-58

Q. 592. All are adulterants of heroin, except
    (a)   Chalk powder
    (b)   Quinine
    (c)   Charcoal
    (d)   Fructose

Ans. (c)

Note
All are adulterants of heroin, except 'Charcoal'.

Q. 593. A 45-year-male with a history of alcohol dependence presents with confusion nystagmus and ataxia. Examination reveals 6th cranial nerve weakness. He is most likely to be suffering from
    (a)   Korsakoff's psychosis
    (b)   Wernicke encephalopathy
    (c)   De Clerambault syndrome
    (d)   Delirium tremens

Ans. (b)

Note
He is most likely to be suffering from 'Wernicke encephalopathy'.

Also see
Wernickes encephalopathy
This is an acute reaction to severe thiamine defiency, the commonest cause being chronic alcohol use. Characteristically the onset occurs after a period of persistent vomiting the important clinical signs are:
1. Occular signs-Coarse nystagmus & ophthalmoplegia with bilateral external rectus paralysis occur early. Pupillary irregularities, retinal hemorrhages & papillary edema can occur causing impairment of vision.
2. Higher mental function disturbance; disorientation confusion, recent memory disturbance, poor attention span &distractibility are common apathy & ataxia are early symptom.

Ref: Neeraj Ahuja 5th Ed, Pg-40, 41

Extended information
Wernicke's encephalopathy is is caused by a lack of thiamine. It is a medical emergency. It is reversible. Untreated it can progress to Korsakov's Syndrome.
Mnemonics for Wernicke's Encehlapathy:

'CANON'
C - Clouded consciousness
A - Ataxia

N - Nystagmus
O - Opthalmoplegia
N – Neuropathy

Q. 594. A 25-year-old female presents with 2 year history of repetitive, irresistible thoughts of contamination with dirt associated with repetitive hand washing. She reports these thoughts to be her own and distressing; but is not able to overcome them along with medications. She is most likely to benefit from which of the following therapies (ALL INDIA/05)
    (a) Exposure and response prevention
    (b) Systematic desensitization
    (c) Assertiveness training
    (d) Sensate focusing

Ans. (a)
Note
She is suffering from OCD and most likely to benefit from exposure and response prevention therapy. It is regarded as first line of technique in behavioural thrapy for patients with OCD.
Also see
Treatment of obsessive compulsive disorder:
Psychotherapy of choice is behaviour therapy:
Thought stopping, behaviour modification is an effective mode of therapy with success rate as high as 80% especially for the compulsive acts.

The techniques used are:
    -Thought stopping
    -Response prevention
    -Systematic desensitization
    -Modeling
Ref: Neeraj Ahuja, 5th Ed, Pg-100

Q. 595. An 18 year old boy came to the psychiatry OPD with a complaint of feeling changed from inside. He described himself as feeling strange as if he is different from his normal self. He was very tense and anxious yet could not point out the precise change in him. This phenomena is best called as
    (a) Delusional mood
    (b) Depersonalization
    (c) Autochthonous delusion
    (d) Over valued idea

Ans. (b)
Note
Depersonalisation
Depersonalization is characterized by alteration in the perception or experience of self, so that feeling of ones own reality is temporarily changed or lost .it is an 'as if' phenomenon.

Ref: Neeraj ahuja, 5th Ed, Pg-113
Also see
Term was introduced by Dugas in 1898.
Characterized by:
Feelings of unreality or strangeness:
    -Feeling of changed personality.
    -Feeling that outside world is unreal.
Loss of or changed conviction of one's own identity.
Withdrawal from reality.
Associated with:
    -Sensation of self-estrangement.
    -Pervasive and distressing feeling of detachment.
    -Disturbances in the body image, e.g. feeling that limbs and other parts of body have changed in size or shape.

Frozen feelings:
 -Inability to form emotional contact or rapport with other people.
Difficulty in concentration:
 -Patient complains that his brain has stopped working.

Q. 596. An 18 year old student complains of lack of interest in studies for last 6 months. He has frequent quarrels with his parents and has frequent headaches. The most appropriate clinical approach would be to (ALL INDIA/05)
 (a) Leave him as normal adolescent problem
 (b) Rule out depression
 (c) Rule out migraine
 (d) Rule out an oppositional defiant disorder

Ans. (b)
Note
The most appropriate clinical approach would be to 'rule out depression'.

Also see
Depressive disorder, clinical or major depression is charecterised by disturbances of mood speech ideas & energy.
However, marked fatigue & headache are the two most common symptoms in depressive illness & may be the first symptom to appear.
Ref: Kumar & Clarke 6th Ed, Pg-288

Extended information
Rule out depression. The features of depression in adolescent may have following features:
 -Loss of interest in socialization and studies
 -loss of pleasure
 -Quick temper
 -Irritability
 -Anger
 -Headache
 -Difficulty in concentration

Q. 597. Preservation is
 (a) Persistent and inappropriate repetition of the same thoughts.
 (b) When a patient feels very distressed about it.
 (c) Characteristic of schizophrenia.
 (d) Characteristic of obsessive compulsive disorder (OCD).

Ans. (a)
Note
Preservation is 'persistent and inappropriate repetition of the same thought'.

Also see

The preservation is persistent and inappropriate repetition of same thought or answers in response to various questions.

Q. 598. One of the following usually differentiates hysterical symptoms from hypochondriacal symptoms (ALL INDIA/05)
 (a) Symptoms do not normally reflect understandable physiological or pathological mechanism.
 (b) Physical symptoms are prominent which are not explained by organic factors.
 (c) Personality traits are significant.
 (d) Symptoms run a chronic course.

Ans. (a)
Note
The differentiating featurs of hysterial from hypochondriacal symptoms is based on that the hystrical symptoms do not reflect understandable physiological / pathological relationship.

Also see
Hysteria
Dissosiative disorders were known as hysteria. It is a condition in which there is a profound loss of awareness or cognitive ability without medical explanation. The term conversion was introduced by Freud to explain how an unresolved conflict would be converted into usually symbolic symptoms as a defence against it
Ref: Kumar & Clarke 6th Ed, Pg-1285

Hypochondriasis

The conspicuous feature is a preoccupation with an assumed serious disease and its consequences. Patient commonly believe that they suffer from cancer or AIDS, or some other serious condition. Characteristically, such patients repeatedly request laboratory & other investigations to either prove they are ill or reassure themselves that they are well.
Ref: Kumar & Clarke 6th Ed, Pg-1285

Q. 599. Signs of organic brain damage are evident on
    (a)   Bender Gestalt test
    (b)   Rorschach test
    (c)   Sentence Completion test
    (d)   Thematic Appercetion test

Ans. (a)
Note
Signs of organic brain damage are evident on 'Bender Gestalt test'.
Also see
Tests for organic brain damage: These assess memory, problem solving and lobe functions. These tests are helpful in dementias, amnesias and other organic dysfunctions. Some of these tests are: the Bender-Gestalt Test, PGI memory scale and neuro-psychological batteries such as Halstead Reitan Battery and Luria Nedraska Battery.

The Bender Gestalt test
In case of Organic psychosis; there is marked difference in verbal and non-verbal tests of intelligence. However, in Functional psychosis there is no marked difference in verbal and non-verbal states of intelligence.

Q. 600. A 25-year old housewife came to the psychiatry out patient department (OPD) complaining that her nose was longer than usual. She felt that her husband did not like her because of the deformity and had developed relationship with the neighboring girl. Further she complained that people made fun of her. It was not possible to convince her that there was no deformity. Her symptoms include
    (a)   Delusion
    (b)   Depersonalization
    (c)   Depression
    (d)   Hallucination

Ans. (a)
Note
Her complaints belong to 'Delusion'.
Also see
Delusions
False, fixed personal beliefs with following characteristics:
Content often bizarre having no rational basis in reality.
Firmly held despite evidence to contrary.
Out of keeping with person's educational and cultural background.
All above features suggest being the feature of persistent delusional disorder, and more specifically the 'Delusional dysmorphobia (body / body part being ugly or mis-shapen) as well as 'Othello syndrome or conjugal paranoia' as is clear from the features presented above as her husband has relationship with the neighbouring girl.
Ref: A Short textbook of Psychiatry by Neeraj Ahuja 4th Edition.

Q. 601. A 30-year old unmarried woman from a low socio-economic status family believes that a rich boy staying in her neighborhood is in deep love with her. The boy clearly denies his love towards this lady. Still the lady insists that his denial is a secret affirmation of his love towards her. She makes desperate attempts to meet the boy despite resistance from her family. She also develops sadness at times when her effort to meet the boy does not materialize. She is able to maintain her daily routine. She, however, remains preoccupied with the thoughts of this boy. She is likely to be suffering from
    (a)   Delusional disorder
    (b)   Depression
    (c)   Mania
    (d)   Schizophrenia

Ans. (a)

Note
She is likely to be suffering from 'Delusional disorder'.

Also see
All above features suggest being the features of Persistant Delusional disorder, and more specifically the 'Erotomanic delusion (Delusion of love). It is a chronic relatively stable behaviour almost normal as far as social and occupational life is concerned. It only becomes obvious when the area of delusions is probed or confronted. Here the content of delusion is erotic which occurs most often in females of young age and she is convinced that a person with higher status is in love with her.

Ref: A Short textbook of Psychiatry By Neeraj Ahuja 4th Edition.

Q. 602. The Non-REM (NREM) sleep is associated with
    (a)   Frequent dreaming
    (b)   Frequent penile erections
    (c)   Increased blood pressure
    (d)   Night terrors

Ans. (d)

Note
The Non-REM (NREM) sleep is associated with 'Night terrors'.

Also see
Night terrors which occur early in the night are a stage 4 Non Rapid Eye Movement disorder and are characterized by complete amnesia.
Ref: Neeraj Ahuja 5th Ed. Pg-148
The night terrors occur in NREM sleep. The patient suddenly gets up screaming and on examination has tachycardia, sweating and hyperventilation. However, in the moning on awakening he not recall the episode.

Sleep EEG shows two distinct features of sleep:
a.   REM sleep: (Rapid eye movement or desynchronizes sleep / active slee/ Paradoxical sleep). Its duration is about 2 hours.
b.   NREM Sleep: (Quiet sleep or Orthodox sleep / Syncronized sleep / S- Sleep) its duration is about 6 hurs. It is further divided into four stages:
    i.   Stage 1 NREM Sleep: characterised by absence of α waves.
    ii.   Stage 2 NREM Sleep: Characterised by (a). Sleep Spindles; Spindle shaped waves of 13-15cycles/sec. (b). K-Complexes; high voltage spikes present intermittently
    iii.   Stage 3 NREM Sleep: Shows high voltage 75 μV, δ waves.
    iv.   Stage 4 NREM Sleep: shows predominant δ activity. Its duration is about 80 minutes.
Ref: A Short textbook of Psychiatry By Neeraj Ahuja 4th Edition.

Q. 603. A 16 year old boy does not attend school because of the fear of being harmed by school mates. He thinks that his classmates laugh at and talk about him. He is even scared of going out to the market. He is most likely suffering from
    (a)   Anxiety neurosis
    (b)   Manic Depressive Psychosis

(c) Adjustment reaction
(d) Schizophrenia

Ans. (d)
Note
He is most likely suffering from 'schizophrenia'.

Also see
The salient features of above case presentation are:
a. Fear of being harmed by school mates – Delusion of persecution / suspicion that his school mates are trying to harm him.
b. He thinks that these classmates laugh at and talk about him - Disturbance of perception.
c. He is scared of going out - Likes to be alone.
The above features are pointers to strong probability of 'Schizophrenia'.

Extended information
Schizophrenia
Schizophrenia is a persistent, mental disorder affecting various aspects of behaviour, thinking, and emotion. Thinking may be disconnected and illogical. Peculiar behaviours may be associated with social withdrawal and disinterest. Patients with delusions or hallucinations may be described as psychotic.
(DSM IV-TR Schizophrenia)

Q. 604. A 41 year old woman working as an Executive Director is convinced that the management has denied her promotion by preparing false reports about her competence and have forged her signatures on sensitive documents so as to convict her. She files a complaint in the police station and requests for security. Despite all this she attends to her work and manages the household. She is suffering from
(a) Paranoid schizophrenia
(b) Late onset psychosis
(c) Persistent delusional disorder
(d) Obsessive compulsive disorder

Ans. (a)
Note
She is suffering from 'Paranoid schizophrenia'.

Also see
The present clinical presentation is of delusion of persecution state and the most suitable diagnostic possibility is paranoid schizophrenia.

Q. 605. All of the following are features of hallucinations, except
(a) It is independent of the will of the observer
(b) Sensory organs are not involved
(c) It is as vivid as that in a true sense perception
(d) It occurs in the absence of a perceptual stimulus

Ans. (c)
Note
All of the above are features of hallucinations, except '(c)'.

Also see
Hallucination: A false perception occurs without external stimuli. Where sensory organs are not involved. It can be of following in nature:
a. Auditory: Most common. Hearing of voices when nobody is around. (Characteristically seen in a psychotic or schizophrenic patient).
b. Visual: Seeing figures, objects, shadows, and ghosts. (Epilepsy, schizophrenia and Organic brain syndrome.)
c. Olfactory: Smelling pleasant or unpleasant odour in the absence of stimuli. (Temporal / Uncinate epilepsy)
d. Gustatory: Peculiar taste in mouth. (Epilepsy / Paranoid disorder)

e. Tactile Hallucination: Feeling of touch or as if insects crawling over the body. (Cocaine bugs, also known as magnan phenomenon. Common in Cocaine addiction.)

Extended information

Hallucinations-healthy people occasionally experience hallucinations, such as in normal grief, or during the transition between sleeping and waking. Hallucinations can be elementary (for e.g. bangs, whistles) or complex (e.g., faces, voices, music) and may affect any of the perceptions: auditory, visual, tactile, gustatory, olfactory or deep sensations.
1. False perception and not a distortion.
2. Perceived as inhabiting objective space.
3. Perceived as having qualities of normal perception.
4. Perceived alongside normal perception.
5. Independent of individual's will.

Ref: kumar & Clarke 6th Ed, Pg-1276

Q. 606. Delirium tremens is characterized by confusion associated with
    (a) Autonomic hyperactivity and tremors
    (b) Features of intoxication due to alcohol
    (c) Sixth nerve palsy
    (d) Korsakoff psychosis

Ans. (a)

Note

Delirium tremens is characterized by confusion associated with 'Autonomic hyperactivity and tremors'.

Also see

Delirium tremens (DTs)

It refers to delirium (mental confusion with fluctuating levels of consciousness) along with a tremor, severe agitation, and autonomic overactivity e.g., marked increases in pulse, blood pressure, and respirations. Fortunately, this serious and potentially life-threatening complication of alcohol withdrawal is rare. Only 5 to 10% of alcohol-dependent individuals ever experience DTs; the chance of DTs during any single withdrawal is less than 1% but is higher if there has been a withdrawal seizure.

Ref: Harrison's 16th Ed. Pg-2565

Q. 607. All of the following are impulse control disorders except
    (a) Pyromania
    (b) Trichotillomania
    (c) Kleptomania
    (d) Capgras' syndrome

Ans. (d)

Note

All of the above are impulse control disorders except 'Capgras syndrome'.

Also see

The Capgras' syndrome belongs to 'Disorder of thought content'. The content specific delusions are observed in Capgras' syndrome and they are as under:
'A significant or usually a family member has been replaced by an identical appearing imposter'.

Extended information

Capgras' Syndrome (The Delusion of Doubles)

A syndrome that is closely related to delusional disorders, it is characterized by a delusional conviction that other persons in the environment are not their real selves but are their own doubles.

There are 4 types:
1. Typical Capgras' Syndrome (Illusion des sosies): Here the person sees a familiar person as a stranger who is imposing as the familiar person.
2. Illusion de fregoli: The person falsely identifies strangers as familiar persons.
3. Syndrome of subjective doubles: The persons own self is perceieved as being replaced by a double.
4. Intermetamorphosis: Here the patient's misidentification is complete (including not only the external appearance as in the previous 3 types, but also the personality).

The syndrome is commonly seen in psychotic conditions with delusional symptomatology like paranoid schizophrenia, delusional disorders and organic delusional disorders.
Ref: Neeraj Ahuja, 5th Ed, Pg-89

The ICD 10 Diagnostic Criteria for Habit and Impulse Disorder includes following conditions:
a. Pathological gambling
b. Pathological fire setting (Pyromania)
c. Pathological stealing (Kleptomania)
d. Trichotillomania (Impulse to pull hair)
Ref; Kaplan & Sadock's Comprehensive Textbook of Psychiatry.

DSMIV- Impulse –Control Disorders not elsewhere classified:
- Intermittent Explosive Disorder
- Kleptomania
- Pathological Gambling
- Pyromania
- Trichotillomania
- Impulse control Disorders NOS (312.30)

Q. 608. A 20-year old man has presented with increased alcohol consumption and sexual indulgence, irritability, lack of sleep and not feeling fatigued even on prolonged periods of activity. All these changes have been present for 3 weeks. The most likely diagnosis is
    (a) Alcohol dependence
    (b) Schizophrenia
    (c) Mania
    (d) Impulsive control disorder

Ans. (c)
Note
The most likely diagnosis is for above 'Mania'.
Also see
The clinical problem presented above has salient features as under:
a. Increased alcohol consumption and sexual indulgence, irritability – suggests lack of impulse control.
b. Lack of sleep and not feeling fatigued even on prolonged period of activity- suggests ceaseless overactivity.
c. All these changes have been present for 3 weeks – suggests an acute phase on onset.

All of the above pointers suggest 'Mania' to be most suitable choice. 'Mania' can be defined as a condition of continuous excitement or restlessness, with elevation of mood, flight of ideas and lack of control.
Features of mania are:

Characteristics	Clinical Appearance
Mood	Elevated or irritable
Talk	Fast, pressurized, flight of ideas
Energy	Excessive
Ideas	Grandiose; self confident; delusion of wealth, power, influence or religious significance, sometimes persecutory
Cognition	Disturbance of registration of memories
Physical	Insomnia, mild to moderate weight loss, increased libido
Behavior	Disinhibition, increased sexual activity, excessive drinking or spending
Hallucinations	Fleeting auditory or, more rarely, visual

Kumar & Clarke 6th Ed, Pg-1294

Q. 609. A 41-year old married female presented with headache for the last 6 months. She had several consultations. All her investigations were found to be within normal limits. She still insists that there is something wrong in her head and seeks another consultation. The most likely diagnosis is
- (a) Phobia
- (b) Psychogenic headache
- (c) Hypochondriasis
- (d) Depression

Ans. (c)

Note
The most likely diagnosis for above is 'Hypochondriasis'.

Also see
The above clinical presentation has following salient features:
a. Patient profile - 41 Year of married female.
b. C/O Headache is since last 6 months
c. Investigative evaluation – Shows all investigations within normal limits.
d. Seeking persistent consultations for her headache.

The patient's history is not consistent with having hypochondriac traits. She is since last 6 months troubled with only one problem 'the headache'. Indian females are known to have low ability to communicate and she is passing through the phase of life where she is nearing menopause, she needs to be looked from 'psychiatric point of view for her headache'.

Her complaint suggests most probable diagnostic choice of 'Depression'. However, masked depression is more appropriate – which can be defined as - 'masked depression' means 'missed depression'. The clinician should always look for underlying features indicative of depression behind physical presenting symptoms.

Q. 610. Behaviour therapy to change maladaptive behaviors using response as reinforcer uses the principles of
- (a) Classical conditioning
- (b) Moneling
- (c) Social learning
- (d) Operant conditioning

Ans. (d)

Note
Behaviour therapy to change maladaptive behaviours using response as reinforcer uses the principles of 'Operant conditioning'.

Also see
Behaviour therapy at times is also referred to as behaviour modification and it involves changing individual response to the environment or altering aspects of the environment that reinforce the individual behaviour.

Operant Conditioning

The reinforcements (e.g., rewards and punishments) are used in order to alter the frequency of behaviour. For example, a child may use the word please more frequently when making a request if he is rewarded with verbal approval each time he does so or, an adult may speak less frequently if he is punished with ridicule each time he does so.

Extended information
Operant conditioning procedures for increasing a behaviour. The common methods for augmenting an adaptive behaviour are:
1. Positive reinforcement- Here the desirable behaviour is reinforced by a reward, material or symbolic.
2. Negative reinforcement- Here on performance of the desirable behaviour, punishment can be avoided.
3. Modeling- The person is exposed to 'model' behaviour and induced to copy it.

Ref: Neeraj Ahuja, 5th Ed, Pg-221

Q. 611. A 15 year old boy feels that the dirt has hung onto him whenever he passes through the dirty street. This repetitive thought causes much distress and anxiety. He knows that there is actually no such thing after he has cleaned once but he is not satisfied and is compelled to think so. This has led to social withdrawal. He spends much of his time thinking about the dirt and contamination. This has affected his studies also. The most likely diagnosis is
(a) Obsessive compulsive disorder
(b) Conduct disorder
(c) Agoraphobia
(d) Adjustment disorder

Ans. (a)
Note
The most likely diagnosis for above is "Obsessive compulsive disorder".
Also see
The above clinical situation has following features:
a. Patient feels that the dirt has gung onto him whenever he passes through dirty streets.
b. This repetitive thought causes much distress and anxiety.
c. He is conscious about the fact that there is no such thing as he became dirty.
d. However, he his compelled to think that he is dirty.
e. This has led to social withdrawal; he spends much time in thinking about the dirt and contamination.
The above features are in favor of 'Obsessive Compulsive Disorder'.
The OCD is characterized by distressing and debilitating obsessional ruminations (recurrent thought intrusion) and compulsive rituals (repetitive unwanted actions), over which patient has no apparent control, though he regards them as absurd, unaccepted and undesirable. Obsessions and compulsions are so persistent and intrusive that they greatly impede patient's functioning.

Extended information
Obsession and compulsion generally occur together and are beyond voluntary control. Obsessions are recurrent, intrusive thoughts, feelings, ideas, images or sensations (fear of contamination, pathological doubt, aggression, sexual thoughts). Compulsions are conscious standardized, recurring patterns of behaviour, such as counting, checking, hoarding and avoidance. Compulsive rituals relieve obsessions induced anxiety. Individual recognizes irrational nature of behaviour. Resisting compulsion increases anxiety.

Ref: API, 7th Ed, Pg-1382

Q. 612. All of the following are features of hallucination, except
(a) Depends on will of the observer.
(b) Occurs in inner subjective space.
(c) It is a vivid sensory perception.
(d) It occurs in absence of perceptual stimulus.

Ans. (a)
Note
All of the above are features of hallucination, except that the hallucination is not dependant on will of the observer.
Also see

Hallucinations-healthy people occasionally experience hallucinations, such as in normal grief, or during the transition between sleeping and waking. Hallucinations can be elementary (for e.g. bangs, whistles) or complex (e.g., faces, voices, music) and may affect any of the perceptions; auditory, visual, tactile, gustatory, olfactory or deep sensations.
1. False perception and not a distortion.
2. Perceived as inhabiting objective space.
3. Perceived as having qualities of normal perception.
4. Perceived alongside normal perception.
5. Independent of individual's will.

Ref: Kumar & Clarke 6th Ed, Pg-1276

Q. 613. Delusion is not present in
  (a) Delirium
  (b) Mania
  (c) Depression
  (d) Compulsive disorder

Ans. (d)

Note
Delusion is not present in compulsive disorder.

Also see
Delusion
The disturbance is not due to the direct physiological effects of a substance (e.g., a drug of abuse, a medication) or a general medical condition. The following types are assigned based on the predominant delusional theme):
Erotomanic Type:
   Delusions that another person, usually of higher status, is in love with the individual.
Grandiose Type:
   Delusions of inflated worth, power, knowledge, identity, or special relationship to a deity or famous person.
Jealous Type:
   Delusions that the individual's sexual partner is unfaithful
Persecutory Type:
   Delusions that the person (or someone to whom the person is close) is being malevolently treated in some way.
Somatic Type:
   Delusions that the person has some physical defect or general medical condition.
Mixed Type:
   Delusions characteristic of more than one of the above types but no one theme predominates.

Q. 614. A patient presented with short lasting episodic behavioural changes which include agitation & dream like state with thrashing movements of his limbs. He does not recall these episodes & has no apparant precipitating factor. The most likely diagnosis is
  (a) Schizophrenia
  (b) Temporal lobe epilepsy
  (c) Panic episodes
  (d) Dissociative disorder

Ans. (b)

Note
The most likely diagnosis is 'Schizophrenia'.

Also see
Schizophrenia
   The peak age of onset is in the early twenties. The diagnostic symptoms of the condition called as first rank symptoms (described by Kurt Schneider). They consist of:
   -Auditory hallucinations in the third person, and/or voices commenting on their behaviour.
   -Thought withdrawal, insertion and broadcast.
   -Primary delusion.
   -Delusional perception.
   -Somatic passivity and feelings - patients believe that thoughts, feelings or acts are controlled by others.
Ref: Kumar & Clark 6th Ed.

Temporal lobe seizures
These partial seizures, either simple or complex, describe feelings of unreality (jamais vu) or undue familiarity (déjà vu) with the surroundings. Absence attacks, vertigo, visual hallucinations (i.e. visions or faces) are other examples of temporal lobe seizures.
Ref: Kumar & Clark 6th Ed Pg- 1221
(The features are in favor of Temporal lobe epilepsy (Complex Partial Seizure).

Panic Episode
Panic disorder is diagnosed when the patient has repeated sudden attacks of overwhelming anxiety, accompanied by severe physical symptoms, and sympathetic nervous system activity. Patients with panic disorder have catastrophic illness beliefs during the panic attack, that they are about to die from a stroke or heart attack.

Q. 615. A young lady presented with repeated episodes of overeating followed by purging after use of laxatives. She is probably suffering from
    (a)   Bulimia nervosa
    (b)   Schizophrenia
    (c)   Aorexia nervosa
    (d)   Binge eating disorder

Ans. (a)
Note
The lady with above presentation is suffering from 'Bulimia nervosa'.
Also see
Bullemia nervosa
-It is an eating disorder characterized by:
-Intense fear of becoming obese.
-Body image disturbance.
-Persistent pre-occupation with eating and an irresistible craving for food.
-There are episodes of over eating in which large amounts of food are consumed with in short periods time.
-There are attempts to counter-act the effects of overeating by induced vomiting, purgative abuse, and periods of starvation.
-Absence of any other psychiatric disorder.

Anorexia nervosa
    The patient has intense fear of becoming obese and indulges in self-imposed dietary restrictions, hides food, breaks food into small bits, involves in vigorous activities. There is body image distortion, and the patient is unable to perceive the body size accurately. Significant loss of weight occurs more than 25% of the original weight.

Binge eating disorder
    Large amounts of food are consumed in a short period of time followed by a severe discomfort and feelings of self-denigration. There is lack of control over eating during the period.
Ref: A Short Textbook of Psychiatry by Niraj Ahuja, 6th Ed, Ch-12, Pg-157,155

Q. 616. An 11 years old boy is all the time so restless that the rest of the class is unable to concentrate. He is hardly ever in his seat and roams around the hall. He has difficulty in playing quietly. The most likely diagnosis is
    (a)   Attention-deficit hyperactivity disorder
    (b)   Conduct disorder
    (c)   Depressive disorder
    (d)   Schizophrenia

Ans. (a)
Note
The features are suggestive of ADHD. The core features of ADHD.
Also see
Attention Deficit Hyperactivity Disorder (ADHD) is characterized by trio of inattention, impulsiveness and hyperactivity, frequently associated with specific learning disabilities, resulting in academic failure and abnormal behaviour.
ADHD was first described in 1902 by English pediatrician George Still. He noticed a group of his patients, mostly boys, had difficult behaviors which had started before the age of 8. Most were inattentive, overactive and were different from other children in their resistance to discipline. He described these children as having poor control of inhibition, being full of aggression and, suffering from, 'lack of moral control'. He perceived this as chronic condition, biological (inborn) in nature, and not caused by poor parenting or adverse environment.

Extended information
Attention deficit disorder with hyperactivity is the commonest type of hyperkinetic disorder. The characteristic clinical features are:
1. Poor attention span with distractibility:
   a) Fails to finish the things started.
   b) Shifts from one uncompleted activity to other.
   c) Does not seem to listen.
   d) Easily distracted by external stimuli.
   e) Often looses things.
2. Hyperactivity:
   a) Fidgety.
   b) Difficulty in sitting still at one place for long.
   c) Moving about here and there.
   d) Talks excessively.
   e) Interference in other people's activities.
3. Impulsivity:
   a) Acts before thinking, on the spur of the moment.
   b) Difficulty in waiting for turn at work or play.
Ref: Neeraj Ahuja, 5th Ed, Pg-173

DERMATOLOGY

Q. 617. A 24 year old male presents to a STD clinic with a single painless ulcer on external genitalia. The choice of laboratory test to look for the etiological agent would be
   (a) Scrappings from ulcer for culture on chocolate agar with antibiotic supplement.
   (b) Serology for detection of specific IgM antibodies.
   (c) Scrappings from ulcer for dark field microscopy.
   (d) Scrappings from ulcer for tissue culture.

Ans. (c)
Note
The choice of laboratory test to look for the etiological agent would be 'Scraping from ulcer for dark field microscopy'.
Also see
The patient seems to be suffering from syphilis and is in the primary stage. It is called as hard chancre. Characteristic features are:
   a. A single painless and hard chancre with an indurated base.
   b. It is usually shallow and oval or round in shape.
   c. It has a raised and hyperemic margin.
The organism cannot be stained and can be demonstrated only by:
   a. Dark ground illumination in fresh preparation.
   b. Fluorescent antibody technique.
   c. Silver impregnation technique.
Ref: Textbook of pathology by Harsh Mohan, 4th edition chapter 5, page 147
Ref: A Concise Textbook of Surgery, S. Das, 3rd Ed, Chapter 11, page 130

Extended information
T. palladium cannot be detected by culture; therefore, other tests are necessary. Dark-field microscopic examination of lesion exudate is useful in evaluating moist cutaneous lesions, such as the chancre of primary syphilis or condylomata of secondary syphilis.
Ref: Harrison's 16th Ed, Pg- 981

Q. 618. A 24 years old female has flaccid bullae in the skin and oral erosions. Histopathology shows intraepidermal acantholytic blister. The most likely diagnosis is
   (a) Pemphigoid
   (b) Erythema multiforme

(c) Pemphigus vulgaris
(d) Dermatitis herpetiformis

Ans. (c)

Note
The most likely diagnosis for above oral erosions and flaccid bullae in skin is 'pemphigus vulgaris'.

Also see
a. *Pemphigoid*: It is of three types:
Localized: This is usually confined to lower extremities.
Vesicular: In which small tense blisters are formed.
Fungating: Wherein verrucous vegetations are found in the axillae and groins.
b. *Erythema multiforme*
This is an acute self limiting disease due to hypersensitivity to certain drugs and infections. These lesions are multiform, i.e.- macular, papular, vesicular and bullous. If severe with involvement of skin and mucous membrane of mouth, conjunctival and genital region it is called as Stevens - Johnson syndrome.
c. *Pemphigus vulgaris*
It is an autoimmune bullous disease of the skin and oral mucosa characterized by acantholysis. There is development of flaccid bullae on skin and oral mucosa which break leaving behind erosions. *Biopsies of early lesions demonstrate intraepidermal vesicle formation secondary to loss of cohesion between epidermal cells i.e.,* **acantholytic** *blisters.*
Ref: Harrison- 15th Edition.
d. *Dermatitis herpetiformis*
Chronic pruritic, vesicular dermatosis found in 3rd and 4th decade. It is associated with gluten sensitive enteropathy. Usually involves the elbow, lower back and buttock. Involvement of mucous membrane is not seen.
Ref: Davidson's Principles and Practice of Medicine, 19th Ed, Ch-21, Pg- 1066
Ref: Textbook of Pathology by Harsh Mohan, 4th Ed, Ch-23, Pg-761-763

Q. 619. Rakesh, a 27-year-old boy had itchy, excoriated papules on the forehead and the exposed parts of the arms and legs for 3 years. The disease was most severe in the rainy season and improved completely in winter. The most likely diagnosis is
(a) Insect bite hypersensitivity
(b) Scabies
(c) Urticaria
(d) Atopic dermatitis

Ans. (a)

Note
The most likely diagnosis is 'insect bite hypersensitivity'.

Also see
Insect-bite: A special type of a beetle called, Paederus, produces a vesiculated chemical which leads to very fine vesicles with intense erythema and tenderness in irregular linear streaks or a smudge. This lesion is usually located on the face, neck, forearm or some other exposed parts of body. This beetle appears only during the rainy season and thus these eruptions also occur during this season.
Ref: Illustrated Textbook of Dermatology by J.S. Pasricha & Ramji Gupta, 1st Ed, Pg 87

Prurigo mitis: This is an allergic response to bites of common insects like mosquitoes and fleas. Multiple pruritic erythematous, edematous papules topped by tiny vesicles characterized the condition. In most instances, central vesical is scrached off by the patient leaving behind a small serosanguinous crusts. Distribution-exposed parts i.e extremities and face.

Ref: Khopkar 5th Ed. Pg-229

Extended information
Bite reactions typically present as intensely pruritic erythematous papules that commonly are excoriated. Vesicular and bullous reactions are not uncommon, and large pseudolymphomatous nodules may occur. Systemic reactions to the insect order Hymenoptera (bees, hornets, wasps, yellow jackets, ants) include fatal anaphylaxis.
Ref: -http://www.emedicine.com/DERM/topic467.htm

Q. 620. A 40 year old male had multiple blisters over the trunk and extremities. Direct immunoflurescence studies showed linear IgG deposits along the basement membrane. Which of the following is the most likely diagnosis?
  (a) Pemphigus vulgaris
  (b) Pemphigus foliaceous
  (c) Bullous pemphigoid
  (d) Dermatitis herpetiformis

Ans. (c)
Note
Above features are in favour of most likely diagnosis the 'Bullous pemphigoid'
Also see
a. *Pemphigus vulgaris*
   Clinical features: Flaccid blisters denuded skin, oro-mucosal lesions.
   Histology: Acantholytic blister formed in suprabasal layer of epidermis.
   Immunopathology: Cell surfaces deposits of IgG on keratinocytes.
b. *Pemphigous foliaceous*
   Clinical: Crusts and shallow erosions on the scalp, central face, upper chest and back.
   Histology: Acantholytic blister formed in superficial layer of epidermis.
   Immunopathology: Cell surface deposits of IgG on keratinocytes.
c. *Bullous pemphigoid*
   Clinical: Large tense blisters on flexor services and trunk.
   Histology: Blister formed in a subepidermal region; usually eosinophil-rich infiltrate.
   Immunopathology: Linear band of IgG and/or C3 in epidermal BMZ.
d. *Dermatitis herpitiformis*
   Clinical: Extremely pruritic small papules and vesicles on elbows, knees, buttocks and posterior neck.
   Histology: Subepidermal blister with neutrophils in dermal papillae.
   Immunopathology: Granular deposits of IgA in dermal papillae.
Ref: Harrison's, 16th Ed, Pg- Pg 312

Q. 621. A 6-month-old infant presented with multiple papules and exudative lesions on the face, scalp, trunk and few vesicles on the palms and soles for 2 weeks. His mother had history of itchy lesions. The most likely diagnosis is
  (a) Scabies
  (b) Infantile eczema
  (c) Infantile seborrheic dermatitis
  (d) Impetigo contagiosa

Ans. (a)
Note
The most likely diagnosis for the above case is 'Scabies'.
Also see

H/O mother having itchy lesions and the infant develops the skin problem. Scabies is caused by Sarcoptes scabiei is the most suspected cause in this case. The infestation spreads in households and environment; there is high frequency of intimate personal contact. In small children the palms and soles can be involved with pustule formation, main symptom is itch. Secondary eczematisation occurs elsewhere in the body. The face and scalp are never involved except in infants. Diagnostic feature is presence of burrow found on the edges of fingers toes or sides of hands and feet.

Ref: Davidson's Principles & Practice of Medicine, 19th Ed, Ch-21, Pg-1085

Q. 622. A 27-year-old male had burning micturition and urethral discharge. After 4 weeks he developed joint pains involving both the knees and ankles, redness of the eye and skin lesion. The most probable clinical diagnosis is
  (a) Psoriasis vulgaris
  (b) Reiter's syndrome

(c) Behcet's syndrome
(d) Sarcoidosis

Ans. (b)

Note
The most likely diagnosis for above condition is 'Reiter's syndrome'.

Also see
Rieter's disease
It is characterized by a triad of urethritis, conjunctivitis and reactive arthritis. It is seen in young men aged 16-35 years. Features are:
- Circinate balanitis
- Keratoderma blenorrhagica
- Nail dystrophy
- Buccal erosions

Behcet's Syndrome
This is a vasculitis of unknown etiology that characteristically targets venules. There is a wide range of clinical features:
- Recurrent oral ulceration- minor aphthous, major aphthous or herpetiform ulceration at least three times in a 12 month period.
- Recurrent genital ulceration
- Eye lesions- anterior uveitis, posterior uveitis
- Skin lesions- erythema nodosum, pseudofolliculitis, or acneiform nodules.

Ref: Davidson's Principles & Practice of Medicine, 19th Ed, Ch-20, Pg-1010, 1044

Q. 623. "Pinch" purpura is diagnostic of
(a) Primary systemic amyloidosis
(b) Secondary systemic amyloidosis
(c) Idiopathic thrombocytopenic purpura
(d) Drug induced purpura

Ans. (a)

Note
"Pinch" purpura is diagnostic of 'Primary Systemic Amyloidosis'.

Also see
Amyloidosis is characterized by deposition of insoluble, fibrillar protein in organs and tissues. Deposits of amyloid in the skin, often appearing as waxy plaques around eyes are prominent in primary systemic amyloidosis and in amyloid associated with multiple myeloma. Pinch purpura appears where the skin is traumatized, it is due to amyloid infiltration of blood vessels.

Ref: Davidson's Principles & Practice of Medicine, 19th Ed, Ch-21, Pg-1097

Extended information

Pink Lesions: The cutaneous lesions associated with primary systemic amylodosis are pink in colour and translucent. Common locations are face, specially, the periorbital and perioral regions and flexural areas. On biopsy, homogeneous deposits of amyloid are seen in the dermis and in the walls of blood vessels, the latter lead to an increase in the vessel wall fragility. As a result, petechiae and purpura develop in clinically normal skin as well as lesional skin following minor trauma, hence the term, pinch purpura.
Ref: Harrison's 16th Edition, Pg-306

Q. 624. A 36-year-old factory worker developed itchy, annular scaly plaques in both groins. Application of a corticosteroid ointment led to temporary relief but the plaques continued to extend at the periphery. The most likely diagnosis is
(a) Erythema annulare centrifugum
(b) Granuloma annulare
(c) Annular lichen planus
(d) Tinea cruris

Ans. (d)

Note
The most likely diagnosis for above presenting features is 'Tinea cruris'.
Also see
However, review the following and use your discretion:
a. *Erythema annulare centrifugum*
It is characterized by a scaling or nonscaling, nonpruritic, annular or arcuate, erythematous eruption. It tends to spread peripherally while clearing centrally. The etiology is uncertain, but it may be due to a hypersensitivity to malignancy, infection, drugs, or chemicals, or it may be idiopathic.
Primary lesion: The eruption begins as erythematous papules that spread peripherally while clearing centrally. These lesions enlarge at a rate of approximately 2-5 mm/d to produce annular, arcuate, figurate, circinate, or polycyclic plaques. The margin, which is usually indurated, varies in width from 4-6 mm, and, often, a trailing scale is present on the inner aspect of the advancing edge. The diameter of the polycyclic lesions varies from a few to several centimeters. Vesiculation may be present.
Distribution: Lesions demonstrate a predilection for the thighs and the legs, but they may occur on the upper extremities, the trunk, or the face. The palms and the soles are spared. EAC is usually self-limited. Topical steroids usually cause involution of the treated lesions, but they do not prevent the occurrence of new lesions.
Ref: http://www.emedicine.com/derm/topic131.htm
b. *Granuloma annulare*
GA is a benign inflammatory dermatosis characterized clinically by dermal papules and annular plaques. Its precise cause is unknown. Women are affected twice as often as men. Localized GA is most commonly found in children and in adults younger than 30 years. Patients with localized GA commonly present with groups of 1- to 2-mm papules that range in color from flesh-toned to erythematous, often in an annular arrangement over distal extremities.

Grouped lesions may expand into arciform or annular plaques measuring 1-5 cm in diameter.
Centers of lesions may be slightly hyperpigmented and depressed relative to their borders, which may be solid or composed of numerous dermal papules.
Lesions most commonly manifest on the dorsal surfaces of the feet, hands, and fingers, and on the extensor aspects of the arms and legs.
GA has traditionally been hypothesized to be associated with tuberculosis, insect bites, trauma, sun exposure, thyroiditis, and viral infections, including HIV, Epstein-Barr virus, and herpes zoster virus. However, these suggested etiologic factors remain unproven. It has a tendency towards spontaneous resolution. Reassurance is often all that is necessary. Painful or disfiguring lesions have been treated by various methods, although the level of evidence supporting these methods is low.
Ref: http://www.emedicine.com/DERM/topic169.htm
c. *Annular lichen planus*
ALP commonly involves the male genitalia but also has a predilection for intertriginous areas such as the axilla and groin folds. Eruptions typically consist of a few lesions localized to one or a few sites. Distal aspects of the extremities, and less commonly the trunk, may also be involved.
Ref: http://www.thedoctorsdoctor.com/diseases/lichen_planus.htm
d. *Tinea cruris*
Tinea or dermatophytes are fungi capable of causing skin infections, when it affects the groin it is called as tinea cruris and caused by Trichophyton rubrum. Itchy erythematous plaques extend from the groin flexures onto the thighs. Inadvertent application of steroid causes worsening of signs and symptom. This is known as tinea incognito.
Ref: Davidson's Principles and Practice of Medicine, 19th Edition, chapter 21, page 1083
The groin is the next most commonly involved area (**tinea cruris**), with males affected much more often than females. It presents as a scaling erythematous eruption that spares the scrotum.
Harrison – 15th Edition.

Q. 625. A 16-year-old boy presented with asymptomatic, multiple, erythematous, annular lesions with a callarette of scales at the periphery of the lesions present on the trunk. The most likely diagnosis is
  (a) Pityriasis versicolor
  (b) Pityriasis alba
  (c) Pityriasis rosea
  (d) Pityriasis rubra pilaris
Ans. (c)

Note
The most likely diagnosis for above presentation is 'Pityriasis rosea'.

Also see
Pityriasis rosea affects the age group between 15-40 yrs and tends to occur in autumn and spring and have an acute onset. It starts as a single herald patch that can occur anywhere on the body but it is usually present on the trunk. This is followed by appearance of similar patches mostly on the trunk in a fir tree pattern. It can also occur on the neck, extremities and flexures. The herald patch tends to persist throughout the eruption and the whole eruption can last for upto three months. Morphology of the rash is well defined erythematous papules and plaques with scaling.
Ref: Davidson's principles and practice of medicine, 19th Edition, chapter 21, page 1060-1061

Q. 626. A 40-year-old woman presents with a 2 year history of erythematous papulopustular lesions on the convexities of the face. There is a background of erythema and telangiectasia. The most likely diagnosis in the patient is
  (a) Acne vulgaris
  (b) Rosacea
  (c) Systemic lupus erythematosus
  (d) Polymorphic light eruption

Ans. (b)

Note
The most likely diagnosis in the patient is 'Rosacea'.

Also see
Rosacea is a persistent facial eruption of unknown cause characterized by erythema and pustules. The disorder is most common in middle age. The cheeks, chin and central forehead are affected. Intermittent blushing is followed by fixed erythema and telangiectasia. Dome shaped papules and pustules are seen.
Ref: Davidson's principles and practice of medicine, 19th Edition, chapter 21, page 1083

Q. 627. An 8-year-old boy from Bihar presents with a 6 months history of an illdefined, hypopigmented slightly atrophic macule on the face. The most likely diagnosis is
  (a) Pityriasis alba
  (b) Indeterminate leprosy
  (c) Morphea
  (d) Calcium deficiency

Ans. (b)

Note
The most likely diagnosis for above presenting feature is 'Indeterminate leprosy'.

Also see
a. *Pityriasis alba*
It is seen in children and presents as asymptomatic hypopigmented ill-defined macules on cheeks and other parts of face. It disappears spontaneously after persisting for a long time. It is rare after puberty.
Textbook of dermatology- Ramji Gupta, chapter 24, page 175
b. *Indeterminate leprosy*
It is an early stage of leprosy and presents as ill defined hypopigmented macules, with doubtful loss of sensation. The nerve supplying the macule is not enlarged. Slit smear from the well stained serial section reveals AFB in dermal N. fibrils infiltrated with lymphocytes. Areas in India where the disease is seen: Tamil Nadu, Bihar, Pondicherry, A.P., Orissa, W. Bengal, Assam
c. *Morphea*
It is a localized form of scleroderma seen in young females and manifests as asymptomatic mildly erythematous plaques with atrophy of the epidermis. Lesions are usually seen on the extremities but may be present on any part of the body.
Ref: Textbook of dermatology- Ramji Gupta, 1st Ed, Chapter 22, Page 165

Q. 628. A 5 year old male child has multiple hyperpigmented macules over the trunk. On rubbing the lesion with the rounded end of a pen, he developed urticarial wheal, confined to the border of the lesion. The most likely diagnosis is
  (a) Fixed drug eruption
  (b) Lichen planus

(c) Urticaria pigmentosa
(d) Urticarial vasculitis

Ans. (c)
Note
The most likely diagnosis for above presentation is 'Uritcaria pigmentosa'.
Also see
Urticaria pigmentosa is a disease that produces skin lesions and intense itching. If the lesions are rubbed, hives may form on the site.
Causes, incidence, and risk factors:

Urticaria pigmentosa is one of several forms of mastocytosis, which is caused by excessive numbers of inflammatory cells (mast cells) in the skin. Other forms include solitary mastocytoma (a single lesion) and systemic mastocytosis (involvement in organs other than the skin).
Urticaria pigmentosa is most often seen in children, but it can occur in adults as well.
Rubbing of a lesion produces a rapid wheal (a hive-like bump). Younger children may develop a fluid-filled blister over a lesion if it is scratched.
Symptoms:
 -Appearance of brownish lesions on skin.
 -Welt or hive formation when lesions are rubbed or scratched.
 -Blister formation over lesion when it is rubbed.
 -Facial flushing.
Ref: http://www.nlm.nih.gov/medlineplus/ency/article/001466.htm

Q. 629. A 25-year-old man presents with recurrent episodes of flexural eczema, contact urticaria, recurrent skin infections and severe abdominal cramps and diarrhea upon taking sea foods. He is suffering from
(a) Seborrheic dermatitis
(b) Atopic dermatitis
(c) Airborne contact dermatitis
(d) Nummular dermatitis

Ans. (b)
Note
The above features promps for the diagnosis of 'Atopic dermatitis'.
Also see
Diagnostic criteria for atopic eczema:
Atopy is a genetic predisposition to form excessive IgE which leads to a generalised and prolonged hypersensitivity to common environmental antigens, including pollen and the house dust mite. Atopic individuals manifest one or more of a group of diseases that includes asthma, hay fever, urticaria, food and other allergies, and this distinctive form of eczema. Although any of these atopic conditions tends to be over-represented in families of persons with any atopic disease, one particular disease type tends to run more strongly in a particular family. A number of operational criteria for the diagnosis of atopic eczema have been proposed for the purpose of research studies.

Diagnostic criteria for atopic eczema are itchy skin with at least 3 of the following:
 -H/O itch in skin creases (or cheeks if <4 yrs)
 -H/O asthma/ hay fever (or in a first- degree relative if < 4 yrs)
 -Dry skin (xeroderma)
 -Visible flexural eczema
 -Onset in first 2 years of life.
Ref: Davidson's principles and practice of medicine, 19th Edition, chapter 21, page 1072.

Q. 630. Acantholysis is characterstic of
(a) Pemphigus vulgaris
(b) Pemphigoid
(c) Erythema multiforme
(d) Dermatitis herpetiformis

Ans. (a)

Note
Acantholysis is characterstic of 'Pemphigus vulgaris'.
Also see
Pemphigus vulgaris
It is an autoimmune bullous disease of the skin and oral mucosa characterized by acantholysis. There is development of flaccid bullae on skin and oral mucosa which break leaving behind erosions.

However other important constellation of Pemphigus includes:
Age group: 40-60yrs
Distribution: torso head
Character of bullae: Flaccid and fragile, many erosions
Mucosal involvement: 100%
Antigen: Desmoglein-3
Antibody: circulating- IgG
Fixed-IgG epidermal
Ref: Davidson's principles and practice of medicine, 19th Edition, chapter 21, page 1066

Q. 631. A 5 year old boy has multiple asymptomatic oval and circular faintly hypopigmented macules with scaling on his face. The most probable clinical diagnosis is
    (a)   Pityriasis versicolor
    (b)   Indeterminate leprosy
    (c)   Pityriasis alba
    (d)   Acrofacial vitiligo

Ans. (c)
Note
The boy in question is suffering from 'Pityriasis alba'.
Also see
Pityriasis alba
It is seen in children and presents as asymptomatic hypopigmented ill-defined macules on cheeks and other parts of face. It disappears spontaneously after persisting for a long time. It is rare after puberty.
Textbook of dermatology- Ramji Gupta, chapter 24, page 175

Pityriasis versicolor
It is a common yeast infection of the body and scalp, trunk and outer upper arms. It is often exacerbated by exposure to sun. The rash is asymptomatic. It presents as a hypo- and hyperpigmented scaly patches.
Ref: Davidson's principles and practice of medicine, 19th Edition, chapter 21, page 1060, 1061

Q. 632. A 40-year old male developed persistent oral ulcers followed by multiple flaccid bullae on trunk and extremities. Direct examination of a skin biopsy immunofluorescence showed intercellular IgG deposits in the epidermis. The most probable diagnosis is
    (a)   Pemphigus vulgaris
    (b)   Bullous pemphigoid
    (c)   Bullous lupus erythematosus
    (d)   Epidermolysis bullosa acquisita

Ans. (a)
Note
The most probable diagnosis for the above presentation is 'Pemphigus vulgaris'.
Also see
Pemphigus vulgaris
It is an autoimmune bullous disease of the skin and oral mucosa characterized by acantholysis. There is development of flaccid bullae on skin and oral mucosa which break leaving behind erosions.
However other important constellation of Pemphigus include:
Age group: 40-60yrs
Distribution: torso head
Character of bullae: Flaccid and fragile, many erosions

Mucosal involvement: 100%
Antigen: Desmoglein-3
Antibody: circulating- IgG
Fixed-IgG epidermal
Ref: Davidson's principles and practice of medicine, 19th Edition, chapter 21, page 1066

Q. 633. Wickham's striae are seen in
(a) Lichen niditus
(b) Lichenoid eruption
(c) Lichen striates
(d) Lichen planus

Ans. (d)

Note
Wickham's striae are seen in 'Lichen Planus'.

Also see
It is a rash characterized by intensely itchy polygonal papules with a voilaceous hue involving the skin, mucosa, hair and nails. Some develop a characteristic fine white network on their surface- Wickham's striae. It is associated with some autoimmune diseases such as myasthenia gravis. The lesions show Kobner's phenomenon, i.e. the new lesions appear at the site of trauma.
Ref: Davidson's principles and practice of medicine, 19th Edition, chapter 21, page 1080

Q. 634. Exfoliative dermatitis can be due to all the following diseases, except
(a) Drug hypersensitivity
(b) Pityriasis rubra
(c) Pityriasis rosea
(d) Psoriasis

Ans. (c)

Note
Exfoliative dermatitis can be due to all the following diseases, except 'Pityriasis rosea'.

Also see
Eczema, psoriasis, drug reactions and lichen planus may occasionally progress to exfoliative dermatitis or erythroderma. It is characterized by wide spread erythema and scaling of all the body surface. Other causes are:
- Cutaneous T-cell lymphoma
- Pityriasis rubra pilaris
- Icthyosis

There is shivering due to loss of temperature regulation and pyrexia. B.P. is low and P.R. is rapid. L.N. may be enlarged due to skin inflammation.
Ref: Davidson's principles and practice of medicine, 19th Edition, chapter 21, page 1061

Q. 635. Genital elephantiasis is caused by
(a) Donovanosis
(b) Congenital syphilis
(c) Herpes genitalis
(d) Lymphogranuloma venereum

Ans. (d)

Note
Genital elephantiasis is caused by ' Lymphogranuloma venereum'.

Also see
Lymphogranuloma venereum (LGV), also known as lymphogranuloma inguinale, tropical bubo, Nicholas-Favre disease, and sixth venereal disease, is an infection caused by a variety of the bacterium *Chlamydia trachomatis*. It primarily causes painful swelling of the lymph nodes located closest to the site of infection. If left untreated, it can cause serious tissue damage, scarring, rectal or intestinal blockages, and extreme swelling of the genitals (elephantiasis). In severe cases, it attacks the central nervous system.
Ref: - http://www.womenshealthchannel.com/std/lymphogranuloma.shtml

Q. 636. A man aged 50 years presents with, alopecia, boggy scalp swelling and easily pluckable hair Next step in establishing the diagnosis would be
  (a) KOH smear
  (b) Culture sensitivity
  (c) Biopsy
  (d) None of the above

Ans. (a)

Note
The next step in above case for establishing the diagnosis is 'KOH smear'.

Also see
Diagnosis of fungal infections is done by microscopy under wood's light. Identification can also be done by mounting the plucked hair in 20% KOH. This allows the keratin to be dissolved and fungal hyphae can be identified.
Ref: Davidson's principles and practice of medicine, 19th Edition, chapter 21, page 1055

Q. 637. Most common organism causing tinea capitis is
  (a) Trichophyton tonsurans
  (b) Microsporum
  (c) Epidermophyton
  (d) Candida albicans

Ans. (a)

Note
Most common organism causing tinea capitis is 'Trichophyton tonsurans'.

Also see
Anthropophillic fungal infection account for majority of cases in urban areas. Fungal infections of the scalp or Tinea capitis cause localized area of hair loss and scaling in the scalp.
Trichophyton tonsurans causes uninflamed patchy baldness with breakage of hair at the surface of skin.
Microsporum dudounii causes minimal inflammation.
Microsporum canis causes more inflammation.
Kerions caused by Trichophyton verrucosum are boggy, inflamed areas of Tinea capitis.
Ref: Davidson's Principles and Practice of Medicine, 19th Ed, Ch-21, Pg- 1070

Q. 638. A young man aged 19 years develops a painless penile ulcer 9 days after sexual intercourse with a professional sex worker. Most likely diagnosis is
  (a) Chancroid
  (b) Herpes
  (c) Primary chancre
  (d) Traumatic ulcer

Ans. (c)

Note
The most likely cause of the above complaint is 'Primary chancer'.

Also see
The patient seems to have contracted syphilis which is caused by Treponema pallidum. The incubation period is usually between 14-28 days with a range of 9-90 days. The preimary lesion or chancre develops at the site of infection usually in the genital region. A dull red macule then develops which becomes popular and erodes to form an indurated ulcer. Both chancre and L.N. are painless and non-tender. Without treatment it resolves in 2-6 weeks to leave a thin atrophic scar. The inguinal L.N. are moderately enlarged, mobile, discreet and rubbery.
Ref: Davidson's principles and practice of medicine, 19th Edition, chapter 1, page 97
The characteristic features of a syphilitic chancre are:
  -A single painless and hard chancre with an indurated base.
  -It is usually shallow and oval or round in shape.
  -It has a raised and hyperemic margin.

Ref: A Concise Textbook of Surgery, S. Das, 3rd Ed, Ch-11, Pg-130

Q. 639. A boy aged 8 years from Tamil Nadu presents with a white, non anesthetic, nonscaly, hypopigmented macule on his face. Most likely diagnosis is
    (a)   Pityriasis alba
    (b)   Pityriasis versicolor
    (c)   Indeterminate leprosy
    (d)   Pure neuritic leprosy

Ans. (c)
Note
The most likely diagnosis for the above presentation is 'Indeterminate leprosy'.
Also see
a.   *Pityriasis alba*
It is seen in children and presents as asymptomatic hypopigmented ill-defined macules on cheeks and other parts of face. It disappears spontaneously after persisting for a long time. It is rare after puberty.
Ref: Textbook of dermatology- Ramji Gupta, Ch-24, Pg-175
b.   *Pityriasis vesicolor*
It is a common yeast infection of the body and scalp, trunk and outer upper arms. It is often exacerbated by exposure to sun. The rash is asymptomatic. It presents as a hypo- and hyperpigmented scaly patches.
Ref: Davidson's Principles and Practice of Medicine, 19th Ed, Ch- 21, Pg- 1060, 1061
c.   *Indeterminate leprosy*
It is an early stage of leprosy and presents as ill defined hypopigmented macules, with doubtful loss of sensation. The nerve supplying the macule is not enlarged. Slit smear from the well stained serial section reveals AFB in dermal N. fibrils infiltrated with lymphocytes. Areas in India where the disease is seen: Tamil Nadu, Bihar, Pondicherry, A.P., Orissa, W. Bengal, Assam
Ref: Textbook of Pathology by Harsh Mohan, 4th Ed, Ch-12, Pg-144

Q. 640. A 20 years old, male patient, from Jaipur presents with an erythematous lesion on the cheek with central crusting. Most likely diagnosis is
    (a)   SLE
    (b)   Lupus vulgaris
    (c)   Chillblains
    (d)   Cutaneous leishmaniasis

Ans. (d)
Note
The most likely diagnosis for the above presentation appear to be 'Cutaneous leismaniasis'.
Also see
The patient seems to be suffering from cutaneous leishmaniasis. It is caused by Leishmania tropica, L. major and L. arthropica.
Lesions are single or multiple on exposed parts of the body, and start as small red papules which gradually increase in size, reaching 2-10 cm in diameter. A crust forms overlying an ulcer with a granular base. Tiny satellite papules are characteristic. If left ubtreated, the lesions heal slowly over many months. Healing produces a depressed mottled scar which may be disfiguring or disabling.
Ref: Davidson's Principles and Practice of Medicine, 19th Ed, Ch-1, Pg- 83, 84

Extended information
Cutaneous leishmaniasis used to occur in the dry, north western states of India bordering Pakistan, extending from Amritsar to Kutch and Gujrat plains. In recent years, one focus of zoonotic cutaneous leishmaniasis (ZCL) has been discovered in the Rajasthan area; in the peak year of 1971.
Ref: Park and Park 18th Ed. Pg-245

Q. 641. A 19 year old pregnant girl presents with light brown pigmentation over the malar eminences. Most likely diagnosis is
    (a)   Chloasma
    (b)   SLE

(c) Melasma
(d) Melanoma

Ans. use your discretion

Note

The most likely cause of light brown pigment ove the malar eminence is due to 'Chloasma / Melasma'
(Please note; Melasma and chloasma are synonymus therefore, both the choices here (a) and (c) are corrent.)

Also see

Melasma is a very common skin disorder. Melasma is a dark skin discoloration found on sun-exposed areas of the face. It is used interchangably with chloasma.
Causes, incidence, and risk factors:
Though it can affect anyone, young women with brownish skin tones are at greatest risk.
Melasma is often associated with the female hormones estrogen and progesterone. It is especially common in pregnant women, women who are taking oral contraceptives ("the pill"), and women taking hormone replacement therapy during menopause.
Ref: http://www.nlm.nih.gov/medlineplus/ency/article/000836.htm
Ref: Davidson's Principles and Practice of Medicine, 19th Ed, Ch-21, Pg- 1087

Ref: Illustrated handbook of skin diseases and sexually transmited infections By Dr. Uday Khopkar 5th Ed. Pg-148

Ref: Illustrated Textbook of Dermatology by J.S. Passrika and Ramji Gupta 1st Ed Pg- 105

Q. 642. A girl aged 19, presents with arthritis and a photosensitive rash on the cheek. Likely diagnosis is:
(a) SLE
(b) Chloasma
(c) Stevens Johnson syndrome
(d) Lyme's disease

Ans. (a)

Note

The most likely diagnosis for above presenting features is 'SLE'.

Also see

SLE:
It is a multisystem disease characterized by a diverse spectrum of antibody production. Its diagnostic features are:
- Malar rash- fixed erythema flat or raised, sparing the nasolabial flod.
- Discoid rash
- Photosensitivity
- Oral ulcers
- Arthritis
- Serositis, pleuritis and pericarditis
- Renal disorders
- Neurological disorders such as seizures
- Hematological disorders
- Abs, such as- ANA, anti-DNA, Anti phospholipids Ab.

Ref: Davidson's principles and Practice of Medicine, 19th Ed, Ch-20, Pg- 1034-1036

Lyme's disease:
It is caused by Borrelia and characterized by a skin reaction around the site of bite of tick (which are the reservoir of infection). This is a red macules or papules which appear around 2-3 days after the bite and enlarges peripherally with central clearing and may persist for months.

Ref: Davidson's Principles and Practice of Medicine, 19th Ed, Ch-1, Pg-21

PAEDIATRICS

Q. 643. A 6-month-old infant presents to the 'diarrhea clinic' unit with some dehydration. The most likely organism causing diarrhea is:
(a) Entamoeba histolytica
(b) Rotavirus
(c) Giardia lamblia
(d) Shigella

Ans. (b)
Note
The most likely cause of diarrhea in above child is 'Rotavirus'.
Also see
Causative agents of acute diarrhea in children in India are: Rotavirus and enterotoxic E. coli. They account for nearly ½ the total diarrheal episodes among children. Shigella and salmonella species are isolated in 3-7% of childhood diarrhea.
Ref: Ghai, Essential Paediatrics, 5th Ed, Ch-12, Pg- 246, 247

Q. 644. The most common underlying anomaly in a child with recurrent urinary tract infections is
(a) Posterior urethral valves
(b) Vesicoureteric reflux
(c) Neurogenic bladder
(d) Renal calculi

Ans. (b)
Note
The most common underlying anomaly in a child with recurrent urinary tract infections is 'Vesicoureteric reflux'.
Also see
Obstructive uropathy, VUR, neurogenic bladder predispose to UTI. These predisposing factors may be found in around 30-40% cases with UTI. Obstructive uropathy is found in usually in boys.

VUR refers to retrograde flow of urine from the bladder to the upper urinary tract. The rise in intravesical pressure occurring during urination is transmitted to the ureter, renal pelvis, papillary collecting ducts and renal tubules. Pathogenic organisms of bladder gain access to renal parenchyma and initiate inflammatory reaction and scarring. It is present in 20-35% of cases with febrile UTI.
Ref: Ghai, Essential Paediatrics, 5th Ed, Ch-16, Pg-374, 375

Q. 645. All of the following are characteristic features of Kwashiorkar, except
(a) High blood osmolarity
(b) Hypoalbuminemia
(c) Edema
(d) Fatty liver

Ans. (a)
Note
All of the following are characteristic features of Kwashiorkar, except 'High blood osmolarity'.
Also see
Markedly retarded growth, psychomotor disturbances and edema of dependant parts are the three essential features of Kwashiorkar. Muscle wasting is masked by subcutaneous tissue preservation and edema.
Edema is caused due to hypoalbuminemia, retention of fluid and water due to increased capillary permeability as a result of infection, potassium deficiency. Face appears moon shaped and puffy.
Child is irritable, peevish and lethargic. Appetite is markedly impaired.
Hepatomegaly, liver is enlarged and with a rounded lower margin, fatty infiltration is seen.
Hair changes- Flag sign.
Skin changes- Large areas of skin show erythema followed by hyperpigmentation. This desquamates leaving behind hypopigmented raw areas- known as flaky paint dermatosis.
Ref: Ghai, Essential Paediatrics, 5th Ed, Ch-4, Pg- 68, 69

Q. 646. All of the following are seen in rickets, except
    (a)   Bow legs
    (b)   Gunstock deformity
    (c)   Pot belly
    (d)   Craniotabes

Ans. (b)
Note
All of the following are seen in rickets, except 'Gunstock deformity'.
Also see
Clinical manifestations of rickets start appearing in the later ½ of 1st year or 2nd year.
a.   Craniotabes: It is the earliest manifestation. Pressure over the soft membranous bones of skull (occipital or post part of parietal bones) is felt like a ping pong ball if compressed and released.
b.   Large anterior fontanelle, delayed closure beyond 18 months.
c.   Frontal and parietal bone bossing becomes evident at 6 months.
d.   Costochondral junction becomes prominent- Rickety rosary.
e.   Pigeon chest
f.   Delayed tething
g.   Widening of epiphyses
h.   Bowing of legs- knock knees, coax vera
i.   Abdomen becomes protuberant and pot bellied because of hypotonia of abdominal walls, visceroptosis, and lumbar lordosis.
Ref: Ghai, Essential Paediatrics, 5th edition, chapter 5, page 83

Q. 647. In neonatal screening programme for detection of congenital hypothyroidism, the ideal place and time to collect the blood sample for TSH estimation is
    (a)   Cord blood at time of birth
    (b)   Heal pad blood at the time of birth
    (c)   Heal pad blood on 4th day of birth
    (d)   Peripheral venous blood on 28th day

Ans. (c)
Note
In neonatal screening for congenital hypothyroidism the ideal plce and time to collect blood sample is 'Heel pad blood on 4th day of birth'.
Also see
Neonatal screening
Done at 3-5 days of birth by beel pick or prickin ear lobe and estimating T4 & TSH usually TSH > 50 mu/L, T4 < 6.5 ug/dl
Ref: Paediatrics Medknow Publications Mumbai revised 2nd Ed. Pg-409

Extended information
Neonatal screening for hypothyroidism- Availability of highly sensitive radioimmunoassay methods for measurement of T_4 and TSH launched the new born thyroid screening using cord blood samples obtained on filter paper. Infants with low T_4 levels and increased TSH are diagnosed as having primary hypothyroidism. Whereas low T_4 and TSH and investigated for thyroid binding globulin deficiency or secondary hypothyroidism.
Ref: Ghai, Essential Paediatrics, 5th edition, chapter 20, page 448

Q. 648. A 3-year old boy is detected to have bilateral renal calculi. Metabolic evaluation confirms the presence of marked hypercalciuria with normal blood levels of calcium, magnesium, phosphate, uric acid and creatinine. A diagnosis of idiopathic hypercalciuria is made. The dietary management includes all, except
    (a)   Increased water intake
    (b)   Low sodium diet
    (c)   Reduced calcium intake
    (d)   Avoid meat proteins

Ans. (c)

Note
For trhe above clinical condition dietary management includes all, except 'reduce calciuim intake'.

Also see
Hypercalciuria is defined by a 24-hour urinary calcium excretion more than 150 mg in an adult female, more than 200 mg in an adult male, or more than 4 mg/kg/d in a child weighing less than 60 kg. In infants younger than 3 months, 5 mg/kg/d is considered the upper limit of normal for calcium excretion. Hypercalciuria can be classified as idiopathic or secondary. Idiopathic hypercalciuria can be diagnosed when clinical, laboratory, and radiographic investigations fail to delineate an underlying cause. Secondary hypercalciuria occurs when a known process produces excessive urinary calcium.

Dietary modifications are important components in treating children with hypercalciuria. General guidelines that are applicable to most children with hypercalciuria include the following:

a. Maintain water intake at 1500 mL/m^2/d.
b. Restrict dietary calcium to the DRI for age. The Food and Drug Administration (FDA) sets the DRI (or recommended daily allowance [RDA]) by doubling the estimated daily need. This was done to ensure an adequate amount of calcium (and other vitamins and minerals) intake for growth and development.
c. Restricting dietary sodium may also be helpful in children with hypercalciuria. As previously mentioned, a direct relationship exists between sodium chloride intake and urinary calcium excretion. Therefore, it seems logical that limiting salt intake would help reduce the amount of urinary calcium. No data indicate that high salt intake alone can induce the clinical syndrome of hypercalciuria. However, evidence may show that lower sodium diets help reduce urinary calcium excretion in children who have idiopathic hypercalciuria. A good target range for dietary sodium intake is 2-3 mEq/kg/d.
d. In children with a history of calcium oxalate stones, lowering dietary oxalate is indicated.
e. Diets high in animal protein may produce a larger metabolic acid load in adults and contribute to stone formation. Studies in children are not available; however, protein intakes higher than the DRI are not necessary and may be harmful.

Ref: http://www.emedicine.com/PED/topic1063.htm

Extended information
Severe dietary calcium restriction is inappropriate. Dietary calcium restriction results in hyperabsorption of oxalate, and so foods containing large amount of oxalate should also be limited. A high fluid intake should be advised as for idiopathic stone-formers. Patients who live in a hardwater area may benefit from drinking softened water.

Ref: Kumar & Clark, 6th Ed, Pg-652

Q. 649. Which one of the following does not produce cyanosis in the first year of life
    (a) Atrial septal defect
    (b) Hypoplastic left heart syndrome
    (c) Truncus arteriosus
    (d) Double outlet right ventricle

Ans. (a)

Note
From the above 'Atrial septal defect' does not produce cyanosis in the first year of life.

Also see
In ASD, VSD and PDA there is communication between the left atrium and right atrium and left ventricle and right ventricle. Since pressure in the right atrium and ventricle is less than the left atrium and ventricle. Therefore the shunt is from right side of heart to the left side. Thus oxygenated blood of the left side mixes with deoxygenated blood on the right side and cyanosis does not occur because the deoxygenated blood does not enter the systemic circulation initially, unless the shunt is reversed. Cyanosis is seen when the deoxygenated blood enters the systemic circulation from a right to left shunt or the blood passing through the lungs is not fully oxygenated.

Ref: Ghai, Essential Paediatrics, 5th Ed, Ch-13, Pg-294-295

Q. 650. One year old male child presented with poor urinary stream since birth. The investigation of choice for evaluation is
   (a)   Voiding cystourethrography (VCUG)
   (b)   USG bladder
   (c)   Intravenous urography
   (d)   Uroflowmetry

Ans. (a)
Note
The investigation of choice for evaluation for the above given case is 'Voiding cystourethrography (VCUG)'.
Also see
Posterior urethral valves constitute an important cause of distal urinary tract obstruction in boys. Dribbling, abnormal urinary stream, palpable bladder and recurrent UTI are the usual presenting featured. The presence of severe obstruction may lead to renal dysplasia. The diagnosis is made on MCU (micturating cystourethrogram) which shows dilated posterior urethral urethra and valvesw at its junction with anterior urethra. Bladder is enlarged and may show diverticuli and trabeculations because of the high pressure in the bladder.
Ref: Ghai, Essential Paediatrics, 5th Ed, Ch-16, Pg-385

Q. 651. Which of the following is the most appropriate method for obtaining a urine specimen for culture in an 8 month old girl?
   (a)   Suprapubic aspiration
   (b)   Indwelling catheter sample
   (c)   Clean catch void
   (d)   Urinary bag sample

Ans. (a)
Note
The appropriate method for obtaining a urine specimen for culture in an 8 month old girl is by 'suprapubic aspiraiton'.
Also see
It is often difficult to obtain a satisfactory specimen in infants below the age of 2 years. Percutaneous supra pubic bladder puncture is a simple and safe technique in these children. After ensuring that the bladder is full, the suprapubic region is cleaned and a sterile syringe with gauge 21 or 22 is used for aspirating urine. No local anesthetic is required.
Urine can also be collected by catheterization of bladder.
Ref: Ghai, Essential Paediatrics, 5th Ed, Ch-16, Pg-363

Q. 652. An 8 year old boy during a routine check up is found to have E coli 1,00,000 cc/ml on a urine culture. The urine specimen was obtained by midstream clean-catch void. The child is asymptomatic. Which is the most appropriate next step in the management?
   (a)   Treat as an acute episode of urinary tract infection
   (b)   No therapy
   (c)   Prophylactic antibiotics for 6 months
   (d)   Administer long term urine alkalinizer

Ans. (a)
Note
The definitive diagnosis of UTI depends on finding 10^5 or more bacteria/ ml on culture.
Management includes:
General measures- child is encouraged to pass urine frequently to prevent stasis of urine and drink plenty of fluids.
In older children prompt institution of treatment is done. The treatment is done for 7-10 days and then cultures are repeated periodically.
Ref: Ghai, Essential Paediatrics, 5th Ed, Ch-16, Pg-374

Q. 653. Congenital hypertrophic pyloric stenosis usually presents
    (a)   Within 2 days after birth
    (b)   Around 1 week after birth
    (c)   Around 2 weeks after birth
    (d)   Around 2 months after birth

Ans. (d)
Note
Congenital hypertrophic pyloric stenosis usually presents 'around 2 months after birth'
Also see
Congenital hypertrophic pyloric stenosis is the commonest surgical disorder of stomach in infancy. The classical presentation is of non-bilious vomiting beginning usually at the age of 3-6 weeks. Vomiting gradually increases in frequency and severity to become gradually projectile. Gradually dehydration and failure to thrive manifest. Persistent vomiting leads to malnutrition, dehydration and hypochloremic alkalosis. Constipation is usual. Vigorous peristalsis moving from left hypochondrium to umbilicus is visible. A small mass due to pyloric thickening might be palpable in the transpyloric plane on the right side.
USG feature are dilation and hypertrophy of stomach, delayed passage of barium through narrow passage gives rise to string sign or double track
Treatment is by Ramstedt's operation.
Ref: Ghai, Essential Paediatrics, 5th Ed, Ch-12, Pg-241,242

Q. 654. 'Weak giants' are produced by
    (a)   Thyroid adenomas
    (b)   Thyroid carcinomas
    (c)   Parathyroid adenomas
    (d)   Pituitary adenomas

Ans. (d)
Note
'Weak giants' are produced by 'Pituitary adenomas'.
Also see
The patient with gigantism in the initial stage does have lot of energy and muscular strength. However lateron on they become very weak.
Hypersecretion of growth hormone in children usually occur due to pituitary adenoma resulting in somatic overgrowth or gigantism. The child is taller than his peers especially at puberty. The peripheral parts like the hands and feet are large and so is the jaw. Nose is broad. There is increased appetite and growth rate. Muscle weakness is seen along with bony and cartilaginous overgrowth; therefore they are called as weak giants.
Treatment involves: complete or partial resection of the tumor
Ref: Ghai, Essential Paediatrics, 5th Ed, Ch-20, Pg-443

Q. 655. Bag and mask ventilation is contraindicated in
    (a)   Cleft lip
    (b)   Meconium aspiration
    (c)   Diaphragmatic hernia
    (d)   Multicentric bronchogenic cyst

Ans. (c)
Note
Bag and mask ventilation is contraindicated in 'Diaphragmatic hernia'.
Also see
Bag and mask ventilation is used after tactile stimulation if:
a.   The infant is apnoeic or gasping.
b.   Respiration is spontaneous but heart rate is less than 100/min.
    In diaphragmatic hernia bag and mask ventilation is contraindicated. In thick meconium stained babies, bag and mask ventilation is carried out after tracheal suction. Three signs indicate improvement in the condition of the patient undergoing resuscitation.
a.   Increased H.R.

b. Spontaneous respiration.
c. Improving color.
Ref: Ghai, Essential Paediatrics, 5th Ed, Ch-7, Pg-119

Q. 656. A neonate develops signs of meningitis at seven days of birth. The presence of which of the following infectious agent in the maternal genital tract can be the causative agent of this disease?
(a) Neisseria gonorrheae
(b) Chlamydia trachomatis
(c) Streptococcus agalactiae
(d) Hemophilus ducreyi

Ans. (c)
Note
The causative agent of this disease is 'Streptococcus agalactiae'.
Also see
Streptococci belonging to Lancefield's group B have since been recognized as a major cause of sepsis and meningitis in human neonates. Lancefield group B consists of single species, S. agalactiae. Early onset infection occurs with in the first week of life, with a median age of 20 h at the onset of illness. Infants have sign of group B streptococcal disease at birth. The infection is acquired during or shortly before birth from organisms colonizing the maternal genital tract. Findings include respiratory distress, lethargy, hypotension, and pneumonia. Late-onset of infections occur in infants between 1 week and 3 months of age, with a mean age at onset of 3 to 4 weeks. The infecting organism may be acquired during delivery (as in early-onset cases) or during later contact with a colonized mother, nursery personal, or another source. Meningitis is the most common manifestation of late-onset infection.
Ref: Harrison's 16th Ed, Pg-829

Extended information
Streptococcus agalactiae belongs to the Group B streptococcus (GBS—predominantly type III) and along with *Escherichia coli* (particularly those strains containing the K1 polysaccharide), and *Listeria monocytogenes* accounts for 75% of neonatal meningitis.
Meningitis due to GBS may occur in the 1st wk of life, accompanying early-onset neonatal sepsis and frequently presenting as a pneumonic illness. Usually, however, GBS meningitis occurs after this period (most commonly in the 1st 3 months of life) as an isolated illness characterized by absence of antecedent obstetric or perinatal complications and the presence of more specific signs of meningitis (e.g., fever, lethargy, seizures).
Ref: http://www.merck.com/mmpe/sec19/ch279/ch279k.html

Q. 657. Oral rehydration mixture contains glucose and sodium because both of them
(a) Are needed to maintain the plasma osmolality.
(b) Are prominent energy sources for the body.
(c) Facilitate the transport of each other from the intestinal mucosa to the blood.
(d) Are required for the activation of sodium potassium ATPase.

Ans. (c)
Note
Oral rehydration mixture contains glucose and sodium because both of them 'facilitate the transport of each other frm the intestinal mucosa to the blood'.
Also see
The aim of oral rehydration is to prevent dehydration and reduce mortality associated with cholera. Composition of ORS-citrate:
a. 1 L water
b. NaCl (3.5g)
c. Trisodium citrate dehydrate (2.9 g)
d. Potassium chloride (1.5 g)
e. Glucose (20 g)
Glucose given orally enhances the intestinal absorption of salt and water and thus is capable of correcting the electrolyte and water deficit. Inclusion of trisodium citrate has made the preparation more stable and results in less stool output.
Ref: Park's & Park, 17th Ed, Ch- 5, Sec-2, Cholera, Pg-171

Q. 658. A 13 year old boy has bilateral gynecomastia. His height is 148 cm, weight 58 kg; the sexual maturity rating is stage 2. The gynecomastia is most likely due to
(a) Prolactinoma
(b) Testicular tumor
(c) Pubertal gynecomastia
(d) Chronic liver disease

Ans. (c)
Note
The bilateral gynecomastia in above case is most likely due to 'Pubertal gynecomastia'.
Also see
Gynecomastia is defined as enlargement of 1 or both breasts during puberty in boys.
In physiological gynecomastia there are no other symptoms. The enlargement tends to spontaneously disappear in 6 months to 2 years.
Pathological gynecomastia, causes are: Deficiency of testosterone (anorchia, klinefelter's syndrome, etc.)
Increased production of estrogen (testicular or adrenal tumor, hCG secreting tumors)
Drugs
Ref: Ghai, Essential Paediatrics, 5th Ed, Ch-2, Pg-44

Q. 659. A 9 year old boy presents with growth retardation and propensity to hypoglycemia. Physical examination reveals short stature, micropenis, increased fat and high-pitched voice. The skeletal survey reveals bone age of 5 years. Which of the following is most appropriate diagnosis?
(a) Malabsorption
(b) Growth hormone deficiency
(c) Adrenal tumor
(d) Thyroxine deficiency

Ans. (b)
Note
The most appropriate diagnosis for above clinical presentation is 'Growth harmone deficinecy'.
Also see
Prime feature of growth hormone deficiency is short stature. Infants with complete deficiency of G.H. may however appear normal at birth. The height is usually less than 3rd percentile for the age and the height velocity is often as low as 1 cm/yr.

C/F:
Children with GH deficiency are short, somewhat overweight for their height with markedly increased subcutaneous fat. Bone age may be delayed.
Other features are:
Crowding of mid-facial features, depressed nasal bridge, single central incisor tooth, prominent philtrum, hypoplastic penis and scrotum. Frontal bossing, high pitched voice.
Diagnostic features are:
 -Height below the third percentile
 -Prepubertal growth velocity <4cm/yr
 -Bone age below chronological age
 -Abnormal 24hr GH secretion pattern
 -Peak GH <10ng/ml during
 -Low IGF 1 and IGFBP 3 levels
Provocation test:
 -Resumption of growth following GH administration.
Ref: Ghai, Essential Paediatrics, 5th Ed, Ch-20, Pg- 441

Q. 660. When does switch over from fetal to adult hemoglobin synthesis begin?
(a) 14 weeks gestation
(b) 30 weeks gestation
(c) 36 weeks gestation
(d) 7-10 days postnatal

Ans. use your discretion

Note
Switch over from fetal to adult hemoglobin synthesis begin around 20th weeks of gestation.

Also see
Hb A appears in the fetal life after 5 months around 20 weeks of intrauterine life, when bone marrow begins to function as a hemopoietic agent.
At 20 weeks of IU life concentration of Hb A is 6% rest of it is Hb F.
At birth- 20%
At 2 months post natal- 50%
At 4 months postnatal -90%
After a year- >99%
Ref: Textbook of Physiology, by A.K. Jain, Volume 1, 2nd Ed, Ch-3,Unit-11, Pg- 54.

Q. 661. A male infant presented with distension of abdomen shortly after birth with passing of less meconium. Subsequently a full-thickness biopsy of the rectum was performed. The rectal biopsy is likely to show
(a) Fibrosis of submucosa
(b) Lack of ganglion cells
(c) Thickened muscularis propria
(d) Hyalinization of the muscular coat

Ans. (b)

Note
In reference to the above clinical presentation the rectal biopsy is likely to show 'Lack of ganglion cells'.

Also see
The patient seems to be suffering from Hirschsprung's disease. It is the congenital absence of ganglion cells in the submucosal and myentric plexuses of the distal intestine. The distal rectum is always aganglionic and the aganglionosis extends proximally usually ending in transition zone in the rectosigmoid colon. As the aganglionic segment is not capable of coordinated peristalsis and fails to relax, this leads to mechanical obstruction. Failure to pass meconium within 36 hours of life, abdominal distention, vomiting and poor feeding are the usual symptoms. Abdominal distention, an empty rectum on digital examination or rectal impaction are the common findings.
The diagnosis is confirmed by rectal biopsy. Recognition of the absence of ganglionic cells in the myentric plexus and submucosal plexus is essential for the diagnosis.
Ref: Ghai, Essential Paediatrics, 5th Ed, Ch-12, Pg-243

Q. 662. A 6 year old boy has been complaining of headache, ignoring to see the objects on the sides for four months. On examination, he is not mentally retarded, his grades at school are good, and visual acuity is diminished in both the eyes. Visual charting showed significant field defect. CT scan of the head showed suprasellar mass with calcification. Which of the following is the most probable diagnosis?
(a) Astrocytoma
(b) Craniopharyngioma
(c) Pituitary adenoma
(d) Meningioma

Ans. (b)

Note
From the choice given above the most probable diagnosis is 'Craniopharyngioma'.

Also see
a. *Astrocytoma*
It is a common tumor of the cerebellar hemisphere. There is ataxia and incoordination more on the side of lesion. Nystagmus is observed on lateral gaze of the child to the affected side. Arreflexia and hypotonia are present. The head is tilted to the side of lesion to relieve the increased intracranial pressure.caused by herniation of tumor or cerebellar tonsils through the foramen magnum.
b. *Craniopharyngioma*
Present at any period throughout childhood. The tumor is congenital and arises from squamous epithelial cell crests of the embryonic Rathke's pouch. The neoplasm is usually cystic and benign. Clinical features are:

growth failure, bitemporal hemianopia, signs of increased intracranial pressure, endocreine abnormalities such as diabetes insipidus and delayed puberty. Bone age is retarded.
Ref for a and b: Ghai, Essential Paediatrics, 5th Ed, Ch-17, Pg-403

c. *Adenomas*
They are the most common pituitary tumors. They are conventionally classified according to hematoxylin-eosin staining into acidophil, basophil and chromophobe. Morphologically they are classified as:
- Lactotroph adenoma : mixed somatotroph-lactotroph
- Somatotrophic adenoma : corticotroph adenoma
- Gonadotroph adenoma : thyrotroph adenoma
- Null cell adenoma : pleurihormonal adenoma.

Clinically it is characterized by a combination of features of Z.E. Syndrome, hyperparathyroidism and hyperpituitarism.
Ref: Textbook of pathology by Harsh Mohan, 4th Ed, Ch-24, Pg-779-780

d. *Meningiomas*
They arise from cap cell layer of arachnoid. The common sites are- in the front ½ of head and include lateral cerebral convexities, midline along falx cerebri adjacent to the major venous sinuses. They are generally single, but may be multiple in Von Recklinghausen's disease usually found in 2nd-6th decade of life with female preponderance.
Ref: Textbook of Pathology by Harsh Mohan, 4th Ed, Ch-27, Pg- 870-871

Q. 663. Which of the following syndromes is best associated with congenital heart disease?
  (a) Lesch-Nyhan syndrome
  (b) Rasmussen syndrome
  (c) Holt-Oram syndrome
  (d) LEOPARD syndrome

Ans. (c)
Note
From the above 'Holt-Oram Syndrome' is best associated with congenital heart disease.
Also see
Lesch-Nyhan syndrome
It is an X-linked recessive disease. LNS is present at birth in baby boys. Patients have severe mental and physical problems throughout life. The lack of HPRT causes a build-up of uric acid in all body fluids, and leads to problems such as severe gout, poor muscle control, and moderate mental retardation, which appear in the first year of life. A striking feature of LNS is self-mutilating behaviors, characterized by lip and finger biting, that begin in the second year of life. Neurological symptoms include facial grimacing, involuntary writhing, and repetitive movements of the arms and legs similar to those seen in Huntington's disease.
Ref: http://en.wikipedia.org/wiki/Lesch-Nyhan_syndrome

Rasmussen syndrome
Rasmussen's syndrome is associated with slowly progressive neurologic deterioration and seizures in children. Seizures are often the first problem to appear. Simple partial motor seizures are the most common type, but in one-fifth of these children, the first seizure is an episode of partial or tonic-clonic status epilepticus. Rasmussen's syndrome usually begins between 14 months and 14 years of age. Recent studies suggest that the cause of Rasmussen's syndrome is an autoimmune disorder (antibodies are produced against the body's own tissues) directed against receptors on the brain cells. The process may be triggered by a viral infection.
Ref: - http://www.epilepsy.com/epilepsy/epilepsy_rasmussens.html

Halt- Oram syndrome
Hereditary is an important factor in the etiology of Congenital Heart Disease. The strongest known familial tendency is known in ASD associated with bony abnormalities: known as Halt Oram Syndrome.
Holt-oram syndrome is an autosomal dominant disorder including upper limb dysplasia and atrial septal defect, often with conduction disturbances in the AV nodes.
Ref: Harrison's 16th Ed, Pg-1138

Leopard syndrome
A genetic syndrome transmitted in an autosomal dominant manner that is named for its characteristic features:
- L - Lentigines (dark freckles) on the head and neck

- E - Electrocardiogram (EKG) abnormalities
- O - Ocular hyperteleorism (wide-spacing of the eyes)
- P - Pulmonary stenosis
- A - Abnormal genitalia
- R - Retardation of growth
- D - Deafness (sensorineural type)

Ref: http://www.medterms.com/script/main/art.asp?articlekey=31833

Q. 664. Which one of the following is the leading cause of mortality in under five children in developing countries?
  (a) Malaria
  (b) Acute lower respiratory tract infections
  (c) Hepatitis
  (d) Prematurity

Ans. (b)

Note
From above 'Acute lower respiratory tract infection' is the leading cause of mortality in under five children in developing countries.

Also see
Under 5 mortality rate or child mortality rate –annual no. of deaths of children under the age of 5 years expressed as a rate/1000 live births. It is calculated by the formula:

No. of deaths of children <5 yrs of age in a given yr X 1000
No of live births in the same yr.

The causes in decreasing order of frequency are:
a. Acute respiratory tract infections
b. Neonatal and perinatal causes
c. Diarrhea
d. Neonatal tetanus
e. T.B
f. Measles
g. Malaria
h. Pertussis
i. Malnutrition
j. HIV
k. Accidents

Ref: Park's & Park, Chapter 9, Page 397

Q. 665. Dengue shock syndrome is characterized by the following except
  (a) Hepatomegaly
  (b) Pleural effusion
  (c) Thrombocytopenia
  (d) Decreased hemoglobin

Ans. (d)

Note
Dengue shock syndrome is characterized by the following except 'Decreased hemoglobin'.

Also see
Dengue hemorrhagic fever is characterized by fever, moderate to marked thrombocytopenia, hemoconcentration and polyserositis. Epigastric tenderness, abdominal pain, tenderness at costal margin is common. Liver becomes palpable. Petechiae are present on the extremities, axillae, face and palate. If severe patient may go into shock and DSS, wherein the skin becomes cool, blotchy, congested, with rapid pulse rate. Patient may become lethargic initially then becomes restless.

Ref: Ghai, Essential Paediatrics, 5th Ed, Ch-9, Pg-189

MCQ's in Practice of Medicine

Q. 666. Which mechanism in phototherapy is chiefly responsible for reduction in serum biliruibin?
    (a)   Photo-oxidation
    (b)   Photo-isomerization
    (c)   Structural isomerization
    (d)   Conjugation

Ans. (b)
Note
'Photo-isomerization' mechanism in phototherapy is chiefly responsible for reduction in serum biliruibin
Also see
Phototherapy has emerged as the most widely used form of treatment in unconjugated hyperbilirubinemia. Mechanism of action is:
    -Geometric photo-isomerisation of the unconjugated bilirubin results in a more soluble form of bilirubin which accounts for 80% of conversion.
    -Conversion of bilirubin through structural isomerization, which can then be excreted into the bile without the need for further hepatic conjugation.
    -Oxidisation results in colorless by products which are excreted by the liver and kidney without the need for conjugation. It is the least important mechanism.
Therefore the correct ans should be (b).
Ref: Ghai, Essential Paediatrics, 5th Ed, Ch-7, Pg-150

Q. 667. Which of the following is the most common inherited malignancy?
    (a)   Infant leukemia
    (b)   Retinoblastoma
    (c)   Wilms' tumor
    (d)   Neuroblastoma

Ans. (b)
Note
'Retinoblastoma' of the above is the most common inherited malignancy
Also see
Retinoblastoma
It is the most commonly occurring tumor in children. It behaves like an autosomal dominant syndrome with complete penetration. F/H is seen in 12% cases. The usual chromosomal anomaly is in chromosome no 13.
Wilm's tumor
This is the second commonest abdominal malignancy. There is some reported suggestion that the tumor may be familial in certain cases.
Neuroblastoma
They are the most common malignant tumor in infancy. Some cases have familial incidence and seem to follow autosomal dominant pattern.
Ref: Ghai, Essential Paediatrics, 5th Ed, Ch-21, Pg- 466,467,473

Q. 668. Which of the following is true of mumps?
    (a)   Salivary gland involvement is limited to the parotids.
    (b)   The patient is not infectious prior to clinical parotid enlargement.
    (c)   Meningoencephalitis can precede parotitis.
    (d)   Mumps orchitis frequently leads to infertility.

Ans. (c)
Note
Form the above (c) is ture of mumps.
Also see
Mumps is a self limiting benign viral infection of the *salivary glands with systemic systemic manifestations*. The virus is localized in the salivary glands and systemic manifestations and may be recovered from saliva, blood, urine and CSF during the acute stage of illness. Incubation period is about 18 days and the *patient may be infectious prior to the onset of clinical signs and symptoms*.

C/F:
Prodrome: Fever, headache, nausea, malaise and loss of appetite.
Salivary manifestations: Child complains of pain near the lobe of ear and difficulty in chewing, obliteration of the mandibular angle. It is bilateral. The opening of stenson's duct is red.
Extrasalivary manifestations: *Meningitis or encephalitis: It may develop before or even in the absence of mumps.*
Other features; Auditory N. damage, cerebellar ataxia, transverse myelitis.
Complications: *Orchitis and epididymitis- B/L involvement is seen in 30% cases and may rarely lead to infertility and sterility.*
Pancreatitis, oophoritis, nephritis are other complications.
Ref: Ghai, Essential Paediatrics, 5th Ed, Ch-9, Pg-181,182

Q. 669. All of the following conditions are observed in marasmus, except
(a) Hepatomegaly
(b) Muscle wasting
(c) Low insulin levels
(d) Extreme weakness

Ans. (a)
Note
All of the following conditions are observed in marasmus, except 'hepatomegaly'.
Also see
Marasmus is characterized by gross wasting of muscle and subcutaneous tissue resulting in emaciation, marked stunting and no edema. Body weight is less than 60% of the average for age. Height is also affected, though to a lesser extent. There is severe depletion of fat. The contour of atrophic muscles is evident under the thin wrinkled skin. Skin folds are prominent over the glutei and the inner side of the thigh. The buccal pad of fat is wasted in the later stages of the disease. The skin is dry, scaly, and inelastic. Hair is hypopigmented and shows flag sign. The abdomen is distended due to wasting of anterior abdominal wall muscles and hypotonia. Midarm circumference is reduced. The baby is alert but irritable.
Ref: Ghai, Essential Paediatrics, 5th Ed, Ch-4, Pg-68

Q. 670. All are true statement about Ductus Arteriosus except
(a) It undergoes anastomotic closure within 24 hours of birth.
(b) Forms the ligamentum venosum in later life.
(c) It is induced to close by high levels of prostaglandins.
(d) May cause a machinery murmur by it patency.

Ans. (c)
Note
All are true statement about Ductus Arteriosus except '(c)'.
Also see
Closure of ductus arteriosus- occurs immediately after birth by contraction of its muscular wall, which is mediated by bradykinin i.e., physiological closure. However, the anatomical closure takes place 1 – 3 months by proliferation of intima. After abolition it is ligamentus arteriosum and not – ductus venosus.
The shut murmur is 'continuous mechaninery murmur'

Q. 671. The chances of having an unaffected baby, when both parents have achondroplasia, are
(a) 0%
(b) 25%
(c) 50%
(d) 100%

Ans. (b)
Note
The chances of having an unaffected baby, when both parents have achondroplasia are 25%.
Also see
Achondroplasia is an autosomal dominant disease. So both heterozygotes and homozygotes suffer from the disease. Therefore the chances of a healthy baby are 25% e.g., if the affected chromosome is A, and normal is N

Ref: Ghai, Essential Paediatrics, 5th Ed, Ch-22, Pg-480

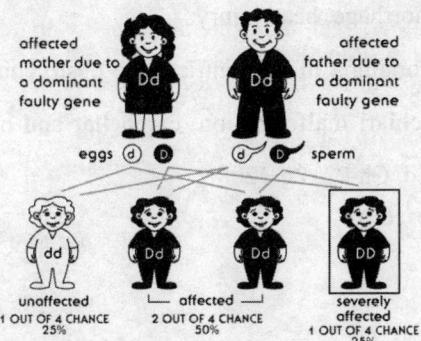

The faulty gene containing a dominant mutation is shown by "D". The correct copy of the gene is shown by "d".

Q. 672. The most common cause of renal scarring in a 3 year old child is
(a) Trauma
(b) Tuberculosis
(c) Vesicoureteral reflux induced pyelonephritis
(d) Interstitial nephritis

Ans. (c)
Note
The most common cause of renal scarring in a 3 year old child is 'Vesicoureteral reflux induced pyelonephritis.

Also see
Reflux of urine from the bladder into 1 or both the ureters during micturition is the major cause of chronic pyelonephritis. It is particularly common in children especially girls due to congenital absence or shortening of the intra vesical portion of the ureter so that the ureter is not compressed during the act of micturition. Reflex leads to increased pressure in the renal pelvis so that the urine is forced into renal tubules which are eventually followed by damage to kidney, loss of concavity of the underlying calyces and scar formation.
Such scarring easily occurs in children because the kidneys are still growing. Formation of fresh scars after the age of 5-6 yrs is uncommon. Reflux nephropathy is an important cause of hypertension and end stage renal failure in children.
Ref: Ghai, Essential Paediatrics, 5th Ed, Ch-16, Pg-376
Ref: Textbook of pathology by Harsh Mohan, 4th Ed, Ch-19, Pg-667

Q. 673. Which one of the following is the common cause of congenital hydrocephalus is?
(a) Craniosynostosis
(b) Intra uterine meningitis
(c) Aqueductal stenosis
(d) Malformations of great vein of Galen

Ans. (c)
Note
From the list give above the common cause of congenital hydrocephalus is 'Aqueductal stenosis'
Also see
Obstruction within the ventricles is the most commonly seen cause of hydrocephalous especially in the narrow channels of the third ventricle and aqueduct, and may be caused by tumor or congenital anomaly such as aqueductal stenosis.

Extended information
Other causes are:
Communicating:

Hydrocephalous is said to be communicating if the obstruction is outside the ventricular system (usually in the basal cisterns)
   -Bacterial meningitis, sarcoidosis, subarachnoid hemorrhage, head injury
Non-communicating:
If the obstruction is in the third ventricle or at the exit foramina of 4th ventricle the obstruction is non-communicating
   -Tumors, colloid cyst, cerebellar abscess, Arnold-chiari malformation, cerebellar and brain stem malformation.
Ref: Davidson's Principles and Practice of Medicine, 20th Ed, Ch-22, Pg-1208

Q. 674. In a child, non-functioning kidney is best diagnosed by
   (a)   Ultrasonography
   (b)   IVU
   (c)   DTPA renogram
   (d)   Creatinine clearance

Ans. (c)

Note
In a child, non-functioning kidney is best diagnosed by DTAP renogram.

Also see
Radionuclide procedures are non invasive, highly sensitive and expose patients to less radiation. The compounds usually labeled with radiosensitive technetium-99 m, commonly used are dimercaptosuccinic acid (DMSA) and diethylenetriamine pentacetic acid (DTPA). DMSA attains a high concentration in the renal cortex and provides very high quality images of renal morphology. This is particularly useful in detection and follow-up of renal parenchyma defects associated with urinary infections. DTPA is freely filtered at the glomerulus with no tubular reabsorption or excretion. A DTPA renogram is useful for evaluating perfusion and function of each kidney. Obstruction to the flow of urine flow can be diagnosed by studying the effect of intravenous frusemide on the renogram. Renal arterial narrowing results in reduced renal blood flow and an abnormal pattern on the DTPA renogram.
Ref: Ghai, Essential Paediatrics, 5th Ed, Ch-16, Pg-364

Q. 675. The most common presentation of a child with Wilms' tumor is
   (a)   An asymptomatic abdominal mass
   (b)   Hematuria
   (c)   Hypertension
   (d)   Hemoptysis due to pulmonary secondary

Ans. (a)

Note
The most common presentation of a child with Wilms' tumor is 'an asymptomatic abdominal mass'.

Also see
Clinical features:
Most common presentation is painless abdominal mass usually discovered by the mother while routinely bathing the baby.
Other presentations are: fever, abdominal pain and haematuria. Rare manifestations may include hypertension, ascites or superficial venous engorgement due to involvement of inferior vena cava.

Extended information
Wilms' tumor is the second most common abdominal neoplasm in children. Tumor occurs in equal frequency in boys and girls. Usual age of diagnosis is 4 months to 6 years with the median age being about 3 years. The tumor is generally unilateral but about 6-7 % of the cases have bilateral disease.
Ref: Ghai, Essential Paediatrics, 5th Ed, Ch-21, Pg-466

Q. 676. All of the following are neural tube defects, except
   (a)   Myelomeningocele
   (b)   Anencephaly
   (c)   Encephalocele
   (d)   Holoprosencephaly

Ans. (d)

Note
All of the above are neural tube defects, except 'Holoprosencephaly'.
Also see
Failure of proper closure of neural tube is known as neural tube defects. It is also known as myelodysplasia. It indicates malformation of the vertebral column (spina bifida), the spinal cord and other portions of the central nervous system may be dysplastic. The spina bifida may be occult and asymptomatic. Examples are:
Myelomeningocele
It presents as a membranous protrusion near the lumbosaccral region and contains meninges, cerebrospinal fluid, nerve roots and a dysplastic spinal cord.
Anencephaly:
It is due to defect in the development of neural axis and is not compatible with life.
Encephalocele
The brain and/or its coverings herniated through a defect in the skull.
Ref: Ghai, Essential Paediatrics, 5th Ed, Ch-7, 17, Pg-155, 406
Holoprosencephaly
It is a type of cephalic disorder. This is a disorder characterized by the failure of the prosencephalon (the forebrain of the embryo) to develop. Holoprosencephaly is caused by a failure of the embryo's forebrain to divide to form bilateral cerebral hemispheres (the left and right halves of the brain), causing defects in the development of the face and in brain structure and function. The most severe of the facial defects (or anomalies) is cyclopia, an abnormality characterized by the development of a single eye, located in the area normally occupied by the root of the nose, and a missing nose or a nose in the form of a proboscis (a tubular appendage) located above the eye. The condition is also referred to as cyclocephaly or synophthalmia.
Ref: http://en.wikipedia.org/wiki/Holoprosencephaly

Q. 677. All of the following can cause a white pupillary reflex, except
 (a) Retinoblastoma
 (b) Cataract
 (c) Retrolental fibroplasias
 (d) Glaucoma

Ans. (d)
Note
All of the above can cause a white pupillary reflex, except 'Glaucoma'.
Also see
Leukokoria (white reflex in pupil) is seen in congenital cataract, retinoblastoma, retrolental fibroplasias, perstent primary hyperplastic vitreous and toxocara endophthalmitis.
Ref: A.K.Khurana 3rd Ed. Pg-23

Extended information
Light reflex normally appears red (red reflex)
Abnormal: Leukokoria (White pupil reflex)
Causes:
 a. Retinoblastoma (most important and urgent)
 b. Corneal opacity
 c. Hyphema or other anterior chamber fluid
 d. Congenital cataract
 e. Vitreous opacity
  -Primary persistent hyperplastic vitreous
 f. Retinal disease
  -Toxocariasis (Dog and Cat roundworms) (granulomas involving retina)
  -Retinal detachment
  -Retinopathy of prematurity
  -Coat's disease (subretinal fluid, lipid collection)
Ref: http://www.fpnotebook.com/EYE32.htm

Q. 678. Retardation of skeletal maturity can be caused by all, except
    (a)   Chronic renal failure
    (b)   Hypothyroidism
    (c)   Protein energy malnutrition (PEM)
    (d)   Congenital adrenal hyperplasia

Ans. (d)
Note
Retardation of skeletal maturity can be caused by all of above, except 'Congenital adrenal hyperplasia'.
Also see
Bone age or epiphyseal development or skeletal maturation is less than the chronological age in cases of constitutional delay in puberty, markedly delayed in hypothyroidism and hypopituitarism. It is moderately delayed in malnutrition and chronic illnesses. Bone age is in advance of the height age in children with genetic short stature, chondrodystrophies, trisomy 21, turner: syndrome, intrauterine infections, storage disorders, seckle syndrome and cockayne syndrome.
Ref: Ghai, Essential Paediatrics, 5th Ed, Ch-3, Pg-49

Q. 679. All of the following are essential features of attention deficit hyperactivity disease (ADHD), except
    (a)   Lack of concentration
    (b)   Impulsivity
    (c)   Mental retardation
    (d)   Hyperactivity

Ans. (c)
Note
All of the above are essential features of attention deficit hyperactivity disease (ADHD), except 'Mental retardation'.
Also see
Attention deficit disorders are characterized by developmentally inappropriate degrees of inattention, impulsiveness and hyperactivity. The cause is an interaction between biologic and psychosocial factors with the clinical expression being considerably modified by the child's environment.
Characteristic signs and symptoms are:
a.   Hyperactivity.
b.   Poor attention and easy distraction.
c.   Impulsive and aggressive behaviour.
d.   Easily frustrated. Irritable, anger, temper tantrums.
e.   Socially inept. Doesn't make friends easily.
f.   Clumsy in dress and behaviour.
g.   Poor sleep habits.
h.   Mild speech disturbances with poor vocabulary.
i.   Isolated learning disabilities with full normal intelligence scores.
j.   Soft but subtle neurologic signs e.g. mild hemiparesis, asymmetry of muscle tones, tight heel cord, difficulty in hoping on one limb, dystonic flexed limb.
Ref: Ghai, Essential Paediatrics, 5th Ed, Ch-3, Pg-54, 55

Q. 680. A two month old child is able to
    (a)   Show a positive parachute protective reflex.
    (b)   Hold head steady in a seated position.
    (c)   Lift head and chest off a flat surface with extended elbows.
    (d)   Sustain head level with the body when placed in ventral suspension.

Ans. (d)
Note
A two month old child is able to 'sustain head level with the body when placed in ventral suspension.

Also see
When a new born baby in prone position is lifted up from the bed with the examiner supporting the chest or abdomen by the palm of his hand, his head flops down. From the age of 4 weeks to 12 weeks, the infant learns to lift and control his head in the horizontal position and then above the horizontal plane. This is known as ventral suspension.
Ref: Ghai, Essential Paediatrics, 5th Ed, Ch-1, Pg-32

Q. 681. A 10 month old child weighing 8 kg has Bitot spots in both eyes which of the following is the most appropriate schedule to prescribe vitamin A to this child?
 (a) 2 lakh units intramuscular (IM) on day 0, 1 amd 4
 (b) 1 lakh units IM on day 0, 1and 4
 (c) 2 lakh units IM on day 0, 1 and 4 weeks
 (d) 1 lakh units IM on day 0, 1 and 4 weeks

Ans. (d)
Note
The most appropriate schedule to prescribe vitamin A to this child is 1 lakh units IM on day, 0, 1 and 14.
Also see
Immediately on diagnosis of Vitamin A deficiency, oral vitamin A is administered in a dose of 50,000, 1 lac and 2 lac IU in children aged <6 months, 6-12 months, and > 1 year respectively. The same dose is repeated next day and 4 weeks later, in cases with impaired absorption, oral intake and vomiting parenteral water soluble Vitamin A administration is recommended.
Ref: Ghai, Essential Paediatrics, 5th Ed, Ch-5, Pg-79

Q. 682. In neonatal cholestasis, if the serum gamma-glutamyl-transpeptidase (gamma GTP) is more than 600 IU/L the most likely diagnosis is
 (a) Neonatal hepatitis
 (b) Choledochal cyst
 (c) Sclerosing cholangitis
 (d) Biliary atresia

Ans. (d)
Note
In neonatal cholestasis, if the serum gamma-glutamyl-transpeptidase (gamma GTP) is more than 600 IU/L the most likely diagnosis is 'biliary atresia'.
Also see
Reference values; Gamma-Glutamyl-Transpeptidase (gamma GTP):
Female: 0 - 60 IU/L
Male: 0 - 65 IU/L
It is a biliary enzyme that is especially useful in the diagnosis of obstructive jaundice, intrahepatic cholestasis, and pancreatitis. GGT is more responsive to biliary obstruction than are aspartate aminotransferase (AST) (SGOT) and alanine aminotransferase (ALT) (SGPT). It is also increased in hepatoma and carcinoma of pancreas and is useful in diagnosis of metastatic carcinoma in the liver.
Very high levels are common in primary biliary cirrhosis. High GGT is found in infants with biliary atresia. It is increased with hyperthyroidism and decreased in those with hypothyroidism.
Ref: http://www.labcorp.com/datasets/labcorp/html/chapter/mono/pr004400.htm

Q. 683. The neonatal kidney achieves concentrating ability equivalent to adult's kidney by
 (a) One year of age
 (b) Eighteen months of age
 (c) Three to six months of age
 (d) Just before puberty

Ans. Use your discretion
Note
The neonatal kidney achieves concentrating ability equivalent to adult's kidney 'After the second year age'.

Also see
The capacity of the kidney to concentrate urine is limited during the neonatal period. An infant can concentrate his urine to a maximum of 700-800 mOsm/kg, whereas the older child can achieve 1200-1400 mOsm/kg. Growing babies utilize most of the proteins for growth rather than catabolise it to urea. Renal function continues to improve during the first two years of life. *After the second year various parameters of renal function approach adult values, if correlated to the standard surface area.*
Ref: Ghai, Essential Paediatrics, 5th Ed, Ch-16, Pg-361

Q. 684. Which of the following is the feature of Y chromosome?
    (a)   Acrocentric
    (b)   Telocentric
    (c)   Submetacentric
    (d)   Metacentric

Ans. (a)
Note
From choices given above the 'acrocentric' is the feature of Y chromosome.

Also see
Acrocentric
Chromosomes have a centromere very near to one end and have very small short arms. *Whereas the autosomes and the X chromosome are telocentric, the Y chromosome is acrocentric.*
Ref: http://jaxmice.jax.org/info/chromosomal_abberati.html
Telocentric
Chromosome whose centromere appears to be at the very tip of the chromosome (Ratio of long arm to short arm is 1:0).
Submetacentric
Chromosomes have short and long arms of unequal length with the centromere more towards one end.
Metacentric
Chromosomes have short and long arms of roughly equal length with the centromere in the middle.

Ref: http://members.aol.com/chrominfo/geninfo.htm

Conditions	Serum calcium (N-9.2-11 mg/dl)	Serum phosphate (N:3-4.5 mg/dl)	Serum alkaline phosphatase (N-3-13 KA units)
Osteoporosis	Normal	Normal	Normal
Osteomalacia	Normal or decreased	Normal or decreased	Increased
Renal osteodystrophy	Decreased	Marked increased	Increased
Primary hyperparathyroidism	Increased	Normal or decreased	Normal or increased

Thus as per the given history:

ESR, blood urea levels are normal.
S. calcium, S. phosphorus and Alkaline phosphatase are elevated.
(S. alkaline phosphatase is elevated in diseases of bone, liver and pregnancy.)
Therefore the most probable diagnosis is primary hyperparathyroidism.

Ref: Textbook of Pathology by Harsh Mohan, 4th Ed, Ch-18, Pg-522
Davidson's Principle and Practice of Medicine, 19th Ed, Ch-20, Pg- 973

Q. 686. A 10 month old child presents with two weeks' history of fever, vomiting and alteration of sensorium. Cranial CT scan reveals basal exudates and hydrocephalus. The most likely etiological agent is
    (a)   Mycobacterium tuberculosis
    (b)   Cryptococcus neoformans
    (c)   Listeria monocytogenes
    (d)   Streptococcus pneumoniae

Ans. (a)
Note
The most likely etiological agent is 'mycobaterium tuberculosis'.
Also see
Tuberculous meningitis is a serious complication of childhood T.B. It may occur at any age but it is most common between 6-24 months of age; usually within a year of primary infection with T.B., the bacillus reaches the meninges by hematogenous route. It may also reach through cervical L.N.
Pathology: The meningeal surface is covered with yellow grey exudates and tubercles. Thus the subarachnoid space and arachnoid villi are obliterated resulting in poor reabsorption of CSF. This leads to hydrocephalus.
Lumbar puncture:
CSF pressure: 30-40 cm H_2O. It may be clear and colorless.
Sugar level reduced to $2/3^{rd}$ of B.S level
Cell count- 100-400/ mm^3
CSF protein- 40 mg/dl
CT scan: Basal exudates, inflammatory granulomas, hypodense lesions or infarcts with hydrocephalus.
Ref: Ghai, Essential Paediatrics, 5th Ed, Ch-17, Pg-394, 395

Q. 687. A 5 year old child presents with history of fever off-and-on for past 2 weeks and petechial spots all over the body and increasing pallor for past 1 month. Examination reveals splenomegaly of 2 cms below costal margin. The most likely diagnosis is
    (a)   Acute leukemia
    (b)   Idiopathic thrombocytopenic purpura
    (c)   Hypersplenism
    (d)   Aplastic anemia

Ans. (a)
Note
The most likely diagnosis is 'Acute Leukemia'.
Also see
Over 95% of leukemias in children of acute type. The peak age of onset is 3-7 years. The peak age of onset is 3-7 years. The disease occurs more frequently in males than in females and this disparity becomes even more obvious with increasing age.
C/F:
Fever, petechiae, bleeding, anorexia, malaise and decreased activity. Bone pains, arthralgia, hepatosplenomegaly and rarely lymphadenopathy may occur.

Extended information
ALL has three subtypes L_1, L_2, and L_3 according to morphology. L_1 has the best prognosis and , L_3 has the worst prognosis.
Other prognostic factors:
    -Children below 12 months of age and older than 9 yrs have poor prognosis
    -WBC count >50,000/cumm
    -Hypogammaglobinemia
    -Hypodiploidy
    -BCR/ABL fusion and chromosomal translocation.
Ref: Ghai, Essential Paediatrics, 5th edition, chapter 21, page 464

Q. 688. An infant develops cough and fever. The X-ray examination is suggestive of bronchopneumonia. All of the following viruses can be the causative agent, except
    (a)   Parainfluenza viruses
    (b)   Influenza virus A
    (c)   Respiratory syncytial virus
    (d)   Mumps virus

Ans. (d)
Note
All of the above viruses can cause pneumonia except 'mumps virus'.
Also see
Pneumonia, etiology:
a.   Viral: RSV, influenza, parainfluenza, adenovirus.
b.   Bacterial: Pneumococcus, staphylococcal, salmonella, klebsiella, H. influenzae.
c.   Chlamydia, mycolasma, pneumocystis carinii.
d.   Fungal: histoplasmosis and coccydiodomycosis.
e.   Metazoal: ascarius.
f.   Aspiration of food.
g.   Hypersensitivity.
C/F:
Insideous onset, URTI or a/c high fever, dyspnea, grunting respiration, increased R.R., flaring of alae nasi, retraction of ribs and lower intercostal spaces.
Signs of consolidation are observed.
Ref: Ghai, Essential Paediatrics, 5th Ed, Ch-15, Pg-346,347

Q. 689. Screening by using maternal serum fetoproteins helps to detect all of the following, except
    (a)   Neural tube defects
    (b)   Duodenal artesia
    (c)   Talipes equinovarus
    (d)   Omphalocele

Ans. (c)
Note

Screening by using maternal serum fetoproteins helps to detect all of the following, except 'talipes equinovarus'.
Also see
MSAFP is used in the detection of following conditions:
1.   Neural tube defects, such as anencephaly - the unborn baby's brain and top of head are not formed completely.
2.   Spina bifida - The unborn baby's spine does not close completely.
3.   Gastroschisis or omphalocele - The unborn baby's intestines are found outside of its abdominal cavity. With gastroschisis, there may be a slightly increase chance of a chromosomal /genetic abnormality
4.   MSAFP is also measured as a part of triple test done for the detection of Down's syndrome. It includes MSAFP, HCG, & UE2. In an affected pregnancy MSAFP & UE2 tend to be low, while HCG is high. (Duodenal atresia is a feature of Down's syndrome).
Ref: Textbook of obstetrics, D.C Dutta, 5th Edition, Cp-11, Pg- 112
Ref: http://www.carle.com/oldsite/LevelIIIPerinatal/PE.MSAFP.pdf

Q. 690. All of the following may occur in Noonan's syndrome except
    (a)   Hypertrophic cardiomyopathy
    (b)   Cryptorchidism
    (c)   Infertility in females
    (d)   Autosomal dominant transmission

Ans. (c)
Note
All of the following may occur in Noonan's syndrome except 'Infertility in females'.

Also see
Noonan's syndrome
Major cardiovascular manifestations: Pulmonic valve dysplasia, cardiomyopathy (usually hypertrophic).
Major non-cardiac abnormalities: Webbed neck, pectus excavatum, and cryptorchidism.
Ref. Harrison's 16th Ed, Pg-382
The sex chromosome is normal and transmission is autosomal dominant, microphalus and delayed puberty are common. Growth hormone secretion is also reduced.
Ref: API, 7th Ed, Pg-086

Extended information
The cardinal features of Noonan's syndrome are unusual facies (ie, hypertelorism, down-slanting eyes, and webbed neck), congenital heart disease (in 50%), short stature, and chest deformity. Approximately 25% of individuals with Noonan's syndrome have mental retardation. Bleeding diathesis is present in as many as half of all patients with Noonan's syndrome. Skeletal, neurologic, genitourinary, lymphatic, eye, and skin findings may be present to varying degrees. Noonan's syndrome occurs in either a sporadic or autosomal dominant fashion. In either case, males and females are affected equally. Features are:

a. Facial features: Triangular-shaped face, Hypertelorism, Down-slanting eyes, Ptosis, Strabismus, Amblyopia, Refractive errors, Low-set ears with thickened helices, High nasal bridge, Short webbed neck
b. Chest/back features: Pectus carinatum/excavatum, Scoliosis
c. Cardiac features: The characteristic lesion is dysplastic/stenotic pulmonic valve, but virtually all types of congenital heart defects have been described in patients with Noonan's syndrome. Hypertrophic cardiomyopathy (obstructive and nonobstructive types) is present in up to 30% of patients.
d. Abdominal features: Hepatosplenomegaly unrelated to cardiac status is present in approximately 25% of patients.
e. Genitourinary features: Renal anomalies, undescended testes.
f. Skeletal features: Joint laxity, Talipes equinovarus, radioulnar synostosis, cervical spine fusion, and joint contractures are less common findings.
g. Skin findings: Lymphedema, Prominent pads of fingers and toes, Follicular keratosis of face and extensor surfaces, Multiple lentigines.
h. Neurologic findings: Hypotonia, Seizure disorder, Unexplained peripheral neuropathy (infrequent).

Ref: http://www.emedicine.com/ped/topic1616.htm

Q. 691. In an single visit, a 9-month old, un-immunized child can be given the following vaccination
(a) Only BCG
(b) BCG, DPT-1, OPV-1
(c) DPT-1, OPV-1, Measles
(d) BCG, DPT-1 OPV-1, Measles

Ans. (c)
Note
In a single visit, a 9-month old, un-immunized child can be given the above vaccination (c).
Also see
BCG:
-BCG can be given with OPV
-BCG can be given with DPT (both administered in different arms)
-4-6 weeks should relapse between BCG and measles vaccination (Measles vaccine can depress cell mediated immunity with less take up of BCG). Similarly BCG and MMR should not be given together.
Though BCG can prevent TB of immunized children, it does not contribute significantly to reduce the overall risk of the infection in the community as a whole.
MMR:
MMR can be given with DPT and OPV simultaneously (but at different sites).
Immunisation for measles later than 9 months means that a significant proportion of children will contract measles in the internal period between wearing off natural protection and introduction of the vaccine. Hence, the most effective compromise is immunization as close to the age of 9 months as possible.
Ref: Paediatrics by Medknow Publications, revised second edition. Pg-354, 359, 360.

Q. 692. A male child of 15 years, with a mental age of 9 years has an IQ of
    (a)   50
    (b)   60
    (c)   70
    (d)   80

Ans. (b)
Note
A male child of 15 years, with a mental age of 9 years has an IQ of 60.

Also see
IQ or intelligence quotient is calculated by:
Mental age X 100
Chronological age
In above case the IQ is = 9/15 x 100 = 60
Levels of intelligence according to IQ:
Idiot: 0-24
Imbecile: 25-49
Moron: 50-69
Borderline: 70-79
Low normal: 80-89
Normal 90-109
Superior: 110-119
Very superior: 120-139
Near genius: 140 and above
Ref: Park & Park, 17th Ed, Ch-11, Pg- 469

Q. 693. Which endocrine disorder is associated with epiphyseal dysgenesis?
    (a)   Hypothyroidism
    (b)   Cushings syndrome
    (c)   Addison's disease
    (d)   Hypoparathyroidism

Ans. (a)
Note
The 'hypothyroidism is the endocrine disorder associated with epiphyseal dysgenesis'.

Also see
Bone age or epiphyseal development is less than the chronological age in cases of constitutional delay in puberty, markedly decreased in hypothyroidism and hypopituitarism. It is moderately delayed in malnutrition and chronic illness.
Ref: Ghai, Essential Paediatrics, 5th Ed, Ch-3, Pg-49

Q. 694. An albino girl gets married to a normal boy. What are the chances of their having an affected child and what are the chances of their children being carriers?
    (a)   None affected, all carriers
    (b)   All normal
    (c)   50% carriers
    (d)   50% affected, 50% carriers

Ans. (a)
Note
For the above 'none will be affected, all carriers'.

Also see
Albinism is an inherited disorder where there are diminished or absent melanin in the skin, hair and eyes due to deficiency of the enzyme tyrosinase. In albinism the melanosomes and melanocytes are normally present but the synthesis of melanin is defective. Generalized albinism is an autosomal recessive trait. Whereas localized is an X- linked recessive trait. Thus for a person to suffer from albinism he/she should be a homozygote i.e. both the chromosomes should carry the gene.

For example the chromosome carrying the gene is represented as A and the normal chromosome as N
AA NN
Albino Normal
AN AN AN AN
Thus all of the offsprings will be carriers of the trait but none will actually suffer from it.
Ref: Ghai, Essential Paediatrics, 5th Ed, Ch-23, Pg-490

Q. 695. Which one of the following is the most common cause of abdominal mass in neonates?
    (a)   Neuroblastoma
    (b)   Wilm's tumour
    (c)   Distended bladder
    (d)   Multicystic dysplastic kidneys

Ans. (d)
Note
Common cause of abdominal mass in neonates is 'Multicystic dysplastic kidneys'.
Also see
Renal dysplasia implies abnormal development of renal parenchyma. It is the commonest cause of renal mass in infants. Here the primitive ducts surrounded by connective tissue, metaplastic cartilage, poorly differentiated glomeruli and cystic dilatation of the tubules are present. A multicystic kidney is a large dysplastic non functioning kidney containing cysts of varying sizes. No intervention is required because it shows progressive involution. At times this kidney may get infected or cause hypertension. Contralateral kidney may show VUR or structural anomalies.
Ref: Ghai, Essential Paediatrics, 5th Ed, Ch-16, Pg-385
Wilm's tumor
This is the second commonest abdominal malignancy. There is some reported suggestion that the tumor may be familial in certain cases.
Neuroblastoma
They are the most common malignant tumor in infancy. Some cases have familial incidence and seem to follow autosomal dominant pattern.
Ref: -Ghai, Essential Paediatrics, 5th Ed, Ch-21, Pg-467,473

Q. 696. Full term, small for date babies are at high risk for
    (a)   Hypoglycemia
    (b)   Intravascular hemorrhage
    (c)   Bronchopulmonary dysplasia
    (d)   Hyperthermia

Ans. (a)
Note
The full term, 'Small for Date Babies' are at high risk for developing *hypoglycemia* as they have poor reserve of glycogen and fat.
Also see
These full term mature infants with intrauterine growth retardation. They are further characterised by certain distinctive features:
-They are exposed to perinatal asphyxia, which leads to; hypoxic injury in the form of ATN, Necrotizing Enterocolitis and Hypoxic Encephalopathy. However, they are less prone to develop Hyaline membrane disease. As the fetal stress in utero, enhances endogenous glucocorticoid production and induced maturation of lung.

    -They have inadequate reserve of brown fat predisposes them to hypothermia.

    -The inadequate reserve of glycogen and Fat predispose them to –Hypoglycemia.

    -Hypocalcemia is frequently develops due to transient hypo-parathyroidism.
    -They are also liable to meconium aspiration, which may lead to pneumo-mediastinum, pneumothorax and pulmonary hemorrhage.
Ref: Ghai 5th Edition Pg-133, 134

697. The following signs would warrant further evaluation of developmental status in a healthy 12 weeks old infant
   (a) Dose not vocalize.
   (b) Dose not babble.
   (c) Dose not raise head up to 90°.
   (d) Dose not transfer a bright red ring from one hand to the other, even when the ring is directly placed in the hand of child.

Ans. (a)
Note
A healty 12 week old infant if 'does not vocalize' would warrant further evaluation of developmental status.
Also see
Key developmental landmarks: Language are:

Age	Milestone
1 month	Turns head to the sound
3 months	Cooing
6 months	Monosyllables (*ma', ba' etc.*)
9 months	Bisyllables (*mama, baba*)
12 months	Two words with meaning
18 months	Ten words with meaning
24 months	Simple sentence
36 months	Telling a story

Ref: Ghai, Essential Paediatrics, 5th Ed, Ch-1, Pg- 32, Table 1.15

Babbling
It is a stage in child language acquisition, during which an infant appears to be experimenting with making the sounds of language, but not yet producing any recognizable words. (Crucially, the larynx or voicebox, originally high in the throat to let the baby breathe while swallowing, descends during 'the first year of life', allowing a pharynx to develop and all the sounds of human speech to be formed Babbling begins around 5 to 7 months of age, when a baby's noises begin to sound like phonemes.
Ref: http://en.wikipedia.org/wiki/Babbling

Q. 698. A 2 years child weighing 6.7 kg presents in the casualty with history of vomiting & diarrhea for last 2 days. On examination skin pinch over the anterior abdominal wall go quickly to its original position. Interpretation of skin pinch test in this child will be
   (a) No dehydration
   (b) Some dehydration
   (c) Severe dehydration
   (d) Skin pinch can not be evaluated in this child

Ans. (a)
Note
The interpretation is 'no dehydration'.
Also see
Skin turgor or elasticity is normally maintained by presence of water and fat in the tissues. Shrinkage of extracellular water in both hypo and isonatremia impairs the elasticity if the skin. The skin appears wrinkled and inelastic like that of the old man. On pinching, it takes a few seconds for the skin fold to return to normal.
Ref: -Ghai, Essential Paediatrics, 5th Ed, Ch-12, Pg-247

MCQ's in Practice of Medicine

Q. 699. Which of the following is not a common manifestation of congenital rubella?
    (a)   Deafness
    (b)   PDA
    (c)   Aortic stenosis
    (d)   Mental retardation

Ans. (c)

Note
From above 'aortic stenosis' is not a common manifestation of congenital rubella.

Also see
Congenital infection with rubella virus is transmitted from mother to the fetus. The risk of infection is higher if the infection is contracted during first trimester; the risk of infection goes on decreasing with advancing pregnancy.
Intrauterine hazards:
    -Abortions
    -Congenital defects:
a.   Unilateral or bilateral sensorineural deafness.
b.   CVS malformations such as PDA, Pulmonary artery branch stenosis, VSD.
c.   Respiratory disorders- interstitial pneumonia and respiratory distress.
d.   Hemopoietic disorders anemia, leucopenia, thrombocytopenia, adenopathies.
e.   Skeletal defects: Micrognathia, linear radiolucent areas and increased bone densities of metaphyses of long bones without periosteal reaction.
f.   Ocular disorders: Retinopathy, nuclear cataract, glaucoma, microphthalmia.
g.   Genitourinary diseases like PCKD.
h.   Esophageal jejunal atresia and hepatitis in GIT.
i.   CNS microcephaly and mental retardation.
j.   IUGR leading to LBW

    -Late sequelae: diabetes, thyroid dysfunction, encephalitis, psychomotor defects, dental abnormalities, language disorders.

Active infection at birth:
The infected infant may be asymptomatic in the neonatal period and develop evidence of congenital rubella syndrome.
Clinical manifestations: Hemolytic anemia, thrombocytopenic purpura, hepatitis, encephalitis, myocarditis, pneumonia, transient radiolucent metaphyseal bone lesions and seizures.
Ref: Ghai, Essential Paediatrics, 5th Ed, Ch-7, Pg-138, 139

Q. 700. Which of the following is not true about atrial septal defect?
    (a)   There is a defect in region of fossa ovalis.
    (b)   Blood flow from left atrium to right atrium.
    (c)   Increased blood flow through lungs lead to pulmonary plethora.
    (d)   There is splitting of first heart sound.

Ans. (d)

Note
From above '(d)' is not true about atrial septal defect.

Also see
Atrial septal defect is an abnormal communication between the two atria. The ostium secondum type is generally anatomically located at the fossa ovalis. The ostium primum type of defect is situated inferior to the fossa ovalis.
Physiologically ASD results in leaking of oxygenated blood from the left to the right atrium at a minor difference in pressure between the two atria. The right atium enlarges in size to accommodate the enormous amount of blood entering it from left atrium. the large volume of blood passes from a normal sized tricuspid valve producing a delayed diastolic murmur. Similiarly the large volume of blood ejected from the pulmonary valve produces a pulmonary ejection systolic murmur. The pulmonary valve closes late and P_2 is delayed. The second sound is therefore widely split and fixed; the P_2 is also accentuated.
Other features: mild to moderate cardiac enlargement. Parasternal impulse is positive.
Ref: Ghai, Essential Paediatrics, 5th Ed. Ch-13, Pg-296

Q. 701. A neonate presents with jaundice and clay white stools. On liver biopsy giant cells are seen. Most likely diagnosis is
- (a) Physiological jaundice
- (b) Neonatal hepatitis with extra biliary atresia
- (c) Neonatal hepatitis with physiological jaundice
- (d) Extra biliary atresia

Ans. (b)
Note
He most likely diagnosis for above is '(b)'.
Also see
On review of above information:
The clay white stools indicate obstructive cause (extra hepatic biliary atresia) and not due to physiological jaundice.
The liver biopsy indicates 'Giants cells'- and neonates respond to hepatic injury by forming Giant cells.
The above findings go more in support of probable diagnosis; Neonatal hepatitis with extra biliary atresia.
Ref: Nelson 15th Ed, Pg- 909

Extended information
Biliary atresia and neonatal hepatitis constitute opposite ends of a spectrum. It can be extrahepatic and intrahepatic. The prime sign of biliary atresia is persistent jaundice. Many times the icterus appears to be a continuation of physiological jaundice. There is absence of bile in stools with the infant passing clay colored stools from the day 4-5 of life. After the neonatal period there is gradual decline in liver function. Liver biopsy may show bile plugs in dilated ducts, fibrosis, inflammatory changes and giant cell transformation.
Ref: -Ghai, Essential Paediatrics, 5th Ed, Ch-7, Pg-152

Q. 702. A newborn has dribbling after feeds. He has respiratory distress and froth at the mouth. Diagnosis is
- (a) Tracheoesophageal fistula
- (b) Tetralogy of Fallot
- (c) Respiratory distress syndrome
- (d) None of the above

Ans. (a)
Note
The clinical presentation is typical of 'tracheoesophageal fistula'.
Also see
Clinical features:
- The new born baby has excessive drooling, saliva is frothy and there is is choking and cyanosis with the first feed.
- Overflow of milk and saliva from esophagus and regurgitation of secretions through the fistulous tract into the lungs results in pneumonia.

Extended information
The five types of tracheoesophageal fistula are known:
a. The commonest variety, the upper part of the esophagus ends blindly and the lower part is connected to the trachea by a fistula.
b. The second type. There is no fistulous connection between either the upper or the lower part of the esophagus and trachea.
c. The third variety there is no esophageal atresia, but there is a fistulous tract between the trachea and esophagus.
d. The fourth variety, where upper segment of esophagus opens into trachea is uncommon.
e. The fifth variety where both segments open into the trachea.
Ref: Ghai, Essential Paediatrics, 5th Ed, Ch-7, Pg-154
Ref: Ghai 4th Ed, Pg-114

Q. 703. Ramu, a 8-years-old boy presents with upper GI bleeding. On examination, he is found to have splenomegaly; there are no signs of ascites, or hepatomegaly; esophageal varices are found on UGIE. Most likely diagnosis is
    (a)   Budd Chiari syndrome
    (b)   Non cirrhotic portal fibrosis
    (c)   Cirrhosis
    (d)   Veno-occlusive disease

Ans. (b)
Note
The salient features are:
Ramu 8 years.
P/Com:
    -Presenting complaint: upper GI Bleed.
O/Eam:
    -Splenomegaly +ve.
    -No ascites, -No hepatomegaly.
O/Inv:
    -Esophagial varices +ve.
The above cinical findings are in favour of 'Non-cirrhotic portal fibrosis'.
Also see
Non-cirrhotic portal fibrosis
It is a group of congenital and acquired diseases in which there is localized or generalized hepatic fibrosis without nodular regenerative activity and there is absence of clinical and functional evidence of cirrhosis. One of the types associated with increased portal fibrosis without definite cirrhosis is seen in idiopathic portal hypertension with splenomegaly, reported from India and Japan. Another variant is congenital hepatic fibrosis seen in polycystic disease of liver. NCPF is characterized by portal hypertension in absence of cirrhosis.
Budd-chiari syndrome
In its pure form it consists of slowly developing thrombosis of hepatic vein and adjacent IVC.
Cause:
    -Polycythemia vera, paroxysmal nocturnal hemoglobinuria, OCP, pregnancy chemotherapy and radiation.
    -The liver is enlarged and swollen.
C/F:
    -Acute: Abdominal pain, vomiting, enlarged liver, ascites and icterus.
    -Chronic: Pain over enlarged liver, ascites and pulmonary hypertension.
Veno-occlusive disease
Intimal thickening, stenosis, obliteration of terminal central vein and hepatic vein. Changes are similar to BCS.
Ref: Textbook of Pathology by Harsh Mohan, 4th Ed., Ch-18, Pg-611
Ref: Ghai, Essential Paediatrics, 5th Ed, Ch-18, Pg-584

Q. 704. A 5-years-old child suffering from nephrotic syndrome is responding well to steroid therapy. What would be the most likely finding on light microscopy?
    (a)   No finding
    (b)   Basement membrane thickening
    (c)   Hypercellular glomeruli
    (d)   Fusion of foot processes

Ans. (a)
Note
The most likely finding on microscopy would be 'No finding'.
Also see
A child well responding to steroid therapy – must be having minimal change disease as it alone - shows most dramatic response to steroids.

The light microscopy for minimal change disease do not show any abnormality – the glomeruli appear normal – that is why; it is called 'minimal change'.
Electron microscope shows; fusion of foot processes.
Ref: Nelson 16th Edition Pg-1636

Q. 705. Most common cause of urinary obstruction in a male infant is
    (a)   Anterior urethral valves
    (b)   Posterior urethral valves
    (c)   Stone
    (d)   Stricture

Ans. (b)
Note
Most common cause of urinary obstruction in a male infant is 'Posterior urethral valves'.
Also see
Posterior urethral valves are the most common cause of urinary obstruction in a male infant. Anterior urethral valve are rarer than posterior urethral valves, but presents with same symptomatology. Renal calculi are not common in infants.
Ref: Nelson 15th Edition Pg-1541
Urethral valve constitute an important cause of urinary obstruction in boys. Dribbling abnormal urinary stream, palpable bladder and recurrent UTI are the usual presenting features. The presence of obstruction in the urinary tract in utero may lead to renal dysplasia. Mild to moderate impairement of renal function may be present at birth. The diagnosis is made on MCU, which shows dilated posterior urethra and valves at its junction with the anterior urethra. The bladder shows diverticuli and trabeculations.
Ref: Ghai, Essential Paediatrics, 5th edition, chapter 16, page 385

Q. 706. A 5-years-old child presents with a calculus of size 2 cm in the upper ureter. He also complains of hematuria. USG shows no further obstruction in the urinary tract. Treatment of choice for this patient would be
    (a)   Ureterolithotomy
    (b)   Endoscopic removal
    (c)   ESWL (Extra Corporeal Shortwave Lithotripsy)
    (d)   Observation

Ans. (c)
Note
The treatment of choice for above patient would be 'Extra Corporeal Shortwave lithotripsy'.
Also see
As a 2 cm stone in this child will not pass on its own therefore surgical intervention is essential. As USG shows no further obstruction in the urinary tract the best choice remains ESWL. This technique is applied in renal and ureteric stones in children with good success rate. The stone fragments will pass down the ureter and a clear passage is a prerequisite for this technique.
Ref: Nelson 15th Edition Pg-552

Extended information
Renal calculi are uncommon in children.
Important causes are:
Idiopathic hypercalciuria, Hyperoxaluria, Distal RTA, Hyperparathyroidism and Cystinuria.
Treatment:
Surgical removal of the calculi is usually required however for small stones ESWL may suffice.
UTI should be treated with large fluid intake.
Ref: Ghai, Essential Paediatrics, 5th edition, chapter 16, page 384

Q. 707. A child aged 2 years presents with nonspecific symptoms suggestive of anemia. On peripheral blood smear target cells are seen. He has hypochromic microcytic picture and Hb of 6 gm%. He also has 'a positive family history'. Next investigation of choice is
    (a)   Hb electrophoresis
    (b)   Coombs' test

(c) Liver function tests
(d) Osmotic fragility test

Ans. (a)
Note
The next investigation of choice in above case is 'Hb Electrophoresis'.
Also see
The salient features in above case are:
Child of 2 years old.
P/C:
    -Anemia.
F/H:
    -Positive family history.
O/Inv:
    -Hb 6gm%
    -P/S: hypochromic microcytic features with target cells.
Impression & Synthesis:
    -The above features are suggestive of thalassemia.
    -Together with hemoglobinopathies, these are hypochromic, microcytic anemias.
    -Thalassemia is a genetic disorder which causes a decreased rate of synthesis of either 1 or 2 globin chains (especially a and ß).
    -Caused by mutations in intergene controlling sites that impairs or prevents gene expression, or by structural gene deletions.
    -No structurally abnormal hemoglobin (Hb) is found.
    -Normally synthesized in the same ratios. Changes in the ratio produces an excess of a or ß chains.
    -a-thal distribution is worldwide, however especially found around the Mediterranean.
    -ß-thal is especially distributed around South East Asia and New Guinea.
    -Also find a, a:ß forms Together with hemoglobinopathies, these are hypochromic, microcytic anemias.

Extended information
Hemoglobin electrophoresis is a test that measures the different types of hemoglobin (Hb) in the blood. This test is performed when a disorder associated with abnormal forms of hemoglobin (hemoglobinopathy) is suspected.
To define the type of hemoglobinopathy, Hb-electrophoresis is the best choice.
Sickle cell syndrome
Here electrophoresis shows no normal Hb A but predominance of HbS and 2-20% HbF
Ref: Harshmohan handbook of pathology, 5th Ed, Pg-273
Thalassaemia major
Here Hb electrophoresis shows presence of increased amounts of HbF, increased amount of HbA2 and almost complete absence or presence of variable amount of HbA.
Thalassaemia minor
Hb electrophoresis is confirmatory for the diagnosis and shows about two fold increase in HbA2 and a slight elevation in HbF (2-3%)
Ref: Harshmohan handbook of pathology, 5th Ed, Pg-276

Q. 708. Most common cause of meningitis in children between 6 months to 2 years of age is
    (a) Pneumococcus
    (b) S. pneumoniae
    (c) H. influenzae
    (d) E. coli

Ans. (b)
Note
The most common cause of meningitis in 6 months to 2 years of age is 'S. Pneumoniae'.

Also see
In developed nations previously H. infleuenzae used to be the most common cause of community acquired meningitis, following the introduction of effective vaccination, the frequency of meningitis caused by this organism has declined by 82%. S. Pneumoniae is now the most common organism responsible for meningitis, both in children and adults.
Ref: Harrison 16th Ed. Pg-485
Ref: API, 7th Ed, Pg-810

Q. 709. Which of the following is true regarding cretinism
(a) Short limbs compared to trunk
(b) Proportionate shortening
(c) Short limbs and short stature
(d) Short limbs and long stature

Ans. (a)
Note
The '(a)' is true regarding cretinism.
Also see
In creatinism birth weight and length are normal, but head size may be slightly increased because of myxedema of the brain. Respiratory difficulty, due in part to the large tongue, includes apnoeic episodes, noisy respiration, and nasal obstruction. Typical respiratory distress syndrome may also occur. Affected infants cry little, sleep much, have poor appetite, and generally sluggish. There is retardation of physical and mental development becomes greater during the following months, and by 36 month of age the clinical picture is fully develop. The child's growth is stunted, *the extremities are short,* and the head size is normal or even increased. The anterior and posterior fontanels are open widely. Development is usually retarded. The voice is hoarse, and they do not learn to talk.
Ref: Nelson Textbook of Pediatrics, 16th Ed, Pg-593

RADIOLOGY

Q. 710. Characteristic finding in CT head in a TB is (ALL INDIA/01)
(a) Exudate seen in basal cistern
(b) Hydrocephalus is non communicating
(c) Calcification commonly seen in cerebellum
(d) Ventriculitis is a common finding

Ans. (a)
Note
The characteristic finding in CT head in a TB is Exudate seen in basal cistern.
Also see
In tubercular meningitis the sub-arachnoid space contains thick exudates, particularly abundant in the sulci and base of brain.
Ref: Harshmohan's Pocket book of Pathology 2nd Ed, Pg-665.

Q. 711. All are seen in right border of heart in chest X-Ray except (K/MD/Ent-II/01)
(a) IVC
(b) SVC
(c) Right atrium
(d) Ascending aorta

Ans. (d)
Note
All are seen in the right border of heart in chest X-Ray except 'Ascending aorta'.
Also see
The right border of mediastinal shadow from above downward consists of the right brachiocephalic vein, the superior vena cava, the right atrium and sometimes inferior vena cava.
Ref: Clinical Anatomy for medical Students, Snell, 6th Ed. Pg-116

Extended information
See the X-ray and its interpretation as under

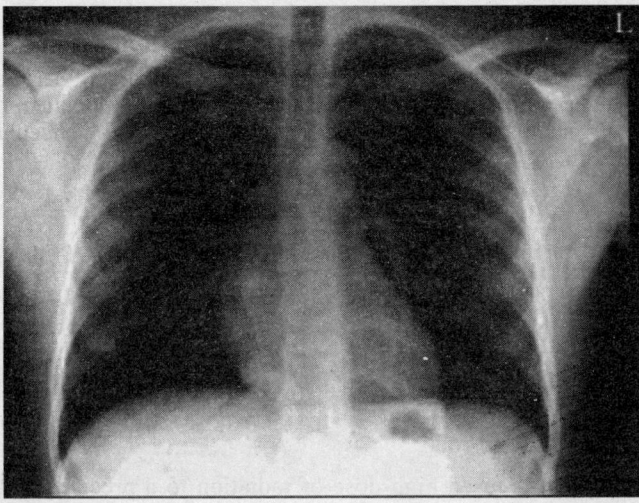

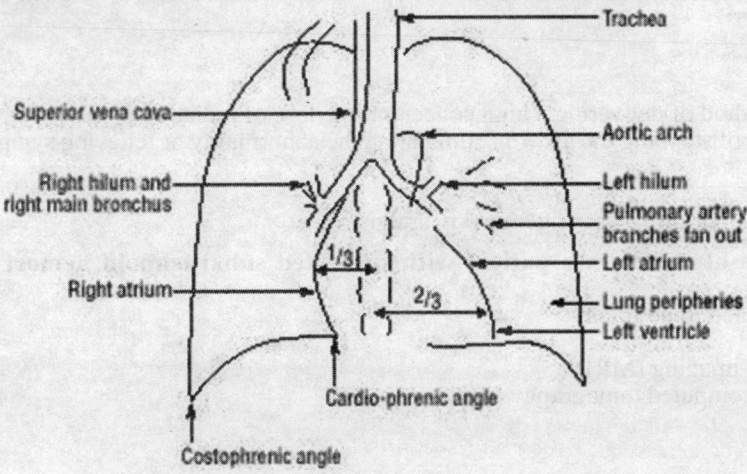

Fig: Normal chest x ray film
Ref: Student BMJ
Ref: http://student.bmj.com/issues/00/09/education/316.php

Q. 712. A young male develops fever, followed by headache, confusional state, focal seizures and a right hemiparesis. The MRI performed shows bilateral frontotemporal hyperintense lesion. The most likely diagnosis is
  (a) Acute pyogenic meningitis
  (b) Herpes simplex encephalitis
  (c) Neurocysticercosis
  (d) Carcinomatous meningitis

Ans. (b)
Note
The most likely diagnosis is 'herpes simplex encephalitis'.

Also see
MRI is the neuroimaging procedure of choice and demonstrates areas of increased T2 signal. Bitemporal and orbitofrontal areas of increased signal are seen in HSV encephalitis.
Ref: Harrison 16th Ed.

Extended information
HSV reaches the brain by cell to cell spread along recurrent branches of trigeminal nere, which innervate the meninges of the anterior and middle fossae. Although this would explain the characteristic localization of the temporal and frontal lobes, it is not clear why such spread is so ratre, with one case of HSV encephalitis occuriring per million in the population per annum.
Ref: Cecil 6th Ed, Pg-850

Q. 713. Stereotactic radio-surgery is a form of
    (a) Radiotherapy
    (b) Radioiodine therapy
    (c) Robotic surgery
    (d) Cryosurgery

Ans. (a)
Note
Stereotactic radio-surgery is a form of 'Radiotherapy'.

Also see
Stereotaxic radiosurgery is the administration of the focused high dose of radiation to a precisely defined volume of tissue in a single treatment. Stereotaxic radiosurgery can potentially achieve tumour ablation within the treated volume.
Ref. Harrison's 16th Ed, Pg-2454

Extended information
Stereotactic radio surgery is a method of delivering a high concentration dose of radiation precisely directed at the abnormality for the purpose of stopping the growth, eliminating the abnormality or relieving symptoms caused by abnormality.
It is used in:
Intracranial tumors, arteriovenous malformation, trigeminal neuralgia.

Q. 714. The first investigation of choice in a patient with suspected subarachnoid hemorrhage should be
    (a) Non-contrast computed tomography
    (b) CSF examination
    (c) Magnetic resonance imaging (MRI)
    (d) Contrast-enhanced computed tomography

Ans. (a)
Note
The first investigation of choice in a patient with suspected subarachnoid haemorrhage should be 'non-contrast computed tomography'.

Also see
CT scan is the incestigation of 1st choice wherever available. The blood from the CSF is rapidly cleared and so the sensitivity of CT sanning falls to 80% at three days, 50% at two weeks, and 30% at three weeks.
Ref: Text Book of Medicine, By Krinshna Das, 4th Ed, Pg-989

Q. 715. Which one of the following imaging modalities is most sensitive for evaluation of extra-adrenal pheochromocytoma?
    (a) Ultrasound
    (b) CT
    (c) MRI
    (d) mIBG scan

Ans. (d)
Note
From above the most sensitive for evaluation of extra-adrenal pheochromocytoma is mIBG scan.

Also see
Scanning with [I31] metaiodobenzylguanidin (mIBG) produces specific uptake in sites of sympathetic activity with about 90% success. It is particularly useful with extra-adrenal tumours.
Ref: Kumar and Clark, 6th Ed, Pg-1098

Extended information
mIBG scan is useful in:
Pheochromocytoma, Neuroblastoma, Ganglioneuroma, Paraganglioma.

Q. 716. Which of the following imaging modality is most sensitive to detect early renal tuberculosis?
    (a)   Intravenous urography
    (b)   Ultrasound
    (c)   Computed tomography
    (d)   Magnetic resonance imaging

Ans. (a)
Note
Intravenous pyelography is most suitable for detecting early renal tuberculosis. Feathery appearance of calyces is the earliest sign.

Also see
Calyceal excavation due to tuberculosis can also be identified on intravenous urography, as can the characteristic small pericalyceal cysts of medullary sponge kidney.
Ref: Radiology and Imaging by David Sutton, 6th Ed, Pg-173

Q. 717. All of the following form radiolucent stones except
    (a)   Xanthine
    (b)   Cysteine
    (c)   Allopurinol
    (d)   Orotic acid

Ans. (b)
Note
All of the above from radiolucent stones except 'Cysteine'.

Also see
The radio-opaque stones are:
    -Struvite, cycteine, oxlate.
The Radiolucent stones are:
    -Xanthine, Uric acid, Uric acid.

Extended information
Oxalate calculus
A calcium oxalte monohydrate stone is very hard and absorbs Xray well, it is easy to see radiologically.
Phosphate calculus
These are large and easy to see on radiographic films.
Uric acid and Urate calculi
These are radiolucent unless they are contaminated with **calcium** salts.
Cystine calculi
They are hexagonal, trancelucent white and **radioopaque because** of sulphur.
Struvite calculi
They are large phosphate calculi, easy to see on radiographic films.
Hereditary oroticaciduria
It is caused by mutation. The disorder is characterized by hypochromic megaloblastic anemia i.e. unresponsive to vitamin B12 and folic acid, growth retardation, and neurologic abnormalities. Increase excretion of orotic acid causes crystalluria and obstructive uropathy.
Hereditary xanthinuria
It is a deficiency of xanthine oxidase causes all purine in the urine to occur in the form of hypoxanthine and **xanthine**. About two third of deficient individuals are asymptomatic. The remainder develops kidney stones **composed** of xanthine.

Ref: Bailey and Love's Short Practice of Surgery, 24th edition. Pg.1316-1317
Ref: Harrison's, 16th edition. Pg. 2312-2313

Q. 718. For the treatment of deep seated tumors, the following rays are used
    (a)   X-rays and gamma-rays
    (b)   Alpha rays and beta-rays
    (c)   Electrons and positrons
    (d)   High power laser beams

Ans. (a)
Note
For the treatment of deep seated tumors the 'X-rays and gamma-rays' are used.

Also see
The gamma rays are very penetrating and not appreciably deflected by magnetic or electric field emitted by radioactive substances. These differ from X-Ray only in being more penetrating.

Extended information
Modern radiotherapy is delivered in the form of mega voltage X-rays or Gamma rays. The main advantages of the high energy are that:
1.   Deep seated tumours can be treated.
2.   Absorption of the radiation is similar in all tissues.
3.   Low energy X-Rays may be used to treat skin cancer and may be of value in palliation.
Ref: Bailey and Love's Short Practice of Surgery, 24th Ed, Pg-220

Q. 719. Maximum permissible radiation dose in pregnancy is
    (a)   05 rad
    (b)   10 rad
    (c)   15 rad
    (d)   30 rad

Ans. (a)
Note
The maximum permissible radiation dose in pregnancy is 05 rad.

Also see
Radiation unit is denoted as 'Rad'.
Rad- Unit of "absorbed dose" – energy absorbed per unit mass of tissue.

Extended information
Radiation related effects (During pregnancy) on the conceptus are as under:
    -Prenatal Death
    -Growth impairment
    -Mental retardation
    -Congenital malformation
    -Childhood cancer

Q. 720. MRI rooms are shielded completely by a continuous sheet or wire mesh of copper or aluminum to shield the imager from external electromagnetic radiations, etc. It is called
    (a)   Maxwell cage
    (b)   Faraday cage
    (c)   Edison's cage
    (d)   Ohm's cage

Ans. (b)
Note
The MRI rooms are shielded completely by a continuous sheet or wire mesh of copper or aluminum and it is called 'Faraday cage'.

Also see
The entire MR scanner installation is enclose in a stainless steel or copper shield known as a Faraday cage that blocks out radio frequency from stations that might influence the MR signals.

Extended information
Other application of Faraday Cage:
- Electromyography (EMG)
- Evoked potential recording (EVP)
- Electroencephalogram (EEG)

Q. 721. For the evaluation of blunt abdominal trauma, which of the following imaging modalities is ideal?
(a) Ultrasonography
(b) Computed tomography
(c) Nuclear scintigraphy
(d) Magnetic resonance imaging

Ans. (b)
Note
The CT scan is the investigation of choice for evaluation of blunt abdominal trauma.
Also see
The definitive radiological investigation of major abdominal trauma in the hemodynamically stable child is a double contrast CT scan, both intravenous and intragastric contrast are given, but the value of the of latter is controversial. Where ultrasound scaning is readily available, it can demonstrate free intraabdominal fluid solid organ injuries, but it is not as sensitive and specific as CT and is more operator dependent.
Ref: Bailey and Love's Short Practice of Surgery, 24th Ed, Pg-1420

Q. 722. The investigation of choice for imaging of urinary tract tuberculosis is
(a) Plain X-ray
(b) Intravenous urography
(c) Ultrasound
(d) Computed tomography

Ans. (b)
Note
The investigation of choice for imaging of urinary tract tuberculosis is IVP.
Also see
IVP is most sensitive and important investigation of urinary tract as it gives excellent anatomical details. In case of renal tuberculosis in the early stage. Feathery appearance of calyces is diagnostic.

Q. 723. "Sunray appearance" on X-rays is suggestive of
(a) A chondrosarcoma
(b) A metastatic tumour in the bone
(c) An osteogenic sarcoma
(d) An Ewing's sarcoma

Ans. (c)
Note
Sunray appearance on X ray is characterstic of osteosarcoma.
Also see
Osteosarcoma
It is characterized by a mixed sclerotic lytic destruction of metaphyseal bone on plain radiography. This is frequently associated with periosteal elevation, which demonstrates sunray-type speculation.
Ewing's Sarcoma
Radiographs of Ewing's sarcoma shows a permeative destruction of bone and typically although not commonly, an 'onion rings' type of periosteal elevation.
Primary chondrosarcoma
Primary chondrosarcoma presents with pain, and radiographs usually demonstrate an area of bone lysis with stippled calcification at its centre.
Multiple myeloma
Multiple myeloma deposits present as purely lytic punched out lesions on radiographs, and bone scan often shows no evidence of bone formation (cold spots).
Ref: Bailey and Love's Short Practice of Surgery, 24th Ed, Pg-436-438

Q. 724. The gold standard for the diagnosis of osteoporosis is
    (a)   Dual energy X-ray absorptiometry
    (b)   Single energy X-ray absorptiometry
    (c)   Ultrasonography
    (d)   Quantitative computed tomography

Ans. (a)
Note
The gold standard for the diagnosis of osteoporosis is Duel energy X-ray absorptionmetry.
Also see
Dual energy X-Ray Absorptiometry (DXA) measures areal bone density (mineral per surface area, rather than a true volumetric density), usually of the lumbar spine and proximal femur. It is precise, accurate, uses low density of radiation and is the gold standard in osteoporosis diagnosis.
Ref: Kumar and Clark, 6th ED, Page-596

Q. 725. What dose of radiation therapy is recommended for pain relief in bone metastases?
    (a)   8 Gy in one fraction
    (b)   20 Gy in 5 fractions
    (c)   30 Gy in 10 fractions
    (d)   Above 70 Gy

Ans. (c)
Note
Dose of radiation therapy is recommended for pain relief in bone metastases is 30 Gy in 10 fractions.
Also see
30 Gy in 10 fractions are for bony metastases in the cervical, lower thoracic and upper lumber spine and for malignant spinal cord compression.

Q. 726. Heberden's nodes are found in
    (a)   PIP joints in osteoarthritis
    (b)   DIP joints in osteoarthritis
    (c)   PIP joint in rheumatoid arthritis
    (d)   DIP joints in osteoarthritis

Ans. (b)
Note
The Haberden's nodes are found in DIP Joints in osteoarthritis.
Also see
Nodal generalized OA is charecterised by:
Herberden's nodes: Bony enlargement of distal IP joint, especially more in females.
Bourchard's nodes: Bony enlargement at proximal IP joints
Ref. API, 7th Ed, Pg-1152

Q. 727. Investigation of choice for detection and characterization of interstitial lung disease is
    (a)   MRI
    (b)   Chest X-ray
    (c)   High resolution CT scan
    (d)   Ventilation perfusion scan

Ans. (c)
Note
Investigation of choice for detection and characterization of interstitial lung disease is 'high resolution CT scan'.
Also see
High resolution CT scan is superior to the chest X-ray for early detection and confirmation of suspected interstitial lung disease.
Ref. Harrison's 16th Ed, Pg-1556

MCQ's in Practice of Medicine

Q. 728. A 40-year-old female patient on long term steroid therapy presents with recent onset of severe pain in the right hip. Imaging modality of choice for this problem is
(a) CT scan
(b) Bone scan
(c) MRI
(d) Plain X-ray

Ans. (c)
Note
The H/O long term steroid therapy in this patient prompts to the probability of avascular necrosis of head of femur. The most specific investigation is MRI having 100% sensitivity and specificity.

Also see
Avascular necrosis of femoral head – This is uncommon but occurs at any age. There is severe hip pain. X rays are diagnostic after a few weeks, when a well demarcated area of increased bone density is visible in femur this lies at the upper pole of femoral head the affected bone may collapse. Early, the x-ray is normal but MRI demonstrates the lesion.
Ref: Kumar and Clark, 6th Ed, Pg-544

Q. 729. Which of the following techniques is the best for differentiating recurrence of brain tumour from radiation therapy induced necrosis?
(a) MRI
(b) Contrast enhanced MRI
(c) PET scan
(d) CT scan

Ans. (c)
Note
From above the 'PET Scan' techniques is the best for differentiating recurrence of brain tumour from radiation therapy induced necrosis.

Also see
Positron emission tomography (PET) and single photon emission tomography (SPECT) have ancillary roles in the imaging of brain tumours, primarily in distinguishing tumor recurrence from tissue necrosis that can occur after irradiation.
Ref. Harrison's 16th Ed, Pg-2452

Q. 730. Which of the following is the most common cause of a mixed cystic and solid suprasellar mass seen on cranial MR scan a 10-year-old child?
(a) Pituitary adenoma
(b) Craniopharyngioma
(c) Optic chiasmal glioma
(d) Germinoma

Ans. (b)
Note
From the choice given above 'Craniopharyngioma' is the most common cause of a mixed cystic and solid suprasellar mass seen on cranial MR scan a 10-year-old child.

Also see
Craniopharyngioma, a usually cystic hypothalamic tumour, which is often calcified, arising from Rathke's pouch often mimics an intrinsic pituitary lesion. It is the most common pituitary tumour in children but may present at any age.
Ref. Kumar and Clark, 6th Ed, Pg-1046

Q. 731. Which of the following is the most common cause of sclerotic skeletal metastasis in a female patient?
(a) Carcinoma breast
(b) Carcinoma ovary
(c) Endometrial carcinoma
(d) Melanoma

Ans. (a)

Note
From the above list 'carcinoma breast' is the most common cause of sclerotic skeletal metastasis of a female patient.
Also see
Bone metastasis occurs in 75% patients with advanced breast and prostate cancer and in 25% of patients with other solid tumours, e.g. lung, GI tract, thyroid, bladder or kidney.
Bone is a frequent site of metastasis due to:
-High blood flow.
-Tumour cell production of adhesions which bind them to marrow stromal cells.
-Growth factors in bone, including insulin like growth factor (ILG)-1 and 2, fibroblastic growth factors.
Ref. Kumar and Clark, 6th Ed, Page-486

Q. 732. Which of the following is the most radiosensitive tumur?
    (a)   Ewing's tumur
    (b)   Hodgkin's disease
    (c)   Carcinoma cervix
    (d)   Malignant fibrous histocytoma

Ans. (a)
Note
Out of above give choice 'Ewing's tumour' most radiosensitive.
Also see
Ewing's sarcoma unlike osteosarcoma, is a radiosensitive tumour, so that it is usually treated with surgery and/ or radiationtherapy in addition to chemotherapy. Sugery is recommended for "expendible bones" such as the fibula and ribs.
Ref: API, 7th Ed, Pg-1030

Extended information
Different tumors and their radio sensitivity is as under:

Highly sensitive	Moderately sensitive	Relatively resistant	Highly resistant
Myeloma	CA Breast	CA Rectum	Melanoma
Wilm's tumor	Basal cell ca.	CA Bladder	CA Pancreas
Lymphoma	CA Ovary	Soft tissue Sarcoma	Osteosarcoma
Ewing's sarcoma	Medulloblstoma	CA Cervix	
Seminoma	Teratoma	Hypernephroma	
	Small Cell Lung ca.	Squamous Cell CA Lung	

Q. 733. Which one of the following is the most preferred route to perform cerebral angiography?
    (a)   Transfemoral route
    (b)   Transaxillary route
    (c)   Direct carotid puncture
    (d)   Transbrachial route

Ans. (a)
Note
From the above 'Transfemoral route' is the most preferred route to perform cerebral angiography.
Also see
Cerebral angiography – Catheter angiography is indicated in the evaluation of the patients with vascular pathology particularly of smaller intracranial vessels. Commonly used femoral arterial puncture provides retrograde access via the aorta to the aortic arch and great vessels. Since the femoral route is used most commonly

the femoral artery must be compressed after the procedure to prevent hematoma from developing.
Ref: Harrison's, 16th Ed, Pg -2356

Extended information
Cerebral angiography or arteriography is a form of medical imaging that visualises the arterial and venous supply of the brain. It was pioneered by Dr Egas Moniz in 1927, and is now the gold standard for detecting vascular problems of the brain.

Any form of angiography involves the passing of a catheter into a large artery (e.g. the femoral artery) and advancing this catheter through the carotid artery. The contrast agent is injected, and a rapid series of radiographs is taken while this radiopaque fluid passes through the vasculature. Another series, taken when the contrast agent has passed through the tissues, visualises the venous supply.

Q. 734. Which one of the following tumors shows calcification on CT scan?
    (a)   Ependymoma
    (b)   Medulloblastoma
    (c)   Meningioma
    (d)   CNS lymphoma

Ans. (c)
Note
Calcificaion on CT scan is best visualized in case of a Meningioma.

Q. 735. Gamma camera in nuclear medicine is used for
    (a)   Organ imaging
    (b)   Measuring the radioiactivity
    (c)   Monitoring the surface contamination
    (d)   RIA

Ans. (b)
Note
Gamma camera in nuclear medicine is use for 'Measuring the radioactivity'
Also see
The gamma camera is an imaging apparatus used to visualize the distribution of radionuclides within the body. The majority of gamma cameras in clinical use operate on the principle devised originally by H.O. Anger at the Donner Laboratory in Berkeley in 1956.

Q. 736. On radiography widened duodenal 'C' loop with irregular mucosal pattern on upper gastrointestinal barium series is most likely due to
    (a)   Chronic pancreatitis
    (b)   Carcinoma head of pancreas
    (c)   Duodenal ulcer
    (d)   Duodenal ileus

Ans. (b)
Note
On radiography widened duodenal 'C' loop with irregular mucosal pattern on upper gastrointestinal barium series is most likely due to 'Carcinoma of head of pancreas'.
Also see
Barium meal X ray of the upper GI tract shows some distortion of the pattern of gastric antrum and duodenum. The barium filled C of the duodenum will be widened in cancer head of pancreas. This is known as Pad sign.
Ref: S Das, Text Book of Surgery. Pg-959
Indirect signs of pancreatic malignancy:
Dilatation of the pancreatic duct proximal to a pancreatic mass is a common finding. It is an important observation since it can lead to detection of small pancreatic carcinoma in the early stages. A normal pancreatic duct usually measures less than 2 – 3 mm and has parallel walls and a straight curse. When it is obstructed, it loses its parallel nature, becomes tortuous, and ends or tapers abruptly.

Q. 737. The radiation tolerance of whole liver is
- (a) 15 Gy
- (b) 30 Gy
- (c) 40 Gy
- (d) 45 Gy

Ans. (b)
Note
The radiation tolerance of whole liver is 40 Gy.
Also see
Radiation tolerance of whole liver is 4000 TD50/5 (100 Rad is equal to 1 gray {Gy})
TD50/5 is the maximal tolerance dose- the dose that, when administered to a given population under a standard set of treatment condition, results in a rate of severe complication s of 50% within 5 yrs of treatment.
Ref: Harrisons 16th Ed. Pg-485

Extended information
The radiation tolerance of the whole liver found by several investigations is in the order of approximately 40 Gy, which seriously restricts its clinical application. The role of whole liver irradiation therefore appears of limited benefit in the palliation of patients with multiple liver metastases.

Q. 738. In which malignancy postoperative radiotherapy is minimally used?
- (a) Head and neck
- (b) Stomach
- (c) Colon
- (d) Soft tissue sarcomas

Ans. (b)
Note
In 'stomach' malignancy postoperative radiotherapy is minimally used.
Also see
Because of the failure of radical surgery to cure advanced gastric cancer, there has been an interest in the use of radiotherapy and chemotherapy. The routine use of radiotherapy has not been supported by clinically trials. There are a number of radiosensitive tissues in the region of the gastric bed, which limits the dose that can be given; this may partly explains the disappointing results. Radiotherapy has a role in the palliative treatment of painful bony metastasis.
Ref: Bailey and Love's Short Practice of Surgery, 24th Ed, Pg-1057

Q. 739. Which of the following is not a CT scan feature of acute pancreatitis?
- (a) Ill defined outline of the pancreas
- (b) Enlargement of the pancreas
- (c) Poor contrast enhancement
- (d) Dilated main pancreatic duct

Ans. (d)
Note
The CT feature from above '**not**' of an acute pancreatitis is 'dilated main pancreatic duct'.
Also see
Computed tomography also gives an indication to acute pancreatitis by changes in the size or shape of the organs, decrease density, loss of sharp peripancreatic soft tissue planes due to extention of the inflammatory process into the adjacent retroperitonum. Appearance of pseudocyst can be easily diagnosed by this technique currently the most widely accepted method used to conform the diagnosis of acute pancreatitis is CT. Pancreatic changes are enlargement, edema, or necrosis with liquifation. Peri-pancreatic changes include thickening of the surrounding tissue planes, presence of fluid collection and blurring.
Ref: S Das, Text Book of Surgery Pg-945

Q. 740. Which of the following is classic CT appearance of an acute subdural hematoma?
    (a)   Lentiform-shaped hyperdense lesion
    (b)   Crescent-shaped hypodense lesion
    (c)   Crescent-shaped hyperdense lesion
    (d)   Lentiform-shaped hypodense lesion

Ans. (c)
The classic CT appearance of an acute subdural hematoma is 'crescent-shaped hyperdense lesion.
Ref: Concise Textbook of Surgery – 3rd Edition – Das Page 546 Fig 31.2

Also see
1. Lentiform-shaped *hyperdense lesion* is Acute Extradural Hemorrahge.
2. Cresent-shaped hypodense *lesion* is Chronic Subdural Hematoma.
3. Cresent-shaped *hyperdense lesion* is Acute Subdural Hematoma.
4. Lentiform-shaped hypodense *lesion* is Chronic Extradural Hematoma.

Explanation
When the blood is between skull and dura, as in the case of extra dural hemorrhage, it is limited by the inner aspect of skull and the dura and gives the classical biconvex or *lentiform shaped*.
When the blood is between dura and arachnoid, as in the case of Sub Dural, it assumes a concavo convex shape, limited by dura on the outer aspect and arachnoid on the inner aspect to produce a crescent shaped lesion.

Extended information
Acute subdural hematomas
These result from torn bridging veins or focal tears of a cortical artery. They can also arise from cortical lacerations and contusions or bleeding from tear in the dural venous sinuses. They are usually associated with more severe, high velocity trauma and thus are associated with a poorer outcome, but they can occur spontaneously as a result of bleeding diathesis or ruptured intracranial aneurysms. Burst temporal lobe is the term sometimes used to describe the appearance of contusional intracerebral hematomas, bleeding out into the subdural space from a disrupted cortical surface. The blood follows the subdural space over the convexity of the brain and appears as a concave hyperdense collection.
Ref. Bailey and Love's Short Practice of Surgery, 24th Ed, Pg-598

Q. 741. High resolution computed tomography of the chest is the ideal modality for evaluating
    (a)   Pleural effusion
    (b)   Interstitial lung disease
    (c)   Lung mass
    (d)   Mediastinal adenopathy

Ans. (b)
Note
High resolution computed tomography of the chest is the ideal modality for evaluating 'Interstitial lung disease'.

Also see
High resolution CT is extremely valuable in detecting interstitial lung disease and assessing the extent and type of involvement, and is also helpful in identifying hilar and para tracheal lymphadenopathy, particularly in sarcoidosis.
Ref: Davidson, 19th Ed, Pg-552

Extended information
HRCT is superior to the chest radiograph in the diagnosis and management of patients with chronic interstitial lung disease. High-resolution studies may demonstrate extensive parenchymal disease when the radiograph is normal and allow for a confident diagnosis when the radiographic findings are nonspecific.

Q. 742. Which one of the following is a recognized X-Ray feature of rheumatoid arthritis?
    (a)   Juxta-articular osteosclerosis
    (b)   Sacroiliitis
    (c)   Bone erosions
    (d)   Peri-articular calcification

Ans. (c)

Note
'Bone erosion' is a recognized X-ray feature of rheumatoid arthritis.

Also see
The complex inflammatory mediators in RA damage the synovial membrane, the articular cartilage and demineralise the underlying the bone producing erosions in the joint margins.
Ref: API, 7th Ed, Pg-1161

Extended information
Juxta-articular osteosclerosis:
 -Above feature is common R.A. as well as seronegative arthropathies.
Sacroiliitis:
 -It is a recognised feature of seronegative arthritis and commonly seen in cases of 'Ankylosing spondylitis
Bone erosion:
 -Recognised feature for RA.
TheAmerican College of Rheumatolgy has defined (1987) the following criteria for the diagnosis of rheumatoid arthritis:
 -Morning stiffness of >1 hour.
 -Arthritis and soft-tissue swelling of >3 of 14 joints/joint groups.
 -Arthritis of hand joints.
 -Symmetric arthritis.
 -Subcutaneous nodules in specific places.
 -Rheumatoid factor at a level above the 95th percentile.
 -Radiological changes suggestive of joint erosion.
At least four criteria have to be met to establish the diagnosis, although many patients are treated despite not meeting the criteria. This is because these criteria are relatively insensitive for early disease. They were primarily intended to categorise patients, especially for research, rather than to help rheumatologists to reach a diagnosis. For example: one of the criteria is the presence of bone erosion on X-Ray. Prevention of bone erosion is one of the main aims of treatment because it is generally irreversible.

Q. 743. A 25 year old man presented with fever, cough, expectoration and breathlessness of 2 months duration. Contrast enhanced computed tomography of the chest showed bilateral upper lobe fibrotic lesions and mediastinum had enlarged necrotic nodes with peripheral rim enhancement. Which one of the following is the most probable diagnosis?
 (a) Sarcoidosis
 (b) Tuberculosis
 (c) Lymphoma
 (d) Silicosis

Ans. (b)

Note
The above clinical presentation suggests most probable diagnosis of 'Tuberculosis'.

Also see
The B/L upper lobe fibrotic lesions point to old tubercular pathology. Active complaints are from last two months with fever, cough, expectoration and breathlessness. Contrast enhance CT shows mediastinal enlarged necrotic nodes with peripheral rid enhancement; it points to most common cause – tuberculosis.

Extended information
The CT scan is used to diagnose mediastinal or hilar lymphadenopathy, cavities and intralesion calcification. Post contrast peripheral enhancement of a lymph node is taken as indirect evidence of tuberculous etiology. High resolution CT scan can be used to differentiate military tuberculosis and other diffuse forms of tuberculosis from other diffuse lung diseases. CT scan is most useful for eliminating the diagnosis of pulmonary or pleural pathology.
Ref: API, 7th Ed, Pg-311

Q. 744. Which of the following is the best choice to evaluate radiologically a posterior fossa tumor?
- (a) CT scan
- (b) MRI
- (c) Angiography
- (d) Myelography

Ans. (b)
Note
The best choice to evaluate radiologically a posterior fossa tumor is MRI.
Also see
Posterior fossa tumor – MRI is of particular value in the investigation of tumors of posterior fossa and brain stems and in delineating the nature and extent of tumors prior to the surgery.
Davidson, 19th Ed, Pg-204

Q. 745. Which of the following radio-isotopes is commonly used as a source for external beam radiotherapy in the treatment of cancer patients?
- (a) Strontium-89
- (b) Radium-226
- (c) Cobalt-59
- (d) Cobalt-60

Ans. (d)
Note
From above Cobalt-60 radio-isotope is commonly used as a source for external bean radiotherapy in treatment of cancer.
Also see
Linear energy transfer and relative biological effectivness value for Cobalt-60 gamma rays is 0.2 keV/μm.
X- rays and gamma rays are the forms of radiation most commonly used to treat cancer. X- rays are generated by linear accelerators, gamma rays are generated from decay of atomic nuclei in radio- isotopes such as cobalt and radium.
Pg 484, Pg 485 Ref: Harrisons 16th Ed

Q. 746. What contrast is needed for proper radiographic image in a heavy built person?
- (a) Increased mA
- (b) Increased kvp
- (c) Increased exposer time
- (d) Increased developing time

Ans. (b)
Note
Obese patients require a high kVP (kilovolt peak) - it determines the beam penetration.

Q. 747. A child with acute respiratory distress shows hyperinflation of unilateral lung in chest X-ray. Most likely cause for above presentation is
- (a) Staphylococcal bronchopneumonia
- (b) Aspiration pneumonia
- (c) Congenital lobar emphysema
- (d) Foreign body aspiration

Ans. (d)
Note
Most likely cause for above presentation is 'Foreign body aspiration'.
Also see
Young child with acute respiratory distress with radiological findings of unilateral hyperinflated lungs is more in tune with foreign body aspitration. Children are at risk of putting small toys, candies, or nuts into their mouth. When the degree of obstruction is less severe or when the aspirated object descends beyond the carina, the presentation is less dramatic. Sudden onset of the classic triad, ie, couging, wheezing and decreased breathing

sounds, is frequently not heatred. In case of complete airway obstruction; respiratory distress, aphonia, cyanosis, loss of of consciousness and death can occur in quick sucession unless the object is dislodged.

Q. 748. Abdominal ultrasonography in a 3 years old boy shows a solid well circumscribed hypoechoic renal mass. Most likely diagnosis is
    (a)   Wilms' tumor
    (b)   Renal cell carcinoma
    (c)   Mesoblastic nephroma
    (d)   Oncocytoma

Ans. (a)
Note
Wilm's tumour imaging by ultrasonography, urography or CT confirms the solid space occupying lesion in the kidney.
Ref. Bailey and Love's Short Practice of Surgery, 24th Ed, Pg-1330
Also see
Wilm's tumor
Wilms tumor (nephroblastoma) accounts for 87% of pediatric renal masses and occurs in approximately 1:10,000 persons. Its peak incidence is at 3–4 years of age, and 80% of patients present before 5 years of age. It is rare in neonates, with less than 0.16% of cases manifesting in this age group. Wilm's tumor is bilateral in 4%–13% of children.
Renal cell carcinoma
Renal cell carcinoma has been reported in patients less than 6 months of age. The tumor is rare in children, accounting for less than 7% of all primary renal tumors manifesting in the first 2 decades of life. Less than 2% of all cases of renal cell carcinoma occur in pediatric patients, with a peak incidence in the 6th decade of life. Wilms tumor outnumbers renal cell carcinoma in childhood by a ratio of 30:1.

Clinical manifestations are similar to those in adults. Gross painless hematuria, flank pain, and a palpable mass are the most common presenting symptoms. Hematuria is more frequent in patients with renal cell carcinoma than in patients with Wilm's tumor.
Mesoblastic nephroma
Mesoblastic nephroma is the most common solid renal tumor in the neonate. Originally thought to represent congenital Wilm's tumor, mesoblastic nephroma has been recognized as a distinct entity, often referred to as fetal renal hamartoma or leiomyomatous hamartoma. It is usually identified within the first 3 months of life, with 90% of cases discovered within the 1st year of life. There is a slight male predominance.

The most common clinical presentation is a palpable abdominal mass, with hematuria less frequent. Some cases are detected at prenatal US and may be associated with polyhydramnios, hydrops, premature delivery, and increased renin levels.
Oncocytoma
Oncocytoma is the most common benign solid renal tumor. More common in males than females. The mean patient age is 62-68 years at the time of resection.
Clinical findings:
Tumors are incidentally detected on imaging studies performed for another indication. However, 17-21% of patients present with symptoms such as hematuria, flank pain, and an abdominal mass. In patients presenting with symptoms, hematuria is more common than mass-like findings.
Prognosis after total or partial nephrectomy is excellent.
Recurrence at the resection site is not reported.

Q. 749. Most radiosensitive tumour of the following is
    (a)   CA kidney
    (b)   CA colon
    (c)   CA pancreas
    (d)   CA cervix

Ans. (d)
Note
Most radiosensitive tumour out of above is 'CA cervix'.

Also see
CA cervix
Radiaton therapy alone is the treatment of CA of uterine cervix.
Web ref: Perez

Q. 750. The EEG cabins should be completely shielded by a continuous sheet of wire mesh of copper to avoid the picking up of noise from external electromagnetic disturbances. Such a shielding is called as (AIIMS/Nov2004)
   (a)   Maxwell cage
   (b)   Faraday cage
   (c)   Edison's cage
   (d)   Ohms cage

Ans. (b)
Note
Such a shielding is called as 'Faraday cage'.
Also see
Michael Faraday invented the above said cage, and was one of the great scientists in history. Some historians of science refer to him as the greatest experimentalist in the history of science. It was largely due to his efforts that electricity became a viable technology.
In his work on static electricity, Faraday demonstrated that the charge only resided on the exterior of a charged conductor, and exterior charge had no influence on anything enclosed within a conductor. This is because the exterior charges redistribute such that the interior fields due to them cancel.

Q. 751. A 55 year old male presents with features of obstructive jaundice. He also reports a weight loss of seven kilograms in last two months. On CT scan, the CBD is dilated till the lower end and the main pancreatic duct is also dilated. Pancreas is also normal. The most likely diagnosis is (AIIMS/Nov2004)
   (a)   Choledocholithiasis
   (b)   Carcinoma gallbladder
   (c)   Hilar cholangiocarcinoma
   (d)   Periampullary carcinoma

Ans. (d)
Note
The most likely diagnosis for above clinical presentation is 'Periampullary carcinoma'.
Also see
In the present case, history of weight loss along with CT scan showing the dilatation of CBD till the lower end and diatation of the main pancreatic duct with normal pancreas is in favor of most likely diagnosis of periampullary carcinoma.

Extended information
Jaundice due to biliary obstruction is found in >80% of patients having tumors in the pancreatic head and is typically accompanied by dark urine, a claylike appearance of stool, and pruritus. In contrast to the "painless jaundice" sometimes observed in patients having carcinomas of the bile ducts, duodenum, or periampullary regions, most icteric individuals with ductal carcinomas of the pancreatic head will complain of significant abdominal discomfort. Although the gallbladder is usually enlarged in patients with carcinoma of the head of the pancreas, it is palpable in <50% (Courvoisier's sign). However, the presence of an enlarged gallbladder in a jaundiced patient without biliary colic should suggest malignant obstruction of the extrahepatic biliary tree.
Ref: Harrison 16th Ed, Pg-537

Q. 752. In which of the following conditions the lead pipe appearance of the colon on a barium enema is seen? (AIIMS/Nov2004)
   (a)   Amoebiasis
   (b)   Ulcerative colitis
   (c)   Tuberculosis of the colon
   (d)   Crohn's involvement of the colon

Ans. (b)

Note
The lead pipe appearance of the colon on a barium enema is seen in 'Ulcerative Colitis'.

Also see
The earliest radiologic change of ulcerative colitis seen on single-contrast barium enema is a fine mucosal granularity. With the progression of disease, mucosa becomes thickened and superficial ulcers are seen. Deep ulcerations appear as "collar-button" ulcers, which indicate that the ulceration has penetrated the mucosa. In mild cases Haustral folds may be normal, but as the disease activity progresses, they become edematous and thickened. *Loss of haustration can occur, especially in patients with long-standing disease. In addition, the colon becomes shortened and narrowed.* Polyps in the colon may be postinflammatory polyps or pseudopolyps, adenomatous polyps, or carcinoma.

Ref: Harrison – Section 1. Disorders of the alimentary tract 287. Inflammatory bowel disease.

Q. 753. Match List – I (X-Ray Features) with List –II (Disease Condition) and select the correct anser using the cods given below the lists (UPSC-04)

List – (X-Ray Features)	List –II (Disease Condition)
A. Sential loop	1. Ischemic Colitis
B. Skip Lesions	2. Ulcerative Colitis
C. Thumb Print	3. Acute Pancreatitis
D. Pipe Stem appearance	4. Crohn's Disease

Code

	A	B	C	D
(a)	3	4	1	2
(b)	1	2	3	4
(c)	3	2	1	4
(d)	1	4	3	2

Ans. (a)

Note
Following is the correct sequence:

List – (X-Ray Features)	List –II (Disease Condition)
A. Sential loop	3. Acute Pancreatitis
B. Skip Lesions	4. Crohn's Disease
C. Thumb Print	1. Ischemic Colitis
D. Pipe Stem appearance	2. Ulcerative Colitis

Also see
Acute pancreatitis
X-ray of the abdomen may reveal pancreatic or biliary calcification, a s ingle dialated paralytic loop of jejunum adjacent to the pancreatic bed known as "sentinel loop sign" only provides contributory evidence to the diagnosis.
Ref: Text book of surgery. By S.Das 3rd Ed. Pg-945

Crohn's disease
The most characteristic feature is that the segments of diseased bowel are separated by apparently normal bowel to form characteristic "Skip lesion". The mucosal surface may vary from grossly normal to slightly oedematous and hyperaemic.

Ref: Text book of Surgery by S.Das, 3rd Ed. Pg-969
Ishemic colitis
Barium enema is diagnostic in stricturing colitis. Marginal "thumb-printing" may be seen due to submucosal hemorrhage and pericolic fat inflammation.
Ref: Text book of surgery by S.Das, 3rd Ed. Pg-1025

Bibliography

Books
1. Davidson 19th Ed.
2. Harrison 15th and 16th Ed.
3. Kumar and Clark 6th Ed.
4. Textbook of Surgery S. Das 3rd Ed.
5. P.J. Mehta's Practical Medicine, 16th Ed.
6. API, 7th Ed.
7. Allen's Key Notes – B. Jain Publishers (P) Ltd., New Delhi.
8. Parasitology by K.D. Chatterjee, 12th Ed.
9. Park & Park 18th Ed.
10. Golwala 15th Ed.
11. Textbook of Pathology – Harsh Mohan (short handbook)
12. A Short book of Psychiatry by Niraj Ahuja, 5th Ed.
13. Ghai, Essential Paediatrics, 5th Ed.
14. Paediatrics by Medknow Publications, revised 2nd Ed.
15. Text Book of Medicine, By Krinshna Das, 4th Ed.
16. Radiology and Imaging by David Sutton, 6th Ed.
17. Color Atlas of Dermatology, by Bhutani 1st Ed.
18. Illustrated Textbook of Dermatology by J.S. Pasricha & Ramji Gupta, 1st Ed.
19. Textbook of dermatology - Ramji Gupta 2nd Ed. – B. Jain Publishers (P) Ltd., New Delhi.
20. Khopkar 5th Ed.
21. Homeopathic Principles of Practice of Medicine – Dr. Chauhan & Meeta Gupta – B. Jain Publishers (P) Ltd., New Delhi.

Websites
www.similima.com
www.fleshandbones.com

Chapter 12
REPERTORY

Q. 1. Remedy for "aversion to onion" in Kent's Repertory is (UPSC-2002)
    (a) Veratrum album
    (b) Thuja occidentalis
    (c) Sabadilla
    (d) Sulphur

Ans. (c)
Note

English Kent

STOMACH-AVERSION to –Onions Sabad.$_k$
Ref: Kent's Repertory (RADAR 10)

Q. 2. Sensation as if heart is suspended from left ribs' – this symptom in 'Synthesis Repertory' is present in the chapter on (UPSC-2002)
    (a) Heart   (b) Chest   (c) Mind   (d) Generalities

Ans. (b)
Note

Schroyens F., Synthesis Treasure Edition Vet   Full Synthesis

CHEST - SUSPENDED –
Heart was suspended from left ribs; as if
kali-c.$_{k,ptk1}$
Ref: Synthesis Repertory (RADAR 10)

Q. 3. In which section of Kent's Repertory is the rubric 'involuntary urination and stool' found? (UPSC2002)
    (a) Bladder   (b) Urethra   (c) Rectum   (d) Stools

Ans. (c)
Note

English Kent

RECTUM - INVOLUNTARY stool - urination, - and stool
Arg-n.$_k$ Arn.$_k$ Ars.$_k$ Chin.$_k$ Hyos.$_k$ Laur.$_k$ **MUR-AC.**$_k$ Olnd.$_k$ Ph-ac.$_k$ Phos.$_k$
Ref: Kent's Repertory (RADAR 10)

Q. 4. In which section of Kent's Repertory do you find the rubric "lies with limbs abducted"? (UPSC2002)
    (a) Generalities   (b) Extremities   (c) Sleep   (d) Mind

Ans. (b)
Note

English Kent

EXTREMITIES - ABDUCTED, lies with limbs
CHAM.$_k$ Psor.$_k$ sulph.$_k$
Ref: Kent's Repertory (RADAR 10)

MCQ's in Repertory

Q. 5. What does the word 'quando' mean in reportorial language? (UPSC2002)
    (a) Personality
    (b) Cause
    (c) Seat of disease
    (d) Time

Ans. (d)
Note
In Boenninghausen's view totality comprised of:
Quis - Peculiar constitution & temperament
Quid - Nature of disease
Ubi - Seat of disease
Quibus auxilius - Concomitants
Cur - Cause of the disease
Quomodo - Modalities of circumstances
Quando - Time modalities

Q. 6. To which chapter in Boenninghausen's Repertory does chlorosis belong? (UPSC-2002)
    (a) Sensation
    (b) Complaints
    (c) Blood
    (d) Circulation

Ans. Use your discretion
Note

> Boger C., Boenninghausen's Repertory

SENSATIONS AND COMPLAINTS IN GENERAL - Chlorosis
Ars.$_{bg2}$ bar-c.$_{bg2}$ **BELL.**$_{bg2}$ **CALC.**$_{bg2}$ carb-an.$_{bg2}$ carb-v.$_{bg2}$ caust.$_{bg2}$ **CHIN.**$_{bg2}$ **COCC.**$_{bg2}$ **CON.**$_{bg2}$ *Dig.*$_{bg2}$ **FERR.**$_{bg2}$ *Graph.*$_{bg2}$ **HELL.**$_{bg2}$ ign.$_{bg2}$ **KALI-C.**$_{bg2}$ **LYC.**$_{bg2}$ *Merc.*$_{bg2}$ **NAT-M.**$_{bg2}$ **NIT-AC.**$_{bg2}$ **NUX-V.**$_{bg2}$ olnd.$_{bg2}$ *Ph-ac.*$_{bg2}$ **PHOS.**$_{bg2}$ **PLAT.**$_{bg2}$ **PLB.**$_{bg2}$ **PULS.**$_{bg2}$ sabin.$_{bg2}$ **SEP.**$_{bg2}$ **SPIG.**$_{bg2}$ *Staph.*$_{bg2}$ sul-ac.$_{bg2}$ **SULPH.**$_{bg2}$ *Valer.*$_{bg2}$ zinc.$_{bg2}$

Ref: BBCR (RADAR 10)
Please note above question has the choice (a) Sensation (b) Complaints, which appear to be ambiguous.

Q. 7. The 'doctrine of analogy' is the philosophical background of (UPSC-2002)
    (a) Knerr's Repertory
    (b) Kent's repertory
    (c) Boericke's Repertory
    (d) Boenninghausen's Repertory

Ans. (d)
Note
Also see the philosophical background of:
a. *Knerr's Repertory*
This belongs to the 'Puritan' group of repertories. This is the repertory which is build up with the symptoms obtained from the provers, in their own language. The Knerr's repertory is based on 'Herings Guiding Symptoms of Materia Medica'. The symptoms are arranged almost in its original form without much change.
b. *Kent's Repertory*
It is based on philosophy of deductive logic, i.e., from general to particulars. Generals are dealt with in depth followed by particulars and minute particulars on concept of individualization. There the structure of repertory, in each rubric, the discussions / descriptions is made about the remedies in general. Thereafter, the rubric is further dissected to arrive at a finer differentiating point on the principles of individualization. Hence rubrics, sub-rubrics and sub-sub-rubrics are found.

c. *Boericke's Repertory*
It is a general clinical repertory. This repertory contain clinical symptoms and conditions covering the whole and also related to different symptoms besides other factors like modalities generalities etc.

Therefore, It has no distinct philosophy in its construction and do not follow any principles, for forming a repertorial totality during the process of repertorisation. They are merely used as reference books and not be used for systematic repertorisation.

d. *Boenninghausen's Repertory*
Doctrine / Concept of Analogy:
Boenninghausen perceived and observed, in materia medica and patients that the manifestations in different localities showed a tendency to resemble each other rather than otherwise. He interpreted conjointly on grounds of analogy and postulated that whenever observations were missing in a particular area, they could validly be inferred from the characteristics expressions (Sensations or Modalities) in other areas. Thereby, it makes it possible for a physician to build up a workable totality for prescribing similimum. His idea was, "what is true of the part is true of the whole".

Here the concept of totality is based on doctrine of analogy and concomitants. Particulars are augmented / upgraded to generals by above concept. No further differentiations of the rubric are made.
Boenninghausen's 'Therapeutic Pocket Book' is based on the concept of generalization.

Q. 8. Prime importance to 'Pathological Generals' has been given by (UPSC-2002)
    (a)   Dr. Boger
    (b)   Dr. Boenninghausen
    (c)   Dr. Kent
    (d)   Dr. Gross

Ans. (a)
Note
Boger's approach:
    -Prime importance to pathological generals
    -Causation
    -Concomitant
    -Modalities
    -Physical generals
    -Use of mentals to differentiate

Q. 9. To which sub-chapter in Boenninghausen's Repertory does 'Abortion' belong? (UPSC-2002)
    (a)   Genitalia female
    (b)   Sexual organs
    (c)   Generalities
    (d)   Menstruation

Ans. (a)
Note
Repertory Boenninghausen's Repertory: Chapter – (Genitalia female) Female Organs abortus.
There is no such chapter like – 'Sexual organs' in Boenninghausen's Repertory.
'Abortus' - the rubric in Boenninghausen's repertory is presented below:

> Boger C., Boenninghausen's Repertory

GENITALIA - Female organs - abortus
acon.$_{bg2}$ ant-c.$_{bg2}$ apis$_{bg2}$ arg-n.$_{bg2}$ **ARN.**$_{bg2}$ *Asar.*$_{bg2}$ **BELL.**$_{bg2}$ borx.$_{bg2}$ **BRY.**$_{bg2}$ **CALC.**$_{bg2}$ *Canth.*$_{bg2}$ caps.$_{bg2}$ carb-an.$_{bg2}$ **CARB-V.**$_{bg2}$ **CHAM.**$_{bg2}$ **CHIN.**$_{bg2}$ cina$_{bg2}$ **COCC.**$_{bg2}$ con.$_{bg2}$ **CROC.**$_{bg2}$ cupr.$_{bg2}$ cycl.$_{bg2}$ **FERR.**$_{bg2}$ *Hyos.*$_{bg2}$ **IP.**$_{bg2}$ **KALI-C.**$_{bg2}$ *Kreos.*$_{bg2}$ lach.$_{bg2}$ **LYC.**$_{bg2}$ *Merc.*$_{bg2}$ nat-c.$_{bg2}$ *Nit-ac.*$_{bg2}$ **NUX-M.**$_{bg2}$ **NUX-V.**$_{bg2}$ op.$_{bg2}$ *Phos.*$_{bg2}$ **PLAT.**$_{bg2}$ plb.$_{bg2}$ **PULS.**$_{bg2}$ **RHUS-T.**$_{bg2,bg2}$ *Ruta*$_{bg2}$ **SABIN.**$_{bg2}$ **SEC.**$_{bg2}$ **SEP.**$_{bg2}$ **SIL.**$_{bg2}$ stram.$_{bg2}$ **SULPH.**$_{bg2}$ *Tril-p.*$_{bg2}$ verat.$_{bg2}$ **VIB.**$_{bg2}$ Zinc.$_{bg2}$

Ref: BBCR (RADAR 10)

MCQ's in Repertory

Q. 10. How many grades do you find in Boenninghausen's Therapeutic Pocket Book (UPSC-2002)
  (a) Three
  (b) Four
  (c) Five
  (d) Six

Ans. (c)
Note
Gradation of Drugs under the rubric:
Boenninghausen evaluated the drugs by introducing a five-grade value system for his repertory.
Latest edition is the Allen's. These grades are given in Allen's Edition of Therapeutic Pocket Book. Pg 25
BTPB- Boeninghausen's Therapeutic Pocket Book.
It is as under:

S. No	Font	Grade
1	CAPITAL	5
2	**Bold face or type**	4
3	*Italics*	3
4	Roman	2
5	(Roman in Parenthesis)	1

Historical
In the early editions we find these gradations were denoted by (Pg 24, BTPB):

S. No	Font	Grade
1	Spaced Italics	5
2	Italics	4
3	Ordinary type Spaced	3
4	Ordinary type	2
5	Ordinary type in Parenthesis	1

However the following information is of significance:
➢ Allen wrongly stated that, *'In this edition, the drugs are divided, as in Boenninhausen's Original, into five ranks;'*. It is a mistake which even modern authors continue to make.
➢ Boenninghausen listed only *'four'* remedy grades, plus a marker of *'uncertainty'* in TT. Every grade (1,2,3,4) within TT indicates a *'characteristic'* (consistency) for that remedy.
➢ Those remedies enclosed in parentheses showed Boenninghausen's uncertainty as to whether they produced such symptom characteristically (consistently) in provings.

The above information is the result of discussion with Dr. D.P. Rastogi.
Ref: From his lecture titled 'TPA; Therapeutic Pocketbook (T. F. Allen) ERRORS'.

Q. 11. How many medicines are there in Boenninghausen's Repertory? (UPSC-2002)
  (a) 347
  (b) 438
  (c) 547
  (d) 638

Ans. NA - Use your discretion
Note
Options appear to be ambiguous. Moreover the MCQ is not clear about which of the following Repertories are to be referred here:
Boger Boenninghausen's Repertory; it contains 464 drugs.

Ref: Essentials of Repertorisaton by Dr S.K. Tiwari Pg-166.
BTPB- Boenninghausen's Therapeutic Pocket Book has 342 drugs.
Ref: Essentials of Repertorisaton by Dr S.K. Tiwari Pg- 42.

Q. 12. The total number of cards in Kishore's Card Repertory is (UPSC-2002)
    (a)   9980
    (b)   9099
    (c)   8899
    (d)   7980

Ans. (a)

Note
Dr. Jugal Kishore's Card Repertory
The most important event in the field of Card Repertory after Dr. Field was that of preparation and publication of Dr. Jugal Kishore's Card Repertory in 1959 which contained 3500 cards. The second edition was published in 1967. It is the biggest and most complete card repertory. There are nearly 10,000 rubric cards which deal with about 600 medicines. This repertory gives the flexibility to work up a case by both the methods i.e., Kent's and Boenninghausen's.
Ref: Essentials of Repertorisation by Dr S.K. Tiwari Pg-380

Q. 13. Choose the correct remedy for the rubric "Perspiration profuse, night, sitting quietly, while (UPSC-2002)
    (a)   Sambucus nigra
    (b)   Psorinum
    (c)   Kali bichromicum
    (d)   Calcerea carbonica

Ans. (c)

Note

> English Kent

PERSPIRATION - PROFUSE - sitting quietly, while
KALI-BI.$_k$
Ref: Kent's Repertory (RADAR 10)

Q. 14. Kent's Repertory is a type of (UPSC-2004)
    (a)   Synthetic Repertory
    (b)   General repertory
    (c)   Regional repertory
    (d)   Particular repertory

Ans. (b)

Note
The construction of the MCQ appears to be faulty. The Choice (a) Synthetic Repertory is defective.
However, Kent's Repertory is based on concept of General to particular; here the generals are given prime importance, then follow the characteristic particulars.
Review:
a.   *Synthetic Repertory*
     It is a type of General repertory, based on concept of individualization on the basis of general to particulars.
b.   *General Repertory*
     The type of Kent's Repertory, based on concept of individualization on the basis of general to particulars.
c.   *Regional repertory*
     These are those repertories which denote a particular Organ / System.
     Example: Repertory of Tongue symptoms – By Douglass, M.B.

d. *Particular repertory*
These are those repertories which denote a particular part of a particular clinical condition.
Example: Homeopathic therapeutic of Diarrhoea – By Bell, B.J.

Also see
Repertories are mainly classified into two main groups:
1. Repertories with principles / philosophy:
It means that the repertories those have a distinct philosophy behind its construction. Again these can be of following two types:
a. Based on concept of concept of individualization:
There the structure of repertory, in each rubric, the discussions / descriptions is made about the remedies in general. Thereafter, the rubric is further dissected to arrive at a finer differentiating point on the principles of individualization. Hence rubrics, sub-rubrics and sub-sub-rubrics are found.

For example:
Repertory of Homeopathic Materia Medica – By Kent J.T.
Synthesis – By Schroyens F.
Synthetic Repertory – By Barthel and Klunker.
b. Based on the concept of generalization:
Here the concept of totality is based on doctrine of analogy and concomitants. Particulars are augmented upgraded to generals by above concept. No further differentiations of the rubric are made.

For example:
Boenninghausen's Therapeutic Pocket Book – By Boenninghausen, C.V.
c. Based on concept of complete symptoms and pathological symptoms:
In this Repertory, attempt have been made to delineate the symptoms / rubrics in various dimensions i.e.,
-Location
-Sensation
-Modalities (Time dimension)
-Concomitant

Example:
Boenninghausen's Characteristics and Repertory – By Boger C.M.
2. Repertories without principles / philosophy:
These are those repertories which have no distinct philosophy in their construction and do not follow any principles, for forming a repertorial totality during the process of repertorisation. They are merely used as reference books and not for systematic repertorisation.

These repertories are further classified as under:
a. Puritan repertories:
These are those repertories which are build up with the symptoms obtained from the provers, in their own language.
Example:
Repertory of Hering's Guiding Symptoms of our Materia Medcia – by Knerr C.B.
The concordance Repertory of the more Characteristic Symptoms of the Materia Medica – By Gentry W. D.
b. Clinical Repertories:
These are those kinds of repertories which contain many clinical symptoms. This type may be sub-classified into further two groups as such:
i. General Clinical Repertories:
These repertories contain clinical symptoms and conditions covering the whole and also related to different symptoms, beside other factors like modalities, generalities, etc.
Example:
Clinical Repertories – By Clarke J.H.
Pocket Manual of Homeopathic Materia Medica comprising the characteristics and guiding symptoms of all remedies – By Boericke, W. and Boericke, O.E.
ii. Particular Clinical Repertories:
These are those repertories which denote a particular part of a particular clinical condition. This type is again sub-divided into following:

- Special Parts / Organs these repertories contain the symptoms related to a particular organ / parts / system.
  Example:
  Repertory of Heart symptoms – By Scander, E.R.
  Repertory of Uterus – By Minton
- Clinical conditions: These repertories describe the individual clinical conditions.
  Example:
  Cough and Expectoration – By Lee and Clarke
  Neuralgia – By Lutze
  Repertory of Intermittent fever – By Allen, H.C.
  Pneumonias – By Douglass, M.B.
  Ref: Text Book of Homeopathic Repertory – By Dr. Niranjan Mohanty 1st Edi, Pg-39, 40, 41.

Q. 15. Von Boenninghausen generalized the symptoms by adopting (UPSC-2004)
    (a) The doctrine of analogy
    (b) The general symptoms
    (c) The conceptual image of the image
    (d) The common symptoms

Ans. (a)
Note
Dr. Boenninghausen introduced the 'doctrine of analogy' and doctrine of 'concomitants' which are even used today.

Also Note
Dr. Boenninghausen's 'Therapeutic pocket Book' was the very first repertory which was based and structured on a philosophical concept', which had a principle of its own for its arrangements as well as use and which was the very first repertory for systemic and full repertorisation.
He was the first man to introduce systematic repertorisation with a definite principles of its own which includes:
a. Doctrine of analogy and doctrine of concomitant
b. Evaluation of drugs
c. Relationship of remedies
This repertory is most suitable for the one sided diseases. Which contains:
    -Complete symptoms
    -Concomitant symptoms
    -Common symptoms
    -Fever totality; cases of fever with all the stages marked
    Ref: Text Book of Repertory By Niranjan Mohanty

Q. 16. In which Chapter of the Kent's Repertory, the rubric 'phimosis' and 'paraphimosis' are found (UPSC-2004)
    (a) Mind
    (b) Skin
    (c) Generalities
    (d) Genitalia

Ans. (d)
Note

> English Kent

MALE GENITALIA - PHIMOSIS
MERC.$_k$ NIT-AC.$_k$

> English Kent

MALE GENITALIA - PHIMOSIS - Paraphimosis
MERC.$_k$ NIT-AC.$_k$
Ref: Kent's Repertory (RADAR 10)

MCQ's in Repertory

Q. 17. In which Chapter of the Kent's Repertory is blood spitting found? (UPSC-2004)
  (a) Respiration
  (b) Expectoration
  (c) Chest
  (d) Cough

Ans. (b)
Note

English Kent

EXPECTORATION - BLOODY, spitting of blood
ACON.$_k$ AM-C.$_k$ ARN.$_k$ ARS.$_k$ CANN-S.$_k$ CROT-H.$_k$ FERR.$_k$ FERR-P.$_k$ IP.$_k$ LAUR.$_k$ LED.$_k$ NIT-AC.$_k$ PHOS.$_k$ PULS.$_k$ SEC.$_k$ STANN.$_k$ SULPH.$_k$
CHEST – HAEMORRHAGE(cross-ref)
Ref: Kent's Repertory (RADAR 10)

Q. 18. In which Chapter of the Kent's Repertory is rubric 'indolence' found? (UPSC-2004)
  (a) Head
  (b) Generalities
  (c) Mind
  (d) Sleep

Ans. (c)
Note

English Kent

MIND - INDOLENCE, - aversion to work
CARBN-S.$_k$ CHEL.$_k$ CHIN.$_{k\ \cdot\ k}$ GRAPH.$_{k\ k}$ LACH.$_k$ NAT-M.$_k$ NIT-AC.$_k$ NUX-V.$_{k\ k}$ SEP.$_{k\ k}$ SULPH.$_k$
Ref: Kent's Repertory (RADAR 10)

Q. 19. In which Chapter of the Kent's Repertory is the sensation of formication in anus found? (UPSC-2004)
  (a) Stool
  (b) Rectum
  (c) Stomach
  (d) Generalities

Ans. (b)
Note

English Kent

RECTUM - FORMICATION in anus
CALC.$_k$ CALC-S.$_k$ KALI-C.$_k$ SULPH.$_{k\ k}$
Ref: Kent's Repertory (RADAR 10)

Q. 20. In which Chapter of the Kent's Repertory is the rubric affectionate found? (UPSC-2004)
  (a) Generalities
  (b) Head
  (c) Mind
  (d) Chest

Ans. (c)

Note

> **English Kent**

MIND - AFFECTIONATE
Croc.$_k$ Ign.$_k$ Nat-m.$_k$ Puls.$_{k\,k}$
(SEE LOVE, INDIFFERENCE)

Ref: Kent's Repertory (RADAR 10)

Q. 21. Which one of the following is not used for grading or evaluation of the medicines in Kent's Repertory? (UPSC-2004)
    (a)   Recording
    (b)   Confirmation by reproving
    (c)   Verification upon the sick
    (d)   Research

Ans. (d)

Note
Gradation of symptoms:
    -The gradation of symptoms of medicine is judged on the basis of following three factors in Kent's Repertory.
    -Recording of the symptoms of the drug proving.
    -Confirmation by re-proving.
    -Verification on the sick.
Grades used in Kent's Repertory are:
Ist Grade:
    First Grade symptoms are those symptoms which:
    -appeared in all or in majority of provers,
    -confirmed by reproving,
    -and verified clinically upon the sick.
II Grade:
    Second grade symptoms are those symptoms which:
    -appeared in few of the provers,
    -confirmed by reproving,
    -and occasionally verified clinically upon the sick.
III Grade:
    Third grade symptoms are those symptoms which:
    -appeared now and then in a proving (symptoms appeared in one or two provers),
    -not yet confirmed by reproving,
    -and it has been verified by having cured sick.
(Ref; A Treatise on Organon of Medicine By A. K. Das Part III, Pg 55)

Q. 22. Delusion is explained as false (UPSC-2004)
    (a)   Thinking
    (b)   Belief
    (c)   Dream
    (d)   Memory

Ans. (b)

Note
Delusions
These are false, fixed, firm personal beliefs with following characteristics:
    -Content is often bizarre having no rational basis in reality.
    -Unshakable despite evidence to the contrary.
    -Related to person's educational, social, and cultural background.

Q. 23. Match List-I (rubric) with List-II (chapter) and select the correct answer using the codes given below the lists (UPSC-2004)

List –I (Ruberic)	List- II (Chapter)
A. Theorising	1. Head
B. Baldness	2. Nose
C. Amaurosis	3. Mind
D. Epistaxis	4. Eye

Code

A	A	B	C	D
	4	1	3	2
B	A	B	C	D
	3	2	4	1
C	A	B	C	D
	4	2	3	1
D	A	B	C	D
	3	1	4	2

Ans. (d)

Note

List –I (Rubric)	List- II (Chapter)
A. Theorising	3. Mind
B. Baldness	1. Head
C. Amaurosis	4. Eye
D. Epistaxis	2. Nose

Q. 24. Author of the Repertory of Hering's Guiding Symptoms of our Materia Medica is (KPSC/Lect/Rep-2004)
(a) Calvin B Knerr
(b) Clara B Knerr
(c) Clavan B Knerr
(d) Carol B Knerr

Ans. (a)
Note
Calvin B Knerr has compiled 'Repertory of Hering's Guiding Symptoms' of our Materia Medica. The symptoms are arranged almost in its original format without any change. 'Repertory of the Hering's guiding symptoms' was published in 1896.

Q. 25. Jahr published the Repertory in the year (KPSC/Lect/Rep-2004)
(a) 1805
(b) 1835
(c) 1833
(d) 1840

Ans. (b)
Note
Jahr initially started to work under the guidance of Hahnemann. His repertory was cut out of the symptoms from Hahnemann's Chronic Disease arranged alphabetically under different headings (sections). It was of nosological approach; with the passage of time Hahnemann had taken to the concept of individualization, and therefore did not appreciate this nosological repertory. Jarh's repertory came out after Boenninghausen's work and was published in 1835.

Q. 26. Gentry's Repertory of Concordance was published in the year (KPSC/Lect/Rep/2004)
    (a)   1886
    (b)   1890
    (c)   1782
    (d)   1990

Ans. (b)
Note
W.D. Gentry's Concordance Repertory of the Materia Medica in 6 Volumes was published in 1890. In this, symptoms were recorded in patient's (Prover's) language and as such a symptom may be found to be recorded at different places. E.g., nausea and nauseating would be found in two different places.

Q. 27. Gentry's Repertory of Concordance consists of volumes (KPSC/Lect/Rep-2004)
    (a)   Two
    (b)   Five
    (c)   Six
    (d)   Eight

Ans. (c)
Note
Gentry's Concordance Repertory of the Materia Medica consists of 6 volumes.

Q. 28. 'Repertory of Hemorrhoids' was written by (KPSC/Lect/Rep-2004)
    (a)   Gentry
    (b)   Kent
    (c)   Guernsey
    (d)   Hering

Ans. (c)
Note
'Repertory of Hemorrhoids' was written by W.J. Guernsey in 1880.
Ref: Essentials of Repertorisation 3rd Edition by Dr. S.K. Tiwari – Pg 21.

Q. 29. Repertory of 'Fevers' was published by (KPSC/Lect/Rep-2004)
    (a)   T.F. Allen
    (b)   H.C. Allen
    (c)   W. A. Allen
    (d)   Milton

Ans. (b)
Note
Repertory of Fever was published by H. C. Allen. In the era of regional repertories from 1880 – 1900.

Q. 30. C.M. Boger's 'Synoptic Key with Repertory' was published in the year (KPSC/Lect/Rep-2004)
    (a)   1931
    (b)   1936
    (c)   1898
    (d)   1930

Ans. (a)
Note
C.M. Boger's 'Synoptic Key with Repertory' was published in the year 1931.
Ref: Essentials of Repertorisation 3rd Edition by S. K. Tiwari – Pg 23.

Q. 31. In 'Boenninghausen's Therapeutic Pocket Book' the gradation of medicines is (KPSC/Lect/Rep-2004)
    (a)   Four
    (b)   Five
    (c)   Three
    (d)   Six

Ans. (b)

MCQ's in Repertory

Note
Refer note at Q. No 10 (Similar question)

Q. 32. In Kent's Repertory 'Urticaria' is in chapter (KPSC/Lect/Rep-2004)
(a) Skin
(b) Generalities
(c) Extremities
(d) All of the above

Ans. (a)
Note

English Kent

SKIN - ERUPTIONS - urticaria
APIS.$_k$ ARS.$_k$ ASTAC.$_k$ CALC.$_k$ CALC-S.$_k$ CARBN-S.$_k$ CAUST.$_k$ CHLOL.$_k$ COP.$_k$ DULC.$_k$ HEP.$_k$ LED.$_k$ NAT-M.$_k$ RHUS-T.$_k$ SULPH.$_k$ URT-U.$_{k\ k}$

Ref: Kent's Repertory (RADAR 10)

Q. 33. In Kent's Repertory "Bubo" is in chapter (KPSC/Lect/Rep-2004)
(a) Stomach
(b) Abdomen
(c) Skin
(d) Genitalia, male

Ans. (b)
Note

English Kent

ABDOMEN - BUBO
BUFO.$_k$ CINNB.$_{k\ k}$ HEP.$_{k\ k}$

Ref: Kent's Repertory (RADAR 10)

Q. 34. In Kent's Repertory 'Lousiness' belongs to chapter (KPSC/Lect/Rep-2004)
(a) Head
(b) Generalities
(c) Skin
(d) None of the above

Ans. (c)
Note

English Kent

SKIN - LOUSINESS
Lyc.$_k$ Merc.$_k$ Psor.$_k$ Sabad.$_k$ Sulph.$_k$
Ref: Kent's Repertory (RADAR 10)

Q. 35. In Kent's Repertory 'Empyema' is in chapter (KPSC/Lect/Rep-2004)
(a) Abdomen
(b) Stomach
(c) Chest
(d) Extremities

Ans. (c)

Note

English Kent

CHEST – EMPYEMA
ARS.$_k$ CALC-S.$_k$ KALI-S.$_{kk}$ MERC.$_{kk}$ SIL.$_k$ SULPH.$_k$

Ref: Kent's Repertory (RADAR 10)

Q. 36. In Kent's Repertory for "Urine Sugar' look in chapter (KPSC/Lect/Rep-2004)
    (a)   Generalities
    (b)   Kidney
    (c)   Urine
    (d)   Bladder

Ans. (c)

English Kent

URINE - SUGAR
BOV.$_{kk}$ HELON.$_k$ LYC.$_k$ PH-AC.$_k$ PHOS.$_{kk}$ PLB.$_k$ TARENT.$_k$ TER.$_k$ URAN-MET.$_{kk}$

Ref: Kent's Repertory (RADAR 10)

Q. 37. Rubric "Addison's disease' in Kent's Repertory is placed under (KPSC/Lect/Rep-2004)
    (a)   Bladder
    (b)   Kidney
    (c)   Ureter
    (d)   Generalities

Ans. (b)

Note

English Kent

KIDNEY-URINARY ORGANS - ADDISON'S disease
CALC.$_{kk}$ IOD.$_k$ NAT-M.$_k$ PHOS.$_{kk}$ SIL.$_{kk}$

Ref: Kent's Repertory (RADAR 10)

Q. 38. In Kent's method of repertorisation more importance is given to (KPSC/Lect/Rep-2004)
    (a)   Physical generals
    (b)   Mental generals
    (c)   Concomitance
    (d)   Modalities

Ans. (b)

Note
The mental generals:
Kent said, 'Man is prior to the organs …..man is the will and the understanding, and the house which he lives in, is his body". What expressed on the part is always preceded by a deviation in the state of health of a person. Such deviations at the highest level can be known through expressions at the level of mental generals.

It includes expressions available at an emotional and intellectual level. So, they reflect the inner self and individuality or the patient, therefore any change in emotional sphere is most important symptom of the patient.

The symptoms of emotions and intellect are taken into consideration in the following order:
    The will:
    -Ailments from anger, bad news, grief, love, joy, reproach, hatred, irritability, jealousy etc.
    The perversions of understanding:
    -Delusions, illusions, ideas, thoughts, and confusion, etc. it also includes symptoms given in repertory like absorbed, clairvoyance, confusion, imbecility etc.
    Perversion of memory:
    -It includes loss of memory, absent-mindedness etc.

MCQ's in Repertory

Q. 39. In Boenninghausen's Repertory rubric 'Ecstasy' is under (KPSC/Lect/Rep-2004)
    (a) Abdomen
    (b) Hunger and thirst
    (c) Intellect
    (d) Sensorium

Ans. (c)

Note
Here the repertory to be referred should be 'Therapeutic Pocket Book' by Boenninghausen rather than the 'Boger Boenninghausen's Characteristics and Repertory (BBCR). Because the Chapter of Intellect is only given in 'Therapeutic Pocket Book' and not in BBCR.
Repertory-Therapeutic Pocket book' – Chapter; Intellect- Rubric; Ecstasy.

Also see
In 'BBCR' the same rubric is as under Mind:

Boger C., Boenninghausen's Repertory

MIND - Ecstasy
Acon.$_{bg2}$ **AGAR.**$_{bg2}$ agn.$_{bg2}$ am-c.$_{bg2}$ ang.$_{bg2}$ **ANT-C.**$_{bg2}$ apis$_{bg2}$ arn.$_{bg2}$ *Bell.*$_{bg2}$ bry.$_{bg2}$ canth.$_{bg2}$ cham.$_{bg2}$ **COFF.**$_{bg2}$ croc.$_{bg2}$ cupr.$_{bg2}$ *Hyos.*$_{bg2}$ *Ign.*$_{bg2}$ jatr-c.$_{bg2}$ **LACH.**$_{bg2}$ olnd.$_{bg2}$ *Op.*$_{bg2}$ ph-ac.$_{bg2}$ *Phos.*$_{bg2}$ *Plat.*$_{bg2}$ puls.$_{bg2,bg2}$ sel.$_{bg2}$ sil.$_{bg2}$ stann.$_{bg2}$ staph.$_{bg2}$ *Stram.*$_{bg2}$ valer.$_{bg2}$ *Verat.*$_{bg2}$

Ref: BBCR (RADAR 10)

Q. 40. In Boenninghausen's Repertory rubric 'Impaired' is under (KPSC/Lect/Rep-2004)
    (a) Intellect
    (b) Complaints
    (c) Head
    (d) Internal head

Ans. (a)

Note
Repertory-Therapeutic Pocket book' – Chapter; Intellect- Rubric; Impaired.
Repertory-BBCR-

Boger C., Boenninghausen's Repertory

MIND - Intellect, impaired, mental exhaustion, weakness of, etc.
abrot.$_{bg2}$ acet-ac.$_{bg2}$ **ACON.**$_{bg2}$ *Agar.*$_{bg2}$ agn.$_{bg2}$ alum.$_{bg2}$ am-c.$_{bg2}$ *Ambr.*$_{bg2}$ **ANAC.**$_{bg2}$ *Ang.*$_{bg2}$ *Ant-c.*$_{bg2}$ arg-met.$_{bg2}$ *Arn.*$_{bg2}$ *Ars.*$_{bg2}$ asar.$_{bg2}$ **AUR.**$_{bg2}$ **BAR-C.**$_{bg2}$ **BELL.**$_{bg2}$ *Bov.*$_{bg2}$ *Bry.*$_{bg2}$ calad.$_{bg2}$ **CALC.**$_{bg2}$ calc-p.$_{bg2}$ camph.$_{bg2}$ *Canth.*$_{bg2}$ caps.$_{bg2}$ *Carb-v.*$_{bg2}$ *Caust.*$_{bg2}$ *Cham.*$_{bg2}$ *Chin.*$_{bg2}$ *Cic.*$_{bg2}$ **COCC.**$_{bg2}$ *Coff.*$_{bg2}$ colch.$_{bg2}$ *Con.*$_{bg2}$ croc.$_{bg2}$ *Cupr.*$_{bg2}$ cycl.$_{bg2}$ dig.$_{bg2}$ dulc.$_{bg2}$ graph.$_{bg2}$ **HELL.**$_{bg2}$ hep.$_{bg2}$ **HYOS.**$_{bg2}$ **IGN.**$_{bg2}$ iod.$_{bg2}$ *Kali-br.*$_{bg2}$ kali-c.$_{bg2}$ **LACH.**$_{bg2}$ laur.$_{bg2}$ led.$_{bg2}$ **LYC.**$_{bg2}$ meny.$_{bg2}$ **MERC.**$_{bg2}$ merc-c.$_{bg2}$ mez.$_{bg2}$ mosch.$_{bg2}$ *Mur-ac.*$_{bg2}$ **NAT-C.**$_{bg2}$ *Nat-m.*$_{bg2}$ nit-ac.$_{bg2}$ **NUX-M.**$_{bg2}$ **NUX-V.**$_{bg2}$ *Olnd.*$_{bg2}$ **OP.**$_{bg2}$ par.$_{bg2}$ *Petr.*$_{bg2}$ **PH-AC.**$_{bg2}$ **PHOS.**$_{bg2}$ *Pic-ac.*$_{bg2}$ **PLAT.**$_{bg2}$ plb.$_{bg2}$ **PULS.**$_{bg2}$ ran-b.$_{bg2}$ rhod.$_{bg2}$ **RHUS-T.**$_{bg2,bg2}$ ruta$_{bg2}$ *Sabad.*$_{bg2}$ sars.$_{bg2}$ *Sec.*$_{bg2}$ *Sel.*$_{bg2}$ seneg.$_{bg2}$ **SEP.**$_{bg2}$ **SIL.**$_{bg2}$ spig.$_{bg2}$ spong.$_{bg2}$ *Stann.*$_{bg2}$ *Staph.*$_{bg2}$ **STRAM.**$_{bg2}$ sul-ac.$_{bg2}$ **SULPH.**$_{bg2}$ tarax.$_{bg2}$ teucr.$_{bg2}$ thuj.$_{bg2}$ *Valer.*$_{bg2}$ **VERAT.**$_{bg2}$ verb.$_{bg2}$ *Viol-o.*$_{bg2}$ zinc$_{bg2}$

Ref: BBCR (RADAR 10)

Comment:
In both The 'Therapeutic Pocket Book' and BBCR; the above rubric is found. However, the question is ambiguous in terms of correct reference to the above repertories.

Q. 41. Rubric 'Cyanosis' in Boenninghausen's Repertory is under (KPSC/Lect/Rep/2004)
    (a) Skin
    (b) Generalities
    (c) Sensations
    (d) Complaints

Ans. (c)

Note
Repertory- Therapeutic Pocket Book' – Chapter; Sensation & Complaints- Rubric; Cyanosis.
Please remember:
The peculiar aspect of 'Therapeutic Pocket Book' is that it contains most of the generalities in the chapter of sensation- which most often are given in chapter of generalities in Kent's Repertory.
For example:
Air, open, aversion to – is given in Generalities in Kent's Repertory.
However, when we look for it in 'Therapeutic Pocket Book it is given as – Air aversion to, open air – in chapter of Sensation.
In reference to BBCR the Cyanosis is given in chapter – Sensation and Complaints in general:

> Boger C., Boenninghausen's Repertory

SENSATIONS AND COMPLAINTS IN GENERAL - Cyanosis, blue face, etc.
ACON.bg2 agar.bg2 alum.bg2 *Am-c.*bg2 *Ang.*bg2 ant-c.bg2 **ANT-T.**bg2 arg-n.bg2 *Arn.*bg2 **ARS.**bg2 asaf.bg2 asar.bg2 *Aur.*bg2 bar-c.bg2 **BELL.**bg2 *Bism.*bg2 *Bry.*bg2 calc.bg2 calc-p.bg2 **CAMPH.**bg2 canth.bg2 carb-an.bg2 **CARB-V.**bg2 caust.bg2 cham.bg2 chel.bg2 chin.bg2 cic.bg2 *Cina*bg2 *Cocc.*bg2 **CON.**bg2 **CUPR.**bg2 **DIG.**bg2 dros.bg2 ferr.bg2 *Glon.*bg2 *Hep.*bg2 **HYOS.**bg2 ign.bg2 iod.bg2 ip.bg2 kali-c.bg2 **LACH.**bg2 led.bg2 lyc.bg2 mang.bg2 *Merc.*bg2 *Merc-c.*bg2 mez.bg2 mosch.bg2 mur-ac.bg2 *Nat-m.*bg2 nit-ac.bg2 nux-m.bg2 *Nux-v.*bg2 **OP.**bg2 ox-ac.bg2 ph-ac.bg2 *Phos.*bg2 phyt.bg2 plb.bg2 *Puls.*bg2 ran-b.bg2 *Rhus-t.*bg2 ruta bg2 sabad.bg2 **SAMB.**bg2 sars.bg2 **SEC.**bg2 seneg.bg2 *Sil.*bg2 *Spong.*bg2 staph.bg2 stram.bg2 sul-ac.bg2 *Sulph.*bg2 thuj.bg2 **VERAT.**bg2 **VERAT-V.**bg2 zinc.bg2

Ref: BBCR (RADAR 10)
Comment:
The above MCQ appears to be ambiguous as it does not qualify for the 'therapeutic Pocket book' or BBCR which one the question is referred to.

Q. 42. In Boenninghausen's Repertory 'Dislocations' is in chapter (KPSC/Lect/Rep-2004)
    (a)   Extremities
    (b)   Joints
    (c)   Complaints
    (d)   Sensations

Ans. (d)
Note
Repertory-Therapeutic Pocket Book' – Chapter; Sensations - Rubric; Dislocation.
Also see
Repertory BBCR (RADAR 10)
Please remember: It has a chapter of lower and upper extremity- and it contains rubrics related to 'Dislocation' i.e`.,:
[Boenning] [Lower extremities] Dislocation, easy:

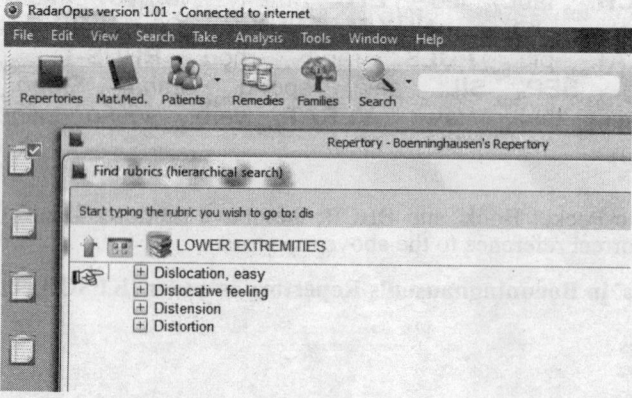

[Boenning] [Upper extremities] Dislocation, easy:

MCQ's in Repertory

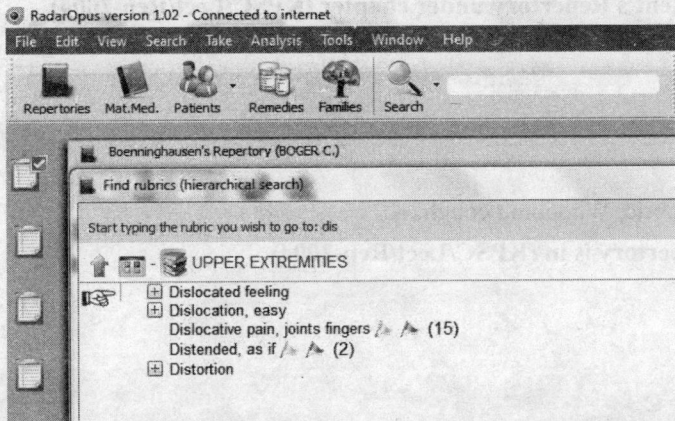

Also see the chapter of Aggravation:

CONDITIONS OF AGGRAVATION AND AMELIORATION IN GENERAL - Dislocations and sprains, agg.
AGN.bg2 *Am-c.*bg2 ambr.bg2 ang.bg2 **ARN.**bg2 bar-c.bg2 bov.bg2 **BRY.**bg2 **CALC.**bg2 **CARB-AN.**bg2 *Carb-v.*bg2 *Caust.*bg2 con.bg2 *Graph.*bg2 hep.bg2 **IGN.**bg2 *Kali-n.*bg2 kreos.bg2 **LYC.**bg2 *M-ambo.*bg2 **MERC.**bg2 mez.bg2 mosch.bg2 **NAT-C.**bg2 **NAT-M.**bg2 **NIT-AC.**bg2 **NUX-V.**bg2 **PETR.**bg2 **PHOS.**bg2 **PULS.**bg2 *Rhod.*bg2 **RHUS-T.**bg2,bg2 **RUTA**bg2 sabin.bg2 **SEP.**bg2 *Sil.*bg2 *Spig.*bg2 stann.bg2 staph.bg2 **SULPH.**bg2 zinc.bg2
Ref: BBCR (RADAR 10)

Q. 43. In Boenninghausen's Repertory 'Emaciation' is in chapter (KPSC/Lect/Rep/2004)
  (a) Generalities
  (b) Face
  (c) Sensations
  (d) None of the above

Ans. (c)

Note
Repertory-Therapeutic Pocket Book' – Chapter; Sensation - Rubric; Emaciation.
Please remember:
The chapter of Sensation in the Therapeutic Pocket Book includes – The type of pain, suffering, and functional or organic changes characterizing the morbid process.
In BBCR the same rubric is as under:

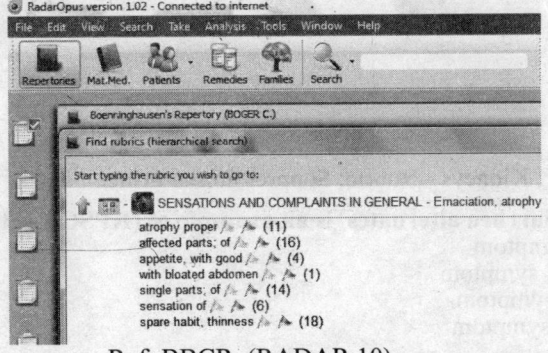

Ref: BBCR (RADAR 10)

Q. 44. For 'Whooping cough' refer Kent's Repertory under chapter (KPSC/Lect/Rep-2004)
    (a) Generalities
    (b) Expectoration
    (c) Chest
    (d) Cough

Ans. (d)
Note
Repertory- Kent – Chapter; Cough - Rubric; Whooping cough.

Q. 45. Rubric "Lochia' in Kent's Repertory is in (KPSC/Lect/Rep-2004)
    (a) Uterus
    (b) Genitalia female
    (c) Generalities
    (d) Menstruation

Ans. (b)
Note
Repertory-Kent – Chapter; Genitalia Female - Rubric; Lochia.

Q. 46. 'Reeling' in Kent's Repertory is placed under (KPSC/Lect/Rep-2004)
    (a) Head
    (b) Mind
    (c) Vertigo
    (d) None of the above

Ans. (c)
Note
Repertory-Kent – Chapter; Vertigo - Rubric; Reeling.

Q. 47. 'Astigmatism' in Kent's Repertory belongs to chapter (KPSC/Lect/Rep-2004)
    (a) Vision
    (b) Eye
    (c) Generalities
    (d) None of the above

Ans. (b)
Note

> English Kent

EYE - ASTIGMATISM
Tub.$_k$
Ref: Kent's Repertory (RADAR 10)

Q. 48. 'Suppression of urine' in Kent's Repertory is placed under (KPSC/Lect/Rep/2004)
    (a) Bladder
    (b) Ureter
    (c) Urethra
    (d) Kidney

Ans. (d)
Note
Repertory-Kent – Chapter; Kidneys - Rubric; Suppression of urine.

Q. 49. 'Headache and diarrhea alternates' is an example of (KPSC/Lect/Rep-2004)
    (a) Common symptom
    (b) Pathological symptom
    (c) Associated symptom
    (d) Alternating symptom

Ans. (d)

MCQ's in Repertory

Note
Definition:
Alternating symptoms are those which manifest the partial picture of a chronic disease in one phase and are replaced by some other manifestations later.
Value:
These help us to obtain the complete picture of a chronic disease.

Q. 50. 'Rheumatism worse from motion' is an example of (KPSC/Lect/Rep-2004)
    (a)   Uncommon symptom
    (b)   Common symptom
    (c)   Peculiar symptom
    (d)   Keynote symptom

Ans. (b)
Note
Definition:
Common symptom is that symptom which is found in many patients, in many diseases and is produced in the provings of many medicines.
Value:
These are important for diagnosis of a disease and sometimes they are also used for palliative treatment.

Q. 51. Hahnemann attempted to prepare a Repertory known as (KPSC/Lect/Rep-2004)
    (a)   Fragmenta viribus
    (b)   Fragmenta de Viribus Medica Mentorum Positivis
    (c)   Repertorium Homeopathica
    (d)   None of the above

Ans. (b)
Note
The 'Fragmenta de Viribus Medica Mentorum Positivis' was published in 1805 by Hahnemann and it contained an index in the second part – which is referred to as Hahnemann's first attempt to prepare a repertory.

Q. 52. Author of Sensation as if is (KPSC/Lect/Rep-2004)
    (a)   Dr. Hahnemann
    (b)   H.A. Roberts
    (c)   W.A. Allen
    (d)   Boenninghausen

Ans. (b)
Note
H. A. Roberts authored 'Sensation as if'. It was published in 1937.
Ref: Essentials of Repertorizaton 3rd Edition By Dr. Shashi Kant Tiwari Pg 23

Q. 53. Systemic Alphabetical Repertory was published in 1888 by (KPSC/Lect/Rep-2004)
    (a)   Robin Murphy
    (b)   Lippe
    (c)   Clofar Muller
    (d)   Jahr.

Ans. (c)
Note
Clofar Muller published 'Systematic Alphabetical Repertory in 1888. It contained 940 pages.
Ref: Essentials of Repertorizaton 3rd Edition By Dr. Shashi Kant Tiwari.

Q. 54. T.F. Allen's Symptom Register was published in the year (KPSC/Lect/Rep-2004)
    (a)   1885
    (b)   1882
    (c)   1880
    (d)   1925

Ans. (c)

Note
T. F. Allen published "Symptom Register' in 1880.
Ref: Essentials of Repertorizaton 3rd Edition By Dr. Shashi kant Tiwari.

Q. 55. Analytical Repertory of Hering was published in (KPSC/Lect/Rep-2004)
    (a)   1881
    (b)   1825
    (c)   1790
    (d)   1921
Ans. (a)
Note
Analytical Repertory of Hering was published in year 1881.
Ref: Essentials of Repertorizaton 3rd Edition By Dr. Shashi Kant Tiwari Pg 20

Q. 56. Repertory of Modalities was published in the year 1880 by (KPSC/Lect/Rep-2004)
    (a)   Worcester
    (b)   Kent
    (c)   Lippe
    (d)   Boricke
Ans. (a)
Note
Repertory of Modalities was published in the year 1880 by Worcester.
Ref: Essentials of Repertorization 3rd Edition By Dr. Shashi Kant Tiwari.

Q. 57. Author of Repertory of Urinary Organs is (KPSC/Lect/Rep04)
    (a)   A.R. Morgan
    (b)   W.C. Allen
    (c)   Possart
    (d)   Lippe
Ans. (a)
Note
Author of 'Repertory of Urinary Organs' is A.R. Morgan.
Ref: Essentials of Repertorizaton 3rd Edition By Dr. Shashi Kant Tiwari.

Q. 58. Hydrocele belongs to the chapter in Kent's Repertory (KPSC/Lect/Rep/2004)
    (a)   Generalities
    (b)   Abdomen
    (c)   Skin
    (d)   None of the above
Ans. (d)
Note
Repertory-Kent – Chapter; Genitalia - Rubric; Hydrocele

Q. 59. In Kent's Repertory rubric Exophthalmic goiter is placed at (KPSC/Lect/Rep-2004)
    (a)   Face
    (b)   External throat
    (c)   Internal throat
    (d)   Generalities
Ans. (b)
Note

English Kent

EXTERNAL THROAT - GOITRE
CALC.$_{k,k}$ IOD.$_k$ SPONG.$_k$
Ref: Kent's Repertory (RADAR 10)

MCQ's in Repertory

Q. 60. In Boenninghausen's Repertory "Haughtiness" is found in the chapter (KPSC/Lect/Rep-2004)
    (a)   Mind
    (b)   Sensorium
    (c)   Complaints
    (d)   Intellect

Ans. (a)
Note

> Boenninghausen C., Therapeutic Pocket Book 3.0
> **MIND AND SENSORIUM - MIND - HAUGHTINESS**
> LYC.$_{b2}$ PLAT.$_{b2.de}$ STRAM.$_{b2.de}$ VERAT.$_{b2}$

Ref: Therapeutic Pocket Book (RADAR 10)

Q. 61. In Boenninghausen's Repertory "Photomania" is found in the chapter (KPSC/Lect/Rep-2004)
    (a)   Mind
    (b)   Eyes
    (c)   Intellect
    (d)   Vision

Ans. (d)
Note

> Boenninghausen C., Therapeutic Pocket Book 3.0
> **PARTS OF THE BODY AND ORGANS - VISION - PHOTOMANIA**
> ACON.$_{b2}$ BELL.$_{b2.b2}$

Ref: Therapeutic Pocket Book (RADAR 10)

Q. 62. Who has published Repertory of Anti Psoric? (KPSC/Lect/Rep-2004)
    (a)   Dr. Samuel Hahnemann
    (b)   Dr. J.T. Kent
    (c)   Dr. Constantine Hering
    (d)   Dr. Boenninghausen

Ans. (d)
Note
The repertory of Antipsoric was published by Boenninghausen in 1832. Ref; Introduction to the 'Therapeutic Pocket Book, Pg18. It was the first repertory developed by Boenninghausen; it contained the preface by Dr. Hahnemann.

Q. 63. Total number of sections in Kent's Repertory (KPSC/Lect/Rep-2004)
    (a)   37
    (b)   07
    (c)   38
    (d)   None of the above

Ans. (a)
Note
The total number of sections in Kent's Repertory are 37.

Q. 64. Total number of sections in Boenninghausen's Therapeutic Pocket Book" (KPSC/Lect/Rep-2004)
    (a)   37
    (b)   07
    (c)   38
    (d)   None of the above

Ans. (b)

Note
Total number of sections in Boenninghausen's 'Therapeutic Pocket Book' are seven. They are as under:
1. Mind and Intellect
2. Parts of the Body and Organs
3. Sensations and complaints
    I. In general
    II. of glands
    III. of bones
    IV. of skin
4. Sleep and Dreams
5. Fever
    I. Circulation of blood
    II. Cold stage
    III. Coldness
    IV. Heat
    V. Perspiration
    VI. Compound fevers
    VII. Concomitant complaints
6. Alterations of the State of Health
    I. Aggravation according to time
    II. Aggravations according to situations and circumstances
    III. Amelioration by positions and circumstances
7. Relationship of Remedies

Ref: Boenninghausen's Therapeutic Pocket Book, Pg-27

Q. 65. Total number of sections in Boger Boenninghausen's Characteristic Materia Medica and Repertory is (KPSC/Lect/Rep-2004)
    (a)   37
    (b)   07
    (c)   38
    (d)   None of the above

Ans. (d)
Note
Total number of sections in Boger Boenninghausen's Characteristic Materia Medica and Repertory are / is 53.
Ref: Essentials of Repertorisaton 3rd edition By Dr. S. K. Tiwari –Pg171-189

Q. 66. Who is the editor of Synthesis Repertory? (KPSC/Lect/Rep-2004)
    (a)   Dr. Fredrick Schroyens
    (b)   Dr. George Vithoulkas
    (c)   Dr. Samuel Hahnemann
    (d)   Dr. Julian Winston

Ans. (a)
Note
Dr. Fredrick Schroyens is the editor of Synthesis Repertory. Synthesis is a product of teamwork. It is a printed version of RADAR (Rapid Aid to Drug Aimed Research) a Computer Programme. It is edited by Dr. Fredrick Schroyens who was born on Jan 12th 1953 at Belgium.
Ref: Essentials of Repertorisaton 3rd edition By Dr. S. K. Tiwari –Pg 421

Q. 67. Total number of chapters in Knerr's Repertory is (KPSC/Lect/Rep-2004)
    (a)   38
    (b)   48
    (c)   47
    (d)   37

Ans. (c)

Note
The number of chapters in Knerr's Repertory are 47.

Q. 68. Outwardly reflected picture of the internal essence of the diseases are (KPSC/Lect/Rep-2004)
    (a)   Objective symptoms
    (b)   Subjective symptoms
    (c)   Totality of symptoms
    (d)   None of the above

Ans. (c)
Note
The Totality of the Symptoms means all the symptoms of the case which are capable of being logically combined into a harmonious and consistent whole, having form, coherency and individuality. Technically, the totality is more (and may be less) than the mere numerical totality of the symptoms. It includes the "concomitance" or form in which symptoms are grouped.

Hahnemann (Organon, 7th aphorism) calls the totality, "this image (or picture) reflecting outwardly the internal essence of the disease, i.e., of the suffering life force."

Q. 69. Factors which affect or modify a symptom are called (KPSC/Lect/Rep-2004)
    (a)   Aggravation
    (b)   Amelioration
    (c)   Causa occasionalis
    (d)   Modality

Ans. (d)
Note
Definition:

By modality we refer to the circumstances and conditions that affect or modify a symptom, of which the conditions of aggravation and amelioration are the most important Dr. William Boericke well said: "The modalities of a drug are the pathognomonic symptoms of the Materia Medica."

Most of these modalities are readily explained-especially those which refer to the circulation of the blood, e.g., the Belladonna headache which is better from cold application to the head and having the head high. The one affect or modify a symptom is called modality.

By "aggravation" is meant an increase or intensification of already existing symptoms by some appreciable circumstance or condition.

"Amelioration" is technically used to express the modification of relief, or diminution of intensity in any of the symptoms, or in the state of the patient as a whole, by medication, or by the influence of any agency, circumstance or condition.

Q. 70. Totality of symptom was introduced in aphorism (KPSC/Lect/Rep-2004)
    (a)   Aphorism 2
    (b)   Aphorism 5
    (c)   Aphorism 7
    (d)   Aphorism 20

Ans. (c)
Note
$ Aphorism 2
The highest ideal of cure is rapid, gentle and permanent restoration of the health, or removal and annihilation of the disease in its whole extent, in the shortest, most reliable, and most harmless way, on easily comprehensible principles.

$ Aphorism 5
Useful to the physician in assisting him to cure are the particulars of the most probable exciting cause of the acute disease, as also the most significant points in the whole history of the chronic disease, to enable him to discover its fundamental cause, which is generally due to a chronic miasm. In these investigations, the ascertainable physical constitution of the patient (especially when the disease is chronic), his moral, and intellectual character, his occupation, mode of living and habits, his social and domestic relations, his age, sexual function, etc. are to be taken into consideration.

$ Aphorism 7
In disease, presenting no manifest exciting cause for removal, the totality of symptoms is the outward image of the inner disease, of the suffering vital force, related as cause and effect. These symptoms alone must constitute the medium through which the disease demands and points out its curative agent. In each case of disease only this totality of symptoms is to be recognized and removed, by the art of healing, that it may be cured and converted into health.
Ref: ORGANON OF ART OF HEALING by BALDWIN

$ Aphorism 20
This spirit-like power to alter man's state of health which lies hidden in the inner nature of medicines can in itself never be discovered by us by a mere effort of reason; it is only by experience of the phenomena it displays when acting on the state of health of man that we can become clearly cognizant of it.
Comment:
Hahnemann in (Organon, Aphorism 7) calls the totality, "this image (or picture) reflecting outwardly the internal essence of the disease."
Ref: Organon Of Medicine

Q. 71. Of the below rubric which is under generalities of Kent's Repertory? (KPSC-Re Exam/Lect/Organon-2004)
    (a)   Awkwardness
    (b)   Feels better when constipated
    (c)   Chilliness from putting hands out of bed -fever chilliness
    (d)   Leprosy, psoriasis eruption

Ans. (b)
Note
In Kent's Repertory:
a. Awkwardness; is found in the chapter of extremities.
b. Feels better when constipated; is found under Chapter of Generalities – Rubric; Constipation amel (2:Calc, 2:Psor).
c. Chilliness from putting hands out of bed-fever chilliness; is found Under chapter – Chill –Rubric; Bed Putting hand out of bed.
d. Leprosy, psoriasis eruption; are given under chapter; Skin – Rubric; Eruption – Leprosy and Psoriasis under eruption.

Q. 72. Of the below in which repertory amelioration is omitted in relationship of remedies? (KPSC-Re Exam/Lect/Organon-2004)
    (a)   Boenninghausen's Therapeutic Pocket book
    (b)   Synthesis
    (c)   Kent's Repertory
    (d)   Complete Repertory

Ans. (a)
Note
The chapter on relationships in BTPB (Boenninghausen's Therapeutic Pocket Book) is divided into sections, each section being devoted to a remedy, in alphabetical order. Each of these remedy sections is subdivided into rubrics, as are all the general sections in the book, but in this chapter we find the rubrics are not particularized as symptoms, but are generalized symptom groups. For instance we find the first rubric in each remedy section to be first Mind, second is Localities, third is Sensations and then glands, bones, skin; Sleep and Dreams; Blood, Circulation and Fever; Aggravations. (Ref; Introduction to BTPB Pg 38) It is obvious from above that the amelioration chapter is omitted in relationship of remedies.

Q. 73. Mind Chapter of Kent's Repertory was prepared by (KPSC/Lect/Physiology & Biochemistory-2004)
    (a)   Lippe
    (b)   Lee
    (c)   Kent
    (d)   Mithel

Ans. (b)

MCQ's in Repertory   1041

Note
History of Kent's Repertory; Taking help from Kent; Lee started working and compiled the Mind and Head sections. Later when Lee became blind, Dr. Kent Took it up, revised and arranged it according to his own plan.
Ref: Essentials of Repertorisation 3rd edition, By Dr. S. K. Tiwari Pg 269

Q. 74. Hypertension is given in (KPSC/Lect/Physiology & Biochemistory-2004)
    (a)   Phatak's Repertory
    (b)   Synthetic Repertory
    (c)   Both
    (d)   None

Ans. (c)
Note
Phatak's Repertory has Rubric of Hypertension (Cross reference) and it is given under blood pressure high. Synthesis has Rubric Hypertension under chapter of Generality.

Q. 75. Illusion of touch is given in the ——————— chapter of Kent's Repertory. (KPSC/Lect/Physiology & Biochemistory-2004)
    (a)   Mind
    (b)   Skin
    (c)   Chill
    (d)   Generalities

Ans. (d)
Note
Repertory: Kent- Chapter; Generalities- Rubric; Touch: illusion of.

Q. 76. "Lump sensation in rectum not ameliorated by stool" is seen in (KPSC/Lect/Physiology & Biochemistory-2004)
    (a)   Anacardium
    (b)   Nux vomica
    (c)   Aesculus Hippocastanum
    (d)   Sepia

Ans. (d)
Note

English Kent

RECTUM - LUMP, sensation of - stool, - not amel. by
SEP.$_k$
Ref: Kent's Repertory (RADAR 10)

Q. 77. Hiccough after alcoholic drink indicates (KPSC/Lect/Physiology & Biochemistry/2004)
    (a)   Sulphuricum acidum
    (b)   Ranunculus bulbosus
    (c)   Nux vomica
    (d)   Lycopodium clavatum

Ans. (b)
Note

English Kent

STOMACH - HICCOUGH - alcoholic drinks, after
RAN-B.$_k$
Ref: Kent's Repertory (RADAR 10)

Q. 78. "White mucous in stool like pieces of popped corn" indicate (KPSC/Lect/Physiology & Biochemistory-2004)
 (a) Cina
 (b) Colchicum
 (c) Cantharis
 (d) Helleborus

Ans. (a)
Note

English Kent

STOOL - MUCOUS, slimy - white - like little pieces of popped corn
CINA$_k$
Ref: Kent's Repertory (RADAR 10)

Q. 79. Necrosis of bones are found in Kent's Repertory in chapter (Kerala MD (Hom) Ent/ Paper 2-2001)
 (a) Generalities
 (b) Extremities
 (c) In (A)&(B)
 (d) Not given

Ans. (a)
Note

English Kent

GENERALS - NECROSIS bones
ARS.$_{k\,k}$
Ref: Kent's Repertory (RADAR 10)

Q. 80. Ist Repertory in English language was published by (Kerala MD (Hom) Ent/ Paper 2-2001)
 (a) J.T. Kent
 (b) Dr. Lippe
 (c) Dr. C. Hering
 (d) Dr. P. Schmidth

Ans. (c)
Note
Ist Repertory in English language was published by Dr C. Hering.

Q. 81. He is the father of Homeopathic repertory (Kerala MD (Hom) Ent/ Paper 2-2001)
 (a) Boenninghausen
 (b) Jahr
 (c) Lippe
 (d) Hahnemann

Ans. (d)
Note
Dr. Hahnemann himself compiled a repertory in 1830-32, which could not be published because of two reasons he himself found the work imperfect and his publisher Mr. Arnold was not in a position to publish it. So, the profession had to look upon other for a useful repertory. (Ref; Essentials of Repertorisation 3rd edition, By Dr. S. K. Tiwari Pg 16) Therefore we can call Hahnemann Father of Homeopathic repertory.

Q. 82. In Kent's Repertory where do we find Milk Absent? (Kerala MD (Hom) Ent/ Paper 2-2001)
 (a) Generalities
 (b) Glands
 (c) Chest
 (d) Not given

Ans. (c)

Note

English Kent

CHEST - MILK - absent
CALC.$_k$ ZINC.$_k$
Ref: Kent's Repertory (RADAR 10)

Q. 83. He was the first person to evaluate remedies (Kerala MD (Hom) Ent/ Paper 2-2001)
    (a)   Boenninghausen
    (b)   Kent
    (c)   Hahnemann
    (d)   Jahr

Ans. (a)
Note
In Boenninghausen's method the individual symptoms are not important but groups are more important. According to Boenninghausen the patients symptoms are to be considered from the group aspect of:
- Location
- Sensation
- Modality
- Concomitants

In Kent's method both symptoms & remedies are graded, while in Boenninghausen's method only remedies are graded and evaluated in therapeutic pocket book. Boenninghausen he produced first repertory as well as gave five grades to the remedies.

Q. 84. Blue Leucorrhoea — in Kent Repertory (Kerala MD (Hom) Ent/ Paper 2-2001)
    (a)   Ambra grisea
    (b)   Sepia
    (c)   Hydrastis
    (d)   Alumina

Ans. (a)
Note

English Kent

FEMALE GENITALIA - LEUCORRHOEA - bluish
ambr.$_k$
Ref: Kent's Repertory (RADAR 10)

Q. 85. First Card Repertory became available to profession in the year (Kerala MD (Hom) Ent/ Paper 2-2001)
    (a)   1892
    (b)   1982
    (c)   1888
    (d)   1891

Ans. (a)
Note
The first card repertory was prepared by William Jefferson Guernsey in 1888 and it was available to the profession in 1892. The number of cards were 2500.
Ref: Essentials of Repertorisation 3rd Edition By Dr. S. K. Tiwari Pg 379

Q. 86. Synthetic Repertory came in the year (Kerala MD (Hom) Ent/ Paper 2-2001)
    (a)   1982
    (b)   1892
    (c)   1897
    (d)   1981

Ans. (a)

Note
Dr. Barthal and Klunker collected data from various possible sources and published the same in the form of 'Synthetic Repertory'. This repertory was originally published by Karl G. Haug Verlag Gmbh and Co., I 1973, which was improved over in 1982. It was published in India in 1987.
Ref: Essentials of Repertorisation 3rd Edition By Dr. S. K. Tiwari Pg 344

Q. 87. In Kent's Repertory - cross-reference given for HUMOROUS is (Kerala MD (Hom) Ent/Paper 2-2001)
    (a)   Mood
    (b)   Jesting
    (c)   Joy
    (d)   Joyous

Ans. (b)
Note
Repertory-Kent – Chapter; Mind – Rubric; Humorus (See Jesting, Mirth).

Q. 88. Awkwardness is found in B.B.C.R. (Kerala MD (Hom) Ent/ Paper 2-2001)
    (a)   Extremities
    (b)   Mind
    (c)   Sensorium
    (d)   Sensation

Ans. (b)
Note
Repertory- BBCR – Chapter; Mind – Rubric; Awkwardness.

Q. 89. Aversion to Husband is present in which chapter of Kent's Repertory? (UPSC-2006)
    (a)   Generalities
    (b)   Female
    (c)   Mind
    (d)   Head

Ans. (c)
Note

> English Kent

MIND - AVERSION, - husband
SEP.$_k$
Ref: Kent's Repertory (RADAR 10)

Q. 90. "Inclination to lie down" is in which chapter of Kent's repertory? (UPSC-2006)
    (a)   Mind
    (b)   Generalities
    (c)   Head
    (d)   Vertigo

Ans. (b)
Note

> English Kent

GENERALS - LIE down - inclination to
ACON.$_k$ **ALUM.**$_k$ **ARAN.**$_k$ **ARS.**$_k$ **CARBN-S.CHAM**$_k$ **FERR.**$_{kk}$ **KALI-AR.**$_{kk}$ **KALI-C.**$_k$ **NUX-V.**$_k$ **SEL.**$_{kk}$ **SIL.**$_{kk}$
Ref: Kent's Repertory (RADAR 10)

MCQ's in Repertory   1045

Q. 91. Stammering is a rubric in which chapter of the Kent's Repertory? (UPSC-2006)
    (a) Larynx and Trachea
    (b) Thorax
    (c) Mouth
    (d) Mind

Ans. (c)
Note

🔖 **English Kent**

MOUTH - SPEECH - stammering
BELL.$_k$ CAUST.$_k$ MERC.$_k$ NUX-V.$_k$ STRAM.$_k$
Ref: Kent's Repertory (RADAR 10)

Q. 92. Concordance Repertories are those (UPSC-2006)
    (a) Written in Prover's language.
    (b) That do not have alphabetical arrangement of chapters and rubrics.
    (c) That do not contain rubrics.
    (d) Having a definite philosophical background.

Ans. (a)
Note
Concordance = In agreement or In harmony
Concordance repertory
Here the medicine is analyzed for its relationship with other medicines at different levels and at different spheres. Logical utilitarian repertories are popular as repertories and the puritan repertories are known as Concordance Repertories or Concordances. These repertories are comprised of mainly of the symptoms in the language of the provers, the whole symptoms expressed by the patient may be obtained as a single unit in these books. The demerit is that the search is very difficult & time consuming.

Q. 93. The abbreviation used in Synthetic Repertory for Aluminium metallicum is (Repertory)
    (a) Alum M
    (b) Alumin.
    (c) Al. met
    (d) Alumin M

Ans. (b)

Q. 94. Match list I with List II and select the correct answer using the code given below the lists (UPSC-2006)

List – I (Type of Case)	List – II (Repertory Most Adopted)
A. Marked Pathology	1. Kent's Repertory
B. Marked Generals	2. Boenninghausen's Repertory
C. Marked Concomitants	3. Boericke's Repertory
D. Marked Causations	4. Clarke's Repertory

Code

	A	B	C	D
(a)	3	2	1	4
(b)	4	1	2	3
(c)	3	1	2	4
(d)	4	2	1	3

Ans. (c)

Note
Following is the correct match:

List – I (Type of Case)	List – II (Repertory Most Adopted)
A. Marked Pathology	3. Boericke's Repertory
B. Marked Generals	1. Kent's Repertory
C. Marked Concomitants	2. Boenninghausen's Repertory
D. Marked Causations	4. Clarke's Repertory

Q. 95. Complaints aggravated while lying on affected side' is a feature of which one of the following? (UPSC-2006)
(a) Aconitum napellus Only
(b) Hepar sulphur Only
(c) Nux Vomica Only
(d) All of above drugs

Ans. (d)
Note

English Kent

GENERALS - LYING - side,on, - painful, - agg.
BAR-C.$_k$ CALAD.$_{k\ k}$ HEP.$_k$ IOD.$_k$ NUX-M.$_k$ RUTA$_k$ SIL.$_k$

Ref: Kent's Repertory (RADAR 10)

Q. 96. Boger was a student of ____ (MD/DACHMH/97/BBSR)
(a) Boenninghausen
(b) Kent
(c) Hahnemann
(d) Jahr

Ans. (a)
Note
Boger was a student of Boenninghausen.

Also see
Probably there has never been a more through student of 'Boenninghausen' than the late Dr Cyrus M. Boger and perhaps one of the greatest pieces of homeopathic literature left by Dr Boger is 'Boenninghausen's Characteristics and Repertory.'
Ref: Essentials of Repertorization, by Shashi Kant Tiwari, page 203, second revised and enlarged edition.

Dr Cyrus Maxwell Boger (1861-1935)
A 1888 graduate of Hahnemann Medical College in Philadelphia, he was one of the earliest teachers at the post-graduate educational programme. He was a follower of the Boenninghausen's method of study, and compiled 'Boenninghausen's Characteristics Materia Medica and Repertory', but he died before completing and publishing his main work.

Dr Cyrus Maxwell Boger (1861-1935)

MCQ's in Repertory

Q. 97. In a particular category of disease condition, 'accessory symptoms' are considered to be a very valuable guide _____ (PSC/WB/93)
- (a) Disease of syphilitic miasm
- (b) One-sided diseases
- (c) Acute disease
- (d) Intermittent diseases

Ans. (b)

Note

In a particular category of disease condition, 'accessory symptoms' are considered to be a very valuable guide in one-sided disease.

Also see

Definition:

Accessory symptom: A symptom that usually but not always accompanies a certain disease. Also called *concomitant symptom*.
Ref: Medical Dictionary
http://medical-dictionary.thefreedictionary.com/accessory+symptom

Aphorism 180

In this case, the medicine, which has been chosen as well as was possible, but which, for the reason above stated, is only imperfectly homoeopathic, will, in its action upon the disease that is only partially analogous to it – just as in the case mentioned above (§ 162, et seq.) where the limited number of homoeopathic remedies renders the selection imperfect – produce accessory symptoms, and several phenomena from it's own array of symptoms are mixed up with the patient's state of health, which are, however, at the same time, symptoms of the disease itself, although they may have been hitherto never or very rarely perceived; some symptoms which the patient had never previously experienced appear, or others he had only felt indistinctly become more pronounced.

Extended information

Aphorism 181

Let is not be objected that the accessory phenomena and new symptoms of this disease that now appear should be laid to the account of the medicament just employed. They owe their origin to it[1] certainly, but they are always only symptoms of such a nature as this disease was itself capable of producing in this organism, and which were summoned forth and induced to make their appearance by the medicine given, owing to its power to cause similar symptoms. In a word, we have to regard the whole collection of symptoms now perceptible as belonging to the disease itself, as the actual existing condition, and to direct our further treatment accordingly.

1. When they were not caused by an important error in regimen, a violent emotion, or a tumultuous revolution in the organism, such as the occurrence or cessation of the menses, conception, childbirth, and so forth.

Aphorism182

Thus the imperfect selection of the medicament, which was in this case almost inevitable owing to the too limited number of the symptoms present, serves to complete the display of the symptoms of the disease, and in this way facilitates the discovery of a second, more accurately suitable, homoeopathic medicine.

Aphorism 183

Whenever, therefore, the dose of the first medicine ceases to have a beneficial effect (if the newly developed symptoms do not, by reason of their gravity, demand more speedy aid – which, however, from the minuteness of the dose of homoeopathic medicine, and in very chronic diseases, is excessively rare), a new examination of the disease must be instituted, the status morbi as it now is must be noted down, and a second homoeopathic remedy selected in accordance with it, which shall exactly suit the present state, and one which shall be all the more appropriate can then be found, as the group of symptoms has become larger and more complete.[1]

1. In cases where the patient (which, however, happens excessively seldom in chronic, but not infrequently in acute, diseases) feels very ill, although his symptoms are very indistinct, so that

this state may be attributed more to the benumbed state of the nerves, which does not permit the patient's pains and sufferings to be distinctly perceived, this torpor of the internal sensibility is removed by opium, and in its secondary action the symptoms of the disease become distinctly apparent.

Concomitant Symptoms

Dr Boenninghausen was the first to realize the importance of the concomitants in prescribing and constructing his repertory. Dr Boger developed the idea fully in Boger's repertory with additions and modifications.

The word concomitant means – existing or occurring together, also known as associated symptoms.

The symptom that accompanies the chief symptom are called concomitant symptoms.

The concomitants bear no relation to the chief complaint than the time association. When these symptoms cannot be explained by pathology, they become characteristic symptoms.

Concomitants arise from the inherent constitutional aspects and tend to remain constant with a patient, irrespective of the nature of the disease.

Rarely found combined with the main affection, here also infrequent under the same condition in the proving.

All these belong to another sphere of the disease than that of the main one.

Finally those which bear the distinctive marks of some drug, even if they have never before noted in the preceding relation.

According to Boger:

Concomitant means accompanying or co-existing The more it belongs to another sphere of the patient's health than the chief complaint – they become an unreasonable attendant.

The peculiar, strange, rare symptoms are indeed concomitants. They cannot be explained on pathology, yet they occur at the same time with the chief complaint.

When a marked peculiar symptom belonging to the disease proper, makes the choice of remedy difficult, a concomitant will decidedly indicate the drug.

Concomitants may far outrank the other symptom of the chief complaint, such a symptom tends individuality to the totality.

Totality is the sum total of the characteristic symptoms. Due attention to concomitants help in finding the simillimum more easily, and with an assurance of accuracy. So concomitants are characteristic symptoms peculiar to the individual patient.

A concomitant having the same modality as the grand symptom, represents a high characteristic feature of the remedy and is of great importance.

Mental concomitant in physical ailments and physical concomitants in mental ailments are an unfailing guide to the simillimum.

In the introduction to Therapeutic Pocket Book, H.A.Roberts says, "The concomitant symptom as to the totality what the condition of < and > is to. Single symptom, it is the differentiating factor."

Accessory Symptoms

These are symptoms produced after the administration of a partially similar remedy. They occur in one-sided diseases where there is a paucity of medicines.

These symptoms are not previously observable in the disease, but at the same time they are symptoms of the disease itself, although they may have been rarely perceived.

Accessory symptoms – can also be explained as – your symptoms improve but in the process, a new one appears for a short period.

What this means:

The remedy only partly matched your symptoms. While it was close enough to trigger an improvement, there was enough difference (and sensitivity) for you to feel one or more of its other effects.

Explanation:

Sometimes a remedy will produce new symptoms while improving those of your original problem. These are called accessory symptoms. They occur when the remedy is only partly similar to your existing problem; the similar part of the remedy makes you feel better while the dissimilar produces a mild dissimilar aggravation.

An example of an accessory symptom would be an itchy scalp triggered during homeopathic treatment for rheumatoid arthrititis.

What to do:

Notify your homeopath. As long as the accessory symptom is not troublesome, your practitioner will probably choose to continue your treatment knowing that the symptom will disappear once the remedy is no longer needed. Until then, your homeopath may prescribe your remedy in a gentler form to minimise any inconvenience from the accessory symptom.

If the accessory symptom is intense or unpleasant, your homeopath will stop treatment and prescribe a new remedy based on the remaining symptoms, including the new accessory ones. This combination will point to a better matching remedy. If the accessory symptom is very unpleasant, your homeopath can antidote it.

Lesser Accessory Symptoms

In chronic diseases, the patients get accustomed to their sufferings and may not feel the necessity of narrating those symptoms with which they had lived for long, which are important for the choice of medicine. They do not consider these symptoms to have anything to do with the prescription that has to be made for the presenting trouble.

Ref: http://www.similima.com/Rep2b.html

Q. 98. 'Grand particularization' is the maxim of (MD/NIH/98)
- (a) Kent
- (b) Hahnemann
- (c) Boenninghausen
- (d) Boger

Ans. (d)

Note

Grand particularization is the maxim of Dr Boger.

Also see

Dr Boger

Boger, while working on Boenninghausen's repertory, subscribed to the priniciple of totality of symptoms, which was orignnally given by Hahnemann. He was fully in agreement with the ideas of what constitutes a complete symptom, which is studied in relation to four factors; viz, location, sensation, modalities and concomitant.

Boger's work Boenninghausen's Characteristics and Repertory is based on the following fundamentals:
(1) Doctrine of complete symptom and concomitant.
(2) Doctrine of Pathological generals.
(3) Doctrine of causation and time.
(4) Clincial rubrics.
(5) Evaluation of remedies.
(6) Fever totality.
(7) Concordances.

In his working of finding the totality, it is seldom necessary to do grand generalization regarding sensation and modalities. Concomitants are given greater importance. Therefore we find that grand particularization is the maxim of Dr Boger.

Ref: Essentials of Repertroization, by Shashi Kant Tiwari, page 167, 168, second revised and enlarged edition.

Extended information

Dr Kent's Repertory

Repertory of Homoeopathic Materia Medica, by J.T. Kent, AM, MD

Concept or philosophy behind the repertory (philosophical background):
1. Individualization of the patient by forming the portrait of the patient taking into consideration:
   - (a) Mental generals
   - (b) Physical generals

(c) Particulars generals
2. Kent has given highest connotation to mental symptoms since they they give you an idea about the individuality of the patient. For example, aversion to company.
3. However, all mental generals do not have the same significance, only characterized mentals are given importance and not the common ones.
4. Then comes the physical generals which are related to the patient as a whole.
5. This is then followed by PQRS.
6. Lastly, the particulars are to be taken into account to determine the simillmum.
7. Kent and Hering have strongly criticized grand generalization by Boenninghausen – the reason being modalities applicable to one part, may not be applicable to the other part/ whole.

For example, Phosphorus craves cold things for his stomach but is chilly (differential modality), but afterwards, Kent found out that this condition is found in few cases and such symptoms became characteristic. Kent says when a modality or a sensation is present at two or more than two places, then only it should be generalized.

The mind recognizes and perhaps names the identity, or describes it's characteristics in comprehensive phrases. Details enter into minor generalizations, and minor generalization into major until one all-inclusive concept or principle is seen and stated.
Ref: Stuart's Logic.

Boger
The greater includes the less; generals are more important than particulars in constructing a case and as a basis for prescribing. The generals, which include and are derived from the particulars, constitute the only reliable basis of a curative prescription. Generalizing therefore is one of the most important functions performed by the homeopathic prescriber in selecting the curative medicine.

Mill, in his *Treatise on Logic,* says : "A general truth is but an aggregate of particular truths; a comprehensive expression by which an indefinite number of individual facts are affirmed or denied at once." Generalization is the process of obtaining a general conception, rule or law, from a consideration of particular facts or phenomena. Generalization is not possible until the mind has grasped and assimilated all the particulars which enter into its formation. Then they take on form and individuality and are seen as a whole. The mind recognizes and perhaps names the identity, or describes its characteristics in comprehensive phrase. Details enter into minor generalizations, and minor generalization into major until one all-inclusive
concept or principle is seen and stated.
Ref: Stuart's Logic.

Q. 99. Boger published his Boenninghausen's Characteristics and Repertory in the year_____ (MD/NIH/98)

(a) 1900
(b) 1905
(c) 1916
(d) 1935

Ans. (b)
Note
Boger published his Boenninghausen's Characterstics and Repertory in the year 1905. Which was published by Boericke and Tafel.
Ref: Esssentials of Repertorization, by S.K. Tiwari, page 211.

Also see
Boenninghausen's Characteristics and Repertory, by C. M. Boger.
Published by Boericke and Tafel (first edition – 1905).
Roy and Co, India (second edition –1937).

Evolution of Boger's Repertory
During the latter part of ninteenth century, with the emergence of Kent's Repertory, the applications of Boenninghausen's Therapeutic Pocket Book were relegated to the back stage. Boger was an ardent follower

of Boenninghausen's school of philosophy which in his view was much closer to the Hahnemannian concept of disease understanding. Boger was a prolific writer on the use of repertories, who was at ease with both Kent's and Boenninghausen's school of philosophy. The construction and information based in Kent's repertory also impressed him. So he embarked on the mission of achieving an integration of the information present in these two repertories.

While Boger was practicing in US, he understood the difficulties faced by the practitioners of his days in finding a simillmum from the materia medica in the shortest possible time. Finding that the practitioners had to depend on the existing faulty translations of the *Repertory of Antipsorics*, he took up the task of translating it in 1899. While doing this translation he was further convinced that the basic principles, plan and construction were sound and the book was comprehensible and practicable. He was also aware of the difficulties faced by practitioners while using the *Therapeutic Pocket Book* as well as the criticisms leveled against its principles and methodology.

So he undertook the rewriting of Boenninghausen's Repertory by adding new chapters, new rubrics and new medicines. Thus, he modified the chapters of Therapeutic Pocket Book by adding modalities and concomitants at the end of each chapter. The outcome was a more useful work and was published by Boericke and Tafel in 1905. Even after the publication of the first edition, Boger continued to work on the repertory. But he could not survive to see the publication of the second edition of his repertory. Later, the manuscripts were published posthumously with the assistance of his wife by Roy and Company in 1937. This can be considered as the first Indian edition of Boger's Repertory.

The second Indian edition was also brought forth by Roy and Company in 1952.

The third Indian edition was published by B. Jain after twenty years in 1972. The entire present editions are reprints of the second edition published in 1937.

Foreword
This is written by H. A. Roberts. He says that it was Boenninghausen who first evaluated the remedies in relation to the individual symptoms and it was he who introduced various relationships of any given remedy to the individual case. The repertory is based on the original Repertory of the Antipsoric Remedies of Boenninghausen.

Q. 100. Repertory of Desires and Aversions was published by_____(MD/NIH/98)
- (a) Guernsey
- (b) Allen
- (c) Doglas
- (d) Knerr

Ans. (a)

Note
Repertory of Desires and Aversions was published by Guernsey.
Ref: Essentials of Repertorization, by S.K. Tiwari, page 25.

Also see
William Jefferson Guernsey 1854 – son of William Fuller Guernsey, MD, and Adilene R. Eastman, Frankford, Philadelphia, Pennsylvania, was born in that city in 1854. His paternal grandmother was a Jefferson, and a relative of the president of that name. His maternal grandfather was Major Ebenezer Eastman of revolutionary fame, and of direct descent, through Governor Winthrop (the pedigree being perfect) from William the Conqueror.

In 1875 he graduated as an MD from Hahnemann Medical College, Philadelphia, and is a conscientious practitioner of homeopathy in its purity, adhering strictly to the principles as enunciated by Hahnemann.

He has made the following contributions to the various repertories : In 1876 the little '*Traveler's Medical Repertory,*' intended for the laity ; in 1877, a '*Repertory on Menstruation;*' in 1882, a repertory under the title of '*The Homœo-Therapeutics of Hæmorrhoids;*' in 1883, '*Repertory of Desires and Aversions*;' in 1889, '*Guernsey's Bœnninghausen,*' a reproduction of the famous '*Bœnninghausen Repertory,*' in the form of adjustable slips, which was sold only on subscription, the entire edition being ordered before publication ; in 1890, '*Repertory on Location and Direction of Pains in the Head;*' in 1892, '*Repertory on Diphtheria;*' in 1892, '*The Homœo-therapeutics of Hæmorrhoids*' (repertory) revised and enlarged, second edition.

For fifteen years he has been at work at intervals upon a repertory on skin diseases, to which he has given particular study, but which is not yet ready for publication.

In 1897 he conceived the idea of combining predigested meat with concentrated malt as a food for invalids and infants, and placed upon the market, in a small way, a preparation containing both the best peptones and malt then obtainable. In 1900, a very much better malt was prepared especially for his food and the designation of 'stronger' was added to the name of 'Perfection Liquid Food,' which is now in demand all over the country and is endorsed by hundreds of leading physicians.

Dr Guernsey married, in 1878, Marion M. Morgan, by whom he has two daughters, Grace K. and Helen R. Guernsey.
Ref: http://homeopathy.wildfalcon.com/archives/2008/04/15/the-guernsey-family-and-homeopath/

Q. 101. Mental general is greater than a physical general symptom, this was told by ____ (PSC/WB/91)
 (a) Boericke
 (b) Kent
 (c) Hahnemann
 (d) Hering

Ans. (b)

Note

Mental general is greater than a physical general symptom was told by Dr J.T. Kent.

Also see

Kent proposed that in order to understand a person he needs to be juged by symptoms at three levels in order of importance. He tells us that, 'Man is prior to his organs,...... man is will and understanding, and the house which he lives in, is his body.' Therefore the symptoms belonging to the mental sphere are of greater value than 'physical generals.' The physical general is a reaction of the body as a whole, that is, I am chilly, I cannot tolerate heat, or I like bathing. 'Pariticular generals' are symptoms which belong to the parts of the body, that is, my knee is swollen, or my head is aching. Local symptoms involving the organs of the body have lesser value as from those of physical generals which in turn is the body as a whole or his organization.
Ref: Essentials of Repertorization, by Dr S. K. Tiwari, page 271, third and revised edition.

Q.102. Repertorization starts from___ (MD/NIH/98)-Repeat (RPSC/08)
 (a) Case taking
 (b) Evaluation
 (c) Calculations
 (d) Rubric hunting

Ans. (a)

Note

Steps to repertorization starts from case taking and ends by finding the simillimum. They are:
 (a) Case taking.
 (b) Recording and interpretation.
 (c) Defining the problem.
 (d) Classification and evaluation of symptoms.
 (e) Erecting a totality.
 (f) Selection of a proper repertory.
 (g) Repertorial result.
 (h) Analysis of repertorial result and prescription.

Case taking

Case taking is the first step, and the outcome of treatment entirely depends upon the success of this first step. Any mistake committed here would certainly interfere in the selection of the drug and planning of the treatment.
Ref: Essentials of Repertorization, by Dr Shashi Kant Tiwari, page 33, 34, third revised and enlarged edition.

Q. 103. The Father of Repertory is _____ (MD/NIH/98) (RPSC/08)
    (a) Hahnemann
    (b) Boenninghausen
    (c) Kent
    (d) Boger

Ans. (b)
The Father of Repertory is Boenninghausen.

Note

In Hahnemann's time, only about 100 drugs were proved and he realized the limitation of the human mind to remember all the symptoms and felt the need for an aid to retrieve the facts. The idea of a repertory was first brought by Dr Hahnemann himself, and the first repertory was born in 1805 as *'Fragmenta de Viribus Medicamentorum Positivis,.'* The first part contains the symptoms observed and the second part contains the index or the repertory. Hahnemann was the first to make a repertory and he was using a repertory for his daily practice.

However, during this time Boenninghaussen had compiled his first repertory – *'Repertory of Antipsorics'*, with a preface by Hahnemann in 1832 under active inspiration from Hahnemann himself. This book had an extremely logical arrangement with an alphabetical order and systematic arrangement. The introduction is of the most useful innovation in the form of gradation and valuation of drugs, and up to this day we follow more or less Boenninghausen's standard of evaluation of drugs.

He continued his work in an attempt to condense the space and in 1835 published *'Repertory of Medicines which are not Antipsoric.'*

In 1836, his great work was published as *'Attempts at Showing the Relative Kinship of Homoeopathic Medicines.'* Thereafter, during 1836 to 1846 he came up with his masterpiece – *'Therapeutic Pocket Book,'* which was published in 1846. This was the culmination of his lifetime work.

He also introduced the doctrine of analogy and doctrine of concomitants which are used even today. He was the first person to introduce:
    (a) Systematic repertorization with a definite principle of its own.
    (b) Doctrine of analogy.
    (c) Doctrine of concomitants.
    (d) Evaluation of drugs.
    (e) Relationship of remedies.

Ref: Essentials of Repertorization by Dr Shashi Kant Tiwari, page 24, 25, third revised and enlarged edition.

Concomitant (auxiliary) Symptoms
Those symptoms that can be explained are of little help in selecting the homeopathic remedy... the auxiliary or concomitant symptoms limit the choice of the simillimum.
Ref: Principles and Art of Cure by Homoeopathy, by Dr A. Roberts.

Ref: http://www.homoeopathicdoctor.com/data.htm

Q. 104. Repertory of Antipsoric remedies was published in the year_____ (MD/NIH/98)
    (a) 1830
    (b) 1832
    (c) 1835
    (d) 1836

Ans. (b)

Note
Repertory of Antipsoric remedies was published in 1832.

Also see
Repertory of Antipsoric Remedies
A Systematic Alphabetical Repertory of Antipsoric Homoeopathic remedies, by Clemens Maria Franz Von Boenninghausen.

History

After Hahnemann's *Materia Medica Pura* was written, it became more and more apparent that some method should be used that would make it possible to find the simillimum more easily and quickly. Records of symptoms developed through proving reached such bulky proportions that medicines were prescribed after referring pages and pages of materia medica. Even Hahnemann who conducted many provings prescribed medicines after much reference to the materia medica. This was a stupendous task even for Hahnemann and he was compelled to make a short repertory of the leading symptoms which were printed in Latin. Later he developed the repertory idea still further but these later repertories are still in manuscript form.

After recovering from purulent tuberculosis in 1828, Boenninghausen developed a firm belief in homeopathy. He started working on the new healing art and came in contact with several physicians from whome he tried to know more and more about homeopathy. Soon he came in contact with Hahnemann in 1830. At that time repertory was a new adventure in homeopathic literature developing under pressure of necessity in indexing many provings that had accumulated or to index the ever enlarging materia medica.

The first repertory from a non-medical person was the culmination of the diligent and labourious work done by Boenninghausen. He undertook the task of compiling a repertory. He meticulously went through the reports of original provings and compared them with the reports of clinical verifications.

It was with the encouragement of Hahnemann, that Boenninghausen developed his first repertory – The *Repertory of Antipsorics Remedies* in 1832.

First edition: 1832
Second edition: 1833
Boger's translation: 1899

Hahnemann, in a footnote to aphorism 153, says, "Dr von Boenninghausen, by the publication of the characteristic symptoms of homoeopathic medicines and his repertory has rendered a great service to homoeopathy..."

Hahnemann's Introduction

Hahnemann writes about – *'On the Repetition of the Homoeopathic Remedy'*. In mild cases, a single small dose is enough to get a cure, especially in cases of small children or delicate or susceptible adults. But in chronic and advanced cases, spoilt by previous treatment with unsuitable remedies and also in grave acute diseases, a single smallest dose of a similar drug is not adequate to produce the curative effects as ordinarily expected from the medicine and hence repetition is required. Action of medicine through inhalation is equal to that of the medicine taken orally and at the same time repetition in the sense, more time he can inhale than the dose taken though orally.

Total number of drugs

52 drugs: 50 antipsoric + Thuja occidentalis (antisycotic) + Mercurius vivus (antisyphilitic)

Gradation

First Edition
    Italics (spaced) - 1st grade
    Italics - second grade
    Roman (spaced) - 3rd grade
    Roman - 4th grade
    Roman in parenthesis - 5th grade

Second edition
    Capital Bold - 1st grade
    Roman bold - 2nd grade
    Italics - 3rd grade
    Roman - 4th grade
    Roman in parenthesis - 5th grade

Plan and construction

    The book comprises of the following chapters:
    Mind

Vertigo
Head, Internal
Head, External
Eyes
Ear
Nose
Face
Teeth and Gums
Mouth
Taste
Appetite
Thirst
Eructation
Waterbrash and Heartburn
Hiccough
Nausea and Vomiting
Hypochondria
Abdomen
External Abdomen
Inguinal and Pubic Region
Flatus
Stool, Evacuation
Anus and Rectum
Perineum
Urine
Urinary Organs
Genitalia
Coryza
Respiration
Cough
Larynx
External Neck
Chest
Back
Upper Extremities
Lower Extremities
Bones and Glands
Skin
Sleep
Dreams
Fever
Compound Fevers
Generalities

Arrangement of rubrics
Location
Sensation
Time
Aggravation
Amelioration
Concomitant
Main rubric – written in bold.
Sub-rubric – written in italic after a space.
Antisycotic and antisyphilitic drugs given at the end of remedies in each rubric after a hyphen.

Features
Hahnemann wrote the Introduction to the repertory.
Duration of action of each remedy is given.
Antidotal relationship of remedies is separately mentioned under each remedy.

Relationship with other books
It was with the encouragement of Hahnemann, that Boenninghausen developed his first repertory: *Repertory of Antipsoric Remedies* in 1832.
In 1835, he published *Repertory of Medicines Which are not antipsoric.*
In 1836, he published *Attempt at Showing the Relative Kinship of Homeopathic Medicines.*
And in 1846 he published, *Therapeutic Manual for Homoeopathic Physicians.* BTP is a combination of all these four books.
Ref: Dr Sumit Goel MD (Hom)
www.homeopathyspace.com

Ref: http://www.homeopathyspace.com/repertory/Repertory%20of%20Antipsoric%20remedies.htm

Q. 105. Catarrhal laryngitis, cough compels child to grasp larynx (MD/ Hyderabad/99)
   (a) Phosphorus
   (b) Iodium
   (c) Allium cepa
   (d) Causticum

Ans. (c)
Note
Allium cepa has symptom – 'Catarrhal laryngitis, cough compels child to grasp larynx.'
Also see

Allium Cepa
Hay fever: in August every year; violent sneezing on rising from bed; from handling peaches. Nasal polypus (Teucr., Sangin-n., Psor.). Catarrhal laryngitis; cough compels patient to grasp the larynx; seems as if cough would tear it. Colic: from cold by getting feet wet; overeating; from cucumbers; salads; haemorrhoidal; of children; < sitting, > moving about.
Ref: Allen's Keynotes.

Q. 106. In comparison to location, sensation is _____ (MD/NIH/98)
   (a) More important
   (b) Less important
   (c) Same
   (d) No relation

Ans. (a)
Note
In comparison to location, sensation is more important.
Also see

Proving of drugs
When a healthy person takes a medicine for experimental reasons, certain effects are produced – changes in body functions, secretions, and sensations – the collective phenomena which is spoken of as a drug proving. When arranged schematically and written down, it is known as a drug's pathogenesis.

Experience with drug proving squads brings out other interesting considerations. Not everyone gives a complete proving. Susceptibility varies materially. Perhaps only 20 per cent of the squad gives comprehensive symptomatology. The same drug will not affect every man in the same manner or in the same parts, and lastly the intensity of sensation is subject to the widest variation. It takes, therefore, considerable experience to evaluate a proving, but there is no question that this is the best way to introduce a student into the study of the homeopathic materia medica.
Ref: Foundation of Homoeopathy.

Extended information

Determinative symptoms, whether encountered in disease or a drug proving are alike and usually consist of:
  (1) Modalities.
  (2) Mental symptoms.
  (3) Qualified basic or absolute symptoms.
  (4) 'Strange, rare, or particular symptoms', as mentioned by Hahnemann.

Homeopathic provings are especially prolific in bringing out such characteristic symptoms. We learn to look for such symptoms in one of the three divisions of the drug's pathogenesis. Thus :
  (1) Location of tissue proclivity (elective affinity).
  (2) Sensation or kind of action.
  (3) Modalities (influences which aggravate or ameliorate).

Locality or seat of action:

Every drug affects some organ or system of organs or tissue or region more decidedly than others, and there especially or primarily expends its power. This specific localization, or seat of a drug, is known as its elective affinity, by which it preferably chooses certain cells, tissues or organs, to manifest its action. In a general way, we see that Belladonna affects principally the brain as its arena for action, and this organ, therefore, has a preferred relationship to Belladonna. So, in the same way, Aconitum napellus affects the heart, Ergotinum the uterus; Bryonia alba the serous membranes; Podophyllum peltatum the duodenum; Rhus toxicodendron the skin; Tellurium metallicum the tympanum; Glonoinum the vasomotor centre in the brain, and so on.

Sensations or kind of action:

While the special seat of action is the first marked fact about the pathogenetic properties of drugs, the special kind of action is the second fact. This may be seen in the sensations and modalities of a drug. Thus, the burning pains of Arsenicum album, the coldness of Camphora officinalis and Veratrum album, the sticking pains of Bryonia alba, the stinging pains of Apis mellifica and Theridion curassavicum, the plug sensation of Anacardium orientale, the soreness of Arnica montana and Hamamelis virginiana, are all characteristic. Frequently, the character of these pains indicates the seat of action and thus points to the elective affinity of the drug, as burning pains in general indicate the mucous membranes; dull, boring, gnawing pains, the bones; sticking, cutting pains, serous membranes, etc. In many drugs, these conditions may be so expressive of their special character, that we nearly always expect them to be present when they are homeopathically indicated and therefore prove to be the curative remedy. Such characteristic conditions are the restlessness and anxiety of Aconitum napellus and Arsenicum album, the chilliness of Pulsatilla nigricans, the thirstlessness of Apis mellifica, the dullness and drowsiness of Gelsemium sempervirens, the hysterical contradiction of its symptoms of Ignatia amara, the melancholy of Aurum metallicum, etc.

Modalities

Modalities are conditions which influence or modify drug action. Just as a plant thrives best in certain conditions of soil, climate, elevation, in short, a suitable environment, so a drug must be similarly situated to enable it to express itself clearly and fully. It is of the greatest importance in drug proving as well as prescribing homeopathically to note the modalities. The main group of modalities are : Time, temperature, weather, motion, menstruation, position, perspiration, eating and emotion. Thus, Lycopodium clavatum has a time aggravation during late afternoon; Sulphur cannot bear heat; Natrium sulphuricum is aggravated by wet weather; Bryonia alba is aggravated by motion, etc.

A practical point is that there are two types of modalities:
  (a) Those that apply to the person as a whole.
  (b) Those that apply to a person's particular complaint or involve an organ.

The first class is by far the most important and a few general modalities should always be present in the outline of symptoms.

Ref: An Analysis of Symptoms.

Q. 107. In Boenninghausen's Repertory, the number of chapters is ____ (MD/NIH/98)
  (a) 5
  (b) 7

(c) 9
(d) 11

Ans. (b)

Note

In Boenninghausen's repertory, the number of chapters is 7.

This is in reference to BTPB that is, 'Boennninghausen's Theraputic Pocket Book', and it contains 7 chapters.

Also see

Ref: Essentials of Repertorisation, by S.K. Tiwari, page 141, third revised and enlarged edition.

Q. 108. Number of cards in Kishore's Card Repertory ---- (MD/NIH/98)
(a) 7000
(b) 8000
(c) 9000
(d) 10,000

Ans. (d)

Note

Number of cards in Kishore's Card Repertory are 10,000.

Also see

Initially it contained 3500 cards. The second edition was published in 1967. The edition was impoved in relation to the number of cards and rubrics. Now has about 10,000 cards.

Ref: Essential of Repertorisation, by S.K. Tiwari, page 380, third revised and enlarged edition.

Q. 109. Repertory of modalities is published by____ (MD/NIH/98)
(a) S. Worchester
(b) Jahr
(c) Lippe
(d) Ruoff

Ans. (a)

Note

Repertory of modalities was published by S. Worchester.

Ref: Essential of Repertorisation, by S.K. Tiwari, third revised and enlarged edition.

Also see

Era of Regional Repertories (1880 - 1900)

Many of them were clinical repertories. Important among these are:
(a) 1880 – Repertory of Fever by H.C. Allen.
(b) Sensation, as if by H.A.Robert.
(c) Repertory of Modalities by Worcester.
(d) Repertory of Intermittent Fever by W.A.Allen.
(e) Repertory of Haemorroids by Guernsey.
(f) 1894. Rheumatism by Porlunins.
(g) 1899 – Repertory of Urinary Organs by Morgan.
(h) 1900 – Repertory of Back by Wilsy.
(i) 1906 – Repertory of Uterine Therapeutics by Minton.
(j) Repertory of Diarrhoea by Bell.
(k) 1906 – Repertory part of Raue's Special Pathology.
(l) Repertory by Boericke.
(m) Clark's Clinical Repertory.
(n) Repertory of Mastitis by W.J. Gurnesy.

MCQ's in Repertory

Q.110. Rubric 'Pulse' is found (Kent Repertory) under Chapter: (MD/NIH/98)
    (a) Extremities
    (b) Chest
    (c) Generalities
    (d) Boils

Ans. (c)

Note

Rubric 'Pulse' is found in Kent's Repertory under chapter Generalities.

Also see

```
[kent ]
[Generalities]Pulse:Frequent,accelerated,elevated,exalted,fast,innumerable,ra
1: Acon     1: Agar     1: Aloe     1: Alum     1: Am-m     1: Ars
2: Aur      1: Bell     1: Benz-ac  1: Bism     1: Cann-i   1: Canth
1: Chin     1: Chin-s   1: Colch    1: Cupr     2: Dig      1: Gels

2 Pulse:                              4 Afternoon:
3 Abnormal:                           4 Evening:
3 Audible:                            4 Midnight,after:
3 Bounding:                           4 Eating,after:
3 Compressible (see soft):            4 Faster than the heart beat:
3 Contracted:                         4 Motion agg:
3 Double:                             4 Noticing,it,when:
3 Empty:                              4 Rest,during:
3 Excited:                            4 Rising up,on:
3 Febrile:                            4 Sitting,when:
3 Fluttering:                         4 Stool,after:
3 Frequent,accelerated,elevated,exalted,fas  4 Thinking of past troubles:
  4 Daytime:                          4 Vexation,after:
  4 Morning:                          4 Warm applications,from:
  4 Forenoon:                         4 And intermittent:
```

Q. 111. The drug for rubric 'Eccentricity' is _____ (MD/NIH/98)
    (a) Rhus toxicodendron
    (b) Sulphur
    (c) Valeriana officinalis
    (d) Veratrum album

Ans. (d)

Note

The drug for rubric 'Eccentricity' is 'Veratrum'.

Also see

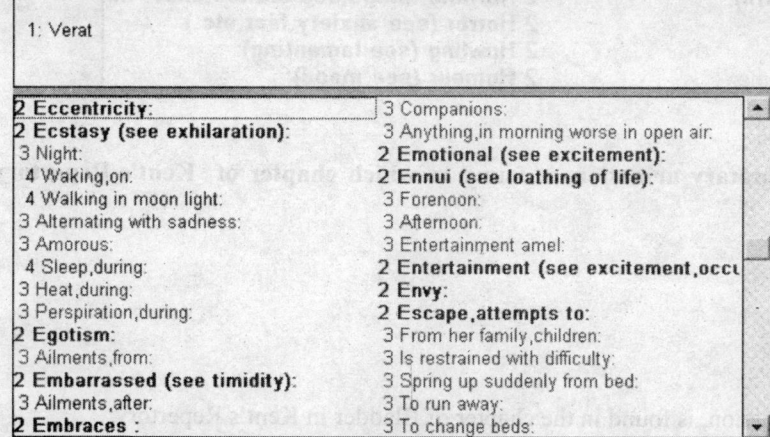

Q.112. Sweat; foetid, axilla; is in which chapter of Boger's Repertory (MD/Hydrabad)
    (a) Sensation and Complaints
    (b) Axilla
    (c) Chest
    (d) Sweat

Ans. (c)

Note
Sweat; foetid, axilla; is in chapter Chest of Boger's Repertory.
Ref: Boger Boenninghausen's Characteristics and Repertory, Chapter Chest-External-Axilla, page 768.

Q.113. The rubric 'haughtiness' found in Chapter in Kent's Repertory (MD/NIH/2000)
    (a) Mind
    (b) Generalities
    (c) Chest
    (d) Head

Ans. (a)

Note
The rubric 'haughtiness' is found in Mind chapter of Kent's Repertory.

Also see

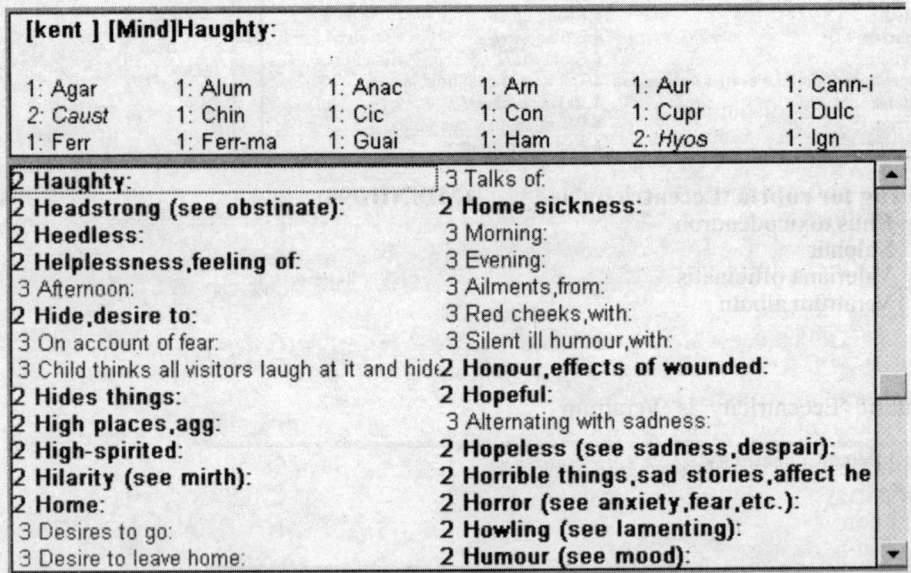

Q.114. Cough with involuntary urination, is found in which chapter of Kent's Repertory (MD/Hydrabad)
    (a) Bladder
    (b) Cough
    (c) Urine
    (d) Kidney

Ans. (a)

Note
Cough with involuntary urination, is found in the chapter of Bladder in Kent's Repertory.

MCQ's in Repertory

Also see

[kent] [Bladder]Urination:Involuntary:Cough,during:
Alum,Anan,*Ant-c*,**APIS**,*Bell,Bry,Caps*,Carb-an,**CAUST**,*Cench,Colch,Dulc,Ferr,Ferr-p*,Hyos,Ign,*Kreos*, Laur,*Lyc*,Mag-c,Murx,**NAT-M**,Nit-ac,*Nux-v,Ph-ac*,**PHOS**,Psor,**PULS**,Rhod,Rhus-t,*Rumx*,Seneg,*Sep*, **SQUIL**,Staph,Sulph,Tarent,*Thuj,Verat*,Vib,*Zinc*,

Q.115. Surrogate means_____ (MD/NIH/98) and (PSC/WB/93)
   (a) Symptoms
   (b) Remedy
   (c) Drug
   (d) Substitute

Ans. (d)
Note
Surrogate means 'substitute'.

Also see
Aphorism 118 and 119. The action of every medicine differs from that of every other.

Note:
There can be no such things as surrogates.
Ref: Organon of Medicine.

Extended intormation

Aphorism 119:
As certainly as every species of plant differs in its external form, mode of life and growth, in its taste and smell from every other species and genus of plant, as certainly as every mineral and salt differs from all others, in its external as well as its internal physical and chemical properties (which alone should have sufficed to prevent any confounding of one with another), so certainly do they all differ and diverge among themselves in their pathogenetic –consequently also in their therapeutic effects.[1]

1. Anyone who has a thorough knowledge of, and can appreciate the remarkable difference of effects on the health of man of every single substance from those of every other, will readily perceive that among them there can be, in a medical point of view, no equivalent remedies whatever, no surrogates. Only those who do not know the pure, positive effects of the different medicines can be so foolish as to try to persuade us that one can serve in the stead of the other, and can in the same disease prove just as serviceable as the other......
   Ref: Organon of Medicine.

Q. 116. Menstruation is _____symptom (PSC/WB/93)- (RPSC/08)
   (a) Particular
   (b) Common
   (c) Peculiar particular
   (d) Peculiar general

Ans. (d) Menstruation is a peculiar general symptom.
Note

Particular (common) symptom
Particular symptoms are localized in the body.

Common general symptom
These are physical symptoms felt throughout the patient's body, such as tiredness, changes in appetite or restlessness.

Peculiar particular symptom
These are symptoms unique to the individual that do not occur in most persons with the acute disease. Homeopaths make note of peculiar symptoms because they often help to determine the remedy.

Peculiar general symptom
These may be present in the mental sphere (love, hate, intellect and memory) or on the physical sphere (heat, cold, colour or discharges, menstrual function).

Also see
The value / rank of symptom is gauged on the following points:

General symptoms
The symptoms which the patient represents with 'I', as at the mental level – I am angry, and at the physical level– I am hungry or I am feeling cold. These also include symptoms belonging to the sexual sphere. These can be:
  (a) Mental generals.
  (b) Physical generals.

When in this sphere, any symptom is unique to that person, it is designated as a 'peculiar general' symptom and it is ranked high; the other symptoms are considered 'common general'.

Symptoms which the patient designates as 'my' are considered as particular general.

For example; my head is aching, this is a 'common particular' symptom. However when modalities are attached to same like headache, location frontal, sensation – throbbing. Modalities–worse in sun, better in a dark room and vomiting (concomitant) it becomes a 'particular peculiar'.

Extended information
Symptoms and their grading according to Kent:

General symptoms include:
  (a) Mental generals (in the declining order of importance):
      (i) Love, hates
      (ii) Intellect
      (iii) Memory
  (b) Physical generals (in declining order of importance):
      (i) Related to blood, colour of discharge, aversions and cravings
      (ii) Menstrual functions (general aggravations related to menses, the character of menses).
      (iii) Environmental factors.

Common symptoms include:
  (a) Particular symptoms (in the declining order of importance):
      (i) Peculiar or unusual symptoms.
      (ii) Discharges.
      (iii) Modalities.
  (b) Common particular symptoms
They become important when they are absent or when intensified.

Q. 117. Full time amelioration with no special relief of patient indicates_____ (MD/NIH/98)
  (a) Palliation
  (b) Suppression
  (c) Cure
  (d) Disease aggravation

Ans. (a)

Note
'Full time amelioration of symptoms with no special relief of patient the is 'seventh observation' of Kent's Twelve Observations.

Also see

Seventh observation:
Full time amelioration of the symptoms, yet no special relief of the patient.
The remedies act favourably, but the patient is not cured, and never can be cured. The patient is palliated in

this instance, and it is a suitable palliation for homeopathic remedies. There are conditions in patients that prevent improvement beyond a certain stage.

(a) A patient with one kidney can only improve to a certain degree; patient with fibrinous structural change in certain places, tubercles that have become encysted and lungs capable of doing only limited work are examples of such cases.

(b) These cases have symptoms, and these symptoms are ameliorated from time to time with remedies, but the patient is only curable to a certain extent; he cannot go beyond and rise above such a state.

(c) After several medicines have been administered – the amelioration of the case has existed the full length of time. But the patient has not risen above his own pitch in this length of time.

Extended information
Kent's twelve obervations:
Prognosis after observing the action of the the remedy
After a prescription has been made, it is important to observe what happens in consequence to the prescription. Not being conversant as to what may happen will result in wrong prescriptions. If the homeopathic physician is not an accurate observer, his observation will be indefinite; and if his observations are indefinite, his prescribing is indefinite.

It is to be understood that after a prescription is made, it has acted. If a medicine is acting, it starts immediately to affect changes in the patient, and these changes are indicated through signs and symptoms. If a prescription is not related to the case, waiting is loss of time, and that should be taken into account among the observations.

The remedy is known to act by the changing of symptoms. The disappearance of symptoms, the increase of symptoms, the amelioration of symptoms, the order of the symptoms and duration are all changes from the remedy, and these changes are to be studied.

Among the commonest things that remedies do is to aggravate or ameliorate.

The aggravation is of two kinds; aggravation of disease, in which the patient grows worse; or aggravation of symptoms, in which the patient grows better. An aggravation of the disease means that the patient is growing weaker, the symptoms are growing stronger, but the homeopathic aggravation, which is the aggravation of the symptoms of the patient while the patient is growing better, is something that the physician observes after a true homeopathic prescription.

The patient should be the aim of the physician, to determine whether he is improving or declining.

First observation
Prolonged aggravation and final decline of the patient.

This is seen in an incurable case, where the antipsoric administered was too deep, and it has established destruction. There is reversal of order of cure.

The patient steadily declines. The symptoms take on an internal phase – vital organs are affected. In this state, vital reaction was impossible.

In incurable and doubtful cases give no higher than the 30 or 200 potency, and observe whether the aggravation is going to be too deep or too prolonged. Begin, in such cases, with a moderately low potency; and the 30 potency is low enough for anybody or anything. Otherwise, the deep acting remedy in high potency results in a killer's aggravation.

Illustration:
A stoop-shouldered patient, with a chronic hacking cough reports for treatment. His face is sickly, he is lean and anxious, he is careworn and poor. An antipsoric seems indicated. Tuberculosis is diagnosed and the patient is steadily declining. On prescribing the antipsoric – he comes back in a few days with quite a sharp aggravation of the symptoms – increased cough, night sweat, and more weakness. This patient returns in a week, and the aggravation is still present and increased – coughing is worse, expectoration is more troublesome, night sweats have been going on; he comes back at the end of the second week and he is still worse, and all the symptoms have been worse since he took that medicine. He was comparatively comfortable before he took that medicine, but at the end of the fourth week he is steadily growing worse. There has been

no amelioration following this aggravation, and he is evidently declining – PROLONGED AGGRAVATION AND FINAL DECLINE.

Second observation
Long aggravation, but final and slow improvement.
Seen in cases that are not so advanced, with not so profound a disturbance – on administration of a high potency.
The aggravation is long and severe and may last for many weeks, yet there is a final amelioration – a slow but sure improvement.
It shows that the disease has not progressed quite so far; the changes have not become quite so marked.
It is always well in doubtful cases to go to the lower potencies, and in this way go cautiously prepared to antidote the medicine if it takes the wrong course.
If, at the end of a few weeks, he is a little better and his symptoms are a little better than when he took the dose, there is some hope that finally the symptoms may have an outward manifestation whereby he will attain final recovery, but for many years you may go along with prolonged aggravations.

Third observation
Aggravation is quick, short and strong with rapid improvement of patient.
Seen in cases where there is no structural change of vital organs or there are superficial structural changes of less vital organs.
Aggravation, that comes quickly, is short, and has been more or less vigorous, then improvement of the patient will be long.
Reaction of the economy is vigorous. There is a difference between organic changes that take place in the organs that are vital, that carry on the work of the economy, and organic changes that take place in structures of the body that are not essential to life.
An aggravation that is quick, short and strong is one that is to be wished for and is followed by quick improvement. Such is the slight aggravation of the symptoms that occurs in the first hours after the remedy in an acute sickness, or during the first few days in a chronic case.

Fourth observation
No aggravation, with recovery of patient
These are cases with very satisfactory cures, where the administration of the remedy is followed by no aggravation whatever.
There is no organic disease, and no tendency to organic disease. The chronic condition itself to which the remedy is suitable is not of great depth, belongs to the functions of nerves rather than to threatened changes in tissues.
If there is no aggravation; the potency just exactly fitted the case. In cures without any aggravation, the potency is suitable, and the remedy is the curative remedy, provided the symptoms go off and the patient returns to health in an orderly way.
It is the highest order of cure in acute affections, yet the physician is sometimes more satisfied if in the beginning of his prescribing he notices a slight aggravation of the symptoms.

Fifth observation
Amelioration comes first and the aggravation comes afterwards.
The patient says he is better, and the symptoms seem to be better; but at the end of a week or four or five days, all the symptoms are worse than when the patient first came.
    (a)   Either the remedy was only a superficial remedy, and could only act as a palliative, or
    (b)   The patient was incurable and the remedy was somewhat suitable.
One of these two conclusions must be arrived at, and this can only be done by a re-examination of the patient and by finding out whether the symptoms relate to that remedy.
The remedy could have been an error. A further study of the case shows that the remedy was only similar to the most grievous symptoms, that it did not cover the whole case, that it did not affect the constitutional state of the patient, and that the patient is incurable and the selection was an unfavourable one.
It is the best thing for the patient if the symptoms come back exactly as they were, but very often they come

back changed, and then one needs to wait through grievous suffering for the picture.

Sixth observation

Too short relief of symptoms.

When a high and right potency acts in curable case – the remedy acts at once and establishes a condition of order, after which there is no need of giving the medicine. This order may continue a considerable length of time, sometimes several months. The patient gets along without any medicine. But, the patient may come back at the end of the first, second and third week and say he has done well, that he has been improving all the time, but at the end of the fourth week he returns back with suffering.

This could be due to some obstacle – something that has spoiled the action of the medicine. This condition is an unfavourable one.

If relief after the constitutional remedy does not last long enough, it is because of some condition that interferes with the action of the remedy; it may be unconscious on the part of the patient, or it may be intentional. A quick rebound means that it is well chosen, that the vital economy is in a good state, and if everything goes well, recovery take place.

In acute cases, when there is too short an amelioration of the symptoms, the remedy has to be repeated. If it is too short an amelioration in acute cases, it is because a high grade inflammatory action is present and that organs are threatened by the rapid processes going on.

If it is too short an amelioration in chronic diseases, it means that there are structural changes and organs are destroyed or being destroyed.

Seventh observation

Full time amelioration of the symptoms, yet no special relief of the patient.

There are conditions in patients that prevent improvement beyond a certain stage.

A patient with one kidney can only improve to a certain degree; patient with fibrinous structural change in certain places, tubercles that have become encysted and lungs capable of doing only limited work are examples of such cases.

These cases have symptoms, and these symptoms are ameliorated from time to time with remedies, but the patient is only curable to a certain extent; he cannot go beyond and rise above such a state.

After several medicines have been administered – the amelioration of the case has existed the full length of time. But the patient has not risen above his own pitch in this length of time.

The remedies act favourably, but the patient is not cured, and never can be cured. The patient is palliated in this instance, and it is a suitable palliation for homeopathic remedies.

Eighth observation

Patients prove every remedy they get.

Patients maybe hysterical, oversensitive to all things.

The patient is said to have an idiosyncrasy to everything, and these oversensitive patients are often incurable.

When administered a dose of a high potency, they go on and prove that medicine, and while under the influence of that medicine they are not under the influence of anything else. Such patients are good provers, they will prove the highest potencies.

For such patients, go back to the 30 and 200 potencies. Many of them are born with this sensitivity and they will die with it.

Ninth observation

Action of the medicines upon the provers.

Healthy provers are always benefited by provings, if they are properly conducted.

It is well to observe carefully the constitutional states of an individual about to become a prover, and to write these down and subtract them from the proving.

These symptoms will not very commonly appear during the proving; if they do, note the change in them.

Tenth observation

New symptoms appearing after the remedy has been administered.

If a great number of new symptoms appear after the administration of a remedy, the prescription will generally prove to be an unfavourable one.

Now and then, the coming of a new symptom will simply be an old symptom coming up that the patient has not observed, and thinks it a new one.

The greater the array of new symptoms coming out after the administration of a remedy, the more doubt there is thrown upon the prescription. The probability is, after these new symptoms have passed away, the patient will settle down to the original state and no improvement takes place. It did not sustain a true homeopathic relation.

Eleventh observation

Is when old symptoms are observed to reappear.

In proportion, as old symptoms that have long been away return, just in that proportion the disease is curable.

They disappeared because newer ones have come up. It is quite a common thing for old symptoms to appear after the aggravation has come, and hence we see the symptoms disappearing in the reverse order of their appearance.

Those symptoms that are present subside, and old symptoms keep coming up.

Old symptoms often come back and go off without any change of medicine. It indicates that the medicine must be let alone. If the old symptoms come back to stay then a repetition of the dose is often necessary.

Twelfth observation

Symptoms take the wrong direction.

If a medicine is prescribed for rheumatism of the joints and relief takes place at once, but the patient now suffers from violent internal distress of the heart, or centers in the spine, there is a transference from circumference to center, and the remedy must be antidoted at once, otherwise structural changes will take place in that new site.

Most gouty patients get along best when their fingers and toes are in the worst condition. To prescribe for this, and see the heart symptoms grow worse is not favourable.

There is a danger in selecting a remedy on external symptoms alone that is, selecting a remedy that corresponds only to the skin and ignoring all the remaining symptoms and general state of the patient; because it is true that the remedy that is related to the skin alone may drive in that skin disease and cause it to appear while the patient himself is not cured. Such a patient will remain sick until that eruption comes back again, or locates in another place.

Ref: Dr Sumit Goel MD (Hom)

www.homeopathyspace.com

Q.118. Accessory symptoms of a drug____ (PSC/WB/93)
    (a)   Are not the symptoms of that drug
    (b)   Are the symptoms of a partial homeopathic drug
    (c)   Are the symptoms which appear after an antipsoric drug
    (d)   Are the symptoms which appear after an allopathic drug

Ans. (b)

Note

Accessory symptoms of a drug are the symptoms of a partial homeopathic drug.

Also see

Accessory symptoms

Aphorism 163

In this case we cannot indeed expect from this medicine a complete, untroubled cure; for during its use some symptoms appear which were not previously observable in the disease, accessory symptoms of the not perfectly appropriate remedy. This does by no means prevent a considerable part of the disease (the

symptoms of the disease that resemble those of the medicine) from being eradicated by this medicine, thereby establishing a fair commencement of the cure, but still this does not take place without those accessory symptoms, which are, however, always moderate when the dose of the medicine is sufficiently minute.
Ref: Organon of Medicine.

Q. 119. Pain in the cervical region is found in which chapter of Kent's Repertory (MD/Hyderabad)
(a) Back
(b) Neck
(c) Head
(d) Cervical

Ans. (a)

Note
Pain in the cervical region is found in 'Back' chapter of Kent's Repertory.

Also see

[kent] [Back]Pain:Cervical region:

1: Abrot	2: Acon	2: Aesc	2: Aeth	2: Agar	1: Ail
1: All-c	1: All-s	2: Alum	1: Alumn	2: Am-c	1: Am-m
1: Ambr	2: Anac	1: Ang	1: Ant-c	2: Apis	1: Arg-m

3 Cervical region:	6 6 p.m. to 4 a.m.:
4 Right side on turning head:	4 Air:
4 Left:	5 A draft of:
4 Morning:	5 Cold,damp:
5 Waking,on:	5 Fresh,amel:
4 Forenoon:	5 Open:
4 Noon:	6 Amel:
4 Afternoon:	4 Alternating with headache:
5 4 p.m.:	4 Ascending steps:
4 Evening:	4 Bending head forward :
5 Going to bed:	5 Amel:
5 Looking up:	5 On:
4 Night:	4 Bending head backward :
5 Midnight:	5 On:
5 Before midnight:	5 Amel:

Q. 120. Anaemia is found in ____ chapter of Boger's Repertory (MD/Hyderabad)
(a) Blood
(b) Circulation
(c) Sensation
(d) Complaints

Ans. (b)

Q. 121. Which is indicated for vertigo after fright____ (PSC/WB/91
(a) Gelsemium sempervirens
(b) Conium maculatum
(c) Silicea terra
(d) Aconitum napellus

Ans. (d)

Note
From the choice of medicines given above, 'Aconitum napellus' covers the above symptom.

Also see
[kent] [Vertigo]Fright.after:
*Acon,*Crot-h,*OP,*
Extended information
The above symptom could not be verified from Allen's Keynotes.

Q. 122. Number of medicines given in Kishore's Card Repertory
   (a) 300
   (b) 400
   (c) 500-
   (d) 600

Ans. (d)

Note
Number of medicines given in Kishore's Card Repertory is more than 600.

Also see
Kishore's Card Repertory
By Dr Jugal Kishore.
Has 10000 cards.
It is based on Kent's work. However, it contains prominent mentals, Physicals or only particulars. Therefore, it is an attempt to substitute both Boenninghausen's as well as Kent's Repertories.
It deals with 600 remedies.
The third edition was published in 1986
Ref: Essentials of Repertorization, by S. K. Tiwari, page 380, third revised and enlarged edition.

Extended information
Kishore's card repertory
By Dr Jugal Kishore.
10000 cards.
Based on Kent's work.
647 drugs are included.
Has gradation of medicines in different types of punched cards.
This card has 80 vertical columns from 1 – 80 from left to right. They are numbered at the bottom in small letters.
First four vertical columns are kept apart and meant for punching the number of the rubrics. They are not divided by vertical lines.
Number of rubrics on the left top corner, in this four column numbers punched so that there is no confusion even if the card is mixed / mutilated.
On the top of the card, rubric name is printed.
The rest of the vertical columns are meant for the coded remedies which have this particular symptom. The remedies are indicated by the punched holes.

Reading : The Punched number (any number from 0-9) is placed against the small digit placed at the bottom of the column of that particular hole. The remedy can be obtained from the list of remedies and their code numbers.
All the grades can be denoted by the shape of the punched hole.
Double hole – 3 marks
Oval – 2 marks
Round – 1 mark
Dr K.R. Mansooor Ali BHMS, MD (Hom)
Government Homeopathic Medical College, Calicut.
Approved practitioner, Ministry of Health, UAE.
Email: info@similima.com
Ref: http://www.similima.com/Rep18.html

MCQ's in Repertory

Q.123. Medicine should not be changed if ____ (MD/NIH/98)
   (a) Patient is improving
   (b) Any discharge or eruption appears
   (c) Patient feels better
   (d) All of the above

Ans. (d)

Note
If all of the above features are present, the medicine should not be changed.

Also see
Ref: The Second Prescription – Lectures on Homoeopathic Philosophy, by J. T. Kent.

Q.124. A complete symptom is characterised by ____ (MD/NIH/98)
   (a) Location, sensation, modalities, concomitant
   (b) Location, time, modalities
   (c) Site, time, extension, modalities
   (d) Rare, uncommon, peculiar

Ans. (a)

Note
A complete symptom is characterised by – location, sensation, modalities and concomitant.

Also see
Concept of a complete symptom
According to Boenninghausen, the following factors are essential for making a complete symptom:
   (1) Locality – the part, organ or tissue involved.
   (2) Sensations – the character of pain, sensation, functional or pathology / organic change characterizing the morbid process.
   (3) Modalities – aggravation and amelioration – the circumstances causing, exciting, increasing, or otherwise affording modification or relief of suffering.
   (4) Concomitant symptoms – was added by him, emphasizing that the doctrine of the totality of the case which must include the concomitants.

According to him, concomitant symptoms are to the totality what the condition of aggravation or amelioration is to the single symptom.
Ref: Essentials of Repertorization, by S. K. Tiwari, second revised and enlarged edition.
Ref: Boenninghausen's Therapeutic Pocket Book, Philosophical Background, page 137.

Q. 125. The drug mentioned under the rubric 'Eccentricity' is _____ (MD/NIH/98)
   (a) Rhus toxicondendron
   (b) Sulphur
   (c) Valeriana officinalis
   (d) Veratrum album

Ans. (d)

Note
The drug mentioned under the rubric 'Eccentricity' is Veratrum album.

Also see
[kent][Mind]Eccentricity:
1: Verat

Q. 126. Desire and aversion are found in _____ chapter of Kent's Repertory (MD/NIH/98)
   (a) Stomach
   (b) Abdomen
   (c) Mind
   (d) Generalities

Ans. (a)

Note
Desire and aversion are found in Stomach chapter of Kent's Repertory.
Also see

[kent] [Stomach]Aversion:

2 Aversion:	3 Breakfast:
3 To acids:	3 Butter:
3 Alcoholic stimulants:	3 Cereals:
3 Ale:	3 Cheese:
3 Apples:	3 Chocolate:
3 Bananas:	3 Coffee:
3 Beef:	3 Cold drinks (see water cold):
3 Beer:	3 Dinner:
4 Morning:	3 Drinks:
4 Evening:	4 Headache, during:
3 Brandy:	4 Heat, during:
4 In brandy drinkers:	4 Hot:
3 Bread:	4 Warm:
4 Brown:	3 Eggs:
4 And butter:	4 To the odour of:

[kent] [Stomach]Desires:

2 Desires:	3 Bananas:
3 Alcoholic drinks:	3 Bitter drinks:
4 Menses, before:	3 Bitter food:
3 Ale:	3 Bread:
3 Beer:	4 And butter:
4 Evening:	4 Dry:
3 Brandy:	4 Rye bread:
3 Whisky:	4 Boiled in milk:
3 Wine:	4 Only:
4 Claret:	3 Butter:
3 Almonds:	3 Chalk (see lime):
3 Apples:	3 Charcoal:
3 Aromatic drinks:	3 Cheese:
3 Ashes:	3 Cheese, strong:
3 Bacon:	3 Cherries:

Q. 127. In comparison to location, sensation is _____ (MD/NIH/98)
    (a)   More important
    (b)   Less important
    (c)   Same
    (d)   No relation

Ans. (b)

Note
In comparision to location, sensation is less important.

Also see
In reference to Boger's concept of totality:

Boger with his long professional experience in evolution of 'protrait of disease'. He re-emphasized the following points to appreciate the whole picture of disease:
    (1)   Change in personality and temperament (Quis).
    (2)   Peculiarities of disease (Quid).
    (3)   Seat of disease (Ubi).
    (4)   Concomitant (Quibus Auxilis).
    (5)   The cause (Cur).
    (6)   Modalities (Quamoda).
    (7)   Time (Qunando).

He instructs while tracing the prortait of the disease to begin with:
    (a)   First to try and elicit the evident cause and course of the sickness down to the least symptom and effect of such influences like – time, temperature, open air, posture, being alone, motion, sleep, eating, drinking, touch, pressure, discharges, etc.
    (b)   Second comes the modalities and consideration of mental state in order of importance.
    (c)   Third comes the entire objective aspect or expression of the sickness including the state of secretions / sensations.
    (d)   Fourth and last is the part affected which must be determined which also brings the investigation in touch with diagnosis. (AQ) He has further advised that by going over the above rubrics in the order named, the contour of the disease picture would be pretty clearly outlined and would point fairly well towards the simillimum and the prescriber has only to keep in mind the fact that the actual differentiating factor may belong to any rubric.

Conclusion
From above it becomes clear that Boger has given importance to causation, modalities, concomitants, general sensations and pathology. Location is given the last place in the order of hierarchy.
Ref: Essentials of Repertorization, by Dr S. K. Tiwari, page 203, 204, second revised and enlarged edition.

Q. 128. Rubric Delirium is seen in _____ Chapter of Boenninghausen's Repertory (MD/NIH/98)
    (a)   Mind
    (b)   Intellect
    (c)   Sensation and Complaints
    (d)   Sleep and Dreams

Ans. (b)

Q. 129. 'Concordance' means_____ (MD/NIH/98)
    (a)   Relationship between two remedies
    (b)   Concomitant
    (c)   Characteristic symptom
    (d)   All

Ans. (a)

Note
'Concordance' means relation between two remedies.

Also see

The word 'concordance' was first used in homeoapthic literature by Boenninghausen in the earlier edition of Therapeutic Pocket Book. This chapter contained various relationships among remedies under different sub-headings. However, the word 'concordance' was replaced by 'relationship of remedies' in later editions by Allen to make the title more comprehensible for this chapter.

Ref: Essentials of Repertorization, by Dr S. K. Tiwari, page 487, second revised and enlarged edition.

Q. 130. 'Nocturnal Enuresis' is found in Kent's Repertory under the chapter____ (MD/NIH/98)
    (a)   Bladder
    (b)   Kidney
    (c)   Urethra
    (d)   Urine

Ans. (a)

Note

Nocturnal enuresis is found in chapter 'Bladder' in Kent's Repertory.

Also see

[kent] [Bladder]Urination:Involuntary:Night (incontinence in bed):
Acon,*Aeth*,*Am-c*,Anac,Anan,APIS,*Apoc*,*Arg-m*,ARG-N,ARN,ARS,*Aur*,Aur-m,Aur-s,Bar-c,Bar-m, BENZ-AC,Bry,Cact,*Calc*,Canth,*Carbn-s*,Carb-v,CAUST,*Cham*,Chin,*Chlol*,Cimx,Cina,Coca,Con,*Crot-c*, Cupr,Dulc,EQUIS,*Eup-pur*,FERR,*Ferr-ar*,Ferr-i,Ferr-p,*Fl-ac*,GRAPH,*Hep*,Hyos,Ign,Kali-c,*Kali-p*, LAC-C,Lac-d,Lyc,Mag-c,*Mag-m*,MAG-P,Mag-s,*Med*,Merc,Mur-ac,*Nat-ar*,Nat-c,NAT-M,*Nat-p*,NIT-AC, Op,Ox-ac,*Petr*,Ph-ac,*Phos*,Plan,Podo,Psor,PULS,RHUS-T,*Ruta*,Sanic,Sars,Seneg,SEP,SIL,Spig, Staph,*Stram*,SULPH,Tab,Ter,*Thuj*,Tub,Uran,Verat,Verb,*Viol-t*,Zinc.

Q. 131. Intermittent fever of malaria is a ____ symptom (MD/NIH/98)
    (a)   Common
    (b)   Particular
    (c)   Local
    (d)   General

Ans. (a)

Note

Intermittent fever of malaria is a common symptom.

Also see

Aphorism 240

But if the remedy found to be the homeopathic specific for a prevalent epidemic of intermittent fever do not effect a perfect cure in some one or other patient, if it be not the influence of a marshy district that prevents the cure, it must always be the psoric miasm in the background, in which case antipsoric medicines must be employed until complete relief is obtained.

Aphorism 241

Epidemics of intermittent fever in situations where none are endemic, are of the nature of chronic diseases, composed of single acute paroxysms; each single epidemy is of a peculiar, uniform character common to all the individuals attacked, and when this character is found in the totality of the symptoms common to all, it guides us to the discovery of the homoeopathic (specific) remedy suitable for all the cases, which is almost universally serviceable in those patients who enjoyed tolerable health before the occurrence of the epidemy, that is to say, who were not chronic sufferers from developed psora.

Ref: Organon of Medicine.

Q. 132. Rubric 'Pulse' is found in the chapter (Kent's Repertory) (MD/Hydrabad/99)
    (a)   Blood
    (b)   Generalities
    (c)   Circulation
    (d)   Chest

Ans. (b)

MCQ's in Repertory

1073

Note
The rubric 'Pulse' in Kent's Repertory is found under chapter generalities.

Also see

[kent] [Generalities]Pulse:Abnormal:

3: Acon	1: Agar	1: Agn	1: Am-c	1: Am-m	1: Am
1: Ant-c	2: *Ant-t*	1: Arg-m	2: *Arg-n*	2: *Arn*	3: A
3: Ars-i	1: Asaf	1: Asar	1: Aur	1: Bar-c	3: B

2 Pulse:	4 Afternoon:
3 Abnormal:	4 Evening:
3 Audible:	4 Midnight, after:
3 Bounding:	4 Eating, after:
3 Compressible (see soft):	4 Faster than the heart beat:
3 Contracted:	4 Motion agg:
3 Double:	4 Noticing, it, when:
3 Empty:	4 Rest, during:
3 Excited:	4 Rising up, on:
3 Febrile:	4 Sitting, when:
3 Fluttering:	4 Stool, after:
3 Frequent, accelerated, elevated, exalted, fas	4 Thinking of past troubles:
4 Daytime:	4 Vexation, after:
4 Morning:	4 Warm applications, from:

Q. 133 Perineum is found in chapter ___ of Kent's Repertory (MD/Hydrabad/99)
(a) Rectum
(b) Abdomen
(c) Stool
(d) Inguinal

Ans. (a)

Note
Reference to 'perineum' is found in chapter Rectum.

Also see

[kent] [Rectum]Pulsation:Perineum:

1: Bov   2: *Caust*   1: Polyg

3 Perineum:	3 Coition, during:
2 Recedes, stool (see constipation):	3 Walking:
2 Redness of anus:	3 With urging to urinate:
2 Relaxed :	2 Straining (see tenesmus):
3 Anus:	2 Stricture:
3 Sensation of, after stool:	2 Swelling of :
2 Retraction:	3 Anus:
3 Painful:	4 Black:
3 Stool, after:	4 Menses, during:
2 Sensitive:	4 Sensation of:
2 Shock, electric-like:	3 Raphe of perineum:
3 Stool, before:	2 Tenesmus (see pain):
2 Slip back, stools (see constipation):	2 Tension:
2 Slow action of rectum (see inactivity)	3 Convulsive:
2 Spasms in:	3 Stool, after:

Q. 134. A quick, short and strong aggravation after the application of the indicated remedy (PSC/WB/91)
   (a)   > will be quick and lasting
   (b)   > will be slow and lasting
   (c)   > will be followed by <
   (d)   > will not ensue

Ans. (a)

Note

A quick, short and strong aggravation after the application of the indicated remedy will produce a quick and lasting amelioration.

Also see

Third observation of Kent's twelve observations

After administering the homeopathic remedy, there is a quick, short and strong aggravation, followed by rapid improvement of the patient. Whenever you find an aggravation coming quickly, is short in duration and has been more or less vigorous, then you will find that the improvement in the condition of the patient will be long lasting. Improvement will be marked, the reaction of the economy will be vigorous, and there is no tendency to any structural change in the vital organs. Any structural change that may be present will be found on the surface, in organs that are not vital; abscesses will form and often glands that can be done without will suppurate in regions that are not important to the life of the patient. Such organic changes are surface changes, and are not like the changes that take place in the liver, in the kidneys, in the heart and in the brain. Make a difference in your mind between organic changes that take place in the organs that are vital, that carry on the work of the economy, and organic changes that take place in structures of the body that are not essential to life. A quick, short and strong aggravation is one that is to be wished for and is followed by quick improvement. Ref: Kent's Lectures – Twelve Observations.

Q. 135. Fissure in larynx. Remedy in Kent's Repertory is_____ (MD/NIH/2000)
   (a)   Staphysagria
   (b)   Selenium metallicum
   (c)   Bufo rana
   (d)   None of the above

Ans. (c)

Note

For fissure in larynx, the remedy in Kent's Repertory is Bufo rana.

Also see

Bufo rana is the single remedy under this rubric in Kent's Repertory.

```
[kent ] [Larynx and Trachea]Fissures in larynx:

1: Bufo

2 Fissures in larynx:                        3 Larynx:
2 Flapping sensation,larynx:                 3 Trachea:
2 Flesh hanging in larynx,sensation o       2 Hemming (see scraping):
2 Food drops into larynx:                    2 Hoarseness (see voice):
2 Foreign substance,sensation,larynx        2 Inflammation :
3 Morning:                                   3 Larynx:
3 Behind larynx:                             4 Evening agg:
3 Trachea:                                   4 Damp weather:
2 Foreign substances drop in larynx w       4 Gangrenous:
2 Fullness,larynx:                           4 Heated,from getting:
3 Morning:                                   4 Recurrent:
3 Evening:                                   4 Singers,in:
2 Grasped (see constriction):                4 Speakers,in:
2 Hair,in trachea,sensation of:              4 Suppressed urticaria:
2 Heat :                                     4 Syphilitic:
```

MCQ's in Repertory

Q. 136. Repertory of causation was published by (MD/NIH/98):
  (a) Bhardwaj
  (b) Curie
  (c) Lutze
  (d) Dr Sarkar

Ans. (a)

Repertory of causation was published by Bhardwaj.

Note

Curie:
- Repertory by P.F. Curie 1906 (A Regional Repertory)

Lutze:
- Repertory of Respiratory Organs by Lutze 1880

Dr Sarkar:
- Repertory by Sarkar 1906

Q. 137. Epileptic convulsions are found in which chapter of Kent's Repertory___.(MD/NIH/(98)
  (a) Extremities
  (b) Generalities
  (c) Abdomen
  (d) Back

Ans. (b)

Note

Rubric 'Epileptic convulsions' are found in the chapter Generalities of Kent's Repertory.

Also see

[kent] [Generalities]Convulsions:Epileptic:
Absin,Acet-ac,Aeth,Agar,Alum,Am-c,Anac,ARG-M,ARG-N,Ars,Art-v,Aster,Bar-c,BAR-M,Bell,BUFO, CALC-AR,Calc-p,Calc-s,Camph,Cann-i,Canth,Carb-an,Carbn-s,Carb-v,CAUST,Cedr,Chin,Chin-s,Cic, Cocc,Con,Crot-c,Crot-h,CUPR,Cupr-ar,Cur,Dig,Form,Gels,Glon,Hell,Hydr-ac,HYOS,Ign,Indg,Iod, Kali-c,Kali-chl,Kali-s,Lach,Laur,Lyc,Lyss,Mag-c,Mag-p,Med,Merc,Mosch,Naja,Nat-m,Nat-s,Nit-ac, Nux-v,OENA,Op,Ph-ac,Phos,Plat,PLB,Psor,Puls,Ran-b,Sec,Sep,SIL,Stann,Staph,Stram,Stry, Syph,Tab,Tarent,Verat,Vip,VISC,

Ref: Kent's Repertory

Q. 138. Patel's Auto-visual Repertory is _____ repertory (MD/NIH/2001)
  (a) Mechanically aided
  (b) Card
  (c) Book
  (d) Computer

Ans. (a)

Note

Patel's Auto-visual repertory is mechanically aided repertory.
Ref: Essentials of Repertorization, by Dr S. K. Tiwari, page 23, second revised and enlarged edition.

Q. 139. 'Delayed talking' is found under which chapter of Kent's Repertory (MD/NIH/98)
  (a) Mind
  (b) Mouth
  (c) Generalities
  (d) Throat

Ans. (a)

Note

'Delayed talking' is found under the chapter Mind in Kent's Repertory.

Also see

[kent][Mind]Talk:Slow learning. to:

1: Agar   1: Bar-c   1: Calc-p   1: Nat-m   1: Nux-m   1: Sanic

Q. 140. If no improvement follows after the administration of a strictly homeopathically selected remedy___(PSC/WB/91)
   (a) Change the remedy instantaneously
   (b) Repeat a fresh and small dose of the same medicine
   (c) Change the potency of the remedy
   (d) Administer a complementary drug

Ans. (c)

Note

In the above situation, change the potency of the remedy.

Also see

If no improvement follows after the administration of a strictly homeopathically selected remedy, the medicine was not similar enough to the patient's illness to have a therapeutic effect. The best aspect here is that the medicine is 'simillimum' then only one possibility remains that the patient is not susceptible to the potency prescribed – therefore, the best next option remains is to change the potency of the remedy.

Q.141. Repertory of 'Sensation As If' published by (MD/NIH/98)
   (a) Dr H.A. Roberts
   (b) W.J. Guernsey
   (c) H.C. Allen
   (d) W.A. Allen

Ans. (a)

Note

Repertory of 'Sensation As If' was authored by Dr H.A. Roberts.

Also see

Sensations As If – A Repertory of Subjective Symptoms, by Herbert A. Robrets, MD, in 1937.

Ref: Essentials of Repertorization, by Dr S. K. Tiwari, page 23, second revised and enlarged edition.
http://www.homeoint.org/books1/robertsasif/neck.htm

Q.142. 'Repertory of the More Characteristic Symptoms of the Materia Medica' was published by (MD/NIH/98)*
   (a) C. Lippe
   (b) C.B. Knerr
   (c) N. M. Chowdhury
   (d) Nash

Ans. (a)

Note

'Repertory of the More Characteristic Symptoms of the Materia Medica' was published by C. Lippe.

Also see

It was published in 1879 and it contained about 332 pages.

Ref: Essentials of Repertorization, by Dr S. K. Tiwari, page 20, second revised enlarged edition.

Q.143. 'Impaired' is found under chapter of _____ Boenninghausen's Therapeutic Pocket Book (MD/NIH/2000)
    (a)   Mind
    (b)   Intellect
    (c)   Sensation
    (d)   Circulation

Ans. (b)

Note

'Impaired' in found under chapter Intellect of BTPB.
Ref: BTPB, Part II, Page 22, B. Jain Publishers, edition 1994.

Also see

Boenninghausen's Therapeutic Pocket Book has seven main chapters:
(1) Mind and Intellect (oldest edition gives it as Mind and Soul).
(2) Parts of the Body and Organs.
(3) Sensations and Complaints:
    (i) In General
    (ii) Of Glands
    (iii) Of Bones
    (iv) Of Skin
(4) Sleep and Dreams
(5) Fever:
    (i) Circulation of Blood
    (ii) Cold Stage
    (iii) Coldness
    (iv) Heat
    (v) Perspitation
    (vi) Compound Fevers
    (vii) Concomitant Complaints
(6) Alterations of the State of Health:
    (i) Aggravation According to Time
    (ii) Aggravation According to Situations and Circumstances
    (iii) Amelioraiton by Position and Circumstances
(7) Relationship of Remedies.
Ref: BTPB, B. Jain Publishers, part-I, page 27, edition 1994.

Q. 144. Boenninghausen's Therapeutic Pocket Book published in the year _____ (MD/NIH/2000)
    (a)   1832
    (b)   1830
    (c)   1836
    (d)   1846

Ans. (b)

Note

BTPB was published in the year 1846.

Also see

Boenninghausen's Therapeutic Pocket Book was published in the year of 1846.
Ref: Essentials of Repertorization, by Shashi Kant Tiwari, page 26, second revised and enlarged Edition.

Q. 145. Which one is the first repertory of Hahnemann_____ (MD/NIH/2000)
    (a)   Fregmenta de viribus
    (b)   Fregmenta de viribus medica mention
    (c)   Fregmenta de viribus medicamentorum positivus
    (d)   None of the above

Ans. (c)

From the choices given above, the first repertory of Hahnemann was 'Fragmenta de viribus Medicamentorum positivus.'

Aphorism 109

I was the first that opened up this path, which I have pursued with a perseverance that could only arise and be kept up by a perfect conviction of the great truth, fraught with such blessings to humanity, that it is only by the homoeopathic employment of medicines[1] that the certain cure of human maladies is possible.[2]

1. It is impossible that there can be another true, best method of curing dynamic diseases (i.e., all diseases not strictly surgical) besides homoeopathy, just as it is impossible to draw more than one straight line betwixt two given points. He who imagines that there are other modes of curing diseases besides it could not have appreciated homoeopathy fundamentally nor practised it with sufficient care, nor could he ever have seen or read cases of properly performed homoeopathic cures; nor, on the other hand, could he have discerned the baselessness of all allopathic modes of treating diseases and their bad or even dreadful effects, if, with such lax indifference, he places the only true healing art on an equality with those hurtful methods of treatment, or alleges the latter to be auxiliaries to homoeopathy which it could not do without! My true, conscientious followers, the pure homoeopathists, with their successful, almost never-failing treatment, might teach these persons better.

2. The first fruits of these labors, as perfect as they could be at that time, I recorded in the Fragmenta de viribus medicamentorum positivis, sive in sano corpore humano observatis, pts. I, ii, Lipsiae, 8, 1805, ap. J. A. Barth; the more mature fruits in the Reine Arzneimittellebre, I Th., dritte Ausg.; II Th., dritte Ausg., 1833; III Th., zweite Ausg., 1825; IV Th., zw. Ausg., 1827 (English translation, Materia Medica Pura, vols i and ii); and in the second, third, and fourth parts of Die chronischen Krankheiten, 1828, 1830, Dresden bei Arnold (2nd edit., with a fifth part, Dusseldorf bei Schaub, 1835, 1839).

Also see

FRAGMENTA DE VIRIBUS

The First Materia Medica and Repertory of Homoeopathy
(Fragmentary observation relative to the positive powers of medicine on the human body)

Fragmenta de viribus as it is most popularly called was one of the first attempts made by Dr Samuel Hahnemann in the direction of a proper materia medica. This work was merely a glimpse of what was to come. It contained the accounts of his first provings, of homeopathic medicines. It was THE PRECURSOR, the forerunner of Homeopathic Materia Medica. It was written in LATIN language and was published in 1805. Publishers were M/S Sumpter Joan Ambrose Barthii of Leipzig.

It was in two volumes:

(i)   The first volume was published in 1805. It was called PARS PRIMA. It had 277 pages comprising of Introduction and the main text of the book.

(ii)   The second volume was the Repertory or Index. It was called PARS SECUNDA. It had 476 pages comprising of Preface and a Repertory of 460 pages.

    In the later editions, the two parts were combined in one volume. In 1834 Dr F.F. Quin, the erstwhile father of British Homoeopathy, called for this book and published it in one volume from London.
    Ref: http://www.homeorizon.com/mainpagegeneral.asp?t=fragmenta.htm#page%20top

Q. 146. 'Carphology' is found under chapter_____ of Boger Boenninghausen's Characteristics and Repertory (MD/Hydrabad/99)
    (a)   Mind
    (b)   Sensation
    (c)   Extremities
    (d)   Generalities

Ans. (b)

Note

'Carphology' is found under chapter Sensation of BBCR Repertory.
Ref: BBCR, page 886, 1990 edition, by B. Jain Publishers.

Q. 147. Kent's Repertory was published in the year____ (MD/NIH/2000)
    (a)   1896
    (b)   1897
    (c)   1899
    (d)   1888

Ans. (b)

Note

Kent's Repertory was published in the year 1897.

Also see

During the last quarter of the nineteenth century, the area of repertory become overcrowded with an unusually large number of repertories of different kinds. This created chaos and confusion in the profession, and prepared a suitable ground for the emergence of a repertory, well organized, systematically planned, and based on a sound philosophy. This was successfully accomplished by Kent in 1897.

Ref: Repertorization Principles and Practice, by Dr S.K. Tiwary, page 20, 21, second revised and enlarged edition.

Extended information

Land marks of Kent's Repertory.

First edition – 1897, it was published in sections and was compiled in 1899.

Second edition – 1908.

Third edition –1916, Dr Kent passed away in the year 1916.

Fourth edition – 1935, published by Dr Ethrhart with the help of Dr Gladvin and Dr J.S. Pugh.

Fifth edition – 1945.

Sixth edition – 1957, the American edition, 1961 Indian edition.

Seventh edition – Dr P. Schmiath combined the Indian edition and American edition (generally called as revised first edition).

Ref: Kent's Repertory – A Comprehensive Study, Dr Sanchoo Balachandran BHMS, MD (Hom), Calicut, Kerala.

http://www.similima.com/Rep31.html

Q. 148. Which symptom is given higher value in Kent's method of repertorisation_____(MD/NIH/2000)
    (a)   Constipation before or during menses
    (b)   Perspiration >
    (c)   Craving sweets
    (d)   Industrious

Ans. (c)

From the choice of symptoms listed above, 'Craving sweets' needs to be given higher value in Kent's method of repertorization.

Note

Treat the patient as a whole, and the symptoms are broken into following areas with grading attached to them:

(1) *Mental Generals*: They have attached value in decling order:
    (a) Love, hates.
    (b) Intellect.
    (c) Memory.

(2) *Physical generals:* their order of significance / values is as:
    (a) Related to blood, colour of discharge, aversions and cravings.
    (b) Menstrual functions (general aggravations related to menses, the character of menses).
    (c) Environmental factors.

(3) *Particular symptoms:* Has the following order of value in decling order:
    (a) Peculiar or unusual symptoms.
    (b) Discharges.
    (c) Modalities.

(4) *Common symptoms:* Their significane is least. These may be given 'importance' if they are absent or intensified.

Also see

The enlisted symptoms in MCQ are analysed and evaluated in in reference to their symptom classification according to the Kent's method and they are as under:

Symptom	Symptom Domain	Value
(a) Constipation before or during menses	Particular general	Low
(b) Perspiration >	Physical general	Medium
(c) Craving sweets	Mental general	High
(d) Ihdustrious	Mental general	Medium

Q. 149. Anaemia is found under chapter _____ of Boger Boenninghausen's Characteristics and Repertory (MD/NIH/2000)
    (a) Circulation
    (b) Blood
    (c) Generalities
    (d) Sensation

Ans. (a)

Note
Anaemia is found under chaper Circulaiton of BBCR.

Also see
BBCR- Circulaiton- Palpitation, Anaemia in.
Ref: BBCR, page 1009, 1990 edition, B. Jain Publishers.

However, we can have an insight into two commonly available and currently used repertories which bear the name of Dr Boenninghausen:
    (a) Theraputic Pocket Book
    (b) Boenninghausen's Characteristic Materia Medica and Repertory, by C.M. Boger:
        There are seven basic Chapters in this repertory. However, these are parts of the body which are further divided into further chapters, including which, the total chapters comes to 57.
    Ref: Essentials of Repertorization, by Shashi Kant Tiwari

Q. 150. Which medicine is found under the rubric 'Benevolence' in Kent's Repertory (MD/NIH/2000)
   (a) Coffea cruda
   (b) Aconitum napellus
   (c) Belladonna
   (d) None of the above

Ans. (a)

Note
Coffea cruda is the remedy found under the rubric 'Benevolence' in Kent's Repertory.

Q. 151. Repertory of Mastitis is written by _____ (MD/NIH/2000):
   (a) Lippe
   (b) Minton
   (c) Guernsey
   (d) None of the above

Ans. (c)

Repertory of Mastitis is written by W.J. Guernsey.

Note
Repertory to the Modalities in Their Relations to Temprature, Air, Water, Winds, Weather and Seasons, By Samuel Worcester.

Introduction:
The above repertory is based on 'Hering's Condensed Materia Medica.' This book was originally compiled to meet a want felt in daily practice by the author so he can decide upon indicated remedy in a few moments, while, without it, a longer search would have been required. This book was originally complied in 1880, and the first Indian edition was published in 1968.

The Construction:
This Repertory is arranged on a different plane. In nearly every instance the exact language of the patient has been given together with associated symptoms thus enabling a more careful discrimination to be made. The starred (*) symptoms are those regarded as characteristic by at least two of the eminent authors.
The repertory has fifteen chapters with sections in each.
Ref: Reperire, by Pro Dr Vidyadhar R. Khanaj, page 917, fourth revised edition.

Also see
Era of Regional Repertories (1880 - 1900)
Many of them were clinical repertories. Important among are:
   a. Repertory of Fever by H.C. Allen (1880).
   b. Sensation, As If by H.A.Roberts.
   c. Repertory of Modalities by Worcester.
   d. Repertory of Intermittent Fever by W.A.Allen.
   e. Repertory of Haemorrhoids by Guernsey.
   f. Rheumatism by Porlunins (1894).
   g. Repertory of Urinary Organs by Morgan (1899).
   h. Repertory of Back by Wilsy (1900).
   i. Repertory of Uterine Therapeutics by Minton (1906).
   j. Repertory of Diarrhoea by Bell.
   k. Repertory part of Raue's Special Pathology (1906).
   l. Repertory by Boericke.
   m. Clarke's clinical repertory.
   n. Repertory of Mastitis by W.J. Guernesy.
Ref: History and Evaluation of Repertory, by Dr K.R. Mansoor Ali.

Q.152. Tinnitus aurium, while lying down, without any defect in that organ is _____ Case Taking and Repertorisation
  (a) A common particular symptom
  (b) A common general symptom
  (c) A peculiar particular symptom
  (d) A peculiar general symptom

Ans. (c)

Tinnutus aurium, while lying down, without any defect in that organ is a peculiar particular symptom.

Note

Kent treats patient as a whole, and the symptoms are broken into following areas with grading attached to them:

  (1) *Mental generals:* They have attached value in decling order:
      (a) Love, hates.
      (b) Intellect.
      (c) Memory.
  (2) *Physical generals:* Their order of significance / values is as:
      (a) Related to blood, colour of discharge, aversions and cravings.
      (b) Menstrual functions (general aggravations related to menses, the character of menses).
      (c) Environmental factors.
  (3) *Particular symptoms:* Has the following order of value in decling order:
      (a) Peculiar or unusual symptoms.
      (b) Discharges.
      (c) Modalities.
  (4) *Common symptoms:* Their significane is least: These may be given importance if they they are absent or intensified.

Q. 153. Pick out the odd one. (MD/NIH/2000)
  (a) Clarke's Repertory
  (b) Kent's Repertory
  (c) Repertory of Intermittent Fever
  (d) Boger's Repertory

Ans. (c)

From the choice given above, the odd one is Repertory of Intermittent Fever.

Note

The Repertory of Intermittent Fever is the odd one and belongs to 'regional / clinical orientation as compared to the all others, which are general repertories.

Q. 154. Sweat on sternum in Kent's Repertory is _____ (MD/BBSR/1999)
  (a) Graphites
  (b) Acidum muriaticum
  (c) Aconitum napellus
  (d) All of the above

Ans. (c)

From the choice of drugs given above, sweat on sturnum in Kent's Repertory is covered by 'Graphites'.

Note

[kent] [Chest] Perspiration:Sternum:
3: Graph

MCQ's in Repertory

Q. 155. Medicine under rubric 'wart on sternum' in Kent's Repertory is_____ (MD/BBSR/99)
    (a)   Nitricum acidum
    (b)   Acidum muriaticum
    (c)   Aconitum napellus
    (d)   Bryonia alba

Ans. (a)
Medicine under rubric 'wart on sternum' in Kent's Repertory is Nitricum acidum.

Note

```
[kent] [Chest] Warts, on sternum:

1: Nit-ac

2 Warmth, sensation of:           3 Cough:
 3 About the heart:                4 From:
2 Warts, on sternum:               4 Impeding:
2 Water :                          4 Menses, before:
 3 Drops, cold, were falling from the heart, sen   3 Eating, while:
 3 Boiling, was poured into chest, sensation       3 Exertion, after:
 3 Sensation of:                   3 Expectoration, after:
  4 In:                            3 Lying :
  4 Hot, in:                        4 Amel:
2 Weakness:                         4 On side:
 3 Morning on waking:              3 Reading:
  4 Lasting until 3 p.m.:           4 Agg:
 3 Evening:                         4 Aloud:
  4 While lying:                   3 Respiration, deep:
 3 Bending forward amel:           3 Singing:
```

Q. 156. Medicine for 'Aura begins from heart', in Kent's Repertory is _____ (MD/Hydrabad/99)
    (a)   Calcarea arsenicosa
    (b)   Lachesis mutus
    (c)   Bufo rana
    (d)   Naja tripudians

Ans. (a)
Note
Medicine for 'Aura begins from heart', in Kent's repertory is Calcarea arsenicosa.

Also see
Aura begans from heart, in Kent's Repertory is Calcarea arsenicosa. However, there are two more medicines also–Lachesis mutus and Naja tripudians, but they are represented in the lowest grade.

Extended Informationa

[kent] [Generalities]Convulsions:Epileptic:Aura:Heart,from:

3: Calc-ar   1: Lach   1: Naja

3 Epileptic:	5 Numbness of brain:
4 Aura:	5 Shocks:
5 Abdomen to head,with:	5 Solar plexus,from:
5 Arms,in:	5 Uterus:
5 Cold air over spine and body:	5 Uterus to throat:
5 Coldness running down spine:	5 Warm air streaming up spine:
5 Coldness on left side before epilepsy:	5 Waving sensation in brain:
5 Drawing in limbs:	3 Epileptiform:
5 Expansion of body,sensation of,before:	3 Errors in diet:
5 General nervous feeling:	3 Eructations amel:
5 Heart,from:	3 Eruptions fail to break out,when:
5 Heel to occiput,right:	3 Exanthemata repelled or do not appear,wl
5 Jerk in nape:	3 Excitement,from:
5 Knees:	3 Exertion,after:
5 Mouse,running like a:	3 Extension of body,forcible,amel:

Bibliography

Books
Repertory of the Homeopathic Materia Medica – Dr. Kent. – B. Jain Publishers (P) Ltd., New Delhi.
Synthetic Repertory – B. Jain Publishers (P) Ltd., New Delhi.
Repertory- BBCR – B. Jain Publishers (P) Ltd., New Delhi.
Therapeutic Pocket Book (BTPB) – B. Jain Publishers (P) Ltd., New Delhi.
A Concise Repertory of Hom. Medicine – Dr. Phatak – B. Jain Publishers (P) Ltd., New Delhi.
Organon Of Medicine – 5th & 6th Ed. – B. Jain Publishers (P) Ltd., New Delhi.
Essentials of Repertorizaton 3rd Edition By Dr. Shashi Kant Tiwari – B. Jain Publishers (P) Ltd., New Delhi.
Repertory of Hering's Guiding Symptoms by Calvin B Knerr – B. Jain Publishers (P) Ltd., New Delhi.
Text Book of Homeopathic Repertory – Dr. Niranjan Mohanty 1st Edition – B. Jain Publishers (P) Ltd., New Delhi.

Websites
www.similima.com

Softwares
RADAR

Chapter 13
QUESTION PAPER
UPSC 2001 (HOMEOPATHY)

Time allocated: 2 Hours **Maximum Mark: 100**
Instructions:
1. All answers must be written in English.
2. This paper consists of 12 Questions in two groups viz. A & B.
3. Attempt any 10 questions taking, however, at least 5 questions from each group.
4. Answer must be brief and to the point.

Group –A

Q. 1. Discuss the difficulties in handling a chronic case. (10)

Ans.
Difficulties involved in taking chronic case:
a) The chronic complaints become part of life and patient may be so acclimatized to these that he fails to communicate them to the physician.
b) Some of the patient does not have the idea of relative significance of their problems, so they give only partial information about the suffering; at times due to chronic long suffering they take then casually.
c) Due to modesty many patients do not communicate to physician or when communicate they put them in vague manner.
d) The concomitant or accessory symptoms, which is important for the homeopaths. However, patients past experience with allopathic physician has just opposite that they ignore the finer details. This preconditions them to ignore these symptoms and therefore, patient fails to mention about these.
e) At times the physician has drawbacks; i.e., he may lack in tact, knowledge of human nature, and patience.

Points of significance in a chronic case:
a) Take particular note of the family H/O and Past H/O to explore the miasmatic background of the patient, and also current predominant miasmatic state, but avoid a very direct question.
b) Delineate the maintaining and exciting cause especially in chronic cases; by exploring the lifestyle of the patient.

Q. 2. What do you mean by 'Constitution' in Homeopathy? Describe in short its various components. (3+7)

Ans.
Definition:
"Constitution is that aggregate of hereditary character, influenced more or less by environment, which determines the individual's reaction, successful or unsuccessful, to the stress of environment". Stuart Close

Constitution is a term, which covers vast dimensions in width depth and intricacy, but it is often inadequately understood. It has two basic factors:
(a) The Endogenous factor
(b) The Exogenous factor

The endogenous factors are innate in the individual incurred from the heredity. They endow the organism with various types of tendencies, susceptibilities, and reaction to the stress of environment.

The exogenous factors are incurred gradually and steadily since birth from the various intimate details of the environmental factors.

Constitution consists of various factors. The brief are:
- (i) Physical make-up of the body
- (ii) Temperament
- (iii) Heat and cold relation
- (iv) Desire and aversion to food
- (v) Predominant miasm
- (vi) Diathesis
- (vii) Susceptibility and responses
- (viii) Addictions, habits, etc.

It also includes all other factors that work in his framing and that make him distinct, definite and different and thus separate from other persons.

Therapeutic Importance:

It has been noticed that every individual drug has a special relative affinity for particular type of constitution. This fact was clearly noticed by Hahnemann while conducting drug proving as well as in his practice.

Types of Constitution

Miasmatic view of constitution:

This classification is based on the puritan miasmatic philosophical base, and on the cardinal clinical manifestations. Traditionally the miasmatic point of view the constitutional disorders are divisible into three main clusters.

1. The Psoric Constitution type:
    a. These are eccentric, philosopher, imaginative.
    b. He is very active, unable to sit still, in one place, starts every work hastily, never satisfied, and all the time formulating new ideas.
    c. Usually their Somatotype is Ectomorphic.
    d. They are prone to itch.
    e. The pathological changes are always reversible.

2. The Sycotic Constitution:
    a. These are mischief oriented beasts.
    b. Full of vitality, has a good memory, and is a bid egoist.
    c. He is intelligent, uncontrolled wild.
    d. Their Somatotype is endomorphic.
    e. Short torso.
    f. These are prone to develop cauliflower like growth on skin.
    g. These ultimately develop growths and tumors.

3. The Syphilitic Constitution:
    a. Low mental IQ or dull. Learns slowly, never takes rapid fire decisions.
    b. He is slow and never in hurry to get anywhere.
    c. They can belong to any somatotype.
    d. Physically they develop deformities and destructions.

Von Grauvogl's Classification of Constitution:

Von Grauvogl arranged the constitutions according to the excess or deficiency of certain elements in the tissue and blood.

The Carbo-Nitrogenoid Constitution:

An excess of Carbon and Nitrogen characterizes it. The Carbo-Nitrogenoid constitution is Hahnemann's Psoric Miasmatic Type.

Examples of the drugs are as:
- a. Sulphur

b. Psorinum.
c. Graphitis.

The Hydrogenoid Constitution:
It is characterized by an excess of Hydrogen and consequently of water in blood and tissues.
The Hydrogenoid constitution corresponds very closely to the Hahnemann's Sycotic Miasmatic Type.
> It covers a much wider area and is not by any means confined to the acquired or inherited results of gonorrhoeal infection.
> Example of drugs:
> a. Thuja occidentalis
> b. Antimonium crudum

The Oxygenoid Constitution:
> It is characterized by an excess of Oxygen, or at least by an exaggerated influence of Oxygen in the organism, this constitution corresponds to the Hahnemann's Syphilitic Miasmatic Type.
> Example of the drugs:
> a. Syphilinum
> b. Mercurius solubilis

There are different types of Constitution, which are carried into homeopathic parlance from old-time pathology. Some of them are:-

I. Scrofulous constitution- Glands remain swollen, general weakness, lack of reaction, wound and inflammations tardy to heal, considered being the result of hereditary combination of Psora and Syphilis.

II. Leucophlegmatic Constitution-Catarrhal, flabby, water-logged constitution, with pale loose skin. Sluggish in all movements and activities. Chilly and susceptible to cold.

Q. 3. Explain the complete process of trituration according to clinical scale. (10)

Ans.
There is no clinical scale however it is probably a typographical mistake for centesimal scale.

TRITURATION

The main object of trituration is to reduce the size of the particles of a a crude medicinal substance to a finer degree and to homogeneously mix them with the vehicle.

Decimal Scale Trituration:
The decimal scale trituration is conducted by adding one part of the drug substance to nine parts of vehicle, milk sugar. (Thus the ratio is 1:10). Take one gramme of the drug substance in a thin porcelain or agate mortar and add to it three grammes of vehicle (1/3 of the total of grammes) and rub it with stage crystal pestle in the mortar for six minutes. Scrape it with a spatula for three minutes and mix it for one minute, thus consuming ten minutes of the process.

The same process of rubbing for six minutes, scraping for three minutes and mixing for one minute is carried out to consume further ten minutes of the process. This complete twenty minutes of the process. Repeat the process by adding next three grammes of the vehicle and complete adding next three grammes of the vehicle and complete adding the second twenty minutes. Repeat the process by adding the last three grammes of the vehicle and working with it for another twenty minutes. Thus it completes one hour of trituration. This thoroughly pulverised and homogeneously mixed preparation has attained the first degree of decimal potency known as 1x, or 1D.

Centesimal Scale Trituration:
An identical process is conduction with one gramme of drug substance and thirty three grammes of milk sugar, at every step of twenty minutes of trituration, adding the second one-third and the third one-third of vehicle to raise the potency by one degree known as 1C

Q. 4. Write the importance of different types of symptoms in Homeopathy. (10)

Ans.
General Symptoms
All sensations or symptoms to which patient uses the first personal pronoun – are general symptoms, e.g., I am weak; I am thirsty etc. These are the symptoms referring to the person as a whole. These include:

(a) **Mental Generals:**
Symptoms referring to mental sphere are classed as mental generals because they reflect the inner self and individuality of the patient.

(b) **Physical generals:**
Symptoms referring to the body as a whole with regard to various physical circumstances etc. It includes-
  I. General Modalities: - Aggravations and Amelioration applying to the patient as a whole.
  II. Hunger/appetite and thirst.
  III. Carving, aversion and intolerance to any food.
  IV. Sleep and Dreams.
  V. Sex Male and Female: Menstruation: - It is so closely related to the whole woman that it becomes a general. The woman says " I menstruate", so and so. She does not attribute it to her ovaries or to her uterus. Her state is, as a rule different when she is menstruating and the whole economy is involved in this matter.
  VI. Tendency to affect a particular side or in a particular direction e.g. Right side - Lyco., Bell., Apis; Left side- Lach., Thuj., Phos. Alternating siders - Lac.-c. Diagonal – Agar., Tarax. and so on.
  VII. Symptoms relating special senses having no pathological condition: - The special senses are often so closely related to the whole man that many of their symptoms are general.

Examples:
Various odorous make sick, the smell of food sickens, or over sensitiveness to sounds, noise, light etc. But if he only experiences a subjective offensive smell in the nose due to some pathological condition, this would merely relate to one organ and consequently would be only particular.

(c) **Particular Symptoms**
Definition-Symptoms which are related to a particular part or organ of the organism are known as particular symptoms.
This term was used by J.T. Kent who comments, "all the things that are predicated of any given organ, are things in particular. If you examine any part alone, you are only examining the particulars."
Example: Headache, sneezing, coated tongue, infected conjunctiva, photophobia, swelling of a single joint etc.
Importance
  1. Helpful in the diagnosis of disease.
  2. These are less important in the selection of Homeopathic remedy.

(d) **Common Symptoms**
Definition: - Common symptoms are those that are found in many patients, in many ailments, and are produced by the proving of many medicines.

Examples:
  I. Common symptoms of disease:- Rash in measles, dragging down sensation in prolapse, stitching pain in chest and rusty expectoration in pneumonia, rice-watery stool and vomiting in cholera, and so on. These are the pathognomonic symptoms of the disease.
  II. Common symptoms of medicine: Diarrhea, fever, loss of appetite, headache, sweat, cough, flatulence, lameness, congestion, swelling etc.

Importance:
  I. It is important for disease diagnosis.
  II. It has no value in homeopathic remedy selection.
  III. In homeopathic prescription it is useful only for palliative treatment, judging the curability of the case, advising diet, management etc.
  IV. It is very important to allopathic physician for treatment because the diagnosis of disease is the only basis of their therapeutics.

(e) **Uncommon, Peculiar Symptoms**
This second group of symptoms is known as uncommon and peculiar symptoms. Those symptoms are uncountable, unexplainable, absurd or paradoxical (contrary to our usual expectations from physiological

and/or pathological point of view). These symptoms are found in few patients and in the provings of few medicines.

Significance:

No two persons are ever alike, be in health or disease. As every man is unique by reason of his individuality, his reactions to the same disease-cause also vary, though suffering from the same disease from the nosological point of view. Hence symptoms vary from individual to individual.

Examples
1) High fever with refusal to uncover.
2) Cold skin with aversion to eat and covering.
3) Dropsy with intense thirst.
4) Palpitation relieved by excertion.
5) Coryza relieved by cold bath.
6) Burning relieved by heat.
7) Moist tongue with great thirst.
8) Dry tongue without thirst.
9) Thirst during chill, no thirst during fever.
10) Pain in different parts of body during coughing.

This type of symptom helps us in individualizing a particular case from others suffering from the same disease. Thus, they are indispensable for selecting homeopathic remedy (i.e. for therapeutic diagnosis).

(f) Concomitant Symptoms

This is a term used with a special significance in homeopathic parlance. It is an innovation of Von Boenninghausen. The word 'Concomitant' means existing or occurring together, attendant.

Definition:

Con (along with) comitant (present) symptoms are those apparently unrelated groups of symptoms present along with the disease symptoms. These groups of symptoms can not be explained on physiological and/or pathological grounds, and yet they exist at the same time in the same individual with the group of symptoms which can be so explained.

This highly valuable doctrine of Boenninghausen has been clearly expounded by Dr. H.A.Roberts in his introduction of the "Therapeutic Pocket Book". According to Dr. Roberts "The concomitant symptoms is to the totality what the conditions of aggravation and amelioration is to the single symptom. It is the differentiating factor".

Example:
(1) Involuntary passage of urine while coughing with pain in hip exp. left-points definitely to Causticum.
(2) Polyuria with coryza, points to Calcerea carbonica.
(3) Pain at distant parts of body while coughing e.g., bladder, legs ears etc- points of Capsicum.

Significance

Each of the symptoms isolately, may be of very common value. But their co-existence definitely characterizes each other and clearly individualizes the totality of the symptoms of the case or drug.

They have no value for disease diagnosis but very important for individualizing patients and drugs. Thus they are important for homeopathic therapeutic diagnosis (i.e. for selecting the remedy homeopathically).

(g) Clinical Symptoms
Definition:

Clinical symptoms are those which do not appear in the proving of a drug, but which were observed as appearing and which were observed disappearing after the administration of the drug in sick persons. These symptoms are to be distinguished from those produced after proving of drugs on healthy human beings which constitute the bulk of the Homeopathic Materia Medica. Dr. Richard Hughes of Britain and his disciples were against the inclusion of these symptoms in Homeopathy. First of all Dr. Constantine Hering of USA incorporated these symptoms in our Materia Medica.

Example:
The pleurisy and pleural pain of Bryonia were not at all marked in the proving, but when Bryonia was given for other symptoms, it was found that Bryonia regularly relieved affections of the pleura, so much so that, undoubtedly, it is the most important drug in these cases. Later on, in animal work it was found that Bryonia readily produces pleurisy.

Importance:
1) These symptoms have lesser importance than the proving symptoms. Its utility is more in acute disease, acute condition of chronic disease and palliative treatment. It has no use in disease diagnosis. (When homeopathic concept of clinical symptom is considered)
2) It helps in the diagnosis of disease when allopathic concept of clinical symptoms is considered.

Q. 5. Write the characteristic symptoms of the following medicines in short (10)
   a. Phosphorus
   b. Sabina
   c. Thuja occidentalis
   d. Kreosotum
   e. Carbolicum acidum

Ans.
a. Phosphorus:
Constitution:
Adapted to tall slender persons of sanguine temperament, fair skin, delicate eyelashes, fine blond, or red hair, quick perception, and very sensitive nature
Young people, who grow too rapidly, are inclined to stoop; who are chlorite or an anemic; old people, with morning diarrhea.
Over-sensitive to all senses to external impressions, light, noise, odors, touch.
Restless fidgety; moves continually, cannot sit or stand still a moment.

Characteristics:
Suddenness of symptoms, sudden prostration, faints, sweats, shooting pains, etc.
Burning in spots.
Hemorrhagic diathesis.
Great weakness and prostration.

Pain:
Acute especially in the chest, aggravated from pressure, even slight, in intercostal spaces, and lying on left side, excited by slightest chill; open air intolerable.
A weak empty, all gone sensation in head, chest, stomach,

Apathetic; unwilling to talk, answers slowly, moves sluggishly.
Eyes; hallow, surrounded by blue rings, lids, puffy, swollen, and edematous.

Desire:
Cold food, and drinks; juicy, refreshing things; ice cream ameliorates gastric pains.
As soon as water becomes warm in stomach it is thrown out.
Heaviness of chest, as if a weight were lying on it.
Perspiration has the odour of sulphur

Modality:
Aggravation:
Evening, before midnight, lying on left or painful side; during the thunderstorm; weather changes, either hot or cold. cold air relieves the head and face symptoms, but aggravates those of chest, throat and neck.

Amelioration:
In the dark, lying on right side, from being rubbed or mesmerized; from cold, cold water, until it gets warm.

b. Sabina:

Constitution:
Females who are predisposed to chronic ailments i.e., arthritic pains; tendency to miscarriages, especially at third month.

Causation:
Ailments; following abortion or premature labor;

Characteristics:
Music is intolerable; produces, nervousness, goes through bone and marrow.
Drawing pains in small of back, from sacrum to pubes in nearly all diseases.
Hemorrhage from the uterus; flow partly pale red, partly clotted; worse from least motion; often relieved by walking; pains extends from sacrum to pubis.
Menses; too early, too profuse, too protracted; partly fluid; partly clotted; in persons who menstruated very early in life; flow in paroxysms; with colic and labor like pains; pains from sacrum to pubes.
Discharge of blood between periods, with sexual excitement.
Retained placenta from atony of uterus; intense after pains.
Menorrhagia; during climacteric, in women who formerly aborted; with early first menses. (Precocious puberty).
Promotes expulsion of moles or foreign bodies from uterus.
Fig-warts with intolerable itching and burning; exuberant granulations.

Modalities:
Aggravation; from least motion; warm air or room.
Amelioration; in cool, open, fresh air.

c. Thuja occidentalis

Constitution:
Best adapted to hydrogenoid constitution; very fleshy persons, dark complexion, black hair, unhealthy skin.

Causation:
Ailments from bad effects of vaccination.

Characteristics:
Fixed ideas; as if a strange person was at his side; as if soul and body was separated; as if a living animal were in abdomen; of being under the influence of a superior power.
Vertigo, when closing the eyes.
Piles swollen pain most severe when sitting.
Coition prevented by extreme sensitiveness of the vagina.
Skin look dirty; brown or brownish-white spots here and there; warts, large, seedy, pedunculated; eruptions only on covered parts, burn after scratching.
Sensation after urinating as of urine trikling in urethra; severe cutting at close of urination.
Sweat; only on uncovered parts; or all over except the head; when he sleeps, stops when he wakes; profuse, sour smelling, fetid, at night.
Perspiration, smelling like honey, on the genitals.
Sensation as if body, especially the limbs, were made of glass and would break easily.
Suppressed gonorrhea; causing articular rheumatism; prostatitis, sycosis, impotence, condylomata and many constitutional troubles.
Nails; deformed brittle.

Modalities:
Aggravation: At night, from heat of bed, at 3 am and 5 pm. From cold damp air, narcotics.
Amelioration:

d. Kreosotum

Constitution:
Dark complexion, slight, lean, ill-developed, poorly nourished.
Overgrown; very tall for her age.
Children: Old looking, wrinkled; scrofulous or psoric affections; **rapid emaciation.**

Causation:
Post climacteric diseases of women.

Characteristics:
Hemorrhagic diathesis; small wounds bleed freely; flow passive.
Bleeding; dark oozing, after the extraction of a tooth.
Roaring and humming in ears, with deafness, before and during menses.
Corrosive, foetid, discharges from mucous membranes
Itching, so violent toward evening as to drive one almost wild.
Painful dentition; teeth begins to decay as soon as they appear.
Gums bluish-red, soft, spongy, bleeding, inflamed, scorbutic, and ulcerated.
Vomiting; of pregnancy, sweetish water.
Severe headache before and during menses.
Menses; too early, profuse. Flow on lying down, ceases on sitting or walking about.
Incontinence of urine; can only urinate when lying.
Urine; copious, pale. Smarting and burning during and after micturation.
Leucorrhea acrid, corrosive, offensive.
Leucorrhea worse between periods; has the odor of green corn, stiffness like starch.
Leucorrhea; stains the linen yellow.
Violent corrosive itching of pudenda and vagina.

Modalities:
Aggravation; In the open air, cold weather, when getting cold; from washing or bathing with cold water, rest, especially when lying.
Amelioration; Generally better from warmth.

e. **Carbolicum acidum**
   Characteristics:
Complaints attended with foul, painless destructive affections.
Stupor, paralysis of sensation and motion.
Feeble pulse and depressed breathing.
Increased olfactory sensibility.
Mental and bodily languor, disinclination to study.
Marked acuteness of smell.
Pains are terrible; come and go suddenly.
Physical exertion brings on abscess somewhere.
Putrid discharges.
Desire for stimulants and tobacco.
Constipation with very offensive breath.
Urine almost black, diabetes; irritable bladder.

Q. 6. Write the cardinal indications of the following medicines in cervical spondylosis (10)
   a. Causticum
   b. Arnica montana
   c. Bryonia alba
   d. Staphysgaria
   e. Sulphur

Ans.
a. **Causticum**
   Cervical Spondylosis:
   -Pain at the nape of the neck.
   -Radiculitis; pain radiates in the distribution of cervical nerve.
   -Associated with muscular weakness.
   -At times features of cervical myelo-compression causing paraplegia.
   -Weakness paralytic.

Constitution:
-Dark hairs, rigid fibers, yellow shallow complexion. Melancholic; sad, hopeless. Extremely sympathetic.

Characteristic:
Thermal sensitivity: Ambithermal.
Laterality: Right lateral affinity.
Sensation: Burning, rawness, soreness.
Pains: Tearing, drawing pains in muscles and fibrous tissue.
Weakness, trembling.
Complaints: appear gradually
Must move constantly but motion does not relieve.
Cannot cover too warmly, but warmth does not relieve.

Modalities:
Aggravation: Clear fine weather.
Amelioration: Damp wet weather.

b. **Arnica montana**
   Cervical Spondylosis:
   Pain in nape of neck.
   Sensation as if bruised or beaten.
   Sprained and dislocated feeling.
   Everything on which he lies seems too hard.

Causation:
Soreness after overexertion; prolonged table work / computer work.
Exposure to cold.
H/O recent or remote trauma or strain to the part affected.

Constitution:
-Nervous; having low pain threshold.
Thermal sensitivity: Ambithermal.
Lateral affinity: Bilateral.

Characteristics:
-Sore, lame, bruised feeling as if beaten.
-Everything on which he lies seems too hard.
-Head is hot, body is cold.

Modalities:
Aggravation: At rest, when lying, wine.
Amelioration: From contact, motion.

c. **Bryonia alba**
   Constitution:
   -Subject having dark complexion, and firm muscular fiber.

Lateral Affinity:
-Right lateral affinity.

Precipitating factors:
-Warm weather after cold. Exposure to heat or cold. Suppression of eruptions. Anger.

Characteristics:
-Onset of complaints is insidious.
-Pains; tearing burning. Better rest and pressure.
-Sensation; heaviness and of pressure.
-Fainting while getting up.
-Desires: Thirst for cold water, large quantities after long intervals.

Aggravation:
- Morning, evening, night, motion, jar, stooping, rising, up, becoming heated, warm room, after eating, lying down.

Ameliorated:
- Pressure, lying on the painful side. Repose, lying down, cold drinks, cold and warm applications.

d. **Staphysagria**

Cervical Spondylosis:
- Sensation of wooden block in the occiput.
- Muscles feel bruised.

Constitution:
- Adapted to mild gentle, sweet person.
- Who are sensitive to rudeness.
- Who are Unable assert for own rights.

Causation / Ailments from:
- Indignation, mortification, disappointments.
- Suppression of emotions, anger, grief.
- Past History of abuse.

Characteristics:
- Desire: Sweets, milk.
- Aversion: Fat, milk.
- <: Milk.
- Colic from anger.
- Dreams; amorous with emissions.

Aggravation:
- Anger, indignation, mortification, onanism, sexual excess, tobacco, least touch of affected parts.

Amelioration:
- After Breakfast. Warmth, rest at night.

e. **Sulphur**

Cervical Spondylosis:
- Stiffness at the nape of neck.
- Drawing pain between the shoulders.
- Rheumatic pain in left shoulder.
- Heaviness and paretic feeling.
- Drawing and tearing pain in arms and hands.

Constitution:
- Lean, thin, tall stooped shouldered person.

Causation:
- Prone for skin affection.
- Poor posture, due constitutional to weakness of muscles.

Characteristics:
- Milk disagrees.
- Great desire for sweets.
- Averse to being washed.
- Skin; dirty, filthy, dry.
- Burning heat.

Aggravation:
- At rest, when standing, warmth in bed, washing, bathing, in morning 11 am.

Amelioration:
- Dry, warm weather, lying on the right side, from drawing up affected side.

Group – B

Q. 7. Write two complications of each of the following:(10)
  [a]. Emphysema.
   - a. Predisposition to lung infections.
   - b. Cor pulmonale.
   - c. Respiratory failure.
   - d. Spontaneous pneumothorax.
  [b]. Gastric Ulcer.
   - a. Hemorrhage.
   - b. Perforation.
   - c. Peritonitis.
   - d. Pyloric stenosis.
   - e. Malignant changes.
  [c]. Bronchial Asthma.
   - a. Status asthmaticus.
   - b. Emphysema.
   - c. Respiratory failure.
   - d. Spontaneous pneumothorax.
  [d]. Chronic Alcoholism.
   - a. Alcoholic Gastritis.
   - b. Alcoholic Hepatitis.
   - c. Alcoholic Cirrhosis.
   - d. Wernicke's Encephalopathy.
  [e]. Hepatic Cirrhosis.
   - a. Portal Hypertension.
   - b. Ascites.
   - c. Hepatic Encephalopathy.
   - d. Hepatocellular Carcinoma.
   - e. Hemorrhage.

Q. 8. Write the importance's of: (10)
   - a. ASO

Ans.
Anti-Streptolysin O: It is a blood test to measure anti-streptolysin O (ADO) antibodies in the blood.
Normal Value:
 -Less than 160 Todd units per milliliter.
ASO testing is a procedure that demonstrates the presence of antibodies generated by the body against infections by group A Strreptococcus. The antibodies may be detected in the blood for weeks or months after the primary source of infection has been eradicated.
Value:
 The test is for detection of poststreptococcal diseases such as glomerulonephritis, rheumatic fever, bacterial endocarditis and scarlet fever.

   - b. **Serum Amylase**

Ans.
 This is a test to measure of amount of amylase in serum.
This test is usually perfomed to diagnose or monitor diseases of pancreas. Amylase is an enzyme that helps digest glycogen and starch. It is produced mainly in the salivary glands and pancreas. When the pancreas is inflamed, amylase escapes into the blood.
 Normal value: 40 – 140 U/L
 Elevated values indicate:
 -Acute Pancreatitis.

-Cancer of Pancreas.
-Mumps.

c. Serum Acid Phosphatase

Ans.

The Serum Acid Phosphatase is also known as Male PAP test.
It is a blood test that measures acid phosphatase (an enzyme found in men in the prostate gland and semen).

Normal Value:
-0. to 08 U/L are normal.
Value: the raised levels are suggestive of:
-Prostate cancer that has spread outside the prostate (mainly to the bones)
-Paget's Disease.
-Multiple myeloma.

d. ESR

Ans. it is known as Erythrocyte Sedimentation Rate.
It is a non-specific screening test for various inflammatory diseases. The test measures the distance (in millimeters) that the RBC settle in unclotted blood in a specially marked test tube.

Normal value:
Men: Less than 15 mm/hr.
Females: less than 20 mm/hr.

Value:
The elevated values commonly seen with:
-Tuberculosis.
-Rheumatoid arthritis.
-Rheumatic fever.
-Typhoid.
Lower than normal values are common with:
-CCF.
-Polycythemia.

e. Casoni's Test.

Ans.

It is a specific test for Hydatid disease (Dog tapeworm).
Adult work develops in small intestine of dog (definitive host). Eggs are passed to intermediate hosts, like sheep, on ingestion it pass from stomach to liver, lung, brain and develop into hydatid cyst. On eating infected sheep meat dog gets worm and cycle is completed. Accidentally while handling dog, humans ingest eggs and develop cyst in brain, liver and lungs.

Q. 9. Discuss briefly the clinical features of:
a. Cerebral Malaria. (5)

Ans.

High fever.
Delirium, drowsiness.
Convulsions, aphasia.
Paralysis, coma.
(These appear within 24 to 72 hours of onset)

b. Acute pyelonephritis. (5)

Ans.
Clinical Features:
Symptoms:
-Onset sudden
-Dysuria
-Frequent urination

-Urgency; urgent need to urinate
-Backache
-Fatigue
-Chill with fever
-Vomiting

Signs:
-Temperature raised
-Pulse fast
-Suprapubic tenderness present
-Tenderness in the renal angles
-Hematuria
-Strong urine odour
-Usually the patient is elderly male who has BHP or a female in the productive age group.

Q. 10. a   Define Leucopenia. (2)
    b   **Discuss two main causes for the same. (2)**
    c   **Discuss two main diagnostic points for each cause. (4)**
    d   **Discuss one complication of each cause. (2)**

Ans.
[a]. Leucopenia. [2]
It is defined as a reduction in the number of leucocytes below the lower limit of 4000/cmm.
[b]. Discuss two main causes for the same.[2]
Bacterial infection; Typhoid, Paratyphoid.
Viral infection; Influenza, measles, infective hepatitis.
Protozoal infections; malaria, kala azar.
[c]. Discuss two main diagnostic points for each cause. [4]
Typhoid:
1. Blood culture.
2. Widhal test.
Paratyphoid:
Same investigations.
[d]. Discuss one complication of each cause. [2]
Complications of Typhoid;
-Intestinal haemorrhage.

Q. 11. In a case of a patient with hepatocellular failure, it is seen that blood-ammonia level is elevated and prothrombin time is prolonged.
    a.   Explain why does the blood ammonia level is elevated in this patient.
    b.   What could be the most serious consequence for prolonged prothrombin time in this case? Explain with reason.

Ans.
    a.   Due to body protein catabolism his blood ammonia level is raised.
    b.   Bleeding may take place and it is the most serious complication in this case.

Q. 12. A seventy five-year-old male is admitted to hospital after sudden loss of consciousness. His signs and symptoms suggest of a 'stroke'. A week later he regains his consciousness, but has difficulty in speaking and cannot move the right side of his body. The stretch reflexes are found to be exaggerated on the affected side of the body and the muscle-tone is elevated.
    a.   Which cerebral hemisphere has been affected by the stroke? (3)
    b.   Which features of the victim's condition suggest this? (7)

Ans.
    a.   The Left Cerebral Hemisphere has been affected by the stroke.
    b.   The cerebral hemisphere control the body on the opposite side therefore all functions including speech is lost indicates the affection of Left cerebral hemisphere.

***

Chapter 14
HISTORY OF HOMEOPATHY IN INDIA

Introduction

Homeopathy today is a rapidly growing system and is being practiced almost all over the world. In India it has become a household name due the safety of its pills and gentleness of its cure. A rough study indicates *that about 10% of the Indian population solely depend on Homeopathy for their Health care needs.*

It is more than a century and a half now that Homeopathy is being practiced in India. It has blended so well into the roots and traditions of the country that it has been recognized as one of the National Systems of Medicine and plays a an important role in providing health care to a large number of people. Its strength lies in its evident effectiveness as it takes a holistic approach towards the sick individual through promotion of inner balance at mental, emotional, spiritual and physical levels.

Origin of Homeopathy

The principle of Homeopathy has been known since the time of *Hippocrates* from Greece, the founder of medicine, around 450 BC More than a thousand years later the Swiss alchemist *Paracelsus* employed the same system of healing based upon the principle that "like cures like". But it was not until the late 18th century that Homeopathy as it is practiced today was evolved by the great German physician, Dr. Samuel Hahnemann. He was appalled by the medical practices of that time and set about to develop a method of healing which would be safe, gentle, and effective. He believed that human beings have a capacity for healing themselves and that the symptoms of disease reflect the individuals struggle to overcome his illness.

Brief About founder of Homeopathy

Dr. Christian Friedrich Samuel Hahnemann

April 10, 1755
Born in Saxony, Meissen

1767 – 1778
Dresden, Meissen to Leipzig – Vienna – Hermannstadt.
Attend School and finished Grammar School.
Paper: The wonderful structure of human hand.

1779
Earlangen, Hettstadt.
Graduated.

1781
Dessau.
Major Event: Married his 1st wife. Henriette, the daughter of Apothecary.
Book: First book on Medicine, which gives the result of his experience of practice in Transylvania.

1789
Lockowitz
Published: Treatise on chemical works – poisoning by Arsenic.
Treatise on Syphilis.
Description of a new preparation – Hahnemann's Soluble Mercury for the treatment of Syphilis.

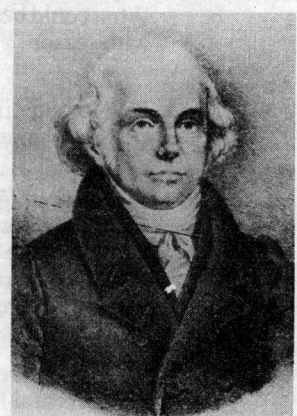

'Non Inutilis Vixi'
(Not lived in Vain)

History of Homeopathy in India

1790
Moved to Leipzig.
Major work: Translated Cullen's Materia Medica.

1792
Georgenthal, in Thuringian Forest.
Duke of Saxe Gotha, offered him to take charge of an asylum for the insane in Georgenthal. Here he cured the Hanoverian Minister: Klockenbring – an insane.

1792
Walschleben.
Published: First part of the "Friend of Health".
First part of his "Pharmaceutical Lexicon".

1795 – 1799
Wolfenbuttel to Konigslutter.
Published: Second part of the "Friend of Health".
Second part of his "Pharmaceutical Lexicon".

1796
Essay on a principle for ascertaining the remedial powers of medicinal substances in Hufeland's Journal.
In Konigslutter – Discovered the prophylactic powers of Belladona in Scarlet fever.
Essay on irrationality of complicated system of diet and regimen, and complex prescriptions.
Essay on antidotes.
Essay on periodical diseases.

1803
Dessau
Published a monograph on the effect of COFFEE which he considered as the source of many chronic diseases.
Preface to translation of a collection of medical prescription.
Translation of the Materia Medica of the great Albert Von Haller.

1805 – 1806
He demolished the time honoured faith in the medicine of 3000 years n his masterly work – 'Aesculapius in the Balance'.
Appearance of 1st Sketch of a 'Pure Materia Medica' in Latin.
The Medicine of Experience – was published in Hufeland's Journal.

1808
Torgau
Published – his strictures on ancient medicine in a magazine of general literature 'Allgemeiner Anzeiger der Deutschen'.
Essay on the value of the soectulative system of medicine, and a touching letter of Hufeland.

1810
Leipzic
Attacked by Prof Hecker of Berlin against the Organon.
1st edition of Organon 'Medicine of Experience', which is put into more methodical, aphoristic form after the model of some of the Hippocratic writing.

1811
Published 1st volume of Pure Materia Medica.
Essay De Helleborismo Veterum.

1811 – 1821
Leipzic
Essay on Typhus (1814).
Treatment of Burns.
2nd edition of Organon

5 more volume of Pure Materia Medica.
1821
3rd, 4th, 5th, edition of Organon.

1827
Coethen
To Dr. Stapf and Dr. Gross, he communicated to them his theory of the origin of Chronic Diseases and published 1st, 2nd volume of his Chronic Diseases, their peculiar nature and Homeopathic treatment.

1829 – 10th August
Coethen
He founded the first Homeopathic society under the name of the "Central Society of German Homeopathists".
1830
Lost his 1st wife.

1831
He published a pamphlet against his foes, entitled 'Allopathy; a Warning to all Sick Persons'.
Cholera invaded Germany from East. He guided by the experience of his therapeutic knowledge and fixed a group of remedies to be used and saved many lives.

1835
Mlle. Melanine d' Hervilly came to Coethen and took him to Paris and influenced upon M. Guizot to let Dr. Hahnemann practice in Paris and later married him also.

1843, 2nd July
At 99 years of age, he died there with full of years and honour.
Buried in the cemetery of Montmartre.

Reference:
Lectures on the Theory and Practice of Homeopathy by R. E. Dudgeon.
Reprint edition 2002.

Historical Evolution of Homeopathy In India
Homeopathy entered India in 1839 when Dr. John Martin Honigberger was called to treat Maharaja Ranjit Singh, the ruler of Punjab, for paralysis of vocal cords and edema. The Maharaja was relieved of his complaints and in return received valuable rewards and later on was made officer-in-charge of a hospital. Dr. Honigberger later on went to Calcutta and started practice there. This royal patronage helped the system to have its roots in India. A large number of missionaries, amateurs in Indian civil and military service personals practiced Homeopathy extensively and spread this system mostly in Bengal and South India.

Recognition of Homeopathy by Government of India
The Government of India soon after Independence started taking keen interest to develop Homeopathic System of Medicine. Govt set up the 'Homeopathic Enquiry Committee' in 1948, the Committee by Planning Commission in 1951 and the Homeopathic Pharmacopoeia Committee in 1962 testify to this. At the instance of the recommendation of these Committees, the Government of India accepted Homeopathy as one of the national System of Medicine and started releasing funds for its development, during the Second five-year Plan. Some of the States also made their own contribution to Homeopathic Education, the employment of Homeopathic practitioners in health services and regulating the practice by forming and enacting States Acts & Rules, etc.

Growth and Development In India
Homeopathy continued to spread and by the beginning of 20th century most of the important cities in India had Homeopathic dispensaries. The popularity of the system led to a mushroom growth of quacks practicing Homeopathy. Seeing this deplorable state of affairs, efforts were made by the Government. It took several steps and in 1948, a Homeopathic Enquiry Committee was set up to evolve a suitable arrangement to regulate teaching and practice of Homeopathy. A Homeopathic Advisory Committee was appointed in 1952 by the Govt. of India and the recommendations of these committees led to passing of a Central Act in 1973 for recognition of this system of medicine. Homeopathy now has been accepted as one of the National Systems of Medicine in India.

History of Homeopathy in India

National Health Policy & Homeopathy:
The National Health Policy as passed by the Indian Parliament assigns to the Indian Systems of Medicine and Homeopathy an important role in the delivery of primary health care and envisages its integration in the over all health care delivery system, specially in the preventive and promotive aspects of health care in the context of the national target of achieving "Health for all by 2000 AD".

Present Set Up:
Homeopathy in India enjoys Government support along with the other systems of medicine because Government is of the view that presence of all these complementary alternative systems of therapeutics offers a much wider spectrum of curative medicine than is available in any other country.

ISM & H in National Health Programmes
The National Health Policy of 1983 envisages integration of ISM & H with the modern system of medicine. The department is exploring the areas of actual involvement in the National Health Programme through ISM & H.
India has a rich heritage by way of its ancient systems of medicine such as Ayurveda, Siddha, Unani, Yoga & Naturopathy. These systems of medicines and its practices are well accepted by the Community and have their own areas of strength. Medicines are easily available and prepared from locally available resources, economical, and comparatively safe from side effects. Because of this fact the Central Government Health Scheme, introduced in 1954 with Allopathic Homeopathic dispensaries was introduced first time in 1967-68.

Homeopathic Education in India:
The important educational regulations as per the Central Council of Homeopathy in respect of homeopathy are as under:
- Homeopathy (Minimum Standards of Education) Regulations, 1983- specifies the standards and infrastructure necessary for Homeopathic colleges.
- Homeopathy (Degree Course) Regulations, 1983 Homeopathy (Graded Degree Course) Regulations, 1983- specifies the course curriculum and syllabus to be followed by every University.
- Homeopathy (Postgraduate course) MD (Hom.) Regulation, 1989-Permits the Universities to conduct a three year PG programme in seven specialties namely Materia medica, Organon of Medicine, Repertory, Pediatrics, Practice of Medicine, Pharmacy and Psychiatry.

Number of Homeopathic institutions at present are as under:

Undergraduate colleges	178
Exclusive PG colleges	2
Postgraduate centers	31
Postgraduate specialties	07
Government institutions	35
Admission capacity / year	13000
Universities conducting UG/PG	40

Strength of Qualified Homeopaths at national level:
Number of qualified Homeopathic doctors in India are about 1,32,356.

Strength of Homeopathic Health care services at national level:
Different State Governments have opened 292 Homeopathic Hospitals with 13694 Bed strength.
Homeopathic dispensaries are 5398.

Indian Homeopathic Drug Industry:
India is the biggest market for Homeopathic drugs and, has 654 drug Manufacturing units. Government has exempted few drugs which could be sold through allopathic outlets. India is exporting homeopathic products to Sri Lanka, Bangladesh, Oman, Malaysia, Switzerland, USA, Mexico, UK, New Zealand and Nepal and many other countries of world.

Definition of Homeopathic Medicine in Drug Rule:
"2(dd) Homeopathic medicine includes any drug which is recorded in Homeopathic provings, the therapeutic efficacy of which has been established through long clinical experience, is recorded in authoritative Homeopathic literature of India /abroad and which is prepared according to the techniques of Homeopathic pharmacy and covers combination of ingredients to such Homeopathic medicines but does not include a medicine which is administered by parental route."

A Homeopathic drug shall be deemed to be misbranded:
- If it is so colored, coated, powdered or polished that damage is concealed or if it is made to appear of better, of greater therapeutic value than it really is; or
- If it is not labeled in the prescribed manner; or
- If its label or container or anything accompanying the drug bears any statement, design or device which makes any false claim for the drug or which is false or misleading in any particular.

A drug shall be deemed to be adulterated:
- If it consists in whole or in part, of any filthy, putrid or decomposed substance; or
- If it has been prepared, packed or stored under insanitary conditions whereby it may have been contaminated with filth or whereby it may have been rendered injurious to health; or
- If its container is composed, in whole or in part, of any poisonous or deleterious substance which may render the contents injurious to health; or
- If it bears or contains, for the purposes of coloring only, a color other than one which is prescribed; or
- If it contains any harmful or toxic substance which may render it injurious to health; or if any substance has been mixed therewith so as to reduce its quality or strength.

A drug shall be deemed to be spurious:
- If it is manufactured under a name which belongs to another drug;
- If it is an imitation of, or is a substitute for, another drug or resembles another drug in a manner likely to device or bears upon its label or container the name of another drug unless it is plainly and conspicuously marked so as to reveal its true character and its lack of identity with such other drugs; or
- If the label or container bears the name of an individual or company purporting to be the manufacture of the drug, which individual or company is fictitious or does not exists; or
- If it has been substituted wholly or in part by another drug or substance; or
- If it purports to be the product of a manufacturer of whom it is not truly a product.

Quality Assurance in Homeopathic Medicines:
- Manufacturing and sale of Homeopathic medicines are governed by the Drugs and Cosmetic Act 1940 and the Drug Rule 1945.
- Manufacturing of Homeopathic medicine needs a License issued by the Drug Controller.
- A separate GMP for Homeopathic medicines has been notified.
- The raw material used in the preparation are scrupulously tested and the process of preparation is standardized.
- Homeopathic medicines are defined under Rule 2(dd) of Drugs and Cosmetics Rules, 1945.
- Standards of Homeopathic medicines to be complied for manufacture, sale, distribution or import are defined under Second Schedule of the Drugs and Cosmetics Act (4a).
- New Homeopathic medicines are covered under Rule 30 aa.
- Ophthalmic preparations, standards and conditions for preparation thereof are covered under Schedule ff (Rule 126 a).
- Anybody can get medicines tested under Section 26.
- Under Section 26-a, Central Government can cancel licence of manufacturing a drug, if therapeutic claims are not genuine.
- Retail sale is covered under Rule 67 c. Application be made under form 20 c. Single drugs.
- Licensing authority for issue of licence for Homeopathic medicines lies with the State Government as per Rule 67 a and 85 b.

References:
Status of Homeopathy in India
By Dr. Eswara Das Deputy Advisor (Homeopathy)

***

Chapter 15
VARIOUS INSTITUTIONS AND ORGANIZATIONS OF HOMEOPATHY IN INDIA

Central Council of Homeopathy

The Central Council of Homeopathy was constituted on December 17th, 1974. It was a significant landmark in the development process of Homeopathy in India.

The main functions of the Central Council are:
1. To lay down minimum standards to be observed in Homeopathic education.
2. To recognize Homeopathic medical colleges & hospitals.
3. To recommend recognition or withdrawal of medical qualification granted by Homeopathic medical institutions in India to Central Govt.
4. To negotiate with institutions located in other countries imparting training in Homeopathy for recognition of their qualification on reciprocal basis.
5. To lay down the standards of professional conduct, etiquette and code of ethics to be observed by the practitioners of Homeopathy.
6. To register qualified homeopaths.

In exercise of the powers conferred by the clauses (i), (j), & (k) of section 33 and sub-section (1) of section 20 of the Homeopathy Central Council Act, 1973, the Central Council has taken expeditious steps towards putting the medical education in Homeopathy and practice on a proper footing keeping in view the national requirements. It has introduced with the prior sanction of the Central Govt. of following educational regulations for Diploma, Degree and post graduate degree courses for maintaining uniformity of medical education at All India level:

Homeopathy (Diploma Course) D.H.M.S Regulations, 1983
DHMS course spreads over a period of four years including compulsory internship of six months duration after passing the final diploma examination. (The Government wide an amendment to this regulation has stopped further admission to the Diploma Course)

Homeopathy (Degree Course) B.H.M.S. Regulations, 1993
BHMS course spreads over a period of five and half years including compulsory internship of one-year duration after passing the final degree examination.
The admission qualification for both the courses is Intermediate Science (10 +2) with Physics, Chemistry and Biology subjects or equivalent.

Homeopathy (Graded Degree Course) B.H.M.S. Regulations, 1983
BHMS Graded Degree course spreads over a period of two years including compulsory internship of six months duration after passing the final degree examination.
This course has been recommended as a bridge or link short terms course for the benefit of diploma holders to raise their educational level to that of a degree.

The Central Council has also laid down minimum standards of education specifying that every college shall provide minimum requirements, norm and standards in regard to teaching as well as hospital staff, equipment, accommodation and other facilities for proper training of the medical students of Homeopathy.

In order to evaluate the standards of medical education being imparted in various Homeopathic medical colleges, the Central Council of Homeopathy has laid down, Homeopathy Central council (Inspectors and Visitors) Regulations, 1982 with the prior approval of Central Government, for inspection of the colleges in terms of teaching facilities, equipment, accommodation, staff provided in the colleges and attached hospitals.

Homeopathy (Post Graduate Degree Course) M.D. (Hom.) Regulations, 1989 which were amended vide Homeopathy post graduate degree course) M.D. (Hom.) (Amendment) Regulations, 1992].
The Central Council has prescribed post graduate degree course in Homeopathic subjects i.e., Materia Medica, Homeopathic Philosophy and Repertory which are spread over 3 year duration including one year of house job or equivalent thereof.

There are about 146 medical colleges of Homeopathy in the country. Out of these, the Central Council permitted 15 colleges to start Post Graduate Degree course in Homeopathic subjects.

CENTRAL COUNCIL OF Homeopathy
Address: 61-66, Institutional Area,
Opp. D Block,
Janakpuri, New Delhi.
Website: www.cchindia.com

Central Council for Research in Homeopathy
Introduction:

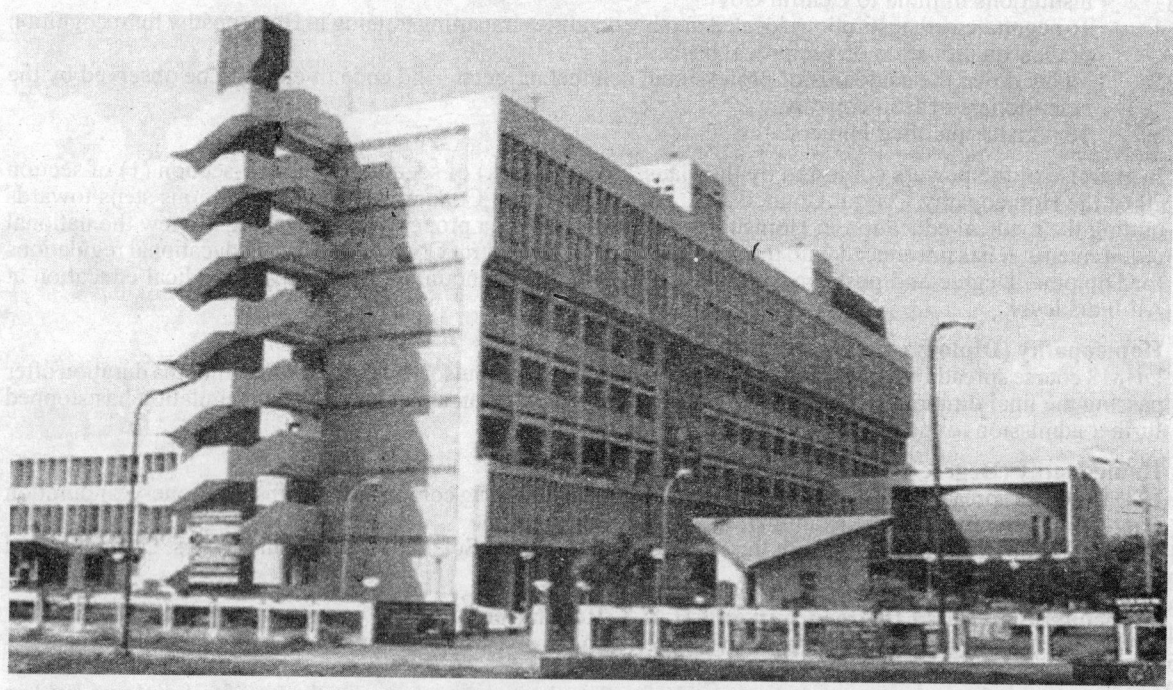

The Central Council for Research in Homeopathy was formally constituted on 30th March, 1978, as an autonomous organisation and was registered under the Societies Registration Act XXI of 1860. It was, however, only in January, 1979 that the Council started functioning as an independent organisation. The policy, directions and overall guidance for the activities of the Council are provided by the Governing Body. The Union Minister of Health and Family Welfare is the President of the Governing Body and has general control on the affairs of the Council and has authority to exercise all the powers.

Various Institutions and Organizations of Homeopathy in India

The Department of Ayurveda, Yoga & Naturopathy, Unani, Siddha and Homeopathy in the Ministry of Health & Family Welfare which is headed by a Secretary, administers various schemes for strengthening of research institutions and renders advice on implementation and monitoring of various research programmes.

Objectives
1. To formulate aims and patterns of research on scientific lines in Homeopathy.
2. To undertake research or other programmes, the prosecution and assistance in research, the propagation of knowledge and experimental measures relating to the cause and prevention of the disease.
3. To initiate, develop and co-ordinate scientific research in fundamental and applied aspects of Homeopathy.
4. To exchange information with other institutions, associations and societies interested in the objects similar to those of the Central Council and especially in observation and study of diseases.
5. To promote and assist institution of research for the study of diseases, their prevention and cure, especially with emphasis for covering the rural population of the country.
6. To prepare, print publish and exhibit papers, posters, pamphlets, periodicals and books for furtherance of the object of the Central Council and to contribute to such literature.
7. To offer prizes and grant scholarships in furtherance of the objectives of the Council.

Research Activities:
The research activities of the council are in the following areas:
1. Clinical Research
2. Clinical Research (Tribal)
3. Clinical Research in Epidemics
4. Drug Proving Research
5. Clinical Verification Research
6. Drug Standardization
7. Drug Research
8. Survey, Collection & Cultivation of Medicinal Plants
9. Literary Research

Clinical Research:
Clinical Research plays an important role in the development of Homeopathic medicines. It helps in clinical validation of the data collected through drug provings on healthy human beings. Clinical studies also facilitate assessment of therapeutic utility of drug substances in specific disease conditions for their optimum utilisation by the profession. It also helps in the elucidation of fundamental principles and their application in the treatment of various diseases. The council has, therefore, laid emphasis on clinical research which has remained an important activity of the council ever since its inception. The Council has taken up clinical evaluation of certain diseases that are common as well as chronic ailments and also in certain diseases of interest from national health point of view viz. Filaria, Malaria, HIV/AIDS, Diabetes, etc.

Total forty one(41) projects, out of which (27) under disease-related, (14) under drug-related clinical research are under progress at six (6) research Institutes, twelve (12) clinical research units and one clinical research unit in tribal area.

Aims And Objectives:
Clinical Research in Homeopathy has a number of objectives such as,
1) Clinical confirmation of drug-pathogenesis.
2) Elicitation of new clinical symptoms.
3) Evaluation of clinical drug pictures.
4) Classification of various complexions, temperaments and constitutions, and
5) To evaluate action of Homeopathic drugs on any given pathological conditions etc.

At present two types of Clinical Research programmes are in progress with the following objectives:

Disease-related Clinical Research:
Aims & Objectives
To evolve a group of most efficacious homeopathic medicines in a given pathological condition, with regard to:

1) Identify their reliable indications.
2) Identify their most useful potencies.
3) Determine their reliable frequency of administration.
4) To deduce the repertorial indices and
5) To determine their relationship with
   a. Other drugs such as which follow-well, complementary, cognate, intercurrent, antidote, incompatible etc.
   b. Improvement in symptoms-sign complex of given pathological conditions.

Drug-related Clinical Research
Aims & Objectives
Certain drug(s) are said to have relation with particular disease such as:
1) Those which have a special affinity for the organ(s) involved in particular disease conditions or
2) Which are traditionally empirically used or
3) Those identified by the various Institutes/Units of the Council through research studies.

Such drugs (discussed later) are tried in order to clinically evaluate them in particular disease(s) with regard to:
1) Identification of their drug pathogenesis
2) Identification of their most useful potencies
3) Determination of their frequency of administration
4) To determine their relationship with
   a. Other drugs such as which follow-well, complementary, cognate, intercurrent, antidote, incompatible, etc.
   b. Improvement in symptoms-sign complex of particular disease.

TRIBAL RESEARCH
Introduction
India being a vast multicultural and multiracial country with a tribal population of 8%, it is foremost to take our tribals towards better health status by providing medical care facilities at the grassroot levels.
CCRH has with a view to deliver health care to this population at their doorsteps established twenty one clinical research units in predominantly tribal areas of the country. These units are catering exclusively to the needs of the tribals besides serving as a potential source for promoting health consciousness. Earlier these units were intended to gather date of prevalence of diseases, food habits, local customs and beliefs, natural resources and folklore concerning medicine and health besides proving medical care to the locals as bye-way of research. At present these units are conducting drug-related clinical research studies on eighteen found prevalent in that particular area during the survey. The homeopathic medicines being tried in these diseases are mostly partially proved or used infrequently in clinical practice but are said to have traditional or empirical use or have a special affinity for the organ(s) in particular disease conditions.

CLINICAL RESEARCH IN EPIDEMICS
Introduction
The Council imparts medical aid-cum-relief operations during the break out of epidemics and natural calamities in the country through its institutes and units. It has rushed to the needs of the affected population in nearly 25 epidemics by providing preventive and medical treatment. Most important ones being MIC Gas Tragedy in Bhopal in December 1984, Plague in Surat in September 1994, Dengue fever in Delhi in October 1996, Japanese Encephalitis in Eastern parts of UP in October - November 1989, October - November 1991 and August 1993, Dropsy in Delhi in 1998, Malaria in some parts of Rajasthan in October 1994, medical relief camps for the victims of Orissa cyclone in October 1999 and Gujarat earthquake in January 2001. The findings of these studies have underlined the utility of homeopathic medicines in acute infections.

DRUG PROVING
(Homeopathic Pathogenetic Trials)
Introduction
Drug Proving now termed as Homeopathic Pathogenetic Trials (HPT) is a process in which drug substances are put into trial over healthy volunteers and their pathogenetic effects are observed and noted for therapeutic

purposes. Therefore, it is the only and unique method which is based on the nature's law of cure i.e. Similia Similibus Curentur which states that likes are cured by likes i.e. a drug's capacity for eradicating a disease, lies in its capacity to produce the same.

Since the emergence of Homeopathy the process & methodology of HPTs has improved greatly. In this effort, Council has also developed a plan & protocol of double blind technique in drug proving which has also been accepted internationally. Process of symptom extraction from HPTs has also been standardised. Success of this methodology can be assessed from the clinical verification studies of proving pathogenesis where many symptoms are repeatedly being verified when prescriptions are based upon them. Such symptoms are being reflected in the reports of clinical verification programme under individual drugs.

Methodology
The proving of drug is conducted under Drysdale's Double Blind Technique where neither the proving master nor the prover knows the name of the drug and its potencies being proved on them. The drug is proved on healthy human beings selected from different regions of the country in order to ascertain whether ecological, socio-economic, climatic, regional factors & food habits, variation in physical constitution of the volunteers affects the pathogenesis in any form. A drug is proved on two different places i.e. two units in order to complete its proving. The healthy volunteers are selected on the basis of pre-trial medical examination conducted by Honorary consultants in the field of Medicine, Psychiatry, Ophthalmology, Otorhinolaryngology, Dermatology, Pathology and Gynecology in case of female provers. Drugs are provided to the provers in coded phials and provers are divided into two groups, one who receive 'placebo' and other 'actual drug' to distinguish between the false and true symptoms. The proving master records the responses of the provers in the prescribed proforma. The data collected during the course of provings is received at the Central Drug Proving-cum-Data Processing Cell at the Hqrs. office of the Council, where, it is processed, analysed and compiled and later on published for the use of the profession.

Drugs Proved so far
1. Abroma augusta folia
2. Acalypha indica
3. Acid butyricum
4. Aegle folia
5. Aegle marmelos
6. Alfalfa
7. Aranea diademe
8. Aranea scinencia
9. Araenicum bromicum
10. Atista indica
11. Azadirachta indica
12. Baryta iodata
13. Bellis perennis
14. Boerrhavia diffusa
15. Calotropis gigantea
16. Carica papaya
17. Cassia fistula
18. Cassia sophera
19. Chelone
20. Chromo kali sulph
21. Cornuus circinata
22. Cup. oxydatum nigrum
23. Curcuma longa
24. Cynodon dactylon
25. Embelia ribes
26. Euphorbia lathyrus
27. Formic acid
28. Glycyrrhiza glabra
29. Holarrhena antidysenterica
30. Hydrocotyle asiatica
31. Icthyolum

32. Kali muriaticum
33. Lapis alba
34. Magnesium sulphuricum
35. Malaria officinalis
36. Mangifera indica
37. Mygale
38. Nictanthes arbortristis
39. Ocimum canum
40. Ocimum sanctum
41. Oxytropis lamberti
42. Paraffin
43. Phyllanthus niruri
44. Rauwolfia serpentina
45. Ricinus communis
46. Senega
47. Staphylococcinum
48. Tarentula cubensis
49. Tarentula hispanica
50. Tela aranea
51. Terminalia arjuna
52. Terminalia chebula
53. Thea chinensis
54. Theridion
55. Thymol
56. Thyroidinum
57. Tribulus terrestris

Publications
Proving data of the drugs proved by the Council is published from time to time for the use of the profession in the form of Monographs or in Quarterly Bulletin.

Monographs
Monographs of following drugs have been published and include the Drug Standardisation studies involving pharmacognostical, pharmacological and studies besides the physio-chemical proving pathogenesis & clinically verified symptoms.
1. Abroma augusta folia
2. Kali muriaticum
3. Cassia sophera
4. Cynodon dactylon
5. Aegle folia
6. Aegle marmelos
7. Hydrocotyle asiatica
8. Atista indica

CLINICAL VERIFICATION RESEARCH
Clinical Verification Research is aimed at making homeopathy more effective and reliable in different disease conditions. In order to establish that homeopathy has real effects, separable from non-specific and placebo effects, priorities have changed in research. Newer methods of clinical trials have emerged, with the adoption of randomized controlled studies. The reliability of earlier provings is in doubt, the most serious flaw being that they were uncontrolled. But even after use of proper methodology with minimum error, symptoms generated during drug proving (Homeopathic Pathogenetic Trials) need to be verified clinically in order to establish their efficacy and the reliability of the proving pathogenesis and to screen out non-beneficial information. Only then the profession will adopt such newer drugs with reliable data. There are many Homeopathic drugs which are mentioned in literature on the basis of empirical use but systematic studies have not been carried out to verify their effectivity.

This study is being continued since last few years and 65 drugs are allotted to Instts./Units engaged in Clinical Verification Research. These sixty five drugs include drugs mainly of indigenous origin or drugs proved by

CCRH. A few of lesser known drugs are also included.
Clinical Verification Studies on sixteen homeopathic drugs (mentioned below) under trial has been concluded has been sufficiently verified. Then compiled of six drugs data after approval of the Scientific Advisory Committeee, has been published in the CCRH Quaterly Bulletin Vol. 19 (3&4), 1997.

1) Abroma augusta folia*
2) Baryta iodata*
3) Berberis vulgaris*
4) Boerrhavia diffusa
5) Caesalpinia bonducella
6) Carica papaya
7) Cassia sophera*
8) Glycosmis pentaphyla (Atista indica)*
9) Hydrocolyte asiatica
10) Jaborandi
11) Justicia adhatoda*
12) Nyctanthes arbortristis
13) Saraca indica
14) Sarsaparilla
15) Terminalia chebula
16) Viscum album

DRUG STANDARDISATION

Success in Homeopathic prescribing is based as much on the purity and uniformity of the prepared drug as on the efficient case taking and repertorization. A sub-standard raw drug will not produce desired results in a sick individual. For this the Council has set up Drug Standardisation Units at Ghaziabad and Hyderabad and a Homeopathic Drug Research Institute at Lucknow. The assignment encompasses a comprehensive evaluation of the homeopathic drugs in respect of their physico-chemical, pharmacological and pharmacognostic in order to study the various qualitative and quantitative characteristics of drugs. The pharmacognostic studies include the macro and miscroscopical characteristics of raw drugs of vegetable origin. The physico-chemical analysis helps to determine the physical and chemical constant of a drug. The pharmacological spectrum of a drug is ascertained through experimental trials on laboratory animals under standard laboratory conditions which include preliminary estimation of dosage, its efficacy and safety, and also the mode of action of homeopathic drugs. Till March 2003, the studies on raw drugs undertaken are Pharmacolognostical - 214, Physico-Chemical- 190 & Pharmacological- 122. The standards of the drugs worked out by the Council are definite gains and will go a long way in making available standard Homeopathic medicines in the market.
In vitro studies with certain homeopathic medicines on animal and human viruses have established their anti-viral activity. This has been a definitive observation corroborated with laboratory findings.
The Unit at Ghaziabad has laid down parameters for determining the standard of crude drugs, mother tinctures and potencies. The methodology for the preparation of biotherapeutic pharmaceutical (nosodes) has also been evolved.

DRUG RESEARCH

Drug Research Program explores the scientific basis of "Potency research and elucidation of mechanism of action of Homeopathic dilutions beyond Avogadro's number" which has posed a challenge in the scientific fraternity globally. Homeopathic Drug Research Institute, Lucknow is undertaking this work scientifically under the existing infrastructural facilities of the institute and has succeeded in enumerating the phenomenon of potentisation, microdoses and the principle of Homeopathic-Similia Similibus Curentur through in-vivo and in-vitro experimental models in biosystems. Active research with experimental approach on animal models using an array of homeopathic drugs for treatment of cholelithiasis, arteriosclerosis, thromboembolism, hypercholesterolemia, diabetes mellitus, hypertension and iodine deficiency diseases have been taken up.

Diabetes Mellitus

Series of homeopathic drugs were attempted to evaluate their Anti-Diabetic Potentiality. Certain drugs like Alloxan, Cephalandra indica and Pterocarpus marsupium etc. and their derivatives in potencies have been extensively studied with parallel experimentation against known oral anti-diabetic drugs of Sulfonylurea and Biguanide groups as well as with insulin. Encouraging results were obtained with Alloxan, Cephalandra indica and Pterocarpus marsupium exhibiting the reactivation and regeneration of Potentiality of damaged beta cells ranging from 50-70 % and proved to be potent Anti-Diabetic Agent. Hormonal profiles have also been attempted while evaluating Anti-Diabetic Potentiality of aforesaid drugs with particular reference to Hormone (GH), Prolactin (Pr) and Adreno-Corticotrophic Hormone (ACTH) Factors.

Iodine Deficiency Disorders And Control (IDDC)
Various homeopathic drugs with potential activity in Iodine Deficiency Disorders are being investigated through Hormonal assay envisaging T3, T4 and TSH hormones.

Cardiovascular Disorders
Homeopathic drugs like Crataegus oxycantha, Cactus grandiflora and Polygonum have been screened to establish their utility in various cardiovascular disorders experimentally and encouraging results were obtained as novel Therapeutic agents. These drugs were specifically attempted as an anti-thromboembolic, anti-arteriosclerotic agents in myocardial infarction and other cardiovascular disorders through well designed in-vitro experimental and clinical trials/studies.

Survey, Collection & Cultivation of Medicinal Plants
Identification and collection of medicinal plats for reference and standardisation studies is an important factor that contributes to the growth of any system. More so in homeopathy where 70% of the medicines used in homeopathy are of vegetable origin. CCRH has accorded due importance to this aspect and has established a survey, collection and cultivation unit at Udhagamandalam (Ooty), Tamilnadu. The unit has a collection of 7752 plant specimens native to areas adjoining Ooty, Nilgiri Hills and has supplied 360 raw drug specimens for standardization studies. Herbarium sheets of 6,307 plant specimens have been prepared.

Literary Research
The study of literature and its revival is an important background material for planning research programmes. The collections, compilation and dissemination thereof is an essential part of scientific activity. Equally important is revision and updating of available data for its optimum and timely utilisation. As such, the Council has undertaken Literary Research as a long term project.

The Literary Research Programme is being carried out on "Review and Revision of Kunzli's (Kent's) Repertory – additions from Boericke's Repertory in relation to other works."

PUBLICATIONS
The Council published the following:

Quarterly Bulletin
Scientific articles covering research activities and achievements of the Council are published in this bulletin. Five volumes from No. 18 to 23 and Vol. 24 (1&2) 2002 were published during this period and a total of 47 articles on the research programmes undertaken by CCRH at its various institutes and units have been published in these issues.

Books
1) A Handbook of Home Remedies in Homeopathy - Reprinted in 1996-97 and 2000-01.
2) Samanya Homeopathy Upchar Pustika - Reprinted in 2000-01,2002-03.
3) A Check list of Homeopathic Medicinal Plants of India Revised and Enlarged Edition.(Under Print)
4) Additions from Boericke's Repertory to Kent's Repertory - Chapter Nose.
5) Additions from Boericke's Repertory to Kent's Repertory - Chapter Mind.
6) Additions from Boericke's Repertory to Kent's Repertory - Chapter Face
7) Additions from Boericke's Repertory to Kent's Repertory - Chapter Throat
8) Booklet on CCRH - A Bird's Eye View printed in 1997-98 and Revised edition printed in 1999-2000.
9) Booklet on 22 common Indian plants used in Homeopathy with their clinically verified data compiled from the data received under the Clinical Verification Research programme of CCRH..
10) Compendium of Research Papers published in various issues of CCRH Quarterly Bulletin.

Monographs
1) A proving of Atista indica (incorporating clinically verified symptoms)
2) A proving of Hydrocotyle asiatica (incorporating clinically verified symptoms)

CENTRAL COUNCIL OF HOMOEOPATHY
Address: 61-66, Institutional Area,
Opp. D Block, Janakpuri, New Delhi
Website: www.ccrhindia.org

Homoeopathic Pharmacopoeia Laboratory Govt. of India
Introduction:
Homeopathic Pharmacopoeia Laboratory, (HPL) Ghaziabad was set up in September 1975. Homeopathic Pharmacopoeia Laboratory, Ghaziabad besides being a sub-ordinate institute to the department of ISM & Homeopathy, Govt. of India, is recognized by the Department of Science and Technology, Govt. of India, as Scientific, Technological and Research Institution.

The laboratory is functioning as standard- setting cum drug testing laboratory at the national level. Standards of homeopathic drugs are covered under Second Schedule of the Drugs and Cosmetics Act, 1940. Standards as worked out by the laboratory and approved by the Homeopathic Pharmacopoeia Committee are published in the from of Homeopathic Pharmacopoeia of India (HPI). So far eight volumes of HPI have been published consisting of standards on 916 basic drugs.

Standards included in HPI, which include information on characterization, identification, testing of standards and preparation of homeopathic medicines are statutory requirement to be followed by all the manufacturers of drugs for maintenance of quality of homeopathic drugs under item 4 A of the Second Schedule under Section 8 and 16 of Drugs and Cosmetics Act, 1940., H.P.L Ghaziabad is set up to test for such standards to ensure and enforcement of such standards with respect to homeopathic drugs. The laboratory is also recognised as Central Drug Laboratory under Drugs Rule 3 A under section 6 for testing of homeopathic drugs.

The laboratory is also functioning as nodal laboratory for testing of homeopathic drugs for States viz. Andhra Pradesh, Delhi, Goa, Karnataka, Orissa, Tripura, Sikkim, Andaman and Nicobar island, Himachal Pradesh, Daman & Diu, Dadar & Nagar Haveli, Maharastra etc. As a regular feature, the laboratory also undertakes testing of such samples as forwarded by these State / Central Government procurement authorities / drug control authorities / port authorities.

Functions of Homeopathic Pharmacopoeia Laboratory:
1. Laying down of standards for identity and purity of homeopathic drugs.
2. Finding out indigenous substitutes for plants.
3. Addition of standards on Nosodes.
4. Verification of standards of drugs included in other Homeopathic Pharmacopoeia and confirmation of work of Pharmacopoeial importance done elsewhere for adoption or improvement of standards already laid down. Revision and updating of standards of Pharmacopoeial importance.
5. Testing of samples referred under different provisions of Drugs Act, which include legal samples forwarded by State Drug Control Authorities; samples referred by Port Authorities; samples referred by State Government Purchase Organisations; consumers etc.
6. Survey and collection of samples of homeopathic drugs for verification of adulteration trends or quality of drugs marketed under such cases, reports are sent to Licensing Authorities for taking remedial measures.
7. Supply of standard drug samples to scientific Organisations.
8. Collection of medicinal plants through survey tours or otherwise for maintenance of reference samples for comparative studies.
9. Maintenance of reference museum and herbarium.
10. Maintenance of a medicinal plant garden which includes cultivation and introduction of medicinal plants of both indigenous and exotic nature.
11. Maintenance of a Germ plasm and Seed Bank of medicinal plants.
12. To impart orientation to all India State Government / Central Govt. Drug Inspectors / Drug Analysts / Pharmacists / Pharmacy incharge of Homeopathic Medical Colleges etc. in methods of standardisation, identification and testing of homeopathic drugs and application of various provisions of Drugs Act and Rules with respect to homeopathic medicines.

13. Documentation and Publication.
14. Guiding students of Homeopathic Medical Colleges in the practice of Homeopathic pharmacy as per syllabus approved by Central Council of Homeopathy.

Equipment facility:
Equipment and other laboratory facility available are as under:
A. Scanning Electron Microscopy.
B. U.V. Spectrophotometer.
C. I.R. Spectrophotometer
D. H.P.L.C.
E. G.L.C.
F. Atomic Absorption Spectrophotometer
G. Nuclear Magnetic Spectrophotometer

Training facility:
The laboratory organises orientation progrmmes twice a year in methods of identity and testing of homeopathic drugs for:
A. All India Drug Control Authorities.
B. Central / State Govt. Drug Inspectors / Pharmacists.
C. Pharmacy lecturers of Homeopathic Medical Colleges.
D. Scientists working in State Government Drug-Testing Laboratories.

The laboratory also provides short-term orientation in Homeopathic pharmacy to students of Homeopathic Medical Colleges on regular basis.

Testing facility:
The laboratory provides facilities for getting tested homeopathic medicines on nominal charges as per provisions covered under Schedule-B for homeopathic medicines under Drugs & Cosmetics Act.

Publications:
The laboratory has brought out the following publications:

A.	A guide to important medicinal poants in Homeopathy vol. I (including 40 plants).
B.	A guide to important medicinal poants in Homeopathy vol. II (including 80 plants).
C.	A photographic album on Medicinal plants used in Homeopathy vol. I (including 150 plants)
D.	A photographic album on Medicinal plants used in Homeopathy vol. II (including 152 plants)

Homoeopathic Pharmacopoeia of India. (Published by Ministry of Health & Family Welfare).

Volume	Number of Monograph	Year
Volume I	180	1971
Volume II	100	1974
Volume III	105	1978
Volume IV	107	1984
Volume V	114	1987
Volume VI	104	1990
Volume VII	105	1999
Volume VIII	101	2000

Other literature available:
A. List of medicinal plants used in Homeopathy.
B. List of generally used Nosodes.

Status of Homeopathic Medicines Under Drugs & Cosmetic Act, 1940 & Rules 1945:

Homeopathic medicines are covered under the provisions of Drugs & Cosmetic Act, 1940 and the Rules made there under:

Some Important Provisions are:
1. Homeopathic medicines are defined under Rule 2(dd) of Drugs and Cosmetics Rules, 1945.
2. Standards of homeopathic medicines to be complied for manufacture, for sale, distribution or import are defined under Second Schedule of the Drugs and Cosmetics Act (item N.4a).
3. New homeopathic medicines are covered under Rule 30 aa.
4. Minimum requirement for good manufacturing are included in Schedule m-1.
5. Ophthalmic preparations, standards and conditions for preparation thereof are covered under Schedule ff (Rule 126 a).
6. Homeopathic Pharmacopoeia Laboratory, Ghaziabad is to function as Central Drugs Laboratory w.r.t. homeopathic drugs, under section 6 of the act under sub-rule 7 of rule 3-a.
7. Anybody can get medicines tested under Section 26.
8. Under Section 26-a, Central Government can cancel licence of manufacturing a drug, if therapeutic claims are not genuine.
9. Procedures for labelling and packing of homeopathic medicines are covered under Rule 32 a, Rule 106 a and 106 b (Part ix-a).
10. Rule 85 b covers manufacture of mother tinctures, potencies or potencies from back potencies. Application for which is made under form 24 c.
11. Rule 85 c and 30 aa covers manufacture of new homeopathic drugs.
12. Individual pharmacists (shop keepers) are allowed to manufacture of potencies only and, that only from back potencies, under Rule 85 d.
13. Retail is covered under Rule 67 c. Application be made under form 20 c. Single drugs.
14. Though whole sale is covered under Rule 67 c, but application is made under form 20-d. Single drugs.
15. Licensing authority for issue of licence for homeopathic medicines lies with the State Government as per Rule 67 a and 85 b.

Homeopathic Pharmacopoeia of India

Homeopathic Pharmacopoeia Committee is constituted with the following objectives:
i. To prepare Pharmacopoeia of Homeopathic drugs whose therapeutic usefulness have been proved on the lines of the American, German and British Homeopathic Pharmacopoeial;
ii. To lay down principles and standards for the preparation of homeopathic drugs;
iii. To lay down test of identity, quality, purity; and
iv. Such other matters as are incidental and necessary for the preparation of a Homeopathic Pharmacopoeia.

Homeopathic Pharmacopoeia Committee has been assigned the above work besides to prepare Homeopathic pharmaceutical codex.

The Homeopathic Pharmacopoeia Committee (HPC) was constituted in September, 1962 on the recommendations of the Homeopathic Advisory Committee and Homeopathic Sub-Committee of the Drugs Technical Advisory Board on the question of control of homeopathic drugs under Drugs and Cosmetics Act, 1940 and Rules, 1945. The source of homeopathic drugs are mostly of natural origin viz. vegetables/plants, animals, minerals, chemicals, nosodes, sarcodes etc. For this purpose the Committee has experts from the Chemistry, Botany, Microbiology/Pharmacology besides manufacturers of homeopathic medicine and eminent homeopaths as well as officials who are concerned with the work of testing and research in drugs.

The term of the Homeopathic Pharmacopoeia Committee was initially for 3 years which was extended from time to time. The Committee was re-constituted on 26th May, 1997 for a period of 3 years.

The Chairman of the Committee has the powers to form sub-Committee whenever required and to co-opt experts from outside.

Work done so far:
The homeopathic drugs are available in the market in mother tincture form and in potency. The priority of the HPC is to fix standards upto the level of mother tincture or equivalent i.e. of the raw materials and method of

preparations. From 1962 onwards the Committee has finalised and recommended standards for Homeopathic Pharmacopoeia of India.

Work in Progress:
The Committee is engaged in laying down the standards of new drugs which are left so far and also revising the earlier volumes. Besides these, the Homeopathic Pharmacopoeial Codex is prepared. Codex is a book on drugs having supplementary information for the purpose of further research work and to keep additional informations on drug materials.

How does it help?
Homeopathic Pharmacopoeia of India (Vol. I-VII) have become official in terms of Schedule-II of the Drugs and Cosmetics Act, 1940 and Rules, 1945. Hence Indian manufacturers are legally bound to manufacture homeopathic medicines as per standards and methodology given in the Homeopathic Pharmacopoeia of India. If some of the drugs are not included in the Homeopathic Pharmacopoeia of India, manufacturers are free to undertake manufacturing as per any recognised Pharmacopoeia of the other countries vis the German Homeopathic Pharmacopoeia, United States Homeopathic Pharmacopoeia, British Homeopathic Pharmacopoeia and French Homeopathic Pharmacopoeia etc. Import and Export of homeopathic medicines should also be based on the standards as laid down in the Pharmacopoeia. HPI also helps in the checking/testing of standards of homeopathic raw-materials and finished product.

Homoeopathic Pharmacopoeia Laboratory
Address: Central Govt. Office Building No. I,
Hapur-Road, Hapur-Chungi, Ghaziabad
Uttar Pradesh, India. **Pin-201002**
http://indianmedicine.nic.in/html/pharma/HPL.htm

National Institute of Homeopathy

Introduction

National Institute of Homeopathy was established on 10th December 1975 in Kolkata as an Autonomous Organisation under the Ministry of Health and Family Welfare, Govt. of India.

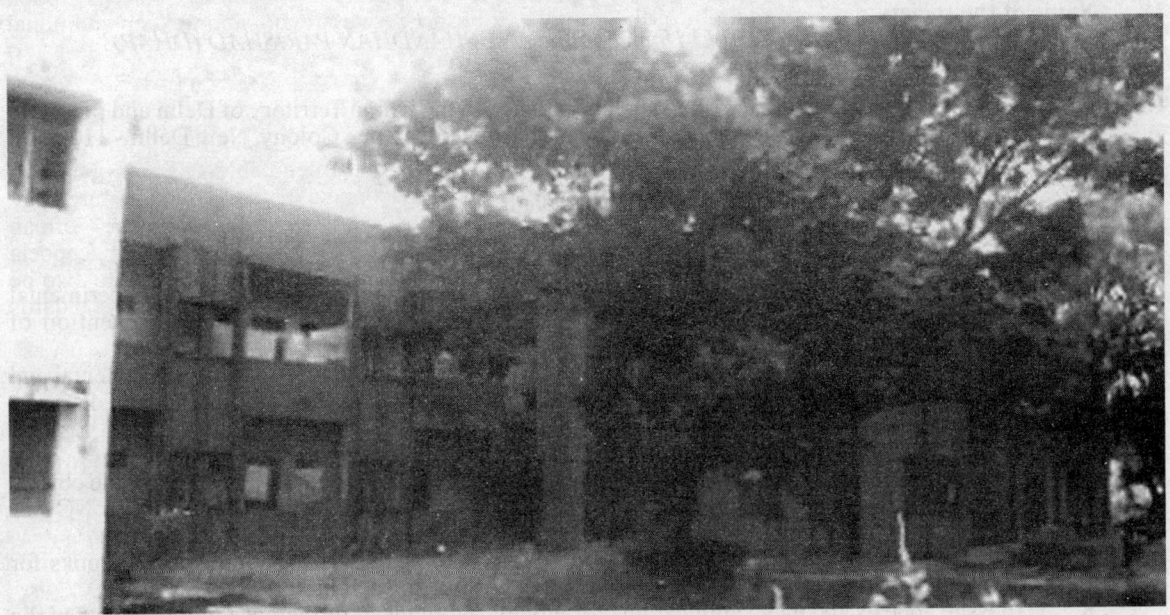

NATIONAL INSTITUTE OF HOMOEOPATHY

Aims & Objectives
- To promote the growth and development of Homeopathy
- To produce graduates and post graduates in Homeopathy
- To conduct research on various aspects of Homeopathy
- To provide medical care through Homeopathy to the suffering humanity
- To provide and assist in providing services and facilities for research, evaluation, training, consultation, and guidance related to Homeopathy
- To conduct experiments and develop patterns of teaching in under - graduate and post - graduate education on various aspects of Homeopathy

The Institute

The Institute is spread over 16 acres of land at Block - GE, Sector - III, Salt Lake, Kolkata. The Institute is affiliated to the West Bengal University of Health Sciences. At present the Institute, conducts the degree course in Homeopathy, Bachelor of Homeopathic Medicine and Surgery [B.H.M.S.] & Post - Graduate course i.e. Doctor of Medicine in Homeopathy [M.D.(Hom.] in three subjects; Organon of Medicine, Repertory and Materia Medica since 1998-99.

A 250 - seated Boys Hostel, a 70 - seated Girls Hostel and a Guest House are also available in the same campus. We also have a Staff Quarters on a plot of land measuring about 9 acres close to the Institute campus within Salt Lake (Block JC).

National Institute of Homoeopathy
Address: GE Block, Sector III,
Salt Lake city,
Kolkata. 700106, India.
Website: www.nih.nic.in

Dilli Homoeopathic Anusandhan Parishad

Dilli Homoeopathic Anusandhan Parishad was established as an autonomous body on 1st July 1998 to initiate, aid, develops and co-ordinate research activities in Homeopathy.

Memorandum of Association And Articles of Association

1. **Name of the society**
   Name of the Parishad shall be *"DILLI Homeopathic ANUSHANDHAN PARISHAD (DHAP)"*

2. **Registered Office:**
   2.1 The Registered Office of the Parishad shall be situated in the Union Territory of Delhi and presently at Nehru Homeopathic Medical College &Hospital, B-Block, Defence Colony, New Delhi - 110024.

3. **Aims, Objectives and Functions:**
   The aims, objectives and functions of the Parishad shall be:

   1. The formulation of aims and patterns of research on scientific lines in Homeopathy.
   2. To undertake research and other programs in Homeopathy.
   3. The prosecution of and assistance in research for propagation of knowledge and experimental measures generally in connection with the causation, mode of spread and prevention of diseases.
   4. To initiate, aid, develop and coordinate scientific research in different aspects, fundamental and applied of Homeopathy and to promote and assist institutions of research for the study of diseases, their prevention, causation and cure.
   5. To finance inquires and researches for the furtherance of objectives of the Parishad.
   6. To exchange information with other institutions, association and societies interested in the objects similar to those of the Parishad and specially in observation and study of diseases in NCT of Delhi.
   7. To prepare, print, publish and exhibit any paper posters, pamphlets, periodicals and books for furtherance of the objects of the Parishad and contribute to such literature.
   8. To issue appeals and make applications for money and funds in furtherance of the objects of the Delhi Parishad and to accept for the aforesaid purpose gifts, donations and subscriptions of cash and securities and of any property whether moveable or immovable.
   9. To borrow or raise moneys with or without security or on security mortgage charge, hypothecation or pledge of all or any of the immovable or movable properties belonging to the Parishad or in any other manner whatsoever.
   10. To invest and deal with the funds and moneys of the Parishad or entrusted to the Parishad not immediately required in such manner as may from time to time be determined by the Governing Body of the Parishad.
   11. To permit the funds of the Parishad to be held by the Government of Delhi. 12. To acquire and hold purchase in the Government of Delhi, whether temporarily or permanently any movable or immovable property necessary or convenient for the furtherance of the objects of the Parishad.
   13. To sell, lease mortgage and exchange and otherwise transfer any of the properties movable or immovable of the Parishad provided prior approval of the Government of Delhi is obtained for the transfer of immovable property.
   14. To undertake and accept the management of any endowment or trust fund for donation the undertaking or acceptance whereof may seem desirable.
   15. To offer prizes and grant of scholarships, including traveling scholarships in furtherance of the objects of Parishad.
   16. To create administrative technical and ministerial and other posts under the Parishad and to make appointments they're to in accordance with the rules and regulations of the Parishad or to appoint, or employ temporarily or permanently, any person that may be required for the purpose of the Parishad and to pay them or other persons in return for services rendered to the Parishad, salaries, wages, honoraria, fees, gratuities, provident fund and pensions.
   17. To do all such other lawful things either alone or in conjunction with others as the Parishad may consider necessary or as being incidental or conducive to the attainment of the above objects
   18. To deal with any property belonging to or vested in he Parishad in any manner which is

considered necessary for promoting the objects as specified in Section 12 of the Societies Registration Act XXI of 1860

19. To build, construct, maintain, repair, alter, improve or develop or furnish any buildings or works necessary or convenient for the purpose of the Parishad.
20. To frame rules and regulations for day to day execution of societies activities and to amend the memorandum of association from time to time if necessary in consultation with the State Govt.

4. Management of Assets

The income and properties of the Parishad howsoever, derived shall be applied towards the objects thereof as set forth in this Memorandum of Association subject to such limitations as the Government of Delhi may from time to time impose. No portion of the income or the properties of the Parishad shall be paid or transferred directly or indirectly by way of dividends bonus or otherwise howsoever, by way of profit to the persons who at any time are, or have been members of the Parishad or to any of them to any person claiming through them or any of them provided that nothing herein contained shall prevent payment in good faith to any individuals in return for the services redeemed by them to the Parishad or for traveling allowance honoraria and other charges.

Parishad is carrying out research in Evaluation of Homeopathic drugs in the treatment of MDRTB/TB and is co-coordinating research activities in Nehru Homeopathic Medical College and Hospital and Dr. B. R. Sur Homeopathic Medical College, Hospital & Research Centre. Special clinics have been established for the research projects.

The evaluation of homeopathic drugs is also been taken in following areas:
- Clinical Research in Tuberculosis/MDRTB
- Clinical Research in Psoriasis
- Clinical Research in Vitiligo
- Clinical Research on Renal Stones and Gall Stones
- Clinical Research in Female Diseases
- Drug Proving Programme
- Clinical Research in Arthritis
- Clinical Research in Respiratory Diseases
- Review of Life Style Diseases OPD
- Review of Psychiatry OPD
- Review of Geriatric OPD
- Functioning of www.delhihomeo.com
- Clinical Research in sub-clinical hypothyroidism
- Review of Children OPD
- Clinical Research in PPRP

To propagate homeopathy, Parishad had hosted its web site "delhihomeo.com" in 2001 and this web site also provides interactive features of online treatment/advice. The site provides informative and flash news about the activities of homeopathy under Govt. of Delhi.

Overcome Hurdles, Accomplish Success

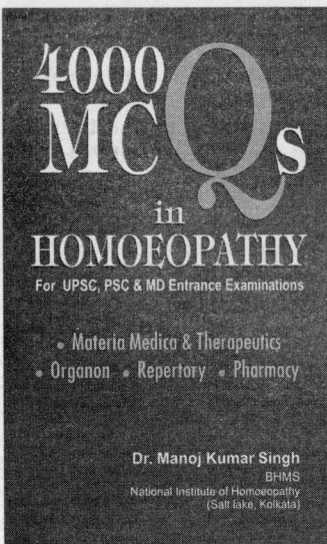

ISBN:978-81-319-**0527-2**
Pages: 496
Price : ₹

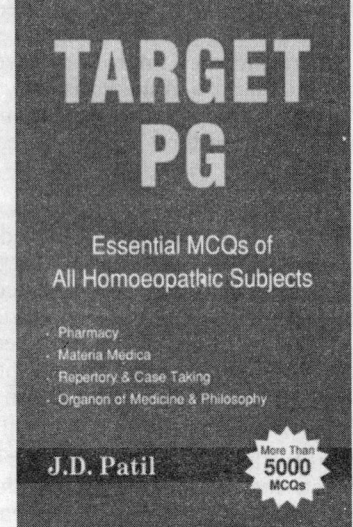

ISBN:978-81-319-**0388-9**
Pages: 552
Price : ₹

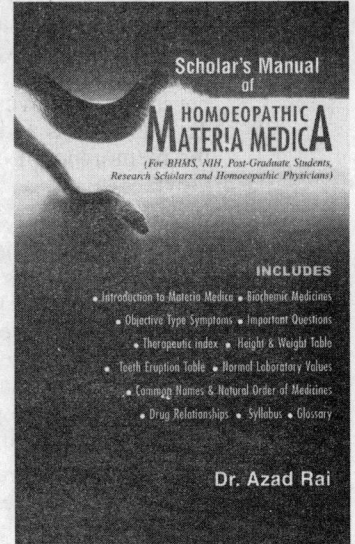

ISBN:978-81-319-**0268-4**
Pages: 1168
Price : ₹ 299.00

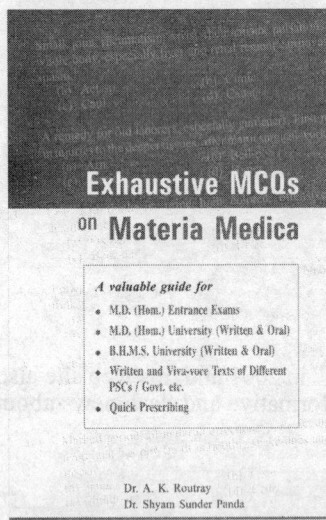

ISBN:978-81-319-**0247-9**
Pages: 344
Price : ₹ 110.00

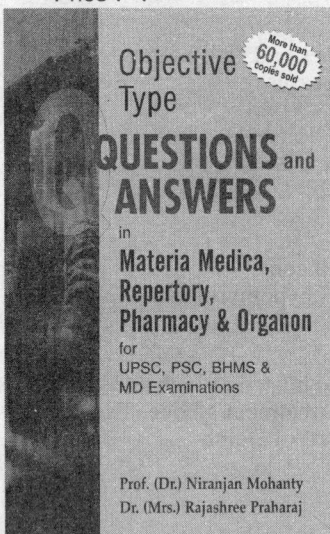

ISBN:978-81-319-**0243-1**
Pages: 400
Price : ₹

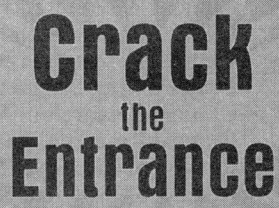

ISBN:978-81-319-**0803-7**
Pages: 614
Price : ₹

Contact your nearest bookstore for a copy

B. Jain PUBLISHERS (P) LTD.

📍 1921, Street No. 10, Chuna Mandi, Paharganj, New Delhi-110055 (India)
📞 +91-11-4567 1000   📠 +91-11-4567 1010   ✉ info@bjain.com   🌐 www.bjain.com

Homoeopathic Pharmacy Hahnemann's Way

MASTER HAHNEMANN *was a person who envisioned an entire system of medicine and then fully developed it into a powerful and practical tool within the span of a single life. This system of medicine he named it as Homoeopathy. In his books at various places he tells us about the various important facts and his observations which he found were important and gave us the cardinal principles of homoeopathy.*

§ 1 Mission of Physician

The physician's high and only mission is to restore the sick to health, to cure, as it is termed[1].

[1] His mission is not, however to construct so-called systems, by interweaving empty speculations and hypotheses concerning the internal essential nature of the vital processes and the mode in which disease originate in.

§ 3 Knowledge of Physician

If the physician clearly perceives what is to be cured in diseases, that is to say, in every individual case of disease *(knowledge of disease, indication)*, if he clearly perceives what is curative in medicines, that is to say, in each individual medicine *(knowledge of medicinal powers)*, and if he knows how to adapt, according to clearly defined principles, what is curative in medicine to what he has discovered to be undoubtedly morbid in the patient, so that the recovery must ensure - to adapt it, as well in respect to the suitability of the medicine most appropriate according to its mode of action to the case before him *(choice of the remedy, the medicine indicated)*, as also in respect to the exact mode of preparation and quantity of a required *(proper dose)*, and the proper period for repeating the dose; - if, finally, he knows the obstacles to recovery in each case and is aware how to remove them, so that the restoration may be permanent, then he understands how to treat judiciously and nationally, and he is a true practitioner of the healing art. [4]

§ 4 Physician as Preserver of health

He is likewise a preserver of health if he knows the things that derange health and cause disease, and how to remove them from persons in health.[a]

§ 6 Unprejudiced observed

The unprejudiced observer - well aware of the futility of transcendental speculations which can receive no confirmation from experience - be his powers of penetration ever so great, takes note of nothing in every individual disease, except the changes in the health of the body and of the mind *(morbid phenomena, accidents, symptoms)* which can be perceived externally by means of the senses; that is to say, he notices only the deviations from

Doctor Hahnemann's say on Mother Tincture and Dilutions

§ 123 Unadulterated Herbs
Each of these medicines must be taken in a perfectly simple, unadulterated form; the indigenous plants in the form of freshly expressed juice, mixed with a little alcohol to prevent it spoiling; exotic vegetable substances, however, in the form of powder, or

B. Jain assures herbs from original source of cultivation or reliable vendors.

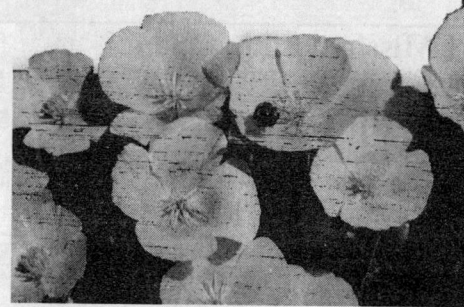

§ 264 Genuine Medicine
The true physician must be provided with genuine medicines of unimpaired strength, so that he may be able to rely upon their therapeutic powers; he must be able, himself, to judge of their genuineness.

At B.Jain we guarantee accurate herb and thus 100% accurate & pure Mother Tincture.

§ 268 Quality control to check genuinity of herb
The other exotic plants, barks, seeds and roots that cannot be obtained in the fresh state the sensible practitioner will never take in the pulverized form on trust, but will first convince himself of their genuineness in their crude, entire state before making any medicinal employment of them.[1]

[1] In order to preserve them in the form of powder, a precaution is requisite that has hitherto been usually neglected by druggists, and hence powders

B.Jain QC Department checks various parameters like TLC, UV, Infrared assuring genuinity of herbs and 100% accurate Mother Tincture.

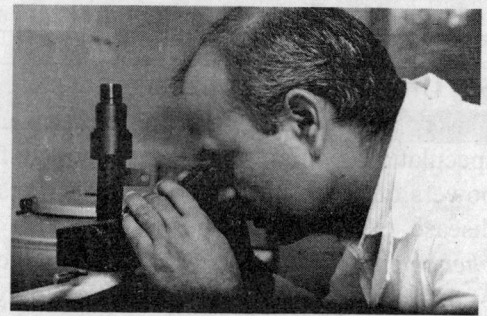

§ 269 Dynamisation/Potentisation

In Sec. § 269 – Another paragraph with foot-notes is added in the Sixth Edition, as follows:

[This remarkable change in the qualities of natural bodies develops the latent, hitherto unperceived, as if slumbering[2] hidden, dynamic (§ 11) powers which influence the life principle, change the well-being of animal life[3]. This is effected by mechanical action upon their smallest particles by means of rubbing and shaking *and through the addition of an indifferent substance, dry or fluid are separated from each other*. This process is called dynamizing, potentizing (development of medicinal power) and the products are dynamizations[4] or potencies in different degrees.']

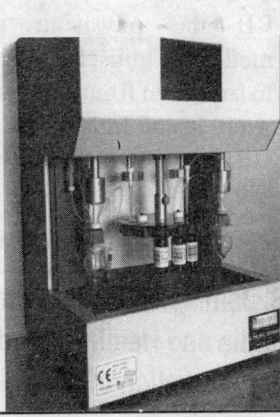

B. Jain latest K-Tronic potentiser for accuracy of potency (99.6% Accuracy) of B. Jain Liquid Dilutions

§ 270 Pure Alcohol

millionth part in powder form. For reasons given below (b) one grain of this powder is dissolved in 500 drops of a mixture of one part of alcohol and four parts of distilled water, of which one drop is put in a vial. To this are added 100 drops of pure alcohol[3] and given one hundred strong succussions with the hand against a hard but elastic body[4]. This is the medicine in the first degree of dynamization with which small sugar globules[5] may then be

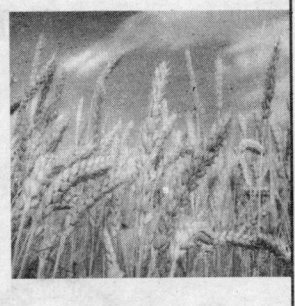

B. Jain uses Grain based ENA for MT and Dilutions which is purest form of alcohol is less bitter thus assuring pure vehicle.

§ 270 Highest Quality Globules

[3] The vial used for potentizing is filled two-thirds full.
[4] Perhaps on a leather – bound book.
[5] They are prepared, under supervision by the confectioner, from starch and sugar and the small globules freed from fine dusty parts by passing them through a sieve. Then they are put through a strainer that will permit only 100 to pass through weighing one grain, the most serviceable size for the needs of a homoeopathic physician.

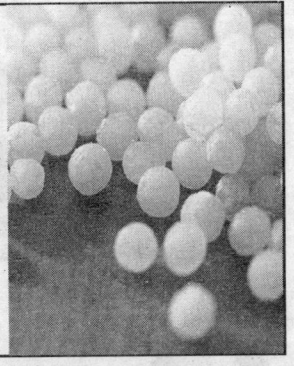

B. Jain uses pharma grade sugar for preparation of globules to assure unadulterated vehicle for you.

§ 271 Medicine preparation method should be reliable

['If the physician prepares his homoeopathic medicines himself, as he should reasonably do in order to save men from sickness,[2], he may use the fresh plant itself, as but little of the crude article is required,

[2] 'Until the State, in the future, after having attained insight into the indispensability of perfectly prepared homoeopathic medicines, will have them manufactured by a competent impartial person, in order to give them free of

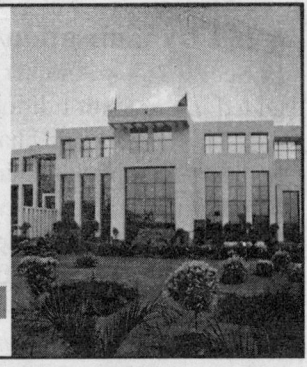

B. Jain has a GMP Certified manufacturing plant with two accrediation (India and Health Canada). B.Jain documents each and every steps followed in preparation of medicine to guarantee the reliability a homeopath needs.

Do You Have Access to all above?

If you want your medicines to comply to above standards

Ask for B. Jain Medicines

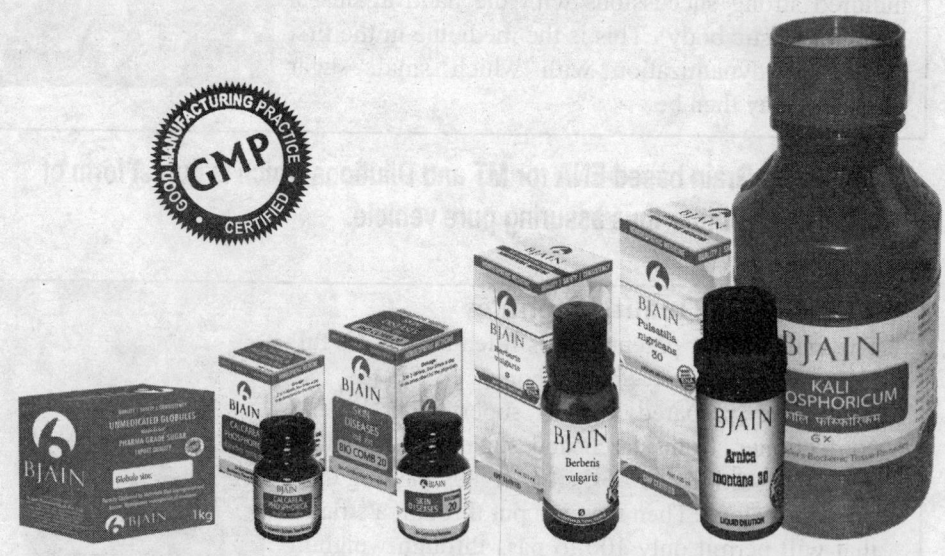

BJAIN Pharmaceuticals (P) Ltd.

Corporate Office: 1921/10, Chuna Mandi, Paharganj, New Delhi - 110055 (INDIA)
Factory Office: E-41/F, RIICO Industrial Area, Khushkhera, District Alwar, Bhiwadi - 301707, India
Tel. +91-11-45671000 Fax: +91-11-45671010 Email: pharma@bjain.com www.pharma.bjain.com